Dr. Michael T. Murray is the author of twenty-three books, including the acclaimed best-seller *The Encyclopaedia of Natural Medicine* (co-authored with Dr. Joseph Pizzorno). He is regarded as the world authority on natural medicine. An educator, lecturer, researcher, and health food industry consultant, Michael also serves as the Director of Product Development and Education at Natural Factors, a health product firm.

Dr. Joseph Pizzorno is a leader in the field of natural medicine and cofounder of Bastyr University, the first-ever accredited, multidisciplinary university of natural medicine in the United States (and the English-speaking world). An international lecturer and ongoing contributor to magazines such as *Natural Health, Better Nutrition,* and *Let's Live,* he also cowrote the acclaimed bestseller *The Encyclopaedia of Natural Medicine* with Dr. Michael Murray.

Lara Pizzorno, M.Div., M.A., is a highly experienced health writer and medical editor, with over twenty years of experience writing and editing articles and books at both the professional and public levels. Mrs. Pizzorno has earned several degrees: M. Div., Yale Divinity, New Haven, CT; M.A., English literature, U.W., Seattle, WA; B.A., Magna cum laude, Wheaton College, MA and is trained and licensed as a massage therapist.

THE ENCYCLOPAEDIA OF
Healing Foods

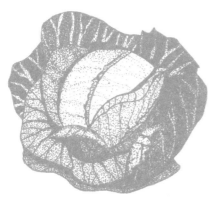

DR MICHAEL MURRAY

and

DR JOSEPH PIZZORNO

with

LARA PIZZORNO, M.A., L.M.T.

TIME WARNER
BOOKS

First published in the United States of America in September 2005 by Atria Books
First published in Great Britain in 2006 by Time Warner Books

The information presented herein is in no way intended as a substitute for medical counseling. You should consult a physician before embarking on any treatment plan. This book has been designed to provide information in regard to the subject matter covered. It is sold with the understanding that the publisher and the author are not liable for the misconception or misuse of information provided.

The moral right of the authors has been asserted.

A CIP catalogue record for this book
is available from the British Library.

ISBN-13: 978-0-316-73190-4
ISBN-10: 0-316-73190-0

Printed and bound in Great Britain by
The Bath Press, Bath

Time Warner Books
An imprint of
Little, Brown Book Group
Brettenham House
Lancaster Place
London WC2E 7EN

A member of the Hachette Livre Group of Companies

www.littlebrown.co.uk

Time Warner Books is a trademark of Time Warner Inc. or
an affiliated company. Used under licence by Little, Brown Book Group,
which is not affiliated with Time Warner Inc.

CONTENTS

PREFACE

There is an ever-growing appreciation of the role of diet in determining our level of health. It is now well established that certain dietary practices cause, as well as prevent, a wide range of diseases. In addition, more and more research is accumulating that indicates certain diets and foods offer immediate therapeutic benefit.

However, as people learn more about the value of proper nutrition, they often become confused by the conflicting opinions they encounter. The purpose of this book is to provide the most up-to-date answers to some important basic questions about nutrition:

What is a healthy diet?

How do I know what to eat and in what quantities?

How much protein, fat, fiber, and other food factors do I need in my diet?

What properties do individual foods possess?

If foods are medicines, which ones offer the greatest benefit for specific health problems?

More important, we hope that this information will inspire you to make healthier food choices. Our belief is that healthier food choices will result in a healthier and happier existence.

The human body is remarkable and truly wondrous, but most Westerners are not feeding the body the high-quality fuel it deserves and needs. When a dynamic living organism does not receive the proper building blocks it needs for energy, maintenance, or repair, it is only a matter of time before it fails to run in an efficient manner. Stated another way, if the body is not fed the full range of nutrients it needs, how can it be expected to stay in a state of good health?

The human body, the vessel of your soul, is something to be cherished. Ralph Waldo Emerson said, "The first wealth is health." We agree with this sentiment and urge you to make eating a healthy diet a lifetime habit. With that goal in mind, we offer you *The Encyclopaedia of Healing Foods: A Comprehensive Guide to the Healing Power of Nature's Best Medicine.*

• • •

May you live in good health, with passion and joy!

Dr Michael T. Murray
Dr Joseph E. Pizzorno
Lara Pizzorno, M.A., L.M.T.

Publisher's note
U.S. cups are used throughout this book as a method to measure the volume of ingredients—liquid or otherwise. Equivalent fluid measurements are: 1 cup = 9 fluid ounces/250 millilitres; ½ cup = 5 fluid ounces/125 millilitres; ⅓ cup = 3 fluid ounces/85 millilitres; ¼ cup = 2 fluid ounces/60 millilitres.

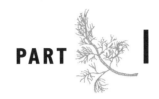

PART I

Basic Principles of a Good Diet

Let your food be your medicine and let your medicine be your food.

—Hippocrates

Human Nutrition:
An Evolutionary Perspective

In order to answer the question "What is a healthy diet?," it is important to first take a look at what our body is designed for. Is the human body designed to eat plant foods, animal foods, or both? Respectively, are we herbivores, carnivores, or omnivores?

While the human gastrointestinal tract is capable of digesting both plant and animal foods, there are indications that we evolved to digest primarily plant foods. Specifically, our teeth are composed of twenty molars, which are perfect for crushing and grinding plant foods, along with eight front incisors, which are well suited for biting into fruits and vegetables. Only our front four canine teeth are designed for meat eating, and our jaws swing both vertically to tear and laterally to crush, while carnivores' jaws swing only vertically. Additional evidence that supports the human body's preference for plant foods is the long length of the human intestinal tract. Carnivores typically have a short bowel,

while herbivores have a bowel length proportionally comparable to humans'.

To answer the question of what humans should eat, many researchers look to other primates, such as chimpanzees, monkeys, and gorillas. These nonhuman wild primates are omnivores. They are also often described as herbivores and opportunistic carnivores in that although they eat mainly fruits and vegetables, they may also eat small animals, lizards, and eggs if given the opportunity. For example, the gorilla and the orangutan eat only 1 percent and 2 percent of animal foods as a percentage of total calories, respectively. The remainder of their diet is derived from plant foods. Since humans are between the weight of the gorilla and orangutan, it has been suggested that humans are designed to eat around 1.5 percent of their diet in the form of animal foods. However, most Americans derive well over 50 percent of their calories from animal foods and the situation is much the same in the U.K. Over the past forty years, Americans' consumption of meat has increased from 89 to 124 kilograms per person per year, while in Europe meat consumption has grown from 56 to 89 kilograms.

Since wild primates fill up on wild fruit and other highly nutritious plant foods, those weighing one tenth the amount of a typical human ingest nearly ten times the level of vitamin C and much higher amounts of many other vitamins and minerals (see Table 1.1). How is this possible? One reason is that the cultivated fruit in a typical Western supermarket is far different from the wild fruit of the primate's diet, which has a slightly higher protein content and a higher content of certain essential vitamins and minerals. Cultivated fruit tends to be higher in sugars and, while very tasty to humans, it is not nearly as nutritious. In fact, it raises blood sugar levels much more quickly than its wild counterparts do.

There are other differences in the wild primate diet that are also important to highlight, such as a higher ratio of alpha-linolenic acid—the essential omega-3 fatty acid—to linoleic acid—the essential omega-6 fatty acid. A higher ratio of omega-3 fatty acid decreases the likelihood of the development of inflammatory and chronic diseases as well as their severity. Finally, the wild primate diet is very high in fiber, while the average American diet is not. A high-fiber diet protects against heart disease and many types of cancer.

Determining what diet humans are best suited for may not be as simple as looking at the diet of wild primates. Humans have some significant structural and physiological differences compared to apes. The key difference may be our larger, more metabolically active brains. In fact, it has been theorized that a shift in dietary intake to more animal foods may have produced

TABLE 1.1

Estimated Mineral Intakes of Wild Monkeys and Humans

Mineral	Total Daily Intake for 7 Kilogram Adult Wild Male Monkey (milligrams)	RDA for 70 Kilogram Adult Human Male (milligrams)
Calcium	4,571	800
Phosphorus	728	800
Potassium	6,419	1,600–2,000
Sodium	182	500
Magnesium	1,323	350
Iron	38.5	10
Manganese	18.2	2.0–5.0
Copper	2.8	1.5–3.0

From: Milton, K., "Nutritional Characteristics of Wild Primate Food: Do the Diets of Our Closest Living Relatives Have Lessons for Us?" *Nutrition* 1999:15; 488–498.

the stimulus for human brain growth. The shift itself was probably the result of limited food availability, which forced early humans to hunt grazing mammals such as antelope and gazelle. Archaeological data support this association—humans' brains started to grow and become more developed at about the same time evidence shows an increase of animal bones being butchered with stone tools at early villages.

While improved dietary quality alone cannot fully explain why human brains grew, it definitely appears to have played a critical role. With their bigger brains, early humans were able to engage in more complex social behavior, which led to improved foraging and hunting tactics, which, in turn, led to even higher quality food intake that fostered additional brain evolution.

Data from anthropologists looking at evidence from hunter-gatherer cultures is providing much insight as to what humans are designed to eat. However, it is important to point out that these cultures were not entirely free to determine their diets. Instead, their diets were molded as a result of what was available to them. For example, the diet of the Inuit Eskimos is far different from that of the Australian Aborigines. Therefore, it may not be appropriate to answer the question "What should humans eat?" simply by looking at these studies alone.

Nonetheless, regardless of whether a hunter-gatherer community relied on animal or plant foods, the rate of diseases of civilization such as heart disease and cancers was extremely low.

How is this possible? One reason is that the meat our ancestors consumed was much different from the meat we find in the supermarket today. Domesticated animals have always had higher fat levels than their wild counterparts, but the desire for tender meat has driven the fat content of domesticated animals to 25 to 30 percent or higher compared to a fat content of less than 4 percent for free-living animals or wild game. In addition, the type of fat is considerably different. Domestic beef contains primarily saturated fats and virtually undetectable amounts of omega-3 fatty acids. In contrast, the fat of wild animals contains over five times more polyunsaturated fat per gram and has desirable amounts of beneficial omega-3 fatty acids (approximately 4 percent).

What conclusions can we draw from the evidence of the wild primate and hunter-gatherer diets about how we should eat today? Overwhelmingly, it appears that humans are better suited to a diet composed primarily of plant foods. This position is supported also by a tremendous amount of evidence showing that deviating from a predominantly plant-based diet is a major factor in the development of heart disease, cancer, strokes, arthritis, and many other chronic degenerative diseases. It is now the recommendation of many health and medical organizations that the human diet should focus primarily on plant-based foods, comprising vegetables, fruits, grains, legumes, nuts, and seeds.

The evidence supporting diet's role in chronic degenerative diseases is substantial. There are two basic facts linking the diet-disease connection:

1. A diet rich in plant foods is protective against many diseases that are extremely common in Western society.
2. A diet providing a low intake of plant

foods is a causative factor in the development of these diseases and provides conditions under which other causative factors became more active.

The Pioneering Work of Denis Burkitt and Hugh Trowell

Much of the link between diet and chronic disease originated from the work of two medical pioneers: Denis Burkitt, M.D., and Hugh Trowell, M.D., editors of *Western Diseases: Their Emergence and Prevention,* first published in 1981. Although now extremely well recognized, the work of Burkitt and Trowell is actually a continuation of the landmark work of Weston A. Price, a dentist and author of *Nutrition and Physical Degeneration.* In the early 1900s, Dr. Price traveled the world observing changes in teeth and palate (orthodontic) structure as various cultures discarded traditional dietary practices in favor of a more "civilized" diet. Price was able to follow individuals as well as cultures over periods of twenty to forty years, and he carefully documented the onset of degenerative diseases as their diets changed.

Based on the extensive studies examining the rate of diseases in various populations (epidemiological data), including the groundbreaking work of Dr. Price and their own observations of primitive cultures, Burkitt and Trowell formulated the following sequence of events:

First stage: In cultures consuming a traditional diet consisting of whole, unprocessed foods, the rate of chronic diseases, such as heart disease, diabetes, and cancer is quite low.

Second stage: Commencing with eating a more "Western" diet, there is a sharp rise in the number of individuals with obesity and diabetes.

Third stage: As more and more people abandon their traditional diet, conditions that were once quite rare become extremely common. Examples of these conditions include constipation, hemorrhoids, varicose veins, and appendicitis.

Fourth stage: Finally, with full Westernization of the diet, other chronic degenerative or potentially lethal diseases, including heart disease, cancer, osteoarthritis, rheumatoid arthritis, and gout, become extremely common.

Since the publication in *Western Diseases* of Burkitt and Trowell's pioneering research, a virtual landslide of data has continually verified the role of the Western diet as the key factor in virtually every chronic disease, but especially in obesity and diabetes. In 1984, in the U.S.A., the Food and Nutrition Board of the National Research Council established the Committee on Diet and Health to undertake a comprehensive analysis on diet and major chronic diseases. Their findings, as well as those of the U.S. surgeon general, the National Cancer Institute, and other highly respected medical groups brought to the forefront the need for Americans (and, by extension, others eating a Western diet) to change their eating habits to reduce their risk for chronic disease. Table 1.2 lists diseases with convincing links to a diet low in plant foods. Many of these now-common diseases were extremely rare before the twentieth century.

TABLE 1.2

Diseases Highly Associated with a Diet Low in Plant Foods

Type of Disease	Diseases
Metabolic	Obesity, gout, diabetes, kidney stones, gallstones
Cardiovascular	High blood pressure, strokes, heart disease, varicose veins, deep-vein thrombosis, pulmonary embolism
Colonic	Constipation, appendicitis, diverticulitis, diverticulosis, hemorrhoids, colon cancer, irritable bowel syndrome, ulcerative colitis, Crohn's disease
Other	Dental caries, autoimmune disorders, pernicious anemia, multiple sclerosis, thyrotoxicosis, psoriasis, acne

---

Trends in U.S. Food Consumption

During the twentieth century, food consumption patterns changed dramatically. Total dietary fat intake increased from 32 percent of calories in 1909 to 43 percent (about 35 percent in the U.K.) by the end of the century; carbohydrate intake dropped from 57 percent to 46 percent (about 48 percent in the U.K.); and protein intake has remained fairly stable at about 11 percent (about 16 percent in the U.K.).

Compounding these detrimental changes are the individual food choices accounting for the changes. There were significant increases in the consumption of meat, fats and oils, and sugars and sweeteners in conjunction with a de-

creased consumption of noncitrus fruits, vegetables, and whole-grain products. But the biggest change in the last hundred years of human nutrition was the switch from a diet with a high level of complex carbohydrates, as found naturally occurring in grains and vegetables, to a tremendous and dramatic increase in the number of calories consumed in the form of simple sugars. Currently, more than half of the carbohydrates being consumed are in the form of sugars such as sucrose (table sugar) and corn syrup, which are added to foods as sweetening agents. High consumption of refined sugars is linked to many chronic diseases, including obesity, diabetes, heart disease, and cancer.

The Government and Nutrition Education

Throughout the years, various governmental organizations in the U.S.A. have published dietary guidelines, but it has been the recommendations of the U.S. Department of Agriculture (USDA) that have become the most widely known. In 1956, the USDA published "Food for Fitness—A Daily Food Guide." This became popularly known as the Basic Four Food Groups. The Basic Four were:

1. The Milk Group: milk, cheese, ice cream, and other milk-based foods
2. The Meat Group: meat, fish, poultry, and eggs, with dried legumes and nuts as alternatives
3. The Fruits and Vegetables Group
4. The Breads and Cereals Group

TABLE 1.3

Quantities of Foods Consumed per Capita in the U.S.A. (pounds/kilograms per year)

Foods	1909	1967	1985	1999
Meat, poultry, and fish:				
Beef	54/25	81/37	73/33	66/30
Pork	62/28	61/27	62/28	50/23
Poultry	18/8	46/21	70/32	68/31
Fish	12/5	15/7	19/9	15/7
Total	146/66	203/92	224/102	199/91
Eggs	37/17	40/18	32/15	32/15
Dairy products:				
Whole milk	223/101	232/105	122/55	112/51
Low-fat milk	64/29	44/20	112/51	101/46
Cheese	5/2	15/7	26/12	30/14
Other	47/21	159/72	190/86	210/95
Total	339/153	450/204	450/204	453/206
Fats and oils:				
Butter	18/8	6/3	5/2	5/2
Margarine	1/½	10/5	11/5	8/4
Shortening	8/4	16/7	23/10	22/10
Lard and tallow	12/5	5/2	4/2	6/3
Salad and cooking oil	2/1	16/7	25/11	29/13
Total	41/18½	53/24	68/30	70/32
Fruits:				
Citrus	17/8	60/27	72/33	79/35
Noncitrus:				
Fresh	154/70	73/33	87/40	115/52
Processed	8/3	35/16	34/15	37/17
Total	179/81	168/76	193/88	231/104
Vegetables:				
Tomatoes	46/21	36/16	38/17	55/25
Dark green and yellow	34/15	25/11	31/14	39/18

Other:				
Fresh	136/62	87/40	96/44	126/57
Processed	8/4	35/16	34/15	39/18
Total	224/102	183/83	199/90	259/118
Potatoes, white:				
Fresh	182/83	67/30	55/25	49/22
Processed	0	19/9	28/13	91/41
Total	182/83	86/39	83/38	140/63
Dry beans, peas, nuts, and soybeans	16/7	16/7	18/8	22/10
Grain products:				
Wheat products	216/98	116/53	122/55	150/68
Corn	56/25	15/7	17/8	28/13
Other grains	19/9	13/6	26/12	24/11
Total	291/132	144/66	165/75	202/92
Sugar and sweeteners:				
Refined sugar	77/35	100/45	63/29	68/31
Syrups and other sweeteners	14/6	22/10	90/41	91/41
Total	91/41	122/55	153/70	159/72

From: Economic Research Service, United States Department of Agriculture, "Food Consumption (per Capita) Data System," www.ers.usda.gov.

One of the major problems with the Basic Four Food Groups model was that it suggested graphically that the food groups were equal in health value. The result was an overconsumption of animal products, dietary fat, and refined carbohydrates and insufficient consumption of fiber-rich foods such as fruits, vegetables, and legumes. This in turn resulted in the diet being responsible for many premature deaths, chronic diseases, and increased health care costs.

To replace the Basic Four Food Groups model, various other government and medical organizations developed guidelines of their own, designed either to reduce a specific chronic degenerative disease such as cancer or heart disease or to reduce the risk for all chronic diseases.

In an attempt to create a new model in nutrition education, the USDA published the "Eating Right Pyramid" in 1992. Since it received harsh criticism from numerous experts and other organizations, it was altered visually in 2005 (see page 10).

One of the main criticisms of the Eating Right

FIGURE 1.1

USDA Eating Right Pyramid

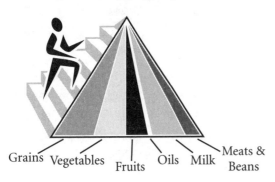

Grains   Vegetables   Fruits   Oils   Milk   Meats & Beans

Pyramid is that it does not stress strongly enough the importance of quality food choices. For example, the USDA thinks foods from the Bread, Cereal, Rice, and Pasta Group should make up the bulk of your diet. Eat six to eleven servings a day from this group, and you are supposedly on your way to a healthier life. What the pyramid doesn't tell you is that you are setting yourself up for insulin resistance, obesity, and adult-onset diabetes if you consistently choose refined products (those containing white flour) rather than whole-grain products in this important category.

You see, the Eating Right Pyramid does not take into consideration how quickly blood sugar levels rise after eating a particular type of food—an effect referred to as the food's glycemic index, or GI. The GI is a numerical scale used to indicate how fast and how high a particular food raises blood glucose (blood sugar) levels. There are two versions of the GI, one based on a standard of comparison that uses glucose scored as 100, while the other is based on white bread. Foods are tested against the results of the selected standard. Foods with a lower glycemic index create a slower rise in blood sugar, while foods with a higher glycemic index create a faster rise in blood sugar.

The glycemic indices of some of the foods the pyramid is directing Americans to eat more of, such as breads, cereals, rice, and pasta, can greatly stress blood sugar control, especially if they are derived from refined grains, and are now being linked to an increased risk for obesity, diabetes, and cancer. As a result, while the goal of the Eating Right Pyramid was to improve the health of Americans and, it was hoped, slow down the growing trend for obesity and diet-related disease, the fact is that because of poor individual food choices within the categories, the pyramid has only worsened the problem.

In light of this, the big question consumers may want to ask is "Is it appropriate to have the USDA making these food recommendations in the first place?" After all, the USDA serves two somewhat conflicting roles. First, it represents the food industry, and second, it is in charge of educating consumers about nutrition. Many people believe that the pyramid was more weighted toward dairy products, red meat, and grains due to the influence of the dairy, beef, and grain farming and processing industries. In other words, the pyramid was not designed as a way to improve the health of Americans but rather to promote the USDA agenda of supporting multinational food giants.

The Optimal Health Food Pyramid

We do like the concept of graphically illustrating what constitutes a healthful diet, so we are offering our version of the Eating Right Pyramid: the Optimal Health Food Pyramid.

The Optimal Health Food Pyramid incorporates the best aspects from two of the most healthful diets ever studied: the traditional Mediterranean diet and the traditional Asian diet. It also more clearly defines what the healthy components within the categories are and stresses the importance of regular consumption of vegetable oils as part of a healthy diet. Let's take a closer look at each category.

Foods to avoid entirely:

- Refined white flour products, including breads, pastas, cakes, muffins, and pretzels.
- Refined sugar-loaded products, including cereals, confectionery, and baked goods.
- Processed foods packed full of empty calories (sugar and fat) and/or salt, for example, canned soups, cinema-style popcorn, and potato crisps.

- Margarine, butter, and shortening.
- Smoked and cured meats, including bacon, hot dogs, smoked luncheon meats, sausages, ham, and Spam.
- Meats cooked at extremely high temperatures or cooked to well done.
- Heavily sweetened or artificially sweetened soft drinks, flavored drinks, and teas.
- Fried foods, including French fries, potato crisps, corn crisps, and doughnuts.

Vegetables: Five to Seven Servings Daily

The word "vegetable" comes from the Latin *vegetare*, meaning "to enliven or animate." Vegetables give us life and should be the main focus of any health-promoting diet. Vegetables provide the broadest range of nutrients of any food class. They are rich sources of vitamins, minerals, carbohydrates, and

FIGURE I.2

The Optimal Health Food Pyramid

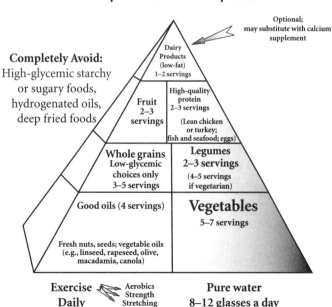

TABLE 1.4 **The Optimal Health Food Pyramid Daily Food Group Recommendations**	
Foods	Number of Daily Servings (2,000-calorie diet)
Vegetables	5–7
Green leafy and cruciferous vegetables	2–4
Low-glycemic vegetables	2–3
Starchy vegetables	1–2
Good oils	4
Nuts and seeds	1
Olive, macadamia, linseed, or rapeseed oil	2–3
Whole grains	3–5
Legumes (beans)	2–3 (4–5 if vegetarian)
High-quality protein	2–3
Fruit	2–3
Dairy products	1–2 (optional)

protein. They also provide high quantities of cancer-fighting phytochemicals.

It is very important not to overcook vegetables. Overcooking will not only result in the loss of important nutrients, it will also drain the flavor. Light steaming, baking, and quick stir-frying are the best ways to cook vegetables. And do not boil vegetables unless you are making soup, as much of the nutrients will leach into the water.

If fresh vegetables are not available, frozen vegetables are preferred over their canned counterparts. The only exception is tomato products, for example, soup, paste, or sauce, because canned products actually provide more absorbable lycopene than do raw tomatoes.

There are three vegetable categories: green leafy and cruciferous; low-glycemic; and starchy. Eating a variety of vegetables from each category daily will help you achieve a "rainbow" assortment and allow you to focus on low-glycemic choices. One vegetable serving equals:

1 cup of raw leafy vegetables (such as lettuce or spinach);
½ cup raw nonleafy, cooked vegetables, or fresh vegetable juice.

GREEN LEAFY AND CRUCIFEROUS VEGETABLES: TWO TO FOUR SERVINGS DAILY

Alfalfa sprouts	Endive
Beet greens	Escarole
Bok choy	Kale
Broccoli	Lettuce (the darker,
Brussels sprouts	the better)
Cabbage	Mustard greens
Cauliflower	Parsley
Chard	Spinach
Chinese cabbage	Turnip greens
Collard greens	Watercress
Dandelion	

LOW-GLYCEMIC VEGETABLES: TWO TO THREE SERVINGS DAILY

Artichoke	Onions
(one medium)	Peas (fresh or frozen)
Asparagus	Radishes
Bean sprouts	Rhubarb
Bell peppers	String beans
Carrots	(green or yellow)
Celery	Summer squash
Courgettes	Tomatoes, tomato
Cucumber	paste, tomato
Fennel	sauce, tomato
Mushrooms	juice, vegetable
Okra	juice cocktail

STARCHY VEGETABLES:
ONE TO TWO SERVINGS DAILY

Beetroot	Winter, acorn,
Potatoes	or butternut
Parsnips	squash
Pumpkin	Yams or sweet
Swedes	potatoes

Good Oils and Fats (Nuts, Seeds, and Vegetable Oils): Four Servings Daily

Nuts and seeds, especially those providing the monounsaturated and medium-chain fatty acids, contain beneficial oils. Regular consumption of nuts has been shown to improve blood sugar regulation and lower the risk for diabetes, heart disease, obesity, and cancer.

Be sure to focus on raw nuts and seeds, avoiding nuts and seeds roasted in oils or coated with sugar. Nuts and seeds are great to add to salads and sautéed greens. Try to mix it up a bit by eating a variety such as almonds, Brazil nuts, linseeds, pecans, sunflower seeds, walnuts, and pumpkin seeds.

Use rapeseed, linseed, macadamia, or olive oil to replace butter, margarine, and shortening, or try them in your homemade salad dressings. However, you never want to cook with linseed oil because it is very rich in omega-3 polyunsaturated fats, which are easily damaged by heat. Coconut and macadamia nut oils are the best cooking oils because of their ability to remain stable at high temperatures, but olive oil is great for sautéed vegetables and rapeseed oil is usually best for baked goods because it has the least "nutty" flavor. Avoid using safflower, sunflower, soy, and corn oil because they contain too much omega-6 fatty acid, which feeds into inflamma-

tory pathways in the body (see discussion on prostaglandins on pages 86–8).

We suggest that you have at least one serving of nuts or seeds (one serving equals ¼ cup) and 3 tablespoons of the healthy oils per day.

Whole Grains: Three to Five Servings Daily

It is very important to choose whole-grain products, such as whole-grain breads, whole-grain flour products, and brown rice, over their processed counterparts, including white bread, white flour products, and white rice. Whole grains provide substantially more nutrients and health-promoting properties. They are a major source of complex carbohydrates, dietary fiber, magnesium and other minerals, and B vitamins. The protein content and quality of whole grains is also greater than that of refined grains. Diets rich in whole grains have been shown to be helpful in both the prevention and treatment of diabetes, heart disease, and cancer.

ONE SERVING OF WHOLE GRAINS EQUALS:

Bread:	
Whole-wheat (wholemeal), rye, or other whole grain	1 slice
Cereals:	
Whole-grain cereal	½ cup
Corn:	
Cooked whole-kernel corn	½ cup
Corn on cob	1 small
Flour and flour products:	
Whole-wheat (wholemeal) flour (unbaked)	2½ tablespoons
Whole-grain pasta (cooked)	½ cup

Whole-grains (cooked):
    Barley, millet, oats, quinoa, ½ cup
       rice, spelt, and
       wheat

Beans (Legumes): Two to Three Servings Daily

Beans, a mainstay in most diets of the world, are second only to grains in supplying calories and protein to the world's population. Compared to grains, they supply about the same number of total calories but usually provide two to four times as much protein and are a richer source of the soluble fiber that lowers cholesterol and stabilizes blood sugar levels. While we do not recommend using canned vegetables or fruit, canned beans retain their fiber content and anticancer flavonoids. Plus, given the long preparation time for cooking beans, canned beans are extremely quick and convenient. A serving size for beans is ½ cup.

Fruits: Three to Four Servings Daily

Fruits are a rich source of many beneficial nutrients, and regular fruit consumption has been shown to offer significant protection against chronic degenerative diseases, including cancer, heart disease, cataracts, diabetes, and stroke. Fruits make excellent between-meals snacks and super desserts. We know it's easy to get into the habit of eating only a few varieties of fruit, so we encourage you to eat a "rainbow" assortment of fruits over the course of a week. Keep in mind that one serving equals one 1 medium fruit or ½ cup of small or cut-up fruit; 4 ounces/125 grams of 100 percent juice; or ¼ cup dried fruit.

High-Quality Protein: Two to Three Servings Daily

The detrimental effects of diets high in saturated fat and cholesterol have been stressed for decades. Likewise, the importance of the omega-3 fatty acids in the battle against chronic disease is now well known. Fish consumption, in particular, has shown tremendous protection against heart disease and cancer because of the high content of omega-3 fatty acids in fish. Choosing smaller species of fatty fish, such as wild salmon, mackerel, herring, and sardines, is best because their smaller size and shorter life span translate into a smaller accumulation of mercury, PCBs, and other environmental toxins. Wild-caught fish have less accumulation than farmed fish. Because of concerns about exposure to mercury and other environmental toxins, we recommend that you consume wild fish at least three, but no more than six, times per week.

We suggest that you limit your intake of red meat (beef, veal, or lamb) to no more than two servings per month and choose the leanest cuts possible. Do not chargrill or cook the meat until well done, as this increases the formation of cancer-causing compounds. Also, consider some of the alternatives to beef, such as venison, rabbit, and ostrich. These emerging beef alternatives are lower in saturated fat and provide higher levels of omega-3 fatty acids.

Chicken and turkey can also provide excellent protein with very little fat, especially if you eat only the white meat (breast) and do not eat the skin. Eggs are also a very good source of high-quality protein and, if produced by free-range hens fed linseed meal, are rich in beneficial omega-3 fatty acids.

One serving is about the size of a deck of cards. That translates to roughly 3 to 4 ounces/ 85 to 125 grams.

Dairy: One to Two Servings Daily (Optional)

Many people are allergic to milk or lack the enzymes necessary to digest dairy products. Even for people who do tolerate dairy foods, milk consumption should be limited to no more than one or two servings per day. Although dairy foods are rich in protein and calcium, they are also high in fat and calories, lacking the wide nutrient spectrum of foods in the categories previously discussed. Dairy foods can also con-tain accumulations of agricultural chemicals and hormones if not organically produced. Use organic, nonfat, or reduced-fat dairy products over whole-milk varieties whenever possible. Also, fermented dairy products such as yogurt, kefir, and acidophilus-fortified milk are preferred over milk due to their content of beneficial bacteria, which predigest the dairy proteins and sugars. If you haven't tried some of the soy milk alternatives to cow's milk, they are delicious, especially the flavored varieties, which include vanilla and chocolate.

One serving equals 1 cup/250 ml of milk, yogurt, or cottage cheese, or 1 ounce/30 grams of cheese. If you do not consume dairy products, we recommend that you take a calcium supplement.

The Optimal Health Food Pyramid and the dietary guidelines given reflect the current scien-

---

FISH CONSUMPTION CAUTION

Fish consumption offers significant protection against heart disease and many forms of cancer, especially the major cancers such as lung, colon, breast, and prostate. While we certainly encourage you to eat more fish, we need to give you some guidelines. Nearly all fish contain trace amounts of methyl mercury. In most cases this is of little concern because the level is so low. The fish most likely to have the lowest level of methyl mercury are salmon (usually nondetectable levels), cod, mackerel, cold-water tuna, farm-raised catfish, and herring. But certain seafood, particularly swordfish, shark, and some other large predatory fish, may contain high levels of methyl mercury. Fish absorb methyl mercury from water and aquatic plants. Larger predatory fish also absorb mercury from their prey. Methyl mercury binds tightly to the proteins in fish tissue, including muscle, and cooking does not reduce the mercury content significantly.

We suggest limiting your intake to no more than about two pounds (one kilogram) of fish per week. This translates to five 7-ounce/200 gram servings per week, maximum. Also, be sure to limit your intake of swordfish, shark, and warm-water tuna to no more than once a week (or once a month if you are a woman of childbearing age who might get pregnant).

tific answer to the ideal diet for most people. They are based upon a 2,000-calorie-a-day diet. If you need to increase your caloric intake, we recommend getting the extra calories you need by increasing the number of servings of vegetables, nuts, and legumes, as these are the best foods for improving blood sugar control. Athletes or people engaged in heavy physical labor or exercise should add another serving of seafood, meat, or poultry to their daily intake or add a soy protein or whey protein smoothie to provide an additional 1 ounce/25 to 30 grams of protein.

The following chapters explain the recommendations of the Optimal Health Food Pyramid in depth and more clearly define the benefits, features, and importance of consuming healing foods.

2

Designing a Healthy Diet

Diet is fundamental to good health, yet few Westerners really spend much thought or time on designing a diet that will promote health. Far too many people have fallen prey to the comforts of modern life, with its physical inactivity and reliance on foods that provide temporary sensory gratification at the expense of true nourishment. As a result, there is an epidemic of diet-related diseases in the United States and other parts of the Western world including Britain.

But it's easy to give your body its best chance of achieving and maintaining good health. Here are seven important principles that will go a long way toward helping you avoid diet-related diseases.

SEVEN KEY PRINCIPLES OF THE
OPTIMAL HEALTH DIET

1. Eat a "rainbow" assortment of fruits and vegetables.
2. Reduce your exposure to pesticides.
3. Eat to regulate your blood sugar level.

4. Do not overconsume meat and other animal foods.
5. Eat the right types of fats.
6. Keep your salt intake low, your potassium intake high.
7. Drink a sufficient amount of water each day.

1. EAT A "RAINBOW" ASSORTMENT OF FRUITS AND VEGETABLES

A diet rich in fruits and vegetables is your best bet for preventing virtually every chronic disease. This fact has been established time and again by scientific studies on large numbers of people. The evidence in support of this recommendation is so strong that it has been endorsed by U.S. and U.K government health agencies and by virtually every major medical organization, including the American Cancer Society. By "rainbow," we simply mean that by selecting fruits and vegetables in a variety of colors, including red, orange, yellow, green, blue, and

TABLE 2.1

The Rainbow Assortment

Red	Dark Green	Yellow and Light Green	Orange	Purple
Apples (red)	Artichokes	Apples (green or yellow)	Apricots	Aubergines
Bell peppers (red)	Asparagus	Avocados	Bell peppers (orange)	Beetroot
Cherries	Bell peppers (green)	Bananas	Butternut squash	Blackberries
Cranberries	Broccoli	Bell peppers (yellow)	Cantaloupe melon	Blueberries
Grapefruit	Brussels sprouts	Bok choy	Carrots	Cabbage (purple)
Grapes (red)	Collard greens	Cabbage	Mangoes	Cherries
Radishes	Cucumbers	Cauliflower	Oranges	Currants
Raspberries	Grapes (green)	Celery	Papaya	Grapes (purple)
Plums (red)	Green beans	Courgettes (yellow)	Pumpkin	Onions (red)
Strawberries	Honeydew melons	Fennel	Sweet potatoes	Pears (red)
Tomatoes	Kale	Kiwifruit	Yams	Plums (purple)
Watermelon	Leeks	Lemons		Radishes
	Lettuce (dark green)	Lettuce (light green)		
	Mustard greens	Limes		
	Peas	Onions		
	Spinach	Pears (green or yellow)		
	Swiss chard	Pineapple		
	Turnip greens	Squash (yellow)		

purple, you'll be giving your body the full spectrum of pigments with powerful antioxidant effects, as well as the nutrients it needs for optimal function and protection against disease.

Fruits and vegetables are so important in the battle against cancer that some experts have said—and we agree—that cancer is a result of a "maladaptation" over time to a reduced level of intake of fruits and vegetables. As a study published in the medical journal *Cancer Causes & Control* put it, "Vegetables and fruit contain the anticarcinogenic cocktail to which we are adapted. We abandon it at our peril."

A vast number of substances found in fruits and vegetables are known to protect against cancer. Some experts refer to these as "chemopreventers," but they are better known as *phytochemicals* (see Table 2.2). Phytochemicals include pigments such as carotenes, chlorophyll, and flavonoids; dietary fiber; enzymes; vitaminlike compounds;

TABLE 2.2

Examples of Anticancer Phytochemicals

Phytochemical	Actions	Sources
Carotenes	Act as antioxidants Enhance immune functions	Dark-colored vegetables such as carrots, squash, spinach, kale, tomatoes, and yams and sweet potatoes; fruits such as cantaloupe melons, apricots, and citrus fruits
Coumarin	Has antitumor properties Enhances immune functions Stimulates antioxidant mechanisms	Carrots, celery, fennel, beetroot, and citrus fruits
Dithiolthiones, glucosinolates, and thiocyanates	Keep cancer-causing compounds from damaging cells Enhance detoxification	Cabbage-family vegetables, such as broccoli, Brussels sprouts, collards, and kale
Flavonoids	Act as antioxidants Have direct antitumor effects Have immune-enhancing properties	Fruits, particularly darker fruits such as berries, cherries, and citrus fruits; also tomatoes, peppers, and greens
Isoflavonoids	Block oestrogen receptors	Soy and other legumes
Lignans	Act as antioxidants Modulate hormone receptors	Linseed and linseed oil; whole grains, nuts, and seeds
Limonoids	Enhance detoxification Block carcinogens	Citrus fruits and celery
Polyphenols	Act as antioxidants Block carcinogen formation Modulate hormone receptors	Green tea, chocolate, and red wine
Sterols	Block production of carcinogens Modulate hormone receptors	Soy, nuts, and seeds

and other minor dietary constituents. Although phytochemicals work in harmony with antioxidants, such as vitamin C, vitamin E, and selenium, phytochemicals exert considerably greater protection against cancer than these simple nutrients. Among the most important groups of phytochemicals are pigments such as chlorophyll, carotenes, and flavonoids.

2. REDUCE YOUR EXPOSURE TO PESTICIDES

In the United States, more than 1.2 billion pounds/500 million kilograms of pesticides and herbicides are sprayed on or added to food crops each year (30 million kilograms per year in the U.K.). That's roughly five pounds/2½ kilograms of pesticides for each man, woman, and child (½ kilogram in the U.K.). There is a

EASY TIPS FOR REACHING THE TEN-SERVINGS-A-DAY GOAL

- *Buy many kinds of fruits and vegetables when you shop, so you have plenty of choices in the house.*
- *Stock up on frozen vegetables for easy cooking so that you can have a vegetable dish with every dinner. You can easily steam frozen vegetables.*
- *Use the fruits and vegetables that go bad quickly, such as peaches and asparagus, first. Save hardier varieties, such as apples, acorn squash, and frozen goods, for later use if you do not shop frequently in a week.*
- *Keep fruits and vegetables where you can see them. The more often you see them, the more likely you are to eat them.*
- *Keep a bowl of cut-up vegetables on the top shelf of the refrigerator.*
- *Make a big tossed salad with several kinds of greens, cherry tomatoes, cut-up carrots, red pepper, broccoli, spring onions, and sprouts. Refrigerate in a large glass bowl with an airtight lid, so a delicious mixed salad will be ready to enjoy for several days.*
- *Keep a fruit bowl on your kitchen counter, table, or desk at work.*
- *Pack a piece of fruit or some cut-up vegetables in your briefcase or backpack and carry wetwipes for easy cleanup.*
- *Add fruits and vegetables to lunch by having them in soup, in salad, or cut up raw.*
- *Increase portions when you serve vegetables. One easy way of doing so is adding fresh greens, such as Swiss chard, collards, or beet greens, to stir-fries.*
- *Add extra varieties of vegetables when you prepare soups, sauces, and casseroles. For example, add grated carrots and courgettes to spaghetti sauce.*
- *Take advantage of salad bars, which offer ready-to-eat raw vegetables and fruits, as well as prepared salads made with fruits and vegetables.*
- *Use vegetable-based sauces such as marinara sauce and juices such as tomato juice.*
- *Choose fresh fruit for dessert. For a special dessert, try a fruit parfait with low-fat yogurt or sherbet topped with lots of berries.*
- *Freeze blueberries. They make a great summer replacement for ice cream, ice lollies, and other sugary foods.*

growing concern that in addition to these pesticides directly causing a significant number of cancers, exposure to these chemicals through food consumption damages your body's detoxification mechanisms, thereby increasing your risk of getting cancer and other diseases.

We are all exposed to pesticides and other toxins in the air that we breathe, the environment, and the food that we eat. To illustrate just how problematic pesticides can be, let's take a quick look at the health problems of the farmer. The lifestyle of farmers is generally healthy. Compared to city dwellers, they have access to lots of fresh food, breathe cleaner air, work harder physically, and have a lower rate of cigarette smoking and alcohol use. Yet studies show that farmers have a higher risk of developing lymphomas, leukemias, and cancers of the stomach, prostate, brain, and skin. In Britain, a Royal Commission on Environmental Pollution report concluded that it was possible that pesticide use could be linked to chronic ill health in "residents and bystanders".

Perhaps the most problematic pesticides are the halogenated hydrocarbon family, such as DDE, PCB, PCP, dieldrin, and chlordane. These chemicals persist in the environment almost indefinitely despite being banned in many European countries. For example, a similar pesticide, DDT, has been banned for nearly thirty years, yet it can still be found in soil and root vegetables, such as carrots and potatoes. Our bodies have a tough time detoxifying and eliminating these compounds, which end up being stored in our fat cells. What's more, inside the body these chemicals can act like the hormone oestrogen. They are thus suspected as a major cause of the growing epidemic of oestrogen-related health problems, including breast cancer. Some evidence also suggests that these chemicals increase the risk of developing lymphomas, leukemia, and pancreatic cancer, as well as playing a role in low sperm counts and reduced fertility in men.

Avoiding pesticides is especially important for preschool-aged children. Children are at greater risk of suffering from the damaging effects of pesticides for two reasons: they eat more food relative to their body mass, and they consume more foods higher in pesticide residues, such as juices, fresh fruits, and vegetables. A recent University of Washington study that analyzed levels of breakdown products of organophosphorus pesticides (a class of insecticides that disrupt the nervous system) in the urine of thirty-nine urban and suburban children two to four years of age found that concentrations of

pesticide metabolites were one sixth as high in the children who ate organic fruits and vegetables as in those eating conventional produce.

After conducting an analysis of U.S. Department of Agriculture residue data for all pesticides for 1999 and 2000, the U.S. Consumers' Union warned parents of small children to limit or avoid conventionally grown foods known to have high residues, such as cantaloupe melons, green beans (including canned and frozen), pears, strawberries, Mexican-grown tomatoes, and winter squash. The University of Washington study added apples to this list.

Here are our recommendations for avoiding pesticides in your diet.

- Do not overconsume foods that have a tendency to concentrate pesticides, such as animal fats, meat, eggs, cheese, and milk. Try to purchase free-range and organic forms of these foods.

- Buy organic produce, which is grown without the aid of synthetic pesticides and fertilizers. Although less than 3 percent of the total produce in the United States is grown without pesticides, organic produce is widely available. In the U.K., around 70 percent of organic food sold in supermarkets is imported, although organic food suppliers also sell directly through 'box' schemes or at farmers' markets. The U.K. government aims to increase the proportion of British organic food to 70 percent by 2010.

- Try to buy local produce, in season.

- Peeling off the skin or removing the outer layer of leaves of some produce may be all you need do to reduce pesticide levels. The downside of this is that many of the nutritional benefits are concentrated in the skin and outer layers. An alternative measure is to remove surface pesticide residues, waxes, fungicides, and fertilizers by soaking the item in a mild solution of additive-free soap, such as pure castile soap. All-natural, biodegradable cleansers are also available at most health food shops. To use, spray the food with the cleanser, gently scrub, and rinse.

For information on the pesticide content of popular fruit and vegetables, see Appendix C, pages 789–91.

3. EAT TO REGULATE YOUR BLOOD SUGAR LEVEL

Refined sugars, white flour products, and other sources of simple sugars are quickly absorbed into the bloodstream, causing a rapid rise in blood sugar. In response, the body boosts secretion of insulin by the pancreas. High-sugar, junk-food diets definitely lead to poor blood sugar regulation, obesity, and ultimately type 2 diabetes. But the stress on the body that they cause, including secreting too much insulin, can also promote the growth of cancer and increase the risk of heart disease. So we will make this simple recommendation: Don't eat "junk foods," and pay attention to the glycemic load of the foods you eat.

In chapter 1, we introduced the term "glycemic index" (GI). The GI refers to how quickly your blood sugar level rises after you eat a certain amount of food based on a referenced amount of carbohydrate. However, since it doesn't tell you how much carbohydrate there is in a typical serving of a particular food, another tool is needed. That is where glycemic load comes in. The glycemic load (GL) is a relatively new way to assess the impact of carbohydrate consumption that takes the glycemic index into account but gives a more complete picture of the effect that a food has on blood sugar levels based on how much carbohydrate you actually eat in a serving. A GL of 20 or more is high, a GL of 11 to 19 is medium, and a GL of 10 or less is low. For example, let's take a look at beetroot, a food with a high GI but a low GL. Although the carbohydrate in beetroot has a high GI, there isn't a lot of it, so a typical serving of cooked beetroot has a glycemic load that is relatively low, about 5. Thus, as long you eat a reasonable portion of a low-glycemic-load food, the impact on blood sugar is acceptable, even if the food is high in its GI. For example, a diabetic can enjoy some watermelon (GI 72) as long as he keeps the serving size reasonable. For example, 4 ounces/120 grams of watermelon has a glycemic load of only 4.

In essence, foods that are mostly water (e.g., apple or watermelon), fiber (e.g., beetroot or carrot), or air (e.g., popcorn) will not cause a steep rise in your blood sugar even if their glycemic index is high as long as you exercise moderation in portion sizes. To help you design your diet, we provide a list of the glycemic index, fiber content, and glycemic load of common foods in Appendix A.

4. DO NOT OVERCONSUME MEAT AND OTHER ANIMAL FOODS

Study after study confirms one basic truth: the higher your intake of meat and other animal products, the higher your risk of heart disease

---

AVOID CONSUMING JUNK FOOD AND SOURCES OF HIDDEN EMPTY CALORIES

According to the third National Health and Nutrition Examination Survey, which studied the eating habits of 15,000 American adults, one third of the average diet in the U.S.A. is made up of unhealthy foods, including potato crisps, crackers, salted snack foods, sweets, gum, fried fast food, and soft drinks. In the U.K., a recent study, the Dietary and Nutritional Survey of British Adults, found similar results, for example that 25 percent of British women eat a diet of predominately convenience foods and a third of men live on beer and fast food. These foods offer little in terms of protein, vitamins, or minerals. What they do have is lots of "empty calories" in the form of sugar and fat. They fill you up so you don't have room for the good stuff—the foods that give your body a fighting chance to prevent cancer and other diseases.

Here are guidelines for making healthier eating choices:

- *Read labels carefully. If sugar, fat, or salt is one of the first three ingredients listed, it is probably not a good option.*
- *Be aware that certain words appearing on the label, such as sucrose, glucose, maltose, lactose, fructose, corn syrup, white grape juice concentrate, or evaporated cane juice, mean that sugar has been added.*
- *Look not just at the percentage of calories from fat but also the number of grams of fat. For every 5 grams of fat in a serving, you are eating the equivalent of 1 teaspoon of fat.*
- *If a snack doesn't provide at least 2 grams of fiber, it's not a good choice.*

---

and cancer, especially for the major cancers such as colon, breast, prostate, and lung cancer.

There are many reasons for this association. Meat lacks the antioxidants and phytochemicals that protect us from cancer. At the same time, it contains lots of saturated fat and other potentially carcinogenic (cancer-causing) compounds, including pesticide residues, as well as heterocyclic amines and polycyclic aromatic hydrocarbons, which form when meat is grilled, fried, or barbecued. The better done the meat, the higher level of amines and hydrocarbons.

Some proponents of a diet high in meats claim that we should eat the way our caveman ancestors did, but that argument doesn't really hold up. The meat of wild animals that early humans consumed was much different from the industrially produced, shrink-wrapped meat we find in supermarkets today. The demand for tender meat has led to the breeding of cattle whose meat contains 25 percent to 30 percent fat, or more. In contrast, meat from free-living animals and wild game has a fat content of less than 4 percent.

It's not just the amount of fat, however, that distinguishes industrially produced meat. Its composition is also different. Domestic beef contains primarily saturated fats and virtually no beneficial omega-3 fatty acids, while the fat of wild animals contains more than five times the polyunsaturated fat per gram and has substantial amounts, about 4 percent, of omega-3 fatty acids. Free-range animals also contain ten times as much conjugated linoleic acid (CLA) as grain-fed animals. CLA is a slightly altered form of the essential fatty acid linoleic acid. It occurs naturally in meat and dairy products. CLA was discovered in 1978 when researchers at the University of Wisconsin were looking for cancer-causing compounds that result from cooking. Instead, they found CLA, which appears to be an anticancer compound. Preliminary studies show that CLA might reduce the risk of heart disease and cancer.

Particularly harmful to human health are cured or smoked meats, such as ham, hot dogs and bacon that contain sodium nitrate and/or sodium nitrites, which are compounds that keep food from spoiling but dramatically increase the risk for cancer. These chemicals react with the amino acids in foods in the stomach to form highly carcinogenic compounds known as nitrosamines.

Research on adults makes a convincing argument to avoid cured or smoked meats. Even more compelling is the evidence linking consumption of nitrates to a significantly increased risk of the major childhood cancers, including leukemias, lymphomas, and brain cancers:

- Children who eat twelve hot dogs per month have nearly ten times the risk of developing leukemia as children who do not eat hot dogs.

- Children who eat hot dogs once a week double their chances of developing brain tumors; eating them twice a week triples the risk.

- Pregnant women who eat two servings per day of any cured meat have more than double the risk of bearing children who have brain cancer.

- Children who eat the most ham, bacon, and sausage have three times the risk of developing lymphoma.

- Children who eat minced meat once a week have twice the risk of acute lymphocytic leukemia as those who eat none; eating two or more hamburgers weekly triples the risk.

Fortunately, vegetarian alternatives to these standard components of the Western diet are now widely available, and many of them actually taste quite good! Consumers can find soy hot dogs, soy sausage, soy bacon, and even soy pastrami at their local health food store as well as in many mainstream supermarkets.

If you choose to eat red meat:

- Limit your intake to no more than 3 or 4 ounces/85 to 125 grams daily—about the size of a deck of playing cards. And choose the leanest cuts available.

- Avoid consuming well-done, chargrilled, and fat-laden meats.

- Don't eat cured meats, including bacon and hot dogs, especially if you are pregnant or a child under the age of twelve.

- Consider buying free-range meats or wild game.

TABLE 2.3

Healthier Food Choices

Reduce Your Intake Of	Substitute
Red meat	Fish, white meat, or poultry
Hamburgers and hot dogs	Soy-based or vegetarian alternatives
Eggs	Egg Beaters and similar reduced-cholesterol products, and tofu
High-fat dairy products	Low-fat or nonfat products
Butter, lard, and other saturated fats	Olive oil
Ice cream, pies, cake, and biscuits	Fruit
Fried foods and fatty snacks	Vegetables and fresh salads
Salt and salty foods	Light salt and low-sodium foods
Coffee and soft drinks	Herbal teas, green tea, and fresh fruit and vegetable juices
Margarine, shortening, and other sources of trans-fatty acids or partially hydrogenated oil	Cook with olive, macadamia nut, or coconut oil, and use vegetable spreads that contain no trans-fatty acids

5. EAT THE RIGHT TYPES OF FATS

There is no room for debate: A diet high in fat, particularly saturated fat and cholesterol, has been linked to numerous cancers. Both the American Cancer Society and the National Cancer Institute recommend a diet that supplies fewer than 30 percent of calories as fat. However, just as important as the amount of fat is the *type* of fat you consume. The goal is to *decrease* your total fat intake, especially your intake of saturated fats, trans-fatty acids, and omega-6 fats, while *increasing* your intake of omega-3 fatty acids and monounsaturated fatty acids.

Some of these terms can be confusing and will be fully explained in chapter 6. What we want to stress in this section is that most Westerners eat way too much of the omega-6 oils found in meats and most vegetable oils, including soy, sunflower, safflower, and corn. And they suffer from a relative deficiency of the monounsaturated fats from nuts, seeds, olive oil, and rapeseed oil, as well as a deficiency of the omega-3 fats found in fish and linseed oil. This situation is associated with an increased risk for cancer and about sixty other conditions, including heart disease, stroke, high blood pressure, skin diseases, and diabetes.

What makes a fat "bad" or "good" has a lot to do with the function of fats in our cellular membranes. Our membranes are made mostly of fatty acids. What determines the type of fatty acid present in the cell membrane is the type of

THE IMPORTANCE OF CONSUMING NUTS

Many people shy away from eating nuts because they believe that nuts are high in calories. Though nuts are high in calories, studies have shown that people who frequently consume nuts actually have less of a problem with obesity than those who do not eat nuts. Frequent nut consumption, particularly of almonds and walnuts, has also been shown to be protective against heart disease. In addition, a recent study has shown that consumption of nuts by women was inversely associated with risk of type 2 diabetes, independent of known risk factors for type 2 diabetes, including age, obesity, and family history of diabetes, physical activity, smoking, and other dietary factors. What the term "inversely associated" means is that the higher the intake of nuts, the less likely it was that a woman would develop type 2 diabetes. What was really amazing was that this relationship was seen even in women who were obese.

In addition to providing beneficial monounsaturated and polyunsaturated fats that improve insulin sensitivity, nuts are also rich in fiber and magnesium and have a low glycemic index. Higher intakes of fiber and magnesium and foods with a low glycemic index have been associated with reduced risk of type 2 diabetes in several population-based studies.

Since nuts are very high in calories—most have about 1,000 calories per cup—we advocate moderation when it comes to eating them in order to promote optimal body weight. We also advocate the use of mostly raw or lightly-roasted fresh nuts and seeds rather than commercially roasted and salted nuts and seeds.

fat you consume. A diet that is composed mostly of saturated fat, animal fatty acids, trans-fatty acids from margarine, shortening, and other sources of hydrogenated vegetable oils and that is high in cholesterol results in membranes that are much less fluid in nature than the membranes in a person who consumes optimal levels of unsaturated fatty acids.

According to modern pathology, or the study of disease processes, an alteration in cell membrane function is the central factor in the development of virtually every disease. As it relates to diabetes, abnormal cell membrane structure due to eating the wrong types of fats leads to impaired insulin action.

Without a healthy membrane, cells lose their ability to hold water, vital nutrients, and electrolytes. They also lose their ability to communicate with other cells and be controlled by regulating hormones, including insulin. Without the right type of fats in cell membranes, cells simply do not function properly. Considerable evidence indicates that cell membrane dysfunction is a critical factor in the development of many diseases.

The type of dietary fat profile that is linked to many diseases is an abundance of saturated fat and trans-fatty acids along with a relative insufficiency of monounsaturated and omega-3 fatty acids, as found in the typical Western diet. Since dietary fat determines cell membrane composition, such a dietary pattern leads to reduced membrane fluidity, which in turn causes reduced insulin binding to receptors on cellular membranes and/or reduced insulin action. Particularly harmful to cell membrane function are margarine, vegetable oil shortening, and other foods containing trans-fatty acids and partially hydrogenated oils. These "unnatural" forms of fatty acids interfere with the body's ability to utilize important essential fatty acids and are now linked to an increased risk for heart disease, diabetes, and cancer. Just the opposite effect has been shown to be created by diets high in monounsaturated fats and omega-3 fatty acids.

One diet that appears to be representative of a way of eating that provides an optimal intake of the right types of fat is the traditional "Mediterranean diet." This term has a specific meaning. It reflects food patterns typical of some Mediterranean regions in the early 1960s, such as Crete, parts of mainland Greece, and southern Italy. The traditional Mediterranean diet has shown tremendous benefit in fighting heart disease and cancer, as well as diabetes. It has the following characteristics:

- Olive oil is the principal source of fat.

- The diet centers on an abundance of plant food, including fruit, vegetables, breads, pasta, potatoes, beans, nuts, and seeds.

- Foods are minimally processed, and there is a focus on seasonally fresh and locally grown foods.

- Fresh fruit is the typical daily dessert, with sweets containing concentrated sugars or honey consumed a few times per week at the most.

- Dairy products, principally cheese and yogurt, are consumed daily in low to moderate amounts and in low-fat varieties.

- Fish is consumed on a regular basis.

- Poultry and eggs are consumed in moderate amounts, about one to four times weekly or not at all.

- Red meat is consumed infrequently and in small amounts.

- Wine is consumed in low to moderate amounts, normally with meals.

Olive oil consists not only of the monounsaturated fatty acid oleic acid, it also contains several antioxidant agents that may account for some of its health benefits. Olive oil is particularly valued for its protection against heart disease, as it lowers harmful LDL cholesterol and increases the level of protective HDL cholesterol. It also helps prevent circulating LDL cholesterol from becoming damaged by free radicals and has been proven to contribute to a better control of the elevated blood triglycerides that are so common in diabetes.

6. KEEP YOUR SALT INTAKE LOW, YOUR POTASSIUM INTAKE HIGH

The electrolytes—potassium, sodium, chloride, and magnesium—are mineral salts that can conduct electricity when dissolved in water. For optimal health, it's important for you to consume these nutrients in proper balance. Too much sodium in the diet from salt (sodium chloride) can disrupt this balance. Many people know that a high-sodium, low-potassium diet can cause high blood pressure, but not as many are aware that such a diet also increases the risk of cancer.

In the U.S., only 5 percent of sodium intake

comes from the natural ingredients in food. Prepared foods contribute 45 percent of our sodium intake, 45 percent is added in cooking, and another 5 percent is added as a condiment. In the U.K., it is thought that the food industry accounts for 80 percent of the average (12 grams) daily intake of salt by men, another 15 percent being added in cooking or at the table.

Here are some tips for reducing your sodium intake:

- Take the salt cellar off the table.

- Omit adding salt when preparing food.

- Learn to enjoy the flavors of unsalted foods.

- If you absolutely must have the taste of salt, try salt substitutes such as Solo or Lo Salt. These products are made with potassium chloride and taste very similar to sodium chloride.

- Try flavoring foods with herbs, spices, and lemon juice.

- Choose low-salt (reduced-sodium) products when available.

- Read food labels carefully to determine the amounts of sodium and learn to recognize ingredients that contain sodium: a food with salt, soy sauce, salt brine, or any ingredient with sodium, such as monosodium glutamate, or baking soda (sodium bicarbonate) as part of its name contains sodium.

- In reading labels and menus, look for words that signal a high sodium content, such as barbecued, broth, marinated, Parmesan, pickled, smoked, and tomato base.

- Prepared sauces and condiments are often high in sodium; these include barbecue sauce, cocktail sauce, Creole sauce, mustard sauce, soy sauce, and teriyaki sauce as well as many salad dressings.

- Don't eat canned foods, particularly vegetables or soups, as these are often extremely high in sodium.

Many of us have already learned to watch our salt intake, but we'd like to encourage you to increase your potassium intake as well. Most Americans have a potassium-to-sodium (K:Na) ratio of less than 1:2. In other words, they ingest twice as much sodium as potassium. (In the U.K., average intakes of sodium are about half as much again as potassium.) But experts believe that the optimal dietary potassium-to-sodium ratio is greater than 5:1—*ten times higher* than the average intake. However, even this may not be optimal. A natural diet rich in fruits and vegetables can easily produce a much higher K:Na ratio, because most fruits and vegetables have a K:Na ratio of at least 50:1. For example, here are the average K:Na ratios for several common fresh fruits and vegetables:

Apples	90:1
Bananas	440:1
Carrots	75:1
Oranges	260:1
Potatoes	110:1

7. DRINK A SUFFICIENT AMOUNT OF WATER EACH DAY

Water is essential for life. The average amount of water in your body is about 10 U.S. gallons/36 liters. We need to drink at least 48 ounces/1½ liters of water per day to replace the water that is lost through urination, sweat, and breathing. If we don't, we are likely to become dehydrated. You need to drink at least six to eight glasses of water (48 to 64 ounces/1½ to 2 liters) each day, though we recommend eight to twelve glasses as optimal. That basically means having a glass of water every two hours while you are awake. Don't wait until you're thirsty; schedule regular water breaks throughout the day instead.

Even mild dehydration results in impaired physiological and performance responses. Here is a list of water's many vital functions:

- Many nutrients dissolve in water so they can be absorbed more easily in your digestive tract.

- Many metabolic processes need to take place in water.

- Water is a component of blood and thus is important for transporting chemicals and nutrients to cells and tissues.

- Each of your cells is constantly bathed in a watery fluid.

- Water carries waste materials from your cells to your kidneys so they can be filtered out and eliminated.

- Water absorbs and transports heat. For example, heat produced by muscle cells during exercise is carried by water in the blood to the surface, helping your body maintain the right temperature balance. The skin cells also release water as perspiration, which helps keep you cool.

Several factors are thought to increase the likelihood of chronic mild dehydration: a faulty thirst "alarm" in the brain; dissatisfaction with the taste of water; regular exercise that increases the amount of water lost through sweat; living in a hot, dry climate; and consumption of the natural diuretics caffeine and alcohol. Diuretics are substances that draw water out of your cells and increase the rate of urination. Surprisingly, if you drink two cups of water and two cups of coffee, cola, or beer, you may end up with a net water intake of zero! Be aware of your "water budget." If you drink coffee or other dehydrating beverages, compensate by drinking an additional glass of water.

A Quick Look at Some Popular Diets

We would be remiss if we did not address our views of some of today's popular diets. While there are literally hundreds of fad diets that have been promoted over the years that we could discuss, we will limit the discussion to the following popular diets:

The Atkins diet
The Blood Type Diet
The Ornish diet
The macrobiotic diet
The vegetarian diet
The Zone diet

We will discuss the background, rationale and principles, and scientific validity of each diet along with our own recommendations.

The Atkins Diet

The Atkins diet is perhaps the most famous weight loss diet of all time. It is a high-protein, low-carbohydrate diet developed by Robert Atkins, M.D., during the 1960s. In the early 1990s, Dr. Atkins brought his diet back into the nutrition spotlight with the publication of his best-selling book *Dr. Atkins' New Diet Revolution.* It is estimated that more than 20 million people worldwide have tried the Atkins diet, which emphasizes the consumption of protein and fat. Individuals following the Atkins diet are permitted to eat unlimited amounts of all meats, poultry, fish, eggs, and most cheeses.

The Atkins diet is divided into four phases: Induction, Ongoing Weight Loss, Premaintenance, and Maintenance. During the Induction phase (the first fourteen days of the diet), carbohydrate intake is limited to no more than 20 grams per day. No fruit, bread, grains, starchy vegetables, or dairy products, except cheese, cream and butter, are allowed during this phase. During the Ongoing Weight Loss phase, dieters experiment with various levels of carbohydrate consumption until they determine the most liberal level of carbohydrate intake that allows them to continue to lose weight. Dieters are encouraged to maintain this level of carbohydrate intake until their weight loss goals are met. Then, during the Premaintenance and Maintenance phases, dieters determine the level of carbohydrate consumption that allows them to maintain their weight. To prevent regaining the weight lost, dieters must stick to this level of carbohydrate consumption, perhaps for the rest of their lives.

While we agree with the underlying principle of the Atkins Diet—that a diet high in sugar and refined carbohydrates causes weight gain and ultimately leads to obesity—we disagree with the solution. One of the big reason why the Atkins diet is so attractive to dieters who have tried unsuccessfully to lose weight on low-fat, low-calorie diets is that while on the Atkins programme dieters can eat as many calories as desired from protein and fat, as long as carbohydrate consumption is restricted. As a result, many Atkins dieters are spared the feelings of hunger and deprivation that accompany other weight loss regimens. However, we simply do not agree that such a diet is conducive to long-term good health.

Despite its enormous popularity, the Atkins programme was not evaluated in a proper clinical trial until 2003. In this initial study, while people following the Atkins Diet did experience initial weight loss, though likely as a result of water loss rather than true fat loss, in the long run they gained it all back plus more. In the study, sixty-three obese men and women were randomly assigned to the Atkins diet or a low-calorie, high-carbohydrate, low-fat diet. Contact with professionals was minimal, to replicate the experience of most dieters. While the subjects on the Atkins diet had lost more weight than subjects on the conventional diet at six months, the difference at twelve months was not significant. Adherence in both groups was poor. Other clinical studies have shown similar results.

The findings from these clinical trials indicate that although adhering strictly to the Atkins diet (dramatically reducing carbohydrate intake while allowing free access to high-fat and high-protein foods) can lead to more weight loss in the first six months, eating a more healthful diet, such as the one we recommend, is associated with equal efficacy in the long run and is considerably more health promoting. Based upon the current evidence, we do not recommend the Atkins diet. Furthermore, since the high protein content of the Atkins diet stresses the liver and kidneys, we do not recommend it for anyone with impaired liver or kidney function.

The Blood Type Diet

The Blood Type Diet is the culmination of nearly four decades of work conducted by Peter D'Adamo, N.D., and his father, James D'Adamo, N.D. It was popularized by the best-selling book by the younger D'Adamo, *Eat Right 4 Your Type.* The principles of the Blood Type Diet are based on the theory that people with different blood types respond differently to specific foods. The concept is also based on evolutionary history and the observation that different blood types emerged as the environmental conditions and eating styles of our ancestors changed. Between 50,000 B.C.E. and 25,000 B.C.E., all humans shared the same blood type: type O. These early humans were skilled hunters and thrived on a meat-based diet. Type A blood type emerged between 25,000 B.C.E. and 15,000 B.C.E. as a necessary adaptation to a more agrarian lifestyle. Climatic changes in the western Himalayan mountains led to the appearance of type B, and the blending of type A and type B blood types in modern civilization resulted in the appearance of the type AB blood type.

According to the Blood Type Diet, the physiological reason why people should eat according to their blood type relates to lectins, proteinlike substances found in many commonly eaten foods. Lectins, also known as phytohemagglutins, were first identified in 1888, at which time it was discovered that lectins interact with sugar-containing molecules on the surface of cells. This discovery allowed certain lectins to be used in blood typing, since blood type is determined by the presence or absence of specific sugar-protein residues on the surface of red blood cells.

Although most of the lectins found in food are destroyed by cooking or digestive enzymes, Dr. D'Adamo believes that as many as 5 percent of the lectins we take in through our diet are absorbed into the bloodstream, and some of these are incompatible with our blood type. Many food lectins look very similar to the antigen that determines one of the four blood types. As a result, when a lectin that looks similar, for example, to the type O antigen is eaten by a person with type A, type B, or type AB blood, the immune system recognizes that lectin as a foreign invader. Dr. D'Adamo implicates this lectin-caused immune response as the origin of many common health complaints and believes that if you want to prevent health problems, it is important to eat foods that are compatible with your blood type.

Since type O was the blood type of the earliest humans, Dr. D'Adamo emphasizes the importance of animal flesh and vegetables for individuals with this blood type. If you are type O, you are encouraged to eat lean beef, lamb, turkey, chicken, and seafood. In addition, adzuki beans, pinto beans, kale, collard greens, and all fruits are considered to be beneficial. Those with type O blood must strictly avoid eggs and dairy foods, breads and pastas made from wheat, cabbage-family vegetables, and corn.

Individuals with type A blood are believed to thrive on a plant-based diet and should consume large amounts of raw or steamed vegetables, lentils, soybeans and soy products, pinto beans, black beans, and whole grains. Berries and plums are also beneficial. Occasional consumption of poultry and fermented dairy products is also well tolerated. Individuals with type A blood should eliminate all meat products, whole-fat dairy products, peppers, tomatoes, and tropical and citrus fruits.

The diet for individuals with type B blood is more varied than the other blood type diets. If you have type B blood, you are encouraged to eat seafood, beef, lamb, and dairy products. Oats and millet, green vegetables, and all fruits are beneficial. Individuals with type B blood are encouraged to avoid chicken, bacon, ham, and shellfish entirely. In addition, it is recommended that individuals with type B blood limit their consumption of beef, wheat, rye, tomatoes, and corn.

Individuals with type AB blood are encouraged to eat lamb, turkey, cultured dairy products such as yogurt and sour cream, eggs, rice, tofu, plums, and cherries. People with type AB blood must strictly avoid all smoked or cured meats and limit their consumption of beef, wheat, corn, tropical fruits, oranges, and bananas.

Our opinion of the Blood Type Diet is that blood type is just one genetic variable. In fact, the ABO system is only one of many different blood-typing methods, and to date, more than

thirty unique markers have been identified on the surface of red blood cells. In addition, one of the key suppositions of this diet is that dietary lectins are actually absorbed, but most of the research on lectins has been performed in test tubes, not humans. Since many food lectins are destroyed by cooking, digestive enzymes, and bacteria in the intestines, it is not really known to what degree, if any, dietary lectins are absorbed. Nonetheless, there is some evidence to support the link between dietary lectins and some disease.

All that being said, we do feel that there appears to be some validity to the programme, especially the idea that our genetics and ancestry are important determinants of what we should eat. We also believe that some people are profoundly benefited by the diet but that the explanation of the observed benefits is probably not strictly related to blood type. For example, all people are encouraged to avoid the high-sugar-content, empty-calorie, processed foods that tend to promote weight gain and poor health in favor of more natural food choices. Furthermore, elimination and avoidance of an allergenic food can result in tremendous relief from conditions linked to food allergies, such as rheumatoid arthritis, eczema, psoriasis, asthma, and food cravings.

The Ornish Diet

Dean Ornish, M.D., is the developer of the Ornish diet. It is quite similar to the diet that Nathan Pritikin developed and popularized in the 1970s. Both diets are basically the opposite of the Atkins diet. While the Atkins regimen is high in fat and protein and low in carbohydrates, the Ornish diet programme is low in fat and protein and high in whole-grain, natural complex carbohydrates. The Ornish prescription is to consume 10 percent of calories as fat, 70 to 75 percent of calories as complex carbohydrates, and 15 to 20 percent of calories as protein. The Ornish diet excludes all animal products, except nonfat milk and nonfat yogurt. It also restricts all plant foods high in fat, such as avocados, nuts, and seeds.

Dr. Ornish and his colleagues have shown quite convincingly in well-designed clinical studies that his diet can reverse heart disease. Our main objections to the Ornish diet are that it is too restrictive and does not provide a sufficient amount of beneficial fats, such as monounsaturated fats and omega-3 fatty acids. In particular, the Ornish diet excludes fish, despite a significant body of research that demonstrates a protective effect of fish (and fish oil) consumption against heart disease.

The Macrobiotic Diet

The macrobiotic diet was developed in the 1920s by a Japanese educator named George Ohsawa. Ohsawa is said to have cured himself of a serious illness by changing to a simple diet of brown rice, miso soup, and sea vegetables. After regaining his health. Ohsawa worked to integrate Eastern and Western philosophy and medicine to form the dietary and lifestyle principles of what is now known as macrobiotics. The following are the key components of the macrobiotic diet and lifestyle:

- Eat only organic foods.

- Eat two or three meals a day.

- Avoid cooking with electricity or microwaves; use a gas or wood stove, and use only cast-iron, stainless-steel, or clay cookware.

- Chew each mouthful of food approximately fifty times to aid digestion and absorption of nutrients.

- Do not eat for at least three hours before bedtime.

- Take short baths or showers as needed with warm or cool water.

- Use grooming, cosmetic, and household products made from natural, nontoxic ingredients.

- Wear only cotton clothing and avoid metallic jewelry.

- Spend as much time as possible in natural outdoor settings and walk at least thirty minutes daily.

- Do aerobic or stretching exercises such as yoga, dance, or martial arts on a regular basis.

- Place large green plants throughout the house to enrich the oxygen content of the air, and keep windows open as much as possible to allow the circulation of fresh air.

- Avoid watching television and using computers as much as possible.

Whole grains, such as brown rice, barley, millet, oats, corn, and rye, make up the bulk of the macrobiotic diet. The diet also emphasizes the consumption of vegetables, especially cabbage, broccoli, cauliflower, kale, bok choy, collards, and mustard greens. Beans, tofu, and sea vegetables should be eaten on a daily basis, and a few servings each week of nuts, seeds, and fresh fish, such as halibut, flounder, cod, or sole, are permissible. All foods should be organically grown, and, ideally, only fresh and locally grown fruits and vegetables should be eaten.

Our view of the macrobiotic diet is that it incorporates many of the same principles that we advocate but falls short in its nutritional completeness and variety of health-boosting foods. Nonetheless, the macrobiotic diet is a health-promoting diet that clinical research has shown to be beneficial for people with cancer and cardiovascular disease.

Vegetarian Diet

The vegetarian diet is defined as one avoiding all animal flesh, including fish and poultry. Vegetarians who avoid flesh but do eat animal products, such as cheese, milk, and eggs, are ovo-lacto-vegetarians (ovo = egg; lacto = milk and cheese). Those who eschew all animal products are referred to as pure vegetarians or vegans.

The vegetarian diet is often promoted as the most beneficial diet and has been advocated by people from philosophers such as Plato to political leaders such as Benjamin Franklin and Gandhi to modern pop icons such as Paul McCartney. There is also considerable scientific research showing the benefits of the vegetarian diet. In fact, it has been shown to be associated with a lower risk of virtually every chronic disease. For example, numerous population-based

studies have shown that vegetarians are nearly 50 percent less likely to die from cancer or heart disease than are nonvegetarians. The vegetarian diet has also been shown to reduce one's chances of developing diabetes, osteoporosis, or high blood pressure or forming kidney stones or gallstones.

While each of us authors has been vegetarian at some point in our lives, we now believe that including fish and small amounts of animal foods in the diet leads to a more optimal nutritional intake. Nonetheless, we recognize the central and tremendous importance that plant foods play in an optimal human diet.

The Zone Diet

The Zone diet was developed by Barry Sears, Ph.D., and popularized in his best-selling book *Enter the Zone*. The basic principle guiding the Zone diet is based on the relationship between the hormone insulin and the ratio of dietary fat, protein, and carbohydrates. The Zone diet proposes a dietary ratio of 40 percent carbohydrate, 30 percent protein, and 30 percent fat.

The Zone diet is popular among people desiring to lose weight, and it definitely works because the actual recommendations of the Zone diet result in the average person taking in only 800 to 1,200 calories per day. Of course, any diet that is low enough in calories will result in weight loss, regardless of its proportions of protein, carbohydrate, and fat. As when following other weight loss programmes, people generally experience good initial weight loss on the Zone diet, but the strict—and confusing—nature of the diet makes it difficult for many to follow. As a result, long-term compliance—and therefore lasting weight loss—with this diet is difficult.

Individuals following the Zone diet are encouraged to consume protein from animal and/or vegetable sources that are relatively low in dietary fat, such as chicken or soy foods. It is also recommended that the diet include a good intake of monounsaturated fats, including olive oil, rapeseed oil, and avocados. Individuals following the Zone diet are encouraged to avoid:

- All refined carbohydrates and most simple sugars, including foods made from white flour (bread, pasta, bagels, tortillas, and breakfast cereals), sweets, fizzy drinks, and desserts.
- Fruits, vegetables, and grains high on the glycemic index, such as rice, papaya, mango, corn, potatoes, and carrots.
- Foods containing saturated fat, most notably red meat and whole-fat dairy products.
- Egg yolks and organ meats.

Our opinion of the Zone diet is that while we agree with many of the goals and principles of the diet, since it does not focus enough on plant foods, the amount of fiber and other important phytochemicals is not sufficient to promote long-term health.

What Is the Best Diet?

The dietary guidelines and principles that we have detailed in this chapter represent our answer to the hotly debated question "What is the best diet?" Over the years, there has been quite a war of opinions as to the diet that best promotes weight loss and health. At one end of the spectrum, although it has become quite popular to restrict carbohydrates of all sorts completely in favor of high-protein and high-fat foods, we simply do not believe that this sort of diet is health-promoting. In fact, we believe that this type of diet has already been proven disastrous to long-term health as it carries with it severe consequences for cardiovascular and kidney function. At the other end of the spectrum is the so-called low-fat, high-complex-carbohydrate diet. This diet is also doomed to fail because it does not differentiate quality of carbohydrate and fails to provide the right type of oils to promote health. We believe that any diet that severely restricts beneficial oils will ultimately fail.

After reviewing every popular diet in detail, as well as thousands of scientific articles on the role of diet in human health, what we offer here is based upon the evolutionary understanding of what constitutes the optimal diet. We believe that it is only a matter of time before what we are recommending will become the accepted answer to the question "What foods should we eat?"

3

Safe Eating

Many consumers are extremely concerned about the safety of the food they eat and the water they drink. In addition to fear of deadly bacteria such as *E. coli,* they are concerned about the effects that food additives, pesticides, pollutants, food irradiation, and genetically modified foods have on their bodies. Are these concerns well founded? Yes. There is much evidence to support that these food issues have the potential to not only harm our health but also alter the composition of the foods we eat in ways that may not be beneficial to us or the environment. In this chapter, we will discuss these food safety concerns in detail.

Foodborne Illnesses

Foodborne illness is caused by consuming contaminated foods or beverages. Many people do not think about food safety until a food-related illness affects them or a family member. While the food supply in the United States is one of the safest in the world, the Centers for Disease Control and Prevention (CDC) estimate that 76 million people get sick, more than 300,000 are hospitalized, and 5,000 Americans die each year from foodborne illnesses. In the U.K. in 2000, just over 1.3 million people reported foodborne illnesses with over 20,000 cases hospitalized and 924 deaths. The microbe or toxin causing foodborne illness enters the body through the gastrointestinal tract and often causes the first symptoms there, so nausea, vomiting, abdominal cramps, and diarrhea are common symptoms. While most cases of foodborne illness are mild, you should consult a physician immediately if you experience any of the following:

- Temperature over 101.5 degrees F./38.5 degrees C., measured orally.
- Blood in the stools.
- Prolonged vomiting that prevents keeping liquids down, which can lead to dehydration.
- Signs of dehydration, including decrease in

urination, dry mouth and throat, and feeling dizzy when standing up.

• Diarrheal illness that lasts more than three days.

More than 250 different organisms have been documented as being capable of causing foodborne illness, including a variety of bacteria, viruses, and parasites. But poisoning can also occur due to ingestion of harmful toxins or chemicals from organisms that have contaminated the food. For example, botulism occurs when the bacterium *Clostridium botulinum* grows in foods and produces a powerful paralytic toxin. The botulism toxin can produce illness even if the bacteria are no longer there.

Most of the common microorganisms that cause foodborne infections are microorganisms commonly present in the intestinal tracts of healthy animals. Meat and poultry can become contaminated during slaughter by contact with even small amounts of intestinal contents, while fresh fruits and vegetables can be contaminated if they are washed or irrigated with water that is contaminated with animal manure or human sewage.

The most common causes of foodborne infections are the bacteria *Campylobacter, Salmonella,* and *E. coli* O157:H7, and the caliciviruses, also known as the Norwalk and Norwalk-like viruses. Undercooked meat and poultry, raw eggs, unpasteurized milk, and raw shellfish are the most common sources of these organisms.

Campylobacter is a bacterial pathogen that causes fever, diarrhea, and abdominal cramps. It is the most commonly identified bacterial cause of diarrheal illness in the world. This bacterium lives in the intestines of healthy birds, and most raw poultry meat has *Campylobacter* on it. Undercooked chicken or other food that has been contaminated with juices dripping from raw chicken is the most frequent source of this infection.

Salmonella is another bacterium that is widespread in the intestines of birds, reptiles, and mammals. It can spread to humans via a variety of different foods of animal origin. The illness it causes, salmonellosis, typically includes fever, diarrhea, and abdominal cramps. In persons with poor underlying health or weakened immune systems, it can invade the bloodstream and cause life-threatening infections.

E. coli O157:H7 is a bacterial pathogen that has a reservoir in cattle and similar animals. Human illness typically follows consumption of food or water that has been contaminated with even microscopic amounts of cow faeces. The illness it causes is often severe and typically provokes bloody diarrhea and painful abdominal cramps, without much fever. In 3 to 5 percent of cases, a complication called hemolytic uremic syndrome (HUS) can occur several weeks after the initial symptoms. This severe complication includes temporary anemia, profuse bleeding, and kidney failure.

Calicivirus, or Norwalk-like virus, is an extremely common cause of foodborne illness, though it is rarely diagnosed because the laboratory test is not widely available. It causes an acute gastrointestinal illness, usually with more vomiting than diarrhea. It usually resolves within two days. Unlike many foodborne pathogens that have animal reservoirs, it is believed that Norwalk-like viruses spread primarily from one infected person to another. Infected kitchen workers can contaminate a salad or sandwich as they prepare it, if they have the virus on their hands. Infected fishermen, for instance, have contaminated oysters as they harvested them.

Preventing Foodborne Illnesses

There is much that you can do to reduce your risk of suffering a foodborne illness. Foremost is to cook meat, poultry, and eggs thoroughly. Using a thermometer to measure the internal temperature of meat is a good way to be sure that it is cooked sufficiently to kill bacteria. For example, minced beef should be cooked to an internal temperature of 160 degrees F./86 degrees C., poultry should reach a temperature of 185 degrees F./72 degrees C., and eggs should be cooked until the yolk is firm.

You can also avoid contaminating foods by being sure to wash hands, utensils, and cutting boards after they have been in contact with raw meat or poultry and before they touch another food. In addition, always put cooked meat on a clean platter, rather than back on one that held the raw meat.

We recommend washing fresh fruits and vegetables in running tap water. Use a soft-bristle brush with a little a mild soap. For greens, we recommend soaking them in cold water as many times as needed to get them clean. Be sure to always wash the knife and cutting board after each use, and avoid leaving cut produce at room temperature for many hours.

Food Irradiation

Food irradiation is the use of ionizing radiation on foods, either packaged or in bulk form, usually in the form of gamma rays from radioactive materials. Food irradiation is used to delay the ripening and extend the shelf life of fruits; to destroy harmful bacteria in fresh meat, poultry, and other foods; and to inhibit the sprouting of certain vegetables such as potatoes, primarily to destroy microorganisms. Food irradiation does not make the food radioactive.

Food irradiation was approved in 1963 by the U.S. Food and Drug Administration (FDA) to rid wheat and flour of insects and to control sprouting of potatoes. In 1983, the FDA approved irradiation of spices and seasonings, and in 1985, it approved irradiation to prevent trichinosis in pork. The following year, approval was extended to fruits and vegetables. In 1990, the FDA approved irradiation of poultry to prevent *Salmonella* and other foodborne bacterial pathogens. And in December 1997, the agency approved its use for red meat to kill *E. coli*. Next on the list of foods approved for irradiation may be fish and shellfish, to kill *Salmonella*, *Vibrio* (the organism that causes cholera), and other bacteria. In the U.K., seven categories of food subjected to specific doses are permitted to be irradiated. Regulations also provide for clear labelling of foods or ingredients that have been irradiated.

While more than forty countries have approved food irradiation, it is an extremely controversial practice. At one end of the spectrum, proponents say that food irradiation is safe and, in fact, necessary to make the food supply safer. In addition to reducing the risk for foodborne illness, food irradiation considerably reduces losses due to spoilage. At the other end of the spectrum, opponents are quick to point out the concern that irradiation produces altered food molecules, destroys most of the vitamins, and alters the fatty acid structures in food.

Even though there is a worldwide standard for food irradiation safety that was accepted in 1963 by the Codex Alimentarius Commission, a joint body of the U.N. Food and Agriculture Organization and the World Health Organization, our feeling is that the science conducted so far on food irradiation is far from complete. In other words, we question how there can be such a strong position on its safety without a more complete evaluation.

One of the real concerns about food irradiation is that it might be used to mask poor sanitation practices in food production. For example, instead of measures being taken to clean up and sanitize production facilities, food irradiation can be used as a way to mask faecal contamination of meat products and poultry.

Irradiated food sold in stores in the United States must, according to federal law, be identified with the green, flowerlike international symbol for irradiation. Labeling also must include the words "Treated with radiation" or "Treated by irradiation." However, there is a move to allow the term "cold pasteurization" to be used instead. Also, since the federal government lacks

jurisdiction over establishments selling prepared foods, irradiated foods are often sold without such labeling. In addition, irradiated ingredients need not be identified as such on labels of prepared and processed foods. Like other label requirements, when an irradiated food is later served at a restaurant or in food service, it does not have to be labeled. In the U.K. the Food Labelling Regulations (1996) state that irradiated foods or ingredients must be clearly labeled as "irradiated" or "treated with ionizing radiation."

Genetically Modified Food

The terms "genetically modified organism" (GMO) and "genetically modified foods" (GM foods) refer to plants or animals whose genes have been changed in the laboratory by scientists. All living organisms have genes written in their DNA. They are the chemical instructions for building and maintaining life. By modifying the genes, scientists can alter the characteristics of an organism. In agriculture, genetic engineering allows simple genetic traits to be transferred to crop plants from wild relatives, other distantly related plants, or virtually any other organism.

Manipulating the genetics of foods is not new. Traditional crop and animal breeding has been practiced since the early domestication of crops and livestock. Through traditional breeding and crossbreeding methods, genes have been transferred with the goal of exhibiting particular desirable traits. Natural breeding techniques are usually a slow process, given the nature of crop growing seasons and animal generation times.

FIGURE 3.1
International Logo for Irradiated Food

With modern genetic engineering techniques, however, changes can be made virtually immediately, and there are much greater manipulation options, including moving genes within or between species. It is the movement of genes between species that is of the greatest concern.

The processes involved in making a transgenic crop are as follows.

- Identification of an organism containing the desired gene; this can be from a plant, animal, or microorganism.
- Isolation of the desired gene from that organism.
- Creation of a modified genetic sequence by the fusion of the desired gene, a promoter sequence which controls the functioning of the gene, and a marker gene, for example, a fluorescent protein or an antibiotic resistance factor that allows the gene's presence to be detected even when the target gene is not being actively expressed.
- Multiplication of the recombinant sequence, usually in bacteria, to produce multiple copies.
- Insertion of the copies of the desired gene into the organism to be modified, using either a particle (gene) gun or a biological agent.
- Selection of those organisms that have successfully taken up the desired gene using a selection test that recognizes only organisms that have adopted the marker gene.
- Multiplication of the modified plants.

The modification made to a crop plant can relate to a factor of the plant that influences its physical characteristics. For example, one of the first GM foods was a tomato, the FlavrSavr tomato developed by Calgene. When natural tomatoes ripen, a gene is triggered to produce a chemical that makes the fruit go soft and eventually rot. With this gene modified, the FlavrSavr tomato has a longer shelf life and firmer fruit.

Do We Need Genetic Engineering?

The argument for genetic engineering of food is that while the world population continues to expand, the area of land available for food production is finite. If the world's population increases, food production must be increased. So proponents of GM foods argue that without its use there will not be enough food to meet the demands of future populations. This argument has some validity, but current techniques are not capable of expanding production that significantly, and the reality is that the primary reason for GM foods is to generate profits for large corporations seeking greater revenues.

Proponents also argue that the development of crops with enhanced resistance to weeds, pests, or diseases will lead to a reduction in the use of pesticide chemicals. The reality is that farmers who grow GM crops actually use more herbicide, not less. For example, Monsanto created Roundup Ready (RR) soy, corn, and cotton specifically so that farmers would continue to buy Roundup, the company's best-selling chemical weed killer, which is sold with RR seeds. Instead of reducing pesticide use, one study of more than eight thousand university-based field trials indicated that farmers who plant RR soy use two to five times more herbicide than farmers who use traditional weed control methods.

Our View of GM Foods

We are concerned about the development of GM foods for several reasons. First of all, there is little scientific data on the long-term safety of GM foods. It may turn out that GM foods cause unexpected health consequences that will not be apparent for years. Second, genes from genetically modified plants have already been shown to be capable of escaping into the environment and contaminating natural crops. And third, manipulating genetic material changes the expression of proteins and antigens in foods, a situation that could lead to allergic reactions.

Since GM has already been shown to contaminate the natural variety of a crop, it is conceivable that they could also cross-fertilize with other plants, resulting in all varieties of a plant being the GM version. GM could also lead to nonproducing crops or even "superweeds" that could wreak havoc and overtake planted crops.

Another concern is that some GM foods, such as GM corn, are being manipulated to resist synthetic pesticides. As a result, more of the pesticide is being used and humans' exposure to toxic pesticides is actually increasing while insects develop resistance to the pesticides' toxic effects. Finally, we also respect the strong sentiment that genetic engineering is morally wrong as it implicates an attempt to modify nature beyond natural laws.

There does not seem to be a strong reason for GM foods, and the GM foods that have currently been introduced have not fulfilled their promise to reduce pesticide use or maintain the integrity of the environment. We therefore recommend choosing non-GM foods.

Food Additives

Food additives are used either to prevent foods' spoiling or to enhance their flavor; they include such substances as preservatives, artificial colors, artificial flavorings, and acidifiers. Although the U.S. government has banned many synthetic food additives, it should not be assumed that all the additives currently used in our food supply are safe. A great number of synthetic food additives remain in use that are being linked to such diseases as depression, asthma or other allergies, hyperactivity or learning disabilities in children, and migraine headaches.

The FDA has approved the use of more than 2,800 different food additives. In Europe, there are between 300 and 400 "E-number" food additives that indicate a substance authorized by the E.U. for human consumption. Other numbered additives may be permitted in individual countries but will not have the "E" designation. It is estimated that the per capita daily consumption of these food additives is approximately 13 to 15 grams. This amount is astounding and leads to many questions: Which food additives are safe? Which should be avoided? An extremist might argue that no food additive is safe. However, many food additives fulfill important functions in our modern-day food supply. Many compounds approved as additives are natural in origin and possess health-promoting properties, while others are synthetic compounds with known cancer-causing effects. In this section, we will help you distinguish between whole, natural foods and foods that are highly processed.

TABLE 3.1

Synthetic Color Additives Certified for Food Use

Name/Common Name	Hue	Common Food Uses
FD&C Blue No. 1/Brilliant Blue FCF/E133	Bright blue	Beverages, dairy products powders, jellies, confections, condiments, icings, syrups, extracts
FD&C Blue No. 2/Indigotine/E132	Royal blue	Baked goods, cereals, snack foods, ice cream, confections, cherries
FD&C Green No. 3/Fast Green FCF (This can be found in the U.K. but has not been certified by E.U. safety tests)	Sea green	Beverages, puddings, ice cream, sherbet, cherries, confections, baked goods, dairy products
FD&C Red No. 3/Erythrosine/E127	Cherry red	Cherries in fruit cocktail and canned fruits for salads, confections, baked goods, dairy products, snack foods
FD&C Yellow No. 5/Tartrazine/E102	Lemon yellow	Custards, beverages, ice cream, confections, preserves, cereals
FD&C Yellow No. 6/Sunset Yellow/E110	Orange	Cereals, baked goods, snack foods, ice cream, beverages, dessert powders, confections
FD&C Red No. 40/Allura Red AC/E129	Orange red	Gelatins, puddings, dairy products, confections, beverages, condiments

Colors

The total annual consumption of food coloring in the United States is approximately 120 million pounds/55 million kilograms for the entire population (the U.K. figures are very similar). Food color additives are officially designated as either certified or exempt from certification. The food color additives that are exempt from certification are primarily natural in origin. This reflects the popular belief that natural compounds are safer. This contention appears to hold up to scientific scrutiny. Table 3.1 lists the current status of food color additives.

One of the most widely used synthetic food colors is FD&C Yellow No. 5, or tartrazine (E102).

Tartrazine is added to almost every packaged food, as well as many drugs, including some antihistamines, antibiotics, steroids, and sedatives. In the United States, the average daily per capita consumption of certified dyes is 15 milligrams, of which 85 percent is tartrazine. Among children, consumption is usually much higher.

Although the overall rate of allergic reactions to tartrazine in the general population is quite low, allergic reactions due to tartrazine range from 20 to 50 percent in individuals sensitive to aspirin as well as other allergic individuals. Like aspirin, tartrazine is a known inducer of asthma, hives, and other allergic conditions, particularly in children. In addition, tartrazine, as well as benzoate and aspirin, increases the

THE FEINGOLD HYPOTHESIS

The hypothesis that food additives can cause hyperactivity in children stemmed from the research of Benjamin Feingold, M.D., and is commonly referred to as the "Feingold hypothesis." According to Feingold, many hyperactive children, perhaps 40 to 50 percent, are sensitive to artificial food colors, flavors, and preservatives as well as to naturally occurring salicylates and phenolic compounds.

Feingold's claims were based on his experience with more than 1,200 cases in which food additives were linked to learning and behavior disorders. Since Feingold's presentation to the American Medical Association in 1973, the role of food additives as a contributing cause of hyperactivity has been hotly debated in the scientific literature. In actuality, however, researchers have focused on only ten food dyes versus the 3,000 food additives with which Feingold was concerned.

At first glance, it appears that the majority of the double-blind studies designed to test this hypothesis have shown essentially negative results. However, upon closer examination of these studies and further investigation into the literature, it becomes evident that food additives do, in fact, play a major role in hyperactivity. In several of the studies, overwhelming evidence was produced. It is interesting to note that, while the U.S. studies have been largely negative, the reports from Australia and Canada have been more supportive. Feingold contended that there is a conflict of interest on the part of the Nutrition Foundation, an organization supported by major food manufacturers, such as Coca-Cola, Nabisco, and General Foods. It appears significant that the Nutrition Foundation has financed most of the negative studies. Feingold contends that the conflict of interest arises because these companies would suffer economically if food additives were found to be harmful. Other countries have significantly restricted the use of artificial food additives because of possible harmful effects discovered in studies conducted outside the United States.

production of a compound that increases the number of mast cells in the body. Mast cells are involved in producing histamine and other allergic compounds. A person with more mast cells in the body will typically be more prone to allergies. For example, examination of patients with hives shows that more than 95 percent have an increase in mast cells.

In studies using provocation tests to determine sensitivity to tartrazine and other food additives in patients with hives, results have ranged from 5 to 46 percent. Diets eliminating tartrazine as well as other food additives in sensitive individuals have, in many cases, been shown to be of great benefit in patients with hives and other allergic conditions such as asthma and eczema. Obviously, people suffering from allergic conditions should eliminate artificial food colors from their diets.

Sweeteners

The three primary artificial sweeteners currently in use are saccharin (Sweet'N Low), aspartame (Equal, NutraSweet), and sucralose (Splenda). These sweeteners are among the most controversial of food additives. Advocates argue that the benefits provided outweigh the potential negative health effects. The perception is that consumption of these sweeteners will lead to a reduction in calories consumed. This, in turn, will lead to weight loss or prevention in weight gain. Unfortunately, this is not the case as detailed studies have not shown these sweeteners to reduce the amount of calories consumed or to have any significant effect on body weight. In fact, aspartame may actually increase appetite.

So if these sweeteners provide no benefits, what are the risks? Saccharin is a known cancer-causing compound in rats. And while these effects have not been noted in humans, it must be pointed out that saccharin has been shown to cause cancer in rats only if it is administered over two generations. Therefore, it might be that future generations may pay for the current consumption of saccharin. This effect on future generations may finally provide the firm evidence the American Medical Association's Council on Scientific Affairs requires. This council has concluded that "until there is firm evidence of its [saccharin's] carcinogenicity in humans, saccharin should continue to be available as a food additive." However, if saccharin poses no benefit to health, as studies have shown, and there is a cloud of doubt that hangs over its safety, why should it be used?

Aspartame is composed of aspartic acid, phenylalanine, and methanol. Aspartame was approved for food use by the FDA in 1981 (1983 in the U.K.), despite the final recommendation of the FDA Advisory Panel on aspartame that no approval be granted until safety issues could be resolved. Richard Wurtman, M.D., the pioneer in the study of nutrition and the brain, cautioned the FDA that, based on his extensive research, aspartame could significantly affect mood and behavior. Wurtman and other researchers have demonstrated that aspartame administration to animals, at levels comparable to those of high human consumption, alters brain chemistry.

While the long-term effects of aspartame are largely unknown, some people are quite sensitive to aspartame and report immediate reactions. Some of the problems associated with aspartame ingestion include seizures, migraine headaches, hives, and disturbances in nerve function. Aspartame is particularly problematic for some individuals who suffer from migraine headaches.

The newest member of the artificial sweetener family is sucralose, popularly known as Splenda. This sweetener is actually made from table sugar, sucrose, with newly attached chlorine molecules. Sucralose is six hundred times sweeter than sucrose and, unlike aspartame, does not break down when heated.

Although sucralose appears safer than either aspartame or saccharin, our top choice for a noncalorie sweetener is stevia, a natural sweetener extracted from the *Stevia rebaudiana* plant. Stevia is currently banned in the U.K.

Stevia contains a molecule known as stevioside that is three hundred times sweeter than sugar. Stevia is used around the world for its incredible sweetening properties. Preliminary studies in animal models show that stevia lowers blood glucose levels and blood pressure—two effects of prime importance in dealing with diabetes. However, since it has not yet passed Food and Drug Administration testing as a food additive, it cannot be advertised as a sweetener in the United States. Since stevia preparations are not likely to be patented (you cannot patent something that exists in nature), no company has been willing to invest in the cost of FDA testing.

Instead, it is sold as a "dietary supplement." There are several different brands of stevia (Stevita, Stevia Plus, SweetLeaf), each with a slightly different taste.

Another new sweetener looks promising: tagatose (Naturlose). It is a low-calorie, natural sugar found in milk that has just attained GRAS (Generally Recognized as Safe) status, allowing it

TABLE 3.2
Ranking the Nonsugar Sweeteners

Sweetener	Other Names	Recommended Use Level	Comments
Stevia	Sweet leaf	Liberal	A natural sweetener extracted from the *Stevia rebaudiana* plant, it is 300 times sweeter than sucrose. Technically Stevia is a dietary supplement because it has not been evaluated or approved by the FDA as a sweetener. It is also currently banned in the E.U. Preliminary studies show blood sugar–lowering and blood pressure–lowering effects.
Tagatose		Moderate	A naturally occurring sugar in milk that is 92 percent as sweet as sucrose but is absorbed poorly. It does have some caloric value, about one third that of sucrose. Studies show that tagatose actually blunts the glycemic response to sucrose.
Xylitol and other polyols (maltitol, sorbitol, mannitol, erythritol)		Moderate	Polyols are roughly 60 percent as sweet as sucrose. They are poorly absorbed sugars that do not break down when heated. Higher dosages—for example, a single dosage of more than 10 to 30 grams or a daily intake of more than 40 to 80 grams—may produce laxative effect.
Sucralose	Splenda	Conservative	Sucralose is composed of sucrose with newly attached chlorine molecules. It is 600 times sweeter than sucrose and does not break down when heated.
Aspartame	NutraSweet	Conservative	A controversial sweetener that is reported to receive more complaints at the FDA than any other food substance. It is made from two amino acids naturally found in foods, phenylalanine and aspartic acid. Aspartame is 200 times sweeter than sucrose but loses sweetness when heated.

(continued on next page)

Sweetener	Other Names	Recommended Use Level	Comments
Acesulphame K	Sunett, Sweet One	Restrictive	Made from vinegar, acesulphame K is not broken down by the body. It is structurally related to saccharin and is 200 times sweeter than sucrose.
Saccharin	Sweet'N Low	Restrictive	Saccharin was initially removed from the market in the U.S. over fears that it was a carcinogen. It is 300 times sweeter than sucrose. Because of safety concerns, it is not recommended during pregnancy.

to be included in foods as a sweetener. (D-Tagatose was recently approved by the Food Standards Agency in the U.K.) Tagatose is a sugar molecule, similar to glucose, that is poorly absorbed. It also appears to be able to actually block the absorption of other sugars, including glucose. When tagatose was given to diabetics prior to an oral glucose tolerance test, their blood glucose levels were significantly reduced. We expect to see tagatose gaining a lot of attention as it enters the crowded sweetener category.

For easy reference, we rank the sweeteners in Table 3.2 and assign each a recommended use level of liberal, moderate, conservative, or restrictive.

Antioxidants

Without antioxidants, many foods would spoil quite rapidly. The two most widely used are butylated hydroxyanisole (BHA) (E320) and butylated hydroxytoluene (BHT) (E321). Like saccharin, these food additives have caused cancers in rats. However, there are other studies showing that these antioxidants actually protect against the development of cancers. In fact,

many so-called experts in life extension have recommended that these substances be taken as a food supplement at very high doses, such as 2 grams per day. Based on extensive research, we feel this recommendation is extremely unwise as it is 100 times the estimated acceptable intake of BHA, BHT, or the sum of both, as set by the Joint Food and Agriculture Organization of the United Nations/World Health Organization Expert Committee on Food Additives. It is also more than 100 times the estimated inhibitory activity of these compounds and may actually promote cancer. While BHA and BHT may be safe at low levels in foods, in the future they will most likely be replaced by naturally occurring antioxidants.

Preservatives

Preservatives, such as sodium benzoate, nitrates, nitrites, and sulphites, work primarily to prevent spoilage by checking the growth of microorganisms. All of these preservatives have come under attack recently. In the case of nitrates and nitrites, these compounds are known carcinogens. Sulphites and benzoates, on the other hand, are capable of producing allergic reactions.

Benzoic acid and benzoates are the most commonly used food preservatives. Although for the general population the rate of allergic response is thought to be less than 1 percent, the frequency of positive challenges in patients with chronic hives or asthma varies from 4 percent to 44 percent. Sulphites pose even more of a problem. Sulphites were once widely used on produce at restaurant salad bars. Since most people were not aware that sulphites were being added and because most people were unaware they had a sensitivity to sulphites, many unsuspecting people experienced severe allergic or asthmatic reactions. For years the FDA refused to even consider a ban on sulphites, even while admitting that these agents provoked attacks in an unknown number of people and in 5 to 10 percent of asthma victims. It was not until 1985, when sulphite sensitivity was linked to fifteen deaths between 1983 and 1985, that the FDA agreed to review the matter. In 1986, the FDA finally banned the use of sulphites on produce and required labeling of other foods, such as wine, beer, and dried fruit, that have had sulphites added. In the E.U., ingredients must include sulphites in concentrations of more than 10 milligrams/kilogram or 10 milligrams/liter. The average person consumes an average of 2 to 3 milligrams of sulphites per day, while wine and beer drinkers typically consume up to 10 milligrams per day. In the U.K. the average man consumes an average of 26 milligrams per day, which is among the highest levels in the world.

From the research, it is clear that all preservatives should be avoided, especially by people prone to allergies. The best way of doing this is to consume fresh, whole foods.

Pesticides

In the United States each year, more than 1.2 billion pounds/½ billion kilograms of pesticides and herbicides are sprayed on or added to our crops (30 million kilograms per year in the U.K.). Although pesticides are designed to work against insects and other organisms, experts estimate that only 2 percent of pesticides actually serve their purpose, while more than 98 percent are absorbed into the air, water, soil, or food supply. Most pesticides in use are synthetic chemicals of questionable safety. The major long-term health risks include the potential to cause cancer and birth defects, while the major health risks of acute intoxication include vomiting, diarrhea, blurred vision, tremors, convulsions, and nerve damage.

The evidence for the cancer-causing capabilities of pesticides in animals is inadequate, and the formal opinion of many "experts" is that they pose no significant risk for the public or the farmer. Yet more and more human evidence is accumulating of increased cancer and birth defect rates after pesticide exposure, which seems to indicate that pesticides are not as safe as the "experts" would like us to believe. This situation reflects a major dilemma to scientists: Which is more valid, studies on laboratory animals or population studies on humans?

The history of pesticide use in the United States is riddled with pesticides that were once widely used and then later banned due to health risks. Perhaps the best-known example of this is

DDT. Widely used from the early 1940s to 1973, DDT was largely responsible for increasing farm productivity in the United States, but at what cost? In 1962, Rachel Carson's classic book *Silent Spring* detailed the full range of DDT's hazards, including its persistence in the food chain and its deadly effects, but it was another ten years before the federal government banned the use of this deadly compound. Unfortunately, although DDT has been banned for nearly thirty years, it is still found in the soil and in root vegetables, such as carrots and potatoes.

The majority of pesticides currently used in the United States are probably less toxic than DDT and other banned pesticides, including aldrin, dieldrin, endrin, and heptachlor. However, many pesticides banned from use in the United States are shipped to other countries, such as Mexico, which then, in turn, send foods treated with pesticide back to the United States.

Although more than 600 pesticides are currently used in the United States, most experts are most concerned about only a relative few. The Environmental Protection Agency (EPA) has identified 64 pesticides as potential cancer-causing compounds, with 80 percent of our cancer risk due to thirteen pesticides that are widely used on fifteen important food crops. The pesticides are linuron, permethrin, chlordimeform, zineb, captafol, captan, maneb, mancozeb, folpet, chlorothalonil, metiram, benomyl, and O-phenylphenol. These pesticides are found in many crops and animal products, but those of greatest concern in descending order are tomatoes, beef, potatoes, oranges, lettuce, apples, peaches, pork, wheat, soybeans, beans, carrots, chicken, corn, and grapes.

In the U.S., pesticide residue levels in food are monitored by both state and federal regulatory agencies. Such monitoring is used to enforce legal tolerance levels. However, there has been increasing public and governmental concern about the adequacy of the residue-monitoring programmes. In theory, here is how the monitoring system is designed to work: The EPA establishes a tolerance level for pesticides in raw or unprocessed foods utilizing available data. The Food and Drug Administration (FDA) is then responsible for enforcing the EPA limits. Individual state organizations, such as departments of health and agriculture, may also be involved in the monitoring of food safety.

Where this system falls short is not simply in the determination of the tolerance level; more important are the facts that (1) probably less than 1 percent of our domestic food supply is screened by the FDA; (2) the FDA does not test for all pesticides; and (3) the FDA does not prevent the marketing of the foods that it finds contain illegal residues. In the U.K., the Pesticides Safety Directorate, part of the Department for Environment, Food and Rural Affairs, provides controls for the use of pesticides and monitors their use, including legal enforcement of regulations. It also works within a larger European Union context.

A number of pesticide poisoning epidemics have been reported over the years in the U.S. The largest to date occurred in 1985. It involved the use of aldicarb, an extremely toxic pesticide, and its illegal use on watermelons. Aldicarb is a systemic pesticide, which means that it permeates the entire fruit. More than one thousand people in the western United States and Canada were struck. Illness ranged from mild

USDA CERTIFIED ORGANIC

The U.S. Department of Agriculture put in place a set of national standards in 2002 for food labeled "organic," whether it is grown in the United States or imported from other countries. Organic food is produced by farmers who emphasize the use of renewable resources and the conservation of soil and water to enhance environmental quality for future generations. Organic meat, poultry, eggs, and dairy products come from animals that are given no antibiotics or growth hormones. Organic food is produced without using most conventional pesticides; fertilizers made with synthetic ingredients or sewage sludge; bioengineering; or ionizing radiation. Before a product can be labeled "organic," a government-approved certifier inspects the farm where the food is grown to make sure the farmer is following all the rules necessary to meet USDA organic standards.

The USDA developed a seal to certify that a food is organic. But the use of the seal is voluntary, so some organic foods may not be labeled with the USDA seal. People who sell or label a product as "organic" when they know it does not meet USDA standards, however, can be fined up to $10,000 for each violation.

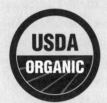

United States Department of Agriculture Logo for Organic Foods

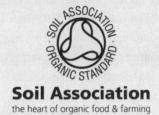

Soil Association
the heart of organic food & farming

In the E.U., under Regulation 2092/91, food products marketed as organic must be certified by an E.U. approved certification body. This includes all food products that are imported from outside the E.U.

In the U.K., the E.U. regulation is interpreted by Defra (the department of environment, food and rural affairs) as the ACOS compendium. Defra accredit certification bodies in the U.K. to carry out inspection and certification. In the U.K., the main body is Soil Association Certification Ltd who certify over 4,300 organic farms and businesses to the Soil Association organic standards. Food certified to these standards can carry the Soil Association symbol, which is the most widely recognised organic symbol in the U.K. For more information about the Soil Association see www.soilassociation.org.

gastrointestinal upset to severe poisoning that included vomiting, diarrhea, blurred vision, tremors, convulsions, and nerve damage.

While the EPA and FDA estimate that excessive pesticide residues are found on about 3 percent of domestic and 6 percent of foreign produce, and acceptable levels are found in 13 percent of domestic produce, other organizations report much higher estimates. For example, the National Resources Defense Council conducted a survey of fresh produce sold in San Francisco markets for pesticide residues and found that 44 percent of seventy-one fruits and vegetables had detectable levels of nineteen different pesticides, with 42 percent of produce with detectable pesticide residues containing more than one pesticide. The sheer number and amount of pesticides showered on certain foods are astounding. For example, more than fifty pesticides are used on broccoli, 110 on apples, and seventy on bell peppers. As many of the pesticides penetrate the entire fruit or vegetable and cannot be washed off, it is obviously best to buy organic foods.

Many supermarket chains and produce suppliers in the U.S. and U.K. are employing their own testing measures for determining the pesticide content of produce and are refusing to stock foods that have been treated with some of the more toxic pesticides, such as alachlor, captan, or EBDCs (ethylene bisdithiocarbamates). In addition, many shops are asking growers to disclose all pesticides used as well as to phase out the use of the sixty-four pesticides suspected of being capable of causing cancers. Ultimately, it will be pressure from consumers that will have the greatest influence on food suppliers. Encouragingly, crop yield studies support the use of organic farming if the risk to human health of using pesticides is added to the equation.

Waxes

In addition to pesticides, consumers must be aware of the waxes applied to many fruits and vegetables to seal in the water contained in the produce, thereby keeping the produce looking fresh. According to FDA law, grocery stores must display a sign noting that waxes or postharvest pesticides have been applied. Unfortunately, most stores do not comply with the law, and the FDA lacks the manpower to enforce it. Adequate labeling of foods remains an issue in the U.K., where it is not easy to ascertain if a food has been waxed. The Food Standards Agency conducted a survey in 2000 which recommended numerous improvements to the information available on food labels, including production methods such as waxing. Legislation has yet to be passed. Currently, the FDA has approved six different waxes for use on produce. Approved compounds include shellac (E904#), paraffin (E905#), palm oil derivatives, such as carnauba wax (E903), and synthetic resins. These same items are used in furniture, floor, and car waxes. Foods to which these compounds may be applied include apples, avocados, bell peppers, cantaloupe melons, cucumbers, aubergines, grapefruits, lemons, limes, melons, oranges, parsnips, passion fruits, peaches, pineapples, pumpkins, swedes, squashes, sweet potatoes, tomatoes, and turnips.

One of the main reasons the waxes are added is to keep the produce from spoiling during the often long period of time from harvest to the supermarket shelves. If supermarket chains bought more local produce, the produce would not require chemicals to keep it looking fresh. Instead the large chains sign contracts with large produce suppliers, regardless of their location. This is why, for example, a grocery store in New York is stocked with Washington State apples and California broccoli.

The waxes themselves probably pose little health risk; however, most waxes have powerful pesticides or fungicides added to them. Since the waxes cannot be washed off with water, the fungicide or pesticide literally becomes cemented to the produce.

How to Reduce Your Exposure

Here are some recommended methods of reducing exposure to pesticides as well as tips on removing the surface pesticide residues, waxes, fungicides, and fertilizers from produce:

1. Buy organic produce. In the context of food and farming, the term organic is used to imply that the produce was grown without the aid of synthetic chemicals, including pesticides and fertilizers. Although less than 3 percent of the total produce grown in the United States is grown without the aid of pesticides, organic produce is widely available. In Europe, the market for organic food grew at 25 percent per year between 1990 and 2000. The U.K. has seen a five-fold increase in five years.

2. If organic produce is not readily available, develop a good relationship with your local supermarket produce manager. Explain to him or her the desire to reduce your exposure to pesticides and waxes. Ask what measures the shop takes to ensure that pesticide residues are within the tolerance limits. Ask where it gets its produce, as foreign produce is much more likely to contain excessive levels of pesticides as well as pesticides that have been banned in the United States or Europe due to suspected toxicity. And try to buy local produce that is in season.

3. To remove surface pesticide residues, waxes, fungicides, and fertilizers, soak the produce in a mild solution of additive-free soap, such as pure castile soap from the health food shop, and then rinse off. Another solution is to use Veggi Wash, a commercially available fruit and vegetable wash.

4. Simply peel off the skin or remove the outer layer of leaves. The downside of this is that many of the nutritional benefits are concentrated in the skin and outer layers.

The Benefits of Organic Foods

While some may say that even whole, organic foods have compounds in them that are poisonous or have been linked to cancer in animal studies, this argument contains some major shortcomings. First of all, while it is true that there are poisonous compounds in nature, rarely are they found in common organic foods. When potentially harmful compounds are contained in an organic food, the whole, organic food also provides a wide range of compounds that protect the body from harm. Potentially harmful food additives, on the other hand, are typically added to artificially preserve freshness in some foods or to nutritionally poor foods, such as cured meats and junk foods. Take nitrates as an example. Many common vegetables, such as celery, radishes, and beetroot, are rich sources of nitrates. The concern about nitrates is that they can be converted to nitrites and then to cancer-causing compounds known as nitrosamines in the gut. However, there are compounds in these vegetables, such as vitamin C and flavonoids, that prevent the conversions from taking place. In contrast, the nitrites and nitrates added to cured meats are easily converted to the cancer-causing nitrosamines. Cured meats are also high in saturated fats and salt and contain other food additives.

Far from being poisonous, organic foods have many benefits. By eating organically grown foods, you:

- *Reduce your exposure to health-robbing toxins* used in conventional agricultural practices, including not only pesticides, but also heavy metals, such as lead and mercury, and solvents, such as benzene and toluene. A number of pesticides have already been recognized as carcinogens, while others have been shown to affect mitochondrial energy production negatively, and still others have been shown to damage cellular membranes, triggering inflammation that has been linked to atherosclerosis. Heavy metals lower IQ and damage nerve function, contributing to neurodegenerative diseases, such as Parkinson's and Alzheimer's diseases and multiple sclerosis. And solvents damage white cells, the immune system defenders that enable the body to resist infections. Not only are these toxic substances harmful singly, but when combined, as they are in commercially grown and processed food, their effects in the human body, where they accumulate, have been found to be magnified as much as a thousandfold.

- *Increase your consumption of health-promoting micronutrients.* A number of studies have demonstrated that organically grown produce contains significantly higher amounts of many vitamins and minerals. In a 1988 review of thirty-four studies that compared organic with conventionally grown foods, organic food was found to have higher protein quality in all comparisons, higher levels of vitamin C in 58 percent of all studies, and 5 to 20 percent higher mineral levels for all but two minerals. In some cases, the mineral levels were dramatically higher in organically

grown foods and were as much as three times higher in one study involving iron content. Organically grown foods also contain higher amounts of plant-protective compounds, such as flavonoids and carotenoids, which are highly desirable for human consumption. Take resveratrol, for example. Resveratrol is a compound produced by grapes in self-defense against environmental stressors, such as attack by insects or fungal infection. Organically grown grapes have been found to produce much higher amounts of resveratrol than conventionally grown grapes, which are already protected by treatment with man-made fungicides.

- *Safeguard your children's health.* Reports from the Natural Resources Defense Council (1989) and the Environmental Working Group (1998) in the U.S.A. found that millions of American children are exposed to levels of pesticides through their food that surpass limits considered safe. Some of these pesticides are known neurotoxins with the potential to harm a developing brain and nervous system. Others, with carcinogenic activity, may wreak even more damage in children and adolescents, whose higher growth rates equal higher rates of cell turnover, particularly as their sexual organs develop.

- *Safeguard the health of the environment.* Residues from toxic chemicals used in conventional farming methods remain in the soil and leach into groundwater. According to the Environmental Protection Agency, pesticides, some known to be carcinogens, now pollute the groundwater—the primary source of drinking water—in thirty-eight states in America, affecting more than half the country's population. The use of chemical-dependent farming methods has not only adversely impacted soil and water but also reduced the biodiversity, nutrient quality, and taste of our foods since synthetic nitrate fertilizers cause nitrate to bind to water, which makes the produce look good but lessens its flavor. Organic farming practices work to preserve and protect the environment by maintaining a restorative and sustainable biosystem, which improves soil quality, preserves water purity, encourages biodiversity, and, by nourishing the soil, produces plants rich in flavor as well as nutrients.

Water

There is currently a great concern about our water supply in the U.S.A. It is becoming increasingly difficult to find pure water. Most of our water supply is full of chemicals, including not only chlorine and fluoride, which are routinely added, but a wide range of toxic and organic compounds and chemicals, such as PCBs, pesticide residues, nitrates, and heavy metals such as lead, mercury, and cadmium. It is estimated that lead alone may contaminate the water of more than 40 million Americans. In an effort to reduce the exposure to these toxic compounds roughly two million home water filtration units are purchased annually. What is the best home filtration unit? It depends on the predominant toxin. For example, if the primary toxin is lead, a carbon filter provides very little benefit. This is significant since carbon filters are the most popular water purification units sold.

To determine the safety of your tap or well water, contact your local water company as they perform routine analyses or contact the Drinking Water Inspectorate. Simply ask for the most recent analysis. There are also private water-testing companies that will test your water for a fee. Once you have your water analyzed and determine the predominant toxin, if any, you can make an informed decision about the water purification unit that's right for you. In the U.K., water quality is regulated by a number of authorities. The Environment Agency is responsible for the quality of fresh and marine, underground and surface water, and for monitoring pollution. The Drinking Water Inspectorate is a national agency with responsibility for drinking water standards, and local authority environmental health departments also have local responsibility.

Water Purification Units

GRANULATED ACTIVATED CARBON

These units tend to be small and attach to the tap. Carbon has been used for centuries as a filtering substance. Activated carbon is specially treated carbon designed to increase the absorptive surface area. Impurities are bound by the carbon as the water passes through.

The major problem with granulated carbon units is that the air spaces between the carbon particles can serve as a breeding ground for bacteria and other organisms. To compensate, many companies impregnate the carbon with silver to kill the bacteria. However, this simply creates additional concerns of silver toxicity and reduced filtration capacity. In short, there are better alternatives to this form of carbon filter.

SOLID CARBON BLOCK

These units alleviate much of the concern over breeding microorganisms. They are quite effective at removing chlorine, bacteria, pesticides, and other organic chemicals, yet maintain dissolved minerals, such as calcium, magnesium, and fluoride. Unfortunately, some of the dissolved minerals, such as lead, mercury, and arsenic, that are detrimental to health are not filtered by these units. A filter should have a pre-filtration unit to remove sediment and should be changed a minimum of every six months.

REVERSE OSMOSIS

These units range from small home units to those of industrial size. In reverse osmosis units the water is filtered through small pores, the size of water molecules, of a special membrane. Often, a solid carbon unit is attached to remove any contaminants that may have passed through the membrane. A reverse osmosis unit eliminates nearly all contaminants, as well as all minerals. The disadvantages of reverse osmosis units are their cost, lack of water conservation (they lose up to 7 gallons/26.5 liters of water for every 1 gallon/4 liters of drinking water obtained), limited water output, and bulky size.

DISTILLED WATER

The purest water is distilled water. The distillation process involves vaporizing water into steam and then cooling it in a separate chamber or through coils. When vaporized, the steam rises and the impurities remain behind. The steam then passes into the cooling chamber, where through condensation the water will once again be in liquid form. Distillation is extremely effective at eliminating most impurities. The only possible exception may be volatile pollutants, which vaporize along with the water. Filtering the water through a carbon filter prior to distillation will overcome this concern.

The disadvantages of distillation are the energy needs of the unit, the cost, and the slow output. There is also the concern that since distilled water has all minerals removed, drinking distilled water may "leach out" minerals such as calcium, magnesium, and fluoride from the body.

More and more evidence is accumulating about the dangerous health effects of pesticides, food additives, and other contaminants of our food supply. In addition, there is growing concern about the potential harm of irradiated and genetically modified foods. The bottom line for a health-promoting diet is to reduce the intake of these potentially harmful substances, foods laden with empty calories, additives, and artificial sweeteners, and replace them with natural foods, preferably organically grown and non-GMO. As for our water supply, its safety is also being scrutinized, for good reason. Check your water supply to make sure it is safe. If it isn't, invest in a home water purification unit that will remove the impurities.

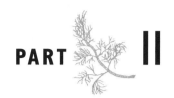

PART II

Food Components

4

Protein

The word "protein" is derived from the Greek *proteios,* or "primary." The name is fitting as, after water, protein is most plentiful component of our body. The body manufactures proteins to make up hair, muscles, nails, tendons, ligaments, and other body structures. Proteins also function as enzymes, hormones, and important components of other cells, such as our genes. The human body contains somewhere between 30,000 and 50,000 unique proteins. The building blocks of all proteins are molecules known as amino acids.

The body strives to make good use of its protein. During a single day, about a pound/½ kilogram of an adult's body protein is broken down into amino acids and reassembled into new proteins. The protein is either broken down or manufactured to allow us to maintain the integrity of the proteins subjected to daily wear and tear. This protein turnover allows us to grow, heal, remodel, and internally defend ourselves on a continual basis. Since there is some loss and although we can manufacture some amino acids, adequate dietary protein intake is essential in providing us with those amino acids that we cannot make, called essential amino acids.

The U.S. government-mandated Recommended Dietary Allowance (RDA) for protein is based on body weight. Take a minute to calculate your protein requirement. The amount is usually considerably less than the amount most people typically take in. The RDA in America is as follows:

Multiply .36 gram by your weight in pounds or .8 gram by your weight in kilograms. This will equal the grams of protein needed each day. For example, a woman who weighs 118 pounds would require 43 grams of protein each day (.36 × 118 = 43 grams). A man who weighs 60 kilograms would require 48 grams of protein each day (.8 × 60 = 48 grams).

The average American easily reaches and often exceeds this protein requirement without even being on a high-protein diet. Actual daily protein consumption ranges from 88 to 92 grams for men and from 63 to 66 grams for women. In the U.K., average daily protein consumption is 88 grams for men (RNI 55.5 to 53.3 grams depending on age) and 64 grams for women (RNI 45 to 46.5 grams). The RNI or Reference Nutrient Intake system used in the U.K. estimates the daily amount of a nutrient required by 97.5 percent of the population (nutrient requirements vary greatly between individuals depending on age, lifestyle, etc.). The RNI for protein is calculated at 0.75 grams per kilogram of bodyweight although the *average* requirement is estimated at only 0.6 grams per kilogram by U.K. authorities.

There are, however, many conditions in which extra protein is needed, including childhood/adolescence (growth), pregnancy, lactation, intense strength and endurance training, and when living with some diseases, such as AIDS and cancer. Elderly persons also may require additional amounts of protein. In these cases, multiply 0.8 grams by your weight in pounds. This will equal the grams of protein needed each day in a high-protein diet.

Since the body does not need or use excess protein, excess protein can become a burden for the kidney and liver—two organs that are in charge of getting rid of wastes. And, contrary to popular belief, you can get fat eating a high-protein diet. Excess protein intake increases the use of amino acids as a daily energy source, which decreases the breakdown and utilization of fat for energy, thereby promoting increased body fat content.

TABLE 4.1 Recommended Dietary Intake of Protein		
	Age	**U.S. RDA (grams)**
Infants	Up to 6 months	13
	6 months–1 year	14
	1–3 years	16
Children	4–6 years	24
	7–10 years	28
Males	11–14 years	45
	15–18 years	59
	19–24 years	58
	25–50 years	63
	51+ years	63
Females	11–14 years	46
	15–18 years	44
	19–24 years	46
	25–50 years	50
	51+ years	50
Pregnant women		60
Lactating mothers	First 6 months	65
	Second 6 months	62

Protein Deficiency

Protein deficiency is still a big problem in developing countries. It affects mainly young children and is the result of both too little food in general and too little protein in the diet. The two most common forms of protein deficiency are marasmus and kwashiorkor.

Marasmus occurs mainly in infants under one year of age who have been weaned off breast milk onto a diet containing too few calories and too little protein. As a result, the child becomes severely underweight and very weak and lethargic.

Kwashiorkor tends to occur in older children who have been weaned onto a diet high in starchy foods but whose diet is still too low in calories and protein. A child with kwashiorkor is severely underweight, but this is often masked by edema (water retention), which makes the face moon-shaped and the arms and legs look plump. The hair is thin and discolored, and the skin may show patches of scaliness and variable pigmentation.

Amino Acids and Protein Structure

As mentioned, proteins are composed of individual building blocks known as amino acids. Amino acids are compounds containing carbon, hydrogen, oxygen, nitrogen, and in some cases sulphur. All amino acids have an acid group and an amino group attached to a carbon atom. Figure 4.1 shows the general structure of an amino acid. The R in the figure signifies a different molecule for every amino acid. In the simplest amino acid, glycine, R is a hydrogen

TABLE 4.2

Essential and Nonessential Amino Acids

Essential Amino Acids	Nonessential Amino Acids
Arginine*	Alanine
Histidine*	Asparagine
Isoleucine	Aspartic acid
Leucine	Cysteine
Lysine	Glutamic acid
Methionine	Glutamine
Phenylalanine	Glycine
Threonine	Proline
Tryptophan	Serine
Valine	Tyrosine

*Essential during growth.

atom, but in other amino acids the R is much more complex.

The human body can manufacture most of the amino acids required for making body proteins. However, there are nine essential amino acids that the body cannot manufacture. The quality of a protein source is based on its level of these essential amino acids along with its digestibility and ability to be utilized by the body.

The amino group of one amino acid can link with the acid group or carboxyl end of another amino acid to form a chain. The link is called a peptide bond. When two amino acids are joined together, a dipeptide is formed; when many amino acids join together, a polypeptide is formed. A typical protein may contain 500 or more amino acids, joined together by peptide bonds. Each protein has its own specific number and sequence of amino acids.

FIGURE 4.1

Basic Amino Acid Structure

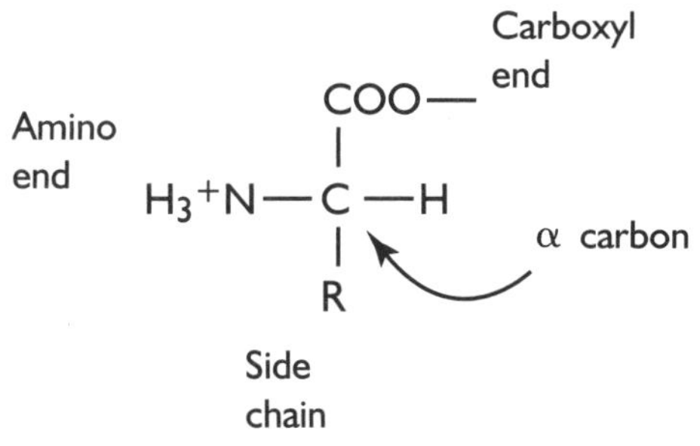

TABLE 4.3
Number and Sequence of Amino Acids

Name	Description
Dipeptide	Linkage of two amino acids
Tripeptide	Linkage of three amino acids
Peptides	Linkage of four to ten amino acids
Polypeptides	Linkage of greater than ten amino acids
Proteins	Very long linkages of amino acids (>100) and/or more than one linkage complexed together

TABLE 4.4
Examples of Substances Made of Individual Amino Acids

Amino Acid	Substances Made of the Amino Acid
Tryptophan	Serotonin
Lysine and methionine	Carnitine
Methionine, glycine, and arginine	Creatine
Methionine	S-adenosylmethionine
Aspartic acid and glutamine	Pyrimidines
Aspartic acid, glutamine, and glycine	Purines
Tyrosine or phenylalanine	Epinephrine (adrenalin) norepinephrine (noradrenalin), thyroid hormone, dopamine

Some smaller proteins exist as a somewhat straight chain of amino acids, but most proteins exist in a complex three-dimensional pattern.

Links between amino acids will contort themselves based upon the sequencing of the amino acids. Some amino acids are attracted to other amino acids in the chain, while others are repulsed. This is due to either opposing or similar charges associated with the side chains of amino acids. Also, as the amino acid chain bends, twists, and warps about three-dimensionally, certain amino acids will bond covalently (the union of two atoms by sharing a pair of electrons), creating a disulphide bond, to other amino acids on another part of the chain. This helps stabilize the final three-dimensional design.

Individual amino acids can also be used to make certain hormones and neurotransmitters, such as epinephrine (adrenalin), serotonin, norepinephrine (noradrenalin), and thyroid hormone. In addition, amino acids are used to make other important substances, such as choline, carnitine, and nucleic acids in our DNA.

Protein Quality

A complete protein source is one that provides all of the nine essential amino acids in adequate amounts. Animal products, such as meat, fish, dairy, and poultry, are examples of complete proteins. Plant foods, especially grains and legumes, often lack one or more of the essential amino acids, but become complete protein sources when they are combined. For example, combining grains with legumes results in a complete protein as the two protein sources complement each other in their amino acid profiles. With a varied diet of grains, legumes, fruits, and vegetables, a person is almost assured complete proteins, as long as the calorie content of the diet is high enough. Nonetheless, when electing to eat less animal food in the diet, it is important to design the diet to provide adequate amounts of protein.

In order to assess the quality of a protein, scientists measure the proportion of the amino acids that are absorbed, retained, and used in the body to determine the protein's *biological value* (BV). The food source that has the highest biological value protein is whey protein. Whey is a natural by-product of the cheese-making process. Cow's milk has about 6.25 percent protein. Of that protein, 80 percent is casein (another type of protein), and the remaining 20 percent is whey. When cheese is made, it uses the casein molecules, leaving the whey behind. Whey protein is made via filtering off the other components of whey, such as lactose, fats, and minerals.

Whey protein is a complete protein because it contains all essential and nonessential amino acids. One of the key reasons why the BV of whey protein is so high is that it has the highest concentrations of glutamine (an amino acid discussed on page 64) and branched-chain amino acids (BCAAs) found in nature. Glutamine and branched-chain amino acids are critical to cellular health, muscle growth, and protein synthesis.

Although whey protein is most popularly used by body builders and athletes looking to increase their protein intake, it can also be used to support recovery from surgery, prevent the "wasting syndrome" of AIDS and cancer, and offset some of the negative effects of radiation therapy and chemotherapy.

Eggs contain the second highest quality food protein known. Some people consider the egg to be a nearly perfect food. In fact, egg protein is

TABLE 4.5
Biological Value of Selected Protein Sources

Food	Biological Value
Whey protein concentrates/isolates	110–159
Whey protein	104
Egg protein	100
Whey (ion-exchange, microfiltered)	100
Whole egg	93.7
Milk	84.5
Fish	76.0
Beef	74.3
Soybeans	72.8
Rice, polished	64.0
Wheat, whole	64.0
Corn	60.0
Beans, dry	58.0

often the standard by which all other proteins are judged.

Animal Protein Versus Plant Protein

In the United States, it is estimated that approximately 72 percent of protein in the diet is from animal products—specifically, 49 percent from meat, fish, and poultry, 18 percent from dairy products, and 4 percent from eggs. In contrast, plant foods account for only 28 percent of protein intake. Grain products provide 18 percent, fruits and vegetables provide about 8 percent, and legumes about 3 percent. In the U.K., approximately 62 percent of protein intake comes from animal products – 36 percent from meat, 7 percent from fish, 16 percent from dairy products, 3 percent from eggs; 23 percent comes from cereals, 4 percent from potatoes and savoury snacks, and only 5 percent from vegetables, including legumes.

It is often difficult to separate the effects of animal protein from the effects of animal fats because they are so highly correlated. That is, when animal protein intake is high, animal fat intake is typically also high. This makes it difficult for researchers to determine what the effects of a high-protein diet are based on population studies, as the source of protein cannot be identified. Despite this obstacle, there is much evidence that reliance on animal proteins to meet protein requirements is linked to the development of several chronic degenerative diseases. For example, there is evidence that the body handles animal proteins differently from plant proteins. This is supported by population studies and animal studies comparing vegetarians to omnivores. Such evidence indicates that it is not simply a matter of protein quantity that is important but that the source of the protein is equally important.

A high intake of animal protein is linked to heart disease, many cancers, high blood pressure, kidney disease, osteoporosis, and kidney stones. Heart disease and high blood pressure are associated with increased intake of animal fats as well as animal protein. Cancer can be caused by proteins that are altered in some cooking processes, such as grilling and blackening, and by the action of gut bacteria on undigested protein. The kidneys are responsible for eliminating the breakdown products of protein, too much of which can have a damaging effect. The last two diseases deal with calcium metabolism as a high-protein diet increases the excretion of calcium in the urine. Simply raising the intake of protein from 47 grams per day to 142 grams per day doubles the excretion of calcium in the urine. A diet this high in protein, common in the United States and Europe, is a significant factor in the increased number of people suffering from osteoporosis and kidney stones. A vegetarian diet is associated with a reduced risk of developing the above-mentioned diseases.

Special Amino Acids

There are special amino acids of specific interest in regard to growth and development, metabolism, and protection from environmental chemicals as well as a variety of diseases. They include arginine, the branched-chain amino acids, glutamine, lysine, methionine and cysteine, and taurine.

Arginine

Arginine is an amino acid that plays an important role in wound healing, detoxification reactions, immune functions, and promoting the secretion of several hormones, including insulin and growth hormone. Recently there has been a considerable amount of scientific investigation regarding arginine's role in the formation of nitric oxide. This compound plays a central role in determining the tone of blood vessels. Specifically, it exerts a relaxing effect on blood vessels, thereby improving blood flow. Normally, the body makes enough arginine, even when the diet is lacking. However, in some instances the body may not be able to keep up with increased requirements and supplementation may prove useful.

Foods high in arginine are chocolate, peanuts, seeds, and nuts such as almonds and walnuts.

CARDIOVASCULAR DISEASE

Arginine supplementation is proving to be beneficial in a number of cardiovascular diseases, including angina pectoris, congestive heart failure, high blood pressure, and peripheral vascular insufficiency (decreased blood flow to the legs or arms). Its beneficial effect in all of these disorders shares a common mechanism: increasing nitric oxide levels. Nitric oxide plays a central role in regulating blood flow. By increasing nitric oxide levels, arginine supplementation improves blood flow, reduces blood clot formation, and improves blood fluidity (the blood becomes less viscous and therefore flows through blood vessels more easily). The degree of improvement offered by arginine supplementation in angina and other cardiovascular diseases can be quite significant as a result of improved nitric oxide levels.

INTERSTITIAL CYSTITIS

Interstitial cystitis is characterized by symptoms typical of a urinary tract infection (pain or burning upon urination, sense of urgency, and increased urinary frequency), but without evidence of an infection. Compared to people without interstitial cystitis, nitric oxide manufacture is decreased in patients with chronic interstitial cystitis.

Nitric oxide plays a role in bladder function. Since arginine is the building block substance for nitric oxide manufacture, researchers have sought to find out if arginine supplementation can improve interstitial cystitis. In a pilot study, good results were observed in ten patients receiving 1,500 milligrams of arginine daily after one month of use. In a follow-up double-blind study, fifty-three interstitial cystitis patients were assigned to receive 1,500 milligrams of arginine daily or a placebo orally for three months. Results indicated that 48 percent of the patients receiving arginine compared to 24 percent of the placebo group experienced a decrease in pain intensity and a tendency toward improvement in urgency and frequency of pain. These results indicate that arginine is helpful in some interstitial cystitis patients. Further research is needed to help identify responders.

MALE INFERTILITY

Arginine supplementation is often, but not always, an effective measure to improve male fertility. The critical determinant appears to be the level of the sperm count. If the sperm count is less than 20 million per milliliter, arginine supplementation is less likely to be of benefit.

In order to be effective for increased fertility, it appears that the dosage of l-arginine should be at least 4 grams a day for three months. In perhaps the most favorable study, 74 percent of

> ### *ARGININE WARNING*
>
> *Because the herpes virus utilizes arginine, diets high in arginine in people harboring the herpes virus may lead to reactivation. For this reason, it is important to balance the intake of arginine by also increasing the intake of lysine. See Table 20.2 on page 735 for more information.*

178 men with low sperm counts had significant improvements in sperm counts and motility.

Please note: l-arginine therapy should be reserved for use after other nutritional measures have been tried; other underlying nutritional requirements may be present and should be addressed as they cannot be corrected by l-arginine therapy alone.

PROMOTION OF GROWTH HORMONE SECRETION

One of the more popular uses of arginine supplementation has been to promote secretion of growth hormone by the pituitary gland. Growth hormone is responsible for stimulating muscle and skeletal growth. Bodybuilders often utilize arginine supplementation in an attempt to boost their natural output of growth hormone.

The fact that arginine increases growth hormone output is generally accepted. In fact, measuring growth hormone levels in the blood after arginine is administered intravenously is used to gauge whether a child or adult is secreting enough growth hormone. However, arginine supplementation *does not* appear to be able to enhance growth hormone release in older subjects, above the age of sixty-five.

Branched-Chain Amino Acids

The branched-chain amino acids (BCAAs) are leucine, isoleucine, and valine. These essential amino acids are very important for the maintenance of muscle tissue and appear to preserve muscle stores of glycogen, a storage form of carbohydrate that can be converted into energy. Some researchers think that a fall in the plasma concentration of BCAAs contributes to fatigue

in endurance events, but attempts to enhance endurance performance with BCAA supplementation have been inconclusive.

BCAAs are found in most high-protein foods, with dairy products and red meat containing the greatest amounts.

Glutamine

Glutamine is the most abundant amino acid in the body and is involved in more metabolic processes than any other amino acid. It is also the most abundant amino acid in the blood and in the free amino acid pool of skeletal muscle. Glutamine stimulates the synthesis and inhibits the degradation of proteins and is an energy source for muscle cell division. Glutamine is also a precursor for the synthesis of amino acids, proteins, nucleotides, glutathione, and other biologically important molecules. Glutamine has an anabolic effect on skeletal muscle.

Glutamine is especially important in serving as a source of fuel for cells lining the intestines and for the proper functioning of white blood cells. It is important to these particular cells because glutamine is utilized at higher rates by these and other rapidly dividing cells. Without glutamine, these cells will not divide properly.

Glutamine is a major amino acid in most foods. In general, the higher the protein content, the higher the glutamine content. Whey protein and eggs are two particularly good sources of glutamine.

ENHANCING ATHLETIC PERFORMANCE

Some evidence suggests that overtraining results in low glutamine levels and that glutamine supplementation can help prevent overtraining in the first place, as well as help an athlete recover from overtraining. Plasma glutamine concentrations increase during exercise. However, during the postexercise recovery period, plasma glutamine concentrations decrease significantly. Several hours of recovery are required before plasma levels are restored to preexercise levels. If recovery between exercise bouts is inadequate, the acute effects of exercise on plasma glutamine concentrations can be cumulative, leading to very low levels of glutamine. This situation can have extremely detrimental effects on athletic performance and muscle growth. Glutamine supplementation has been shown to boost muscle levels of glutamine and promote muscle protein synthesis. However, it does not appear to enhance exercise performance. Instead, the clearest benefit of glutamine supplementation in athletes is in prevention of infections.

IMPROVING IMMUNE FUNCTION

Glutamine supplementation has been shown to boost immune function and fight infection. These effects have been best demonstrated in endurance athletes (extreme exercise suppresses the immune system) and critically ill subjects. In fact, its importance is becoming well appreciated in conventional medical circles, as it is an extremely important component of intravenous feeding mixes in hospitals. Double-blind studies have shown supplementation with glutamine to dramatically increase survival in critically ill subjects. However, it is not known if glutamine supplementation enhances immune function in healthy individuals.

PEPTIC ULCERS

Glutamine promotes the healing of peptic ulcers. In a double-blind study of fifty-seven patients with peptic ulcers, twenty-four took 1.6 grams of glutamine per day, and the rest used conventional therapies, such as antacids and antispasmodics. Glutamine proved to be the more effective treatment. According to X-ray analysis, half of the glutamine patients showed complete healing within two weeks, and twenty-two of the twenty-four showed complete relief and healing within four weeks. In addition, cabbage juice, which has been shown to be so beneficial in the healing of ulcers, is quite high in glutamine.

PREVENTION OF CHEMOTHERAPY SIDE EFFECTS

Glutamine, given its importance to the cells of the lining of the gastrointestinal tract and immune system, has been shown to prevent the mouth ulcers (stomatitis), muscle and joint pain, and suppression of the immune system in cancer patients receiving some types of chemotherapy, most notably 5-fluorouracil and paclitaxel (Taxol).

Lysine

Lysine is an essential amino acid required for many body functions, including growth and bone development in children; calcium absorption and maintenance of the correct nitrogen balance in the body; maintenance of lean body mass; production of antibodies, hormones, and enzymes; collagen formation and repair of tissue.

Since lysine helps with the building of muscle protein, higher intakes of lysine are useful for patients recovering from injuries or operations, and lysine supplementation may be used to help maintain healthy blood vessels.

The most popular use of lysine is in fighting herpes infections and cold sores. Herpes viruses require arginine to replicate; in fact, the very presence of arginine appears to simulate replication. In contrast, lysine appears to block the effects of arginine and thus has antiviral activity.

Foods high in lysine include most vegetables, legumes, fish, turkey, and chicken. See Table 20.2 on page 735 for more information.

Methionine and Cysteine

Methionine and cysteine are interconvertible sulphur-containing amino acids. Methionine is considered an essential amino acid; cysteine is not. These sulphur-containing amino acids are very important to the health of connective tissue, joints, hair, skin, and nails. They are also utilized by the body in detoxification reactions, helping the body to excrete heavy metals, and reducing bladder irritation by regulating the formation of ammonia in the urine.

Methionine is also converted in the body to S-adenosyl-l-methionine (SAM, or SAMe). This compound is involved in more than forty biochemical reactions in the body. It functions closely with folic acid and vitamin B12 in "methylation" reactions. Methylation is the process of adding a single carbon unit (a methyl group) to another molecule. SAMe is many times more effective in transferring methyl groups than other methyl donors. Methylation reactions are critical in the manufacture of many body components, especially brain chemicals, as well

as in detoxification reactions. SAMe is also required in the manufacture of all sulphur-containing compounds in the human body, including glutathione (see page 149) and various sulphur-containing cartilage components, such as chondroitin sulphate. SAMe supplementation has been shown to produce positive results in the treatment of depression, osteoarthritis, fibromyalgia, liver disorders, and migraine headaches.

Cysteine is a key component in the important tripeptide glutathione (see page 149), an important antioxidant in cells. The N-acetyl form of cysteine (NAC) can be used to increase glutathione levels in well-nourished people. However, if malnourishment is a concern, NAC should be combined with glutamine to increase glutathione levels. NAC is also used to thin secretions in chronic mucus-forming conditions.

Methionine and cysteine are found mainly in meat, fish, eggs, and dairy products.

Taurine

Taurine is a sulphur-containing amino acid that can be derived from the diet or produced in the body from methionine and cysteine. Taurine is different from other amino acids in two other key ways:

1. It is not utilized in protein synthesis but rather is found unbound or existing in small peptide chains.
2. Its structure is different from that of other amino acids in that a sulphur group replaces the carboxylic acid element found in other amino acids.

TABLE 4.6		
Food Sources of Taurine		
Food	Amount	Taurine (milligrams)
Cheese	3 ounces/85 grams	1,000
Cheese, cottage	1 cup	1,700
Granola	1 cup	650
Wild game	3 ounces/85 grams	600
Pork	3 ounces/85 grams	540
Oatmeal flakes	1 cup	500
Milk, whole	1 cup	400
Chocolate	1 cup	400
Yogurt	1 cup	400
Wheat germ, toasted	¼ Cup	350
Egg	1 (medium size)	350
Turkey	3 ounces/85 grams	240
Chicken	3 ounces/85 grams	185

As an important regulator of cellular charge, taurine plays a critical role in maintaining cell membrane stability. It regulates heartbeat, helps prevent brain cell overactivity, and is essential in the visual process.

Taurine supplementation of 1 to 4 grams per day has been shown in small double-blind studies to be effective in improving heart function in congestive heart failure; lowering blood pressure; and reducing seizures in people with epilepsy whose disease is poorly controlled with antiseizure drugs.

The average intake of taurine, via foods, varies widely, from 40 to 2,500 milligrams daily.

Generally speaking, taurine is found in greater concentrations in animal products.

Tryptophan

Tryptophan is an essential amino acid that plays many vital roles. One of its most important roles is as the starting point in the manufacture of the neurotransmitters serotonin and melatonin. Serotonin is particularly important as it is kind of a "master control chemical." The activities of many other important brain compounds, including those that govern your muscle movements, your state of alertness, your mental activity, and even your ability to fall asleep, depend upon serotonin.

Serotonin was first discovered about fifty years ago. Since then, an enormous amount of research has been done to unlock the secrets of this multitalented molecule. In the past few decades, findings in the laboratory have led to the development of many potent serotonin-active drugs. Among these are Prozac, the popular antidepressant, which enhances the mood-regulating activity of serotonin; Imitrex, a treatment for migraine headaches, which works by activating serotonin nerve pathways to constrict blood vessels; and Redux, which controls eating by delivering a dose of serotonin to the appetite control centers in the brain (known as Adifax in the U.K.—it was withdrawn from use). Other serotonin-altering drugs relieve anxiety, enhance sleep, and ease muscular and skeletal pain.

Melatonin is another primary hormone involved in sleep regulation. In fact, melatonin determines your sleep-wake cycle, also called the circadian rhythm. Melatonin is secreted from a small gland in the brain called the pineal gland as daylight begins to decline. Melatonin is also a potent antioxidant that has protective effects against many types of cancer. As we age as adults, there is a tendency to produce less melatonin.

Fortunately, there may be a better way to overcome serotonin and melatonin deficiency by providing the right sort of support to tryptophan metabolism. A poor diet, lack of exercise, use of harmful substances such as caffeine or alcohol, and overall physical and emotional stress can rob your brain of the ability to make enough serotonin and melatonin to meet your body's demands. The main determinant of tryptophan metabolism is the balance of other amino acids in the bloodstream, which, in turn, is determined by the types of foods in your diet. Compared to other amino acids, tryptophan is found in foods only in small quantities. A few

hours after you eat a high-protein meal, such as one containing meat, there will be high levels of many different amino acids, all competing for entry into the brain on the few available transport molecules. On the other hand, if you eat a high-carbohydrate meal, there will be relatively higher levels of tryptophan and lower levels of other amino acids. In that case, the tryptophan enters the brain more quickly, and the level of serotonin rises. The same thing happens if you eat foods rich in tryptophan, such as turkey, milk, cottage cheese, chicken, eggs, red meats, soybeans, tofu, and nuts, especially almonds.

Protein is necessary for the structure of almost every molecule in the body, particularly many hormones, neurotransmitters and all enzymes. Adequate protein from a variety of high-quality sources with high biological value ensures a good supply of essential amino acids, as well as special amino acids and peptides.

5

Carbohydrates and Dietary Fiber

Dietary carbohydrates play a central role in human nutrition because they provide the primary source of the energy we need to fuel bodily functions. Carbohydrates are classified into two basic groups: simple and complex. Most dietary fiber is composed of indigestible carbohydrates, so fiber and related compounds are discussed in this chapter as well.

Many in the medical and research communities now believe that excessive consumption of carbohydrates—specifically, carbohydrates that have been refined and stripped of their supportive nutrients—is a major contributing factor in a wide variety of diseases and premature aging. Virtually all of the fiber, phytochemical, vitamin, and trace element content has been removed from white sugar, white breads and pastries, and many breakfast cereals. Even the natural simple sugars in fruits and vegetables have an advantage over sucrose (white sugar) and other refined sugars in that they are balanced by fiber and a wide range of nutrients that aid in the utilization of the sugars.

Eating too many carbohydrates, particularly simple sugars, can be harmful to blood sugar control, especially if you are insulin-resistant, experience reactive hypoglycemia, or are diabetic. Carbohydrate excess, especially consuming too many refined carbohydrates, is also associated with increased risk for obesity, heart disease, and some forms of cancer. Currently, more than half of the carbohydrates being consumed in the United States are in the form of simple sugars being added to foods as sweetening agents. In the U.K., just over 30 percent of carbohydrates consumed take the form of sugar, confectionery, drinks and snacks.

The consumption of sweeteners in the United States increased from about 14 million tons in 1979 to about 22 million tons in 1999. Included in the category of sweeteners are sugar, corn sweeteners, honey, maple syrup, and other edible syrups. The per capita consumption just of added sugars went from 27 teaspoons (108 grams) per person per day in 1970 to 32 teaspoons (128 grams) per person per day in 1996, according to U.S. food supply data. In the U.K., the average daily intake of sugar is about 72 grams, but this doesn't include other sweeteners such as corn syrups. What is staggering to consider is that noncaloric sweeteners are not included in these calculations.

The large increase in the use of corn sweetener, or high-fructose corn syrup (HFCS), in the past thirty years is directly related to the overall increase in sugar consumption in the United States. In spite of its name, there is no more fructose in high-fructose corn syrup than there is sucrose. HFCS is simply sweet and is much less expensive than sucrose.

Many different products can use HFCS as an ingredient. Some of these include beverages, cereals and baked goods, dairy products, sweets, and many other processed foods. Production of HFCS in the United States increased from 2.2 million tons in 1980 to 9.4 million tons in 1999. The production of HFCS in 2000 consumed about 5.3 percent of the total American corn crop. The consumption of sugar-sweetened beverages has played the largest role in the increase of added sweeteners in the American diet. Food consumption studies have found that the recent increases in energy intake coincide with increased consumption of soft drinks. The U.K. has also seen a significant rise in the consumption of soft and fizzy drinks giving rise to health concerns for children in particular.

Simple Carbohydrates

Simple sugars are either monosaccharides composed of one sugar molecule or disaccharides composed of two sugar molecules. The principal monosaccharides that occur in foods are glucose and fructose. The major disaccharides are sucrose, also known as white sugar, which is composed of one molecule of glucose and one molecule of fructose; maltose, which is composed of two molecules of glucose; and lactose, which is composed of one molecule of glucose and one molecule of galactose.

Glucose is not particularly sweet-tasting compared to fructose and sucrose. It is found in abundant amounts in fruits, honey, sweet corn, and most root vegetables. Glucose is also the primary repeating sugar unit of most complex carbohydrates (starches).

Fructose, or fruit sugar, is the primary carbohydrate in many fruits, maple syrup, and honey. Fructose, which is very sweet, is roughly one and a half times sweeter than sucrose (white sugar). Although fructose has the same chemical formula as glucose, its structure is quite different. In order to be utilized by the body, fructose must first be converted to glucose within the liver.

Sucrose, which is common table sugar, is found in a large number of processed foods and some fruits. Maltose is found in malted grain products and syrups derived from grains such as barley and sorghum. Lactose is the sugar found in milk. Humans have an enzyme called lactase to digest lactose as infants but later start to lose this enzyme. By age four, most of our lactase production is absent. In some people, particularly those of Afro-Caribbean descent, lactase production is completely absent, causing lactose intolerance with symptoms of wind, bloating, and diarrhea when dairy products are consumed. Lactase enzyme can be supplemented for the occasional consumption of dairy foods by people who are lactose-intolerant.

Sucrose, maltose, and lactose are broken down into their constituent sugars in the small intestine. Glucose is the primary form of sugar that enters the bloodstream. In fact, most of the content of other sugars is converted to glucose at the surface of the intestine or in the liver.

Complex Carbohydrates

Complex carbohydrates, or starches, are composed of many simple sugars joined together by chemical bonds. These bonds can be linked in a serial chain, one after the other, as well as side to side, creating branches. Basically, the more chains and branches, the more complex the carbohydrate. The more complex a carbohydrate is, the more slowly it is broken down. Some carbohydrates are complex in a way that the body cannot digest them. These carbohydrates are a major component of fiber, discussed below, and generally pass through the digestive tract unabsorbed. In general, as long as complex carbohydrates are present in high-fiber foods, the body breaks down complex carbohydrates into simple sugars more gradually, which leads to better blood sugar control. More and more research on heart disease, various forms of cancer, and diabetes indicates that complex carbohydrates,

including high-fiber foods, should form a major part of the diet. For example, the Dietary Approaches to Stop Hypertension, or DASH, diet focuses on a whole-food diet made up of vegetables, legumes, and whole grains, which are excellent sources of complex carbohydrates, high in fiber.

Glycemic Index and Glycemic Load

More important than labeling a carbohydrate simple or complex is to consider its "glycemic index" and "glycemic load." As described in chapter 1, the glycemic index (GI) provides a numerical value that expresses the rise of blood glucose after eating a particular food. The GI is computed in two ways due to the fact that there are two standards of comparison. The first standard to be developed was based on the rise in blood sugar seen with the ingestion of glucose, which was given a value of 100. Today, this glucose standard has largely been abandoned by the scientific community in favor of the more accurate starch standard. In the starch standard, a 50 gram portion of white bread made using refined flour (the bread most commonly eaten in the United States and accounting for nearly 70 percent of the bread eaten in the U.K.) is given the value of 100. White bread was selected as the new standard because the glycemic response to white bread is more reliable than the response to glucose. This is because glucose attracts water, an effect called osmolarity, that can delay gastric emptying and misrepresent the insulin response. In addition, white bread stimulates more insulin activity than glucose. Using either

TABLE 5.1

**Glycemic Index of
Some Common Foods**

Food	Glycemic Index
Sugars:	
Fructose	20
Glucose	100
Honey	75
Maltose	105
Sucrose	60
Fruits:	
Apples	39
Bananas	62
Oranges	40
Orange juice	46
Raisins	64
Vegetables:	
Beetroot	64
Carrot, raw	31
Carrot, cooked	36
Potato, baked	98
Potato (new), boiled	70
Grains:	
Bran cereal	51
Bread, white	100
Bread, whole grain (wholemeal)	72
Corn	59
Cornflakes	80
Oatmeal	49
Pasta	45
Rice	70
Rice, puffed	95
Wheat cereal	67
Legumes:	
Beans	31
Lentils	29
Peas	39
Other foods:	
Ice cream	36
Milk	34
Nuts	13

standard, the glycemic index ranges from about 20 for fructose and whole barley to about 98 for a baked potato. The insulin response to carbohydrate-containing foods is similar to the rise in blood sugar.

The glycemic load (GL) takes the glycemic index into account, but gives a more complete picture of the effect that a food has on blood sugar levels because it also takes into consideration the amount of carbohydrate in the food. Appendix A provides a more complete table of the GI, GL, and carbohydrate and fiber content of selected foods, but the table shown here will provide some immediate food for thought.

Dietary Fiber

Originally, the definition of dietary fiber was restricted to the sum of plant compounds that are not digestible by the secretions of the human digestive tract. But this definition is vague since it depends on an exact understanding of what exactly is not digestible. For our purposes, the term "dietary fiber" will be used to refer to the

TABLE 5.2

Classification of Dietary Fiber

Fiber Class	Chemical Structure	Plant Part	Food Sources	Physiological Effect
I. Cellulose	Unbranched 1-4-beta-D-glucose polymer	Principal plant wall component	Wheat bran	Increases faecal weight and size
II. Soluble fibers				
A. Hemicelluloses	Mixture of pentose and hexose molecules in branching chains	Plant cell walls	Oat bran, guar gum (E412)	Increases faecal weight and size, binds bile acids
B. Gums	Branched-chain uronic acid containing polymers	Endosperm of plant seeds, plant exudates	Karaya (E416), locust bean (E410), tragacanth (E413), gum Arabic	Bulk laxative
C. Mucilages	Similar to hemicelluloses	Endosperm of plant seeds	Legumes, psyllium, konjac root, slippery elm bark, marshmallow root	Hydrocolloids that bind cholesterol and delay gastric emptying; chelate out heavy metals
D. Pectins	Mixture of methyl esterified galacturan, galactan, and arabinose in varying proportions	Plant cell walls	Citrus rind, apple and onion skin	As above
E. Algal polysaccharides	Polymerized D-mannuronic acid and L-glucuronic acid	Algin (E400), agar (E406), carrageenan	Seaweeds	As above
III. Lignans	Noncarbohydrate polymeric phenylpropene	Woody part of plant	Wheat (25%), apple (25%), cabbage (6%), linseeds, other nuts and seeds	Antioxidant, anticarcinogenic

components of the plant cell wall as well as the indigestible residues.

The composition of the plant cell wall varies according to the species of plant. In general, most plant cell walls contain 35 percent insoluble fiber, 45 percent soluble fiber, 15 percent lignans, 3 percent protein, and 2 percent ash. It is important to recognize that dietary fiber is a complex of these constituents, so supplementation of a single component cannot substitute for a diet rich in high-fiber foods. Some of these components, including inositol hexaphosphate and fructooligosaccharides, are discussed below.

Cellulose and Insoluble Fibers

The best example of an insoluble fiber is wheat bran. Wheat bran is rich in cellulose. Although it is relatively insoluble in water, it has the ability to bind water. This ability accounts for its effect of increasing faecal size and weight, thus promoting regular bowel movements. Although cellulose cannot be digested by humans, it is partially digested by beneficial microflora in the gut, for which it is the primary food source. The natural fermentation process, which occurs in the colon, results in the degradation of about 50 percent of the cellulose and is an important source of the short-chain fatty acids that nourish our intestinal cells.

Soluble Fibers

The majority of fibers in most plant cell walls are water-soluble compounds. Included in this class are hemicelluloses, gums, mucilages, pectin, and algal polysaccharides. It is these fiber compounds that exert the most beneficial effects.

HEMICELLULOSES

Hemicelluloses, such as those found in oat bran, also promote regular bowel movements by increasing hydration of the stool. Hemicelluloses also directly bind cholesterol in the gut, preventing cholesterol absorption. Bacteria in the gut digest hemicelluloses, increasing the number of beneficial bacteria in the gut and creating short-chain fatty acids (discussed on page 79), which colon cells use as fuel and which decrease cholesterol.

GUMS AND MUCILAGES

Structurally, gums and mucilages resemble the hemicelluloses, but they are not classed as such due to their unique location in the seed portion of the plant. They are generally found within the inner layer (endosperm) of grains, legumes, nuts, and seeds. Also, some gums are exuded on the surface of plants, such as gum arabic, gum karaya, and gum tragacanth. Guar gum, which is technically a mucilage and not a gum, is found in most legumes (beans) and is the most widely studied plant mucilage. Commercially, guar gum is used as a stabilizing, thickening, and film-forming agent in the production of cheese, salad dressings, ice cream, soups, toothpaste, pharmaceutical jelly, skin cream, and tablets. Guar gum is also used as a laxative.

Gums and other mucilages, including psyllium seed husk and konjac root glucomannan, are perhaps the most potent cholesterol-lowering agents of the gel-forming fibers. In addition, mucilage fibers have been shown to reduce fast-

---

PECTIN FIGHTS THE SPREAD OF CANCER

Modified citrus pectin (MCP), also known as fractionated citrus pectin, is a complex sugar (polysaccharide) obtained from the peel and pulp of citrus fruits. Modified citrus pectin is rich in short, nonbranched, galactose-rich carbohydrate chains. These shorter chains dissolve more readily in water and are better absorbed and utilized by the body than ordinary long-chain pectin.

MCP appears to reduce the risk of metastasis, the spread of cancerous cells from one tumor to other sites in the body. For metastasis to occur, cancer cells must first clump together. Protein molecules called galectins appear on the surface of cancer cells and bind the cells to molecules of glucose. The more galectins present, the easier it is for the cancer cells to clump together and metastasize. According to preliminary research, MCP binds to the galectins. By doing so, it blocks the cancer cells' ability to clump and spread.

Lab studies suggest that MCP is best used in preventing the metastasis of breast cancer, prostate cancer, lung cancer, and melanoma. Not many human data are available yet, but initial results appear promising. In one of the few human studies, MCP was shown to decrease the cancer growth rate in four of seven men with prostate cancer as measured by a reduced rate of increase in PSA levels (a sign of prostate cancer severity).

The typical dosage recommendation for adults is 6 to 30 grams daily in divided doses. MCP powder is usually dissolved by blending in water or juice.

---

ing and after-meal glucose and insulin levels in both healthy and diabetic subjects; and mucilage has decreased body weight and hunger ratings when taken with meals by obese subjects.

PECTINS

Pectins are found in all plant cell walls as well as in the outer skin and rind of fruits and vegetables. For example, the rind of an orange contains 30 percent pectin, an apple peel 15 percent, and onion skins 12 percent. The gel-forming properties of pectin are well known to anyone who has made jelly or jam. These same gel-forming qualities are responsible for the cholesterol-lowering effects of pectin. Pectin lowers cholesterol by binding the cholesterol and bile acids in the gut and promoting their excretion.

ALGAL POLYSACCHARIDES

Algal polysaccharides, or seaweed gums, are derived from brown seaweeds, such as alginates, and red seaweeds, such as agar and carrageenan, which is also known as Irish moss. Alginates form insoluble gels that are used as emulsifiers, thickeners and binders in food production. Agar forms a gel that is soluble in hot water, but not cold water. Agar is used as a culture medium for microbes as well as a stabilizer in many foods. Carrageenan can be broken into components that do and do not form gels. Carrageenan is used in many foods to thicken them and create a smooth texture.

Lignans

Lignans are compounds found in high-fiber foods that show important properties, such as anticancer, antibacterial, antifungal, and antiviral activity. Plant lignans are changed by the gut flora into enterolactone and enterodiol, two compounds protective against cancer, particularly breast cancer. Lignans bind to oestrogen receptors and interfere with the cancer-promoting effects of oestrogen on breast tissue. Lignans also increase the production of a compound known as sex hormone–binding globulin, or SHBG. This protein regulates oestrogen levels by escorting excess oestrogen from the body.

Linseeds are the most abundant source of lignans. Additional good sources of lignans are other seeds, grains, and legumes.

Inositol and Inositol Hexaphosphate (Ip6 or Phytic Acid)

Inositol is an "unofficial" member of the B vitamins that functions as a primary component of cell membranes and, with phosphate groups attached, acts as an important regulator of cell division. Although inositol has not been shown to be essential in the human diet, supplementation has been shown to exert some beneficial effects in cases of depression, panic attacks, and diabetes.

Inositol is required for the proper action of several brain neurotransmitters, including serotonin and acetylcholine. It is currently thought that a reduction of brain inositol levels may induce depression as inositol levels in the cerebrospinal fluid have been shown to be low in patients with depression. In double-blind studies, inositol at a dosage of 12 grams per day has demonstrated therapeutic results, such as reduction in the Hamilton Depression Scale. The results are similar to those of tricyclic antidepressant drugs, but without their side effects.

The major source of inositol in nature is found in the form of inositol hexaphosphate (Ip6), which is a component of fiber from whole grains and legumes and not a fiber class on its own. In the plant, Ip6 is responsible for storing minerals, such as calcium, phosphorus, magnesium, and potassium, as phytates. There is some concern that Ip6 can adversely affect the uptake and utilization of many minerals in the body, including calcium, iron, and zinc; however, this does not seem to be the case. Phytates are destroyed by heat and by the enzyme phytase during the leavening of bread.

Although naturally occurring Ip6 exerts impressive antioxidant and antitumor effects, it may be better to take supplements containing purified Ip6 plus inositol. The supplement form offers several advantages. In grains and beans, Ip6 binds to molecules of protein and minerals, such as calcium, magnesium, or potassium, to form phytate. The body has trouble absorbing this complex. Studies have shown that pure Ip6 is significantly more bioavailable than the Ip6 found in foods as phytates. Supplemental Ip6 should be taken on an empty stomach away from other mineral-containing substances to avoid phytates forming in the digestive tract, as we do not produce our own phytase to break these down.

Fructooligosaccharides (FOS)

Fructooligosaccharides (FOSs) are another fiber component found in many vegetables, and consist of short chains of fructose molecules. The term "oligosaccharide" refers to a short chain of sugar molecules ("oligo" means "few"; "saccharide" means "sugar"). Galactooligosaccharides (GOSs), which also occur naturally, consist of short chains of galactose molecules. Inulin is one of the better-researched FOS molecules that is derived from elecampane root *(Inula helenium)*, as well as the roots of other plants such as chicory. These compounds can be digested by humans only partially. When oligosaccharides are consumed, the undigested portion serves as food for "friendly" bacteria, such as *Bifidobacterium* and *Lactobacillus* species. Clinical studies have shown that FOS, GOS, and inulin can increase the number of these friendly bacteria in the colon while simultaneously reducing the population of harmful bacteria. Other benefits noted with FOS, GOS, or inulin supplementation include increased production of beneficial short-chain fatty acids such as butyrate, increased absorption of calcium and magnesium, and improved elimination of toxic compounds.

Several double-blind studies have looked at the ability of FOS or inulin to lower blood cholesterol and triglyceride levels. These studies have shown that in individuals with elevated total cholesterol or triglyceride levels, including people with non-insulin-dependent diabetes, FOS or inulin in amounts ranging from 8 to 20 grams daily can produce meaningful reductions in these blood lipids. But in individuals with normal or low cholesterol or triglyceride levels, FOS or inulin produces little effect.

FOS and inulin are found naturally in Jerusalem artichoke, burdock, chicory, dandelion root, leeks, onions, and asparagus. FOS can be synthesized by enzymes of the fungus *Aspergillus niger* acting on sucrose. GOS is naturally found in soybeans and can be synthesized from lactose (milk sugar). FOS, GOS, and inulin are available as prebiotic or probiotic nutritional supplements in capsules, as tablets, and as a powder.

The Physiological Effects of Dietary Fiber

It is beyond the scope of this chapter to detail all the known effects of dietary fiber on humans. Instead, we will concentrate on the effects of greatest significance: stool weight and transit time, digestion, lipid metabolism, short-chain fatty acids (SCFA), and intestinal bacterial flora. We will also review a selection of diseases that are highly correlated with lack of dietary fiber, namely, colon diseases, obesity, and diabetes.

BENEFICIAL EFFECTS OF DIETARY FIBER

- Decreased intestinal transit time.

- Delayed gastric emptying resulting in reduced after-meal blood sugar levels.

- Increased satiety.

- Increased pancreatic secretion.

- Increased stool weight.

- More advantageous intestinal microflora.

- Increased production of short-chain fatty acids.

- Decreased serum lipids..

- More soluble bile.

Stool Weight and Transit Time

Fiber has long been used in the treatment of constipation. Dietary fiber, particularly the water-insoluble fibers, such as cellulose, increase stool weight as a result of their water-holding properties. Transit time, the time taken for passage of material from the mouth to the anus, is greatly reduced on a high-fiber diet.

People who consume a high-fiber diet (100 to 170 grams per day) usually have a transit time of thirty hours and a faecal weight of 500 grams. In contrast, Europeans and Americans, who typically eat a low-fiber diet (20 grams per day) have a transit time of greater than forty-eight hours and a faecal weight of only 100 grams. The increased intestinal transit time associated with the Western diet allows prolonged exposure to various cancer-causing compounds within the intestines.

Fiber should be thought of not only in the treatment of constipation, but also in the treatment of diarrhea due to irritable bowel syndrome. When fiber is added to the diet of subjects with abnormally rapid transit times of less than twenty-four hours, it causes slowing of the transit time. Dietary fiber acts to normalize bowel movements.

Dietary fiber's effect on transit time is apparently directly related to its effect on stool weight and size. A larger, bulkier stool passes through the colon more easily; it requires less pressure to

be produced during defecation and consequently less straining. This results in less stress on the colon wall and therefore avoids the ballooning effect that creates diverticuli, which are sacs or pouches in the wall of the intestinal tract. Diverticuli can become lodged with faeces, causing inflammation, which is called diverticulitis. Dietary fiber also prevents the formation of hemorrhoids and varicose veins.

Digestion

Although dietary fiber increases the rate of transit through the gastrointestinal tract, it slows gastric emptying. This effect means that the food is released more gradually into the small intestine, and as a result, blood glucose levels rise more gradually. Pancreatic enzyme secretion and activity also increase in response to dietary fiber.

A number of research studies have examined the effects of fiber on mineral absorption. Although the results have been somewhat contradictory, it now appears that large amounts of dietary fiber (i.e., more than 50 grams daily) may result in impaired absorption and/or negative balance of some minerals, and supplemental fiber at higher dosages (e.g., greater than 5 grams) of insoluble fiber, especially wheat bran, may result in mineral deficiencies. However, dietary fiber at usual levels or supplementation with soluble forms of dietary fiber does not appear to interfere with mineral absorption from other foods.

Lipid Metabolism

The water-soluble gels and mucilagenous fibers, such as oat bran, guar gum, and pectin, are capable of lowering serum cholesterol and triglyceride levels by greatly increasing their faecal excretion as well as preventing their manufacture in the liver. The water-insoluble fibers, such as wheat bran, have much less effect in reducing serum lipid levels.

Short-Chain Fatty Acids (SCFA)

The fermentation of dietary fiber by the intestinal flora produces three main end products: short-chain fatty acids, various gases, and energy. Of these, the SCFAs, including acetic, proprionic, and butyric acids, have many important physiological functions.

Proprionate and acetate are transported directly to the liver and utilized for energy production. Proprionate may also help lower elevated cholesterol levels as it is a natural inhibitor of the key enzyme for cholesterol synthesis within the liver (HMG Co A reductase inhibitor).

Butyrate provides an important energy source for the cells that line the colon. In fact, butyrate is the preferred source for energy metabolism in the colon. Butyrate production may also be responsible for the anticancer properties of dietary fiber. Butyrate has been shown to possess impressive anticancer activity and is being used in enemas for ulcerative colitis.

Certain fibers appear to be more effective than others in increasing the levels of SCFAs in the colon. Pectins (both apple and citrus), guar gum, and other legume fibers produce more SCFAs than beet fiber, corn fiber, or oat bran.

Intestinal Bacterial Flora

Dietary fiber improves all aspects of colon function. Of central importance is the role it plays in maintaining a suitable bacterial flora in the colon. A low fiber intake is associated with both an overgrowth of endotoxin-producing bacteria (bad guys) and a lower percentage of *Lactobacillus* (good guys) and other acid-loving bacteria. A diet high in dietary fiber promotes the increased synthesis of short-chain fatty acids, which reduce the colon pH, creating a friendly environment for the growth of acid-loving bacteria.

Although dietary carbohydrates provide the primary source of the energy we need to fuel bodily functions, the type of carbohydrate we choose to perform this task has consequences, both good and bad, that reverberate throughout the body. In particular, it is quite clear that too much carbohydrate, particularly simple carbohydrates and high-glycemic foods, is a major contributing factor in a wide variety of diseases and premature aging.

Diseases Associated with a Low-Fiber Diet

Because of the important physiological effects of dietary fiber, a diet low in dietary fiber will obviously lead to altered physiology or disease. The diseases with the strongest correlation with a lack of dietary fiber are diseases of the colon and gastrointestinal tract, heart disease, obesity, and diabetes. Each of these will be discussed briefly below.

Diseases of the Colon and Gastrointestinal Disorders

The data documenting the protective effect of dietary fiber on colon cancer are well known. There is evidence for similar strong links with other common diseases of the colon: diverticulitis, diverticulosis, irritable bowel syndrome, ulcerative colitis, and appendicitis as well as hemorrhoids, peptic ulcers, and hiatal hernia.

Heart Disease

Increasing fiber intake is a safe and inexpensive dietary strategy to reduce the risk of heart disease. A diet high in dietary fiber is known to reduce total cholesterol and triglyceride levels while increasing HDL cholesterol levels.

Obesity

A dietary-fiber-deficient diet is an important causative factor in the development of obesity.

Dietary fiber plays a role in preventing obesity by

- Increasing the amount of necessary chewing, thus slowing the eating process.
- Increasing faecal caloric loss.
- Improving blood sugar control.
- Inducing satiety (the feeling of fullness).

Diabetes

Population-based studies clearly show type 2 diabetes to be one of the diseases most clearly related to inadequate dietary fiber intake. Clinical trials that have demonstrated the beneficial therapeutic effect of increased dietary fiber through diet and/or supplementation on diabetes have further substantiated this association. Soluble fiber sources significantly outperform insoluble forms in this application.

6

Fats

Dietary fat plays several important roles in the body. First, fat is the most concentrated source of calories as it provides 9 calories per gram. Carbohydrate and protein provide less than half that amount, at 4 calories per gram each. Second, fat is the preferred energy source to fuel the body. And third, fats are used in the body as structural components in cell membranes and as the backbone for hormonelike compounds known as prostaglandins.

Despite these important roles, fat is often given a bad rap as any extra dietary fat is converted to body fat and stored in fat cells. Since the human body has an almost unlimited capacity to store fat, eating a diet too high in fat can lead to obesity. We recommend a diet that supplies less than 30 percent of calories as fat. However, just as important as the amount of fat is the *type* of fat you consume. The goal is to *decrease* your total fat intake, especially your intake of saturated fats, trans–fatty acids (also called hydrogenated fats), and omega-6 fats, while *increasing* your intake of omega-3 fatty acids and monounsaturated fatty acids.

Fat Nomenclature

Fat molecules are made of atoms of carbon, hydrogen, and oxygen. Each of the separate atoms attaches to the others only in precise predetermined ways. The backbone of a fat is a chain of carbon atoms (C):

```
  |   |   |   |
– C – C – C – C –
  |   |   |   |
```

Hydrogen (H) and oxygen (O) atoms can then attach to the carbon. A *saturated fat* is a fat molecule in which all of the available binding sites are occupied by another atom. In other words, the carbons are *saturated* with all of the atoms they can hold:

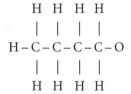

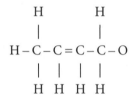

An *unsaturated fat* has one or more bonding sites left unoccupied. The two neighboring carbon atoms will take up the slack by forming a double bond:

A fat molecule with one double bond is called a *monounsaturated fat*. Molecules with more than one double bond are called polyunsaturated fats. *Mono-* means "one"; *poly-* means

TABLE 6.1
Fatty Acid Composition
(Percentage of Total Fat) of Selected Oils*

	SF†	OA†	LA†	GLA†	Alpha-LA†
Cooking oils:					
Rapeseed	8	54	30	0	8
Coconut	92	7	1	0	0
Corn	17	24	59	0	0
Olive	16	76	8	0	0
Macadamia nut	19	59	3	0	1
Safflower	7	11	82	0	0
Soy	15	26	50	0	9
Medicinal oils:					
Evening primrose	10	9	72	9	0
Black currant	8	10	52	17	13
Borage	14	16	48	22	0
Linseed	9	19	14	0	58

* "Vegetable oil" generally refers to a combination of various vegetable-derived oils such as corn, rapeseed, safflower, and soy.

† SF = saturated fats
  OA = oleic acid (an omega-9 monounsaturated fat)
  LA = linoleic acid (an omega-6 polyunsaturated fat)
  GLA = gamma-linolenic acid (an omega-6 polyunsaturated fat)
  Alpha-LA = alpha-linolenic acid (an omega-3 polyunsaturated fat)

COOKING OILS

The best oils to cook with in baking recipes, stir-fries, and sautés are the monounsaturated oils and coconut oil. While olive oil and rapeseed oil are by far the most popular monounsaturated oils, macadamia nut and coconut oils are superior to cook with because of their lower level of polyunsaturated oil: 1 percent for coconut, and 3 percent for macadamia nut oil versus 8 percent for olive and 30 percent for rapeseed. Because of their higher mono- and polyunsaturated contents, olive oil and rapeseed oil can form lipid peroxides (rancid by-products created through oxidation) at relatively low cooking temperatures, while coconut and macadamia nut oils are stable at much higher temperatures, in fact, more than twice as stable as olive oil and four times as stable as rapeseed. In addition, macadamia nut oil, like olive oil, is very high in natural antioxidants. In fact, it contains more than four and a half times the amount of vitamin E as olive oil.

Even more stable for cooking than monounsaturated fats are the saturated fats from coconut oil. The saturated fats from coconut oil are different from the ones found in animal products because they are shorter in length. Coconut oil contains what are referred to as short- and medium-chain triglycerides, while the saturated fats in animal products are long-chain triglycerides. Being shorter in length, short- and medium-chain triglycerides are processed by the body differently and are preferentially sent to the liver to be burned as energy. In fact, these fats actually have been shown to promote weight loss by increasing the burning of calories (thermogenesis); some research suggests that they lower cholesterol as well.

"many." When an unsaturated fat contains the first double bond at the third carbon, it is referred to as an omega-3 fatty acid. If the first double bond is at the sixth carbon, it is an omega-6 fatty acid, and if it occurs at the ninth carbon it is an omega-9 fatty acid.

Essential Fatty Acids

The only two official essential fatty acids are linoleic acid (an omega-6 fat) and alpha-linolenic acid (an omega-3 fat), but other fats are clearly beneficial. Although not considered essential, since they can be formed from alpha-linolenic acid, the longer-chain omega-3 fatty acids, such as eicosapentaenoic acid (EPA) and docosahexaneoic acid (DHA) found in fish, especially cold-water fish, such as salmon, mackerel, herring, and halibut, are gaining tremendous acceptance in the scientific community as vital components of good health. The role of the omega-9 oil oleic acid is also gaining recognition.

Cell Membrane Function

The primary answer to the question "What makes saturated fats and most margarines 'bad' and monounsaturated and omega-3 fatty acids 'good'?" is related to the function of fats in cellular membranes. Every human cell has a protective, permeable membrane. Membranes contain two layers, each made mainly of proteins,

FIGURE 6.1

Cis **Versus** *Trans*

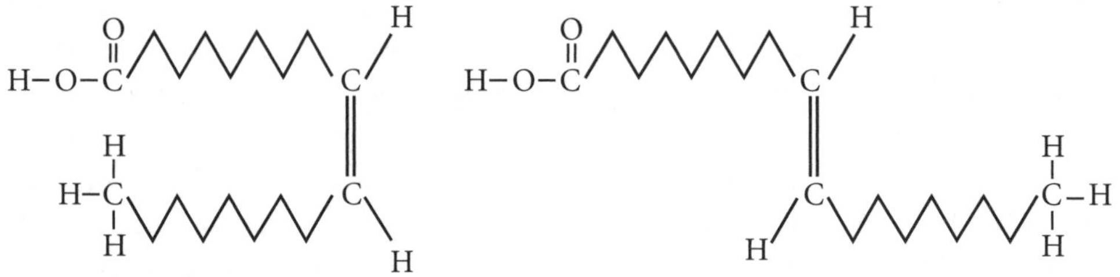

cis–fatty acid	trans–fatty acid
The H's are on the same side of the double bond, forcing the molecule to assume a horseshoe shape.	The H's are on opposite sides of the double bond, forcing the molecule into an extended position.

cholesterol, and fats in the form of phospholipids. Phospholipids are almost the same as triglycerides, except that one of the three fatty acid units has been replaced with a molecule that contains phosphorus.

What determines the type of fatty acid present in the cell membrane is the type of fat you consume. A diet that is high in cholesterol and composed mostly of saturated fat, animal fatty acids, and trans–fatty acids (from margarine, shortening, and other sources of hydrogenated vegetable oils) results in cell membranes that are much less fluid in nature than the cell membranes found in a person who consumes optimal levels of unsaturated fatty acids.

According to modern pathology, or the study of disease processes, an alteration in cell membrane function is the central factor in the development of virtually every disease. As it relates to diabetes, abnormal cell membrane structure due to eating the wrong types of fats leads to an impairment in the action of insulin.

Without a healthy membrane, cells lose their ability to hold water, vital nutrients, and electrolytes. Without the right type of fats in cell membranes, cells simply do not function properly. In particular, they lose their ability to communicate with other cells and be controlled by regulating hormones. To highlight the impact of having the right type of fat in the cell membranes, let's look at the effects of different diets on insulin action. Insulin is a hormone produced by the pancreas that plays a critical role in blood sugar regulation. Loss of sensitivity to the effects of insulin is linked to obesity and type 2 diabetes. While margarine and saturated fats dampen insulin sensitivity, clinical studies have shown that monounsaturated fats and omega-3 oils improve insulin action. Adding further support to these studies is the fact that population studies have indicated that frequent consumption of monounsaturated fats, such as olive oil, nuts and nut oils, and omega-3 fatty acids from fish protect against the development of type 2 diabetes. Similar associations are seen with more than fifty health conditions, including heart disease, cancer, and arthritis; see the list below.

Margarine and Other Foods Containing Trans–Fatty Acids and Partially Hydrogenated Oils

Margarine and shortening are manufactured from vegetable oils through "hydrogenation." This means that a hydrogen molecule is added to the natural unsaturated fatty acid molecules of the vegetable oil to make it more saturated. Hydrogenation, the addition of hydrogen molecules, changes the structure of the natural fatty acid to many "unnatural" fatty acid forms, as well as from the *cis,* or U-shaped, configuration to the *trans,* or Z-shaped, configuration. The resulting hydrogenated vegetable oil becomes solid or semisolid.

Margarine, vegetable oil shortening, and other foods containing trans–fatty acids and partially hydrogenated oils are particularly harmful to cell membrane function. These "unnatural" forms of fatty acids interfere with the body's ability to utilize important essential fatty acids. For example, one study estimated that substituting polyunsaturated vegetable oils for margarine containing hydrogenated vegetable oil would reduce the likelihood of developing type 2 diabetes by a whopping 40 percent.

HEALTH CONDITIONS LINKED TO INSUFFICIENT INTAKE OF OMEGA-3 FATTY ACIDS

Acne	Dementia	Multiple sclerosis
AIDS	Depression	Osteoarthritis
Allergies	Dermatitis	Postviral fatigue
Alzheimer's disease	Diabetes	Pregnancy complications
Angina	Eczema	Premenstrual syndrome
Angioplasty recovery	Heart disease	Psoriasis
Arthritis	High blood pressure	Refsum's syndrome
Atherosclerosis	Hyperactivity	Reye's syndrome
Asthma	Hypertension	Rheumatoid arthritis
Attention deficit disorder	Hypoxia	Schizophrenia
Autoimmune diseases	Ichthyosis	Sepsis
Breast cancer	Immune disorders	Sjögren-Larsson syndrome
Breast cysts	Inflammatory bowel	Stroke
Breast pain	disease	Vascular disease
Cancer	Inflammatory conditions	Vision development
Cartilage destruction	Kidney dysfunction	impairment
Coronary bypass recovery	Learning difficulties	
Cystic fibrosis	Menopausal symptoms	

Arthritis

Constipation

Cracked nails

Depression

Dry, lifeless hair

Dry mucous membranes (tear ducts,
    mouth, vagina, etc.)

Dry skin

Fatigue, malaise, low energy

Forgetfulness

Frequent colds and sickness

High blood pressure

History of cardiovascular disease

Immune weakness

Indigestion, wind, bloating

Lack of endurance

Lack of motivation

* These symptoms are not specific to a deficiency of
essential fatty acids. They may also be caused by other
diseases or dietary insufficiencies.

Prostaglandins

Essential fatty acids are transformed into regulatory compounds known as prostaglandins. These compounds carry out many important tasks in the body including playing a role in the regulation of

Allergic response

Blood clotting and platelet aggregation

Blood pressure

Gastrointestinal function and secretions

Heart function

Inflammation

Inflammation, pain, and swelling

Kidney function and fluid balance

Nerve transmission

Steroid production and hormone synthesis

Prostaglandins are assigned to either the 1, 2, or 3 series based upon the number of double bonds in the fatty acid. Series 1 and 2 prostaglandins come from the omega-6 fatty acids, with linoleic acid serving as the starting point. Linoleic acid is changed to gamma-linolenic acid and then to dihomo-gamma-linolenic acid (DHGLA), which contains three double bonds and is the precursor of prostaglandin of the anti-inflammatory 1 series.

Dihomo-gamma-linolenic acid can also be converted to arachidonic acid, which contains four double bonds and is precursor to the proinflammatory 2 series prostaglandins. However, because the delta-5-desaturase enzyme responsible for the conversion of DHGLA to arachidonic acid prefers the omega-3 oils, in humans the greatest source of arachidonic acid is from the diet. Arachidonic acid is found almost entirely in animal foods, along with saturated fats.

The omega-3 prostaglandin pathway can begin with alpha-linolenic acid, which can eventually be converted to eicosapentaenoic acid (EPA) and docosahexaenoic acid (DHA), the precursors to the anti-inflammatory 3 series prostaglandins, but the process is much more efficient when the EPA and DHA are already preformed, as they are, for example, in fish oils.

Prostaglandins of the 1 and 3 series are generally viewed as "good" prostaglandins, while prostaglandins of the 2 series are viewed as "bad." This labeling is most evident by looking at their effects on platelets. Prostaglandins of the

FIGURE 6.2
Prostaglandin Metabolism

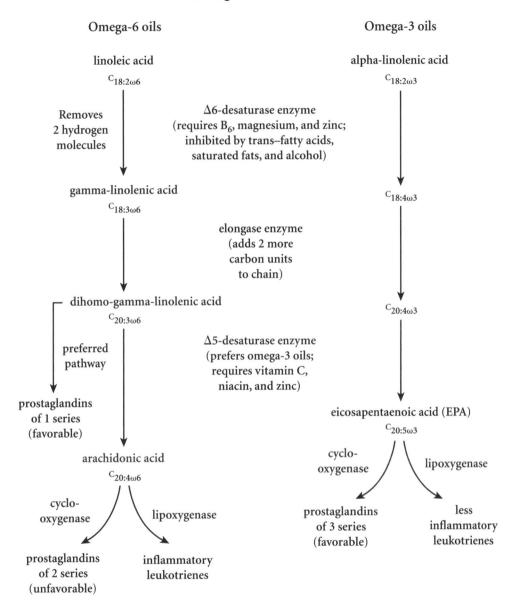

Omega-6 oils

linoleic acid
$C_{18:2\omega6}$

Removes 2 hydrogen molecules

Δ6-desaturase enzyme (requires B_6, magnesium, and zinc; inhibited by trans–fatty acids, saturated fats, and alcohol)

gamma-linolenic acid
$C_{18:3\omega6}$

elongase enzyme (adds 2 more carbon units to chain)

dihomo-gamma-linolenic acid
$C_{20:3\omega6}$

preferred pathway

prostaglandins of 1 series (favorable)

Δ5-desaturase enzyme (prefers omega-3 oils; requires vitamin C, niacin, and zinc)

arachidonic acid
$C_{20:4\omega6}$

cyclo-oxygenase   lipoxygenase

prostaglandins of 2 series (unfavorable)   inflammatory leukotrienes

Omega-3 oils

alpha-linolenic acid
$C_{18:2\omega3}$

$C_{18:4\omega3}$

$C_{20:4\omega3}$

eicosapentaenoic acid (EPA)
$C_{20:5\omega3}$

cyclo-oxygenase   lipoxygenase

prostaglandins of 3 series (favorable)   less inflammatory leukotrienes

2 series promote platelet stickiness, a factor that leads to hardening of the arteries, heart disease, and strokes. In contrast, the 1 and 3 series prostaglandins prevent platelets from sticking together, improve blood flow, and reduce inflammation.

By altering the type of dietary oils consumed and stored in cell membranes, prostaglandin metabolism can be manipulated. Prostaglandin manipulation can be extremely powerful in the treatment of inflammation, allergies, high blood pressure, and many other health conditions. The basic goal in most situations is twofold: to (1) reduce the level of arachidonic acid and (2) increase the level of DHGLA and EPA/DHA. This goal can best be achieved in most circumstances by reducing the intake of sources of omega-6 fatty acids and animal foods, while increasing the intake of omega-3 fatty acids, particularly fish oils. Although linseed oil provides alpha-linolenic acid, which can be converted by the enzyme delta-6-desaturase into stearidonic acid and then elongated into EPA and DHA, this cumbersome conversion process is obviously not as effective in increasing tissue concentrations of EPA and DHA as fish oil supplements.

These following steps will help you gain the optimal ratio of essential fatty acids for healthy cell membranes and balanced and efficient production of prostaglandins:

1. Be aware of the fat content of foods. Limit total dietary fat intake to no more than 30 percent of calories consumed. That's 400 to 600 calories a day from fat, based on a standard 2,000-calorie-a-day diet (see the list below). Reduce the amount of saturated fats and total fat in the diet. In general, animal products are high in fat, while most plant foods are very low in fat. However, while most nuts and seeds are relatively high in fat, the calories they supply come mostly from monounsaturated fats.

2. Reduce the intake of meat and dairy products, while increasing the intake of fish. Particularly beneficial are the cold-water fish, such as wild salmon, mackerel, herring, and halibut, because of their high levels of omega-3 fats.

3. Cook with rapeseed, coconut, macadamia nut, or olive oil.

4. Eliminate margarine and other foods containing trans–fatty acids and partially hydrogenated oils. These "unnatural" forms of fatty acids interfere with the body's ability to utilize important essential fatty acids.

5. Take a high-quality fish oil supplement providing 600 to 1,200 milligrams of omega-3 fatty acids. Vegetarians may take 1 tablespoon of linseed oil daily.

THE FAT CONTENT OF SELECTED FOODS

Meats

Sirloin steak, with bone, lean	83%	Frankfurters	80%
Pork sausage	83%	Lamb rib chops, lean	79%
T-bone steak, lean	82%	Duck meat, w/skin	76%
Porterhouse steak, lean	82%	Salami	76%
Bacon, lean	82%	Liverwurst	75%
Rib roast, lean	81%	Rump roast, lean	71%
Bologna sausage	81%	Ham, lean	69%
Country-style sausage	81%	Stewing beef, lean	66%
Spareribs	80%	Goose meat, w/skin	65%

Minced beef, lean	64%	Chuck rib roast, lean only	50%
Veal breast, lean	64%	Chuck steak, lean only	50%
Leg of lamb, lean	61%	Sirloin steak, lean	47%
Chicken, dark meat w/skin, roasted	56%	Turkey, dark meat w/skin	47%
Round steak, lean	53%	Chicken, light meat w/skin roasted	44%

Fish

Tuna, chunk, oil-packed	63%	Caviar, sturgeon	52%
Herring	58%	Mackerel, Pacific	50%
Anchovies	54%	Sardines, Atlantic, in oil, drained	49%
Bass, black sea	53%	Salmon, sockeye (red)	49%
Perch, ocean	53%	Halibut	45%

Vegetables

Mustard greens	13%	Celery	6%
Kale	13%	Courgette	6%
Beet greens	12%	Cucumber	6%
Lettuce	12%	Turnip	6%
Turnip greens	11%	Carrots	4%
Mushrooms	8%	Green peas	4%
Aubergine	7%	Artichokes	3%
Cabbage	7%	Onions	3%
Cauliflower	7%	Beetroot	2%
Asparagus	6%	Chives	1%
Green bean	6%	Potatoes	1%

Legumes

Tofu	49%	Lima bean	4%
Soybeans	37%	Mung bean sprouts	4%
Soybean sprouts	28%	Lentils	3%
Chickpeas	11%	Broad bean	3%
Kidney bean	4%	Mung bean	3%

Dairy products

Butter	100%	Cream, light	85%
Cream, light whipping	92%	Egg yolks	80%
Cream cheese	90%	Half and half	79%

Blue cheese	73%	Cow's milk	49%
Brick cheese	72%	Yogurt, plain	49%
Cheddar cheese	71%	Ice cream, low-fat	48%
Swiss cheese	71%	Cottage cheese	35%
Ricotta cheese, whole-milk type	66%	Milk, low-fat (2%)	31%
Eggs, whole	65%	Yogurt, low-fat (2%)	31%
Ice cream	64%	Ice milk	29%
Mozzarella cheese, part-skimmed type	55%	Cottage cheese, nonfat (1%)	22%
Goat's milk	54%		

Fruits

Olive	91%	Banana	4%
Avocado	82%	Cherry	4%
Grapes	11%	Orange	4%
Strawberry	11%	Cantaloupe melon	3%
Apple	8%	Pineapple	3%
Blueberry	7%	Grapefruit	2%
Lemon	7%	Papaya	2%
Watermelon	5%	Peach	2%
Apricot	4%	Prune	1%

Grains

Oatmeal	16%	Bulgur wheat	4%
Buckwheat, dark	7%	Barley	3%
Rye, dark	7%	Buckwheat, light	3%
Corn, flour	5%	Rye, light	2%
Rice, brown	5%	Rice, wild	2%
Wheat, whole	5%		

Nuts and Seeds

Coconut	85%	Sunflower	71%
Walnut	79%	Cashew	70%
Almond	76%	Peanut	69%
Sesame	76%	Chestnut	7%
Pumpkin seeds	71%		

Other Fatty Substances

Phospholipids

Phospholipids are the predominant form of fats in our cell membranes. The major phospholipid of the human body is phosphatidylcholine. Commercially available phosphatidylcholine supplements are derived from soy lecithin, an excellent source of phosphatidylcholine. These preparations are used in the treatment of Alzheimer's disease, bipolar disorder, elevated cholesterol levels, and liver disorders. The beneficial effects are most likely due primarily to the essential fatty acid components of phosphatidylcholine and the soy lecithin preparations, because the body primarily breaks down phospholipids into free fatty acids, which benefit the body. These free fatty acids are used directly as fuel by the cells of the body. As previously discussed, free fatty acids can be long, short, saturated, or unsaturated. The free fatty acids in soy lecithin are beneficial medium- and short-chain, unsaturated fatty acids.

Phosphatidylcholine has many important functions in the body, including increasing the solubility of cholesterol, thereby decreasing its ability to induce atherosclerosis. Phosphatidylcholine also aids in lowering cholesterol levels and removing cholesterol from tissue deposits. In a total of fifteen clinical trials with a duration of treatment with phosphatidylcholine ranging from one to twelve months, total serum cholesterol was lowered by 8.8 to 28.2 percent, triglyceride levels decreased by 25 percent, and HDL cholesterol levels increased by 13.4 to 20 percent. The typical dosage was 1.5 to 2.7 grams daily.

Phosphatidylcholine is a component of many foods, such as whole grains, legumes (especially soy), meat, and egg yolks. Phosphatidylcholine supplements are available as soy lecithin and phosphatidylcholine isolated and purified from soy lecithin ranging in content from 10 percent to 55 percent phosphatidylcholine.

Cholesterol

Cholesterol is often portrayed as an evil compound, but it serves many important roles as it is the starting point for the manufacture of many hormones and bile acids, and serves as an important component of cell membranes as well. While the liver is the major source of blood cholesterol, dietary cholesterol can be an important contributor. Diets high in cholesterol are associated with an increased risk for heart disease, cancer, and strokes. However, it may turn out that the level of saturated fats in these diet foods is more relevant than the cholesterol content. This opinion is supported by a statistical analysis of 224 dietary studies carried out over the past twenty-five years that investigated the relationship between diet and blood cholesterol levels in more than 8,000 subjects. What investigators found was that saturated fat in the diet, not dietary cholesterol, is what influences blood cholesterol levels the most.

Cholesterol is transported in the blood on carrier molecules known as *lipoproteins.* The major categories of lipoproteins are very-low-density lipoprotein (VLDL), low-density lipoprotein (LDL), and high-density lipoprotein (HDL). Since VLDL and LDL are responsible for transporting fats (primarily triglycerides and cholesterol) from the liver to body cells while HDL is responsible for returning fats to the liver for use as energy and for excretion, elevation of either VLDL or LDL is associated with an increased risk of developing atherosclerosis, the primary cause of a heart attack or stroke. In contrast, elevations of HDL are associated with a low risk of heart attacks.

It is currently recommended in the U.S.A. that the total blood cholesterol level be less than 200 milligrams per deciliter. In addition, it is recommended that the LDL cholesterol be less than 130 milligrams per deciliter, the HDL cholesterol be greater than 35 milligrams per deciliter, and triglyceride levels be less than 150 milligrams per deciliter. In the U.K., cholesterol levels are measured using a different system. The recommended level of total blood cholesterol is less than 5 mmol/l (millimoles per liter), a LDL level under 3 mmol/l, and triglyceride levels below 2 mmol/l.

The ratio of total cholesterol to HDL cholesterol and the ratio of LDL to HDL are also important and are referred to as the cardiac risk factor ratios because they reflect whether cholesterol is being deposited into tissues or broken down and excreted. The total cholesterol-to-HDL ratio should be no higher than 4:1, and the LDL to HDL ratio should be no higher than 2.5:1. The risk of developing heart disease can be reduced dramatically by lowering the LDL cholesterol level while simultaneously raising the HDL cholesterol level. It has been concluded that for every 1 percent drop in the LDL cholesterol level, the risk for a heart attack drops by 2 percent. Conversely, for every 1 percent increase in HDL level, the risk for a heart attack drops by 3 to 4 percent.

Cholesterol levels and ratios can be improved by dietary changes undertaken to reduce your overall cholesterol and dietary fat intake (see Table 6.2).

Conjugated Linoleic Acid

Conjugated linoleic acid (CLA) is a slightly altered form of the essential fatty acid linoleic acid. It is found naturally occurring in meat and dairy products from grass-fed cows. It was discovered in 1978, when researchers at the University of Wisconsin were seeking to find possible cancer-causing compounds in meat that are produced with cooking. Instead, they found what appears to be the anticancer compound CLA. In preliminary animal and test-tube studies, CLA has shown evidence that it might reduce the risk of cancers at several sites, including breast, prostate, colon, lung, skin, and stomach. Whether CLA will produce a similar protective effect in humans has yet to be determined. Human studies have focused on its ability to help promote lean body mass during weight loss programmes, which have been somewhat promising. For example, researchers from the University of Wisconsin recruited eighty obese people and had half of them take 3,000 milligrams of CLA (Tonalin) daily, while the other half took a placebo. They were all put on a diet programme and encouraged to exercise. Weight loss was about the same for both groups, an average of 5 pounds/2¼ kilograms. So why take CLA? Those taking CLA reported less fatigue, dizziness, and nausea than those on the placebo. But the real advantage was that while the people taking the placebo put the weight back on mainly as fat, the people taking CLA who put weight back on put it on primarily as lean muscle, not as fat. In other words, CLA

TABLE 6.2

Cholesterol and Fat Content of Selected Foods

Food	Serving Size (grams)	Total Fat (grams)	Saturated Fat (grams)	Monounsaturated Fat (grams)	Polyunsaturated Fat (grams)	Cholesterol (milligrams)
Beef, lean	85	7.9	3.0	3.3	0.3	73
Beef liver, braised	85	4.2	1.6	0.6	0.9	331
Chicken, breast, roasted	85	3.0	0.9	1.1	0.6	72
Chicken, leg, roasted	85	7.2	2.0	2.6	1.7	79
Egg yolk	1 large	5.1	1.6	1.9	0.7	213
Fish, cod	85	0.7	0.1	0.1	0.3	40
Lobster, boiled	85	0.5	0.1	0.1	0.1	61
Pork, lean	85	11.1	3.8	5.0	1.3	79
Prawn, boiled	85	0.9	0.2	0.2	0.4	166
Turkey, dark, roasted	85	6.1	2.1	1.4	1.8	73
Turkey, light, roasted	85	2.7	0.9	0.5	0.7	59
Butter	1 tablespoon	11.5	7.2	3.3	0.4	31
Cheese, cheddar	30	9.4	6.0	2.7	0.3	30
Ice cream, regular	125 ml	7.2	4.5	2.1	0.3	30
Milk, low-fat (2%)	250 ml	4.7	2.9	1.4	0.2	18
Milk, skimmed	250 ml	0.4	0.3	0.1	neg	4
Milk, whole	250 ml	8.2	5.1	2.4	0.3	33

promoted an increase in lean muscle mass and a decrease in percentage of body fat.

In another study, supplementation with CLA (Tonalin) at a dosage of 4.5 grams per day was shown in a twelve-month double-blind study to help overweight adults decrease body fat mass and increase lean body mass by as much as 9 percent. This 2004 study was the first to clearly establish the efficacy of CLA supplementation over an extended time period without changes in exercise or diet.

Ferulic Acid Derivatives

Ferulic acid derivatives include gamma-oryzanol, a growth-promoting substance found in grains and isolated from rice bran oil. Gamma-oryzanol has been used in Japan as a medicine since 1962. Initially it was used in the treatment of minor anxiety, and later it became approved for the treatment of menopausal symptoms (1970) and elevated cholesterol and triglyceride levels (1986).

Gamma-oryzanol was first shown to be effective for menopausal symptoms, including hot flushes, in the early 1960s. Clinical studies demonstrated that 67 to 85 percent of the women who took gamma-oryzanol had a 50 percent or greater reduction in their menopausal symptoms.

Gamma-oryzanol has been shown to be quite effective in lowering blood cholesterol and triglyceride levels in several double-blind studies, lowering total cholesterol levels by 8 to 12 percent and triglycerides by 15 percent within the first four weeks. Gamma-oryzanol's cholesterol-lowering action appears to involve a combination of effects in that it increases the conversion of cholesterol to bile acids and inhibits the absorption of cholesterol.

Double-blind studies have also shown supplemental gamma-oryzanol to increase lean body mass, increase strength, improve recovery from workouts, and reduce body fat and post-exercise soreness.

Octacosanol

Octacosanol is a waxy substance that is naturally present in wheat germ oil, rice bran, and the wax layer of many plants. Animal research indicates that it shares many common features with vitamin E and plays a role in enhancing energy production within cells. Early research suggested that octacosanol may help in improving amyotrophic lateral sclerosis (Lou Gehrig's disease), but this possible treatment was subsequently disproved. More recent research has focused on octacosanol as an ergogenic (exercise performance–promoting) agent. Preliminary studies have found that octacosanol has promising effects on endurance, reaction time, and other measures of exercise capacity. In one study, a dosage of only 1 milligram per day of octacosanol for eight weeks was found to improve grip strength and visual reaction time but had no effect on chest strength, auditory reaction time, or endurance.

Octacosanol is also one of the key components of policosanol, a mixture of fatty substances isolated and purified from the wax of sugarcane *(Saccharum officinarum)*. Policosanol has exceptional clinical documentation demonstrating its efficacy, safety, and tolerability in lowering cholesterol and triglyceride levels. The clinical studies have included comparative studies versus conventional cholesterol-lowering drugs, such as pravastatin, simvastatin, gemfibrozil, and probucol. In these studies, policosanol in dosages ranging from 5 to 20 milligrams per day has demonstrated significant improvements in lowering cholesterol levels on a par with these drugs, typically 20 to 30 percent.

In addition to its effects on cholesterol levels, policosanol exerts additional positive effects in the battle against atherosclerosis. It prevents excessive platelet aggregation without affecting coagulation and exerts good antioxidant effects in preventing against LDL oxidation. Better news still is that these benefits of policosanol may be present in other waxy substances that coat most fruits and vegetables.

Conclusions

Dietary fats and fatty substances are important dietary components that have many roles, including being the primary fuel of the body as well as being critical in cellular structures, hormone precursors, and regulators of normal metabolism. The types of fats we consume have a significant influence on our health and well-being.

7

Vitamins

Vitamins are essential nutrients required for normal chemical processes to occur in the body. They serve as essential components in enzymes and coenzymes. Enzymes are molecules involved in speeding up chemical reactions necessary for human bodily function such as energy production or the assembling of tissue components. Coenzymes are molecules that help the enzymes in their chemical reactions.

Enzymes and coenzymes work either to join molecules together or split them apart by making or breaking the chemical bonds that link them together. Most enzymes are composed of a protein along with an essential mineral and possibly a vitamin. If an enzyme is lacking the essential mineral or vitamin, it cannot function properly.

There are thirteen vitamins divided into two primary classes. Those that dissolve in fat (are fat-soluble) are the vitamins A, D, E, and K. Those that dissolve in water (are water-soluble) are vitamin C, the B vitamins, biotin, and folic acid.

Fat-soluble vitamins can be stored in fat

cells. For this reason your body is able to keep a supply of these vitamins available for use on demand. The downside is that toxic levels can be built up in the body, leading to potentially severe side effects. Water-soluble vitamins, on the other hand, are stored in the body only in small amounts. Normally, any quantity of these vitamins that your body does not use is excreted in the urine. However, while it is harder to build up toxic amounts of water-soluble vitamins, it is also easier to develop deficiencies of them.

The RDA and DRI, and the RNI and RDA

Included in the description of each vitamin is the Recommended Dietary Allowance (RDA). The RDAs for vitamins and minerals have been prepared by the Food and Nutrition Board of the National Research Council in the U.S.A. since 1941. These guidelines were originally developed to reduce the rates of severe nutritional deficiency diseases such as scurvy (deficiency of vitamin C), pellagra (deficiency of niacin), and beriberi (deficiency of vitamin B1). Another critical point is that the RDAs were designed to serve as the basis for evaluating the adequacy of diets of groups of people, not individuals, because individuals simply vary too widely in their nutritional requirements. As stated by the Food and Nutrition Board, "Individuals with special nutritional needs are not covered by the RDAs." Statistically speaking, RDAs prevented deficiency diseases in 97 percent of a population, but there was no scientific basis that RDAs met the needs of any individual person.

In 1993, the Food and Nutrition Board put the RDA revision process into motion by holding a symposium and asking for scientific and public comment on how the RDAs should be revised. Utilizing feedback from this conference and other sources, the Food and Nutrition Board developed an ambitious framework for revamping the old RDAs. Rather than having a single group of scientists revise the existing set of RDAs, they had expert panels review nutrient categories in much more detail than had ever been done before. The Food and Nutrition Board partnered with Health Canada, the Canadian government agency responsible for nutrition policy, and the two groups jointly appointed the Standing Committee on the Scientific Evaluation of Dietary Reference Intakes of the Food and Nutrition Board.

As a result, not only did the definition of RDAs change, but three new values were also created: the Estimated Average Requirement (EAR), the Adequate Intake (AI), and the Tolerable Upper Intake Level (UL). All four values are collectively known as Dietary Reference Intakes, or DRIs.

The RNI or Reference Nutrient Intake system used in the U.K. estimates the daily amount of a nutrient required by 97.5 percent of the population (as nutrient requirements vary

---

Dietary Reference Intakes *(DRIs)* is the umbrella term that includes the following values:

- Estimated Average Requirement (EAR): *A nutrient intake value that is estimated to meet the requirement of half the healthy individuals in a group. It is used to assess the nutritional adequacy of intakes in population groups. In addition, EARs are used to calculate RDAs.*
- Recommended Dietary Allowance (RDA): *This value is a goal for individuals and is based upon the EAR. It is the daily dietary intake level that is sufficient to meet the nutrient requirement of 97 to 98 percent of all healthy individuals in a group. If an EAR cannot be set, no RDA value can be proposed.*
- Adequate Intake (AI): *Used when a RDA cannot be determined, this is a recommended daily intake level based on an observed or experimentally determined approximation of nutrient intake for a group (or groups) of healthy people.*
- Tolerable Upper Intake Level (UL): *The highest level of daily nutrient intake that is likely to pose no risks of adverse health effects to almost all individuals in the general population. As intake increases above the UL, the risk of adverse effects increases.*

U.S. RDA/DRI TIME LINE

1941: First edition of the Recommended Dietary Allowances (RDAs) is published.

1941–1989: RDAs are periodically updated and revised based on cumulative scientific data. Tenth edition is published in 1989.

1993: The Food and Nutrition Board (FNB) holds a symposium on the subject "Should the Recommended Dietary Allowances Be Revised?" Based on comments and suggestions from this meeting, FNB proposes changes to the development process of RDAs.

1995: The Standing Committee on the Scientific Evaluation of Dietary Reference Intakes (DRI) announces that seven expert nutrient group panels will review major nutrients, vitamins, minerals, antioxidants, electrolytes, and other food components.

1997: First DRI report, on calcium, phosphorus, magnesium, vitamin D, and fluoride, is issued.

1998: Second DRI report, on thiamine, riboflavin, niacin, vitamin B6, folate, vitamin B12, pantothenic acid, biotin, and choline, is issued.

2000: DRI report on vitamins C and E, beta-carotene, and selenium is issued.

2001: DRI report on vitamin A, vitamin K, arsenic, boron, chromium, copper, iodine, iron, manganese, molybdenum, nickel, silicon, vanadium, and zinc is issued.

---

so much between individuals). Nutritionists use other Dietary Reference Values (DRVs) too, including the Estimated Average Requirement (EAR) and the Lower Reference Nutrient Intake (LRNI) for the 2.5 percent of people with very low nutrient needs.

There is also the European Union Recommended Daily Amount (RDA), an overall value which is based on meeting the nutritional demands of groups of adults and not reflecting individual differences according to age, sex, physiological states, etc., and reflecting the variation of opinion across the Community.

The DRIs reflect a shift in emphasis from preventing deficiency to decreasing the risk of chronic disease through nutrition and proper nutritional supplementation. The RDAs were based on the amounts needed to protect against deficiency diseases. Where adequate scientific data exist, the DRIs strive to include levels that can help prevent certain cancers, cardiovascular disease, osteoporosis, and other diseases that are diet-related.

The DRIs are intended to apply to the healthy general population. They do not apply to individuals who are deficient in a particular nutrient and need to restore proper levels, nor do they apply to individuals with diseases associated with increased nutritional requirements or individuals whose genetic inheritance gives them a higher need for certain vitamin or mineral cofactors for the proper function and activity of various enzymes.

Fat-Soluble Vitamins

Vitamin A

Vitamin A was the first fat-soluble vitamin to be recognized. The initial discovery of vitamin A in 1913 was made almost simultaneously by two groups of research workers, Elmer McCollum and Marguerite Davis at the University of Wisconsin, and Thomas Osborne and Lafayette Mendel at Yale University. They found that young animals fed a diet deficient in natural fats became very unhealthy, as evidenced by their inability to grow and poor immune function. These researchers also noted that the animals' eyes became severely inflamed and infected on the restricted diet and that this could be quickly relieved by the addition to the diet of either butterfat or cod-liver oil. Today, we know that these foods are excellent sources of vitamin A. Once known as the "anti-infective vitamin," vitamin A has recently regained recognition as a major determinant of immune status.

The best understood role of vitamin A, however, is its effects on the visual system. The human retina has four kinds of vitamin A-containing compounds that function in the visual process. Night blindness or poor dark adaptation is an early consequence of vitamin A deficiency.

Vitamin A is also necessary for proper growth and development, and is particularly important in maintaining the health and structure of the skin. Many skin disorders, including acne and psoriasis, are often responsive to vitamin A. Other body functions aided by vitamin A include reproduction; adrenal and thyroid hormone manufacture and activity; maintaining structure and function of nerve cells; immunity; and cell growth.

Vitamin A was originally measured in international units (IU). In 1967, however, an FAO/WHO Expert Committee recommended that vitamin A activity be referred to in terms of retinol (vitamin A) equivalents rather than in IU, with 1 microgram of retinol being equivalent to 1 retinol equivalent (RE). The amount of beta-carotene required for 1 RE is 6 micrograms, while the amount required for other provitamin A carotenoids is 12 micrograms. In 1980, The Food and Nutrition Board of the NRC/NAS adopted this recommendation. The Recommended Dietary Allowance (RDA) for vitamin A is now stated in both micrograms and RE. For the adult male, the RDA is set at 1,000 RE (750 as retinol and 250 as beta-carotene, or 5,000 IU), while the RDA for women is lower, at 800 RE (4,000 IU). Children need 400 to 1,000 RE (2,000 to 5,000 IU), with the dosage increasing from infancy to fourteen years. In the U.K., the RNI for adult males is 700 micrograms, for adult females 600 micrograms and for children up to four 363 micrograms. The E.U. RDA is 800 micrograms.

The most concentrated sources of preformed vitamin A are liver, whole milk, and fortified skimmed milk. Vitamin A can also be formed from beta-carotenes and other carotenes. The leading sources of provitamin A carotenes are dark green leafy vegetables, such as collards and spinach, and yellow-orange vegetables, such as carrots, sweet potatoes, yams, and squash. Toxicity to vitamin A has been reported in people who supplement with excessive doses (over 10,000 RE for many months) or eat 6 to 24 pounds/2½ to 11 kilograms per week of liver. In contrast, beta-carotene exerts no toxicity.

VITAMIN A CONTENT OF SELECTED FOODS,
IN INTERNATIONAL UNITS (IU) PER 100 GRAM
SERVING (UNLESS OTHERWISE NOTED)

Liver, ox	43,900
Liver, calf's	22,500
Chili peppers	21,600
Dandelion root	14,000
Chicken liver	12,100
Carrots	11,000
Apricots, dried	10,900
Collard greens	9,300
Kale	8,900
Sweet potatoes	8,800
Parsley	8,500
Spinach	8,100
Mustard greens	7,000
Mangoes	4,800
Hubbard squash	4,300
Cantaloupe melon	3,400
Apricots	2,700
Broccoli	2,500
Nonfat milk (fortified), 250 ml	500
Whole milk, 250 ml	227

Vitamin D

Since vitamin D can be produced in our bodies by the action of sunlight on the skin, many experts consider it to be more of a hormone than a vitamin. In the skin, sunlight changes the precursor of vitamin D, 7-dihydrocholesterol, into vitamin D3 (cholecalciferol). It is then transported to the liver and converted by an enzyme into 25-hydroxycholecalciferol (25-OHD3), which is five times more potent than cholecalciferol (D3). The 25-hydroxycholecalciferol is then converted by an enzyme in the kidneys to 1,25-dihydroxycholecalciferol (1,25-$(OH)_2$D3), which is ten times more potent than cholecalciferol and the most potent form of vitamin D3.

Disorders of the liver or kidneys result in impaired conversion of cholecalciferol to more potent vitamin D compounds. In many patients with osteoporosis, the level of 25-OHD3 is high, while the level of 1,25-$(OH)_2$D3 is quite low. This signifies an impairment of the conversion of 25-OHD3 to 1,25-$(OH)_2$D3 in osteoporosis. Many theories have been proposed to account for this decreased conversion, including relationships to oestrogen and magnesium deficiency. Recently, the trace mineral boron has been theorized to play a role in this conversion as well.

Vitamin D deficiency results in rickets in children and osteomalacia in adults. Rickets and osteomalacia are characterized by an inability to calcify the bone matrix. This results in softening of the skull bones, bowing of legs, spinal curvature, and increased joint size. Once common, these diseases are now extremely rare.

Vitamin D is best known for its ability to stimulate the absorption of calcium. As such, it is added to milk and other foods. More natural sources of vitamin D are cod-liver oil; cold-water fish, such as mackerel, salmon, and herring; butter; and egg yolks. Vegetables are low in vitamin D, but the best plant sources are dark green leafy vegetables. Vitamin D has the greatest potential to cause toxicity in comparison to other fat-soluble vitamins. Supplementation greater than 400 IU per day, the RDA for children, appears to be unwarranted. In the U.K. there is no established RNI for adults but children up to the age of four are recommended to take 7 micrograms. The E.U. RDA is 5 micrograms.

FIGURE 7.1

Vitamin D Metabolism

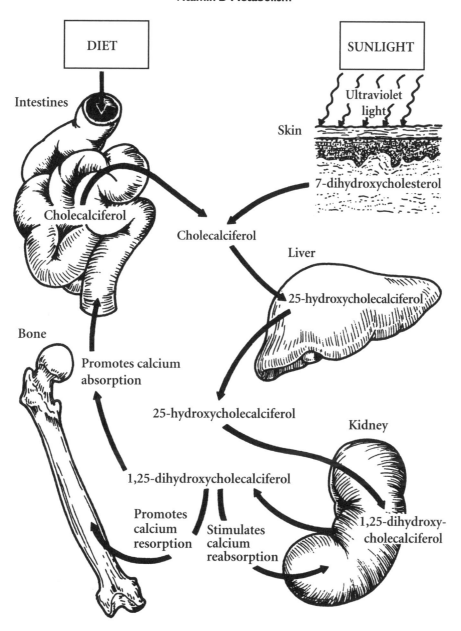

VITAMIN D CONTENT OF SELECTED FOODS,
IN INTERNATIONAL UNITS (IU) PER 100 GRAM
SERVING (UNLESS OTHERWISE NOTED)

Cod-liver oil, 1 tablespoon	1,360
Sardines, canned in oil, drained	500
Salmon, cooked	360
Mackerel, cooked	345
Tuna fish, canned in oil	200
Milk, vitamin D fortified, 250 ml	98
Egg, 1 whole	20
Liver, ox, cooked	154
Cheese, Swiss, 30 grams	12

Vitamin E

Vitamin E is required by most animal species, including humans. It was discovered in 1922, when rats fed a purified diet without vitamin E became unable to reproduce. Wheat germ oil added to their diet restored their fertility. Later, vitamin E was isolated and was originally called the "antisterility" vitamin or tocopherol. The word tocopherol comes from the Greek words *tokos,* meaning "offspring," and *phero,* meaning "to bear." Hence, tocopherol literally means "to bear children," a reference to the rats' renewed ability to reproduce. Alpha-tocopherol is the chemical name for the most active form of vitamin E, at least in rats. In humans, new research suggests that the gamma and delta fractions and the tocotrienols may be much more important for cardiovascular health.

Vitamin E functions primarily as an antioxidant in protecting against damage to cell membranes. Without vitamin E, the cells of the body would be quite susceptible to damage. Nerve cells would be particularly vulnerable. Severe vitamin E deficiency is quite rare, but there are a number of conditions in which low levels of vitamin E have been reported, including acne, anemia, some cancers, gallstones, Lou Gehrig's disease, muscular dystrophy, Parkinson's disease, and Alzheimer's disease.

Vitamin E and diets high in Vitamin E have been shown to exert a protective effect in many common health conditions, including heart disease, cancer, strokes, fibrocystic breast disease, and viral infections. Typically, vitamin E is used at a dose of 400 to 600 IU per day. It is extremely well tolerated, even at these high doses. However, if you decide to take a vitamin E supplement, we recommend that you choose one containing mixed tocopherols rather than simply alpha-tocopherol. Also, the D form is the active form and the D form is not used in the body.

In the U.K. an RNI has not been established but the E.U. RDA is 10 milligrams. Although the RDA for vitamin E is set at 10 milligrams (roughly 15 IU), the amount of vitamin E required is largely dependent upon the amount of polyunsaturated fats in the diet. The more polyunsaturated fats are consumed, the greater the risk that they will be damaged. Since vitamin E prevents this damage, as the intake of polyunsaturated fatty acids increases, so does the need for vitamin E. Fortunately, in nature, where high levels of polyunsaturated fatty acids are found they are accompanied by higher levels of vitamin E. The best sources of vitamin E are wheat germ oil and polyunsaturated vegetable oils, seeds, and nuts. Good sources are asparagus, avocados, green leafy vegetables, tomatoes, and whole grains.

FIGURE 7.2

Activation of Osteocalcin

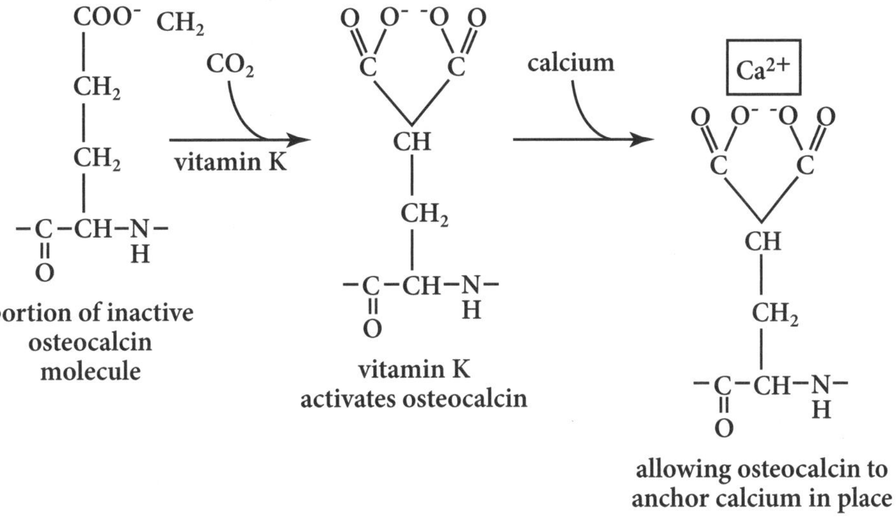

Vitamin E Content of Selected Foods,
in International Units (IU) per 100 gram
serving

Wheat germ oil	63.6
Sunflower seeds	26.8
Safflower oil	19.5
Sunflower oil	18.3
Almonds	12.7
Wheat germ	6.0
Whole-wheat (wholemeal) flour	3.6
Spinach	2.2–3.3
Peaches, canned	2.1–2.4
Dried prunes	1.61–1.85
Tomato	1.5
Cabbage	1.5
Asparagus	1.1–1.6
Avocados	0.95–2.0
Broccoli	0.8–3.4
Whole-wheat cereal	0.4–0.6
Beef	0.33–1.0
Turkey	0.09
Milk, whole	0.01

Vitamin K

One vitamin that is often neglected is vitamin K. Natural vitamin K from plants is called vitamin K1, phylloquinone, or phytonadione. Vitamin K2, or menaquinone, is derived from bacteria in the gut, and vitamin K3, or menadione, is a synthetic derivative.

The three vitamin Ks function similarly in helping with blood clotting, but for other important functions, vitamin K1 appears to be substantially superior. For example, vitamin K1 plays an important role in bone health as it is responsible for converting the bone protein osteocalcin from its inactive to its active form. Osteocalcin is the major noncollagen protein found in our bones. As shown above, vitamin K is necessary for allowing the osteocalcin molecule to join with calcium and hold it in place within the bone.

A deficiency of vitamin K1 leads to impaired mineralization of the bone due to inadequate active osteocalcin levels. Very low blood levels of vitamin K1 have been found in patients with fractures due to osteoporosis. The severity of the fracture strongly correlated with the level of circulating vitamin K: the lower the level of vitamin K, the greater the severity of the fracture. Vitamin K1 is found in green leafy vegetables and may be one of the protective factors of a vegetarian diet against osteoporosis.

Rich sources of vitamin K are dark green leafy vegetables, green tea, spinach, broccoli, lettuce, and cabbage. Good sources are asparagus, oats, whole wheat, and fresh green peas. The RDA for vitamin K is 1 microgram per 2.2 pounds/1 kilogram of body weight. There is no RNI or E.U. RDA.

VITAMIN K CONTENT OF SELECTED FOODS, IN MICROGRAMS PER 100 GRAM SERVING

Kale	729
Green tea	712
Turnip greens	650
Spinach	415
Broccoli	200
Lettuce	129
Cabbage	125
Watercress	57
Asparagus	57
Oats	20
Green peas	19
Whole wheat	17
Green beans	14

Water-Soluble Vitamins

Thiamine (Vitamin B1)

Thiamine, or vitamin B1, was the first B vitamin discovered. It has an interesting history that is told on page 323. Thiamine functions as part of the enzyme thiamine pyrophosphate, or TPP, which is essential for energy production, carbohydrate metabolism, and nerve cell function. A deficiency of thiamine usually results initially in fatigue, depression, pins and needles sensations or numbness in the legs, and constipation. Severe thiamine deficiency results in a deficiency syndrome known as beriberi. Symptoms include mental confusion, muscle wasting (dry beriberi), fluid retention (wet beriberi), high blood pressure, difficulty walking, and heart disturbances.

Although severe thiamine deficiency is relatively uncommon, except in alcoholics, many Americans do not consume the RDA of 1.5 milligrams, and subclinical thiamine deficiency is very common. In the U.K., thiamine is added by law to all flour, except wholemeal. In addition, diuretics, such as furosemide (Lasix), are known to induce thiamine deficiency, and digoxin (Lanoxin) interferes with thiamine in the heart muscle. Individuals taking these drugs require thiamine supplementation (200 to 240 milligrams daily). In the U.K., the RNI for adult males is 1 milligram, for adult females 0.8 milligrams, and for children up to the age of four 0.3 milligrams. The E.U. RDA is 1.4 milligrams.

Rich plant sources of thiamine are sunflower seeds, peanuts, and soybeans. Good sources are whole wheat and nuts. It should be noted that thiamine is extremely sensitive to alcohol and sulphites. In the presence of either, thiamine is destroyed or made useless. Thiamine is also destroyed by antithiamine factor in uncooked freshwater fish and shellfish, and in tea. There is no known toxicity due to thiamin.

THIAMINE CONTENT OF SELECTED FOODS, IN MILLIGRAMS PER 100 GRAM SERVING

Yeast, brewer's	15.61
Yeast, torula	14.01
Wheat germ	2.01
Sunflower seeds	1.96
Rice polishings	1.84
Pine nuts	1.28
Peanuts, with skins	1.14
Soybeans, dry	1.10
Peanuts, without skins	.98
Brazil nuts	.96
Pecans	.86
Soybean flour	.85
Beans, pinto and red	.84
Split peas	.74
Millet	.73
Wheat bran	.72
Pistachio nuts	.67
Haricot beans	.65
Buckwheat	.60
Oatmeal	.60
Whole-wheat (wholemeal) flour	.55
Whole-wheat grain	.55
Lima beans, dry	.48
Hazelnuts	.46
Wild rice	.45
Cashews	.43
Whole-grain rye	.43
Mung beans	.38
Cornmeal, whole ground	.38
Lentils	.37
Green peas	.35
Macadamia nuts	.34
Brown rice	.34
Walnuts	.33
Chickpeas	.31
Garlic, cloves	.25
Almonds	.24
Lima beans, fresh	.24
Pumpkin and squash seeds	.24
Chestnuts, fresh	.23
Soybean sprouts	.23
Peppers, red chili	.22
Sesame seeds, hulled	.18

Riboflavin (Vitamin B2)

Riboflavin, or vitamin B2, was first recognized as a yellow-green pigment in milk in 1879. Ingesting an excess of riboflavin results in an increased urine content of riboflavin, which can give urine a yellow-green fluorescent glow. Riboflavin functions in two important enzymes involved in energy production, flavin mononucleotide (FMN) and flavin adenine dinucleotide (FAD).

Riboflavin deficiency results in decreased energy production, particularly in cells that replicate frequently, such as the skin and mucous membranes. Early riboflavin deficiency is characterized by cracking of the lips and corners of the mouth; an inflamed tongue; visual disturbances, such as sensitivity to light and loss of visual acuity; cataract formation; burning and itching of the eyes, lips, mouth, and tongue; and other signs of disorders of mucous membranes.

The RDA for riboflavin is 1.7 milligrams for males and 1.3 milligrams for females. In the U.K., the RNI for adult males is 1.3 milligrams, for adult females 1.1 milligrams, and for children up to age four 0.5 milligrams. The E.U. RDA is 1.6 milligrams. Rich sources of riboflavin are yeast and organ meats, such as liver, kidney, and heart. Good plant sources are almonds, mushrooms, whole grains, soybeans, and green leafy vegetables. Riboflavin is destroyed by light but is not destroyed by cooking.

RIBOFLAVIN CONTENT OF SELECTED FOODS
IN MILLIGRAMS PER 100 GRAM SERVING

Yeast, torula	5.06
Yeast, brewer's	4.28
Liver, calf's	2.72
Almonds	.92
Wheat germ	.68
Wild rice	.63
Mushrooms	.46
Millet	.38
Soy flour	.35
Wheat bran	.35
Collards	.31
Soybeans, dry	.31
Split peas	.29
Kale	.26
Parsley	.26
Rice bran	.25
Broccoli	.23
Pine nuts	.23
Sunflower seeds	.23
Haricot beans	.23
Beet and mustard greens	.22
Lentils	.22
Prunes	.22
Rye, whole grain	.22
Beans, pinto and red	.21
Black-eyed peas	.21

Niacin (Vitamin B3)

Since niacin, or vitamin B3, can be made in the body by the conversion of tryptophan, many nutritionists do not consider niacin an essential nutrient as long as tryptophan intake is adequate. Niacin functions in the body as a component in the coenzymes nicotinamide adenine dinucleotide (NAD) and nicotinamide adenine dinucleotide phosphate (NADP), which are involved in well over fifty different chemical reactions in the body. These niacin-containing coenzymes play an important role in energy production; fat, cholesterol, and carbohydrate metabolism; and the manufacture of many body compounds, including sex and adrenal hormones.

Niacin was discovered during the search for the cause of pellagra. Pellagra was a common disease in Spain and Italy in the eighteenth century. In Italian, *pellagra* means "rough skin." It is characterized by the "three Ds" of pellagra: dermatitis, dementia, and diarrhea. The skin develops a cracked, scaly dermatitis; the brain does not function properly, leading to confusion and dementia; and diarrhea results from the impaired manufacture of the mucous lining of the gastrointestinal tract. Pellagra is now known to be due to a severe deficiency of niacin and tryptophan. Although the RDA for niacin is based on caloric intake, an intake of at least 18 milligrams per day is recommended by many authorities. In the U.K., the RNI for adult males is 17 milligrams, for adult females 13 milligrams, and for children up to age four 5 milligrams. The E.U. RDA is 18 milligrams. However, additional niacin has been shown to exert a favorable effect on many health conditions. Supplemental niacin is available as either nicotinic acid or niacinamide. Each form has different applications. In the nicotinic acid form, niacin is an effective agent for lowering blood cholesterol levels, while in the niacinamide form, niacin is useful in treating arthritis. In the field of orthomolecular psychiatry, large doses of niacin in the form of nicotinic acid or niacinamide are often utilized in the treatment of schizophrenia. Doses in excess of 50 milligrams of niacin as nicotinic acid typically produce a transient flushing of the skin. Also, high doses—2 to 6 grams per day—of either nicotinic acid or niacinamide should be monitored by a physician as they may result in liver disorders, peptic ulcers, and glucose intolerance.

Rich food sources of niacin as nicotinic acid include liver and other organ meats, eggs, fish, and peanuts. All of these foods are also rich sources of tryptophan. Good sources of niacin include legumes and whole grains (except corn).

NIACIN CONTENT OF SELECTED FOODS,
IN MILLIGRAMS PER 100 GRAM SERVING

Yeast, torula	44.4
Yeast, brewer's	37.9
Rice bran	29.8
Rice polishings	28.2
Liver, ox	21.4
Wheat bran	21.0
Peanuts, with skin	17.2
Peanuts, without skin	15.8
Swordfish	10.2
Wild rice,	6.2
Sesame seeds	5.4
Sunflower seeds	5.4
Brown rice	4.7
Pine nuts	4.5
Buckwheat	4.4
Peppers, red chili	4.4
Whole-wheat grain	4.4
Whole-wheat (wholemeal) flour	4.3
Wheat germ	4.2
Barley	3.7
Almonds	3.5
Split peas	3.0
Egg, whole	2.6

Pantothenic Acid (Vitamin B5)

Pantothenic acid, or vitamin B5 (please note, there is no vitamin B4), is a component of coenzyme A (CoA), which plays a critical role in the utilization of fats and carbohydrates in energy production, as well as in the manufacture of adrenal hormones and red blood cells. Pantothenic acid is particularly important for optimal adrenal function and has long been considered the "antistress" vitamin because of its central role in adrenal function and cellular metabolism.

A deficiency of pantothenic acid is believed to be quite rare in humans as pantothenic acid is found in a large number of foods. In fact, its name is derived from the Greek word *pantos,* meaning "everywhere." However, additional pantothenic acid is often used to support adrenal function, and pantethine, the most active stable form of pantothenic acid, is used to lower blood cholesterol and triglyceride levels.

Pantothenic acid is found in highest concentrations in liver and other organ meats, milk, fish, and poultry. Good plant sources of pantothenic acid include whole grains, legumes, broccoli, cauliflower, and nuts. There is no official RDA for pantothenic acid, but a daily intake of 4 to 7 milligrams is believed to be adequate. There is no RNI for pantothenic acid but the E.U. RDA is 6 milligrams.

PANTOTHENIC ACID CONTENT OF SELECTED FOODS, IN MILLIGRAMS PER 100 GRAM SERVING

Yeast, brewer's	12.0
Yeast, torula	11.0
Liver, calf's	8.0
Peanuts	2.8
Mushrooms	2.2
Soybean flour	2.0
Split peas	2.0
Pecans	1.7
Soybeans	1.7
Oatmeal, dry	1.5
Buckwheat flour	1.4
Sunflower seeds	1.4
Lentils	1.4
Rye flour, whole	1.3
Cashews	1.3
Chickpeas	1.2
Wheat germ	1.2
Broccoli	1.2
Hazelnuts	1.1
Brown rice	1.1
Whole-wheat (wholemeal) flour	1.1
Peppers, red chili	1.1
Avocados	1.1
Black-eyed peas, dry	1.0
Wild rice	1.0
Cauliflower	1.0
Kale	1.0

Pyridoxine (Vitamin B6)

Pyridoxine, or vitamin B6, is an extremely important B vitamin involved in the formation of body proteins and structural compounds, chemical transmitters in the nervous system, red blood cells, and prostaglandins. Vitamin B6 is also critical in maintaining hormonal balance and proper immune function.

Deficiency of vitamin B6 is characterized by depression, convulsions (especially in children), glucose intolerance, and impaired nerve function. Although extreme deficiency of vitamin B6 is believed to be quite rare, numerous clinical studies have demonstrated the importance of vitamin B6 in a number of health conditions that typically respond to B6 supplementation, including asthma, premenstrual syndrome (PMS), carpal tunnel syndrome, depression, morning sickness, and kidney stones. It is of interest to note that the increased rate of these disorders since the 1950s parallels the increased levels of vitamin B6 antagonists found in the food supply and used as drugs during the same period. These antagonists to vitamin B6 include the hydrazine dyes, such as FD&C Yellow No. 5; certain drugs, such as isoniazid, hydralazine, dopamine, and penicillamine; oral contraceptives; alcohol; and excessive protein intake. The intake of Yellow No. 5, also called tartrazine (E102), is especially problematic, as it is often consumed in greater quantities, with a per capita intake of 15 grams per day, than the RDA for vitamin B6, which is 2 milligrams for males and 1.6 milligrams for females. The U.K. RNI for adult males is 1.4 milligrams, for adult females 1.2 milligrams and for children up to four 0.4 milligrams. The E.U. RDA is 2 milligrams.

Good plant sources of vitamin B6 include whole grains, legumes, bananas, seeds and nuts, potatoes, Brussels sprouts, and cauliflower. Also, vitamin B6 levels inside the cells of the body appear to be intricately linked to the magnesium content of the diet: see "Magnesium" in the next chapter.

PYRIDOXINE CONTENT OF SELECTED FOODS, IN MILLIGRAMS PER 100 GRAM SERVING

Yeast, torula	3.00
Yeast, brewer's	2.50
Sunflower seeds	1.25
Wheat germ, toasted	1.15
Soybeans, dry	.63
Walnuts	.73
Soybean flour	.63
Lentils, dry	.60
Lima beans, dry	.58
Buckwheat flour	.58
Black-eyed peas, dry	.56
Haricot beans, dry	.56
Brown rice	.55
Hazelnuts	.54
Chickpeas, dry	.54
Pinto beans, dry	.53
Bananas	.51
Avocados	.42
Whole-wheat (wholemeal) flour	.34
Chestnuts, fresh	.33
Kale	.30
Rye flour	.30
Spinach	.28
Turnip greens	.26
Peppers, sweet	.26
Potatoes	.25
Prunes	.24
Raisins	.24
Brussels sprouts	.23
Barley	.22
Sweet potatoes	.22
Cauliflower	.21

Folic Acid

Folic acid, also known as folate, folacin, and pteroylmonoglutamate, functions together with vitamin B12 in many body processes and is critical to cellular division because it is necessary in DNA synthesis. Without folic acid, cells do not divide properly. In the case of folic acid deficiency, all cells of the body are affected, but it is the rapidly dividing cells, such as red blood cells and cells of the gastrointestinal and genital tracts, that are affected the most. Folic acid deficiency is characterized by poor growth, diarrhea, anemia, gingivitis, and an abnormal Pap (cervical) smear in women. Folic acid is critical to the development of the nervous system of the fetus and deficiency of folic acid during pregnancy has been linked to several birth defects, including neural tube defects such as spina bifida.

Folic acid, vitamin B12, and betaine also function to reduce body concentrations of homocysteine, an intermediate in the conversion of the amino acid methionine to cysteine. A higher-than-average homocysteine level has been implicated in a variety of conditions, including atherosclerosis and osteoporosis. Homocysteine is thought to promote atherosclerosis by directly damaging the arteries as well as reducing the integrity of the vessel walls. In osteoporosis, elevated homocysteine levels lead to a defective bone matrix by interfering with the proper formation of collagen, the main protein in bone.

Despite its wide occurrence in food, folic acid deficiency is the most common vitamin deficiency in the world. The reason reflects food choices: animal foods, with the exception of liver, are poor sources of folic acid, while plant foods, which are rich sources, are not as frequently consumed. In addition, alcohol and many prescription drugs, such as oestrogens, sulphasalazine, and barbiturates, impair folic acid metabolism; and folic acid is extremely sensitive to and easily destroyed by light or heat. The RDA for folic acid is 200 micrograms for males and 180 micrograms for females. In the U.K., the RNI for folic acid is 200 micrograms with an extra 100 micrograms during pregnancy and 60 micrograms during lactation. Recommended preconception levels are 400 micrograms until the twelfth week of pregnancy. The E.U. RDA is 200 micrograms.

Folic acid received its name from the Latin word *folium*, meaning "foliage," because it is found in high concentrations in green leafy vegetables, such as spinach, kale, beet greens, and Swiss chard. Other good sources of folic acid include whole grains, legumes, asparagus, broccoli, and cabbage.

FOLIC ACID CONTENT OF SELECTED FOODS, IN MICROGRAMS PER 100 GRAM SERVING

Yeast, brewer's	2,022
Black-eyed peas	440
Rice germ	430
Soy flour	425
Wheat germ	305
Liver, ox	295
Soybeans	225
Wheat bran	195
Kidney beans	180
Mung beans	145
Lima beans	130
Haricot beans	125
Chickpeas	125
Asparagus	110
Lentils	105
Walnuts	77
Spinach, fresh	75
Kale	70
Filbert nuts (hazelnuts)	65
Various greens	60
Peanuts, roasted	56
Peanut butter	56
Broccoli	53
Barley	50
Split peas	50
Whole-wheat cereal	49
Brussels sprouts	49
Almonds	45
Whole-wheat (wholemeal) flour	38
Oatmeal	33
Cabbage	32
Dried figs	32
Avocado	30
Green beans	28
Corn	28
Coconut, fresh	28
Pecans	27
Mushrooms	25
Dates	25
Blackberries	14
Orange	5

Vitamin B12 (Cobalamin)

Vitamin B12, or cobalamin, was isolated from liver extract in 1948 and identified as the nutritional factor in liver that prevented pernicious anemia. The crystallized compound of vitamin B12 is bright blue due to its high content of the mineral cobalt. Vitamin B12 works with folic acid in many body processes, including the synthesis of DNA. Since Vitamin B12 reactivates folic acid, a deficiency of B12 will result in a folic acid deficiency if folic acid levels are only marginal. More specifically, vitamin B12 deficiency results in impaired nerve function, which can cause numbness, "pins and needles" sensations, or a burning feeling in the feet, as well as impaired mental function, which in the elderly can mimic Alzheimer's disease. In addition to depression or mental confusion, vitamin B12 deficiency can present as anemia; a smooth, beefy red tongue; and diarrhea. Vitamin B12 deficiency is thought to be quite common in the elderly.

Vitamin B12 is necessary in only very small quantities. The RDA is 2 micrograms. The U.K. RNI for adult males is 1.5 micrograms, for adult females 1.5 micrograms, and children up to age four 0.4 micrograms. The E.U. RDA is 1 microgram. Vitamin B12 is found in significant quantities only in animal foods. The richest sources are liver and kidney, followed by fish, eggs, meat, and cheese. Strict vegetarians (vegans) are often told that fermented foods such as tempeh are excellent sources of vitamin B12, and, depending upon the medium on which it is grown, nutritional brewer's yeast may also provide B12. However, in addition to the tremendous variation in B12 content in fermented foods and brewer's yeast, there is some evidence that the form of B12 in these foods is not exactly the form that meets our bodily requirements. Although the vitamin B12 content of certain cooked sea vegetables is in the same range as beef, it is not known if this form is utilized in the

same manner either. Therefore, at this time it appears to be an extremely good idea for vegetarians to supplement their diets with vitamin B12.

VITAMIN B12 CONTENT OF SELECTED FOODS, IN MICROGRAMS PER 100 GRAM SERVING

Liver, lamb	104.0
Clams	98.0
Liver, ox	80.0
Kidneys, lamb	63.0
Liver, calf's	60.0
Kidneys, beef	31.0
Liver, chicken	25.0
Oysters	18.0
Sardines	17.0
Trout	5.0
Salmon	4.0
Tuna	3.0
Lamb	2.1
Eggs	2.0
Whey, dried	2.0
Beef, lean	1.8
Edam cheese	1.8
Swiss cheese	1.8
Brie cheese	1.6
Gruyère cheese	1.6
Blue cheese	1.4
Haddock	1.3
Flounder	1.2
Scallops	1.2
Cheddar cheese	1.0
Cottage cheese	1.0
Mozzarella cheese	1.0
Halibut	1.0
Perch, fillets	1.0
Swordfish	1.0

Biotin

Biotin is a B vitamin that functions in the manufacture and utilization of fats and amino acids. Without biotin, metabolism is severely impaired. However, since biotin is manufactured in the intestines by intestinal bacteria, it is not discussed very much. For adults, a vegetarian diet has been shown to alter the intestinal bacterial flora in such a manner as to enhance the synthesis and promote the absorption of biotin. There is no official RDA for biotin, but a daily intake of 30 to 100 micrograms is believed to be adequate. There is no RNI in the U.K. but the E.U. RDA is 150 micrograms.

A biotin deficiency in adults is characterized by dry, scaly skin; nausea; anorexia; and seborrhea. In infants under six months of age, the symptoms are seborrheic dermatitis (cradle cap) and alopecia (hair loss). In fact, the underlying factor for cradle cap in infants appears to be a biotin deficiency. Cradle cap is a common condition that may be associated with excessive oiliness (seborrhea) and scales. Since a large portion of the human biotin supply is provided by intestinal bacteria, it has been postulated that the absence of normal intestinal flora in the newborn may be responsible for cradle cap. A number of studies have demonstrated successful treatment of cradle cap with biotin when given as a supplement of 2 to 10 micrograms per day or as liver or egg yolk to the nursing mother and/or the infant.

The best sources of biotin are brewer's yeast, organ meats, and soybeans. Good sources are peanuts, oatmeal, cauliflower, and mushrooms. *Note:* Raw egg whites contain avidin, a protein that binds biotin and prevents its absorption. Avidin is destroyed by cooking.

BIOTIN CONTENT OF SELECTED FOODS, IN MILLIGRAMS PER 100 GRAM SERVING

Yeast, brewer's	200
Liver, ox	96
Soy flour	70
Soybeans	61
Rice bran	60
Rice germ	58
Rice polishings	57
Peanut butter	39
Walnuts	37
Peanuts, roasted	34
Barley	31
Pecans	27
Oatmeal	24
Black-eyed peas	21
Split peas	18
Almonds	18
Cauliflower	17
Mushrooms	16

Choline

Choline is often referred to as an "unofficial member" of the B vitamin family. Although choline can be manufactured in the body from either the amino acid methionine or serine, it has recently been designated an essential nutrient. Choline works very closely with other B vitamins, performing a vital function in the proper metabolism of fats. Without choline, fats become trapped in the liver, where they block metabolism. Specifically, it is required for the export of fat from the liver. Technically, this is referred to as a lipotropic effect. Choline is also required to make the important neurotransmitter acetylcholine and main components of our cell membranes such as phosphatidylcholine (lecithin) and sphingomyelin. Good dietary sources of choline include egg yolks, organ meats, legumes, and lecithin.

CHOLINE CONTENT OF SELECTED FOODS PER SERVING, IN MILLIGRAMS

Food	Free Choline	Phosphatidylcholine	Total Choline
Ox liver, 100 grams	60.64	3,362.55	532.28
Egg, 1 large	0.22	2,009.80	282.32
Beefsteak, 100 grams	0.78	466.12	68.75
Orange, 1 medium	13.24	107.35	27.91
Cauliflower, ½ cup	6.79	107.06	22.15
Potato, 1 medium	5.95	25.97	9.75
Milk, whole, 250 ml	3.81	27.91	9.64
Grape juice, 175 grams	8.99	2.11	9.37
Iceberg lettuce, 30 grams	8.53	2.86	9.06
Tomato, 1 medium	5.50	4.94	6.58
Apple, 1 medium	0.39	29.87	4.62
Banana, medium	2.85	3.26	3.52
Whole-wheat (wholemeal) bread, 1 slice	2.52	6.57	3.43
Cucumber, ½ cup	1.18	3.06	1.74

Vitamin C (Ascorbic Acid)

Vitamin C is perhaps the most publicized vitamin. The primary function of vitamin C is the manufacture of collagen, the main protein substance of the human body. Specifically, vitamin C is involved in the joining of a portion of molecule to the amino acids lysine and proline to form hydroxylysine and hydroxyproline. The result is a very stable collagen structure. Since collagen is such an important protein in the structures that hold our body together, including cartilage, connective tissue, ligaments, and tendons, vitamin C is vital for wound repair, healthy gums, and the prevention of easy bruising. In addition to its role in collagen manufacture, vitamin C is also critical to immune function, the manufacture of certain nerve transmitting substances and hormones, and the absorption and utilization of other nutritional factors. Vitamin C is also a very important nutritional antioxidant.

Numerous experimental, clinical, and population studies have shown increased vitamin C intake to result in a number of beneficial effects, including reducing cancer rates; boosting immunity; protecting against pollution and cigarette smoke; enhancing wound repair; increasing life expectancy; and reducing the risk of developing cataracts. Many claims have also been made about the role of vitamin C in enhancing the immune system, especially regarding the prevention and treatment of the common cold. However, despite numerous positive clinical and experimental studies, for some reason this effect is still hotly debated. But from a biochemical viewpoint, there is considerable evidence that vitamin C plays a vital role in many immune mechanisms. Specifically, vitamin C has been shown to increase many different immune functions, including enhancing white blood cell function and activity; and increasing interferon levels, antibody responses, antibody levels, secretion of thymic hormones, and the integrity of ground substance, the basic material that adheres cells together. Vitamin C also possesses many biochemical effects very similar to those of interferon, the body's natural antiviral and anticancer compound. The high concentration of vitamin C in white blood cells, particularly lymphocytes, is rapidly depleted during infection, and a relative vitamin C deficiency may ensue if vitamin C is not regularly replenished.

During times of chemical, emotional, psychological, or physiological stress, the urinary excretion of vitamin C is increased, signifying an increased need for vitamin C during these times. Examples of chemical stressors include cigarette smoke, pollutants, and allergens. Extra vitamin C in the form of supplementation or increased intake of vitamin C–rich foods is often recommended to keep the immune system working properly during times of stress. In certain instances, vitamin C supplementation is the only way to meet the concentrations needed for many health conditions. The RDA for vitamin C is 60 milligrams per day. The U.K. RNI for adult males is 40 milligrams, for adult females 40 milligrams, and for children up to age four 26 milligrams. The E.U. RDA is 60 milligrams.

In the case of scurvy or severe vitamin C deficiency, the classic symptoms are bleeding gums, poor wound healing, and extensive bruising. In addition to these symptoms, susceptibility to infection, hysteria, and depression are hallmark features of vitamin C deficiency. Only 10 to 20 milligrams per day is required to prevent scurvy and severe vitamin C deficiency, although this amount is too low to support optimal health.

While most people think of citrus fruits as the best source of vitamin C, vegetables also contain high levels, especially peppers, broccoli, and Brussels sprouts. Vitamin C is destroyed by exposure to air, so eating fresh foods as quickly as possible is best. Although a salad from a salad bar is a healthy lunch choice, the vitamin C content of the fruits and vegetables is only a fraction of what it would be if the salad were made fresh. For example, freshly sliced cucumbers, if left standing, lose between 41 and 49 percent of their vitamin C content within the first three hours. A sliced cantaloupe melon, left uncovered in the refrigerator, loses 35 percent of its vitamin C content in less than twenty-four hours.

VITAMIN C CONTENT OF SELECTED FOODS, IN MILLIGRAMS PER 100 GRAM SERVING

Acerola	1,300
Peppers, red chili	369
Guavas	242
Peppers, red sweet	190
Kale leaves	186
Parsley	172
Collard leaves	152

Turnip greens	128	Cantaloupe melons	33
Peppers, green sweet	128	Swiss chard	32
Broccoli	113	Green onions	32
Brussels sprouts	102	Liver, ox	31
Mustard greens	97	Okra	31
Watercress	79	Tangerines	31
Cauliflower	78	New Zealand spinach	30
Persimmons	66	Oysters	30
Cabbage, red	61	Lima beans, young	28
Strawberries	59	Black-eyed peas	29
Papayas	56	Soybeans	29
Spinach	51	Green peas	27
Oranges and juice	50	Radishes	26
Cabbage	47	Raspberries	25
Lemon juice	46	Chinese cabbage	25
Grapefruit and juice	38	Yellow summer squash	25
Elderberries	36	Loganberries	24
Liver, calf's	36	Honeydew melons	23
Turnips	36	Tomatoes	23
Mangoes	35	Liver, pig's	23
Asparagus	33		

8

Minerals

The human body utilizes minerals for the proper composition of bone and blood and the maintenance of normal cell function. Minerals function along with vitamins as essential components in enzymes and coenzymes. If an enzyme is lacking the necessary mineral, it cannot function properly no matter how much of the vitamin is available. For example, zinc is necessary for the enzyme that activates vitamin A in the visual process. Without zinc in the enzyme, vitamin A cannot be converted to its active form. This deficiency can result in what is known as night blindness. Only when it is supplied with both zinc and vitamin A is the enzyme able to perform its vital function.

The minerals are classified into two categories: major and minor. This classification is determined by the amount of the mineral needed by the body, not by how essential it is to good health. If a mineral is required at a level greater than 100 milligrams per day, it is considered to be a major mineral.

MAJOR MINERALS
  Calcium
  Phosphorus
  Potassium
  Sulphur
  Sodium
  Chloride
  Magnesium

MINOR (ALSO KNOWN AS "TRACE") MINERALS
  Zinc
  Iron
  Manganese
  Copper
  Boron
  Silicon
  Molybdenum
  Vanadium
  Chromium
  Selenium
  Iodine

NONESSENTIAL MINERALS

The following minerals have not been shown to be important in human nutrition. In fact, many of them are considered toxic chemicals and should be avoided.

Aluminium	Niobium
Antimony	Osmium
Arsenic	Palladium
Barium	Platinum
Beryllium	Praseodymium
Bromine	Rhenium
Cadmium	Rhodium
Cerium	Rubidium
Cesium	Ruthenium
Cobalt	Samarium
Dysprosium	Scandium
Erbium	Silver
Europium	Tantalum
Gallium	Tellurium
Gandolinium	Terbium
Gold	Thallium
Hafnium	Thorium
Holmium	Thullium
Indium	Tin
Iridium	Titanium
Lanthanum	Tungsten
Lead	Vanadium
Lithium	Ytterbium
Lutetium	Yttrium
Mercury	Zirconium
Nickel	

Dietary Sources of Minerals

Because plants incorporate minerals from the soil into their own tissues, fruits, vegetables, grains, legumes, nuts, and seeds are often excellent sources of minerals. The minerals, as they are found in the earth, are inorganic. However in plants, most minerals are complexed with organic molecules. This usually means better mineral absorption, but there are some plant compounds, such as phytates and tannins, that bind minerals so tightly that they cannot be absorbed. For this reason, juicing is thought to provide even better mineral absorption compared to the intact fruit or vegetable because juicing liberates the minerals into a highly bioavailable medium and separates the minerals from some of the fiber constituents, which can interfere with absorption. The green leafy vegetables are the best sources of many of the minerals, especially calcium, and this source is made more available by juicing.

Major Minerals

Calcium

Calcium is the most abundant mineral in the body. It constitutes 1.5 to 2 percent of total body weight, with more than 99 percent of the calcium being present in the bones. In addition to its major function in building and maintaining bones and teeth, calcium is important in the activity of many enzymes in the body. The contraction of muscles, release of neurotransmitters, regulation of heartbeat, and clotting of blood are all dependent on calcium.

The current U.S. RDA for calcium is 1,000 milligrams for adults. However, there has been considerable concern that this recommendation may be inadequate to maintain the integrity of the bone. This is especially true during the

FIGURE 8.1

Average Total Body Content of Major and Selected Trace Minerals

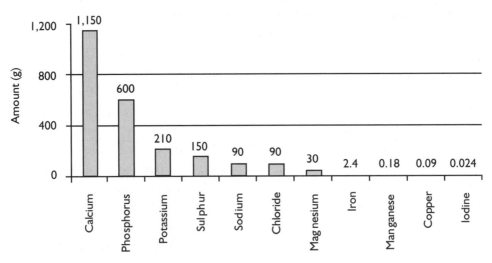

periods of growth, pregnancy, and lactation. Preadolescent children may need even more calcium than adults. The recommendation for this group is 1,200 milligrams of calcium per day. During pregnancy and lactation, the recommendation is also 1,200 milligrams per day.

RECOMMENDED DIETARY ALLOWANCE
OF CALCIUM (U.K. RNIs IN BRACKETS)

Infants

0–0.5 year	400 mg	}(525 mg)
0.5–1 year	600 mg	

Children

1–3 years	800 mg	(350 mg)
4–6 years	800 mg	(450 mg)
7–10 years	800 mg	(550 mg)

Young Adults and Adults

Males 11–24 years	1,200 mg	(1,000 mg age 11–18)
Males 25+ years	800 mg	(700 mg age 19+)
Females 11–24 years	1,200 mg	(800 mg age 11–18)
Females 24+ years	800 mg	(700 mg age 19+)
Pregnant	1,200 mg	(700–800 mg depending on age)
Lactating	1,200 mg	(1,200 mg)

Calcium deficiency in children may lead to rickets, which results in bone deformities and growth retardation. In adults, calcium deficiency may result in osteomalacia, which is a softening of the bones. Extremely low levels of calcium in the blood may result in muscle spasms and leg cramps. It is also generally well accepted that low calcium intake contributes greatly to high blood pressure and osteoporosis.

Foods high in calcium are kelp and other seaweeds, cheddar cheese, and leafy green vegetables, such as collards, kale, and turnip greens. Good sources of calcium are nuts and seeds, such as almonds and sesame seeds, yogurt, tofu, and apricots. The following list shows the calcium content of selected foods.

CALCIUM CONTENT OF SELECTED FOODS, IN MILLIGRAMS PER 100 GRAM SERVING

Food	mg	Food	mg
Kelp	1,093	Soybeans, cooked	73
Cheddar cheese	750	Pecans	73
Carob flour	352	Wheat germ	72
Dulse	296	Peanuts	69
Collard greens	250	Miso	68
Kale	249	Romaine lettuce	68
Turnip greens	246	Apricots, dried	67
Almonds	234	Swedes	66
Yeast, brewer's	210	Raisins	62
Parsley	203	Black currant	60
Dandelion greens	187	Dates	59
Brazil nuts	186	Green beans	56
Watercress	151	Artichokes	51
Goat's milk	129	Prunes, dried	51
Tofu	128	Pumpkin seeds	51
Figs, dried	126	Beans, cooked	50
Buttermilk	121	Cabbage	49
Sunflower seeds	120	Soybean sprouts	48
Yogurt	120	Wheat	46
Wheat bran	119	Orange	41
Whole milk	118	Celery	41
Buckwheat, raw	114	Cashews	38
Sesame seeds, hulled	110	Rye grain	38
Olives, ripe	106	Carrot	37
Broccoli	103	Barley	34
Walnuts	99	Sweet potato	32
Cottage cheese	94	Brown rice	32

Phosphorus

Phosphorus is one of the most essential minerals, as it ranks second only to calcium in total body content. About 80 percent of the phosphorus in the human body is found as calcium phosphate crystals in bones and teeth. However, phosphorus participates in many other body functions, including energy metabolism, DNA synthesis, and calcium absorption and utilization.

Phosphorus is readily available in most foods, especially high-protein foods. However, more important than the total phosphorus content of a food is its ratio of calcium to phosphorus. Too little calcium and too much phosphorus have been linked to osteoporosis. Foods low in calcium but high in phosphorus include red meats, poultry, and soft drinks. The ratio of calcium to phosphorus in red meats and poultry is generally 1:20, while the level of phosphorus per serving in soft drinks is typically 500 milligrams, with virtually no calcium to offset it. In order to maintain proper calcium balance, the dietary calcium-to-phosphorus ratio should be close to 2:1. The higher the phosphorus level is compared to the calcium, the greater the amount of calcium lost in the urine.

The RDA for phosphorus is equal to the RDA for calcium. The main food sources of phosphorus are meat, milk, and whole grains, nuts and seeds (though the phosphorus is in a bound form in these foods and is about 50 percent less bioavailable than phosphorus from other meat and milk sources).

PHOSPHORUS CONTENT OF SELECTED FOODS, IN MILLIGRAMS PER SERVING

Yogurt, plain, nonfat, 200 grams	383
Lentils, ½ cup, cooked	356
Salmon, 85 grams, cooked	252
Milk, skimmed, 250 ml	247
Halibut, 85 grams, cooked	242
Beef, 85 grams, cooked	173
Turkey, 85 grams, cooked	173
Chicken, 85 grams, cooked	155
Almonds, 30 grams	139
Mozzarella cheese, part skimmed, 30 grams	131
Egg, 1 large, cooked	104
Peanuts, 30 grams	101
Bread, whole wheat, (wholemeal) 1 slice	64
Carbonated cola drink, 425 ml	44
Bread, enriched, white, 1 slice	24

Magnesium

Magnesium is an extremely important mineral. Next to potassium, it is the most predominant mineral within our cells. Magnesium also functions very closely with calcium and phosphorus. Approximately 60 percent of the magnesium in the body is found in bone, 26 percent in muscle, and the remainder in soft tissue and body fluids. The functions of magnesium primarily center around its ability to activate many enzymes. Like potassium, magnesium is also involved in maintaining the electrical charge of cells, particularly in muscles and nerves. In addition, magnesium is involved in many cellular functions, including energy production, protein formation, and cellular replication.

Magnesium deficiency is characterized by symptoms quite similar to those of potassium deficiency, including mental confusion, irritability, weakness, heart disturbances, and problems in nerve conduction and muscle contraction. Other symptoms of magnesium deficiency may include muscle cramps, headaches, loss of appetite, insomnia, and a predisposition to stress.

Magnesium deficiency is extremely common in the geriatric population and in women during the premenstrual period. Magnesium deficiency is often secondary to factors that reduce absorption or increase secretion, such as high calcium intake, alcohol consumption, surgery, diuretic use, liver disease, kidney disease, and oral contraceptive use.

The RDA for magnesium is 350 milligrams per day for adult males and 300 milligrams per day for adult females. For pregnant and lactating women, the recommended allowance is 450 milligrams per day. In the U.K. the RNI is 300 milligrams for men and 270 milligrams for women. Many nutritional experts feel the ideal intake for magnesium should be based on body weight (6 milligrams per kilogram of body weight). For a 110-pound/50 kilogram person, the recommendation would be 300 milligrams; for a 154-pound/70 kilogram person, 420 milligrams; and for a 200-pound/91 kilogram person, 540 milligrams.

The average intake of magnesium by healthy adults in the United States ranges between 143 and 266 milligrams per day. This is obviously far below the RDA. Similarly in the U.K., a survey concluded that 42 percent of adult men and 72 percent of adult women were consuming less than the daily RNI for magnesium. What is the result of this low dietary magnesium? Food choices are the main reason. Since magnesium occurs abundantly in whole foods, most nutritionists and dieticians assume that most Westerners get enough magnesium in the diet. But most Westerners are not eating whole foods; they are consuming large quantities of processed foods. Since food processing refines out a very large portion of magnesium, most Westerners are not getting the RDA or RNI of magnesium. Low levels of magnesium in the diet and our bodies increase susceptibility to a variety of diseases, including heart disease, high blood pressure, kidney stones, cancer, insomnia, PMS, and menstrual cramps.

Magnesium's role in preventing heart disease and kidney stones is the most widely accepted. Individuals dying suddenly of heart attacks have been shown to have very low levels of magnesium in their heart. Magnesium is extremely important to the heart, in terms of both energy production and heart muscle contraction. A magnesium deficiency may cause a heart attack by producing a spasm of the coronary arteries, thereby reducing the flow of blood and oxygen to the heart. Magnesium also increases the solubility of calcium in the urine, thereby preventing stone formation. Supplementing magnesium to the diet has demonstrated effectiveness in preventing recurrences of kidney stones.

The best dietary sources of magnesium are kelp and other seaweeds, nuts, whole grains, and tofu. Fish, meat, milk, and most commonly eaten fruits are quite low in magnesium.

MAGNESIUM CONTENT OF SELECTED FOODS, IN MILLIGRAMS PER 100 GRAM SERVING

Food	mg	Food	mg
Kelp	760	Parsley	41
Wheat bran	490	Prunes, dried	40
Wheat germ	336	Sunflower seeds	38
Almonds	270	Beans, cooked	37
Cashews	267	Barley	37
Molasses	258	Dandelion greens	36
Yeast, brewer's	231	Garlic	36
Buckwheat	229	Raisins	35
Brazil nuts	225	Green peas, fresh	35
Dulse	220	Potato with skin	34
Filberts (hazelnuts)	184	Crab	34
Peanuts	175	Banana	33
Millet	162	Sweet potato	31
Wheat grain	160	Blackberry	30
Pecan	142	Beetroot	25
English walnuts	131	Broccoli	24
Rye	115	Cauliflower	24
Tofu	111	Carrot	23
Coconut meat, dried	90	Celery	22
Soybeans, cooked	88	Beef	21
Brown rice	88	Asparagus	20
Figs, dried	71	Chicken	19
Apricots	62	Green pepper	18
Dates	58	Winter squash	17
Collard greens	57	Aubergine	16
Prawns	51	Cantaloupe melons	16
Corn, sweet	48	Tomato	14
Avocado	45	Milk	13
Cheddar cheese	45		

Potassium, Sodium, and Chloride

Potassium, sodium, and chloride are electrolytes, mineral salts that can conduct electricity when they are dissolved in water. They are so intricately related that they are most often discussed together in nutrition textbooks, and we will follow that tradition in this discussion.

Electrolytes are always found in pairs. A positive molecule, such as sodium or potassium, is always accompanied by a negative molecule, such as chloride. Together, electrolytes function in the maintenance of

- Water balance and distribution.
- Kidney and adrenal function.
- Acid–base (alkaline) balance.
- Muscle and nerve cell function.
- Heart function.

More than 95 percent of the potassium in the body is found within cells. In contrast, most of the sodium in the body is located outside the cells in the blood and other fluids. How does this happen? Cells actually pump sodium out and potassium in via the "sodium-potassium pump." This pump is found in the membranes of all cells in the body. One of its most important functions is preventing the swelling of cells. If sodium is not pumped out, water accumulates within the cell, causing it to swell and ultimately burst.

Sodium levels are regulated by the kidney and adrenal gland. The adrenal gland produces a hormone called aldosterone that tells the kidneys how much sodium to retain. When either sodium or potassium becomes unbalanced, the kidney may expend the other electrolyte to maintain a balance. In kidney disease, this balancing function is lost and electrolyte imbalance occurs, causing problems with electrical conduction throughout the body, including the muscles, nerves, and heart.

The sodium-potassium pump is integral in maintaining the acid–base (alkaline) balance as well as in healthy kidney function. Energy is derived from pumping sodium outside the cell, where it becomes concentrated, wanting to push its way back in. This energy is used to remove acid from the body.

The sodium-potassium pump also functions to maintain the electrical charge within the cell. This is particularly important to muscle and nerve cells. During nerve transmission and muscle contraction, potassium exits the cell and sodium enters, resulting in a change in electrical charge that causes a nerve impulse or muscle contraction. Therefore, it is not surprising that a potassium deficiency affects muscles and nerves first.

The balance of sodium, potassium, and chloride is extremely important to human health. Too much sodium in the diet can lead to disruption of this balance. Numerous studies have demonstrated that a high-sodium, low-potassium diet plays a major role in the development of cancer and cardiovascular diseases. Conversely, a diet high in potassium and low in sodium is protective against these diseases, and in the case of high blood pressure it can be therapeutic.

Excessive consumption of dietary sodium chloride (table salt), coupled with diminished dietary potassium consumption, is a common cause of high blood pressure. Numerous studies have shown that sodium restriction alone does not improve blood pressure control in most people; it must be accompanied by a high potassium intake. In the U.S. only 5 percent of sodium intake comes from the natural ingredients in food. Prepared foods contribute 45 percent of our sodium intake, 45 percent is added in cooking, and another 5 percent is added as a condiment. In the U.K., it is thought that the food industry accounts for 80 percent of the average (12 grams) daily intake of salt by men; another 15 percent is added in cooking or at the table. However, all that the body requires in most instances is the salt that is supplied in the food.

As a result, most Americans have a potassium-to-sodium (K:Na) ratio of less than 1:2. This means that most people ingest more than twice as much sodium as potassium. In the U.K., average intakes of sodium are up to half as much again as potassium (50–150 mmol of potassium: 85–145 mmol of sodium). Researchers recommend a dietary potassium-to-sodium ratio of greater than 5:1 to maintain optimal health. This is a ten times larger proportion of potassium than in the average intake. However, even this may not be optimal. A natural diet rich in fruits and vegetables can produce a K:Na ratio greater than 100:1, as most fruits and vegetables have a K:Na ratio of at least 50:1. For example, here are the average K:Na ratios for several common fresh fruits and vegetables:

Apples	90:1
Bananas	440:1
Carrots	75:1
Oranges	260:1
Potatoes	110:1

POTASSIUM AND SODIUM CONTENT OF SELECTED FOODS, IN MILLIGRAMS PER SERVING

Food	Potassium	Sodium
Fresh Vegetables		
Asparagus, ½ cup	165	1
Avocado, ½	680	5
Carrot, raw, 1	225	38
Corn, ½ cup	136	Trace
Lima beans, cooked, ½ cup	581	1
Potato, 1 medium	782	6
Spinach, cooked, ½ cup	292	45
Tomato, raw, 1 medium	444	5
Fresh Fruits		
Apple, 1 medium	182	2
Apricots, dried, ½ cup	318	9
Banana, 1 medium	440	1
Cantaloupe, ½ melon	341	17
Orange, 1 medium	263	1
Peach, 1 medium	308	2
Plums, 5	150	1
Strawberries, ½ cup	122	Trace
Unprocessed Meats		
Chicken, light meat, 85 grams	350	54
Lamb, leg, 85 grams	241	53
Pork, 85 grams	219	48
Roast beef, 85 grams	224	49

Fish

Cod, 85 grams	345	93
Flounder, 85 grams	498	201
Haddock, 85 grams	297	150
Salmon, 85 grams	378	99
Tuna, 85 grams	225	38

Although sodium and chloride are important, potassium is the most important dietary electrolyte. In addition to functioning as an electrolyte, potassium is essential for the conversion of blood sugar into glycogen, which is the storage form of blood sugar found in the muscles and liver. A potassium shortage results in a lower level of stored glycogen. Because glycogen is used by exercising muscles for energy, a potassium deficiency will produce great fatigue and muscle weakness. These are typically the first signs of potassium deficiency.

A potassium deficiency is also characterized by mental confusion, irritability, weakness, heart disturbances, and problems in nerve conduction and muscle contraction. Dietary potassium deficiency is typically caused by a diet low in fresh fruits and vegetables but high in sodium. It is more common to see dietary potassium deficiency in the elderly. Dietary potassium deficiency is less common than deficiency due to excessive fluid loss, such as sweating, diarrhea or urination, or the use of diuretics, laxatives, aspirin, and other drugs.

The amount of potassium lost in sweat can be quite significant, especially if exercise is prolonged in a warm environment. Athletes and people who exercise regularly have higher potassium needs. Because up to 3 grams of potassium can be lost in one day by sweating, a daily intake of at least 4 grams of potassium is recommended for these individuals.

The estimated safe and adequate daily dietary intake of potassium, as set by the Committee on Recommended Daily Allowances, is 1.9 to 5.6 grams. In the U.K., the RNI for adults is 3,500 milligrams and 765 milligrams for children up to the age of four. If body potassium requirements are not being met through diet, supplementation is essential to good health. This is particularly true for the elderly and the athletic. Potassium salts are commonly prescribed by physicians in the dosage range of 1.5 to 8.0 grams per day. However, potassium salts can cause nausea, vomiting, diarrhea, and ulcers. These effects are not seen when potassium levels are increased through the diet only. This highlights the advantages of using juices, foods, or food-based potassium supplements to meet the human body's high potassium requirements.

Can you take too much potassium? Of course, but most people can handle any excess of potassium. The only exception is people with kidney disease. These people do not handle potassium in the normal way and are likely to experience heart disturbances and other consequences of potassium toxicity. Individuals with kidney disorders usually need to restrict their potassium intake and follow the dietary recommendations of their physicians.

Sulphur

Sulphur is a component of four amino acids: methionine, cysteine, cystine, and taurine. As part of the sulphur-containing amino acids, it performs a number of important functions, such as providing a place for these amino acids to bond together, thus solidifying a protein structure. It is found in high concentrations in the protein structure of the joints, hair, nails, and skin. In the case of arthritis, cartilage can be repaired by adequate sulphur intake through supplementation.

The hormone insulin is a protein-based hormone rich in sulphur-containing amino acids. The detoxifying compound glutathione is also a sulphur-containing compound, where sulphur, as cysteine, is a beneficial nutrient in liver disorders. As part of taurine, it aids in digestion, as taurine is a bile acid component. As a part of methionine and cysteine, it is utilized in the metabolism of homocysteine.

Although there is no official RDA (nor RNI) for sulphur, it is a critical nutrient. Daily intake is usually 800 to 900 milligrams of sulphur per day. Certain health conditions, such as arthritis and liver disorders, may be improved by increasing the intake of sulphur to 1,500 milligrams per day in supplemental form (nost commonly as methyl-sulphonylmethane, or MSM). Sulphur-rich foods include eggs, legumes, whole grains, garlic, onions, Brussels sprouts, and cabbage.

Trace Minerals

Boron

Vegetarians are at a lower risk of developing osteoporosis because, in addition to vitamin K1 and the high levels of many minerals found in plant foods, their increased consumption of the trace mineral boron helps reduce their risk. Boron has been shown to have a positive effect on calcium and active oestrogen levels in postmenopausal women, the group at highest risk for developing osteoporosis. In one study, supplementing the diet of postmenopausal women with 3 milligrams of boron per day reduced urinary calcium excretion by 44 percent and dramatically increased the levels of 17-beta-oestradiol, the most biologically active oestrogen. It appears that boron is required to activate certain hormones, including oestrogen and vitamin D. Both oestrogen and vitamin D are important for building and maintaining healthy bone structure.

Boron has also been shown to be of benefit in arthritis; its mechanism of action is not yet understood, although it appears to play a role in calcium metabolism similar to that seen in osteoporosis prevention.

No RDA is set for boron, and requirements vary from 1 to 6 milligrams per day, though most diets provide only 1 to 3 milligrams per day. (There is no RNI in the U.K. but the estimated requirement is 2 milligrams.) Dried fruit, nuts, bananas, apples, and other fruits and vegetables are good sources of boron. Since nuts, fruits, and vegetables are the main dietary sources of boron, diets low in these foods may be deficient in boron.

BORON CONTENT OF SELECTED FOODS,
IN MILLIGRAMS PER 100 GRAM SERVING

Prunes	2.7
Raisins	2.5
Almonds	2.3
Peanuts	1.8
Hazelnuts	1.6
Banana	.372
Apple, red, with peel, raw	.273
Apple juice	.241
Grape juice	.202
Peaches, canned	.187
Broccoli	.185
Orange juice	.159
Cherries, dark	.147

Chromium

Chromium functions in the "glucose tolerance factor," a critical enzyme system involved in blood sugar regulation. A lack, as well as an excess, of blood sugar (glucose) in the body can be devastating. For this reason, the body strives to maintain blood sugar levels within a narrow range with the help of hormones, such as insulin and glucagon. Considerable evidence now indicates that chromium levels are a major determinant of insulin sensitivity. If chromium levels are low, blood sugar levels may remain high due to a lack of sensitivity to insulin. Insulin promotes the absorption and utilization of glucose by the cells. Insulin insensitivity is a classic feature in obesity and diabetes.

Reversing a chromium deficiency by supplementing the diet with chromium has been demonstrated to lower body weight yet increase lean body mass and to improve glucose tolerance as well as decrease total cholesterol and triglyceride levels. All these effects appear due to increased insulin sensitivity.

Although there is no RDA (nor RNI) for chromium, it appears that we need at least 200 micrograms each day in our diet. In the U.K., the average diet provides 13.6 to 47.7 micrograms per day, leaving some people deficient in this mineral. Chromium levels can be depleted by use of refined sugars and white flour products, and lack of exercise.

CHROMIUM CONTENT OF SELECTED FOODS,
IN MICROGRAMS PER 100 GRAM SERVING

Yeast, brewer's	112
Liver, calf's	55
Whole-wheat (wholemeal) bread	42
Wheat bran	38
Rye bread	30
Potatoes	24
Wheat germ	23
Green pepper	19
Apple	14
Butter	13
Parsnips	13
Cornmeal	12
Banana	10
Spinach	10
Carrots	9
Haricot beans, dry	8
Orange	5
Blueberries	5
Green beans	4
Cabbage	4

Copper

Copper functions as an important factor in the manufacture of hemoglobin; collagen structures, particularly joints and arteries; and energy. Copper deficiency is characterized by anemia, fatigue, poor wound healing, elevated cholesterol levels, and poor immune function.

Since a deficiency of copper produces a marked elevation of cholesterol, copper deficiency has been suggested to play a major role in the development of atherosclerosis. There is additional evidence to support this as recent surveys indicate that less than 25 percent of Americans appear to be meeting the RDA of 2 milligrams of copper. (The RNI in the U.K. is 1.2 milligrams for adults and a survey in 1990 indicated that the average daily intake of copper for men was 1.6 milligrams and 1.2 milligrams for women. However, certain age groups were failing to reach the RNI: over 80 percent of fifteen to eighteen year olds and over 60 percent of over sixty-five year olds.) There is also evidence that because of copper-lined water pipes, many Americans are getting too much copper in their diets. (Copper piping in the U.K. is thought to provide up to 6 milligrams of copper per day.) Excessive copper levels have been linked to schizophrenia, learning disabilities, premenstrual syndrome, and anxiety.

Many of the problems of copper can be offset by zinc because zinc and copper compete for absorption sites. If there is too much zinc, copper absorption will be decreased and vice versa. In nature, foods rich in copper are typically even higher in zinc. Nuts and legumes are a good example of this.

COPPER CONTENT OF SELECTED FOODS, IN MILLIGRAMS PER 100 GRAM SERVING

Brazil nuts	2.3
Almonds	1.4
Hazelnuts	1.3
Walnuts	1.3
Pecans	1.3
Split peas, dry	1.2
Buckwheat	0.8
Peanuts	0.8
Sunflower oil	0.5
Butter	0.4
Rye grain	0.4
Barley	0.4
Olive oil	0.3
Carrot	0.3
Coconut	0.3
Garlic	0.3
Millet	0.2
Whole wheat	0.2
Corn oil	0.2
Gingerroot	0.2
Molasses	0.2
Turnips	0.2
Green peas	0.1
Papaya	0.1
Apple	0.1

Iodine

The thyroid gland adds iodine to the amino acid tyrosine to create thyroid hormones. A deficiency of iodine results in the development of an enlarged thyroid gland, commonly referred to as a goiter. When the iodine level in the diet and blood is low, it causes the cells of the thyroid gland to become quite large, and eventually the entire gland at the base of the neck swells.

Goiters are estimated to affect more than 200 million people the world over. In all but 4 percent of these cases, the goiter is caused by iodine deficiency. Iodine deficiency is now quite rare in the United States and other industrialized countries, due to the addition of iodine to table salt. Adding iodine to table salt began in Michigan, where, in 1924, the goiter rate was an incredible 47 percent.

Few people in the United States are now considered iodine-deficient, yet the rate of goiter is still relatively high (5 to 6 percent) in certain high-risk areas (the so-called goiter belt of the midwestern and Great Lakes states). The goiters in these populations are probably a result of the excessive ingestion of foods that block iodine utilization. These foods, known as goitrogens, include cabbage, cassava root, millet, mustard, peanuts, pine nuts, soybeans, and turnips. Cooking usually inactivates goitrogens. (In the U.K., goiters are found in 8 percent of women and 2 percent of men—95 percent are benign lumps.)

The RDA for iodine for adults is quite small, 150 micrograms. In the U.K. the RNI is 140 micrograms for adults, and the E.U. RDA is 150 micrograms. Seafood, including clams, and seaweeds, such as kelp, are nature's richest sources of iodine. However, in the United States, the majority of iodine is derived from the use of iodized salt, which contains 30 micrograms of iodine per gram of salt. Sea salt, in comparison, has little iodine. Due to the high salt intake in the United States, the average intake of iodine is estimated to be more than 600 micrograms per day.

However, too much iodine can actually inhibit thyroid gland synthesis. For this reason, and because the only function of iodine in the body is for thyroid hormone synthesis, it is recommended that dietary levels or supplementation of iodine not exceed 1 milligram (1,000 micrograms) per day for any length of time.

IODINE CONTENT OF SELECTED FOOD CATEGORIES, IN MICROGRAMS PER 100 GRAM SERVING

Salt (iodized)	3,000
Seafood	66
Vegetables	32
Meat	26
Eggs	26
Dairy products	13
Bread and cereals	10
Fruits	4

Iron

Iron is critical to human life. It plays the central role in the hemoglobin molecule of our red blood cells (RBCs), where it functions in transporting oxygen from the lungs to the body's tissues and carbon dioxide from the tissues to the lungs. In addition, iron functions in several key enzymes in energy production and metabolism, including DNA synthesis.

Iron deficiency is the most common nutrient deficiency in the United States, the U.K., and worldwide. The groups at highest risk for iron deficiency are infants under two years of age, teenage girls, women of childbearing age, pregnant women, and the elderly. Studies have found evidence of iron deficiency in 30 to 50 percent of people in these groups. For example, some degree of iron deficiency occurs in 35 to 58 percent of young, healthy women of childbearing age.

During pregnancy, the figure is even higher. In the U.K. iron deficiency is the most common nutrient deficiency among children—one study found 27 percent of a group of eight month olds were deficient.

Iron deficiency may be due to an increased iron requirement, inadequate dietary intake, diminished iron absorption or utilization, blood loss, or a combination of these factors. Increased requirements for iron occur during the growth spurts of infancy and adolescence, as well as during pregnancy and lactation. Currently, the vast majority of pregnant women are routinely given iron supplements during their pregnancy, as the dramatic increased need for iron during pregnancy cannot usually be met through diet alone. In the U.K., monitoring of iron levels continues throughout pregnancy and supplementation is given as necessary. In infants and adolescents, inadequate dietary iron necessitates iron supplementation as well.

Inadequate dietary intake of iron is common in many parts of the world, especially in populations that consume primarily vegetarian diets. Typical infant diets in developed countries, which are high in milk and cereals, are also low in iron. The adolescent consuming a "junk food" diet is at high risk for iron deficiency, too. However, the population at greatest risk for a diet deficient in iron is the low-income elderly population. This is complicated by the fact that decreased absorption of iron is extremely common in the elderly. Decreased absorption of iron is often due to a lack of hydrochloric acid secretion in the stomach, an extremely common condition in the elderly. Other causes of decreased absorption include chronic diarrhea or malabsorption, the surgical removal of the stomach, and antacid use.

Blood loss is the most common cause of iron deficiency in women of childbearing age. This is most often due to excessive menstrual bleeding. Interestingly enough, iron deficiency is a common cause of excessive menstrual blood loss. Other common causes of blood loss include bleeding from peptic ulcers, hemorrhoids, and donating blood.

The negative effects of iron deficiency are due largely to the impaired delivery of oxygen to the tissues and the impaired activity of iron-containing enzymes in various tissues. Iron deficiency can lead to anemia, excessive menstrual blood loss, learning disabilities, impaired immune function, and decreased energy levels and physical performance.

Anemia is a condition in which the blood is deficient in red blood cells or the hemoglobin (iron-containing) portion of red blood cells. As noted, the primary function of the red blood cells (RBCs) is to transport oxygen from the lungs to the tissues of the body in exchange for carbon dioxide. The symptoms of anemia, such as extreme fatigue, reflect a lack of oxygen being delivered to tissues and a buildup of carbon dioxide.

Iron deficiency is the most common cause of anemia; however, it must be pointed out that anemia is the last stage of iron deficiency. Iron-dependent enzymes involved in energy production and metabolism are the first to be affected by low iron levels. Serum ferritin is the best laboratory test for determining body iron stores.

Several researchers have clearly demonstrated that even slight iron-deficiency anemia leads to a reduction in physical work capacity and productivity. Nutrition surveys done in the

United States have indicated that iron deficiency is a major impairment of health and work capacity and, as a consequence of this, an economic loss to the individual and the country. Supplementation with iron has shown rapid improvements in work capacity in iron-deficient individuals. Impaired physical performance due to iron deficiency is not dependent on anemia. Again, the iron-dependent enzymes involved in energy production and metabolism are impaired long before anemia occurs.

In the developing child, even slight iron deficiency can lead to learning disabilities. The developing nervous system is undergoing significantly more energy-consuming activity than a mature nervous system. Adequate iron is imperative to provide adequate energy for proper growth and development.

The RDA for iron is 10 milligrams for males and 15 milligrams for females. In the U.K., the RNI for adult males is 8.7 milligrams (11.3 milligrams for boys aged eleven to eighteen) and for adult menstruating women (aged eleven to fifty) 14.8 milligrams (8.7 milligrams over the age of fifty). The E.U. RDA is 15 milligrams. It must be pointed out that there are two forms of dietary iron, "heme" iron and "nonheme" iron. Heme iron is iron that is bound to hemoglobin and myoglobin. It is found in animal products and is the most efficiently absorbed form of iron. Nonheme iron is found in plant foods. Compared to heme iron, it is poorly absorbed.

IRON CONTENT OF SELECTED FOODS, IN MILLIGRAMS PER SERVING

Clams, cooked, 85 grams	23.8	Sirloin steak, cooked, 85 grams	2.9
Soybeans, cooked, 1 cup	8.8	Spinach, cooked, 1 cup	2.9
Lentils, cooked, 1 cup	6.6	Potato, 1 medium	2.8
Tofu, firm, 100 grams	6.6	Beet greens, cooked, 1 cup	2.7
Tofu, regular, 100 grams	0.7–6.6	Soy yogurt, plain, 1 cup	2.7
Blackstrap molasses, 2 tablespoons	6.4	Prawns, cooked, 85 grams	2.6
Ox liver, fried, 85 grams	5.3	Sesame seeds, 2 tablespoons	2.6
Quinoa, cooked, 1 cup	5.3	Tahini, 2 tablespoons	2.6
Kidney beans, cooked, 1 cup	5.2	Peas, cooked, 1 cup	2.5
Chickpeas, cooked, 1 cup	4.7	Lima beans, cooked, 1 cup	2.3
Pinto beans, cooked, 1 cup	4.5	Sunflower seeds, ¼ cup	2.3
Black-eyed peas, cooked, 1 cup	4.3	Figs, dried, 5 medium	2.1
Swiss chard, cooked, 1 cup	4.0	Cashews, ¼ cup	2.0
Tempeh, 1 cup	3.8	Apricots, dried, 10 halves	2.0
Black beans, cooked, 1 cup	3.6	Chicken breast, skinless, ½ breast	0.9
Turnip greens, cooked, 1 cup	3.2	Turkey breast, 85 grams	0.9
Prune juice, 250 ml	3.0		

Manganese

Manganese functions in many enzyme systems, including the enzymes involved in blood sugar control, energy metabolism, and thyroid hormone function. Manganese also functions in the antioxidant enzyme superoxide dismutase, or SOD. This enzyme is responsible for preventing the deleterious effects of the superoxide free radical from destroying cellular components. Without SOD, cells are quite susceptible to damage and inflammation. Manganese supplementation has been shown to increase SOD activity, indicating increased antioxidant activity. Clinically, manganese is used for strains, sprains, and inflammation. There is evidence that patients with rheumatoid arthritis and presumably other chronic inflammatory diseases have an increased need for manganese. No trials have yet been done with manganese and rheumatoid arthritis, but supplementation appears to be indicated.

Low manganese has also been linked to epilepsy. This link was first suggested in 1963, when it was observed that manganese-deficient rats were more susceptible to seizures than manganese-replete animals, and that manganese-deficient animals exhibited epileptic-like brain wave tracings. This prompted researchers to look at manganese concentrations in epileptics. Low whole blood and hair manganese levels have been found in epileptics, and those with the lowest levels typically have the highest seizure activity.

Manganese plays a significant role in cerebral function as it is a critical metal for glucose utilization within the neuron, adenylate cyclase activity, and neurotransmitter control. For optimal central nervous system function, proper manganese levels must be maintained. A high-manganese diet or manganese supplementation may be helpful in controlling seizure activity for some patients.

Although there is no specific RDA (nor RNI) for manganese, it is estimated that most people require between 2 and 5 milligrams per day. This can easily be met by regularly consuming nuts and whole grains, as these are the best sources of manganese. In the U.K., it is thought that tea provides half the amount of manganese in the average diet.

MANGANESE CONTENT OF SELECTED FOODS, IN MILLIGRAMS PER 100 GRAM SERVING

Pecans	3.5
Brazil nuts	2.8
Almonds	2.5
Barley	1.8
Rye	1.3
Buckwheat	1.3
Split peas, dry	1.3
Whole wheat	1.1
Walnuts	0.8
Spinach, fresh	0.8
Peanuts	0.7
Oats	0.5
Raisins	0.5
Turnip greens	0.5
Rhubarb	0.5
Beet greens	0.4
Brussels sprouts	0.3
Oatmeal	0.3
Cornmeal	0.2
Millet	0.2
Carrots	0.16
Broccoli	0.15
Brown rice	0.14
Bread, whole-wheat (wholemeal)	0.14

Molybdenum

Molybdenum functions as a component of several enzymes, including those involved in alcohol detoxification as the cofactor of aldehyde oxidase. In uric acid formation, molybdenum is the cofactor of xanthine oxidase. In sulphur metabolism, molybdenum plays a role in the metabolism of the sulphur-containing amino acids cysteine and methionine as well as sulphites. A molybdenum deficiency has been suggested as a cause of sulphite sensitivity since the enzyme that detoxifies sulphites, sulphite oxidase, is molybdenum-dependent. However, molybdenum deficiency is rare, likely due only to a genetic sulphite oxidase defect or during long-term total parenteral nutrition therapy, where nutrients are administered intravenously only.

The average diet contains 50 to 500 micrograms of molybdenum per day. Legumes and whole grains are the richest sources.

MOLYBDENUM CONTENT OF SELECTED FOODS, IN MICROGRAMS PER 100 GRAM SERVING

Lentils	155
Split peas	130
Cauliflower	120
Green peas	110
Yeast, brewer's	109
Wheat germ	100
Spinach	100
Brown rice	75
Garlic	70
Oats	60
Rye bread	50
Corn	45
Barley	42
Whole wheat	36
Bread, whole-wheat (wholemeal)	32
Potatoes	30
Onions	25
Peanuts	25
Coconut	25
Green beans	21
Molasses	19
Cantaloupe melons	16
Apricots	14
Raisins	10
Butter	10
Strawberries	7
Carrots	5
Cabbage	5

Selenium

Selenium, as a component of the antioxidant enzyme glutathione peroxidase, works with vitamin E in preventing free-radical damage to cell membranes. Low levels of selenium render people at higher risk for cancer; cardiovascular disease; inflammatory diseases, such as asthma; and other conditions associated with increased free-radical damage, including premature aging and cataract formation. Selenium supplementation of 100 to 250 micrograms or more per day is often used in the treatment of these disorders.

Although there is no specific RDA for selenium in the U.S., a daily intake of 200 micrograms is often recommended. In the U.K., the RNI for adult males is 75 micrograms and for adult females 60 micrograms. Whole grains, fish, meat, and eggs are the richest sources. However, be aware that a daily intake in excess of 2,000 micrograms can be toxic.

SELENIUM CONTENT OF SELECTED FOODS,
IN MICROGRAMS PER 100 GRAM SERVING

Wheat germ	111
Brazil nuts	103
Bread, whole-wheat (wholemeal)	66
Tuna, canned in water	65
Wheat bran	63
Calf's liver	57
Swiss chard	57
Oats	56
Loin chops	47
Brown rice	39
Salmon	37
Pork loin, lean	35
Top sirloin, lean	33
Turkey, breast, without skin	32
Egg, whole	30
Minced beef, lean	29
Chicken, breast	27
Lamb, lean	26
Garlic	25
Barley	24

Silicon

Silicon is responsible for cross-linking collagen strands, thereby contributing greatly to the strength and integrity of the connective tissue matrix of bone. Since silicon concentrations are increased at calcification sites in growing bone, this process may be dependent upon adequate levels of silicon. It is not known whether the typical Western diet provides adequate amounts of silicon. In patients with osteoporosis, or where accelerated bone regeneration is desired, silicon requirements may be increased.

Although no official RDA (nor RNI) for silicon has been set, 20 to 50 milligrams per day has been recommended to meet fundamental requirements. An increased need for silicon is best met by increasing the consumption of unrefined grains, as they are a rich source of absorbable silicon (silicic acid).

Vanadium

Vanadium was named after the Scandinavian goddess of beauty, youth, and luster. It is a controversy as to whether vanadium is an essential trace mineral in human nutrition. Although it has been suggested to function in hormone, cholesterol, and blood sugar metabolism, no specific deficiency signs have been reported. Some researchers have speculated that a vanadium deficiency may contribute to elevated cholesterol levels and faulty blood sugar control manifesting as either diabetes or hypoglycemia. Making things more difficult is the fact that vanadium exists in five different forms, with the most biologically significant being either vanadyl or vanadate.

Since vanadium can be a relatively toxic mineral its use as a dietary supplement should be limited to dosages reflective of dietary intake (e.g., 500–1,000 micrograms daily). The major concern is that excessive levels of vanadium have been suggested to be a factor in manic depression, as increased levels of vanadium are found in hair samples from manic patients, and these values fall towards normal levels with recovery. Vanadium, as the vanadate ion, is a strong inhibitor of the sodium-potassium pump. Lithium, the drug of choice for manic depression, has been reported to reduce this inhibition, too.

There is no established RDA (nor RNI) for

vanadium and no consistent recommendation for the vanadium content of the diet. Although the following list shows the vanadium content of some selected foods, it is not known how meaningful these data are, as some studies have shown that most ingested vanadium (greater than 95 percent) is not absorbed.

VANADIUM CONTENT OF SELECTED FOODS, IN MICROGRAMS PER 100 GRAM SERVING

Buckwheat	100
Parsley	80
Soybeans	70
Safflower oil	41
Sunflower seed oil	41
Oats	35
Olive oil	30
Sunflower seeds	15
Corn	15
Green beans	14
Peanut oil	11
Carrots	10
Cabbage	10
Garlic	10
Tomatoes	6
Radishes	5
Onions	5
Whole wheat	5
Beetroot	4
Apples	3
Plums	2
Lettuce	2
Millet	2

Zinc

Zinc is a component of more than 200 enzymes in our bodies. In fact, zinc functions in more enzymatic reactions than any other mineral. Although severe zinc deficiency is very rare in developed countries, many individuals in the United States have marginal zinc deficiency. This is particularly true in the elderly population. Marginal zinc deficiency may be reflected by an increased susceptibility to infection, poor wound healing, a decreased sense of taste or smell, low sperm count, prostate enlargement, or skin disorders. In the U.K., a 1990 survey found the average intake of zinc in men was 11.4 milligrams per day, and 8.4 milligrams in women (which is greater than the RNI), but also that a significant proportion of the population—especially women, the elderly, and children and teenagers—were failing to consume adequate amounts of zinc.

Adequate zinc levels are necessary for proper immune system function, and zinc deficiency results in an increased susceptibility to infection. Zinc appears to be vital for normal thymus gland functioning in the synthesis and secretion of thymic hormones, and in the protection of the thymus from cellular damage. Several defects in immune function related to aging are reversible upon zinc supplementation, again highlighting the importance of this nutrient for the elderly. As well as stimulating the immune system, zinc has displayed virus-inhibiting activity. In one double-blind clinical study, zinc supplementation significantly reduced the average duration of colds by seven days.

Zinc is also required for protein synthesis and cell growth, and therefore for wound healing. Zinc supplementation has been shown to decrease wound-healing time, while a zinc deficiency leads to prolongation of the wound. A high zinc intake is indicated to aid protein synthesis and cell growth following any sort of trauma, including burns, surgery, and wounds.

Zinc is essential for the maintenance of vision, taste, and smell, too. Zinc deficiency results in impaired functioning of these special senses, and night blindness is often due to a zinc deficiency. The loss of the sense of taste and/or smell is a common complaint in the elderly. Zinc supplementation has been shown to improve taste and/or smell acuity in some individuals.

Zinc may be critical to healthy male sex hormone and prostate function, as well. Male infertility may be caused by a decreased sperm count due to zinc deficiency, and zinc supplementation may increase sperm count and motility, particularly in men with low testosterone. Zinc deficiency may be a contributing factor in the high rate of prostate enlargement in the U.S.A. It is estimated that 50 to 60 percent of the men between the ages of 40 and 59 have prostate enlargement. In the U.K. about 33 percent of men over the age of fifty are thought to be affected by benign prostatic hyperplasia, and the NHS estimates that about 25 percent of men over sixty-five have moderate to severe symptoms from prostate enlargement. Zinc supplementation has been shown to reduce the size of the prostate in the majority of the patients.

The importance of zinc in normal skin function is well known. Typically, serum zinc levels are lower in thirteen-to-fourteen-year-old males than in any other age group. This group is also the most susceptible to acne. During puberty there is an increased requirement for zinc due to increased hormonal production. One group of researchers believes that low levels of zinc are responsible for acne during puberty. Several double-blind studies have confirmed this hypothesis, as zinc supplementation has been shown to be as effective as tetracycline for the treatment of acne, but without the side effects. It appears that zinc is able to normalize some of the hormonal factors responsible for acne.

Optimal zinc levels must be attained if optimal health is desired. Although severe zinc deficiency is quite rare in the U.S.A., many individuals consume a diet that is low in zinc. The RDA is 15 milligrams for men and 12 milligrams for women. In the U.K., the RNI for adult males is 9.5 milligrams and for adult females (including pregnant women) 7 milligrams. For lactating women the RNI is 9.5 to 13 milligrams. The E.U. RDA is 15 milligrams. In addition to oysters, zinc is found in good amounts in seeds, nuts, legumes, and whole grains.

ZINC CONTENT OF SELECTED FOODS,
IN MILLIGRAMS PER 100 GRAM SERVING

Oysters, fresh	148.7
Pumpkin seeds	7.5
Gingerroot	6.8
Pecans	4.5
Split peas, dry	4.2
Brazil nuts	4.2
Whole wheat	3.2
Rye	3.2
Oats	3.2
Peanuts	3.2
Lima beans	3.1
Almonds	3.1
Walnuts	3.0
Buckwheat	2.5

Hazelnuts	2.4
Green peas	1.6
Turnips	1.2
Parsley	0.9
Potatoes	0.9
Garlic	0.6
Carrots	0.5
Whole-wheat (wholemeal) bread	0.5
Black beans	0.4

Final Comment

Minerals function along with vitamins as essential components in many metabolic processes as well as to maintain the structure and integrity of the body, constituting up to 5 percent of our body weight. Mineral deficiencies are common but can easily be avoided by focusing on a whole-food diet in order to provide both major and trace minerals in abundant amounts.

9

Accessory Nutrients and Phytochemicals

This chapter describes nutrients that are not considered essential in the same manner that vitamins and minerals are. Included in this section are amino acids and their derivatives—essential fatty acids, phospholipids, compounds that exert "vitaminlike" activity, and substances that are part of normal physiology. More and more research indicates that accessory nutrients, although most are not considered "essential" in the classical sense, play a major role in preventing and treating illness. In this chapter we will also discuss phytochemicals. Some of the most important phytochemicals are plant pigments, such as carotenes, chlorophyll, and flavonoids. Although these phytochemicals work in harmony with antioxidants, such as vitamin C, vitamin E, and selenium, they also exert considerably greater protection against cancer than these simple nutrients do.

Betaine

Betaine (trimethylglycine) functions very closely with choline, folic acid, vitamin B12, and a form of the amino acid methionine known as SAMe (*S*-adenosyl-methionine). All of these compounds function as "methyl donors." They carry and donate methyl molecules to facilitate necessary chemical reactions. The donation of methyl groups by betaine is very important to proper liver function, cellular replication, and detoxification reactions.

Betaine is closely related to choline. The difference is that choline (tetramethylglycine) has four methyl groups attached to it. When choline donates one of these groups to another molecule, it becomes betaine (trimethylglycine). If betaine donates one of its methyl groups, it becomes dimethylglycine.

Betaine has been reported to play a role in reducing blood levels of homocysteine, a toxic breakdown product of amino acid metabolism that is believed to promote atherosclerosis and osteoporosis. While the main nutrients involved in controlling homocysteine levels are folic acid, vitamin B6, and vitamin B12, betaine has been reported to be helpful in occasional individuals whose elevated homocysteine levels did not improve with these other nutrients, as well as in individuals with certain rare genetic disorders involving cysteine metabolism. In normal situations, however, or with supplementation of the other methyl donors, betaine is not likely to produce any lowering effect on homocysteine levels. Instead, its primary use as a nutritional supplement is in supporting proper liver function in the dosage range of 50 to 100 milligrams daily.

Betaine is often referred to as a "lipotropic factor" because of its ability to help the liver process fats (lipids). In animal studies, betaine supplementation has been shown to protect against chemical damage to the liver. The first stage of liver damage as a result of alcohol is the accumulation of fat in the liver (alcohol-induced fatty liver disease). Betaine, because of its lipotropic effects, has demonstrated significant protective benefits to the liver in both animal models and human clinical studies. For example, betaine has been studied in clinical trials conducted in Germany, Italy, and France in the treatment of alcohol-related liver disease. Some success was noted in these studies, but the popularity of betaine for alcohol-related liver disease has been supplanted by SAMe and milk thistle extract. However, it has recently been suggested that betaine may be a more cost-effective method as a first-step therapy for alcohol-induced fatty liver disease.

The best dietary sources of betaine (trimethylglycine) mirror those of free choline (tetramethylglycine) such as beetroot, fish, and legumes (see page 112).

Carnitine

Carnitine is a vitaminlike compound that stimulates the breakdown of long-chain fatty acids by mitochondria (tiny energy-producing organelles in our cells). Carnitine is essential in the transport of fatty acids into the mitochondria. A deficiency in carnitine results in a decrease in fatty acid concentrations in the mitochondria and reduced energy production for the cell.

Carnitine is synthesized from the amino acid lysine in the liver, kidney, and brain. It also requires adequate levels of iron and vitamin C. A deficiency of any of these factors will lead to a deficiency of carnitine.

Carnitine has been shown to offer significant support to people with heart disease. Since long-chain fatty acids are the preferred energy source in well-oxygenated heart tissue, normal heart function is dependent on adequate concentrations of carnitine within the heart. Carnitine also increases HDL (good) cholesterol levels, while decreasing triglyceride and LDL (bad) cholesterol levels.

Carnitine deficiency is linked to a large number of heart disorders, including familial endocardial fibroelastosis, cardiac enlargement, congestive heart failure, and cardiac myopathies. All of these disorders respond to carnitine supplementation.

Dietary sources richest in carnitine are red meats, particularly lamb and beef, and dairy products. Vegetables, fruits, and grains contain little or no carnitine, but the human body can make carnitine from the amino acid lysine, and legumes are a very good dietary source of lysine.

There is no established RDA (nor RNI) for carnitine; however, the average diet contains 5 to 10 milligrams of carnitine per day. Carnitine is supplemented from 500 to 4,000 milligrams per day.

Carnosine

Carnosine is a small protein composed of the amino acids histidine and alanine. It is found in relatively high concentrations in several body tissues, most notably in skeletal muscle, heart muscle, and the brain. The exact biological role of carnosine is still under investigation, but numerous animal studies have demonstrated that it possesses strong and specific antioxidant properties, protects against radiation damage, improves the function of the heart, and promotes wound healing. Carnosine has been suggested to be the water-soluble counterpart to vitamin E in protecting cell membranes from oxidative damage. Other suggested roles for carnosine include actions such as a neurotransmitter, modulator of enzyme activities, and chelator of heavy metals.

Many claims have been made in respect to the therapeutic actions of carnosine, including exerting antihypertensive, immune-enhancing, wound-healing, and anticancer effects. These claims are based primarily on preliminary Russian research. Unfortunately, the claims have not been convincingly documented or subjected to rigorous clinical evaluation. Furthermore,

although carnosine is absorbed intact from the gastrointestinal tract, it is broken down extensively in the blood, especially in people who exercise regularly.

Dietary sources of preformed carnosine include meat, poultry, and fish. The average daily intake of carnosine from foods is estimated to be in the range of 50 to 250 milligrams depending upon the amount of meat, poultry, or fish in the diet. Typical dosages of carnosine supplementation range from 100 to 300 milligrams daily.

Carotenes

The carotenes are a highly colored group of fat-soluble plant pigments ranging from red to violet in hue. All organisms that rely on the sun for energy, whether bacteria or plants, contain carotene molecules. Due to their antioxidant effects, these compounds play a crucial role in protecting organisms against damage during the process of photosynthesis, which is the process of converting sunlight into chemical energy.

In humans, carotenes play two primary roles: some are converted into vitamin A, and all exert antioxidant activity. Of the 600 carotenes that have been identified, about thirty to fifty are believed to have vitamin A activity. Carotenes that the body is able to convert to vitamin A are referred to as "provitamin A" carotenes. The best known of this group are beta-carotene and alpha-carotene. Some of the better-known carotenes without provitamin A activity but with very high antioxidant activity are lutein, lycopene, and zeaxanthin.

Preliminary and experimental studies suggest that a higher dietary intake of carotenes offers protection against developing certain cancers, such as lung, skin, uterine, cervix, and gastrointestinal tract; heart disease; macular degeneration; cataracts; and other health conditions linked to oxidative or free-radical damage. However, one of the major problems with much of the research on carotenes in cancer and cardiovascular disease protection has been the focus on beta-carotene. Beta-carotene is likely of less importance than many other carotenes, especially lycopene and lutein, because it does not exert the same degree of antioxidant protection.

Carotenes are found in all plant foods. In general, the greater the intensity of color, the higher the level of carotenes. In green leafy vegetables, beta-carotene is the predominant carotene. Orange-colored fruits and vegetables, such as carrots, apricots, mangoes, yams, and squash, are excellent sources of alpha-, beta-, and gamma-carotenes, but in most plant foods, other non–provitamin A carotenes typically predominate. For example, yellow vegetables have higher concentrations of yellow carotenes (xanthophylls), hence a lowered provitamin A activity, but these compounds, including lutein, are showing significant health benefits due to their antioxidant effects. And red and purple vegetables and fruits, such as tomatoes, red

TABLE 9.1

Carotenes, Vitamin A Activity, and Food Sources

Carotene	Vitamin A Activity, %	Food Sources
Beta-carotene	100	Green plants, carrots, sweet potatoes, squash, spinach, apricots, green peppers, mangoes, yams
Alpha-carotene	50–54	Green plants, carrots, squash, corn, watermelons, green peppers, potatoes, apples, peaches
Gamma-carotene	42–50	Carrots, sweet potatoes, corn, tomatoes, watermelons, apricots
Beta-zeacarotene	20–40	Corn, tomatoes, yeast, cherries
Cryptoxanthin	50–60	Corn, green peppers, persimmons, papayas, lemons, oranges, prunes, apples, apricots, paprika, poultry
Lycopene	0	Tomatoes, carrots, green peppers, apricots, pink grapefruit, red cabbage, berries, plums
Zeaxanthin	0	Spinach, paprika, corn, most fruits
Lutein	0	Green plants, corn, potatoes, spinach, carrots, tomatoes, most fruits
Canthaxanthin	0	Mushrooms, trout, crustaceans
Crocetin	0	Saffron
Capsanthin	0	Red peppers, paprika

FOOD OR PILLS?

Increasing your levels of lutein, lycopene, and zeaxanthin can play a central role in protecting against the development of macular degeneration. Although lutein and lycopene supplements are entering the marketplace, they are relatively expensive, especially when you compare them to food sources. Before you check out at the health food shop till, check this out:

Lycopene Source	Total (milligrams)	Cost	
Tomato paste/purée, 30 gram can	16	$0.065	£0.85 (70 gram tube)
Lycopene supplement, three 5 milligram capsules	15	$1.25	£0.30
Tomato paste/purée, 375 gram can	192	$0.69	£0.69 (312 gram jar, organic)
Lycopene supplement, one bottle of 30 capsules	150	$7.95	£10.49 (fifty 10 milligram capsules

In short, it looks as if the cheapest and healthiest way to boost lycopene levels as well as lutein and zeaxanthin levels is through diet. The twenty foods richest in these important carotenes are:

Corn	Green grapes
Kiwifruit	Brussels sprouts
Red grapes	Spring onions
Squash (courgettes, pumpkin, butternut, etc.)	Green beans
Bell peppers (red > orange > green > yellow)	Orange
Greens (spinach, kale, chard, etc.)	Broccoli
Cucumber	Apple
Peas	Mango
Honeydew melon	Peach
Celery	Tomato paste or juice

cabbage, berries, and plums, contain a large portion of non–vitamin A–active carotenes such as lycopene, that are also showing health benefits.

Legumes, grains, and seeds are also significant sources of carotenes. Carotenes are found in various animal foods, such as salmon and other fish, egg yolks, milk, and poultry. Good supplemental forms of mixed carotenes include palm oil carotene products, algal products,

carrot oil, and the various "green drinks" on the market, such as dehydrated barley greens and wheat grass.

In regard to carotene supplements, there are five primary sources on the market:

• Synthetic all-*trans* beta-carotene.
• Beta- and alpha-carotene from *Dunaliella* algae.

- Mixed carotenes from palm oil.
- Lutein.
- Lycopene.

Of the three sources of beta-carotene, mixed carotenes from palm oil carotenes seem to be the best form as they more closely mirror the pattern in high-carotene foods. In particular, unlike the synthetic version, which provides only the *trans* configuration of beta-carotene, natural carotene sources provide beta-carotene in both *trans* and *cis* configurations:

- 60 percent beta-carotene (both *trans* and *cis* isomers).
- 34 percent alpha-carotene.
- 3 percent gamma-carotene.
- 3 percent lycopene.

Palm oil carotenes have also been shown to be absorbed about four to ten times better than synthetic all-*trans* beta-carotene. Carotenes from *Dunaliella* algae have also been shown to be well absorbed.

For beta-carotene sources, a daily dosage of 15 milligrams of beta-carotene (25,000 IU of vitamin A activity) appears to be reasonable for general health. Again, mixed carotene preparations are preferred to isolated beta-carotene supplements. For lutein and lycopene the usual dosages range from 2 to 5 milligrams for general health and from 15 to 30 milligrams for specific applications (e.g., lutein in the treatment of macular degeneration and lycopene in prostate cancer).

Chlorophyll

Chlorophyll is the green pigment of plants found in the chloroplast compartment of plant cells, where electromagnetic energy (light) is converted to chemical energy in the process known as photosynthesis. The chlorophyll molecule is essential for this reaction to occur.

The natural chlorophyll found in green plants is fat-soluble. The majority of the chlorophyll products found in health food shops, however, contain water-soluble chlorophyll. In order to produce water-soluble chlorophyll, the natural chlorophyll molecule must be altered chemically. The fat-soluble form, the natural form of chlorophyll as found in green vegetables and other plants, offers several advantages over water-soluble chlorophyll. Most important, fat-soluble chlorophyll can stimulate hemoglobin and red blood cell production, while water-soluble chlorophyll cannot. In fact, it is interesting to note that the chlorophyll molecule is very similar to the heme portion of the hemoglobin molecule of our red blood cells.

Because water-soluble chlorophyll is not absorbed from the gastrointestinal tract, its use is limited to soothing the gastrointestinal tract and reducing faecal odor. It is approved for use in reducing the faecal odor associated with a colostomy, which is the removal of the colon and replacement with a small collection bag outside the body. The beneficial effect of water-soluble chlorophyll in this case is largely due to its astringent qualities, that is, its ability to attract water.

Good dietary sources of chlorophyll include

green leafy vegetables, broccoli, wheat grass juice, and algae, such as spirulina and chlorella.

Ellagic Acid

Ellagic acid is a phenolic compound related to flavonoids. It is present in plants in the form of complexes called ellagitannins. When these complexes are broken down, they yield ellagic acid.

Ellagic acid exhibits significant anticancer activity. A potent antioxidant, ellagic acid protects against damage to the chromosomes. It also blocks the cancer-causing actions of many pollutants, such as the polycyclic aromatic hydrocarbons (PAHs) found in cigarette smoke and toxic chemicals such as benzopyrene.

Ellagic acid is not destroyed by freezing or freeze-drying, but it is destroyed by heat. For example, while fresh, whole apples and fresh or frozen apple juice contain approximately 100 to 130 milligrams of ellagic acid per 100 grams, the amount found in cooked or commercial apple products is at or near zero. The ellagic acid content in fresh or frozen raspberries and blackberries is exceptionally high, up to 1.5 milligrams per gram of fruit. In fact, these levels are approximately five to six times higher than the levels found in other foods. Other good sources of ellagic acid are other berries, fruit, and nuts such as walnuts and pecans.

Enzymes

Fresh fruits and vegetables, as well as juices made from them, are often referred to as "live" foods because they contain active enzymes. Enzymes are found in higher amounts in raw foods because they are extremely sensitive to heat and are destroyed during cooking and pasteurization.

There are two major types of enzymes: *synthetases* and *hydrolases*. The synthetases help build body structures by making or synthesizing larger molecules. The synthetases are also referred to as metabolic enzymes. The hydrolases work to break down large molecules into smaller ones by adding water to the larger molecule. This process is known as hydrolysis. The hydrolases are also known as digestive enzymes.

There is little doubt that some food enzymes are absorbed intact and are active in the human body. Specifically, various hydrolases have been shown to be active when given orally. The best-known example is bromelain, the protein-digesting enzyme in pineapples. Introduced as a medicinal agent in 1957, bromelain has since been the subject of more than 250 scientific papers, and there is definite evidence that, in both animals and man, up to 40 percent of bromelain given by mouth is absorbed intact, without being broken down. This provides some evidence that other plant enzymes may also be absorbed intact and exert beneficial effects as well. Bromelain has been reported in these scientific studies to exert a wide variety of beneficial effects, including

- Assistance in digestion.
- Reduction of inflammation in cases of arthritis, sports injury or trauma.
- Prevention of swelling (edema) after trauma or surgery.
- Inhibition of blood platelet aggregation; enhancement of antibiotic absorption.
- Relief of sinusitis.

- Inhibition of appetite.
- Enhancement of wound healing.

Although most studies have utilized commercially prepared bromelain in pills, it is conceivable that fresh pineapple or its juice could exert similar benefits.

Flavonoids

The flavonoids are a group of plant pigments that exert antioxidant activity that is generally more potent and effective against a broader range of oxidants than the traditional antioxidant nutrients vitamins C and E, beta-carotene, selenium, and zinc. Besides lending color to fruits and flowers, flavonoids are responsible for many of the medicinal properties of foods, juices, herbs, and bee pollen. Flavonoids are sometimes called "nature's biological response modifiers" because of their anti-inflammatory, antiallergic, antiviral, and anticancer properties.

Flavonoids are sometimes considered "semi-essential" nutrients, but in our view they are as important to human nutrition as the so-called essential nutrients. Because they have a broader range of antioxidant activity, as well as other important anticancer effects, we recommend including as many different types of flavonoids as possible in your diet. Doing so will provide extra insurance that your body can mop up any type of free radical or oxidant that escapes the other protective systems.

Recent research suggests that flavonoids may be useful in the support of many health conditions. Different flavonoids will provide different health benefits. For example, the flavonoids responsible for the blue to purple colors of blueberries, blackberries, cherries, grapes, hawthorn berries, and many flowers are termed "anthocyanidins" and "proanthocyanidins." These flavonoids are found in the flesh of the fruit as well as the skin and possess very strong "vitamin P" activity. Among their effects is an ability to increase vitamin C levels within our cells, decrease the leakiness and breakage of small blood vessels, protect against free radical damage, and support our joint structures.

Flavonoids also have a very beneficial effect on collagen. Collagen is the most abundant protein of the body and is responsible for maintaining the integrity of ground substance, which is responsible for holding together the tissues of the body. Collagen is also found in tendons, ligaments, and cartilage. It is destroyed during inflammatory processes that occur in rheumatoid arthritis, periodontal disease, gout, and other inflammatory conditions involving bones, joints, cartilage, and other connective tissue. Anthocyanidins and other flavonoids affect collagen metabolism in many ways:

- They have the unique ability to cross-link collagen fibers, resulting in reinforcement of the natural cross-linking of collagen that forms the so-called collagen matrix of connective tissue, including ground substance, cartilage, and tendon.
- They prevent free-radical damage with their potent antioxidant and free-radical scavenging action.
- They inhibit destruction to collagen structures by enzymes secreted by white blood cells during inflammation.
- They prevent the release and synthesis of

TYPES OF FLAVONOIDS

Flavonoids are a subgroup of a large class of molecules called phenols. More than eight thousand phenolic compounds have been characterized and classified according to their chemical structures. Polyphenols are complexes of phenols found in such foods as green tea, red wine, and even chocolate. These substances are potent antioxidants that offer significant protection against heart disease and various cancers, especially in the gastrointestinal tract. They work by blocking the formation of cancer-causing chemicals, such as nitrosamines.

Each subgroup of phenols has a common biosynthetic origin based on the same structural skeleton.

- *The anthocyanidins and PCOs (short for proanthocyanidin oligomers) are the blue or purple pigments found in grapes, blueberries, and other foods. They can also be extracted from pine bark. These substances increase vitamin C levels within our cells, decrease the leakiness and breakage of small blood vessels, protect against free-radical damage, and help prevent destruction of collagen, an important protein for healthy skin and connective tissue. Extracts of grape seeds and pine bark are popular supplements that provide anthocyanidins and PCOs.*
- *4-oxo-flavonoids comprises the subgroups of flavonones, flavones, and flavonols, which account for more than 90 percent of all flavonoids. Quercetin is a flavonol found in many foods. One of the best dietary sources is onions. Besides serving as an antioxidant, quercetin helps reduce the effects of inflammation and promotes activity of hormones such as insulin. Quercetin is a popular flavonoid supplement often used in the treatment of allergies.*
- *Citrus bioflavonoids, formed by two flavonoids joined together, are found in oranges, limes, lemons, and grapefruit. Besides providing antioxidant activity, they appear to improve blood circulation and increase the integrity of capillaries. Citrus bioflavonoids are often included in vitamin C supplements because they enhance the activity of vitamin C.*
- *Isoflavonoids are another category with a similar structure to the 4-oxo-flavonoids and some have oestrogenic activity. However, most oestrogenic activity occurs only after metabolism by beneficial bacteria in the digestive tract. Isoflavonoids are found in soy and red clover.*

For simplicity, we will refer to all of these subgroups as flavonoids since this is the most commonly used term to describe these compounds.

compounds that promote inflammation, such as histamine.

These useful effects on collagen structures and their potent antioxidant activity make these flavonoids extremely useful in cases of arthritis and hardening of the arteries. As atherosclerotic processes are still the major killers of Americans and Britons, foods rich in anthocyanidins and proanthocyanidins appear to offer significant prevention against, as well as a potential reversal of, these processes.

Several studies have shown that people who have a high intake of plant flavonoids are less

RED WINE, WHITE WINE, OR GRAPE JUICE?

The French consume more saturated fat than Americans yet have a lower incidence of heart disease. This is referred to as the "French paradox." Many experts suspect that the French are less vulnerable to heart disease because they consume more red wine. Presumably the protective effect is the result of the flavonoids in red wine, which protect against oxidative damage from LDL cholesterol.

Grape juice also contains flavonoids and may offer similar protection. However, while some studies show benefit with grape juice, a recent study indicated that it did not provide the same level of support as red wine in protection against damage to LDL. In addition, the study showed that consumption of white wine actually increased LDL oxidation. Red wine contains mainly single molecules of flavonoids, primarily quercetin. In contrast, grape juice flavonoids are usually complexed with other flavonoids and are bound to various sugars that may reduce their bioavailability. Also, the flavonoid content in white wine is significantly lower than that in red wine.

The bottom line is that for women, one glass, and for men, one or two glasses, of red wine per day appears to be a good prescription for a healthy heart.

likely to die from heart disease or develop some cancers or other chronic diseases. In one of the largest studies, when researchers studied the diets of more than 10,000 men and women, they found that those who ate fruits and vegetables rich in different flavonoids had a lower risk of overall mortality and of several chronic diseases, including heart disease, stroke, and lung and prostate cancer, type 2 diabetes, and asthma.

Still other flavonoids are remarkable anti-allergic compounds, modifying and reducing all phases of the allergic response. Specifically, they inhibit the formation and secretion of potent inflammatory compounds that produce the allergic response. Several prescription medications developed for allergic conditions were actually patterned after flavonoid molecules. An example of an antiallergy flavonoid is quercetin, which is available in many fruits and vegetables. Quercetin

TABLE 9.2
Flavonoid Content of Selected Foods, in Milligrams per 100 gram Serving

Foods	4-oxo-flavonoids*	Anthocyanins	Catechins†	Biflavans
Fruits:				
Apple juice				15
Apples	3–16	1–2	20–75	50–90
Apricots	10–18		25	

(continued on next page)

Foods	4-oxo-flavonoids*	Anthocyanins	Catechins†	Biflavans
Blueberry		130–250	10–20	
Cherries, sour		45		25
Cherries, sweet			6–7	15
Cranberries	5	60–200	20	100
Currant juice		75–100		
Currants, black	20–400	130–400	15	50
Grapefruit juice	20			
Grapefruit	50			
Grapes, red		65–140	5–30	50
Hawthorn berries			200–800	
Orange juice	20–40			
Oranges, Valencia	50–100			
Peaches		1–12	10–20	90–120
Pears	1–5		5–20	1–3
Plums, blue		10–25	200	
Plums, yellow		2–10		
Raspberries, black		300–400		
Raspberries, red		30–35		
Strawberries	20–100	15–35	30–40	
Tomatoes	85–130			
Vegetables:				
Cabbage, red		25		
Onions	100–2,000	0–25		
Parsley	1,400			
Rhubarb		200		
Miscellaneous:				
Beans, dry		10–1,000		
Chocolate, dark semisweet				170
Sage	1,000–1,500			
Tea	5–50		10–500	100–200
Wine, red	2–4	50–120	100–150	100–250

* The sum of flavanones, flavones, and flavonols (including quercetin).

† Including proanthocyanins.

is a potent antioxidant that inhibits the release of histamine and other allergic compounds.

Our recommended daily intake for flavonoids for good health from dietary sources is at least 300 milligrams per day. There is a variety of flavonoid supplements on the market, such as citrus bioflavonoids, grape seed extract, quercetin, and bilberry extract. Dosages of these preparations are based upon the results observed in clinical trials. For therapeutic purposes, proper dosages for the various flavonoid preparations are as follows.

Flavonoid-rich extract	Typical daily dosage	Indication
Green tea extract (60–70% total polyphenols)	150–300 mg	Systemic antioxidant. May provide the best protection against cancer, best choice if there is a family history of cancer. Also protects against damage to cholesterol.
Quercetin	150–300 mg	Allergies, symptoms of prostate enlargement or bladder irritation, eczema.
Grape seed extract (95% procyanidolic oligomers)	50–100 mg	Systemic antioxidant; best choice for most people under age 50. Also specific for the lungs, diabetes, varicose veins, and protection against heart disease.
Ginkgo biloba extract (24% ginkgo flavonglycosides)	120–240 mg	Best choice for most people over the age of 50. Protects brain and vascular lining.
Milk thistle extract (70% silymarin)	100–300 mg	Best choice for additional antioxidant protection of liver or skin needs.
Bilberry extract (25% anthocyanidins)	80–160 mg	Best choice to protect the eyes.
Hawthorn extract (10% proanthocyanidins)	150–300 mg	Best choice in heart disease or high blood pressure

Glutathione

Glutathione is a small protein composed of three amino acids: cysteine, glutamic acid, and glycine. It is involved in detoxification and antioxidant mechanisms. Many toxins are dealt with by "handcuffing" the toxin to another molecule so it can be escorted out of the body. The process of adding one molecule to another is called *conjugation*. Glutathione is one of the most important conjugating compounds in helping the body eliminate fat-soluble toxins, such as heavy metals, solvents, and pesticides, transforming them into a water-soluble form in order to allow more efficient excretion via the kidneys.

The combination of detoxification and free-radical protection results in glutathione being one of the most important anticancer and anti-aging agents in our cells. Dietary glutathione intake is associated with protection against some forms of cancer.

The greater the exposure to toxins, the faster the body uses up its supply of glutathione. Without the protection of glutathione, cells die at a faster rate, making people age more quickly and putting them at risk for toxin-induced diseases, including cancer.

People who smoke; are chronically exposed to toxins; suffer from inflammatory conditions, such as rheumatoid arthritis; or suffer from chronic conditions, such as diabetes, AIDS, or cancer typically have lower levels of glutathione. It's a vicious cycle: health problems deplete the supply of glutathione, and reduced levels of glutathione increase the risk of health problems.

In addition to its dietary role in enhancing detoxification and protecting against cancer, studies using intravenous glutathione have found it to be useful in preventing clot formation during operations; reducing the side effects and increasing the efficacy of chemotherapy drugs such as cisplatin; treating Parkinson's disease; and increasing sperm counts in men with low sperm counts. A small study in eight patients with liver cancer showed modest effects when glutathione was supplemented at a daily dosage of 5,000 milligrams orally. However, whether increasing dietary intake with glutathione is effective in any of these conditions is unknown at this time.

Fresh fruits and vegetables provide excellent levels of glutathione, but cooked foods contain far less. Asparagus, avocado, and walnuts are particularly rich dietary sources of glutathione.

TABLE 9.3

Comparison of Glutathione Content of Fresh and Cooked Foods

Glutathione Amount (Dry Weight), in Milligrams per 100 gram Serving

Food	Uncooked	Cooked
Apples	21	0.0
Carrots	74.6	0.0
Grapefruit	70.6	0.0
Spinach	166	27.1
Tomatoes	169	0.0

Terpenes

The term "terpene" probably conjures up images of cleaning solvents. While it is true that naturally occurring terpenes are used as alternatives to synthetic terpenes in many natural cleaning products, the primary health benefits of terpenes revolve around some impressive anticancer effects, in both prevention and possibly treatment. D-limonene and perillyl alcohol are the most widely tested terpenes and in animal studies have been shown to provide considerable benefits against a wide number of cancers. Both of these terpenes are being investigated in humans with advanced cancers; the preliminary results are encouraging.

The best dietary sources of terpenes are citrus fruits and volatile herbs, such as peppermint, thyme, and rosemary.

DIETARY GLUTATHIONE IS BETTER THAN SUPPLEMENTS

Don't look to supplements containing glutathione to boost body levels of glutathione. While dietary forms of glutathione appear to be absorbed into the blood efficiently, the same does not appear to be true for oral glutathione supplements. Although supplemental glutathione may reach the liver, when healthy subjects were given a single dose of up to 3,000 milligrams of glutathione, researchers found that there was no increase in blood glutathione levels. The authors of the study concluded, "It is not feasible to increase circulating glutathione to a clinically beneficial extent by the oral administration of a single dose of 3,000 mg of glutathione." In contrast, blood glutathione levels rose by nearly 50 percent in healthy individuals taking 500 milligrams of vitamin C. Vitamin C raises glutathione by helping the body manufacture it. In addition to vitamin C, dietary sources of glutathione and several other nutritional compounds can help increase glutathione levels, including N-acetylcysteine (NAC), alpha-lipoic acid, glutamine, methionine, and whey protein. Also, vitamin B6, riboflavin, and selenium are required for the manufacture of glutathione.

Conclusions

Although the nutrients discussed in this chapter are not considered essential in the same manner that vitamins and minerals are, clearly they play an important part in normal physiology. Furthermore, a considerable amount of research indicates that accessory nutrients and phytochemicals are critical in the battle against the development of many chronic degenerative diseases, such as heart disease and cancer. Although some of these valuable food components are available as dietary supplements, in many cases accessory nutrients and phytochemicals are even more bioavailable in foods. This fact once again shows the tremendous healing power of a whole-food diet.

PART 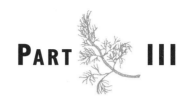 III

Compendium of Healing Foods

The Healing Power of Vegetables

The word "vegetable" comes from the Latin *vegetare,* meaning "to enliven or animate." The name is appropriate, as vegetables do truly give us life. More and more evidence is accumulating showing that vegetables can prevent, as well as treat, many diseases, especially chronic degenerative diseases such as heart disease, cancer, diabetes, and arthritis. Vegetables provide the broadest range of nutrients and phytochemicals, especially fiber and carotenes, of any food class. They are rich sources of vitamins, minerals, carbohydrates, and protein, and the little fat they contain is in the form of essential fatty acids.

What Is the Difference Between a Vegetable and a Fruit?

In 1893, this question came before the U.S. Supreme Court. The court ruled that a vegetable refers to a plant grown for an edible part that is generally eaten as part of the main course, while a fruit is a plant part which is generally eaten as an appetizer, a dessert, or out of hand. Some typical parts of plants used as vegetables are: bulbs, such as garlic and onion; flowers, such as broccoli and cauliflower; fruits, such as pumpkins and tomatoes; leaves, such as spinach and lettuce; roots, such as carrots and beetroot; seeds, such as legumes, peas, and corn; stalks, such as celery; stems, such as asparagus; and tubers, such as potatoes and yams.

The USDA Grading System

The U.S. Department of Agriculture has established a set of voluntary grade standards for fruit and vegetables. The official USDA grades are as follows:

U.S. Fancy: Premium quality, the top quality range.

U.S. No. 1: The chief trading grade; good quality.

U.S. No. 2: Intermediate quality.

U.S. No. 3: Low quality.

The USDA grading is largely visually determined not only on the external qualities but also on the internal appearance of the fruits and vegetables. Models, color guides, and color photographs are available for graders to check samples for shape, degree of coloring, and degree of defects or damage.

In the U.K., the grading, marketing and labeling of fruits and vegetables are regulated by British and European Union law. For details, contact the Food Standards Agency: www.foodstandards.gov.uk.

How Should We Eat Vegetables?

One answer to this question is: It doesn't matter! What's important is to make sure you're eating *enough* vegetables, in whatever form. Vegetables should play a major role in your diet. The U.S. National Academy of Science, the U.S. Department of Health and Human Services, and the National Cancer Institute plus many U.K. healthcare agencies recommend that people consume a minimum of three to five servings of vegetables per day.

Another answer to the question "How should we eat vegetables?" is: Raw. In their raw form, vegetables provide many important phytochemicals in much higher concentrations. However, some of the most beneficial carotenes, such as lycopene and lutein, are better absorbed from cooked foods. In addition, it may not be wise to consume more than four servings per week of raw cabbage-family vegetables, including broccoli, cauliflower, and kale, because these foods in their raw state contain compounds that can interfere with thyroid hormone production.

When cooking vegetables, it is very important not to overcook them. Overcooking will not only result in the loss of important nutrients, it will also alter the flavor of the vegetables. Light steaming, baking, and quick stir-frying are the best ways to cook vegetables. Do not boil vegetables unless you are making soup or stock, as many of the nutrients from the vegetables remain in the water. If fresh vegetables are not available, frozen vegetables are preferable to their canned counterparts.

Although pickled vegetables are quite popular, they may not be healthy choices. Not only are they high in salt, they may also be high in cancer-causing compounds. Pickled vegetables contain high concentrations of *N*-nitroso compounds. Once ingested, these compounds can form potent, cancer-causing nitrosamines. Several population studies have suggested an association between consumption of pickled vegetables and cancer of the oesophagus.

In Western countries generally, we are fortunate to have a great variety of vegetables to choose from. Many varieties of vegetables from cultures all over the world have made their way to different countries by way of the immigrants bringing them. Table 10.1 highlights many of these vegetables and their places of origin.

TABLE 10.1

Origins of Modern Vegetables

Northern Europe	Mediterranean	Africa	Middle East	India and Asia	North America	Central America	South America
Beetroot	Artichoke	Okra	Cabbage	Aubergine	Jerusalem artichoke	Jicama	Pepper
Broccoli	Asparagus	Yam	Carrot	Beetroot		Peppers	Potato
Brussels sprouts	Celery		Cauliflower	Bok choy		Pumpkin	Sweet potato
Cabbage	Chard		Cucumber	Carrot		Squash	Tomato
Chives	Chickpea		Lettuce	Chives		Sweet potato	
Collards	Endive		Mustard	Garlic		Tomato	
Fennel	Kale		Radish	Leek			
Horseradish	Kohlrabi		Spinach	Onion			
Mustard	Olive		Watercress	Shallot			
Peas	Parsley		Yam	Turnip			
Swede	Parsnip			Water chestnut			
Turnip							
Watercress							

Common Vegetables

Artichoke

Long considered a delicacy, the globe artichoke is actually the unopened edible flower bud of a thistlelike plant whose Latin name is *Cynara scolymus*. Each green, sphere-shaped bud is fully enclosed by overlapping, leaflike scales that are fibrous and inedible at the tip but whose flesh is sweet and tender at the base. These bright green outer "leaves" surround an inedible thistle, or "choke," enclosed by a tiny cone of pale rose or green immature leaves. The round, firm-fleshed bottom of the choke, the "heart" of the artichoke, has a similar consistency as the base of the outer leaves and is often considered the artichoke's most delectable morsel.

The base of the outer leaves and the heart are normally the only parts eaten, although in some areas, the tender young leaf stalk is also consumed. As the flower bud matures, all parts become too fibrous and tough to consume.

Eventually, the buds develop into six-inch bluish thistlelike flower heads.

Mature plants normally grow to a height of 4 to 5 feet (1.2–1.5 meters) with a similar spread. Artichokes of varying sizes all grow on the same plant. Large entrée-sized specimens weighing a pound/½ kilogram or more grow on the central stalk, while midsized buds develop on the side branches and "baby" artichokes, typically weighing only 2 ounces/60 grams, are found at the base. These tiny artichokes have no choke; their bottoms and tender centers are all heart.

Large artichokes, their choke removed, are typically filled with a stuffing that qualifies them to be served as an entrée. Midsized artichokes usually appear with a dip as an appetizer, and the tiny "baby" artichokes are canned or used to produce the marinated artichoke hearts that are so delicious as a topping on pizza and in salads and antipastos.

Artichokes also vary in shape. In the market, a spherical or oval shape is preferred, but a cylindrical shape is also common, and a conical shape has also been produced.

HISTORY

The globe artichoke, one of the world's oldest cultivated vegetables, has a noble history. Artichokes are referenced in the writings of the Greek historian Dioscorides, who noted their large-scale cultivation near Carthage, and the early Roman scholar Pliny, who remarked that they were more esteemed and commanded a higher price than any other garden vegetable. In the fifteenth century, artichokes were ardently cultivated in Florence and were taken to France by Catherine de Médicis, when she became the wife of France's Henry II. French and Spanish explorers first took artichokes to the United States, but significant cultivation did not occur until the nineteenth century, first in Louisiana and then along the midcoastal regions of California, where the cool, foggy climate is ideally suited to their propagation.

Today, 99 percent of all the globe artichokes grown in the United States are produced in the area of Castroville, California, self-named the "Artichoke Capital of the World." Eighty percent of the world's artichoke crop is, however, produced by Italy (486,000 tons), Spain (444,000 tons), and France (93,000 tons), all countries that border the Mediterranean Sea and have a similar climate. Next in artichoke production is Argentina (72,000 tons), followed by the United States, where 58,000 tons of globe artichokes are grown annually.

NUTRITIONAL HIGHLIGHTS

Globe artichokes are an excellent source of dietary fiber, magnesium, and the trace mineral chromium; a very good source of vitamin C, folic acid, biotin, and the trace mineral manganese; and a good source of niacin, riboflavin, thiamine, vitamin A, and potassium. A medium-sized globe artichoke delivers all these nutrients for a mere 60 fat-free calories and also provides 4.2 grams of protein, no cholesterol, 0.2 gram of fat, and 11.2 grams of carbohydrate with 5.4 grams of fiber.

HEALTH BENEFITS

Fresh artichokes are very low in calories because most of the carbohydrate is in the form of inulin, a polysaccharide or starch that is handled by the body differently than other sugars. In fact, inulin is not utilized by the body for energy metabolism. This makes artichokes extremely beneficial to diabetics, as inulin has actually been shown to improve blood sugar control in diabetes. However, it is important that the artichoke be as fresh as possible, as inulin is broken down into other sugars when artichokes are stored for any length of time. For more information about the health benefits of inulin, see page 77.

The artichoke has a long folk history in treating many liver diseases. Recent scientific evidence supports this longtime use. The active ingredients in artichoke are caffeoylquinic acids, such as cynarin. These compounds are found in highest concentrations in the leaves, but are also found in the bracts and heart. Artichoke leaf extracts have demonstrated significant liver-protecting and -regenerating effects. They also have a choleretic effect, meaning they promote the flow of bile and fat to and from the liver. This is very important, because if the bile is not transported adequately to the gallbladder, the liver is at increased risk of damage. Choleretics are very useful in the treatment of hepatitis and other liver diseases via this "decongesting" effect.

Choleretics typically lower cholesterol levels too, since they increase the excretion of cholesterol and decrease the manufacture of cholesterol in the liver. Consistent with its choleretic effect, artichoke leaf extract has been shown to lower blood cholesterol and triglyceride levels in both human and animal studies. In one experimental double-blind study, thirty patients given 500 milligrams of pure cynarin per day for fifty days had an average 20 percent reduction in total cholesterol along with an average 15 percent reduction in triglycerides compared to a matched group who received a placebo.

Artichoke leaf extracts have been shown to improve the functioning of the cells that line the arteries—the endothelial cells. Dysfunction of the endothelial cells represents the first stage of atherosclerotic disease. In one clinical trial, twenty-eight men and women with elevations of LDL cholesterol were given 20 ml per day of frozen artichoke juice. In addition to lowering cholesterol levels, the artichoke extract demonstrated a clear ability to improve endothelial function, thereby establishing another mechanism for its benefits against atherosclerosis.

Caffeoylquinic acids from artichokes have also demonstrated potent activity against the human immunodeficiency virus (HIV). Specifically, these compounds inhibit the HIV integrase enzyme, which is essential to the virus's ability to reproduce.

HOW TO SELECT AND STORE

Regardless of its shape, an artichoke should be compact and heavy for its size. Its outer leaves should be thick, firm, fleshy, and tightly closed. Avoid artichokes whose leaves have begun to spread apart or appear dry and woody. These are signs that the artichoke is past its prime. Turn the artichoke over and check the stem end; tiny holes are evidence of worm damage, which may be extensive inside.

Spring artichokes should be a softer green than the autumn and winter crop, which are typically olive green and may have what growers call a "winter-kissed" appearance: bronze-tipped leaves or a lightly blistered, whitish outer surface. These changes are caused by light frost exposure in the fields and do not affect the artichoke's taste or tenderness. However, avoid those with blackened, wilted leaves or dark spots; these artichokes are not "bronzed" but damaged and deteriorating. Lastly, give your prospective purchase a squeeze; the plump, crisp leaves of a fresh artichoke will reply with a squeaky sound.

In addition to fresh, whole artichokes, baby artichokes and artichoke hearts are also available in cans and jars or frozen. All the inedible parts have been removed from these products, so they're practically ready to enjoy. Canned artichokes are usually packed in brine. To reduce their high sodium content, drain the brine and rinse them with cool water. Similarly, with marinated artichokes, which are usually sold in jars, you can significantly lessen the hefty calorie tally supplied by the seasoned oil mixture in which they are preserved by pouring off the oil and letting them drain in a colander for a few minutes, then rinsing with cold water if sodium is a concern. Frozen artichoke hearts are uncompromised by added ingredients; simply cook them briefly until heated through.

Despite their sturdy appearance, artichokes are quite perishable. Place them in a plastic bag, sprinkle in a few drops of water to maintain moisture, and store in the vegetable crisper of your refrigerator, where they will keep for no more than four to five days. Do not rinse, wash, or trim artichokes before storing. To store cooked artichokes, allow them to cool, wrap them in cling film or place them in a plastic bag, and refrigerate. Thus treated, they should keep for four to five days.

TIPS FOR PREPARING

Rinse each artichoke well under cold running water or, holding it by the stem, swish it vigorously in a large bowl or basin of water. If the artichoke is not organically grown, soak in cold water with a mild solution of additive-free soap or use a produce wash (see page 50) and rinse. Once properly cleaned, with a large, sharp knife (don't use a carbon steel knife as it will cause cut parts to turn black), cut off the artichoke's topmost inch to remove the upper inedible leaf tips. Trim the tips of the remaining outer leaves with kitchen shears. To prevent cut parts from darkening, rub them with lemon juice or place the entire artichoke into a bowl of cold water with a tablespoon of either lemon juice or vinegar added. Immediately before cooking, clip or pull off any short, coarse leaves at the bottom, and cut the stem flush with the base. This will enable the artichoke to rest upright in the pot as it cooks and also makes for a more attractive presentation when it is served.

Artichokes can be steamed, baked, or boiled and are delicious eaten either hot or cold. Artichoke hearts can also be sautéed or stir-fried alone or with other vegetables in a small amount of broth or oil.

To steam artichokes, stand trimmed artichokes, stem end down, in a vegetable steamer and cook over boiling water. Or, in a nonreactive pot, stand enough artichokes together that they hold one another upright. Add an inch of boiling water and 2 tablespoons of vinegar or lemon juice or a lemon wedge to prevent darkening. Cover and simmer until you can easily pull out one of the inner leaves and a sharp knife easily pierces the base of the artichokes. The cooking time needed ranges from 25 to 40 minutes. If the artichokes are not done the first time you test, cook them an additional 5 minutes and test again. Before serving or stuffing, invert and drain the artichokes for a few minutes.

To boil artichokes, follow the same procedure given for steaming, but instead of using a vegetable steamer, fill the pot with water and bring to a boil. The addition of 1 tablespoon of either lemon juice or vinegar per litre of water will flavor the artichokes and prevent darkening. Lifting the lid a few times during cooking will also help the artichokes retain their color. Cooking time ranges from 20 to 40 minutes. Test as you would when steaming. Thoroughly drain the artichokes immediately after cooking by inverting them in a colander.

To bake artichokes, prepare them by steaming or boiling first. If desired, make "cups" as described below, and fill with stuffing. Stand filled artichokes upright in a baking dish and add some vegetable stock, white wine, or tomato sauce to prevent the vegetables from drying out. Cover with foil and bake for 20 to 30 minutes, until heated through.

If a recipe calls for the removal of the choke, so the artichoke provides a "cup" for stuffing, cook the vegetable by steaming or boiling first, and allow it to cool. Gently spread the outer leaves apart and pull out the thin rose or pale green petals covering the choke and the tuft of slender, hay-colored fibers resembling corn silk. Scrape out the choke with a teaspoon, and the artichoke cup is ready to be filled with stuffing (you may wish to use the choke in the stuffing). Either serve as is or bake to serve hot.

If a recipe uses only artichoke hearts or bottoms, remove all the leaves from the cooked artichoke and either save them to eat separately, or scrape off the flesh from the base of each leaf to mix in with the other ingredients. Remove the delicate petals covering the choke by scraping off with a teaspoon or paring knife. If desired, use a knife to trim the edges of the heart.

QUICK SERVING IDEAS

- Serve whole artichokes or quartered artichoke bottoms with a healthy dipping sauce. Try an olive oil and balsamic vinaigrette either as is, or with added garlic. To prepare the garlic, simply add several unpeeled cloves to the pot when cooking the artichokes. Mash the cloves to create a paste and add to the vinaigrette. For a sauce with an Asian flair, combine soy sauce, lemon juice or rice vinegar, minced garlic, and grated fresh ginger, and top with a dash of rich, dark sesame oil. For a rich creamy dip, plain whole yogurt makes an excellent base. Flavor it with puréed roasted red peppers; roasted aubergine, lemon juice and garlic; or a rich blue cheese- or buttermilk-based salad dressing.

- Stuff steamed or boiled artichokes with a mixture of cooked brown rice or quinoa, pine nuts or walnuts, and chopped vegetables, such as onions, mushrooms, sweet peppers, and broccoli. They can also be chilled after cooking and filled with tuna, prawns, salmon, or chicken salad.

- Quartered artichoke hearts can be used as a vegetable topping for whole-wheat pizza, as a filling for omelets, or as an addition to tossed salads, pasta, rice pilaf, tuna or chicken casseroles, or warm potato salad.

SAFETY

As a member of the Compositae (Asteraceae) family, the globe artichoke is related to daisies. Allergic hypersensitivity reactions may occur in individuals sensitive to daisies or other Compositae flowers, such as yarrow, calendula, chamomile, and dandelion.

Asparagus

Asparagus is a member of the lily family. Native to the Mediterranean, asparagus is now grown all over the world. Surprisingly, there are about 300 varieties of asparagus, but only twenty are edible. Asparagus has fleshy spears topped with budlike, compact heads. It is usually harvested in the spring when it is 6 to 8 inches/15 to 20 centimeters tall. Normally green or greenish purple in color, white asparagus is grown underground to inhibit its development of chlorophyll content in order to provide a more delicate flavor and color for a unique culinary experience.

HISTORY

Asparagus originated in the eastern Mediterranean region, as well as in northern and southern Africa. There is evidence that it was first cultivated in ancient Egypt, where it was prized not only as a food but also for its medicinal properties. Today, asparagus is cultivated in most subtropical and temperate parts of the world including Britain, with the majority of commercially available asparagus grown in the United States, Mexico, Peru, France, Spain, and other Mediterranean countries.

NUTRITIONAL HIGHLIGHTS

Asparagus is low in calories and carbohydrates, but relatively rich in protein compared to other vegetables. One cup of asparagus supplies only 24 calories, almost half of which are derived from protein. Asparagus is an excellent source of potassium, vitamin K, folic acid (263 micrograms per cup), vitamins C and A, riboflavin, thiamine, and vitamin B6; and it has an excellent ratio of potassium (288 milligrams per cup) to sodium (19.8 milligrams per cup). Asparagus is also a very good source of dietary fiber, niacin, phosphorus, protein, and iron.

HEALTH BENEFITS

Asparagus has historically been used in the treatment of arthritis and rheumatism, and as a diuretic. The diuretic effect of asparagus may be due to the amino acid asparagine, which when excreted in the urine gives off a strong, characteristic odor. The benefit in arthritis may be the result of recently identified unique phytochemical antioxidants (racemofuran, asparagamine A, and racemosol) as well as inhibitors of the COX-2 enzyme, which produces inflammatory compounds.

HOW TO SELECT AND STORE

The best-quality asparagus is firm and the tips are closed. In general, the darker the stalk, the higher the concentration of nutrients. Once trimmed and cooked, asparagus loses about half its total weight, so buy about half a pound/250 grams per person when purchasing this vegetable fresh for use as part of a main dish.

Asparagus is perishable and loses many nutrients, as well as its flavor, if it is not used within a day or two after purchasing. To maintain freshness as long as possible, store in the refrigerator with the ends wrapped in a damp paper towel.

TIPS FOR PREPARING

Wash asparagus under cold running water and gently scrub with a vegetable brush. If it is not organically grown, soak in cold water with a mild solution of additive-free soap or use a produce wash (see page 51) and rinse.

Asparagus is most often prepared by lightly

steaming the entire spear, or cutting the spear diagonally and stir-frying. Snap off the tough stem ends of the asparagus by holding a spear in both hands and bending; it will break where the tender and tough parts meet. Be sure to wash asparagus under cold water to remove any sand or soil residues before cooking.

If you love asparagus and eat it often, invest in an asparagus steamer, a tall, narrow steamer that allows asparagus to be cooked to perfection. Avoid cooking asparagus in an iron pot, as the tannins in the asparagus can react with the iron and cause the stalks to become discolored. After cooking, asparagus can be served hot or cold. If your recipe calls for cold asparagus, plunge the stalks into cold water immediately after cooking, then remove them quickly; letting them soak too long can cause them to become soggy.

Roasting asparagus is another simple and flavorful technique. Simply mix asparagus with an oil or oil-based vinaigrette and your favorite herbs and spices. Place it in a roasting dish and bake at 400 degrees F./200 degrees C./gas 6 for 10 minutes. If other vegetables are added, be sure that they cook quickly or are thinly sliced, given the short cooking time of this dish.

QUICK SERVING IDEAS

- Asparagus can be roasted alone or along with other vegetables, such as yams, squash, and potatoes.
- Chilled, steamed asparagus served with a light lemon vinaigrette makes a delightfully refreshing salad.
- Steamed asparagus can be puréed with stock and seasoning to make a delicious soup.
- Add steamed asparagus to freshly cooked

pasta and toss along with haricot beans, olive oil, thyme, tarragon, and rosemary.
- Finely chopped raw asparagus makes a flavorful and colorful addition to omelets.
- Stir-fry asparagus with garlic, shiitake mushrooms, and chicken (or tofu).

SAFETY

People not familiar with asparagus are often alarmed by the strong odor coming from their urine after eating it. Several different chemicals contribute to the smell, most notably asparagine. Different people form different amounts of these chemicals after eating asparagus, and many people cannot smell the odor, even when they produce the chemicals.

Asparagus contains low amounts of oxalate. Individuals with a history of oxalate-containing kidney stones should avoid overconsuming this food. For more information, see Appendix D, page 793.

Asparagus contains a moderate amount of purines, so individuals with gout should limit their consumption of this food.

Aubergine

Aubergine (*Solanum melongena*) belongs to the nightshade plant family (Solanaceae) along with the tomato and potato. In fact, aubergines grow in a manner much like tomatoes, hanging

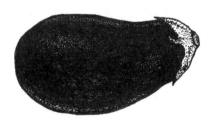

from the vines of a plant that grows several feet in height.

The most popular variety of aubergine looks like a large, pear-shaped egg, hence the American name "egg plant." It has a deep purple, glossy skin encasing a flesh that is cream-colored, with seeds arranged in a conical pattern and a spongy consistency. In addition to this classic variety, aubergine is available in other colors, including lavender, jade green, orange, and yellow-white, as well as in sizes and shapes that range from that of a small tomato to that of a large courgette.

HISTORY

The modern aubergine owes its origin to the wild version that grew in India. Around the fifth century B.C.E., the plant was first cultivated in China, and prior to the Middle Ages it was introduced in Africa, then in Italy. It then spread throughout Europe and the Middle East. The aubergine was brought to the Western Hemisphere by European explorers.

For centuries after its introduction to Europe, aubergine was used more as a decorative garden plant than as a food. Not until new varieties were developed in the eighteenth century did aubergine lose its bitter taste and bitter reputation. Although the aubergine is now cultivated worldwide, China is still the world's leading producer, followed by Japan, Turkey, and Italy.

NUTRITIONAL HIGHLIGHTS

Aubergine is an excellent source of dietary fiber, with 2.5 grams per 100 gram serving. It's also a very good source of vitamins B1 and B6 and potassium. In addition, aubergine is a good source of copper, magnesium, manganese, phosphorus, niacin, and folic acid.

HEALTH BENEFITS

Research on aubergine has focused on an anthocyanin flavonoid found in aubergine skin called nasunin. A potent antioxidant and free-radical scavenger, nasunin has been shown to protect cell membranes from damage. In animal studies, nasunin has been found to protect the lipids (fats) in brain cell membranes. Cell membranes are almost entirely composed of lipids and are responsible for protecting the cell from free radicals, letting nutrients in and wastes out, and receiving instructions from messenger molecules that tell the cell which activities it should perform.

Nasunin is not only a potent free-radical scavenger, but it also helps move excess iron out of the body. Although iron is an essential nutrient and is necessary for oxygen transport, normal immune function, and collagen synthesis, too much iron is not a good thing. Excess iron increases free-radical production and is associated with an increased risk of heart disease and cancer. Menstruating women, who lose iron every month in their menstrual flow, are unlikely to be at risk, but in postmenopausal women and men, iron, which is not easily excreted, can accumulate. By helping to bind excess iron, nasunin lessens free-radical formation with numerous beneficial results, including protecting blood cholesterol (which is also a type of lipid or fat) from becoming a highly reactive toxic form; preventing cellular damage that can promote cancer; and lessening free-radical damage in joints, which is a primary factor in arthritis.

Aubergine may also help to lower cholesterol levels. When rabbits with high cholesterol were given aubergine juice, their blood cholesterol, the cholesterol in their artery walls, and the cholesterol in their aortas (the aorta is the main artery that carries blood from the heart) was significantly reduced, while the walls of their blood vessels relaxed, improving blood flow. These positive effects were likely due not only to nasunin but to other phytochemicals in aubergine known as terpenes.

HOW TO SELECT AND STORE

On visual inspection, the skin color should be vivid, shiny, and free of discoloration, scars, and bruises, which usually indicate that the flesh beneath has become damaged and possibly decayed. The stem and cap on the end of the aubergine should also be free of discoloration. Choose aubergines that are firm and heavy for their size. To test the ripeness of an aubergine, gently press the skin with the pad of your thumb. If it springs back, the aubergine is ripe; if an indentation remains, it is not.

Aubergines are actually very perishable, being sensitive to both heat and cold. Store them whole in a plastic bag and store in the refrigerator, where they will keep for a few days. If you cut an aubergine before you store it, it will decay quickly. Once cooked, aubergine can be stored in the refrigerator for up to three days.

TIPS FOR PREPARING

Wash the aubergine first under cold running water and gently scrub with a soft vegetable brush. If it is not organically grown, peel away the outer peel and soak in cold water with a mild solution of additive-free soap or use a produce wash and rinse thoroughly. After washing it, cut off the ends. It is important to use a stainless-steel knife, as carbon steel will react with the phytochemicals and cause the aubergine to turn black.

Most aubergines can be eaten either with or without their skin. However, the skin of larger aubergines is generally a bit tough and unpalatable. To remove skin, you can peel it before cutting, or if you are baking it, you can scoop out the flesh once it is cooked.

It is often recommended to tenderize aubergine to reduce some of its bitter taste by salting it. After cutting the aubergine into the desired size and shape, sprinkle it with salt and allow it to rest for about 30 minutes. This process pulls out some of the aubergine's water content and along with it some of the bitter components. If you need to restrict your sodium intake, simply rinse the salt off.

Aubergine can be baked, stir-fried, steamed, or grilled. If baking it whole, pierce the aubergine several times with a fork to make small holes for the steam to escpe. Bake at 350 degrees F./180 degrees C./gas 4 for 15 to 25 minutes, depending upon size. The aubergine is done when a knife or fork can easily pass through it.

QUICK SERVING IDEAS

- Add cubed aubergine to your next stir-fry.
- Mix 2 cups cubed, roasted aubergine with 2 grilled peppers, 1 cup cooked lentils, ½ cup diced red onion, and 1 clove raw, mashed garlic and top with a balsamic vinaigrette.
- For homemade baba ganoush, mix 1 - medium puréed roasted aubergine, 2 cloves garlic, 3 tablespoons tahini, 2 tablespoons lemon juice, and 1 tablespoon olive oil. Use it as a dip for vegetables or as a sandwich filling.

- Create an easy grilled sandwich by melting mozzarella cheese over sliced roasted aubergine placed on crusty whole-grain bread.
- Stuff roasted aubergine boats with a mixture of equal parts of feta cheese, pine nuts, and roasted peppers.

SAFETY

Aubergine is one of the vegetables in the nightshade (Solanaceae) family, which includes bell pepper, tomatoes, and potatoes. Anecdotal case histories link improvement in arthritic symptoms with removal of these foods. Although no case-controlled scientific studies confirm these observations, some individuals consuming nightshade-family vegetables experience an aggravation of arthritic symptoms and may benefit from limiting or avoiding these foods.

Aubergine contains significant amounts of oxalate. Individuals with a history of oxalate-containing kidney stones should avoid over-consuming them. For more information, see Appendix D, page 793.

Beans: See Chapter 13, "The Healing Power of Legumes."

Beets

The beet *(Beta vulgaris)* or beetroot belongs to the same family as chard and spinach (Chenopodiaceae). However, unlike these greens, both the root and the leaves of beets are eaten. Beet leaves have a lively, bitter taste similar to that of chard. Attached to the beet's green leaves is a round or oblong root. Although typically a reddish purple hue, beets also come in varieties that feature white or golden roots. Because of their high sugar content, beets are delicious when eaten raw but are more typically cooked or pickled. Beets are the main ingredient in borscht, a traditional eastern European soup.

HISTORY

The wild beet originated in North Africa and grew along Asian and European seashores. Like many modern vegetables, beets were first cultivated by the ancient Romans. The tribes that invaded Rome were responsible for spreading beets throughout northern Europe.

The commercial value of beets grew in the nineteenth century, when it was discovered that they could be converted into sugar. When access to sugarcane was restricted by the British, Napoleon decreed that the beet be used as the primary source of sugar. Today the leading commercial producers of beets include the United States, the Russian Federation, France, Poland, and Germany.

NUTRITIONAL HIGHLIGHTS

Beet greens are higher in nutritional value than beetroots, as they are richer in calcium, iron, and vitamins A and C. Beetroots are an excellent source of folic acid and a very good source of fiber, manganese, and potassium. Beet greens and roots are a good source of magnesium, phosphorus, iron, and vitamin B6.

A 100 gram serving of beet greens contains 27 calories and 3 grams of fiber, while the same serving of cooked beetroot provides 44 calories with 10 grams of carbohydrate, primarily as 8 grams of sugars.

HEALTH BENEFITS

Beetroots have long been used for medicinal purposes, primarily for disorders of the liver, given their stimulating effects on the liver's detoxification processes. Beets have also gained recognition for their reported anticancer properties. The pigment that gives beets their rich, purple-crimson color, betacyanin, is a powerful cancer-fighting agent. Beet fiber has been shown to have a favorable effect on bowel function and cholesterol levels, too.

The combination of their betacyanin and fiber content is probably responsible for the protective role of beets against colon cancer. In animal studies, beet fiber has been shown to increase the level of the antioxidant enzymes, specifically glutathione peroxidase and glutathione-*S*-transferase, as well as increase the number of special white blood cells responsible for detecting and eliminating abnormal cells. In a study of patients with stomach cancer, beet juice was found to be a potent inhibitor of the formation of nitrosamines (cancer-causing compounds derived primarily from the ingestion of nitrates from smoked or cured meats) as well as the cell mutations caused by these compounds.

HOW TO SELECT AND STORE

Good-quality beets should have their greens intact. The greens should be fresh-looking, with no signs of spoilage. Slightly flabby greens can be restored to freshness if stored in the refrigerator in water; if it is too late, you can simply cut off the greens. The beetroot should be firm, smooth, and a vibrant red-purple, not soft, wrinkled, and dull-colored. Fresh beets with the greens attached can be stored for three to five

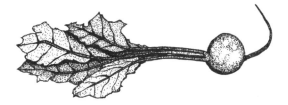

days in the refrigerator, but beets with the greens removed can be stored in the refrigerator for two to four weeks.

If you will be storing beets for longer than a couple of days, cut the majority of the greens and their stems from the roots, so they do not pull moisture away from the root. Leave about two inches of the stem attached to prevent the roots from "bleeding." Store the unwashed greens in a separate perforated plastic bag, where they will keep fresh for about four days.

Raw beets do not freeze well since they tend to become soft upon thawing. Freezing cooked beets is fine; they'll retain their flavor and texture.

TIPS FOR PREPARING

Wash beets gently under cool running water, taking care not to tear the skin—this tough outer layer helps keep most of the beets' pigments inside the vegetable. If the beets are not organically grown, soak them in cold water with a mild solution of additive-free soap or use a produce wash and rinse (see page 51).

Beet greens are typically prepared by steaming. Be sure to cook them lightly to retain their anticancer effects. When boiling beetroots, leave the beets with their root ends and one inch of stem attached; and don't peel them until after cooking since beet juice can stain your skin. If your hands become stained during the cleaning and cooking process, rubbing some lemon juice on them will remove the stain.

The color of beets can be altered during cooking if desired. Adding an acidic ingredient, such as lemon juice or vinegar, will brighten the color, while an alkaline substance, such as bicarbonate of soda, will often cause them to turn a deeper purple. Salt will blunt beets' color, so add it only at the end of cooking, if needed.

QUICK SERVING IDEAS

- Raw beetroot can be grated for use in salads and as a garnish for soups. Not only does it add excellent nutrition, it also adds flavor and color.
- Beet greens can also be used in salads in place of lettuce.
- Beetroots can be roasted with other vegetables in the oven or under the grill.
- Lightly sauté beet greens with other greens, such as chard and mustard greens.
- Swirl puréed cooked beetroot and stewed apples together with cinnamon and nutmeg to make a colorful and delicious snack or dessert.
- Beet juice is a delicious way to increase your nutrient intake. However, start with a small amount of juice, such as ½ to 1 fluid ounce/15 to 30 milliliters, mixed with other juices, such as carrot and apple. Larger amounts of beet juice may cause an upset stomach.

SAFETY

Some people eating beets may experience beeturia, a red or pink color in the urine or stool; it is a totally harmless condition.

Beet greens and, to a lesser extent, the roots contain high levels of oxalate. Individuals with a history of oxalate-containing kidney stones should avoid overconsuming beetroot and beet greens. For more information, see Appendix D, page 793.

Bell Peppers

The bell pepper (*Capsicum annuum*) is a member of the Solanaceae, or nightshade, family of vegetables, which includes potatoes, aubergines, and tomatoes. Bell peppers are native to Central and South America. They are available in several colors: green and purple peppers have a slightly bitter flavor, while red, orange, and yellow peppers are sweeter and almost fruity. Red bell peppers are actually green peppers that have been allowed to ripen on the vine; hence they are much sweeter. The spices pimento and paprika are both prepared from red bell peppers.

HISTORY

Like many other nightshade vegetables, bell peppers originated in South America at least 7,000 years ago. Like many of the other foods native to the Americas, bell peppers were spread to Europe and throughout the world by Spanish and Portuguese explorers. Because bell peppers adapt very well to different climates, they grow in both tropical and temperate climates, and their cultivation and adoption into varying cuisines spread rapidly throughout many parts of the world. In fact, they have become an integral ingredient in both Spanish and Portuguese cuisines. Currently, the main producers of bell peppers are China, Turkey, Spain, Romania, Nigeria, and Mexico.

NUTRITIONAL HIGHLIGHTS

Bell peppers are one of the most nutrient-dense foods available. Though a 100 gram serving of raw bell pepper provides only 20 calories (mostly as carbohydrate and fiber), it is a good source of a large number of nutrients, including vitamin C, beta-carotene, vitamin K, thiamine, folic acid, and vitamin B6. Bell peppers are also a very good source of phytochemicals with exceptional antioxidant activity, such as chlorogenic acid, coumeric acid, and zeaxanthin. Red bell peppers have significantly higher levels of nutrients than green. Red bell peppers also contain lycopene, a carotene that offers protection against cancer and heart disease.

HEALTH BENEFITS

Studies have shown that bell peppers exert a protective effect against cataracts, possibly due to their vitamin C and beta-carotene content. However, like other nutrient-dense vegetables, they contain many different powerful phytochemicals. In one study, Italian researchers compared the presurgery diets of 207 hospital patients who had cataracts removed with 706 patients who did not have to have the operation. Consumption of bell peppers was associated with a reduced risk for cataract surgery.

Bell peppers also contain substances, including capsaicin, flavonoids, and vitamin C, which have been shown to prevent blood clot formation and reduce the risk of heart attacks and strokes. Although they are not as rich in these compounds as chili peppers, nonetheless bell pepper consumption should be promoted for individuals with elevated cholesterol levels. For more information on chili peppers, see "Cayenne," page 474.

HOW TO SELECT AND STORE

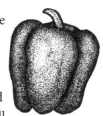

Bell peppers are available throughout the year but are usually more abundant during the summer months. They should be fresh, firm, and bright in appearance. Avoid bell peppers that appear dry, are wrinkled, or show signs of decay, including injuries to the skin or water-soaked areas. Bell peppers should be heavy for their size and firm enough that they gently yield to slight pressure. Be aware that the shape of the bell pepper does not generally affect the quality.

Unwashed bell peppers stored in the vegetable compartment of the refrigerator will keep for up to one week. Bell peppers can be frozen without first being blanched, but it is better to freeze them whole since there will be less exposure to air, which can degrade both their nutrient content and their flavor.

TIPS FOR PREPARING

Wash bell peppers thoroughly under cold running water with a soft vegetable brush before coring and/or cutting. If the pepper has been waxed or is not organically grown, you will need to spray it with or soak it in a mild solution of additive-free soap or use a produce wash before washing. To remove the stem, use a paring knife to cut around it and then pull it out. Bell peppers can be cut into various shapes and sizes or left whole to be stuffed after carefully removing the seeds from the inner cavity.

QUICK SERVING IDEAS

- Raw bell peppers can be used in vegetable juices, salads, and vegetable trays.

- Bell peppers can be used in casseroles, stir-fries, and other recipes.
- Finely chopped bell peppers can be added to tuna or chicken salad.
- Steam cored bell peppers for 5 minutes, stuff them with your favorite rice salad or grain pilaf, and bake in a 350 degree F./180 degrees C./gas 4 oven until they are hot.
- For a simple Louisiana Creole dish: Lightly sauté chopped bell peppers, celery, and onions, then combine with tofu, chicken, or seafood.
- Grill bell peppers marinated in olive oil, garlic, lemon juice, and black pepper.

SAFETY

Buy organic bell peppers whenever possible, as bell peppers are among the top foods on which pesticide residues have been most frequently found. Bell peppers are one of the vegetables in the nightshade (Solanaceae) family, which includes aubergine, tomatoes, and potatoes. Anecdotal case histories link improvement in arthritic symptoms with removal of these foods. Although no case-controlled scientific studies confirm these observations, some individuals consuming nightshade family vegetables experience an aggravation of arthritic symptoms and may benefit from limiting or avoiding these foods.

Bell peppers contain low to moderate amounts of oxalate. Individuals with a history of oxalate-containing kidney stones should avoid overconsuming them. For more information, see Appendix D, page 793.

Bitter Melon

Bitter melon (*Momordica charantia*) is a green cucumber-shaped fruit with gourdlike bumps all over it. In fact, it looks like an ugly cucumber. And, like the cucumber, bitter melon is a member of the Cucurbitaceae, or gourd family, along with squash and watermelon. The name of the plant's genus, *Momordica,* comes from the Latin word meaning "to bite," a reference to its seeds, whose edges are serrated as if they had been chewed or bitten.

Bitter melon is a fast-growing, slender, climbing vine with long-stalked leaves. It produces yellow flowers in July and/or August. Bitter melon is native to the tropical areas of Asia, Africa, India, the Caribbean, and South America.

The fruit of the bitter melon is also known as the balsam pear. Inside it is filled with large seeds loosely packed in its white, spongy flesh. The fruit appears from September to October. It is light to emerald green when young, turning yellow-orange as it ripens. At maturity, the fruit tends to split open, revealing orange flesh with a bright red placenta to which numerous tan or white seeds are attached.

Usually the bitter-flavored unripe fruit is used as a vegetable. Although it is one of the most popular vegetables in China, Taiwan, Vietnam, India, and the Philippines, bitter melon is an acquired taste for most Westerners.

HISTORY

Bitter melon grows well in warm temperatures and is thought to have originated in Africa or Asia, but it is now a relatively common food in tropical regions around the world. Virtually everywhere it grows, bitter melon has been used medicinally. Native healers in the Amazon to Ayurvedic doctors in India have used bitter melon to treat diabetes as it is a natural hypoglycemic (blood sugar–lowering) agent. In the Amazon, fruit juice and/or a tea made from the leaves is also employed to treat colic, sores and wounds, infections, worms and parasites, measles, hepatitis, fevers, and as an emmenogogue (a medication that brings on or increases a woman's menstrual flow). In India, the plant is used to treat hemorrhoids, abdominal discomfort, fever, warm infections, and skin diseases, especially scabies (a skin disease caused by a mite that burrows into the skin). To treat scabies, practitioners of Ayurvedic medicine extract the juice from the leaf of bitter melon and apply it externally to the affected area.

In the Philippines, bitter melon has been used for centuries as a remedy for diabetes, leukemia, asthma, insect bites, menstrual cycle problems, and stomach problems. And in traditional Chinese medicine, it is used as an appetite stimulant; as a treatment for gastrointestinal infection, dry coughs, bronchitis, and throat problems; and to combat breast cancer. The seeds are also applied topically for skin swellings caused by sprains and fractures, and for sores that are slow to heal.

NUTRITIONAL HIGHLIGHTS

Bitter melon is low in calories—a whole cup of cooked bitter melon is only 23.5 calories—but dense in nutrients. Bitter melon is an excellent source of vitamin C, folic acid, zinc, potassium, and dietary fiber; a very good source of thiamine, riboflavin, vitamin E, magnesium, and manganese; and a good source of pantothenic acid and copper.

HEALTH BENEFITS

The hypoglycemic effect of the fresh juice of the unripe bitter melon has been confirmed in scientific studies in animals and humans. Bitter melon contains a compound known as charantin that is even more potent than the drug tolbutamide, which is often used in the treatment of diabetes to lower blood sugar levels. Bitter melon also contains an insulinlike compound referred to as polypeptide P, or vegetable insulin. Since polypeptide P and bitter melon appear to have fewer side effects than insulin, they have been suggested as replacements for insulin in some patients. However, it may not be necessary to inject these insulin alternatives, as the oral administration of as little as 2 fluid ounces/60 millilitres of bitter melon juice has shown good results in clinical trials in patients with diabetes.

Bitter melon has also been found to contain antiviral proteins. Two of these proteins, which are present in the seeds, fruit, and leaves of bitter melon, have been shown to inhibit the AIDS virus *in vitro* (in test-tube studies). In 1996, the scientists conducting this research filed a U.S. patent on a novel protein they found and extracted from the fruit and seeds of bitter melon, which they named "MAP 30." Their patent states that MAP 30 is "useful for treating tumors and HIV infections." MAP 30 has also demonstrated powerful antiviral activity against other viruses, including the herpes simplex virus.

In addition, the ripe fruit of bitter melon has been shown to exhibit some rather profound anticancer effects, especially against leukemia.

HOW TO SELECT AND STORE

Unripe bitter melon is available primarily at Asian greengrocers. The unripe fruit should be firm, like a cucumber. Avoid fruits that have turned orange or have soft spots. Growers are advised to harvest young bitter melon fruits eight to ten days after the flowers open, while the fruits are still firm and light green. The fruits at this stage are typically 4 to 6 inches/10 to 15 centimeters long. Beyond this stage, fruits will turn yellow-orange and become spongy and excessively bitter.

Bitter melon can be stored in the fruit bin of the refrigerator covered and unwashed for four to five days. This fruit is delicate and should be handled with care. It is sensitive to cold and should not be stored below 50 degrees F./10 degrees C. Symptoms of cold exposure include pitting, discolored areas, and a high incidence of decay. On the other hand, fruits stored at temperatures greater than 55 degrees F./13 degrees C. tend to continue to ripen, turning yellow and splitting open.

Store bitter melon away from apples, pears, potatoes, and other fruits and vegetables that produce ethylene gas, since it will cause the fruit to continue to ripen and become more bitter.

TIPS FOR PREPARING

Wash bitter melon thoroughly under cold running water with a soft vegetable brush. If it has been waxed or is not organically grown, you will need to spray it with or soak it in a mild solution of additive-free soap or use a produce wash before eating. Slice bitter melon lengthwise and scoop out the seeds as you might with a cucumber. Unlike cucumbers, however, the seeds of a bitter melon should always be removed. To lessen the bitter flavor, soak bitter melon in salt water or parboil with a little salt before cooking.

QUICK SERVING IDEAS

- Bitter melon is often very difficult to make palatable for Westerners. As its name implies, it is quite bitter. If you desire the medicinal effects, it is best to simply take a 2 fluid ounce/60 milliliter shot of the juice.
- Bitter melon is typically used as a flavor-enhancing addition in recipes, as all parts of the plant, as its name suggests, have a very bitter taste and add an astringent sour quality to a dish.
- Bitter melon dishes are a favorite in Bengal, where they are eaten at the start of a meal with plain boiled rice, since serving bitter foods at the beginning of a meal is thought to get the digestive juices flowing.
- The most famous Bengali way of eating bitter melon is in a stew of bitter melon and other vegetables known as *shukto*. To make *shukto*, dice about 1 cup each of bitter melon, potato, plantain (green banana), aubergine, onion, and taro (kalo), along with about ½ cup of radish. Stir-fry the vegetables in a little rapeseed oil. Add 1 teaspoon each of grated ginger and mustard seed. Then add 2 cups cooked lentils, and stir to mix the ingredients well. Next, add salt and sugar to taste, enough water to form a thick-soup consistency, and bring to a boil. Cover and simmer until heated through. Serve with rice.

- In any vegetable stew, bitter melon accentuates the mix of flavors, especially when combined with blander vegetables, such as okra, onions, potatoes, and aubergine.
- Bitter melons are also enjoyed as part of other vegetable curries, for example, stir-fried with potatoes or curried with aubergine and onions. *Thito* is a popular bitter melon curry dish. To prepare it, heat some rapeseed oil in a deep pot or wok and stir-fry three large or four medium sliced onions. Add liberal amounts of chili, cumin, and turmeric powders and stir well. Add equal amounts (1 to 2 cups each) of cubed aubergine and bitter melon. Stir-fry for several minutes, then add salt and a little water if needed. Cover and simmer until the vegetables are cooked through. Serve with plain cooked rice.
- Another delicious way to enjoy bitter melon is to slice it into ¼-inch/6mm slices (after it has been cut in half lengthwise and seeded) and then sauté it briefly with sliced onions and tomatoes. Add scrambled eggs and other seasonings to taste.
- Try *korola bhaté* (mashed bitter melon): Parboil green bitter melons until soft, slice in half lengthwise and scoop out the seeds, then mash. Add an equal amount of mashed boiled potatoes. Saute a handful of dried red chili peppers in olive oil and add to the mashed bitter melon/potato mixture. Mix well, salt to taste, and serve with rice.

SAFETY

Consuming excessive amounts of bitter melon—several melons or 6 to 8 ounces/175 to 250 millilitres of fresh juice—may cause mild abdominal pain or diarrhea. When bitter melon is prescribed as a therapeutic agent in diabetes, patients are told to eat one small melon or take no more than 60 milliliters (30 milliliters = 1 fluid ounce) per day. Diabetics taking hypoglycemic drugs, such as chlorpropamide, glibenclamide, or metformin, may need to alter the dosage of these drugs if they consume bitter melon on a daily basis.

Bitter melon should not be eaten by pregnant women because the active constituents (alpha- and beta-monorcharins) in bitter melon have been shown to stimulate the uterus and may cause preterm labor.

In animal studies, bitter melon seed extracts have been shown to have male antifertility effects, specifically, reduction of sperm production. Such adverse effects have not been reported in humans, however, despite widespread consumption of the fruits.

Broccoli

Broccoli is a member of the cruciferous, or cabbage, family of vegetables. Its name is derived from the Latin *brachium,* meaning "branch" or "arm," a reflection of its treelike shape featuring a compact head of florets attached by small stems to a larger stalk. Broccoli provides a complex of tastes and textures, ranging from the soft and flowery florets to the fibrous and crunchy stem and stalk. Its color can range from deep sage to dark green to purplish green, depending upon the variety. The most popular type of broccoli sold in the United States and the U.K. is known as Italian green, or Calabrese, named after the Italian province of Calabria, where it first grew.

Other vegetables related to broccoli are broccolini, a mix of broccoli and kale, and broccoflower, a cross between broccoli and cauliflower. Broccoli sprouts have also recently become popular as a result of research disclosing their high concentration of the anticancer phytochemical sulphoraphane.

HISTORY

Broccoli developed from a wild cabbage native to Europe. There are indications it has been known in Europe for 2,000 years. It was improved upon by the Romans and later-day Italians and is now cultivated throughout the world. Broccoli was introduced to the United States in colonial times and popularized by Italian immigrants who brought this prized vegetable with them to the New World. But it was not a popular vegetable until the 1920s.

In 1923 D'Arrigo Bros. Company planted trial fields of Italian sprouting broccoli near San Jose, California, and later shipped the first ice-packed broccoli to eastern markets via railroad in the autumn of 1924. In 1929, D'Arrigo started what is thought to be the first direct advertising programme for broccoli with a cooperative radio programme in Italian and space in some Italian-language newspapers. Development of the broccoli industry within California was rapid after this renewed popularity in the Italian communities on the East Coast.

NUTRITIONAL HIGHLIGHTS

Though low in calories, broccoli is one of the most nutrient-dense foods. It is especially rich in vitamin C. A one-cup serving of broccoli provides about the same amount of protein as a cup of corn or rice but less than one third the amount of calories. Broccoli is an excellent source of vitamins K, C, and A, as well as folic acid and fiber. It is a very good source of phosphorus, potassium, magnesium, and the vitamins B6 and E. It also contains glucosinolates, phytochemicals with tremendous anticancer effects, and the carotenoid lutein.

A 100 gram serving of cooked broccoli provides 35 calories, 2.3 grams of protein, no cholesterol, 0.4 grams of fat, 7.2 grams of carbohydrate, and 3.3 grams of fiber.

HEALTH BENEFITS

Broccoli, like other members of the cabbage family (see "Cabbage," page 178), demonstrates remarkable anticancer effects, particularly in breast cancer. Compounds in broccoli known as glucosinolates, specifically indole-3-carbinol and sulphoraphane, increase the excretion of the form of oestrogen (2-hydroxyestrone) linked to breast cancer.

Sulforaphane was first identified in broccoli sprouts grown in plastic laboratory dishes by scientists at the Johns Hopkins University School of Medicine in Baltimore, Maryland. These researchers were investigating the anticancer compounds present in broccoli when they discovered that broccoli sprouts contain anywhere from thirty to fifty times the concentration of protective chemicals that are found in mature broccoli plants. In fact, feeding sulphoraphane-rich broccoli sprout extracts to laboratory rats exposed to a standard carcinogen dramatically reduced the frequency, size, and number of tumors they developed. Human studies with sulphoraphane have shown that these compounds stimulate the body's production of detoxification enzymes and exert antioxidant effects.

Indole-3-carbinol is also an important cancer-fighting compound, as it has been shown to arrest growth of both breast and prostate cancer cells in preliminary studies. It also increases the ability of the liver to detoxify toxic compounds as well as decreases the growth of human papillomavirus (a virus linked to cervical cancer).

Preliminary studies suggest that, in order to cut the risk of cancer in half, the average person would need to eat about 2 pounds/1 kilogram of broccoli or similar vegetables per week. Because the concentration of sulphoraphane is much higher in broccoli sprouts than in mature broccoli, the same reduction in risk theoretically might be had with a weekly intake of just a little over an ounce/30 grams of sprouts.

Sulphoraphane may also be proven to be effective in helping the body get rid of *Helicobacter pylori.* This bacterium is responsible for most peptic ulcers and also increases a person's risk of getting gastric cancer three- to sixfold. It is also a causative factor in a wide range of other stomach disorders, including gastritis, oesophagitis, and acid indigestion.

Broccoli is also a rich source of lutein, which has also shown anticancer effects. It may also be helpful in preventing the development of age-related macular degeneration, as this carotenoid is concentrated in the retina, where it acts to protect it from damage.

HOW TO SELECT AND STORE

Broccoli should be deep sage, dark green, or purplish green depending on the variety. The stalks and stems should be firm. Yellowed or wilted leaves indicate loss of much of the nutritional value. Avoid wilted, soft, and noticeably aged broccoli.

Broccoli is very perishable and should be stored in an open plastic bag in the refrigerator crisper, where it will keep for about four days. Since water on the surface will encourage its degradation, do not wash broccoli before refrigerating, or else use washed broccoli the same day you wash it. Broccoli that has been blanched and then frozen can be stored for up to one year. Leftover cooked broccoli should be placed in a tightly covered container and stored in the refrigerator, where it will keep for a few days.

Broccoli sprouts should have green tops and white stalks. They are usually sold in covered packages to keep them from drying out. Be sure to smell them, as growth without good water circulation causes bacterial growth. Well-grown sprouts of any kind should smell fresh, without any unpleasant odor. Sprouts do not keep very long, so use within four days of purchasing. As a rule, sprouts do not withstand freezing.

TIPS FOR PREPARING

Wash broccoli under cold running water and gently scrub with a vegetable brush. If it is not organically grown, soak in cold water with a mild solution of additive-free soap or use a produce wash and rinse.

Broccoli can be eaten raw or cooked and served hot or cold. Since the fibrous stems take longer to cook, they can be cooked separately for a few minutes before adding the florets. For quicker cooking, make lengthwise slits in the stems. While people do not generally eat the leaves, they are perfectly edible and contain concentrated amounts of nutrients.

Broccoli sprouts are eaten raw and can be added to cooked dishes just before serving.

QUICK SERVING IDEAS

- Layer broccoli sprouts on top of salads and vegetable dishes for an added cancer-fighting action.
- Add broccoli florets and chopped stalks to salads or omelets, or simply use as a crudité.
- Broccoli can be lightly steamed for 9 to 12 minutes, sautéed, or stir-fried.
- Sprinkle lemon juice and sesame seeds over lightly steamed broccoli.
- Sauté broccoli florets in olive oil with pine nuts, and garlic and toss with pasta. Add salt and pepper to taste.
- Purée cooked broccoli and cauliflower, then add seasonings of your choice to make a simple, yet delicious soup. Add vegetable stock if required.

SAFETY

Members of the cabbage family contain goitrogens, naturally occurring substances that can interfere with the functioning of the thyroid gland. Dietary goitrogens are usually of no clinical importance unless they are consumed in large amounts or there is coexisting iodine deficiency. Cooking helps to inactivate the goitrogenic compounds. Individuals with already existing and untreated thyroid problems may want to avoid consumption of cabbage-family vegetables in their raw form for this reason. (See "Cabbage," page 178, for more information.)

Brussels Sprouts

Like broccoli, Brussels sprouts developed from the wild cabbage. They resemble miniature cabbages, with a diameter of about 1 inch/2.5 cm. Brussels sprouts grow in groups of twenty to forty along the stems of plants that grow as high as three feet/one meter tall. Brussels sprouts are typically sage green in color, although some varieties feature a red hue. They are normally sold separately but can be found in farmers' markets still attached to the stem.

HISTORY

The first mention of Brussels sprouts occurred in the late 1500s near Brussels, Belgium. They remained primarily a local crop in this area until their use spread across Europe during World War I, though Thomas Jefferson introduced Brussels sprouts to North America in 1812. Brussels sprouts are now cultivated throughout Europe and the United States. In the United States, almost all Brussels sprouts are grown in California.

NUTRITIONAL HIGHLIGHTS

Brussels sprouts are similar in nutritional quality to broccoli. They are an excellent source of folic acid, vitamins C and K, and beta-carotene. Brussels sprouts are a very good source of vitamin B6, fiber, thiamine, and potassium. In addition to these nutrients, Brussels sprouts contain numerous cancer-fighting phytochemicals in the form of glucosinolates.

A 100 gram serving of cooked Brussels sprouts provides 35 calories, 2.3 grams of protein, no cholesterol, 0.4 grams of fat, 7.2 grams of carbohydrate, and 3.3 grams of fiber.

HEALTH BENEFITS

As a member of the cabbage family, Brussels sprouts are being investigated for their anticancer properties (see "Cabbage" and "Broccoli"). Researchers in the Netherlands investigated the effect of a diet high in Brussels sprouts on DNA damage. They compared two groups of healthy male volunteers. Five men ate a diet that included 300 grams (about 10 ounces) of cooked Brussels sprouts daily, while the other five men ate a diet free of cruciferous vegetables. After three weeks, the group that ate Brussels sprouts had a 28 percent decrease in measured DNA damage. Reduced DNA damage may translate to a reduced risk of cancer since mutations in DNA are what lead to the development of cancerous cells.

In addition, since one cup of Brussels sprouts contains more than 4 grams of fiber, they are an excellent food to reduce the appetite, promote bowel regularity, and prevent colon cancer.

HOW TO SELECT AND STORE

Brussels sprouts should be firm and fresh in appearance, with a good green color. Avoid dull, wilted, or yellow Brussels sprouts. If they are sold loose, choose those of equal size to ensure that they will cook evenly. Brussels sprouts are available year-round, but their peak growing period is autumn to early spring.

Keep unwashed and untrimmed Brussels sprouts stored in a perforated plastic bag in the vegetable compartment of the refrigerator. They can be kept for three to four days. Cooked Brussels sprouts will keep for three days refrigerated. If you want to freeze Brussels sprouts, blanch them first for three to five minutes. They will keep in the freezer for up to one year.

TIPS FOR PREPARING

Before washing Brussels sprouts, remove stems and any yellow or discolored leaves. Wash the sprouts well under cold running water or soak them in a bowl of water to remove any insects and dirt that may reside in the inner leaves. If they are not organically grown, soak them in cold water with a mild solution of additive-free soap or use a produce wash and rinse.

Brussels sprouts are usually cooked whole. To allow the heat to permeate throughout all of the leaves and better ensure an even texture, cut an "X" in the bottom of the stem before cooking. Brussels sprouts are best prepared by lightly steaming for 5 to 7 minutes.

QUICK SERVING IDEAS

- Top steamed Brussels sprouts with your favorite hard grated cheese and grill for a few minutes.
- Chilled, steamed Brussels sprouts make a nice addition to green salads.
- Drizzle hazelnut or toasted sesame oil onto cooked Brussels sprouts for a simple, light side dish.
- Braise Brussels sprouts in liquid infused with basil, thyme, or other aromatic herbs.
- Combine quartered cooked Brussels sprouts with sliced red onions, walnuts, and your favorite mild-tasting cheese, such as a goat cheese or feta. Toss with olive oil and balsamic vinegar for an exceptionally healthy side dish.

SAFETY

Members of the cabbage family contain goitrogens, naturally occurring substances that can interfere with the functioning of the thyroid gland. Dietary goitrogens are usually of no clinical importance unless they are consumed in large amounts or there is coexisting iodine deficiency. Cooking helps to inactivate the goitrogenic compounds. Individuals with already existing and untreated thyroid problems may want to avoid consumption of cabbage-family vegetables in their raw form for this reason. (See "Cabbage," below, for more information.)

Cabbage

Cabbage is the "king" of the cruciferous family of vegetables, which also includes broccoli, Brussels sprouts, cauliflower, collards, kale, mustard greens, radishes, swedes, turnips, and other common vegetables. The members of this family of vegetables are currently receiving much attention for their impressive anticancer properties.

The three major types of cabbage are green, red, and Savoy. The color of green cabbage ranges from pale to dark green, while red cabbage has leaves that are either crimson or purple with white veins running through. Both green and red cabbage have smooth-textured leaves, while the leaves of Savoy cabbage are more ruffled and yellowish green in color. The flavor of Savoy cabbage is more delicate and mild than the characteristic definite taste and crunchy texture of red or green.

Because cabbage's inner leaves are protected from the sunlight by the surrounding leaves, they are often lighter in color.

HISTORY

The modern-day cabbage developed from wild cabbage brought to Europe from Asia by roving bands of Celtic people around 600 B.C.E. Because cabbage is well adapted to growing in cooler climates, has high yields per acre, and can be stored over the winter in cold cellars, it quickly spread as a food crop throughout northern Europe. The Russian Federation, Poland, China, and Japan are a few of the leading producers of cabbage today.

Cabbage and sauerkraut, which is fermented cabbage, were introduced into the United States by early German settlers. As a result of this affiliation, people of German descent are often referred to as "krauts."

NUTRITIONAL HIGHLIGHTS

Cabbage is a nutrient-dense, low-calorie food providing an excellent source of many nutrients, especially vitamin C, potassium, folic acid, vitamin B6, biotin, calcium, magnesium, and manganese. But perhaps more important than the nutrient content of cabbage is its phytochemical content. In particular, cabbage contains powerful anticancer compounds known as glucosinolates. A 100 gram serving of cooked cabbage provides 35 calories, 2.3 grams of protein, no cholesterol, 0.4 grams of fat, 7.2 grams of carbohydrate, and 3.3 grams of fiber.

HEALTH BENEFITS

One of the American Cancer Society's key dietary recommendations to reduce the risk of cancer is to include cruciferous vegetables, such as cabbage, broccoli, Brussels sprouts, and cauliflower, in the diet on a regular basis. The reason for this recommendation? The cabbage family of vegetables contains more phytochemicals with demonstrable anticancer properties than any other vegetable family. Most of these compounds are glucosinolates. Those receiving the most attention are indole-3-carbinol, sulphoraphane, di-indolmethane, and isothio-cyanates.

The anticancer effects of cabbage-family vegetables have been noted in population studies. Consistently, the higher the intake of cabbage-family vegetables, the lower the rates of cancer, particularly colon, prostate, lung, and breast cancer. The glucosinolates in cabbage work primarily by increasing antioxidant defense mechanisms, as well as improving the body's ability to detoxify and eliminate harmful chemicals and hormones. Specifically, indole-3-carbinole (I3C), has been shown to increase the rate at which oestrogen is broken down through the liver's detoxification pathway by nearly 50 percent.

Cabbage has also been shown to be extremely effective in the treatment of peptic ulcers. Dr. Garnett Cheney from the Stanford University School of Medicine and other researchers in the 1950s clearly demonstrated that fresh cabbage juice is extremely effective in the treatment of peptic ulcers, showing measurable effect usually in less than seven days. The antiulcer component of cabbage was initially referred to as "vitamin U" but later identified as the amino acid glutamine, a critical factor in the growth and regeneration of the cells that line the gastrointestinal tract.

HOW TO SELECT AND STORE

Cabbage should be fresh and crisp with no evidence of decay or worm injury. Choose cabbage heads that are firm and dense with shiny, crisp, colorful leaves free of cracks, bruises, and blemishes. There should be only a few outer loose leaves attached to the stem. If not, it may be an indication of undesirable texture and taste. Avoid buying precut cabbage, either halved or shredded, since once cabbage is cut, it begins to lose its valuable vitamin C content.

Keeping cabbage cold will keep it fresh and help it retain its vitamin C content. Put the whole head in a perforated plastic bag in the crisper of your refrigerator. Red and green cabbage will keep this way for about two weeks, while Savoy cabbage will keep for about one week. If you need to store a partial head of cabbage, cover it tightly with cling film and refrigerate. Since the vitamin C content of cabbage degrades quickly once it has been cut, you should use the remainder within a couple of days.

TIPS FOR PREPARING

Even though the inside of a cabbage is usually clean because the outer leaves protect it, you must still wash it before eating. Remove the thick fibrous outer leaves, cut the cabbage into pieces, and then wash under cold running water. If the cabbage is not organically grown, soak it in cold water with a mild solution of additive-free soap or use a produce wash (see page 51) and rinse thoroughly.

To cut cabbage into smaller pieces, first quarter it and remove the core. Cabbage can be cut into slices of varying thickness, grated by hand, or shredded in a food processor. To preserve its vitamin C content, cut and wash the cabbage right before cooking or eating it. Since phyto-chemicals in the cabbage react with carbon steel and turn the leaves black, use a stainless-steel knife to cut it.

If you notice any signs of worms or insects, which sometimes appear in organically grown cabbage, soak the head in salt water or vinegar water for 15 to 20 minutes first.

QUICK SERVING IDEAS

- Raw cabbage can be juiced, or shredded and made into coleslaw or added to salads.
- Use ¼ cup shredded raw cabbage as a garnish for sandwiches.
- Combine 1 cup each shredded red and white cabbage with 3 to 4 tablespoons soy or rapeseed mayonnaise and seasonings, such as turmeric, cumin, coriander, and black pepper, to make coleslaw with an Indian twist.
- Braise 2 cups sliced red cabbage with 1 chopped apple, ½ cup red wine, salt, and pepper. This is a child-friendly dish, since the alcohol, but not the flavor or the flavonoids, will evaporate.
- Sauté equal amounts of cabbage and onions in olive oil and serve over cooked buckwheat for a hardy side dish.
- For a twist on the traditional Reuben sandwich (corned beef, sauerkraut, swiss cheese, dressing on rye), place grilled tempeh on a slice of whole-grain bread, layer with sauerkraut, top with cheese or "meltable" soy cheese, and then grill for a few minutes until the sandwich is hot and toasty. Top with Russian dressing (mayonnaise-based, with chili sauce, Worcestershire sauce and ketchup) and enjoy.

SAFETY

Cabbage-family vegetables contain goitrogens, compounds that can interfere with thyroid hormone action in certain situations, primarily when iodine levels are low. The goitrogens are largely isothiocyanates, which block the utilization of iodine; however, despite our warning here, there is no evidence that these compounds in cruciferous vegetables interfere with thyroid function to any significant degree when dietary iodine levels are adequate. Furthermore, cooking may help inactivate the goitrogenic compounds found in cabbage and other cruciferous vegetables.

If large quantities of raw cruciferous vegetables—more than four servings per week—are being consumed, it is a good idea that the diet also contain adequate amounts of iodine. Iodine is found in kelp and other seaweeds, vegetables grown near the sea, seafood, iodized salt, and food supplements.

Carrots

The carrot is a plant with a thick, fleshy, deeply colored root that grows underground and feathery green leaves that emerge above ground. It is known scientifically as *Daucus carota*, a name that can be traced back to ancient Roman writings of the third century B.C.E. Carrots belong to the Umbelliferae family, named after the umbrellalike flower clusters common to plants in this family, including parsnips, parsley, fennel, and dill. There are more than a hundred different varieties of carrot that vary in size and color. Carrots can be as short as 2 inches/5 cm or as long as 3 feet/1 meter, ranging in diameter from ½ inch/1 cm to over 2 inches/ 5cm. Carrot roots have a crunchy texture and a sweet, minty, aromatic taste, while the greens are fresh-tasting and slightly bitter. While carrots are generally associated with the color orange, they also grow in a host of other colors, including white, yellow, red, and purple, the last being the color of the original variety.

HISTORY

Carrots are believed to have originated in the Middle East and Asia. The earlier varieties were not orange but mostly purple and black. Apparently the modern-day carrot was originally a mutant variety lacking certain purple or black pigments. In pre-Hellenic times, a yellow-rooted carrot variety appeared in Afghanistan; it was further cultivated and developed into an earlier version of the carrot we know today. Both types of carrots spread throughout the Mediterranean region and were adopted by the ancient Greeks and Romans for medicinal uses.

The carrot did not become popular in Europe until the Renaissance, however, probably due to the fact that the early varieties had a tough, fibrous texture. By the 1600s several different types of carrots had been developed, including the orange-colored carrot, which had a more appealing texture. Carrots were introduced into North America by European colonists. As a sign of its heightened popularity, in the early 1800s the carrot became the first vegetable to be canned. The world's largest producers of carrots today are the United States, France, Britain, Poland, China, and Japan.

NUTRITIONAL HIGHLIGHTS

The carrot provides the highest source of provitamin A carotenes of the commonly consumed vegetables. Two carrots provide roughly 4,050 retinol equivalents, or roughly four times the RDA of vitamin A. Carrots also provide excellent levels of vitamin K, biotin, and fiber and very good levels of vitamins C and B6, potassium, and thiamine.

A 100 gram serving of carrots provides 41 calories with 9.6 grams of carbohydrate as 4.5 grams of sugars and 3 grams of fiber.

HEALTH BENEFITS

Carrots are an excellent source of antioxidant compounds that help protect against cardiovascular disease and cancer. In one study that examined the diets of 1,300 elderly persons in Massachusetts, those who had at least one serving of carrots and/or squash each day had a 60 percent reduction in their risk of heart attacks compared to those who ate less than one serving of these carotenoid-rich foods per day.

High carotene intake has been linked with a 20 percent decrease in postmenopausal breast cancer and up to a 50 percent decrease in the incidence of cancers of the bladder, cervix, prostate, colon, larynx, and oesophagus. Extensive human studies suggest that a diet including as little as one carrot per day could conceivably cut the rate of lung cancer in half.

Carrots also promote good vision, especially night vision. In fact, beta-carotene, which is present in high levels in carrots, provides protection against macular degeneration and the development of senile cataracts—the leading cause of blindness in the elderly.

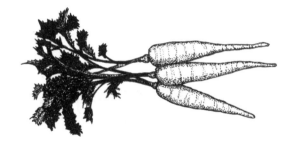

HOW TO SELECT AND STORE

Carrots are available throughout the year. The inspection of carrots begins with how they look; avoid carrots that have cracks, are bruised, or have mold growing on them. The carrots should be deep orange in color and fresh-looking. If the tops are not attached, look at the stem end and ensure that it is not darkly colored, as this is also a sign of age. Next, evaluate the physical characteristics; avoid carrots that are limp or rubbery. The carrots should feel hard, crisp, and smooth.

Since carrots are efficient at maintaining their water content, they will keep longer than many other vegetables. To maximize storage time, store them in the coolest part of the refrigerator in a perforated plastic bag or wrapped in a paper towel. This will reduce the amount of condensation that is able to form. Stored this way, carrots will stay fresh for up to two weeks.

If carrots are purchased with attached green tops, the tops should be cut off before storing in the refrigerator, as if they remain attached they will pull moisture from the roots and cause the carrots to wilt prematurely. The carrot tops will need to be used right away, as they are quite fragile and wilt quickly.

Carrots should be stored away from apples, pears, potatoes, and other fruits and vegetables that produce ethylene gas, since this gas will cause them to become bitter.

TIPS FOR PREPARING

Wash carrots under cold running water and gently scrub them with a vegetable brush. If the carrots are not organically grown, definitely peel them. The same is true if they are a bit old or cracked. If the stem end is green, it should be cut away, as it will be bitter. Carrots can be left whole, julienned, grated, shredded, or sliced into sticks or rounds depending upon the need or your personal preference.

Though carrots are delicious when eaten raw, cooking actually enhances the bioavailability of their beta-carotene by breaking down the fiber and making it easier for the body to utilize the beta-carotene.

QUICK SERVING IDEAS

- Carrot juice is perhaps the most popular juice prepared in home juice extractors. Its sweetness blends well with other vegetables.
- Lightly steamed carrots are delicious on their own.
- Grated carrots can be added to many fruit salads, such as chopped apples, raisins, and pineapple; chopped or sliced carrots can be added to vegetable salads.
- Carrots can be added to baked goods, such as carrot cakes and muffins, soups, casseroles, and other recipes.
- To make spiced carrot sticks, soak 2 cups carrot sticks in 2 cups hot water with ¼ to ½ teaspoon cayenne, 1 teaspoon ground coriander seeds, 1 teaspoon ground cumin seeds, 2 teaspoons rice vinegar, and salt. Soak until cool, drain, and serve.
- For a quick, nutritious soup that can be served hot or cold, purée 2 cups boiled carrots, ½ cup celery, 1 roasted onion, and 1 teaspoon ginger in a blender or food processor. Add ¼ cup olive oil and enough vegetable stock to thin to a creamy soup. Season with other herbs and spices to taste.

SAFETY

Carotenes are stored in adipose tissue, the liver, other organs (the adrenals, testes, and ovaries have the highest concentrations), and the skin. Ingesting large quantities of carotenes can lead to a yellowing of the skin known as carotenodermia. This occurrence is not serious; in fact, it may be beneficial in protecting against sun damage to the skin. Sometimes carotenodermia is not directly attributable to dietary intake or supplementation, as it may be indicative of a deficiency in a necessary factor in the conversion of beta-carotene to vitamin A, such as zinc, thyroid hormone, vitamin C, or protein. The ingestion of large amounts of carrots or carrot juice—0.45 to 1 kilogram of fresh carrots per day for several years—has, however, been shown to cause a decrease in the number of white blood cells, as well as menstrual disorders. Although the blood carotene levels of these patients did reach levels (221 to 1,007 micrograms per deciliter) similar to those of patients taking high doses of beta-carotene (typically 800 micrograms per deciliter), the disturbances have been due to some other factor in carrots, as neither of these effects nor any others have been observed in subjects consuming very high doses of pure beta-carotene equivalent to 4 to 8 pounds/2 to 4 kilograms of raw carrots per day over long periods of time.

Since carrots are among the foods on which pesticide residues have been most frequently found, we recommend choosing carrots grown organically.

Cauliflower

Cauliflower is a member of the cruciferous vegetable family, which includes broccoli, kale, and cabbage. Cauliflower has a compact head called a "curd," which is composed of undeveloped flower buds. The curd averages 6 inches/15 cm in diameter. The flower buds are attached to a central stalk, and when the buds bloom, cauliflower looks like a little tree.

Cauliflower is white because its ribbed, coarse green leaves protect the curd from sunlight, thereby impeding the development of chlorophyll. While this process contributes to the white coloring of most varieties, cauliflower can also be found in light green and purple.

Raw cauliflower is firm yet a bit spongy in texture. It has a slightly sulphurous and faintly bitter flavor.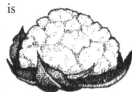

HISTORY

Like broccoli and Brussels sprouts, cauliflower developed from the wild cabbage, thought to have originated in ancient Asia. Cauliflower has gone through many changes since then, with the current version appearing in Turkey and Italy around at least 600 B.C.E. During the mid-1500s, it gained popularity in France, which led it to be extensively cultivated in northern Europe and Britain. Today, the United States, France, Italy, India, and China produce significant amounts of cauliflower. California produces 80 percent of the U.S. crop (cauliflower needs a stable, temperate climate, as it is susceptible to both frost and hot weather).

NUTRITIONAL HIGHLIGHTS

Cauliflower is not as nutrient-dense as many of the other cabbage-family vegetables, but it is still power-packed with nutrition. One cup of raw cauliflower is an excellent source of vitamin K (476.2 percent of the RDA) and vitamin C and is a very good source of fiber, potassium, phosphorus, and B vitamins. Its white color is a sign that it has much less of the beneficial carotenes and chlorophyll found in other cruciferous vegetables; however, cauliflower is almost always a good source of the trace mineral boron, as it will not grow well in boron-deficient soil.

A 100 gram serving of cooked cauliflower provides 35 calories, 2.3 grams of protein, no cholesterol, 0.4 grams of fat, 7.2 grams of carbohydrate, and 3.3 grams of fiber.

HEALTH BENEFITS

Cauliflower and other cruciferous vegetables, such as broccoli, cabbage, and kale, contain compounds that may help prevent cancer. These compounds appear to stop enzymes from activating cancer-causing agents in the body, and they increase the activity of enzymes that disable and eliminate carcinogens. For more information on the anticancer properties of cauliflower, see "Cabbage," page 178.

HOW TO SELECT AND STORE

Visual inspection goes a long way in the selection of cauliflower. The head should be fresh-looking, with clean white flower heads and crisp green leaves. Avoid cauliflower with wilted leaves, dirty flower heads, or obvious signs of decay.

Cauliflower is best stored with the stem side down in a perforated paper or plastic bag in the refrigerator to prevent moisture from developing in the floret clusters. It will generally keep for about a week if stored in this manner.

When purchasing cauliflower as precut florets, keep in mind that you must consume them within one to two days, as they lose their freshness quickly. Cooked cauliflower also spoils quickly, so consume cooked cauliflower within one to two days of storing it in the refrigerator.

TIPS FOR PREPARING

Wash cauliflower under cold running water and gently scrub with a vegetable brush. If the cauliflower is not organically grown, soak in cold water with a mild solution of additive-free soap or use a produce wash (see page 51) and rinse.

In addition to the florets, the stem and leaves are edible and are especially good for adding to soup stocks.

To cut cauliflower, first remove the outer leaves and then slice the florets at the base where they meet the stalks. You can further cut them, if you desire pieces that are smaller or of uniform size. Trim any brown coloration that may exist on the edges.

Cauliflower contains phytochemicals that release odorous sulphur compounds when heated. These odors become stronger with increased cooking time. If you want to minimize odor, retain the vegetable's crisp texture, and reduce nutrient loss, cook the cauliflower for only a short time, such as steaming large chunks for 5 minutes or sautéing thin slices for 1 to 2 minutes.

Some phytochemicals may react with iron in cookware and cause the cauliflower to take on a brownish hue. To prevent this, add a bit of lemon juice to the water in which you blanch the cauliflower.

QUICK SERVING IDEAS

- Cauliflower can be prepared in ways similar to broccoli (see page 176).
- Raw cauliflower florets can be added to green salads or used as a crudité for dipping in sauces.
- Sauté 2 cups of cauliflower in ¼-inch/½ cm slices with 2 cloves sliced garlic, ½ inch/1 cm peeled, minced ginger, 1 tablespoon rapeseed oil, and 1 tablespoon tamari.
- For cauliflower with a vivid yellow color, prepare it with a spoonful of turmeric or a generous pinch of saffron. An entire head can be boiled with either spice for a decorative and nutritious centerpiece.
- Slice a cauliflower head into thin slices, brush with oil, and cook in the oven or on the barbecue.
- Boil 2 cups cauliflower in just enough stock to cover it until soft. Purée the cauliflower with its liquid, adding 2 teaspoons ground fennel seeds, other favorite herbs and spices, and 2 tablespoons olive oil, and serve as soup, either hot or cold.
- For a pasta dish that not only tastes Italian but bears the colors of Italy's flag, serve spinach pasta with freshly chopped tomatoes, basil, and small steamed cauliflower florets.

SAFETY

Members of the cabbage family contain goitrogens, naturally occurring substances that can interfere with the functioning of the thyroid gland. Dietary goitrogens are usually of no clinical importance unless they are consumed in large amounts or there is coexisting iodine deficiency. Cooking helps to inactivate the goitrogenic compounds. Individuals with already existing and untreated thyroid problems may want to avoid consumption of cabbage family vegetables in their raw form for this reason. (See "Cabbage," page 178, for more information.)

Celery (and Celeriac)

Celery is a member of the Umbelliferae family, along with carrots, parsley, and fennel. It is a biennial vegetable, meaning it has a normal growing cycle of once every two years. While most people associate celery with its stalks, its leaves, roots, and seeds are also used as food and seasoning.

Celery grows to a height of 12 to 16 inches/30 to 40 cm and is composed of leaf-topped ribs arranged in a conical shape and joined at a common base (the collection of ribs forms the stalk). The ribs have a crunchy texture and a delicate but mildly salty taste. The ribs in the center are called the heart and are the most tender. In the United States, we are used to celery being different shades of green, but Europeans also enjoy a variety that is white in color. Like white asparagus, this type of celery is grown shaded from direct sunlight, so its production of chlorophyll, and hence its green color, are inhibited.

HISTORY

Modern celery originated from wild celery, native to the Mediterranean, where its seeds were once widely used as a medicine, particularly as a diuretic. The initial mention of the medicinal properties of celery leaves dates back to the ninth century B.C.E., when celery made an appearance in the *Odyssey,* the famous epic by the Greek poet Homer. The Ancient Greeks used the leaves as laurels to decorate their renowned athletes, while the ancient Romans used celery as a seasoning, a tradition that has been carried on through the centuries.

The use of celery as a food was expanded beyond medicine and as a seasoning in Europe during the 1700s. Celery was introduced in the United States early in the nineteenth century and is now produced throughout the world.

NUTRITIONAL HIGHLIGHTS

Celery is an excellent source of vitamin C and fiber. It is a very good source of potassium, folic acid, and vitamins B6 and B1. Celery is a good source of calcium and vitamin B2. While it is true that celery contains more sodium than most other vegetables, the sodium is offset by very high levels of potassium. Furthermore, the amount of sodium is not significant even for the most salt-sensitive individuals. One celery stalk contains approximately 32 milligrams of sodium and 104 milligrams of potassium and only 20 calories as carbohydrate.

HEALTH BENEFITS

Celery contains phytochemical compounds known as coumarins, which are being shown to be useful in cancer prevention and capable of enhancing the activity of certain white blood cells. Coumarin compounds also tone the vascular system, lower blood pressure, and may be useful in cases of migraines.

Two researchers at the University of Chicago Medical Center have performed studies on a coumarin compound found in celery, 3-*n*-butyl-

phthalide (3nB), and found that it can indeed lower blood pressure. In animal studies, a very small amount of 3nB consumed daily lowered blood pressure by 12 to 14 percent and also lowered the cholesterol level by about 7 percent. The equivalent dose for humans can be supplied by four ribs of celery. The research was prompted by the father of one of the researchers, who after eating quarter of a pound/115 grams of celery every day for a week, observed that his blood pressure dropped from 158 over 96 to a normal reading of 118 over 82.

Celery is also rich in potassium and sodium. In fact, celery-based juices consumed after a workout serve as great electrolyte replacement drinks. And celery may also help lower cholesterol and prevent cancer by improving detoxification.

A celery extract standardized to contain 85% 3nB has also been shown to produce significant benefits in the treatment of "rheumatism"—the general term used for arthritic and muscular aches and pain. In two clinical studies the efficacy of celery seed extract was evaluated by well-established clinical protocols used to measure the effectiveness of conventional drugs used in arthritis and muscular pain. Study participants included patients suffering from osteoarthritis or gout.

In the first study, the subjects had joint pain present for approximately ten years in a remittent or continual form leading to a lack of joint mobility and pain that prevented the carrying out of household duties, hobbies, and activities involved in these subjects' jobs. The subjects were given only 34 milligrams of the celery extract twice daily. Nonetheless, the results of the study were extremely positive and quite statistically significant. The chance that such a positive effect in reducing pain in these subjects was a placebo effect was less than one in 1,000. Subjects experienced significant pain relief after three weeks of use, with an average reduction in pain scores of 68 percent, and some subjects experiencing 100 percent relief from pain. Most subjects achieved maximum benefit after six weeks of use, although some did notice more improvement the longer the extract was used.

In a second study, a similar group of patients received 75 milligrams of the celery extract twice daily for three weeks. At this higher dosage, the subjects reported even better results than in the first study. Statistically and clinically significant reductions were noted in pain scores, mobility, and quality of life. As in the first study, no side effects were noted other than a diuretic effect.

When the data on the subset of patients with gout were analyzed, it was clear that they responded extremely well. Subsequent evaluation to explain the benefits noted in these patients indicates that 3nB lowers the production of uric acid by inhibiting the enzyme xanthine oxidase. Eventually celery seed extract lowers blood uric acid levels; however, quite interestingly, the initial blood uric acid measurements may increase in people with gout as uric acid crystals begin to dissolve—a very good sign.

HOW TO SELECT AND STORE

Celery should be light green, fresh-looking, and crisp—the ribs should be hard and firm. Limp, pliable celery should be avoided. Avoid celery that looks damaged or has any signs of discoloration. Also, make sure that the celery does not have a seed stem—a round stem in place of the smaller, tender stalks that should reside in the center of the celery. Celery with seed stems is often more bitter in flavor.

Celery root (celeriac) is light brown on top and becomes darker toward the bottom where the rootlets extend. Celery root should be firm when fresh.

To store celery stalks or roots, place them in a sealed container or wrap in a perforated plastic bag or damp cloth and store them in the refrigerator. If you are storing cut celery or peeled celeriac, ensure that it is dry and free from water residue, as this can drain some of its nutrients. Freezing will make celery wilt and should be avoided unless you will be using it in a future cooked recipe.

TIPS FOR PREPARING

Prior to washing celery, cut off the base and leaves, then wash the leaves and stalks under cold running water. If the celery is not organically grown, soak in cold water with a mild solution of additive-free soap or use a produce wash and rinse thoroughly. Cut the stalks into pieces of desired length. Remove any fibrous strings by making a thin cut into one end of the stalk and peeling away the fibers. Try to utilize the leaves as well as the ribs, as the leaves contain the most vitamin C, calcium, and potassium.

Due to its high water content and tendency to wilt quickly, celery should not be kept at room temperature for too long. If you have celery that has wilted, sprinkle it with a little water and place it for several hours in the refrigerator, where it will regain its crispness.

Celeriac should be peeled before preparing, particularly the bottom, as the skin around the rootlets is hairy and thick, creating an unpleasant texture in finished dishes.

QUICK SERVING IDEAS

- Raw celery can be eaten whole, juiced, or used in salads.
- Add chopped celery to your favorite tuna or chicken salad recipe.
- Celery, although it can be served on its own after lightly steaming, is an excellent addition to soups, stews, and vegetable stir-fries.
- Braise chopped celery, radicchio, and onions, and serve topped with walnuts and your favorite soft cheese.
- Celeriac can be chopped into ½-inch/1 cm cubes along with other root vegetables, given a light coat of oil, and roasted at 350 degrees F. /180 degrees C./gas 4 for 30 to 40 minutes.

SAFETY

Since celery is among the foods on which pesticide residues have been most frequently found, we recommend choosing celery that has been organically grown.

Chard: See Swiss Chard.

Chicory: See Endive.

Chili Pepper: See Cayenne Pepper and Paprika in chapter 15.

Collards: See Kale.

Corn: See chapter 12.

Courgettes: See Squash, Summer.

Cucumbers

Cucumbers *(Cucumis sativus)* are cylindrical in shape and commonly range in length from about 6 to 9 inches/15 to 20 cm, although they can be smaller or much larger. Their skin ranges in color from green to white and may be either smooth or ridged, depending upon the variety. Inside a cucumber is a very pale green flesh that is dense yet aqueous and crunchy at the same time, as well as numerous edible fleshy seeds. The seedless, thin-skinned, and longer varieties are most often grown in greenhouses.

More than 70 percent of the U.S. cucumber crop is used to make pickles. Cucumbers that are cultivated to make pickles are usually of the smaller varieties. For example, the gherkin is one popular variety of cucumbers cultivated for this purpose.

HISTORY

The cucumber is a tropical plant that originated in Southeast Asia more than 10,000 years ago. Early explorers and travelers from India and other parts of Asia brought it back with them, and its popularity spread to the ancient civilizations of Egypt, Greece, and Rome. During ancient times, it was used not only as a food, but also for its beneficial skin-healing properties. During the seventeenth century, greenhouse cultivation of cucumbers was developed. Cucumbers were introduced to the United States by the early colonists.

The pickling process of cucumbers is thought to have originated in Spain, as pickles were said to be valued by Roman emperors.

NUTRITIONAL HIGHLIGHTS

Fresh cucumbers are composed primarily of water but still pack a lot of nutritional value.

The flesh of cucumbers is a very good source of vitamins C and A and folic acid. The hard skin is rich in fiber and contains a variety of important minerals, including silica, potassium, magnesium, and molybdenum. A 100 gram serving of cucumber provides only 12 calories as carbohydrate.

HEALTH BENEFITS

Cucumber is an excellent source of silica, a trace mineral that contributes to the strength of our connective tissue. Connective tissue is what holds our body together. It includes the intracellular cement, muscles, tendons, ligaments, cartilage, and bone. Without silica, connective tissue would not be properly constructed, leaving it impaired. Cucumber is often recommended as a source of silica.

Cucumbers are also used topically for various types of skin problems, including swelling under the eyes and sunburn. Two compounds in cucumbers, ascorbic acid and caffeic acid, prevent water retention, which may explain why cucumbers applied topically are often helpful for swollen eyes, burns, and dermatitis.

HOW TO SELECT AND STORE

Cucumbers should be fresh-looking, well shaped, and medium to dark green in color. Avoid cucumbers that are yellow or puffy, have sunken, water-soaked areas, or are wrinkled at their tips. Thinner cucumbers will generally have fewer seeds than those that are thicker.

Store cucumbers in the refrigerator, where they will keep for several days. If you do not use an entire cucumber during one meal, wrap the remainder tightly in plastic or place it in a sealed container to retain its freshness, but even then it should be used within one to two days. Cucumbers should not be left out at room temperature for too long, as this will cause them to wilt and become limp.

TIPS FOR PREPARING

Wash cucumbers under cold running water and gently scrub them with a vegetable brush. If waxed or not organically grown, the cucumber should also be peeled. Cucumbers can be sliced, diced, or cut into sticks. While the seeds are edible and nutritious, some people prefer not to eat them. To remove them easily, cut the cucumber lengthwise and use the tip of a spoon to gently scoop them out.

QUICK SERVING IDEAS

- Mix 1 cup diced cucumbers with 1 cup sugar snap peas and ½ cup chopped mint leaves, and toss with a rice wine vinaigrette.
- For a quick and easy cold gazpacho soup, simply purée 1 peeled cucumber, 1 cup fresh tomatoes, 1 green pepper, and ½ red onion, then add salt and pepper to taste.
- To make a cucumber compote: Sauté cubed cucumbers with dill in a little vegetable stock for a few minutes; remove from heat; chill; and then top with a dollop of plain yogurt and a sprig of dill or parsley before serving.
- Make cucumber tempura by dredging cucumber slices in a beaten egg and then in whole-wheat (wholemeal) flour. Bake on a baking tray at 300 degrees F./150 degrees C./gas 2 until crispy and serve with a dipping sauce or dressing of your choice.

SAFETY

Since cucumbers are among the foods on which pesticide residues have been most frequently found, we recommend choosing cucumbers that have been organically grown. In addition, cucumbers are often waxed to protect them from bruising during shipping. Plant-, insect-, animal-, or petroleum-based waxes may be used. Since you may not be able to determine the source of these waxes, again, we recommend choosing organically grown cucumbers.

Dandelion

The dandelion is a perennial plant with an almost worldwide distribution. While many individuals consider the dandelion to be an unwanted weed, herbalists all over the world have revered this valuable herb. Its common name, dandelion, is a corruption of the French for "tooth of the lion" *(dent-de-lion)*. This name describes the herb's leaves, which have several large, pointed teeth. Its scientific name, *Taraxacum,* is from the Greek *taraxos* (disorder) and *akos* (remedy). This alludes to dandelion's ability to correct a multitude of disorders.

A hardy perennial that grows in all temperate areas of the Northern Hemisphere, dandelion

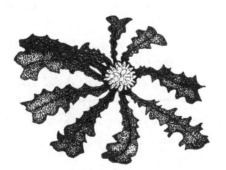

reaches 1¼ to 14 inches/3 to 35 centimeters in height and is easily recognized by its deeply toothed, hairless leaves, measuring 2 to 12 inches/5 to 30 centimeters long and ½ to 4 inches/1 to 10 centimeters wide, which form a rosette at ground level, and the single golden yellow flower that emerges from the rosette's center on a straight, purplish, leafless, hollow stem.

The flower, which is actually a collection of tiny florets, appears from early spring until late autumn. When the florets mature, they produce downy seeds that are easily dispersed by the wind, giving rise to dandelion's aliases of "puff-ball" and "blowball." Although its flowers are most evident in early summer, dandelion may be found in bloom, and consequently prolifically dispersing its seeds, throughout most of the year.

As anyone who has ever removed one from the lawn knows, dandelion plants have a long, dark brown taproot, tapering from 1 inch/2 to 3 centimeters wide and at least 6 inches/15 centimeters in length. The whole plant, including the root, contains a milky white sap or latex. On top of the root, but still below the surface, is a crown of blanched leaf stems, which dandelion aficionados consider the tastiest part of the plant. They can be used in salads or as a cooked vegetable. Next is found the rosette of leaves. These are the dandelion greens, which must be gathered before the plant blooms or they will become quite bitter and tough. The young greens, which have a slightly bitter, tangy flavor that adds interest to salads and which can also be cooked like spinach, are the part most often consumed, but dandelion roots can also be eaten as a root vegetable or roasted and ground to make "coffee," and the flowers can be used to make dandelion wine and tea.

HISTORY

From ancient times to the present, dandelion has been valued as a healthful food and a medicine. According to legend, Theseus ate a dandelion salad after killing the Minotaur. The Gauls and Celts ate the plant, as did the Romans when they invaded the North. The Anglo-Saxon tribes of Britain and the Normans of France also ate dandelion and used the plant to control scurvy, and as a diuretic.

Dandelion was planted in the medicinal gardens of monasteries and appears in the writings of the famous Arab physician Avicenna (980–1037 C.E.), who used it to regulate menstruation and spoke of it as a sort of wild endive, under the name of *Taraxacum.*

Allusion is made to the use of dandelion as a medicine by the Welsh in the thirteenth century. In the fifteenth century, Master Wilhelmus, a surgeon, provided another reason for its common name, writing that dandelion was as powerful as a lion's tooth in fighting off certain diseases. The dandelion continued to be extensively used in Europe for its medicinal effects as a diuretic and tonic helpful in digestive, kidney, and liver complaints. As a food, however, dandelion did not become popular until the early nineteenth century, when several very palatable varieties were developed in Europe.

In Britain at this time, not only were the leaves considered a delicacy in salads, but dandelion roots were roasted, ground and used to make "coffee," a process described with much approval by Grieve in *A Modern Herbal,* the first comprehensive encyclopaedia of herbs, published in 1931 in Great Britain:

The prepared powder is said to be almost indistinguishable from real coffee, and is claimed to be an improvement to inferior coffee, which is often an adulterated product. Of late years, Dandelion Coffee has come more into use in this country, being obtainable at most vegetarian restaurants and stores. Formerly it was used occasionally for medicinal purposes, generally mixed with true coffee to give it a better flavor. The ground root was sometimes mixed with chocolate for a similar purpose. Dandelion Coffee is a natural beverage without any of the injurious effects that ordinary tea and coffee have on the nerves and digestive organs. It exercises a stimulating influence over the whole system, helping the liver and kidneys to do their work and keeping the bowels in a healthy condition, so that it offers great advantages to dyspeptics and does not cause wakefulness.

Grieve also notes that dried dandelion leaves were used as an ingredient in many digestive drinks and herb beers. She describes "dandelion stout," a drink made from dandelions, nettles, and yellow dock, as "an agreeable and wholesome fermented drink" that was a favorite of workmen in the furnaces and potteries of the industrial towns of the Midlands, who had "frequent resource to many of the tonic Herb Beers, finding them cheaper and less intoxicating than ordinary beer." And finally, Grieve provides a recipe using dandelion flowers to make dandelion wine, which she gives as follows:

This is made by pouring a gallon of boiling water over a gallon of the flowers. After being well stirred, it is covered with a blanket and allowed to stand for three days, being stirred again at intervals, after which it is strained and the liquor boiled for 30 minutes, with the addition of 3½ lbs. of loaf sugar, a little ginger sliced, and the rinds of 1 orange and 1 lemon sliced. When cold, a little yeast is placed in it on a piece of toast, producing fermentation. It is then covered over and allowed to stand two days until it has ceased "working," when it is placed in a cask, well bunged down for two months before bottling. This wine is suggestive of sherry slightly flat, and has the deserved reputation of being an excellent tonic, extremely good for the blood.

The dandelion was brought to America by the early colonists, who used all parts of the plant but favored the roots, which they used to make dandelion coffee. On the frontier, dandelions undoubtedly saved lives. Frontier healers recommended dandelion greens as a spring tonic, and we now know they provide significant amounts of vitamins A and C, as well as other important nutrients unavailable to pioneers during the winter.

NUTRITIONAL HIGHLIGHTS

Dandelion's calorie count is exceptionally low—a cup is only 25 calories—while its nutrient content is exceptionally high. In fact, the dandelion contains greater nutritional value than many other vegetables. It is particularly high in vitamins and minerals, protein, choline, inulin, and pectin. Its carotenoid content is extremely high, as is reflected by its higher vitamin A content than carrots'—dandelion has 14,000 IU of vitamin A per 100 grams compared to 11,000 IU for carrots. In addition, dandelion is an excellent source of vitamin C, riboflavin, B6, and thiamine, as well as calcium, copper, manganese, and iron.

HEALTH BENEFITS

Dandelion is a rich source of nutrients and other compounds that may improve liver functions, promote weight loss, possess diuretic activity, and improve blood sugar control. Overall, dandelion is a rich source of medicinal compounds that have a "toning" effect on the body, and both the greens and the roots can be used for this purpose. The digestive tonic properties attributed to dandelion are now thought to be due to a bitter principle researchers have named "taraxacin" and identified as belonging to a class of active substances called guaianolides, which have intestinal antiseptic, germicidal, and expectorant effects.

Dandelion root is regarded as one of the finest liver remedies, as both food and medicine. Studies in both humans and laboratory animals have shown that dandelion root enhances the flow of bile, improving such conditions as liver congestion, bile duct inflammation, hepatitis, gallstones, and jaundice. Dandelion's action on increasing bile flow is twofold: it has a direct effect on the liver, causing an increase in bile production and flow to the gallbladder (choleretic effect), and a direct effect on the gallbladder, causing contraction and release of stored bile (cholagogue effect).

Dandelion's historical use in such a wide variety of conditions is probably closely related to its ability to improve the functional ability of the liver. For example, in one animal study, dandelion significantly improved the liver's ability to clear toxins by 244 percent. Dandelion's effectiveness in improving the liver's ability to clear potentially toxic agents was also demonstrated in a study in which rats were given the antimicrobial drug ciprofloxacin. In those rats that also received dandelion, levels of the drug were rapidly and significantly lowered by 73 percent.

Dandelion has also historically been used as a weight loss aid in the treatment of obesity. This fact prompted researchers to investigate dandelion's effect on the body weight of experimental animals. When these animals were administered a fluid extract of dandelion greens for one month, they lost as much as 30 percent of their initial weight. Much of the weight loss appeared to be a result of significant diuretic activity.

Research has also revealed that dandelion root contains a very high concentration—up to 40 percent—of an indigestible carbohydrate called inulin (see page 76), which serves as a food source for, and thus promotes the growth of, the "friendly" colonic bacteria species *Bifidobacterium* and *Lactobacillus*. When these beneficial bacteria are encouraged to proliferate, they crowd out other harmful bacteria, thus acting like a natural protective antibiotic and improving the health of the digestive tract.

Inulin is also helpful in improving blood sugar control and diabetes. In one study, dandelion, given to diabetic rats in the form of a water extract, significantly improved the rats' production of antioxidant liver enzymes while decreasing their blood sugar, total cholesterol, and triglyceride levels and raising their level of beneficial HDL cholesterol.

HOW TO SELECT AND STORE

Wild dandelion is plentiful in most parts of the United States and United Kingdom. Dandelion greens are available commercially as well from specialist herb growers. The fresher the dandelion, the better. Though dandelion greens are available until winter in some places, the best, most tender greens are harvested early in the spring, before the plant begins to flower. Choose brightly colored, tender-crisp leaves; avoid those with yellowed or wilted tips or brown spots. Usually, the lighter green the leaf, the more tender the taste.

Store dandelion greens unwashed and wrapped in damp paper towels in a plastic bag in the vegetable bin of your refrigerator, where they should remain fresh for three to five days.

Commercial growers debate about the optimum time to harvest dandelion root. Some believe the roots are more bitter when harvested in autumn, while others consider the roots to be more bitter in spring. The *British Herbal Pharmacopoeia* (BHP) recommends harvesting the roots in autumn. One reason may be that, in the spring, food reserves from the root, primarily inulin, have been used up for the production of leaves and flowers. In autumn, the inulin content of dried root is up to 40 percent, while in spring it is only 2 percent. However, dandelion root in the spring is still a nutritious raw or cooked vegetable.

TIPS FOR PREPARING

The best time to gather dandelion greens is in the very early spring, even before the last frost, when the bloom bud appears but before the stalk grows. After blooming, dandelion greens become too bitter and tough to eat. The long taproot can be used as a vegetable or roasted and used as a coffee substitute. You also may find the beginnings of the blossoms in the center of the crown. These will appear as a yellowish, closely packed mass and can be cut out and cooked. If the plant has already bloomed, the blossoms can be used to make delicious wine and the roots can be roasted and ground for "coffee."

Like other greens, even if dandelion leaves look clean, they should be washed thoroughly. Trim off any remaining roots, and then, holding the greens by the stems, gently swish them around in a large bowl of cool water. Lift them out and rinse and refill the bowl. Repeat this process until no sand or grit settles in the bottom of the bowl.

If using the greens for cooking, leave them damp. If serving them in salads, dry them well. To remove remaining water, a salad spinner is easiest, as it dries delicate leaves quickly and thoroughly. If you do not have a salad spinner, hold the greens by the stems and shake off excess water, then blot gently with clean paper towels. Store them for up to five days in the refrigerator. Cooked dandelion greens should be eaten within two days.

Smaller, pale leaves are more delicate in flavor and thus best for salads. The more robust flavor of the larger, darker leaves makes these best for cooking. Also, the center ribs of more mature leaves should be removed, as it becomes tough and quite bitter.

To retain the best flavor, the leaves should always be torn to pieces, rather than cut.

To reduce bitterness in more mature leaves, soak the leaves in a bicarbonate of soda solution (one teaspoon of bicarb to 1 cup water) for 1 hour.

Dandelion flowers can also be eaten, but they require parboiling to reduce their bitterness.

QUICK SERVING IDEAS

- Young dandelion leaves make an excellent spring salad, either alone or in combination with other greens, lettuces, shallot tops, or chives.

- For an exceptional wilted dandelion green salad, try the following: Take 2 large bunches of dandelion greens (about 2 pounds/1 kilogram), remove the tough stems, tear the remaining greens into ¾-inch/1½ cm pieces, and reserve in a large serving bowl. Coarsely chop ¼ cup hazelnuts and 3 cloves garlic or 1 medium onion, and cook in 2 tablespoons of virgin olive oil in a heavy skillet over moderate heat, stirring until the onion or garlic is golden. Stir in 1 tablespoon balsamic vinegar, and add salt and pepper to taste. Pour the hot vinaigrette over the greens and toss to combine.

- Young dandelion leaves are also delicious steamed or boiled, thoroughly drained, seasoned with fresh ground pepper and salt, moistened with olive oil or butter, and served hot. For a very delicate flavor, young dandelion can be prepared in the same way as endive (see page 197). When using more mature leaves, mix with half spinach to lessen the bitterness, but cook the dandelion partially first, as it takes longer to cook than spinach. Grated nutmeg or garlic, or a teaspoonful of chopped onion or grated lemon peel, can be added to the greens after cooking.

- Instead of watercress, try young dandelion leaf sandwiches. Layer the tender leaves on slices of lightly buttered bread and sprinkle with salt. If desired, add a sprinkle of lemon juice and a dash of pepper to vary the flavor.

- The white crown of the leaf stems is an especially delicious part of the dandelion plant and can be eaten raw in salads or cooked. Slice the crowns off the roots just low enough that they all stay together, then slice again where the leaves start getting green. Wash well to remove all the dirt, then soak in salt water until you are ready to use them. To make a salad, cut the crowns finely and use them as you would lettuce in a wilted lettuce salad, or toss them with enough vinaigrette dressing to just coat the leaves, then garnish with slices of hard-boiled egg. To cook them, boil in a lot of water for about 5 minutes, drain, and season with butter, salt, and fresh ground pepper. Put the pot back on the stove and shake just long enough to dry the greens out slightly and melt the butter.

- Young, tender dandelion roots are delicious cooked. Peel them with a potato peeler. Slice thinly crosswise and boil in water to which you've added a pinch of bicarbonate of soda. Pour off the water, cover with fresh water, and boil again. Drain and season with salt, pepper, and butter.

- Old, tough roots can be used to make "coffee." Scrub them well and let dry completely. When thoroughly dry, roast in a slow oven (200 to 250 degrees F./100 to 120 degrees C./gas ¼ to ½) for 4 hours or more until they are deep brown and break with a snap. Allow to cool and grind coarsely. Store the dried coffee substitute as is in sealed containers, or blend first with chicory. Use one teaspoon of ground root for one cup of coffee.

- Dandelion tea can be made from the plant's leaves, roots, or flowers. To make dandelion leaf or flower tea, add 2 to 3 tablespoons of dried leaves or buds to one cup of boiling water and allow to steep for 3 to 5 minutes. If using the roots, scrub them, add 1 cup of them to 4 cups of boiling water, cover, and let simmer for 10 to 15 minutes. The tea is strongest if left to steep overnight.

SAFETY

Individuals with allergies to daisies or other members of the Compositae family may wish to avoid dandelion. If picking wild dandelion greens from lawns or meadows, be sure the area has not been treated with weed killer or fungicides and that it is not located close to a heavily traveled road, where it will be exposed to pollutants from automobile exhaust.

Endive

Much more appreciated in Europe than in the United States, the endive family is a large one. Belgian endive, curly endive, escarole, and radicchio are all members of this chicory family of greens. Each differs considerably in appearance, color, and to some extent, flavor, although all share a slightly bitter taste, and most produce a root that can be roasted, ground, and combined with coffee to create the chicory coffee beloved in French/Creole cultures. Chicory itself is a member of the sunflower (Compositae) family, the same family to which not only lettuce but artichokes, calendula, dandelions, and Jerusalem artichokes belong.

Belgian endive is actually a preflowering growth stage of chicory called a "chicon." This blanched, elongated head of tightly folded leaves is produced by "forcing" defoliated chicory rootstocks to grow buds in a darkened environment.

The growing of Belgian endive, so named since the process was discovered in Flanders in the 1800s, involves sowing seed in early spring in soil fertilized with generous amounts of phosphorus and potassium but limited nitrogen, to ensure that the plant's roots, rather than its foliage, develop fully. After about four months of growth, the roots are harvested and stored outdoors for several months to activate the enzyme inulase, which converts carbohydrate stored in the roots in the form of inulin to the more readily utilized sugar fructose. The roots are then trimmed of any foliage and extraneous branches and placed in specially prepared beds, where they are kept in darkness and warmth to force the growth of the cones of pale, succulent leaves, each of which is often wrapped in purple paper to prevent greening. After three to four weeks, the bullet-shaped heads of tightly closed leaves are typically large enough to harvest.

HISTORY

A native of the Mediterranean region, chicory has been used since ancient Greek and Roman times, when it grew abundantly along roadsides and as a weed in cultivated fields. Pliny the Elder (23–79 C.E.) praised the plant for both its food value and curative powers. In 1616, chicory was actively cultivated in Germany. Other European countries soon followed suit, and chicory became so popular that immigrants to the United States brought the vegetable with them for their gardens.

In the mid-1800s, in Flanders, a part of western Belgium along the North Sea, the technique for producing the tender, mild-flavored chicons was accidentally discovered, which is why this form of chicory is usually called Belgian endive (although it is also referred to as French endive or Witloof chicory since the French became the leading producers of chicons and used primarily the Witloof variety of chicory). In 1830, the head horticulturist at the Brussels Botanical Gardens, M. Brezier, neglected some chicory plants set in a dark warehouse. The plants blanched for lack of light, and the resulting 4 to 6 inch/10 to 15 cm cones of creamy white or pale yellow petals were discovered to be a delicious new vegetable. Thirty years later, Belgian endive was introduced into Paris's haute cuisine, whereupon the French immediately dubbed it "white gold."

In Europe, chicory's cultivation increased dramatically when someone discovered that its roasted and ground roots could be used as a coffee extender. This practice of mixing chicory with coffee was brought by the French to Louisiana, where it became a standard feature in Creole cuisine. Today, Belgian endive is gourmet fare grown on almost every continent.

NUTRITIONAL HIGHLIGHTS

Delectable yet a dieter's friend, each leaf of Belgian endive contains only one calorie. Belgian endive is an excellent source of vitamin A and a good source of fiber and vitamin C. A 100 gram serving provides 17 calories, mostly as carbohydrate and fiber.

HEALTH BENEFITS

Belgian endive has a 95 percent water content and a very low calorie content of 7.5 calories per cup. It is an excellent source of carotenes. Pliny recommended chicory for insomnia and to "purify the blood."

HOW TO SELECT AND STORE

When purchasing Belgian endive, look for firm, plump, crisp, smooth white heads with pale yellow leaf tips. If the tips are green rather than the desired yellow, the endive isn't fresh and will taste very bitter. Short, fat heads are preferable to those that are long and thin.

Avoid heads that are blemished or have limp, withered leaves or brown, dark, or slimy spots.

Belgian endive is quite fragile and must be kept dry. If cleaning is necessary, wipe each endive gently with a damp paper towel or cloth.

Belgian endives are best consumed soon after purchase, for they increase in bitterness with age. If you must hold them over, wrap them in a dry paper towel and place inside a plastic bag in the back of the vegetable crisper, where they will be kept cool (38 degrees F./3½ degrees C. is ideal). Kept this way, they can be stored for no more than three days.

TIPS FOR PREPARING

Wash endive thoroughly under cool running water to remove any sand or dirt that may remain in the leaves. If not organically grown, soak the endive in a mild solution of additive-free soap or use a produce wash, rinse thoroughly, and dry with paper towels or a salad spinner.

When serving raw endive leaves, slice about ⅛ inch/¼ cm from the stem end. Then, with a paring knife, cut a small cone shape about ¼ inch/½ cm deep from the stem end. This will enable you to easily peel off each leaf. If cutting leaves for a salad, do so immediately before serving, for their edges brown quickly. In cooked preparations, use the entire head.

QUICK SERVING IDEAS

- Smaller, boat-shaped chicons, or petals, are best for hors d'oeuvres. Carefully separate the leaves as described above and serve with a delicately flavored dip or fill with smoked salmon, goat cheese, spiced walnuts, baby prawns, salmon roe, or pâté.
- Belgian endive's color and slightly bitter flavor really dress up any salad. Try combining it with rocket, oak-leaf or Boston lettuce, watercress, and radicchio; then toss with olive oil and balsamic vinegar.
- Another salad favorite combines Belgian endive with pears, Gorgonzola cheese, and walnuts. Toss with a raspberry vinaigrette.
- The tangy flavor of Belgian endive changes subtly when it is steamed, stewed, grilled, or baked. Use it to add a particularly nice touch to cream soups.
- Lightly sauté the leaves of one head in 3 to 4 tablespoons butter in a shallow pan over a hot stove, turning after 1 to 2 minutes to sauté both sides. Sprinkle with Parmesan cheese, or, for a sweet, lemony flavor, add 3 tablespoons lemon juice, 2 teaspoons honey, and ½ teaspoon salt. Cover the pan and let simmer for about 25 minutes.

SAFETY

Individuals with allergies to daisies or other members of the Compositae family may wish to avoid Belgian endive.

Fennel

Fennel (*Foeniculum vulgare dulce*) is a member of the Umbelliferae family along with carrots, celery, and parsley. Fennel is composed of a white or pale green bulb on which closely super-imposed stalks are arranged. The stalks are topped with feathery green leaves, near which flowers grow and produce fennel seeds. The bulbs, stalks, leaves, and seeds are all edible.

Fennel's aromatic taste is unique, but still quite similar to licorice and anise, while its texture is similar to that of celery, being crunchy and striated.

HISTORY

Fennel has a long history of use as a medicinal plant in the Mediterranean region. Greek myths state that not only was fennel closely associated with Dionysus, the Greek god of food and wine, but that a fennel stalk carried the coal that passed down knowledge of fire from the gods to men. The ancient Greeks knew fennel by the name "marathon." It grew in the field in which one of the great ancient battles was fought, and which was subsequently named the Battle of Marathon after this revered plant. Fennel was also awarded to Pheidippides, the runner who delivered the news of the Persian defeat to Athens.

Fennel has traditionally been used in Europe for digestive ailments. For this reason, fennel has been grown throughout Europe, especially areas surrounding the Mediterranean Sea, and the Near East since ancient times. Today, the United States, France, India, and the Russian Federation are among the leading cultivators of fennel.

NUTRITIONAL HIGHLIGHTS

Fennel is an excellent source of vitamin C, potassium, and dietary fiber. It is also a very good source of phosphorus and folic acid. In addition, fennel is a good source of the minerals magnesium, manganese, iron, calcium, and molybdenum. A 100 gram serving provides only 31 calories as carbohydrate with 3.1 grams of fiber.

HEALTH BENEFITS

Fennel is often consumed for its medicinal effects. Among herbalists, fennel is referred to as (1) an intestinal antispasmodic, or compound that relieves intestinal spasms or cramps; (2) a carminative, or compound that relieves or expels wind; (3) a stomachic, or compound that tones and strengthens the stomach; and (4) an anodyne, or compound that relieves or soothes pain. Fennel also contains phytoestrogens, making it useful as a remedy for many female complaints, especially symptoms of menopause.

Fennel extract may also turn out to be effective in the treatment of idiopathic hirsutism, the occurrence of excessive male-pattern hair growth in women who have a normal ovulatory menstrual cycle and normal levels of serum androgens. In a double-blind study, thirty-eight patients were treated with creams containing 1 percent and 2 percent of fennel extract or placebo (0 percent). Hair diameter and the rate of growth were measured to judge effectiveness. The mean value of hair diameter reduction was 7.8 percent, 18.3 percent, and −0.5 percent for patients receiving the creams containing 1 percent, 2 percent, and 0 percent (placebo) respectively. These results clearly show fennel to exert an antitestosterone action.

Fennel is also very high in anticancer coumarin compounds, such as anethole, the primary component of its volatile oil. In animal studies, anethole has repeatedly been shown to reduce inflammation and to prevent cancer development. Researchers have also proposed a biological mechanism that may explain these anti-inflammatory and anticancer effects. This mechanism involves the shutting down of an intercellular signaling system that prevents activation of potentially strong gene-altering and inflammation-triggering molecules (e.g., NF-kappa-B).

HOW TO SELECT AND STORE

It is best to select fennel with both the bulb and stems attached to ensure maximum freshness. It should be whitish or pale green in color, and, like celery, its branches should be hard and firm as opposed to limp or bending. Look for signs of flowering buds, a sure indicator that the fennel is past maturity. Also, take time to smell the plant, as fresh fennel should have a fragrant smell of licorice or anise. Fennel is usually available from autumn through early summer.

It is best to use fennel soon after purchase to take advantage of its aromatic fragrance. It should be stored in the refrigerator crisper, where it can stay fresh for up to three days.

Dried fennel seeds should be stored in an airtight container in a cool and dry location, where they will keep for about six months. Storing fennel seeds in the refrigerator will help to keep them fresh for up to one year.

TIPS FOR PREPARING

As with celery, all of the components of fennel can be used in cooking. To clean fennel, cut off the base and leaves, then wash the leaves, bulb, and stalks under cold running water. If it is not organically grown, soak in cold water with a mild solution of additive-free soap or use a produce wash and rinse thoroughly. Cut the stalks away from the bulb at the place where they meet.

Cut the fennel in any manner based upon preference or recipe. The best way to slice it is to do so vertically through the bulb; when preparing chunked, diced, or julienned fennel, it is best to first remove the harder core that resides in the center of the bulb before cutting it. The stalks can be used for soups, stocks, and stews, while the leaves can also be used as an herb seasoning.

Fennel seeds may be ground, crushed, or used whole. Whole seeds should be lightly bruised with a mortar and pestle or lightly roasted to bring the flavorful oils out.

QUICK SERVING IDEAS

- Sliced raw fennel with avocados, oranges, and haricot beans creates a colorful, healthful salad.
- Braised fennel is a wonderful complement to any fish or seafood entrée.
- Add sliced fennel to any sandwich as an addition to or substitute for the traditional toppings of lettuce and tomato.
- Layer baked potato and fennel slices, top with your favorite grated hard cheese, and grill until the gratiné becomes hot and melted.
- Mix thinly sliced fennel and minced mint leaves with plain yogurt.

SAFETY

No safety issues are known for fennel.

Garlic

Garlic (*Allium sativum*) is a member of the lily family that is cultivated worldwide. The garlic bulb is the most commonly used portion of the plant and is composed of individual cloves enclosed in a white, parchmentlike skin. The teardrop-shaped garlic bulbs vary in size; however, they usually average around two inches/5cm in height and two inches/5 cm in width at their widest point. Elephant garlic has larger cloves and is more closely related to the leek.

HISTORY

Native to Central Asia, garlic is one of the oldest cultivated plants in the world. Its usage predates written history. Sanskrit records document the use of garlic remedies approximately 5,000 years ago, while the Chinese have been using it for at least 3,000 years. The Ebers Codex, an Egyptian medical papyrus dating to about 1550 B.C.E., mentions garlic as an effective remedy for a variety of ailments. Hippocrates, Aristotle, and Pliny cited numerous therapeutic uses for garlic. Garlic has been used throughout the world to treat atherosclerosis, coughs, dandruff, diarrhea, diphtheria, dysentery, earache, hypertension, hysteria, toothache, vaginitis, and many other conditions.

Stories, verse, and folklore, such as its alleged ability to ward off vampires, give historical documentation to garlic's power. Sir John Harrington, in *The Englishman's Doctor*, written in 1609, summarized garlic's virtues and faults:

Garlic then hath power to save from death
Bear with it though it maketh unsavory
   breath,
And scorn not garlic like some that think
It only maketh men wink and drink and
   stink.

Currently, China, South Korea, India, Spain, and the United States are among the top commercial producers of garlic.

NUTRITIONAL HIGHLIGHTS

Garlic is an excellent source of vitamin B6. It is also a very good source of manganese, selenium, and vitamin C. In addition, garlic is a good source of other minerals, including phosphorus, calcium, potassium, iron, and copper. A 100 gram serving provides 149 calories with 6.4 grams of protein, 0.5 grams of fat, and 33.1 grams of carbohydrate, mostly complex, with 2.1 grams of fiber.

HEALTH BENEFITS

It is beyond the scope of this book to detail all of the wonderful properties of this truly remarkable medicinal plant. Many of the therapeutic effects of garlic are thought to be due to its volatile factors, which are composed of the sulphur-containing compounds allicin, diallyl disulphide, diallyl trisulphide, and others. Additional constituents of garlic include other sulphur-containing compounds; high concentrations of trace minerals, particularly selenium and germanium; glucosinolates; and enzymes. Chopping or crushing garlic stimulates the enzymatic process that converts the phytochemical alliin into allicin, a compound to which many of garlic's health benefits are attributed. The compound allicin is also mainly responsible for the pungent odor of garlic.

Garlic appears to provide protection against atherosclerosis and heart disease. Many studies have shown that garlic decreases total serum cholesterol levels while increasing serum HDL-cholesterol levels. HDL cholesterol, often termed "good" cholesterol, is a protective factor against heart disease. Garlic has also demonstrated blood pressure-lowering action in many studies. It has typically decreased the systolic pressure by 8 mm Hg and the diastolic pressure by 5 mm Hg in patients with high blood pressure.

In a 1979 study, three populations of vegetarians in the Jain community in India that consumed differing amounts of garlic and onions were studied. Numerous favorable effects on blood lipids, as shown in Table 10.2, were observed in the group that consumed the largest quantities of garlic and onions. The study is quite significant because the subjects had nearly identical diets, differing only in garlic and onion ingestion.

Garlic also has a long history of use as an infection fighter. In fact, it has been referred to as "Russian penicillin" to denote its antibacterial properties. The antimicrobial activity is due to allicin. Allicin has been shown to be effective not only against common infections, such as colds, flu, stomach viruses, and *Candida* yeast, but also against powerful pathogenic microbes, including tuberculosis and botulism.

Garlic also appears to offer protection against some cancers. For example, studies have shown that as few as two or more servings of garlic a week may help protect against colon cancer. Substances found in garlic, such as allicin, have been shown not only to protect

TABLE 10.2

Effects of Garlic and Onion Consumption on Serum Lipids Under Carefully Matched Diets

Garlic/Onion	Cholesterol	Triglycerides
None	208 mg/dl	109 mg/dl
10/200 grams per week	172 mg/dl	75 mg/dl
50/600 grams per week	159 mg/dl	52 mg/dl

colon cells from the toxic effects of cancer-causing chemicals but also to stop the growth of cancer cells once they develop.

The beneficial effects of garlic are clearly quite extensive. Its use as a food should be encouraged, despite its odor, especially by individuals with elevated cholesterol levels, heart disease, high blood pressure, diabetes, *Candida* infections, asthma, infections (particularly respiratory tract infections), and gastrointestinal complaints.

HOW TO SELECT AND STORE

For best flavor and maximum health benefits, buy fresh garlic, as it is widely available. Purchase garlic that is plump, with unbroken skin. Do not buy garlic that is soft, shows evidence of decay, such as mildew or darkening, or is beginning to sprout. Garlic in flake, powder, or paste form is convenient, but it is simply not as good as fresh garlic.

Fresh garlic should be stored at room temperature in an uncovered (or loosely covered) container in a cool, dark place away from exposure to heat and sunlight. Storing in this manner will help prevent sprouting, which reduces its flavor and uses up the clove.

Depending upon its age and variety, a whole garlic bulbs will keep fresh from two weeks to two months. Inspect the bulb frequently and remove any cloves that appear to be dried out or mouldy. Note: Once you break the head of garlic, it greatly reduces its shelf life, to just a few days.

TIPS FOR PREPARING

Unless you are roasting the entire bulb, when using garlic you will need to separate the individual cloves from the bulb. You will next need to separate the skin from the individual cloves. There are kitchen tools that will do this for you, or you can do it with either your fingers or a small knife.

When juicing garlic, it is best to remove the garlic clove from the bulb and wrap it in a green vegetable such as parsley. This accomplishes two things: (1) it prevents the garlic from popping out of the juicer, and (2) the chlorophyll helps bind some of the odor. It is a good idea to juice the garlic first, as the other vegetables will remove the odor from the machine.

QUICK SERVING IDEAS

- Garlic, either chopped, sliced, or crushed, is a valuable addition to many foods, sauces, and soups to improve the nutritional benefits as well as the flavor.
- Macerate garlic in olive oil for one week and use this flavored oil in dressings and marinades.
- Purée two or more cloves fresh garlic, 12 ounces/350 grams canned chickpeas, 2 tablespoons sesame butter, 2 tablespoons olive oil, and 2 to 3 tablespoons lemon juice to make a quick and easy hummus dip.

- Purée the cloves from two heads roasted garlic, 3 cups cooked potatoes, and ½ cup olive oil together to make delicious garlic mashed potatoes. Season to taste.
- Stuff pitted olives with pieces of garlic and serve as hors d'oeuvres or mix into salads.

SAFETY

Garlic poses little safety issue. Allergies to garlic are extremely rare.

Jerusalem Artichoke (Sunchoke)

The Jerusalem artichoke is neither from Jerusalem nor an artichoke. It is the edible tuber, or underground stem, of a Native American plant belonging to the daisy family (Compositae) that is actually a variety of sunflower.

The Jerusalem artichoke resembles a small knobby potato or piece of gingerroot 3 to 4 inches/7½ to 10cm long and 1 to 2 inches/2½ to 5 cm in diameter with light brown mottled skin, which may have a yellow, red, or purple tinge, depending upon the soil in which it is grown. It has a flavor and sweet aftertaste similar to those of the globe artichoke, hence its "artichoke" designation. A versatile vegetable, these sweet, crunchy, nutty-tasting tubers can be enjoyed raw or cooked. With a crispness similar to water chestnuts, they can even stand in for water chestnuts, served raw in salads or lightly cooked in stir-fries.

HISTORY

A native of North America, the Jerusalem artichoke grew wild along the eastern seaboard, from the lakes region of Canada south to Georgia, and was cultivated by Indians living along the coast of what was to become Massachusetts. The Indians called the perennial tubers "sun roots" and introduced them to the Pilgrims, who quickly adopted them as a staple food.

In 1605, the French explorer Samuel de Champlain is said to have first encountered Jerusalem artichokes growing in an Indian vegetable garden in Cape Cod. After sampling the vegetable, he likened its taste to that of an artichoke, a name he carried back with the tubers to France. Shortly thereafter, the exotic vegetable from the Americas was being sold by Parisian street vendors, who named them *topinambours* after a Brazilian Indian tribe of the same name, of which six members had been brought back to the curious French in 1613 after an expedition.

The "artichokes" then made their way across Europe, reaching England in 1617 and Germany in 1632, by which time "Jerusalem" had been affixed to their name, the result of an English corruption of either Ter Neuzen, the town in the Netherlands that provided the English with their first taste of the plant, or the Italian name they were given, *girasole,* whose literal meaning is "turning to the sun," which this sunflower relative does throughout the day.

The French readily accepted the Jerusalem artichoke in the early 1600s, probably because it was introduced under the name "artichoke." The potato, on the other hand, was regarded with suspicion. When the Irish potato finally won acceptance, the Jerusalem artichoke fell into disrepute both because the potato produced higher yields and because the Jerusalem artichoke's irregular shape and brown mottled skin, which resembles the deformed fingers of lepers, gave rise to an old wives' tale linking the tuber to leprosy.

In times of desperation, however, the value of the Jerusalem artichoke again became appreciated. In 1805, during a time when they had difficulty finding adequate food, the explorers Meriwether Lewis and William Clark were sustained by Jerusalem artichokes prepared by the Indians in what is now North Dakota. When a famine occurred throughout Europe in 1772, it was discovered that Jerusalem artichokes could be quickly and easily grown to provide nourishment. During World War II, because they could be bought without a ration card, the tubers again gained popularity in Europe, along with a reputation as a poor man's vegetable. Today, Jerusalem artichokes are an important cash root crop with more than two hundred varieties cultivated in Europe and Asia, as well as the Americas, where they are also marketed as sunchokes.

NUTRITIONAL HIGHLIGHTS

The Jerusalem artichoke provides a rich source of minerals, such as iron, copper, potassium, molybdenum, and magnesium. It also provides an array of B vitamins, being an excellent source of thiamine and pantothenic acid, a very good source of niacin, and a good source of vitamin B6 and riboflavin. Freshly harvested, raw Jerusalem artichokes contain 114 calories in a one-cup serving. As their starch converts to sugar with increased storage time, this calorie count increases slightly.

HEALTH BENEFITS

Jerusalem artichokes, like globe artichokes, are a rich source of inulin. Inulin is a polysaccharide, or starch, that is handled by the body differently from other sugars. In fact, inulin is not utilized by the body for energy metabolism. This makes

Jerusalem artichokes extremely beneficial to diabetics. In fact, Jerusalem artichoke polysaccharides have actually been shown to improve blood sugar control. Since the body does not utilize the primary carbohydrate of Jerusalem artichoke, the effective calorie content is virtually nil.

Although inulin is not utilized by the human body, it does provide nutrition to health-promoting bacteria in the intestinal tract. Specifically, inulin promotes the growth of bifidobacteria, a cousin of *Lactobacillus acidophilus* and the primary organism in live yogurt cultures. Bifidobacteria are the primary organisms found in mother's milk and it is believed they are critical to maintaining a healthy balance of intestinal microflora throughout an individual's lifetime. Bifidobacteria are effective inhibitors of many disease-causing organisms; exhibit antitumor activity; help to reduce serum cholesterol levels; and may provide some B vitamins. Bifidobacteria dairy products and supplements are available in the marketplace. However, consumption of Jerusalem artichokes and flour made of them has been shown to effectively promote bifidobacteria growth in the intestinal tract.

Jerusalem artichokes may also have some immune-enhancing activity, as inulin also has the ability to enhance a component of our immune system known as complement. Complement is responsible for increasing host defense mechanisms, such as neutralization of viruses, destruction of bacteria, and increased movement of white blood cells (neutrophils, monocytes, eosinophils, and lymphocytes) to areas of infection. Many medicinal plants, such as echinacea and burdock, owe much of their immune-enhancing effects to inulin. Jerusalem artichoke is one of the richest sources of inulin available.

One caveat: Since the majority of carbohydrate in Jerusalem artichoke is inulin, these tubers may, like beans, cause flatulence in some people, so try them in small amounts initially. For those sensitive to wind-producing foods, a good deal of the inulin Jerusalem artichokes contain can be leached out by either boiling or freezing the tubers before cooking.

HOW TO SELECT AND STORE

Although Jerusalem artichokes are available all year round in the fresh produce department of most supermarkets, their prime season is from October to March. If you're planning to cook them whole, try to choose tubers of similar size, so they will finish cooking at the same time. Choose smooth, plump, clean, unblemished tubers with a minimum of bumps, although protrusions and unevenness on the skin are fine. Farmers are attempting to breed out the bumps in newer varieties, so some are less knobby than others. Avoid any that are limp or spongy or have wrinkled skins, soft spots, a greenish tinge, or sprouts.

Handle Jerusalem artichokes with care, as they bruise easily. Raw Jerusalem artichokes are best stored in the vegetable crisper of the refrigerator, wrapped in paper towels to absorb humidity and sealed in a plastic bag. Their sweetness is known to increase when they are refrigerated after harvesting, so refrigerate them for a day or two before consuming.

Depending upon how long they have been sitting in the shop, raw Jerusalem artichokes can be stored from one to three weeks but, for maximum flavor and nutrition, are best eaten within one week. After that, they may begin to wither.

Cooked Jerusalem artichokes should be refrigerated and consumed within two days. Canning and freezing are not recommended due to discoloration and deterioration of texture.

TIPS FOR PREPARING

Scrub these root vegetables thoroughly but gently under running cold water with a vegetable brush to remove any dirt or grit. If they are not organically grown, soak them in a mild solution of additive-free soap or use a produce wash before washing and scrubbing. Peeling is not only difficult, due to their knobby nature, but unnecessary, since not only are the peels quite thin and edible, but many nutrients are stored just under the skin. If you still wish to peel Jerusalem artichokes and will be eating them raw, slice off the smaller bumpy areas and use a vegetable peeler to remove the skin. If you will be eating them cooked, it's easier to boil, steam, or microwave them whole before peeling.

Once cut, the flesh of Jerusalem artichokes will darken with exposure to air just as potatoes will, so prepare them close to serving time or cut them and immerse them in water with a little added lemon or vinegar to prevent oxidation.

Cooking them with their skins on may cause the skins to darken due to their high iron content. Even after cooking, the high level of iron found in Jerusalem artichokes may cause cooked, stored tubers to turn an unappealing gray. A bit of acid in the form of lemon juice or vinegar in the cooking water will prevent this. Add 1 tablespoon of vinegar or lemon juice per litre of water. Since the acid will also strengthen the Jerusalem artichokes' texture, if you want to mash them or simply prefer a softer result, add the lemon juice or vinegar during the last 5 minutes of cooking.

Avoid aluminum or iron pans. Either of these metals will produce oxidation and turn the vegetable an unappetizing dark grey.

Jerusalem artichokes can be baked, boiled, steamed, fried, or stewed. They cook faster than potatoes and can easily turn to mush in a matter of minutes, so monitor them closely and remove from the heat as soon as they can easily be pierced with a fork or skewer.

QUICK SERVING IDEAS

- Extremely versatile, Jerusalem artichokes can be eaten cooked or raw, whole, diced, sliced, or julienned.
- Jerusalem artichokes can be boiled whole or cut as desired. Add to a pot of boiling water, cover, and boil for 10 to 15 minutes if whole, 5 to 8 minutes if cut up. Season as desired or mash like potatoes.
- Mashed Jerusalem artichokes can be used as a sweet substitute for mashed potatoes or a thickener for soups and stews.
- For a wonderful creamy soup, cook 2 pounds/1 kilogram of Jerusalem artichokes in simmering water for 30 to 40 minutes, until tender. Drain and discard the cooking liquid. Peel and mash, then place in a large saucepan. Stir in 6 cups of vegetable or chicken stock and 1½ cups of spring onions. Simmer about 15 minutes. Season to taste with salt and pepper, and serve sprinkled with a tablespoon or two of basil or dill.
- Coarsely chop, then steam Jerusalem artichokes over high heat for 5 to 7 minutes, and add your favorite seasonings. In addition to

seasoning them with virgin olive oil, sea salt, and coarsely ground black pepper, you can also partner them with cinnamon, nutmeg, cloves, onion, and/or yogurt.

- Shredded Jerusalem artichokes can provide a delicious variation for your favorite potato pancake recipe.
- Toss sliced Jerusalem artichokes in a bowl with a little virgin olive oil, place on a baking sheet, and bake at 375 degrees F./190 degrees C./gas 5 for 20 to 25 minutes, turning them halfway through. Season with salt and pepper to taste.
- Jerusalem artichokes can be substituted for turnips or parsnips in most any recipe.
- Add diced Jerusalem artichokes to your favorite vegetable medley in stir-fry dishes. For a tender-crisp consistency, stir-fry 2 to 4 minutes. For a softer consistency, stir-fry 4 to 6 minutes.
- Sliced raw Jerusalem artichokes add a sweet crunch to green salads; can be served with crudités and dips; shredded into a slaw; or diced and added to other chopped vegetables, such as carrot, celery, and onion, for a delicious chopped salad.

SAFETY

Jerusalem artichokes contain starch in the form of inulin (see page 76), a beneficial fiberlike polysaccharide. Because it can produce excess wind or a loose stool in certain cases, it is important to introduce it to the diet in moderate amounts (one or two servings per day). Also, those who suffer from allergies to daisies or other members of the Compositae family may wish to avoid Jerusalem artichokes. There has been one unusual case of an allergic reaction involving swelling and breathing difficulties linked to inulin.

Jicama

Jicama, pronounced "HEE-ka-ma," is a turnip-shaped root vegetable native to Mexico and Central America. A member of the morning glory family (Convolvulaceae), the jicama plant is a vine that grows to a length of 20 feet/6 meters or more and produces beautiful sprays of mauve flowers that resemble butterflies, but these are rarely seen in the United States because the vines are usually killed by frost before they bloom. The roots are light brown and can reach weights of up to 50 pounds/23 kilograms, although those in the markets usually weigh from 1 to 3 pounds/½ to 1½ kilograms.

Jicama is related to the sweet potato but resembles the water chestnut in color, texture, and flavor, with a thin brown skin that encloses crisp, juicy, white flesh. In fact, many Oriental restaurants substitute jicama for the more expensive water chestnut.

HISTORY

Jicama, also known as yam bean, Mexican potato, or Mexican turnip, has been eaten in Central America for many centuries. From its native Mexico, where it is sometimes called *bejuco blanco*, meaning "white vine," jicama has recently been brought, along with Mexican cuisine, to the southwestern United States.

Jicama is now being grown on a small scale in the Southwest of the United States. The crop is cultivated in frost-free climates, where the vine is grown in rows from seeds and harvested within a year for its large taproot. The rest of the plant, a legume with trifoliate leaves and reportedly poisonous seeds, is inedible and is thrown away. In Britain, jicama comes mainly from Asian sources and is likely to be found in Asian greengrocers and supermarkets.

Although in California jicama is commonly added raw to salads or sliced into strips like carrots, in Mexico the ivory-colored flesh is marinated with lime and then served topped with chili powder. On the streets, fruit salad vendors hawk jicama mixed with chunks of cantaloupe melon, watermelon, and papaya.

Residents of Mexico also know jicama as one of the four elements used in "The Festival of the Dead," celebrated on November 1. The other foods are sugarcane (from southern Asia), tangerines (from eastern Asia), and peanuts (from Bolivia), so this is a festival with international flair. During the festival, "jicama dolls" are cut from strips of paper.

Jicama is also enjoyed in the Philippines, where it is called *singkamas* and is eaten raw in salad dressed with a vinaigrette as an accompaniment for fish or eaten plain, sprinkled with salt.

NUTRITIONAL HIGHLIGHTS

A cup of raw, sliced jicama provides 27 percent of the recommended daily intake (RDI) of fiber, plus 35 percent of the RDI for vitamin C, all for a mere 49 calories. In addition to being an excellent source of fiber and vitamin C, jicama is a very good source of the trace mineral molybdenum and a good source of potassium.

HEALTH BENEFITS

A fiber-rich, low-carbohydrate Mexican "potato," jicama's nutritional profile makes it the perfect "baked potato" for those wishing to lose excess weight. Eaten raw, jicama's high vitamin C content also translates into good insurance against colds and flu.

HOW TO SELECT AND STORE

High-quality jicama is firm and heavy for its size. Jicama that is shriveled, soft, or particularly large is likely to be tough and woody and contain less water. The younger and smaller the tuber, the sweeter and more mild it will be.

Jicama is also frequently sold in pieces, which may be more practical as this root vegetable often weighs 3 to 5 pounds/1½ to 2¼ kilograms. Choose pieces that are tightly wrapped in plastic and have a clean white flesh. Store pieces, wrapped in plastic, in the refrigerator crisper, where they will keep for up to one week.

Whole jicama can be kept in a cool, dark place for up to two weeks and will store for up to three weeks refrigerated, uncovered in the vegetable crisper. However, if it is not stored properly, jicama will quickly mould. If you do not use all of the jicama, peel it, cut in slices or cubes, place in an airtight container, cover with water to maintain crispness, and store refrigerated for up to three days. Cooked jicama will keep for three days refrigerated.

TIPS FOR PREPARING

Always remove the peel, as it is inedible. Then remove the first layer of flesh directly under the skin since, except in young jicama, it is often too fibrous. Slice into uniform sticks, dice, or shred.

If not serving cut jicama immediately, refrigerate cut pieces in a container of cold water.

Jicama's delicate flavor enables it to be used in a variety of ways. Since it does not turn brown, peeled, sliced jicama can have a starring role in a raw vegetable platter. Diced or sliced, it also makes a sweet, crunchy addition to salads.

In addition to being eaten raw, jicama can be prepared in some of the same ways as the potato, but it is less starchy and has half the calories found in a potato.

Be sure to size up your jicama. A one-pound/½ kilogram jicama yields about 3 cups of chopped or shredded flesh. If you are not going to use all of it for the recipe you are preparing, cut the jicama in half or quarters, wrap the unused portion in cling film, and refrigerate.

QUICK SERVING IDEAS

- Jicama's high water content makes it a fantastic vegetable to juice.
- In Mexico, raw sliced jicama is a favorite hors d'oeuvre, either served with salsa or sprinkled with lime juice and chili powder.
- For exceptional black beans, mix ½ cup diced jicama, 1 medium chopped tomato, ½ red sweet pepper, 2 cloves minced garlic, ½ cup corn, 4 tablespoons chopped fresh coriander, 1 teaspoon ground cumin, 2 tablespoons olive oil, 2 tablespoons lime juice, and 1 pound/½ kilogram cooked black beans.
- Combine jicama with another Mexican favorite, avocado. Cut jicama into slices, then thin strips, and toss with a balsamic vinegar and olive oil dressing. Top with slices of avocado, a squeeze of lime juice, and a little minced red onion.

- Use jicama as a less expensive but equally delicious substitute for water chestnuts in Asian dishes. Since it retains its crispness when cooked, slivers of jicama can add crunch and texture when stir-fried with other vegetables; chopped eggs, fish, meats or poultry; and various seasonings.
- Jicama can also be boiled or baked and enjoyed like a potato.

SAFETY

Unlike the Irish potato's, the skin of the "Mexican potato" is inedible. Also, the seeds of the jicama plant are reputed to be poisonous. The vines are also considered inedible and are discarded.

Kale (Collards)

Kale (*Brassica oleracea acephala*) is a green leafy vegetable that is a member of the cruciferous or cabbage family. In fact, kale is probably the closest relative of wild cabbage in the entire cabbage family. Kale and collards are essentially the same vegetable, only kale has leaves with curly edges and is less tolerant to heat. Other greens of the cabbage family, such as mustard greens, turnip greens, kohlrabi, and watercress, offer similar benefits as kale and collards and can be used similarly.

There are several varieties of kale, known commonly as curly kale, ornamental kale, and dinosaur kale, all of which differ in taste, texture, and appearance. Curly kale has ruffled leaves and a fibrous stalk and is usually deep green in color. It has a lively, pungent flavor with delicious bitter, peppery qualities. Ornamental kale is a more recently cultivated species that is often referred to as salad savoy in the U.S.A. Its leaves may be green, white, or purple, and its stalks coalesce to form a loosely knit head. Ornamental kale has a more mellow flavor and tender texture. Dinosaur kale is the common name of the kale variety known as Lacinato. It is better known as cavolo nero or Tuscan kale in Europe. It features dark blue-green leaves that have an embossed texture. It has a slightly sweeter and more delicate taste than curly kale.

HISTORY

Kale is a descendant of the wild cabbage, a plant thought to have originated in Asia Minor and to have been brought to Europe around 600 B.C.E. Curly kale was a significant crop in ancient Rome and a popular vegetable eaten by peasants throughout the Middle Ages. Kale was brought to the United States by English settlers in the 1600s. Today in the United States, kale and collards are grown primarily on the East Coast from Delaware to Florida.

NUTRITIONAL HIGHLIGHTS

Kale is among the most highly nutritious vegetables. It is an excellent source of carotenes, vitamins C and B6, and manganese. In fact, one cup of kale supplies more than 70 percent of the RDI for vitamin C, with only 20 calories. It is also a very good source of dietary fiber, as well as many minerals, including copper, iron, and calcium. In addition, it is a very good source of vitamins B1, B2, and E.

HEALTH BENEFITS

Kale has almost three times as much calcium as phosphorus, which is a very beneficial ratio since high phosphorus consumption has been linked to osteoporosis because it reduces the utilization and promotes the excretion of calcium.

As members of the cabbage family, kale and collards exhibit the same sort of anticancer properties as other members (see "Cabbage," page 178). Kale is also extremely high in chlorophyll and carotenes, especially beta-carotene, lutein, and zeaxanthin.

HOW TO SELECT AND STORE

High-quality kale and collards, as well as other "greens," are fresh, tender, and dark green. Avoid greens that show dry or yellowing leaves, evidence of insect injury, or decay. Smaller-sized leaves are not only easier to handle, they will be more tender and have a milder flavor than those with larger leaves. Kale is available throughout the year, although it is more widely available, and at its peak, from the middle of winter through the beginning of spring.

Kale should be stored in the refrigerator crisper wrapped in a damp paper towel or placed in a perforated plastic bag. Do not wash before storing, as this will cause it to become limp. Kale can be kept in the refrigerator for several days, although it is best when eaten within one to two days after purchase since the longer it is stored, the bitterer its flavor will become. Cooked kale will keep for two days refrigerated.

TIPS FOR PREPARING

Wash kale leaves thoroughly under cool running water to remove any sand or dirt that may remain in the leaves. If not organically grown, soak them in a mild solution of additive-free soap or use a produce wash (see page 51), rinse thoroughly, and dry with paper towels or a salad spinner. Both the leaves and the stem of kale can be eaten; simply cut the leaves and stem into the shape and size you desire.

If your recipe calls for the leaves only, take a leaf in hand and fold it in half lengthwise, then hold the remaining folded leaves near the base where they meet the stem and gently pull on the stem of the single leaf you're holding. You can also use a knife to separate the leaves from the stem.

While people are accustomed to eating kale only when it is cooked, this leafy green vegetable has a strong but delightful taste when eaten raw. Cut into small pieces, it adds a spark, both flavor-wise and nutritionally, to vegetable or grain salads.

Kale leaves make an excellent addition to fresh vegetable juices, too. Typically one third of the volume of the juice should be composed of kale, as it can be quite strong. Usually the leaves can be fed into the juicer intact, but large leaves may need to be cut.

QUICK SERVING IDEAS

- Perk up your dinner salad by using chopped kale as a salad green.
- Lightly sauté kale with fresh garlic and sprinkle it with lemon juice before serving.
- Braise chopped kale and apples, then sprinkle with balsamic vinegar and chopped walnuts just before serving.
- Combine chopped kale, pine nuts, and feta cheese with whole-grain pasta drizzled with olive oil.

- The taste and texture of steamed kale make it a wonderful topping for homemade pizzas.
- Purée cooked kale and potatoes together and season with salt, pepper, cayenne pepper, and cumin for a delicious soup. Add vegetable stock if needed.

SAFETY

Members of the cabbage family contain goitrogens, naturally occurring substances that can interfere with the functioning of the thyroid gland. Dietary goitrogens are usually of no clinical importance unless they are consumed in large amounts or there is coexisting iodine deficiency. Cooking helps to inactivate the goitrogenic compounds. Individuals with already existing and untreated thyroid problems may want to avoid consumption of cabbage-family vegetables in their raw form for this reason. (See "Cabbage," page 178, for more information.)

Kale also contains significant amount of oxalate. Individuals with a history of oxalate-containing kidney stones should avoid overconsuming kale and other oxalate-containing greens. For more information, see Appendix D, page 793.

Kohlrabi: See Kale.

Leeks

The leek (*Allium ampeloprasum porrum*) is related to onions and garlic. However, while the bulbs of garlic and onions are typically the edible portion, with leeks it is the leaves and stems that are eaten rather than the long, narrow

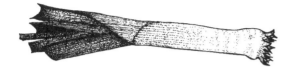

bulb. Leeks have a long white cylindrical stalk of superimposed layers that flows into green, tightly wrapped, flat leaves. Leeks are about 12 inches/30 cm in length and 1 to 2 inches/2 to 5 cm in diameter and feature a characteristic fragrant flavor similar to onions, but sweeter and more subtle. Wild leeks, known as "ramps" and similar to mild garlic, are much smaller in size but have a stronger, more intense flavor.

HISTORY

Leeks are native to Central Asia, and they have been cultivated in this region and in Europe for thousands of years. Leeks were prized by the ancient Greeks and Romans for their beneficial effect upon the throat. The Greek philosopher Aristotle credited the clear voice of the partridge to a diet of leeks, while the Roman emperor Nero supposedly ate leeks every day to make his own voice stronger.

The Romans are thought to have introduced leeks to Britain, where they were able to flourish because they could withstand cold weather. In addition, leeks have attained an esteemed status in Wales, where they are the country's national emblem. The high regard that the Welsh hold for leeks can be traced back to their being placed under the caps of Welsh soldiers to differentiate themselves from the Anglo-Saxons during a successful battle in 620. Leeks are still an important vegetable in the diet of many northern European countries.

NUTRITIONAL HIGHLIGHTS

Leeks have a similar caloric and nutritional profile as onions. They are a good source of vitamins B6 and C and folic acid. They are also a good source of the minerals manganese and iron. In addition, leeks are a good source of dietary fiber.

HEALTH BENEFITS

Leeks provide many of the same health benefits as onions and garlic. However, since they are less dense than garlic and onion, larger quantities of leeks need to be consumed to produce effects similar to those of onions and garlic. Presumably, leeks can lower cholesterol levels, improve the immune system, and fight cancer just as onions and garlic can.

HOW TO SELECT AND STORE

A leek should have broad, dark, solid leaves and a thick, white neck, with a bulb about 1 inch/2½ cm in diameter. Leeks with yellowing, wilted, or discolored leaves should be avoided. Choose smaller leeks (bulb diameter of 1 to 1½ inches/2½ to 3 cm or less), as when they are overly large they tend to be more fibrous in texture. If you are planning to cook leeks whole, try to purchase leeks that are of similar size to ensure more consistent cooking. Leeks are available throughout the year, although they are in greater supply from the autumn through to the early part of spring.

Fresh leeks should be stored unwashed and untrimmed in the refrigerator, where they will keep fresh for one to two weeks. Keeping them in perforated or loosely wrapped plastic will help them to retain moisture. Cooked leeks are highly perishable and, even when kept in the refrigerator, will stay fresh for only up to two days. Leeks may be frozen after being blanched for 2 to 3 minutes, although they will lose some of their desirable taste and texture. Leeks will keep in the freezer for about three months.

TIPS FOR PREPARING

To prepare leeks, clean them thoroughly under running cold water to remove any soil that may have become caught within the overlapping layers. If they are not organically grown, soak in cold water with a mild solution of additive-free soap or use a produce wash (see page 51) before washing. Then trim off the rootlets and a portion of the green tops and remove the outer layer. For all preparations, except cutting into cross sections, make a lengthwise incision to the centerline, fold it open, and rinse the leek under cool water. If your recipe calls for cross sections, first cut the leek into the desired pieces, then place the slices in a colander and rinse under cool water.

QUICK SERVING IDEAS

- Leeks can be utilized in ways similar to onions (see page 216).
- Add finely chopped leeks to salads, soups, or omelets.
- Lightly sauté equal parts leeks and fennel for 3 to 4 minutes. Garnish with fresh lemon juice and thyme.
- Make vichyssoise, a cold soup made of puréed cooked leeks and potatoes.
- Braised leeks sprinkled with fennel or mustard seeds make a wonderful side dish for fish, poultry, or steak.

SAFETY

Leeks contain a small amount of oxalate. Individuals with a history of oxalate-containing kidney stones should avoid overconsuming them. For more information, see Appendix D, page 793.

Lettuce

Lettuce varieties are members of the daisy or sunflower family (Compositae). Most varieties of lettuce exude small amounts of a white, milky liquid when their leaves are broken. This "milk" gives lettuce its slightly bitter flavor and its scientific name, *Lactuca sativa.* "Lactuca" is derived from the Latin word for "milk."

Lettuce can be classified into four categories:

- Iceberg/crisphead: With green leaves on the outside and whitish leaves on the inside, this variety of head lettuce has a crisp texture and a watery, mild taste. The best-known variety of crisphead lettuce is iceberg.

- Romaine: Also known as cos, this variety of head-forming lettuce has deep green, long leaves with a crisp texture and deep taste.

- Butterhead: These types of lettuce feature tender, large leaves that form a loosely arranged head that is easily separated from the stem. They have a sweet flavor and a soft texture. In the U.K. the best known variety of butterhead lettuce is Roundhead.

- Loose-leaf: Featuring broad, curly-leaf varieties that are green and/or red, loose-leaf lettuce offers a delicate taste and a mildly crispy texture. In the U.K. the best-known varieties of loose-leaf lettuce include lollo rosso, lollo bianco, frisee and oak leaf.

Although vegetables such as rocket, mizuna, and watercress are not technically lettuce, these greens are often used interchangeably with lettuce in salads. (See "Rocket" and "Mustard Greens.")

HISTORY

Lettuce is native to the eastern Mediterranean region and western Asia. The ancient Greeks and Romans hailed it as a medicinal plant, and Augustus Caesar went so far as to erect a statue in honor of lettuce based on his belief that it had aided his recovery from illness.

In China, where lettuce has been growing since the fifth century, lettuce represents good luck. It is served on birthdays, New Year's Day, and other special occasions. Christopher Columbus introduced varieties of lettuce to North America during his second voyage in 1493. Lettuce was first planted in California (now the major U.S. producer) by Spanish missionaries in the seventeenth century. In the twentieth century, with the development of refrigeration and railway transportation, the popularity of lettuce grew tremendously.

NUTRITIONAL HIGHLIGHTS

In general, the darker the lettuce, the greater the nutrient content; therefore, romaine > loose-leaf > butterhead > iceberg. All lettuce is a good source of chlorophyll and vitamin K. Iceberg lettuce is a surprisingly good source of choline.

Romaine lettuce is generally the most nutrient-dense lettuce and is an excellent source of vitamin A, folic acid, and vitamins C, B1, and B2. It is also an excellent source of the minerals manganese and chromium.

HEALTH BENEFITS

Due to its extremely low calorie content, 15 calories per 100 gram serving, and high water volume, lettuce is probably the most famous diet food. In fact, the term "salad" is often synonymous with "lettuce." Since it is primarily water, lettuce provides little health benefit beyond its nutrient content.

HOW TO SELECT AND STORE

Good-quality lettuce is fresh, crisp, and free of any evidence of decay. Avoid lettuce that has a rusty appearance and signs of decay. A salad spinner is a great way to dry the leaves and prepare them for use in salads and for storage. Lettuce should be washed and dried before storing in the refrigerator to remove excess moisture. Crisphead and romaine lettuce will keep for five to seven days, butterhead and loose-leaf lettuce for two to three days.

TIPS FOR PREPARING

To clean lettuce, first remove the outer leaves and with one slice cut off the tips of the lettuce, which tend to be bitter. Chop the remaining lettuce to the desired size and discard the bottom root portion. Rinse and pat dry, or, if you have one available, use a salad spinner to remove the excess water.

For rocket and watercress, trim their roots and separate the leaves, placing the leaves in a large bowl of cold water or mild solution of additive-free soap or use a produce wash, swishing them around with your hands. This will allow any sand to become dislodged. Remove the leaves from the water, empty the bowl, refill with clean water, and repeat the process until no dirt remains in the water—usually two or three times will do the trick.

QUICK SERVING IDEAS

- Give sandwiches extra crunch and nutrients by garnishing with lettuce leaves.
- When it comes to salads, the only limitation is your imagination. Be creative. Use a variety of different lettuce types and add your favorite foods, whether they be vegetables, fruits, seeds, nuts, whole grains, soy products, meats, or cheeses; almost every food goes well with lettuce.
- For an interactive meal that is both unusual and fun, arrange nuts, diced vegetables, chicken and/or baked tofu, and romaine lettuce leaves on a large plate. Diners can then make their own lettuce pockets by placing the favorite fillings in a lettuce leaf and making a breadless sandwich wrap.
- For a unique side dish, simmer lettuce in liquid seasoned with your favorite herbs and spices. To help preserve the lettuce's color, blanch the leaves for a few minutes before simmering.
- Lettuce makes a good addition to soups made with other leafy greens. Add toward the end of cooking.

SAFETY

Lettuce is generally not associated with any specific safety issues. After all, it is primarily water. The key is to wash it thoroughly and focus on organically grown.

Mustard Greens

Mustard greens are the leaves of the mustard plant (Brassica juncea), which is a member of the cabbage, or cruciferous, family. In addition to providing nutritious greens, this plant also produces the acrid-tasting brown seeds that are used to make Dijon mustard (see page 494).

There are several different varieties of mustard greens. Most are emerald green in color, and some are not green at all but rather shades of dark red or deep purple. The other major variant is the nature of the leaves, as they can have either a crumpled or flat texture and may have toothed, scalloped, frilled, or lacy edges.

HISTORY

Mustard greens are native to the Himalayan region of India, where they have been cultivated for more than 5,000 years. Mustard greens are a notable vegetable in many different cuisines, ranging from Chinese to southern African-American. The popularity of mustard and turnip greens in southern U.S. cuisine can be traced to the substitution of these greens for the greens that were an essential part of the traditional West African diet. The United States is a major grower of mustard greens, as are India, Nepal, China, and Japan.

NUTRITIONAL HIGHLIGHTS

Mustard greens are a low-calorie, antioxidant-dense food. They are an excellent source of carotenes, vitamin C, folic acid, manganese, vitamin E, copper, dietary fiber, vitamin B6, and calcium. They are a very good source of phosphorus, vitamin B2, potassium, magnesium, protein, vitamin B1, and iron. A 100 gram serving of cooked mustard greens provides 35 calories, 2.3 grams of protein, no cholesterol, 0.4 grams of fat, 7.2 grams of carbohydrate, and 3.3 grams of fiber.

HEALTH BENEFITS

Mustard greens, a member of the cruciferous vegetable family, are best known for their anticancer effects (see "Cabbage"). This benefit relates to their high content of antioxidant compounds, including vitamins C and E, and carotenes, as well as their high content of the glucosinolates.

Mustard greens are also an especially good food choice for women going through menopause, due to their ability to protect against breast cancer and heart disease and their high content of nutrients that are supportive of bone health, such as calcium, magnesium, and folic acid.

HOW TO SELECT AND STORE

Like other greens, purchase mustard greens that look fresh and crisp and are a lively green, dark red, or deep purple color. They should be unblemished and free from any yellowing or brown spots.

Mustard greens should be stored in a perforated plastic bag in the refrigerator, where they should keep fresh for about three to four days. Cooked mustard greens will keep for two days when refrigerated.

TIPS FOR PREPARING

The easiest way to clean the leaves of dirt and debris is to place them in a large bowl of cold water or mild solution of additive-free soap or use a produce wash and swish them around with your hands to dislodge any dirt or debris. Remove the mustard greens from the water, empty the bowl, refill it with clean water, and repeat the process until no sand or dirt remains in the water—usually two or three times will do the trick.

To prepare mustard greens for most dishes, after washing them fold them in half along the stem. Since the thicker part of the stem is much tougher than the softer leaves, it is best to remove it by cutting the folded leaf along the stem and then discarding the stem. If you are planning to use mustard greens in soup, you can keep the leaves intact with their center stem, as the long cooking time is sufficient to soften them.

QUICK SERVING IDEAS

- Like kale, young mustard greens can be added to virtually any green salad.
- A simple but nutritious side dish can be prepared quickly by sautéing mustard greens with olive oil, walnuts, and lemon juice.
- For a simple meal with southern U.S. flair, serve cooked mustard greens with red beans and rice.
- Lightly sauté mustard greens, sweet potatoes, and tofu and serve alongside your favorite grain.

SAFETY

Members of the cabbage family contain goitrogens, naturally occurring substances that can interfere with the functioning of the thyroid gland. Dietary goitrogens are usually of no clinical importance unless they are consumed in large amounts or there is coexisting iodine deficiency. Cooking helps to inactivate the goitrogenic compounds. Individuals with already existing and untreated thyroid problems may want to avoid consumption of cabbage-family vegetables in their raw form for this reason. (See "Cabbage" for more information.)

Mustard greens also contain significant amounts of oxalate. Individuals with a history of oxalate-containing kidney stones should avoid overconsuming them. For more information, see Appendix D, page 793.

Onions

The onion *(Allium cepa),* like garlic, is a member of the lily family. There are numerous forms and varieties of onions, as they are cultivated worldwide. Common varieties are white globe, yellow globe, red globe, and green. With globe onions, the part used is the fleshy bulb, while with green or spring onions, both the long slender bulb and the green leaves are used.

Onions differ in their size, color, and taste. There are two main types of large globe-shaped onions: spring/summer and storage onions. Spring/summer onions are grown in warm-weather climates and have a characteristically mild or sweet taste. Included in this group are the Walla Walla, Vidalia, and Maui Sweet onions. Storage onions are grown in colder-weather climates and, after harvesting, are dried out for a period of several months, during which they attain dry, crisp skins. They generally have a more pungent flavor and are usually named by their color: white, yellow, or red. The Spanish onion is an example of a storage onion.

Smaller onions also come in many types, such as the green or spring onion, chives, leeks (see page 210), and shallots; and the pearl onion.

HISTORY

Onions originated in Central Asia, from Iran to Pakistan and northward into the southern part of Russia. Onions have been revered throughout time not only for their culinary use but also for their therapeutic properties. In fact, as early as the sixth century B.C.E., onions were used as a medicine in India.

Although onions were popular with the ancient Greeks and Romans, they were often dressed with extra seasonings since many people did not find them spicy enough. Yet it was their pungency that made onions popular among poor people throughout the world, who could freely use this inexpensive vegetable to spark up their meals. Onions were a key component in the cuisines of many European countries during the Middle Ages and were even served as a breakfast food. Early explorers to North America, including Christopher Columbus, brought onions to the Western Hemisphere. The leading producers of onions today are China, India, the United States, the Russian Federation, and Spain.

NUTRITIONAL HIGHLIGHTS

Onions are a very good source of vitamins C and B6, biotin, chromium, and dietary fiber. In addition, onions are a good source of folic acid and vitamins B1 and K. A 100 gram serving provides 44 calories, mostly as complex carbohydrate, with 1.4 grams of fiber.

HEALTH BENEFITS

Onions contain a variety of organic sulphur compounds that provide health benefits. Like

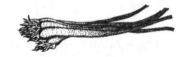

garlic, onions also have the enzyme alliinase, which is released when an onion is cut or crushed, causing the conversion of trans-*S*-(1-propenyl)cysteine sulphoxide to the so-called lacrimatory, or crying, factor, propanethial *S*-oxide. Other constituents include flavonoids (primarily quercetin); phenolic acids, such as ellagic, caffeic, sinapic, and *p*-coumaric; sterols; saponins; pectin; and volatile oils.

Although not nearly as valued a medicinal agent as garlic, onion has been used almost as widely. Onions possess many of the same positive effects as garlic (see "Garlic"). There are, however, some subtle differences that make one more advantageous than the other for certain conditions.

Like garlic, clinical studies have shown onions and onion extracts to decrease blood lipid levels, prevent clot formation, and lower blood pressure. Onions have also been shown to have a significant blood sugar-lowering action, comparable to that of the prescription drugs tolbutamide and phenformin, which are often given to diabetics. The active blood sugar-lowering principle in onions is believed to be allyl propyl disulphide (APDS), although other constituents, such as flavonoids, may play a significant role as well. Experimental and clinical evidence suggests that APDS lowers glucose by competing with insulin (also a disulphide molecule) for breakdown sites in the liver, thereby increasing the life span of insulin. Other mechanisms, such as increased liver metabolism of glucose and increased insulin secretion, have also been proposed.

Onion has historically been used to treat asthma, too. Its action in asthma is due to its ability to inhibit the production of compounds that cause the bronchial muscle to spasm and to relax the bronchial muscle.

In addition, an onion extract was found to destroy tumor cells in test tubes and to arrest tumor growth when tumor cells were implanted in rats. The onion extract was shown to be unusually nontoxic, since a dose as high as forty times that of the dose required to kill the tumor cells had no adverse effect on the host. In addition, shallots have been shown to exhibit significant activity against leukemia in mice.

The liberal use of the *Allium* species, including garlic, leeks, and onions, appears particularly indicated, considering their healing effects for the major disease processes, such as atherosclerosis, diabetes, and cancer, that are dominant today.

HOW TO SELECT AND STORE

Globe onions should be clean and hard and have dry, smooth skins. Avoid onions in which the seed stem has developed. Also, avoid those that are misshaped and/or show evidence of decay. Green or spring onions should have fresh-looking green tops and a white neck. Yellowing, wilted, or discolored tops should be avoided.

Onions should be stored at room temperature, away from bright light, and in an area that is well ventilated. To best accomplish this goal, place them in either a wire hanging basket or a perforated bowl with a raised base so that air can circulate underneath. The length of storage capability varies with the type of onion. Those that are more pungent in flavor, such as yellow onions, will keep longer than those with a sweeter taste, such as white onions, since the compounds that produce the sharp taste are natural preservatives as well. Green or spring onions should be stored in a perforated plastic bag in the refrigerator, where they will keep for about a week. All onions should be stored away from potatoes, as they will absorb their moisture and ethylene gas, causing them to spoil more readily.

The remainder of cut onions should be wrapped tightly in cling film or stored in a sealed container. They oxidize quickly, so you will need to use them within one to two days. Cooked onions will maintain their taste best in an airtight container but still will hold their flavor and freshness for only a day or two. Do not store them in metal bowls or storage containers, as this will cause them to discolor. Peeled, chopped onions can be frozen, but this process will cause them to lose much of their flavor.

TIPS FOR PREPARING

Several of the sulphur-containing compounds of onions are responsible for producing tears when an onion is cut. The compound allyl sulphate, which is produced when sulphur compounds released by the onion's ruptured cells are exposed to air, is especially irritating. To reduce the production of this compound, chill the onions for an hour or so before cutting. Chilling will reduce the activity of the enzyme that produces the allyl sulphate. Also, always use a very sharp knife, and cut the onions while standing so your eyes will be as far away as possible.

QUICK SERVING IDEAS

- Onions can be eaten on their own, either steamed or boiled, although some people do eat raw sweet onions like apples. However, onions are usually utilized to flavor and enhance other recipes.
- Sautéed chopped onions can be added to almost any vegetable dish to enhance its nutritional content and taste.
- For instant vegetarian chili, heat together 1 medium chopped sautéed onion with a 12-ounce/350-gram can of kidney beans, 12 ounces/350 grams of chunky tomato sauce, and 2 tablespoons olive oil, and season to taste with chili powder.
- Combine 1 chopped red onion, 2 Roma tomatoes, 2 avocados, and 1 jalapeño for an all-in-one guacamole salsa dip.
- Place chunks of onion or small pearl onions on a skewer, either alone or with other vegetables, coat lightly with olive oil, and grill for approximately 10 minutes.

SAFETY

Onions contain small amounts of oxalate. Individuals with a history of oxalate-containing kidney stones should avoid overconsuming them. For more information, see Appendix D, page 793.

Parsley

Parsley *(Petroselinum crispum)* is a member of the Umbelliferae family, just like carrots and celery. But while carrots and celery are used as staple vegetables, parsley is most often used as a garnish of or complement to other foods. In fact, the high chlorophyll content of parsley can help mask the odor and taste of many other foods, such as garlic and onions.

The two most popular types of parsley are curly parsley and Italian flat-leaf parsley. Both varieties are a vibrant green color. The curly variety has bright green, compact, furled leaves, while the Italian flat-leaf parsley has darker, smooth leaves, similar to and darker than those of coriander. The Italian variety has a more fragrant and less bitter taste with an overall stronger "parsley" flavor than the curly variety.

HISTORY

Parsley is native to the Mediterranean region. The ancient Greeks held parsley to be sacred, using it not only to adorn victors of athletic contests but also to decorate the tombs of the deceased. The practice of using parsley as a garnish actually has a long history that can be traced back to the civilization of the ancient Romans. Parsley has now been cultivated for more than 2,500 years and was regarded as an important medicine prior to being consumed as a food.

NUTRITIONAL HIGHLIGHTS

Parsley is extremely rich in a large number of nutrients, chlorophyll, and carotenes. Parsley is a very good source of vitamin C, folic acid, and iron. It is also a good source of minerals, including magnesium, calcium, potassium, and zinc. In addition, parsley is a good source of dietary fiber. A 100 gram serving provides 36 calories, mostly as carbohydrate, with 3.6 grams of fiber.

HEALTH BENEFITS

Ingesting parsley has been shown to inhibit the increase in the appearance of mutagens excreted in the urine of humans following the consumption of fried foods. This is most likely due to its chlorophyll content, but other compounds in parsley, such as vitamin C, flavonoids, and carotenes, have also been shown to inhibit the cancer-causing properties of fried foods. In particular, parsley's volatile oil components—myristicin, limonene, eugenol, and alphathujene—have all shown anticancer effects.

Parsley has benefits well beyond its chlorophyll content. It has long been used for medicinal purposes and is regarded as an excellent "nerve stimulant." Empirical evidence seems to support this claim and is probably responsible for so many juice enthusiasts labeling parsley-containing juices "energy drinks."

HOW TO SELECT AND STORE

Parsley can be grown at home or purchased fresh from the supermarket or greengrocers. Whenever possible, choose fresh parsley over dried. Parsley should be vibrant green, fresh, and free from yellowed leaves or signs of decay.

Fresh parsley should be kept in the refrigerator in a perforated plastic bag for no more than a week. If the parsley is slightly wilted, either sprinkle it lightly with some water or wash it without completely drying it before storing in the refrigerator.

TIPS FOR PREPARING

Place the parsley in a suitably sized bowl containing cold water in a mild solution of additive-free soap or commercial produce wash and swish it around with your hands to dislodge any dirt or debris. Remove the parsley from the bowl, empty the bowl, refill it with clean water, and repeat the process until no dirt or debris remains in the water.

Since Italian flat-leaf parsley has a stronger flavor than the curly variety, it holds up better to cooking and therefore is usually the type preferred for hot dishes. It should be added toward the end of the cooking process so that it can best retain its taste, color, and nutritional value.

If you are making a light-colored sauce, use the stems from the Italian variety as opposed to the leaves, so the sauce will take on the flavor of the parsley but will not be imbued with its green color.

QUICK SERVING IDEAS

- Fresh parsley is often used in vegetable juices.
- Chopped parsley can be added to salads, soups, sauces, vegetable sautés, and grilled fish.
- To make the classic Middle Eastern dish tabbouleh: Combine chopped parsley with bulgur wheat, chopped garlic, mint leaves, lemon juice, and olive oil.
- Add parsley to pesto sauce to add more texture and green color.
- Combine chopped parsley, garlic, and lemon zest and use it as a rub for chicken, lamb, or beef.
- Make a colorful salad of chopped fennel, orange, cherry tomatoes, pumpkin seeds, and parsley leaves.

SAFETY

Parsley is not associated with any safety issues.

Parsnips

The parsnip (*Pastinaca sativa,* from *pastinvu,* the name of a tool for digging), like parsley, carrots, and celery, is a member of the Umbelliferae family. It resembles the carrot in the shape of its long, fleshy, edible root, while its green leafy top is similar to that of Italian flat-leaf parsley. Unlike carrots' trademark orange color, however, parsnips are creamy white. They can also grow larger than carrots, to up to 15 inches/38 cm in length and 3 to 4 inches/7½ to 10 cm across the top. The roots have a mild celerylike fragrance and a sweet, nutty flavor. Although parsnips can be harvested after the first frost of autumn, wintered parsnips taste best, because the long exposure to cold causes almost all of their starch to convert to sugars. In fact, part of the parsnip's attraction to farmers is that it can be left in the frozen ground all winter, thawed out in the soil in spring, and then eaten.

Since young parsnip roots contain both sugar and starch, beer and spirits can be prepared from them. In Northern Ireland, parsnips are often brewed with malt instead of hops and fermented with yeast to produce a pleasant drink, and in Wales, parsnip wine was once considered a gourmet's delight.

HISTORY

The parsnip is reported to have originated in the Mediterranean area, where wild forms were cultivated by the Romans for their edible root. According to Pliny, parsnips were held in such repute by the Emperor Tiberius that he had them brought annually from the banks of the Rhine to Rome, where they were then successfully cultivated.

In the Middle Ages, the parsnip held an eminent place on Lenten tables because it is both filling due to its high fiber and carbohydrate content and delectably sweet, having been harvested after the winter and its starches turned to sugars. Today, we know that it is also highly nutritious.

By the sixteenth century, parsnips were culti-vated in Germany and England. They were then brought to New World by the colonists and in-troduced to the Indians, who grew them along-side their hillocks of beans and corn as a source of food in winter.

Parsnips were a major staple food in Europe until the late nineteenth century, when they were finally upstaged by a new vegetable from the Americas: the blander and more versatile potato. Meanwhile, during the colonial period through the nineteenth century in America, the parsnip was much more popular than the po-tato. In the dead of winter, the parsnip, its starch turned to sugar by a good freeze, was paired with salted fish to feed many a starving Protes-tant Pilgrim, just as the parsnip had satiated the appetites of Europe's Catholics during Lent.

Colonists with plenty to eat also enjoyed parsnips, turning them into pancakes and pud-dings by following "receipts," such as that in-scribed by William Penn's first wife, Gulielma, in mid-seventeenth-century England. She wrote, "Too make a Parsnep puding. Take sum parsnips and boyle them till thay bee very soft, then mash them very small and picke out the hard peces." The hard, woody pieces of which Gulielma warned are found only in roots well past their prime. Worst-case scenario: Should you discover that you have purchased an old parsnip, the hard pieces of the core can be easily scooped out after cooking.

Today, parsnips are commonly grown in Eu-rope and many northern areas of the United States but are not a popular vegetable in the South, as the weather rarely gets cold enough to induce the production of their sweet flavor.

NUTRITIONAL HIGHLIGHTS

Parsnips are an excellent source of fiber, vitamin C, folic acid, pantothenic acid, manganese, and copper. They are also a very good source of thi-amine, niacin, potassium, and magnesium, and a good source of riboflavin, and vitamins B6 and E. A 100 gram serving provides 71 calories, mostly as 17.1 grams of carbohydrate with 3.6 grams of fiber.

HEALTH BENEFITS

Parsnips provide similar nutritional value as po-tatoes, though parsnips are lower in calories and contain only about 50 percent of the protein and vitamin C content of potatoes. However, parsnips are higher in fiber than potatoes. Also, while both parsnips and potatoes provide sig-nificant amounts of a number of B vitamins, the parsnip is a much better source of folic acid. One cup of cooked parsnip supplies 23 percent of the RDI of folic acid, in comparison to only 5 percent of the RDI for this critical nutrient pro-vided by a cup of cooked potato.

HOW TO SELECT AND STORE

Although fresh parsnips are available all year round, they are best harvested after exposure to winter's frost or a stay in a grower's cold storage vault, during which time their starch is con-verted to sugars. Parsnips left in the ground until early spring will also be rich in natural sugars.

Choose well-shaped young (small to me-dium) roots. Avoid limp, flabby, shriveled, or spotted parsnips.

Parsnips can be stored in the refrigerator in a plastic bag for up to two weeks. Should you buy parsnips with their greens attached, be sure to snip off this foliage before storing, or the greens will pull nutrients from the roots. Cooked parsnips will keep for three to five days refrigerated.

TIPS FOR PREPARING

Parsnips can be baked, boiled, sautéed, or steamed, but perhaps the easiest and most nutritious way to cook them is to parboil them with the skin on, then plunge them in cold water, after which the skins will slip off like wet paper. Once the skins are removed, you can slice the parsnips crosswise into "coins" or lengthwise into narrow strips and toss the slices in olive oil or butter and parsley or glaze them with a little honey or maple syrup. If you choose not to parboil them, be sure to use a mild solution of additive-free soap or use a produce wash and scrub the parsnips well, since parsnip roots tend to shrivel easily in storage.

Much like a potato, the parsnip's dry texture is greatly improved by moisturizing accompaniments, such as olive oil, butter, milk, or yogurt. Like the sweet potato, parsnip's natural sweetness also combines well with other natural sweeteners, such as honey or maple syrup, and spices, such as cinnamon, nutmeg, allspice, and cloves.

Four medium parsnips typically weigh about 1 pound/½ kilogram, which will produce about 2½ cups of the vegetable when cooked and diced.

QUICK SERVING IDEAS

- Parsnips are most often prepared as potatoes are in that they are puréed, mashed, whipped, or added to soups and stews.
- For a healthful modern version of parsnip fritters, make a batter by combining cooked and puréed parsnips with flour, egg, a little butter, and some ground nuts. Form the batter into balls and bake on a baking tray at 350 degrees F./180 degrees C./gas 4 for 20 minutes for a delectable and very different hors d'oeuvre.
- One popular way of preparing parsnips is to parboil or steam them in their skins, then peel them, slice them lengthwise, and pan-glaze them with butter and a touch of brown sugar and nutmeg. This treatment results in a taste much like that of candied sweet potatoes.
- Purée boiled parsnips, then mix in peas and spring onions along with a little olive oil or butter and whole-milk yogurt, top with bread crumbs, and bake for 10 to 15 minutes at 325 degrees F./170 degrees C./gas 3 to heat through.
- Parsnips are excellent roasted along with turkey, lamb, or chicken.
- Parsnips are also delicious roasted with other vegetables, such as potatoes, celery, sweet potatoes, carrots, onions, and garlic. Toss all the vegetables with olive oil, salt, and pepper. Place a few tablespoons of water and another bit of olive oil into a roasting pan, scatter chopped onion, parsley, thyme, and dill in the bottom of the pan, and cover with your assortment of vegetables. Cover and bake for 30 minutes, then uncover and bake for another 20 minutes, or until tender.

SAFETY

Parsnips are susceptible to moisture loss and tend to shrivel when placed by growers in cold storage to convert their starch to sugar. To prevent this, they are often heavily waxed. The FDA has approved six different wax compounds for use on produce, including shellac, paraffin, palm oil derivatives, and synthetic resins. Although the waxes themselves likely pose little health risk, powerful pesticides or fungicides are frequently added to them. Since the waxes cannot be washed off with water, the fungicide or pesticide becomes cemented to the produce. To remove it, soak parsnips in a mild solution of additive-free soap, such as Ivory or pure castile soap from a health food store, or use one of the biodegradable fruit and vegetable cleansers now available, such as Fit (for more information, go to www.tryfit.com). You can also peel off the skin, but the downside of this technique is that many nutrients are concentrated in the plant's skin and outer layers.

Should you decide to try harvesting and cooking wild parsnip, exercise caution. Cases have been reported of people being poisoned by what they thought were wild parsnips, when what they had actually eaten was water hemlock, a plant that belongs to the same botanical family as the parsnip and has a very similar appearance.

Peas: See chapter 13.

Peppers: See Bell Peppers.

Potatoes

The potato *(Solanum tuberosum)* is a member of the Solanaceae or nightshade family, whose other members include tomatoes, aubergines, and bell peppers. Potatoes vary in size, shape, color, starch content, and flavor. Surprisingly, there are about 100 varieties of edible potatoes. They are often classified as either mature potatoes, which are the large potatoes that we are generally familiar with, or new potatoes, which are the smaller varieties that are harvested before maturity. Some of the popular varieties of mature potatoes in the U.S. include the Russet Burbank, the White Rose, and the Katahdin, while the Red LeSoda and Red Pontiac are two types of new potatoes. In the U.K., 75 percent of the potato crop comes from seventeen varieties, four of which account for half of the crop: Maris Piper, Cara, Record, and Pentland Dell. The Jersey Royal is, of course, the most well-known new potato. There are also delicate fingerling varieties of potatoes, which, as their name suggests, are finger-shaped.

The skin of potatoes is generally brown, red, or yellow and may be smooth or rough; the flesh is yellow or white. There are also other varieties that feature purple-gray skin and a deep violet flesh.

As potatoes have a neutral starchy flavor, they serve as a good complement to many meals. Their texture varies slightly depending upon their variety and preparation, but it can be generally described as rich and creamy.

HISTORY

Potatoes are native to the Andes mountains of Bolivia and Peru, where they have been cultivated for more than 7,000 years. Sometime during the early part of the sixteenth century, potatoes were taken to Europe by Spanish explorers. Potatoes are a hearty crop and became a favorite food in Ireland, largely as a result

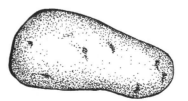

of the tremendous rise in population in Ireland in the 1800s coupled with the declining economy. Because 1½ acres of land could produce enough potatoes to feed a family of five, most Irish families came to depend upon potatoes for food. Then, tragically, the Irish Potato Famine of 1846–1850 took as many as one million lives from hunger and disease and changed the social and cultural structure of Ireland in profound ways. It also spurred new waves of emigration, thus shaping the histories of the United States and Britain as well.

The potato was brought to the United States in the early eighteenth century by Irish immigrants who settled in New England. By the nineteenth century it was extensively cultivated. Today, the potato is the vegetable that Americans consume more of pound for pound than any other. Interestingly, more than 40 percent of all potatoes grown in the United States are sold to fast-food companies such as McDonald's for French fries. In the U.K., potatoes are equally popular, each person eating on average 226 pounds/103 kilograms of potatoes a year, second only to the Portuguese and Irish in Europe. Currently, joining the United States (Idaho and Washington are the top growers) as the main producers of potatoes are the Russian Federation, Poland, India, and China.

NUTRITIONAL HIGHLIGHTS

Potatoes are a very good source of many nutrients, including potassium, vitamins B6 and C, niacin, pantothenic acid, and dietary fiber. The protein quality in potatoes is actually moderate, too, with 2.5 grams in a medium potato. Although the protein in potatoes is about the same in terms of content as corn or rice, potatoes contain lysine, an essential amino acid often lacking in grains. It is important to note, however, that most of the nutrients, fiber, and protein are found in the skins.

Potatoes are actually low in calories; a medium-sized potato contains only 115 calories. Unfortunately, most people eat potatoes in the form of French fries or chips, hash browns, potato crisps, or baked potatoes smothered with butter or sour cream. In these forms, potatoes become a very-high-calorie food.

HEALTH BENEFITS

The health benefits of potatoes relate to their nutrient content, though they may possess other healing properties as well. As an interesting side note, boiled potato peel dressings may be an effective treatment for skin wounds in some third-world countries where modern skin graft procedures are not available. Preliminary studies conducted at a children's hospital in Bombay, India, using a dressing prepared from boiled potato peelings attached to standard gauze bandages, have demonstrated good therapeutic effect in promoting healing and keeping a burn from becoming infected. Patients noted pain relief, while physicians noted reduced levels of bacterial contamination and faster healing with the use of boiled potato peel dressings.

HOW TO SELECT AND STORE

Use only high-quality potatoes that are firm and display the characteristic features of their variety. Avoid wilted, leathery, sprouting, or discolored potatoes, especially those with a green tint. Green coloration indicates that the toxic alkaloid solanine may be present. Solanine has not only been found to impart an undesirable taste, but it can also cause a host of different health conditions, such as circulatory and respiratory depression, headaches, and diarrhea. Since new potatoes are harvested before they are fully mature, they are much more susceptible to the toxic alkaloid solanine. Be especially observant when purchasing new potatoes, inspecting them carefully for discoloration and injury.

The ideal scenario for storing potatoes is in a dark, dry place between 45 and 50 degrees F./7 and 10 degrees C., as higher temperatures, even room temperature, will cause the potatoes to sprout and dehydrate prematurely. Unfortunately, this sort of environment is hard to find in most modern houses, so most people simply store them in their pantry or cupboard. Keep the potatoes in a burlap, paper, or perforated plastic bag to allow moisture to escape. Potatoes should not be stored in the refrigerator, as their starch content will turn to sugar, giving them an undesirable taste. Also, try not to store potatoes near onions, as the gases that they each emit will cause each other's degradation. If stored properly, potatoes can keep for up to two months. Check on the potatoes frequently, removing any that have sprouted or shriveled, as spoiled ones can quickly affect the quality of the others. New potatoes are much more perishable and will keep for only one week.

Cooked potatoes will keep fresh in the refrigerator for several days; however, potatoes do not freeze well.

TIPS FOR PREPARING

If you are using organically grown potatoes, wash under cold running water and gently scrub with a soft vegetable brush right before cooking. If organically grown potatoes are not being used, soak them in a mild solution of additive-free soap or produce wash, then either peel or scrub them thoroughly with a natural bristle vegetable brush under cool running water. Remove any deep eyes or bruises with a paring knife. If you elect to peel the potatoes, do so with a vegetable peeler and try to remove only a thin layer of the skin to retain as much nutritional value as possible.

Potatoes without their peel or those that have been cut are easily discolored (oxidized) when exposed to air. If you cannot cook them immediately after cutting or peeling, place them in a bowl of cold water with a little bit of lemon juice. Also, avoid cooking potatoes in iron or aluminum pots, and avoid using a carbon-steel knife to cut them, as these metals can also cause them to discolor.

QUICK SERVING IDEAS

- Potatoes can be boiled, baked, mashed, or fried.
- Quarter two medium-sized potatoes and brush them with olive oil, then place them on the barbecue and cook them at medium-high heat for 5 to 7 minutes on each side.
- For healthy French fries, cut potatoes into the desired stick shapes, toss them with a little olive oil, place on a baking tray, and bake at 350 degrees F./180 degrees C./gas 4 for 20 minutes, then turn with a spatula and bake for another 15 to 20 minutes. Season with your favorite spices and enjoy.
- Brush new potatoes with olive oil, sprinkle fresh rosemary leaves on top, and bake at 350 degrees F./180 degrees C./gas 4 for 45 minutes.
- To make delicious garlic mashed potatoes: purée roasted garlic, cooked potatoes, and olive oil together. Season to taste.

• For salade niçoise, combine chunks of new potatoes with chunks of tuna fish and steamed green beans; dress lightly with olive oil and balsamic vinegar.

SAFETY

Since potatoes are among the foods on which pesticide residues have been most frequently found, choose organic varieties when available. If organic potatoes are not available, soak them in a mild solution of additive-free soap or produce wash, then either peel or scrub thoroughly with a natural bristle vegetable brush under cool running water.

Potatoes are one of the vegetables in the nightshade (Solanaceae) family, which includes aubergine, peppers, and tomatoes. Anecdotal case histories link improvement in arthritic symptoms with removal of these foods. Although no case-controlled scientific studies confirm these observations, some individuals consuming nightshade-family vegetables experience an aggravation of arthritic symptoms and may benefit from limiting or avoiding these foods.

Pumpkins: See Squash, Winter.

Radishes

The radish (*Raphanus sativus*) is a root vegetable whose white flesh resembles that of turnips in its texture but whose sharp biting flavor is unique. Like other members of the cruciferous family, which includes such nutritional superstars as broccoli, cabbage, Brussels sprouts, and mustard, radishes contain a characteristic oil, the source of their pungency.

The radish has been developed in many varieties, each with its own distinctive color, mostly variations of red, white, and black; length, from 1 inch/2½ cm to as long as 3 feet/nearly 1 meter; size, from 1 ounce/30 grams up to 100 pounds/45 kilograms; and level of pungency, from mild to searingly sharp. Like many other root vegetables, the radish also produces green leafy tops that are edible and add a peppery zest to salads.

Some varieties of radish are quick-growing spring roots. The most popular spring varieties are those that have bright red or red-and-white round roots, such as Champion, Cherry Belle, Comet, Early Scarlet Globe, Red Boy, and Sparkler White Tip. These are small round or oval-shaped radishes with crisp white flesh. They range from 1 to 4 inches/2½ to 10cm in diameter. White Icicle, the most popular long-rooted spring variety of radish, is a tapered root that grows up to 6 inches/15 cm long. Its flesh is less pungent than that of the round varieties.

The other varieties of radish are slow-growing summer and winter vegetables. The winter varieties produce long, large roots whose flavor is usually more biting and whose texture is more fibrous and less crisp than the spring and summer varieties. The winter varieties—April Cross, Long Black Spanish, Omny, and Round Black Spanish—take twice as long to mature as the spring radishes and are usually grown as an autumn crop for winter storage. One exception among the winter varieties is the

California Mammoth White. The flesh of this 8-inch/20 cm long oblong root is even milder than that of the White Icicle.

The daikon radish, the favored variety in Asian cultures, is a very large carrot-shaped root, growing up to 3 feet/1 meter long and weighing up to 100 pounds/45 kilograms, although it is typically 12 to 18 inches/30 to 45 cm in length and weighs 1 to 3 pounds/½ to 1½ kilograms. The flavor of the white flesh of the daikon, which is also called the Japanese radish, is typically more pungent than the spring but milder than the winter radish.

Lo bok is a Chinese radish that forms large, oval roots. Like other radishes, its flesh is firm and crisp, but depending upon its season of growth, its flavor ranges from sweet and mild to pungent.

HISTORY

The modern radish is thought to have come from southern Asia and may be descended from the wild radish of the eastern Mediterranean. Radishes were cultivated in Egypt during the rule of the Pharaohs (2780 B.C.E.), were mentioned by the Chinese philosopher Confucius (479 B.C.E.), and were highly esteemed in ancient Greece, where they were carried on golden platters as vegetable sacrifices to the gods.

The earliest cultivars of the radish were long, tapering, and black. In 1547, the radish appeared in Britain, and in 1598 the historian Gerard recorded four varieties being cultivated, including white radishes. In the 1700s, red radishes were developed and were soon imported to the New World.

Today, Mexican artists carve the long white radishes that grow in Oaxaca into elaborate sculptures for La Noche de los Rabanos (the Night of the Radishes), an annual celebration that commemorates the introduction of the radish by the Spanish colonists. The radishes of this region usually grow to the size of yams and, due to the rocky soil, are twisted and gnarled. Local artists carve them into scenes from the Bible, history, and Aztec legends. Cash prizes are awarded to the best ones, and a fireworks display ends the event.

The predominant radish in Asia, the daikon, which is often pickled and eaten after the rice portion of the meal, is said to be the number one pickled vegetable in Japan. Another Japanese radish variety, the Sakurajima radish, which originates from the peninsula of the same name in southern Japan, is characterized by immense radishes, like daikon, that can reach a weight of up to 100 pounds/45 kilograms!

In India, the Mougri radish is grown not for its root but for its long, edible seed pods, which, it is claimed, can grow to a length of more than 3 feet/1 meter, although 8 to 24 inches/10 to 60 cm is a more normal range.

In the United States, radishes are grown in virtually all states, with the largest crops coming from Florida and California.

NUTRITIONAL HIGHLIGHTS

All varieties of radishes and their greens are very low in calories and an excellent source of vitamin C. Radish leaves contain almost six times the vitamin C of the root and are also a good source of calcium. In addition, some varieties are a very good source of the trace mineral molybdenum and a good source of folic acid and potassium. Daikons are also a very good source of copper and potassium. A 100 gram serving of radish provides only 16 calories as carbohydrate and fiber.

HEALTH BENEFITS

As a member of the cruciferous vegetable family, the radish shares the cancer-protective actions of its cousins broccoli, cabbage, kale, and Brussels sprouts.

It has also been used as a medicinal food for liver disorders throughout history. Radishes contain a variety of sulphur-based chemicals that increase the flow of bile, thus helping to maintain a healthy gallbladder and liver and improving digestion.

In India, both radish roots and greens are used not only to prevent vitamin C deficiency but as a diuretic, as an expectorant, to treat gastric discomfort, and as a laxative. Radish seeds are also used for cosmetic purposes. An emulsion of radish seeds, applied to the face, is said to remove blackheads and freckles.

Cooking destroys radish root's vitamin C content. Radish greens, which can be added to green salads, have more vitamin C, calcium, and protein than the roots.

HOW TO SELECT AND STORE

Good-quality red radishes have intact greens. The greens should be fresh-looking, with no signs of spoilage. Slightly flabby greens can be restored to freshness if stored in the refrigerator in water; if it is too late to save them, simply cut them off. The radish root should be firm, smooth, and vibrant red versus soft, wrinkled, and dull-colored. Fresh radishes with the greens attached can be stored for three to five days in the refrigerator, but radishes with the greens removed can be stored in the refrigerator for two to four weeks. Black radishes with the greens removed will store for months if they remain dry. Store all radishes in perforated bags in the vegetable crisper of your refrigerator. Cooked radishes will keep for one to two days refrigerated.

Red and white radishes are sold all year round, although supplies are best in spring. Black radishes are at their peak in winter and early spring. Daikons are most flavorful in autumn and winter.

TIPS FOR PREPARING

Soak radishes in a mild solution of additive-free soap or produce wash, then scrub them thoroughly with a vegetable brush under cool running water; trim off the root tip and stem end. Although White Icicle radishes are fairly mild, you may wish to use a vegetable peeler to remove the daikon's thin but very pungent skin. The skin of black radishes is often thin and can be left on, but be warned that sometimes it is thick and very hot.

Red radishes are most often used to add a spicy accent to salads, but they can also be added to casseroles, stir-fries, and soups; roasted whole with other vegetables; or pickled. To prepare any radishes, scrub them as you would carrots, peel if desired, then slice, chop, or grate as required for your recipe. All varieties can be used raw and also stand up to long cooking times. To keep radishes crisp when using them in cooked dishes, sprinkle them with a little salt after peeling and let stand for 20 minutes, then rinse well before adding to your recipe.

QUICK SERVING IDEAS

- For a festive, tangy salad, combine grated red radishes with segments of navel oranges. Mix together with a little honey and lemon juice and marinate for 30 minutes.
- Red radishes and cucumber can also team up to produce a zesty Chinese variation on the typical cucumber salad, called "Smashed Radishes." Slice both radishes and cucumber thinly. Use the bottom of a heavy glass to lightly smash the radish slices. Combine the smashed radish and cucumber slices and marinate in vinaigrette made from tamari or soy sauce, sherry, toasted sesame oil, and honey.
- For milder-tasting radishes, try red radishes boiled. Boil ½ inch/1cm of water, add sliced radishes, cover, and simmer 5 to 10 minutes until tender. Drain and toss with a little olive oil, salt, and pepper.
- Steaming also results in milder-tasting radishes and, in the case of red roots, a pale pink flesh. Try steaming whole radishes and baby carrots together for 8 to 12 minutes, and glaze with orange juice.
- To tame their strident flavor, black radishes can be sliced or shredded, then steamed or boiled for 15 to 30 minutes until barely tender. Serve with vegetable dip or in salads. You can also bake black radishes whole and eat them as you would turnips. For a striking black-and-white pattern, peel off thin strips of skin before baking.
- Daikon and lo bok radishes can be cut into chunks and used like turnips to flavor vegetable soups and stews and to provide a pungent contrast to sweet carrots and bland potatoes. Julienne strips of these Asian radishes can also be used to enliven any meat or vegetable broth; add them during the last 10 minutes of cooking.
- Daikon is especially good shredded and steamed with shredded carrot for 5 minutes, then dressed with a vinaigrette using a small amount of dark sesame oil and sprinkled with sesame seeds.
- Sliced radishes or julienne strips of daikon or lo bok radishes add zest to stir-fries. Add as one of the last vegetables and cook no longer than 3 to 5 minutes to retain their crispness.

SAFETY

Radishes are not associated with any safety issue. Theoretically, because radishes help increase the flow of bile, individuals with gallbladder disease (stones or obstructions) should not consume large amounts of this vegetable.

Rocket

Rocket is a powerfully charismatic, mustardlike leafy green. Its pungent flavor adds a distinctive energy to any salad, a quality that has endeared rocket to legions of salad aficionados. The combination of various mineral salts combined in rocket, including manganese, calcium, magnesium, potassium, copper, iron, and zinc, contributes to this green's exceptionally lively flavor.

Rocket's peppery, woodsy, and earthy flavors explode in your mouth, which may be one reason for rocket's name. It's also a corruption of the French "roquette," which derives from the Old Italian *rochetta*, a diminutive form of *ruca*, which in turn is derived from the Latin *eruca*, meaning "caterpillar," most likely a Roman reference to the plant's somewhat hairy stems.

In the dialect of southern Italy, the Latin *eruca* became *arugula,* the name that traveled across to America with the huge influx of immigrants from this region about a hundred years ago and became the primary American name for this spicy green, although it may also be found under other names such as rugola, rucola, roquette, garden rocket, Mediterranean rocket, Roman rocket, and Italian cress.

With its small flat leaves on long stems, rocket resembles dandelion greens and is sometimes displayed with its roots attached. A native of the Mediterranean region, rocket grows wild in parts of southern Europe and also in the Far East.

Domestic rocket *(Eruca vesicaria sativa)* is typically thought of as a salad green, a zestier cousin of lettuce, but rocket is actually a crucifer, a member of the health-enhancing Brassica family, which also includes broccoli, Brussels sprouts, cabbage, mustard, and kale. Like other crucifers, rocket's flavors are both sweetened and enhanced by light steaming or a quick sauté.

Wild rocket is an experience best reserved for true rocket fanatics. It has smaller, finely cut leaves on a willowy stem, small yellow flowers, and a seriously pungent flavor that makes ordinary rocket seem tame. Lightly cooked is definitely the way to go with wild rocket *(Eruca sylvatica),* as a light steam or sauté softens the bite of this particularly spicy variant.

HISTORY

Rocket's enlivening properties were noted by the ancient Romans and Egyptians, who considered the green a potent aphrodisiac and consecrated it to Priapus, one of Rome's minor fertility gods and the protector of gardens and domestic animals. Modern herbalists rarely mention rocket's aphrodisiac qualities, instead recommending its warming nature as an aid to the fires of digestion.

Rocket has been cultivated in Britain for centuries and was brought to America by the colonists, who planted it in the earliest gardens in New England. Today, in addition to its growing popularity in the United States and the U.K., rocket is a favored green in Italy, France, Spain, Greece, and Egypt. In India, rocket leaves are not used, and the plant is grown primarily for the oil derived from its seeds.

NUTRITIONAL HIGHLIGHTS

Rocket is an excellent source of vitamin A, vitamin C, folic acid, manganese, calcium, and magnesium; a very good source of riboflavin, potassium, copper, and iron; and a good source of zinc. A 100 gram serving of raw rocket provides 25 calories, 2.3 grams of protein, no cholesterol, 0.7 grams of fat, and 3.7 grams of carbohydrate with 1.6 grams of fiber.

HEALTH BENEFITS

Like other cruciferous vegetables, rocket contains a group of anticancer compounds known as glucosinolates. These compounds exert antioxidant activity, but, more important, they are potent stimulators of natural detoxifying enzymes in the body. For more information on the anticancer benefits of these compounds, see "Cabbage," page 178.

Like other "greens," rocket is rich in many essential vitamins and minerals, as well as important phytochemicals, such as carotenes and chlorophyll, making it an excellent source of antioxidants.

HOW TO SELECT AND STORE

Rocket is available all year long, but production peaks from June through to December. Rocket thrives in the cooler weather of late spring and autumn, which are the best seasons to purchase this tangy green treat since, in the heat of late summer, rocket tends to bolt and to develop a very sharp flavor.

Like all greens, rocket is highly perishable and should be displayed under refrigeration or on ice. Also, like other greens, rocket should be fresh and crisp, especially the stems. The leaves should be dark green, never yellow. Avoid wilted greens or leaves that have brown or yellow edges, or dark or slimy spots.

Rocket should be kept cool and moist and used within one to two days of purchase. It keeps best if the roots are first wrapped in damp paper towels, then the whole bunch is placed in a plastic bag. Alternatively, rocket, with its roots attached, can be placed upright in a glass of water (as one would do with a bunch of flowers), covered with a plastic bag, and refrigerated. If the roots have been removed, the best way to maintain rocket's crispness is either to rinse the leaves, spin them dry in a salad spinner, then wipe dry the outer bowl of the salad spinner, replace the inner bowl containing the rocket, and store in the refrigerator; or rinse the leaves, layer them in clean paper towels, place them in a plastic bag, and refrigerate in the crisper drawer until serving time—optimally, later the same day.

Store rocket and other greens away from apples, bananas, and pears since, as they ripen, these fruits give off ethylene gas, which will cause the leaves to develop brown spots, an indication of decay.

TIPS FOR PREPARING

Wash rocket under cold running water and, if it is not organically grown, soak in cold water with a mild solution of additive-free soap or use a produce wash (see page 51); then spin dry in a salad spinner. Rocket grown in summer may have too much peppery fire unless lightly cooked. Wild rocket *(Eruca sylvatica)* should also be lightly steamed or sautéed to soften its potentially excessive spicy bite. Always taste a little rocket before you prepare it, as it can range in intensity from mild if it is greenhouse-grown or heavily irrigated to extremely peppery if grown in late summer or in a dry year. Adjust the amount of rocket you wish to use to the strength of your particular batch and your palate.

Even if rocket leaves look clean, they should be washed. Cut off the roots, and then, holding the greens by the stems, gently swish them around in a large bowl of cool water. Lift them out, rinse out and refill the bowl with water, and repeat the process until no sand or grit settles in the bottom of the bowl.

To remove remaining water, a salad spinner dries delicate leaves quickly and thoroughly. If you do not have a salad spinner, hold the greens by the stems and shake off excess water, then blot gently with clean paper towels.

The best time to use rocket raw in salads or in tomato dishes is when the serrated leaves measure two to three inches long.

Rocket can be added to soups, steamed or sautéed and served as a side dish, or puréed and added to sauces or used to make pesto. The leaves can also be frozen for later use.

QUICK SERVING IDEAS

- Because rocket has such a potent, peppery flavor, it is often mixed with milder greens to produce an interesting, yet balanced salad. Served raw in mixed salads, rocket leaves complement both bland butterhead lettuce and bitter chicories. Rocket can be substituted for virtually any green but is closest in temperament to Belgian endive, escarole, and dandelion greens.
- Rocket makes a memorable tossed salad when combined with a soft, buttery lettuce such as Bibb or Boston leaf.
- As a salad green, rocket can also stand on its own, holding center stage in dressier salads, such as a combination of rocket, blood oranges, and avocado.
- For a spectacular first course at your next dinner party, serve the classic Italian rocket salad with porcini mushrooms and Parmesan cheese. Toss chopped rocket leaves, thinly sliced porcini mushrooms, and walnuts with a balsamic olive oil vinaigrette, then top with shavings of Parmesan cheese and freshly ground black pepper.
- Make rocket pesto: Blend together 2 bunches (about 2 packed cups) of rocket with three garlic cloves, ¼ cup walnuts, ¼ cup freshly ground Parmesan cheese, ½ cup olive oil, and salt, pepper, and lemon juice to taste. Use as a vegetable dip, or, for delectable crostini, use this pesto to top toasted baguette slices and bake at 400 degrees F./200 degrees C./gas 6 for about 5 minutes.
- Lightly steamed or sautéed along with some onion or garlic in olive oil, rocket makes a delectable side dish or addition to pasta or rice. For example, toss rocket sautéed in olive oil with just-cooked pasta. Add freshly ground black pepper, then sprinkle with pine nuts and Gorgonzola cheese and serve immediately.

SAFETY

Leafy greens, such as rocket, contain low amounts of oxalate. Individuals with a history of oxalate-containing kidney stones should avoid overconsuming this food. For more information, see Appendix D, page 793.

Shallots: See Onions.

Spinach

Spinach *(Spinacia oleracea)* belongs to the same family (Chenopodiaceae) as beets and chard. It shares a similar taste profile with these two other vegetables—it has the bitterness of beet greens and the slightly salty flavor of chard. There are three different types of spinach generally available: Savoy has crisp, creased, curly dark green leaves that have a springy texture. Semi-Savoy is similar in texture and color to Savoy but is not as crinkled in appearance. And Smooth-leaf has flat, unwrinkled, spade-shaped, medium-green leaves.

HISTORY

Spinach originated in southwestern Asia or Persia as a wild plant. It has been cultivated in China and many areas of the other areas of Asia and the Middle East for at least 2,000 years. It was used as an important medicinal plant in many traditional systems of medicine. Spinach grows very well in temperate climates.

Spinach cultivation in Europe has a more recent history, however, as it began only in the eleventh century, when the Moors introduced it into Spain. In fact, for a while, spinach was known as "the Spanish vegetable" in England.

One of the classic uses of spinach is using it as a bed to place entrées upon. This popular use owes its origin to Catherine de Médicis in the sixteenth century. When she left her home in Florence to marry the king of France, she brought not only spinach seeds to plant, but also her own cooks who prepared spinach in the ways she preferred. Since this time, dishes prepared on a bed of spinach have been referred to as "à la Florentine."

The United States and the Netherlands are among the largest commercial producers of spinach today.

NUTRITIONAL HIGHLIGHTS

A one-cup serving of spinach has only 41 calories, but it is extremely nutrient-dense. It is an excellent source of vitamin K, carotenes, vitamin C, and folic acid. It is also a very good source of manganese, magnesium, iron, and vitamin B2. In addition, spinach is a good source of vitamins B6, E, and B1.

HEALTH BENEFITS

There is much lore regarding spinach (e.g., the source of Popeye's strength). Historically, it was regarded as a plant with remarkable abilities to restore energy, increase vitality, and improve the quality of the blood. There are sound reasons why spinach would produce such results, primarily the fact that spinach contains twice as much iron as most other greens. Spinach is also one of the most alkaline-producing foods (see

Appendix B), making it useful in helping to regulate body pH.

Spinach is one of the richest dietary sources of lutein (see page 140) making it an especially important food for promoting healthy eye-sight and preventing macular degeneration and cataracts.

Spinach, like other chlorophyll and carotene containing vegetables, is a strong protector against cancer. In addition to carotenes such as lutein, researchers have identified at least thirteen different flavonoid compounds in spinach that function as antioxidants and as anticancer agents. Many of these substances fall into a category of flavonoids known as methylenedioxyflavonol glucuronides. The anticancer properties of these spinach flavonoids have been sufficiently impressive to prompt researchers to create specialized spinach extracts that can be used in controlled studies. These spinach extracts have been shown to slow down cell division in human stomach cancer cells (gastric adenocarcinomas) and, in studies on mice, to reduce skin cancers (skin papillomas). A study on adult women living in New England in the late 1980s also showed intake of spinach to be inversely related to incidence of breast cancer. In other words, the higher the intake of spinach, the lower the incidence of breast cancer.

HOW TO SELECT AND STORE

Fresh spinach should be medium to dark green, fresh-looking, and free from any evidence of decay. Fresh spinach should be stored loosely packed in a sealed plastic bag in the refrigerator crisper, where it will keep for about four days. Do not wash spinach before storing, as the moisture will cause it to spoil. Cooked spinach does not store too well, certainly no longer than one day in the refrigerator. Spinach can be frozen after being blanched for two minutes, although this will cause its texture to become very soft, so do not completely thaw it before cooking.

TIPS FOR PREPARING

Spinach, whether bunched or prepackaged, should be washed very well, since the leaves and stems tend to collect sand and soil. Before washing, trim off the roots and separate the leaves. Place the spinach in a large bowl of cold water in a mild solution of additive-free soap or commercial produce wash and swish the leaves around with your hands, as this will allow any dirt to become dislodged. Remove the leaves from the water, empty the bowl, refill with clean water, and repeat this process until no dirt remains in the water—usually two to three times will do the trick. Cut away any overly thick stems for more even cooking. If you are going to use the spinach in a salad, you can dry it by shaking it in a colander or using a salad spinner. If you are going to steam the spinach, don't worry about drying it.

Slightly wilted spinach can be revived to freshness by placing it in cold water.

QUICK SERVING IDEAS

- Instead of, or in addition to, lettuce, use raw spinach leaves in your dinner salad.
- Lightly sauté spinach with garlic in olive oil. Top with lemon juice and pine nuts.
- Add layers of spinach to any lasagna recipe.
- Use spinach leaves as a garnish for sandwiches.

- Serve sautéed spinach topped with red onion slices and goat cheese and sprinkled with balsamic vinegar as a warm spinach salad.

SAFETY

Spinach contains a high amount of oxalate. Individuals with a history of oxalate-containing kidney stones should avoid overconsuming it. For more information, see Appendix D, page 793.

Spinach also contains purines and should be consumed in moderation by people with gout.

Since spinach is among the foods on which pesticide residues have been most frequently found, we recommend choosing spinach grown organically. If not, then be sure to prepare it as described above.

Squash, Summer

Squash belong to the gourd or melon family (Cucurbitaceae). There are many types of squash, but, in general, there are two major categories: summer and winter. While each type varies in shape, color, size, and flavor, all squash share some common characteristics: The entire vegetable, including its flesh, seeds, and skin, is edible. In addition, some varieties of the squash plant produce edible flowers.

Unlike winter squash, summer squash are more fragile and cannot be stored for long periods of time. Varieties of summer squash include:

- *Courgette:* The best known of the summer squashes, courgette is a type of narrow squash that resembles a cucumber in size and shape. It has smooth, thin skin that is either green or yellow in color and can be striped or speckled. Its tender flesh is creamy white in color and features numerous seeds. Its edible flowers are often used in French and Italian cooking.

- *Crookneck and straightneck squash:* Both of these summer squashes have creamy white flesh and generally have yellow skins, although sometimes you can find them with green skin. Crookneck squash is partially straight, with a swanlike neck. It was genetically modified to produce its straightneck cousin, which is shaped as its name implies.

- *Pattypan squash:* This small, saucer-shaped squash features skins that can be either pale green or golden yellow in color. Its cream-colored flesh is denser and slightly sweeter than that of the courgette.

HISTORY

Native to Central America, squash has been consumed for more than 10,000 years. Squash was first cultivated specifically for its seeds, since early squash did not contain much flesh and what it did contain was very bitter and unpalatable. Over time, the cultivation of squash spread throughout both North and South America. Cultivation led to the development of varieties with a greater quantity of sweeter-tasting flesh. Early explorers to the Western Hemisphere, including Christopher Columbus, brought squash back to Europe, where it was subsequently extensively cultivated. Today, the largest commercial producers of squash include China, Japan, Romania, Turkey, Italy, Egypt, and Argentina.

NUTRITIONAL HIGHLIGHTS

Due to their 95 percent water content, summer squash are not as nutrient-dense as the winter varieties, which have an 81 percent water content. However, summer squash are excellent diet foods as they are very low in calories, with only 14 calories per 100 grams. Summer squash also provide fair amounts of potassium, carotenes, and vitamin C.

HEALTH BENEFITS

It appears that the anticancer effects of squash rival those of some of the more popular cancer fighters. In laboratory studies, the juices made from summer squash are equal to juices made from pumpkin, leeks, and radishes in their ability to prevent cell mutations.

Summer squash appear to be particularly healthful during the summer months due to their high water content (to protect against dehydration) and carotenes (to protect against the damaging effects of the sun).

HOW TO SELECT AND STORE

When selecting summer squash, make sure the squash selected exhibits the color, firmness, and other qualities or characteristics of the variety selected. Look for summer squash that are heavy for their size and have shiny, unblemished rinds. Additionally, the rinds should not be very hard, since this indicates that the squash is overmature and will have hard seeds and stringy flesh. Purchase summer squash that is of average size, since those that are overly large may be fibrous, while those that are overly small may be inferior in flavor.

Summer squash is very fragile and should be handled with care, as even small punctures will lead to decay. It should be stored unwashed in a perforated plastic bag in the refrigerator crisper, where it will keep for about seven days. While summer squash can be frozen, this will make the flesh much softer. Blanch slices of summer squash for 2 minutes before freezing.

TIPS FOR PREPARING

Wash summer squash thoroughly under cold running water with a vegetable brush. If it has been waxed or is not organically grown, you will need to soak in cold water with a mild solution of additive-free soap or use a produce wash (see page 51) and then gently scrub with a vegetable brush and rinse. Summer squash are usually left unpeeled and cooked whole, sliced, or cubed.

QUICK SERVING IDEAS

- Grated courgette or other summer squash can be sprinkled on top of salads and sand-wiches.
- Steam summer squash slices in a vegetable steamer and then season with cumin and lemon juice.
- Serve raw summer squash slices with your favorite dips.
- Cut courgettes lengthwise and remove some of the center core. Stuff with whole-wheat bread crumbs, top with tomato sauce and grated cheese, then bake.
- Courgettes or other summer squash can be added to your favorite muffin or bread recipe by decreasing the amount of liquid in the recipe by about one third to compensate for the moisture present in the squash.

SAFETY

Summer squash does contain high levels of oxalates. Individuals with a history of oxalate-containing kidney stones should avoid overcon-suming it. For more information, see Appendix D, page 793.

Squash, Winter

Winter squash include pumpkins and acorn, butternut, and spaghetti squash. These mem-bers of the Cucurbitaceae family vary in shape, color, size, and flavor, but they do share some common characteristics. Their shells are hard and difficult to pierce, enabling them to have long storage periods of one to six months. Their flesh is mildly sweet in flavor and finely grained in texture. Additionally, all have seed-containing hollow inner cavities.

Varieties of winter squash include:

- *Acorn squash:* This squash has harvest green skin speckled with orange patches, and pale yellow-orange flesh. It has a very unique sweet, nutty, and peppery flavor.

- *Butternut squash:* Shaped like a large pear, this squash has cream-colored skin, deep or-ange-colored flesh, and a sweet flavor.

- *Hubbard squash:* A larger-sized squash that can be dark green, grey-blue, or orange-red in color, the Hubbard's flavor is less sweet than many other varieties'.

- *Pumpkins:* Small sugar pumpkins are the culi-nary variety, weighing only a few pounds, as opposed to the larger vari-eties used to carve jack-o'-lanterns.

- *Spaghetti squash:* A larger-sized, yellow squash with light colored flesh that pulls away in strands resembling spaghetti when cooked.

- *Turban squash:* Green in color and either speckled or striped, this squash has an orange-yellow flesh whose taste is reminiscent of hazelnuts.

HISTORY

See Squash, Summer.

NUTRITIONAL HIGHLIGHTS

Winter squash, like other richly colored vegetables, are excellent sources of carotenes—the richer the color, the richer the concentration. They are also a very good source of vitamins C and B1, folic acid, pantothenic acid, potassium, and dietary fiber. In addition, winter squash is a good source of vitamin B6 and niacin.

HEALTH BENEFITS

Winter squash, especially the darker-fleshed varieties such as pumpkin and acorn, provide exceptional amounts of carotenes. Like other carotene-rich vegetables, winter squash have been shown to exert a protective effect against many cancers, particularly lung cancer. In addition to cancer and heart disease, diets rich in carotenes also appear to offer protection against developing type 2 diabetes, with pumpkin consumption being the most protective.

Pumpkin seeds have also been shown to be helpful in reducing symptoms of benign prostatic hyperplasia (BPH).

HOW TO SELECT AND STORE

Winter squash is prone to decaying easily, so it is important to inspect it carefully before purchase. Choose winter squash that are firm, heavy for their size, and have dull, not glossy, rinds. The rind should be hard, as a soft rind may indicate that the squash is watery and lacking in flavor. Avoid those with any signs of decay, which will manifest in spots that are water-soaked or mouldy.

Winter squash has a much longer storage life than summer squash. Depending upon the variety, it can be kept for between one and six months. It should be kept away from direct exposure to light and should not be subject to extreme heat or extreme cold. The ideal temperature for storing winter squash is between 50 and 60 degrees F./10 to 16 degrees C. Once it is cut, cover the pieces of winter squash in cling film and store them in the refrigerator, where they will keep for one to two days. The best way to freeze winter squash is to first cut it into pieces of suitable size for individual recipes. Cooked winter squash will keep for three to five days refrigerated.

TIPS FOR PREPARING

Wash winter squash thoroughly under cold running water with a vegetable brush. If it has been waxed or is not organically grown, you will need to soak the squash in cold water with a mild solution of additive-free soap or use a produce wash and then gently scrub with a vegetable brush and rinse.

After washing winter squash, cut it in half and remove the seeds and fibrous material in the cavity. Depending upon the recipe preparation, you can use the winter squash either peeled or unpeeled.

QUICK SERVING IDEAS

- To cook halved squash, pierce it in several locations with a knife to allow any steam to escape, and then bake in a 350 degree F./180 degree C./gas 4 oven for 45 minutes to one hour, until a knife can be easily inserted near the stem. Top with a little butter and maple syrup or brown sugar.
- Spaghetti squash is often prepared as a substitute for spaghetti by baking or steaming it until the rind softens, usually 30 to 45 minutes; then it is cut in half lengthwise and the spaghetti strands are removed. You can top the "strings" of spaghetti squash with pasta sauce.
- Pumpkin and other varieties of winter squash, such as acorn and butternut, are often mashed like potatoes and either eaten as such or used in bread, cake, muffin, and pie recipes.
- Top puréed, cooked winter squash with cinnamon and honey.
- Combine puréed, cooked winter squash with stewed apple and serve alone as a pudding-like dessert, or as a topping for pancakes, waffles, and oatmeal.
- Steam cubes of winter squash for five minutes, and then dress with olive oil, tamari, ginger, and pumpkin seeds.
- Add cubes of winter squash to your favorite vegetable soup recipe.

SAFETY

Winter squash is not associated with any safety issues.

Sunchoke: See Jerusalem Artichoke.

Swedes: See Turnips and Turnip Greens.

Sweet Potatoes

The sweet potato *(Ipomoea batatas)* is not a member of the potato (Solanaceae) family but rather of the Convolvulaceae, or morning glory, family. In the United States, the darker, sweeter sweet potato is often called a yam. In actuality it is not a yam, but is in fact a variety of sweet potato.

There are nearly 400 sweet potato varieties. Their flesh may be white, yellow, or orange, and the thin skin may be white, yellow, orange, red, or purple. Some are shaped like a potato, being short and blocky with rounded ends, while others are longer with tapered ends.

Sweet potatoes are grouped into two different categories depending upon the texture they have when cooked: firm, dry, and mealy, or soft and moist. In both types, the taste is starchy and sweet, but different varieties have different, unique tastes.

HISTORY

Sweet potatoes are native to Central America. They have been consumed since prehistoric times, as is evidenced by sweet potato relics dating back 10,000 years that have been discovered in Peruvian caves, making them one of the oldest vegetables known.

As with other foods indigenous to the Western Hemisphere, Christopher Columbus was the first to bring sweet potatoes to Europe. Spanish and Portuguese explorers in the sixteenth century took sweet potatoes to Africa, India, Indonesia, and southern Asia. Early settlers in the southeastern United States began cultivating sweet potatoes, making them a staple food in this region even today.

In the mid–twentieth century, the orange-fleshed sweet potato was introduced to the United States and given the name "yam" to distinguish it from the white-fleshed sweet potato to which most people were accustomed. The name "yam" was adopted from *nyami,* an African word for the root of the *Dioscorea* genus of plants, which are considered to be true yams. The U.S. Department of Agriculture mandates that the moist-fleshed, orange-colored sweet potatoes that are labeled as "yams" also be accompanied by the label "sweet potatoes" in an attempt to distinguish between the two, but for many people this does not help to clarify the distinction between these very different root vegetables. Yet once you experience the distinct taste and texture of a real yam, you will definitely know the difference, appreciating each of these root vegetables for their unique qualities.

Sweet potatoes are a featured food in many Asian and Latin American cuisines. Today, the main commercial producers of sweet potatoes include China, Indonesia, Vietnam, Japan, India, and Uganda.

NUTRITIONAL HIGHLIGHTS

Sweet potatoes are an excellent source of carotenes. In general, the darker the variety of sweet potato, the higher the concentration of carotenes. Sweet potatoes are also a very good source of vitamins C and B6. In addition, sweet potatoes are a good source of manganese, copper, biotin, pantothenic acid, vitamin B2, and dietary fiber. A 100 gram serving provides 90 calories, 2 grams of protein, 20.7 grams of carbohydrate, and 3.3 grams of fiber, but only 8.4 grams of sugars.

HEALTH BENEFITS

Sweet potatoes contain unique root storage proteins, which have been shown to exert significant antioxidant effects. In one study, these proteins had about one third the antioxidant activity of glutathione—one of the body's most important internally produced antioxidants. The presence of these proteins, along with the high content of carotenes and vitamin C, makes sweet potatoes a valuable food for boosting antioxidants in your body.

Unlike many other starchy vegetables, sweet potatoes are classified as an "antidiabetic" food. Animal studies have shown that sweet potatoes actually help stabilize blood sugar levels and improve the response to the hormone insulin.

HOW TO SELECT AND STORE

Use only high-quality sweet potatoes that are firm and display the characteristic features of their variety. Remember, the darker the variety, the higher the carotene content. Avoid wilted, leathery, or discolored sweet potatoes, especially those with a green tint. Green coloration indicates that the toxic alkaloid solanine may be present. Solanine has not only been found to impart an undesirable taste, but it can also cause a host of different health conditions, such as circulatory and respiratory depression, headaches, and diarrhea.

Sweet potatoes should be stored in a cool, dark, well-ventilated place, where they will keep fresh for up to ten days. They should be stored loose and not kept in a plastic bag. Keep them away from exposure to sunlight or temperatures above 60 degrees F./16 degrees C., since this will cause them to sprout or ferment. Uncooked sweet potatoes should not be kept in the refrigerator, as they will easily mould. Cooked sweet potatoes will keep for three to five days refrigerated.

TIPS FOR PREPARING

If using organically grown sweet potatoes, wash them under cold running water and gently scrub with a soft vegetable brush right before cooking. If organically grown sweet potatoes are not being used, soak them in a mild solution of additive-free soap or produce wash, then either peel or scrub thoroughly with a natural bristle vegetable brush under cool running water. Remove any deep bruises with a paring knife. If you elect to peel the sweet potato, do so with a vegetable peeler and try to remove only a thin layer of the skin to retain as much nutritional value as possible.

If you cannot cook them immediately after cutting or peeling, place them in a bowl of cold water with a little lemon juice to prevent discoloration. Also, avoid cooking potatoes in iron or aluminum pots and avoid using a carbon-steel knife to cut them, as these metals can also cause them to discolor.

QUICK SERVING IDEAS

- Sweet potatoes can be prepared in ways similar to potatoes.
- For a delicious hot dessert, purée cooked sweet potatoes with bananas, maple syrup, and cinnamon. Top with chopped walnuts.
- Thinly slice sweet potatoes, then lightly coat with olive oil and your favorite seasonings. Bake the sweet potato chips at 300 degrees F./150 degrees C./gas 2 until crispy, or approximately 20 minutes.
- Spread mashed sweet potatoes on a piece of whole-wheat bread and top with a layer of peanut butter and sliced apples.
- Cubed sweet potatoes can be added to any vegetable stir-fry.

SAFETY

Sweet potatoes contain high levels of oxalate. Individuals with a history of oxalate-containing kidney stones should avoid overconsuming this food. For more information, see Appendix D, page 793.

Swiss Chard

Chard *(Beta vulgaris cicla)* is commonly referred to as Swiss chard and belongs to the same family as beets and spinach (Chenopodiaceae). Swiss chard has a thick, crunchy stalk to which fan-like wide green leaves are attached. The leaves may be either smooth or curly, depending upon the variety, and feature lighter-colored ribs running throughout. The stalk, which can measure almost two feet/60 cm in length, comes in three colors: white, red, and yellow. Sometimes, in the market, all three varieties will be bunched together and labeled "rainbow chard." Both the leaves and stalk of Swiss chard are edible and their taste resembles the bitterness of beet greens and the slightly salty flavor of spinach leaves. Some popular varieties include the following:

- *Bright Lights* has brilliant multicolored leaves and stems.

- *Fordhook Giant* has huge glossy leaves with white veins and stems. It is tasty and high-yielding, producing bumper crops even during high temperatures.

- *Lucullus* produces pale yellow-green leaves with fleshy midribs.

- *Perpetual spinach,* or *spinach beet,* produces narrower stems and dark, fleshy leaves. It is a good one for regrowing for the occasional meal once the stem has been harvested.

- *Rhubarb chard,* or *ruby chard,* is noted for its magnificent bright crimson leaf stalks and dark green ruffled leaves. It is often used as an ornamental border.

- *Vulcan* produces beautiful red stems and dark green, sweet-tasting leaves.

HISTORY

Chard is native to the Mediterranean region. The ancient Greeks and Romans honored chard for its medicinal properties. Historically, the juice from chard was used as a decongestant, and the leaves were said to neutralize acid and have a powerful laxative (purgative) effect.

Chard got its common name from another Mediterranean vegetable, cardoon, a celerylike plant with thick stalks that resemble those of chard. The French got the two confused and called them both "carde." Apparently, in the nineteenth century seed catalogues added "Swiss" to the name, presumably to distinguish it from cardoon.

NUTRITIONAL HIGHLIGHTS

Swiss chard is rich in nutrition. It is an excellent source of carotenes, vitamins C, E, and K, dietary fiber, and chlorophyll. It is also an excellent source of many minerals, including magnesium, potassium, iron, and manganese. In addition, Swiss chard is a good source of many other nutrients, including vitamin B6, calcium, protein, thiamine, zinc, niacin, folic acid, and selenium.

HEALTH BENEFITS

The combination of traditional nutrients; phytochemicals, particularly carotenes, chlorophyll, and other plant pigments; and soluble fiber makes Swiss chard one of the most powerful anticancer foods, particularly against digestive tract cancers. Several research studies on Swiss chard focus specifically on colon cancer, where the incidence of precancerous lesions in animals has been found to be significantly reduced following dietary intake of Swiss chard extracts.

In addition, the vitamin K provided by Swiss chard—388.9 percent of the daily value in one cup of cooked Swiss chard—is important for maintaining bone health. Vitamin K1 activates osteocalcin, the major noncollagen protein in bone. Osteocalcin anchors calcium molecules inside the bone. Therefore, without enough vitamin K1, osteocalcin levels are inadequate, and bone mineralization is impaired.

HOW TO SELECT AND STORE

Choose Swiss chard that is held in a chilled display, as this will help to ensure that it has a crunchier texture and sweeter taste. Look for leaves that are vivid green in color and that do not display any brown or yellow spots. The leaves should be unwilted and free of tiny holes, which may have been caused by insect damage. The stalks should look crisp and be unblemished.

To store, place unwashed Swiss chard in the refrigerator in a perforated plastic bag. It will keep fresh for several days. If you have large batches of chard, you can blanch the leaves and then freeze them. Cooked Swiss chard will keep for one to two days refrigerated.

TIPS FOR PREPARING

Swiss chard must be washed very well, since the leaves and stems tend to collect sand and soil. Before washing, trim off the thick stems on the bottom and separate the leaves. Place the Swiss chard in a large bowl of cold water in a mild solution of additive-free soap or commercial produce wash and swish the leaves around with your hands, as this will allow any dirt to become dislodged. Remove the leaves from the water, empty the bowl, refill with clean water, and repeat this process until no dirt remains in the water—usually two to three times will do the trick. Cut away any overly thick stems for more even cooking. If you are going to use the Swiss chard in a salad, you can dry it with paper towels or using a salad spinner. If you are going to steam the Swiss chard, don't worry about drying it.

Do not cook Swiss chard in an aluminum pot, since the oxalates contained in the Swiss chard will react with the metal and cause the pot to discolor.

QUICK SERVING IDEAS

- Swiss chard adds unique color and taste to green salads.
- Sprinkle chopped walnuts over braised Swiss chard and top with a little freshly squeezed orange juice.
- Toss penne pasta with olive oil, lemon juice, garlic, haricot beans, and shredded steamed Swiss chard.
- Add zest to omelets and frittatas by adding some chopped Swiss chard.
- Use Swiss chard in place of, or in addition to, spinach when preparing vegetarian lasagna.

SAFETY

Swiss chard contains high amounts of oxalate. Individuals with a history of oxalate-containing kidney stones should avoid overconsuming Swiss chard. For more information, see Appendix D, page 793.

Tomatoes

The tomato is a member of the Solanaceae or nightshade family, along with bell peppers, aubergine, and potatoes. Tomatoes have fleshy internal segments filled with slippery seeds surrounded by a watery matrix. They can be red, yellow, orange, green, or brown in color. In fact, there are over a thousand different varieties that vary in shape, size, and color. There are small cherry tomatoes, bright yellow tomatoes, Italian pear-shaped tomatoes, and the green tomato, famous for its fried preparation in southern American cuisine.

Although tomatoes are fruit in a botanical sense, since they don't have the sweet quality of other fruit they are commonly thought of as a vegetable. For this reason, they are included in this chapter.

HISTORY

The tomato, like many other members of the nightshade family, originated in Central and South America. The first type of tomato grown is thought to have resembled the smaller-sized cherry tomato more than the larger varieties. The tomato was first cultivated in Mexico, supposedly because the Mexican Indians were intrigued by this fruit since it resembled the tomatillo, which was a staple in their cuisine. The Spanish conquistadors who came to Mexico shortly after Columbus's discovery of the New World "discovered" tomatoes and took the seeds back to Spain, beginning the introduction of the tomato into Europe.

Although the tomato spread throughout Europe and made its way to Italy by the sixteenth century, it was originally not a very popular food because many people held the belief that it was poisonous since it was a member of the deadly nightshade family. They were wise to fear that the tomato plant was poisonous, but their fear was not entirely accurate as it is the leaves of the tomato plant, but not its fruit, that contain toxic alkaloids. Yet, due to this belief, tomatoes were more often grown as an ornamental garden plant than as a food for several more centuries in some European countries.

The name the tomato was given in various languages reflects some of the history and mystery surrounding it. The Latin name, *Lycopersi-con,* means "wolf peach" and refers to the former belief that, like a wolf, this fruit was dangerous. The French called it *pomme d'amour,* meaning "love apple," since they believed it to have aphrodisiac qualities, while the Italians named it *pomodoro,* or "golden apple," probably owing to the fact that the first known species with which they were familiar were yellow in color.

Tomatoes made their way to North America with the colonists who first settled in Virginia, yet did not readily gain popularity until the late nineteenth century. Part of the reason may have been the widely held belief in North America that tomatoes were poisonous, even though by that time they had become a dietary staple in many parts of Europe. It wasn't until 1820, when Robert Gibbon Johnson ate a tomato on the courthouse steps in Salem, Indiana, that the "poisonous tomato" barrier was broken.

Since new varieties have been developed and more efficient means of transportation established, tomatoes have become one of the top-selling vegetables in the United States. Today, the United States, the Russian Federation, Italy, Spain, China, and Turkey are among the top-selling commercial producers of tomatoes.

NUTRITIONAL HIGHLIGHTS

The tomato is a low-calorie food packed with nutrition, especially when fully ripe. For example, red tomatoes have up to four times the amount of beta-carotene as green tomatoes. Tomatoes are an excellent source of vitamin C, carotenes (especially lycopene), biotin, and vitamin K. They are also a very good source of vitamin B6, pantothenic acid, niacin, folic acid, and dietary fiber. A 100 gram serving of cooked tomato provides 32 calories with 2 grams of fiber.

HEALTH BENEFITS

The health-promoting ability of tomatoes has received a lot of attention recently because of their lycopene content. This red carotene has been shown to be extremely protective against breast, colon, lung, skin, and prostate cancers. It has also been shown to lower the risk of heart disease, cataracts, and macular degeneration. Lycopene helps prevent these diseases and others by neutralizing harmful oxygen free radicals before they can do damage to cellular structures.

In one of the more detailed studies, Harvard researchers discovered that men who consumed the highest levels of lycopene (6.5 milligrams per day) in their diet showed a 21 percent decreased risk of prostate cancer compared with those eating the lowest levels. Men who ate two or more servings of tomato sauce each week were 23 percent less likely to develop prostate cancer during the twenty-two years of the study than men who ate less than one serving of tomato sauce each month. In another study, lycopene supplementation (15 milligrams per day) given to patients with existing prostate cancer was shown to slow tumor growth, shrink the tumor, and lower the level of PSA (prostate-specific antigen, a marker of cancer activity) by 18 percent.

The amount of lycopene in tomatoes can vary significantly, depending upon the type of tomato and how ripe it is. In the reddest strains, lycopene concentration is close to 50 milligrams per kilogram, compared with only 5 milligrams per kilogram in the yellow strains. Lycopene appears to be relatively stable during cooking and food processing. In fact, you actually get up to five times as much lycopene from tomato paste or juice as you do from raw tomatoes, because processing "liberates" more lycopene from the plant's cells. Eating a lycopene source with oil, such as olive oil, can also improve its absorption. That's one reason why a Mediterranean diet (see page 27) has so many healthful properties.

HOW TO SELECT AND STORE

Good-quality tomatoes are well formed and plump, fully colored, firm, and free from bruise marks. Avoid tomatoes that are soft or show signs of bruising or decay. They should not have a puffy appearance, since this indicates that they will be of inferior flavor and will also cause excess waste during preparation due to their higher water content. Ripe tomatoes will yield to slight pressure and will have a noticeably sweet fragrance.

When buying canned tomatoes, it is often better to buy those that are produced in the United States or E.U., as many countries do not have strict standards for lead content in containers. This is especially important with a fruit such as tomatoes, whose high acid content can cause corrosion and subsequent migration into the foods of the metal with which it is in contact.

Since tomatoes are sensitive to cold and it will impede their ripening process, store them at room temperature and out of direct exposure to sunlight. They will keep for up to one week, depending upon how ripe they are when purchased. To hasten the ripening process, place them in a paper bag with a banana or apple, since the ethylene gas that these fruits emit will hasten the tomatoes' maturation. If the tomatoes begin to become overripe but you are not yet ready to eat them, place them in the refrigerator (if possible, in the butter compartment, which is a warmer area), where they will keep for one to two more days. Removing them from the refrigerator about thirty minutes before using will help them to regain their maximum flavor and juiciness. Whole tomatoes, chopped tomatoes, and tomato sauce freeze well for future use in cooked dishes. Sun-dried tomatoes should be stored in an airtight container, with or without olive oil, in a cool dry place. Cooked tomatoes will keep for five to seven days refrigerated.

TIPS FOR PREPARING

Soak tomatoes in cold water with a mild solution of additive-free soap or produce wash, rinse under cool running water, and pat dry. It is better to cut tomatoes vertically, rather than horizontally, as this process will allow them to better retain their juice and seeds.

Sometimes recipes call for peeled tomatoes. The easiest way to do this is to first blanch the tomatoes in boiling water for 15 to 30 seconds. After carefully removing them, place them in a colander in the sink and rinse them briefly under cold running water. Use a paring knife to gently remove the skin, which should now come off rather easily.

If your recipe requires seeded tomatoes, cut the fruit in half horizontally and gently squeeze out the seeds and the juice. Any remaining seeds can be extracted by hand or with a small spoon.

It is especially important when cooking tomatoes not to use aluminum cookware, since the high acid content of tomatoes will interact with the metal. This may result in the migration of the aluminum into the tomatoes, which will not only impart an unpleasant taste but, more important, may have deleterious effects on your health.

QUICK SERVING IDEAS

- Tomatoes are a nutritious addition to salads and soups. To make things colorful, use yellow, green, and purple tomatoes in addition to the red varieties.
- Slice a variety of tomatoes (red, yellow, and orange) and top with balsamic vinegar and olive oil for a quick and nutritious salad.
- For a quick salsa dip, combine chopped onions, tomatoes, and chili peppers.
- Purée tomatoes, cucumbers, bell peppers, and spring onions together in a food processor and season with herbs and spices of your choice to make the refreshing cold soup gazpacho.
- Add tomato slices to sandwiches and salads.

SAFETY

Tomatoes are one of the foods most commonly associated with allergic reactions.

Tomatoes are one of the vegetables in the nightshade (Solanaceae) family, which includes aubergine, peppers, and potatoes. Anecdotal case histories link improvement in arthritic symptoms with removal of these foods. Although no case-controlled scientific studies confirm these observations, some individuals consuming nightshade-family vegetables experience an aggravation of arthritic symptoms and may benefit from limiting or avoiding these foods.

Tomatoes contain moderate amounts of oxalate. Individuals with a history of oxalate-containing kidney stones should avoid over-consuming them. For more information, see Appendix D, page 793.

Finally, since tomatoes are among the foods on which pesticide residues have been most frequently found, we recommend choosing tomatoes that have been grown organically.

Turnips and Turnip Greens

The turnip (*Brassica rapa rapifeera*) is a member of the cruciferous vegetable family, which also includes cabbage and broccoli. Both the root and the greens of turnips are edible. Turnip greens are smaller and tenderer than their cousin collards, and they have a slightly bitter flavor.

Swedes, which are similar to turnips, are actually a cross between turnips and kale.

HISTORY

Turnips were cultivated almost 4,000 years ago in Asia. The Greeks and Romans further cultivated turnips into several new varieties. They were widely grown throughout Europe during the Middle Ages and enjoyed wide popularity there until the potato was introduced to Europe in the eighteenth century. Turnips were introduced into North America by the early European settlers and colonists. They grew well in the South and became a popular food in the local cuisine of this region.

Turnip greens became an integral part of southern African-American cuisine when during the time of slavery the slave owners would reserve the turnip roots for themselves, leaving the turnip greens for the slaves. The slaves did not mind, however, as the traditional West African cuisine utilizes a wide variety of green leaves in its cooking, so they quickly adopted turnip greens.

NUTRITIONAL HIGHLIGHTS

Although turnips are considered a "starch" vegetable, they provide only one third the amount of calories as an equal amount of potatoes, having only 22 calories per 100 gram serving, with 2 grams of fiber.

Turnips are an excellent source of fiber, vitamin C, folic acid, pantothenic acid, manganese, and copper. They are also a very good source of thiamine, niacin, potassium, and magnesium and a good source of riboflavin, and vitamins B6 and E.

Turnip greens supply many times the nutrient content of the root. They are an excellent source of many vitamins, including vitamins A, C, E, and B6 and folic acid. They are also an excellent source of the minerals calcium, copper, and manganese. In addition, they are an excellent source of dietary fiber.

HEALTH BENEFITS

As a cabbage-family vegetable, turnips provide numerous health benefits (see "Cabbage").

HOW TO SELECT AND STORE

Turnip roots should be firm and smooth with no visible signs of mould or decay. Avoid soft, shriveled, or large turnips, as they will not be as nutritious or as tasty.

Turnip greens are usually available with their roots attached. Look for greens that are unblemished, crisp, and deep green in color.

If you have purchased turnip greens with

roots attached, remove them from the root. Store them in the refrigerator separately wrapped in a perforated plastic bag. They should keep fresh for about four days.

TIPS FOR PREPARING

Scrub turnips under running cold water with a vegetable brush to remove any dirt or grit. If they are not organically grown, soak them in a mild solution of additive-free soap or use a produce wash and rinse thoroughly. If you elect to peel the turnip, do so with a vegetable peeler and try to remove only a thin layer of the skin to retain as much nutritional value as possible.

For basic turnip green preparation, follow the same preparation as for mustard greens (see page 215).

QUICK SERVING IDEAS

- Turnips are most often prepared by boiling diced turnips in water and then mashing them. Mashed turnips can be served on their own or mixed with an equal amount of mashed potatoes.
- Turnips are great in soups, stews, and vegetable casseroles.
- Turnip greens can be added to any green, mixed salads.
- Serve sautéed turnip greens seasoned with lemon juice and cayenne pepper.
- Lightly sauté turnip greens, sweet potatoes, and tofu, and serve alongside your favorite grain.
- Use turnip greens with an equal amount of spinach when making vegetarian lasagna.

SAFETY

Members of the cabbage family contain goitrogens, naturally occurring substances that can interfere with the functioning of the thyroid gland. Dietary goitrogens are usually of no clinical importance unless they are consumed in large amounts or there is coexisting iodine deficiency. Cooking helps to inactivate the goitrogenic compounds. Individuals with already existing and untreated thyroid problems may want to avoid consumption of cabbage-family vegetables in their raw form for this reason. (See "Cabbage" for more information.)

Turnip greens also contain high amounts of oxalate. Individuals with a history of oxalate-containing kidney stones should avoid overconsuming them. For more information, see Appendix D, page 793.

Watercress: See Kale.

Yams

True yams are members of the Dioscoreaceae family and are different from the sweet potatoes labeled "yams" in the United States, having their own distinct taste and texture. The word "yam" comes from *nyami*, an African word for the root of the *Dioscorea* genus of plants.

Depending upon the yam variety, of which there are about 200, the flesh may be of varying colors, including white, ivory, yellow, or purple, while the thick skin may be white, pink, or brownish black. Yams are long and cylindrical, often having offshoots referred to as "toes," while their exterior texture is rough and scaly. Yams have a very starchy and slippery texture and, when cooked, will be either creamy or firm, depending upon the variety. Their taste is earthy and hardy, with most varieties having minimal, if any, sweetness. Specific types of yams include *Dioscorea alata* (Hawaiian yam), *Dioscorea batatas* (Korean yam), and *Dioscorea esculenta* (sweet yam).

HISTORY

Although it is uncertain in which country yams originated, they are one of the oldest food plants known. They have been cultivated in Africa and Asia since 50,000 B.C.E. In addition to these continents, yams also currently grow in the tropical and subtropical regions of North and South America.

Yams are one of the most popular and widely consumed foods in the world. They play a staple role in the diets of many different countries, most notably those in South America, Africa, the Pacific Islands, and the West Indies.

NUTRITIONAL HIGHLIGHTS

Yams are a very good source of dietary fiber and potassium. They are also a good source of several vitamins, including vitamins B1, B6, and C. In addition, yams are a good source of manganese and carbohydrates. A 100 gram serving provides 116 calories, mostly as 27.6 grams of carbohydrate, with 3.9 grams of fiber.

HEALTH BENEFITS

Yams contain a unique phytoestrogen called diosgenin that is used as a starting material for the synthesis of the hormones oestrogen and progesterone by drug manufacturers. Contrary to some popular claims, the human body cannot convert diosgenin into the human hormone

progesterone; however, yams are still a superfood for women, especially since they possess phytoestrogen activity and are a good source of vitamin B6. One cup of baked cubed yam contains 24 percent of the daily value of B6, which is required by the liver, along with folic acid and other B vitamins, to detoxify excess oestrogen. This action is particularly beneficial in helping women improve symptoms of premenstrual syndrome. At least a dozen double-blind, placebo-controlled trials have demonstrated positive effects of vitamin B6 in relieving PMS symptoms, including fibrocystic breast disease.

HOW TO SELECT AND STORE

Yams are not widely available in the United States nor in British supermarkets. If they are available, it will be at Asian or African food markets. Choose yams that are firm and do not have any cracks, bruises, or soft spots. Avoid those that are displayed in the refrigerated section of the produce department, since cold temperature negatively alters their taste.

Yams should be stored in a cool, dark, well-ventilated place, where they will stay fresh for up to ten days. They should be stored loose and not kept in a plastic bag. Keep them from exposure to sunlight or temperatures above 60 degrees F./16 degrees C., since this will cause them to sprout or ferment. Uncooked yams should not be kept in the refrigerator.

TIPS FOR PREPARING

See "Sweet Potatoes."

QUICK SERVING IDEAS

- Thinly slice yams, then lightly coat with olive oil and your favorite seasonings. Bake the yam chips at 300 degrees F./150 degrees C./gas 2 until crispy, or approximately 20 minutes.

- Slice open a baked yam and top with a drizzle of maple syrup and a few walnuts.
- Purée cooked yam with a little milk and season with tamari, coriander, cumin, and cayenne.
- As yam has an earthy, deep taste, it nicely complements darker meats, such as venison.
- Add grated yams to recipes that feature potatoes, such as potato pancakes and hash browns.

- Add chunks of yam to your next stir-fry or pan of roasted vegetables. For example, roasted yams, fennel, onions, and mushrooms make a delicious combination.

SAFETY

No significant safety issues are associated with yams.

The Healing Power of Fruits

When most people think of fruit, they think of sweet, soft, succulent, refreshing, and delicious natural foods such as apples, oranges, berries, and melons. However, by strict definition, a fruit is the ripened ovary of a female flower. This scientific definition covers both what the lay person calls fruit, as well what most people consider as nuts and some vegetables, such as squash, pumpkins, and tomatoes. But for our purposes in this chapter, we include only fruit that fits within the layperson's definition.

Fruit, in general, is an excellent source of many vital antioxidant nutrients and phytochemicals, such as vitamin C, carotenes, flavonoids, and polyphenols. Regular fruit consumption, like regular vegetable consumption, has been shown to offer significant protection against many chronic degenerative diseases, including cancer, heart disease, cataracts, and strokes. Although most fruit is seasonal, with modern transportation methods a wide variety of healthful fresh fruit is now available to most people year-round.

Since fruit contains a fair amount of natural fruit sugars, such as fructose, it is generally recommended to limit your intake to no more than four servings, or two 8-ounce/250 ml glasses, of fresh fruit juice per day. If you suffer from hypoglycemia, diabetes, candidiasis, or gout, it is probably best for you to eat fruit in its whole form or drink fresh fruit juice with food or dilute it with an equal amount of pure water. Eating whole fruit and drinking diluted juice decreases the rate at which sugar enters your bloodstream compared to drinking concentrated fruit drinks.

Although fructose and other sugars are as much as one and a half times sweeter than sucrose (white sugar), they are handled by the body in a different manner. For example, in order to be utilized, fructose must be changed to glucose in the liver. As a result, blood sugar (glucose) levels do not rise as rapidly after fructose consumption compared to other simple sugars. Sucrose, which is composed of one molecule of glucose and one molecule of fructose, results in immediate elevations in blood sugar levels. While most diabetics cannot tolerate sucrose, most can tolerate moderate amounts of fruit and fructose without loss of blood sugar control. In fact, fruit is much better tolerated and has a lower glycemic index than white bread and other refined carbohydrates (see page 22 for more information on the glycemic index).

Regular fruit consumption may also help control the appetite and promote weight loss. While aspartame (NutraSweet), glucose, and sucrose may increase the appetite, fructose has actually been shown to decrease the amount of calories and fat consumed in several studies. Typically, the studies give the subjects food or drink containing an equivalent amount of fructose or other sweetener 30 minutes to 2½ hours before allowing them to consume as much food as they desired at a dinner buffet. The studies were designed in a double-blind fashion so that neither the observers nor participants knew who had been given what. Consistently, subjects receiving the fructose-sweetened food or drink consumed substantially fewer calories and fat than the groups receiving aspartame, sucrose, or glucose.

Since fruit contains fructose in a natural form, consuming a serving of fruit or fruit juice at least 30 minutes before dinner may result in significantly fewer calories being consumed during the meal. When fewer calories are consumed, weight loss is much easier to achieve. Thus, fruit makes an excellent between-meal snack.

The fruit options we have today come from all over the world, as numerous varieties of fruit were brought by migrants from many countries. The table on page 252 illustrates the diverse origins of the fruits commonly seen in the supermarket.

Common Fruits

Apple

The apple *(Malus pumila)* is a member of the rose family, along with the pear. It is a crisp, white-fleshed fruit with a red, yellow, or green skin.

In the United States, more than twenty-five varieties of apples are available; they vary not only in color and appearance but also in sweetness, flavor, and tartness. For example, Golden and Red Delicious apples are mild and sweet, while Pippins and Granny Smith apples are notably brisk and tart. Tart apples are better able to retain their texture during cooking, while sweeter varieties, such as Delicious, Braeburn, and Fuji apples, are usually eaten raw. Most supermarkets in the U.K. sell about eight varieties (and about 70 percent of apples sold) but there are approximately 2,040 varieties at the National Fruit Collection at Brogdale. The most popular varieties are Royal Gala, Jonagold, Braeburn, Fiesta and Cox's Orange Pippin.

HISTORY

The original apple tree is thought to have grown in eastern Europe and southwestern Asia but has now spread to most temperate regions of the world. There are now over 7,000 varieties of apples in the market as a result of cultivation and hybridization.

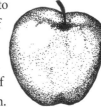

TABLE 11.1
Origins of Modern Fruits

Europe	Africa	Middle East	India	China	Central Asia	South Pacific	North America	Central America	South America
Blueberry (Bilberry)	Cantaloupe and other melons	Apple	Cantaloupe and other melons	Apricot	Cranberry	Banana	Blueberry	Acerola cherry	Pineapple
Cranberry	Watermelon	Cantaloupe and other melons	Lemon	Kiwifruit	Currant	Plantain	Cranberry	Avocado	Strawberry
Currant		Cherry	Lime	Lemon			Currant	Grapefruit	
Plum and prune		Date	Mango	Nectarine			Plum and prune	Papaya	
Raspberry		Fig		Orange			Raspberry		
Strawberry		Grape and raisin		Peach			Strawberry		
		Pear		Plum					
		Raspberry		Tangerine					

The apple holds a special place in many historical and mythical realms, beginning with the biblical story of Adam and Eve. In Norse mythology, apples were believed to keep people young forever. The apple has been used as a symbol in many classic stories (e.g., "Snow White"). One story that is based on irrefutable fact is the legend of Johnny Appleseed—a real person named John Chapman, who in the 1800s walked barefoot across an area of 100,000 square miles in the United States planting apple trees that provided food and a livelihood for generations of settlers.

NUTRITIONAL HIGHLIGHTS

Apples are an excellent source of vitamin C, pectin, and other fibers. They are also a good source of potassium. Most of the apple's important nutrients are contained in its skin, and raw apples are higher in many nutrients and phytochemicals as well. If apples are raw and unpeeled, they are a great source of many important phytochemicals, such as ellagic acid and flavonoids (especially quercetin). For example, fresh whole apples and fresh apple juice contain approximately 100–130 milligrams per 100 grams of ellagic, chlorogenic, and caffeic acids. The content of these compounds in cooked or commercial apple products, however, is at or near zero.

A 100 gram serving of apple is one small apple (four per pound/½ kilogram) and provides 52 calories, 0.3 grams of protein, 0.2 grams of fat, and 12.8 grams of carbohydrate with 2.4 grams of fiber and 10.4 grams as natural sugars. For comparison, a medium-sized apple (three per pound/½ kilogram) provides 72 calories, 0.4 grams of protein, 0.2 grams of fat, and 19.1 grams of carbohydrates with 3.3 grams of fiber and 14.3 grams of sugars.

A 100 gram serving of dried apple provides 243 calories, 0.9 grams of protein, 0.3 grams of fat, and 65.9 grams of carbohydrate with 8.7 grams of fiber and 57.2 grams of sugars; this serving also provides a whopping 450 milligrams of potassium.

HEALTH BENEFITS

The old saying "An apple a day keeps the doctor away" appears to be true. In an analysis of more than eighty-five studies, apple consumption was shown to be consistently associated with a reduced risk of heart disease, cancer, asthma, and type 2 diabetes compared to other fruits and vegetables. In one of the studies evaluated, researchers in Finland followed more than 5,000 Finnish men and women for more than twenty years. Those who ate the most apples and other flavonoid-rich foods, such as onions and tea, were found to have a 20 percent lower risk of heart disease than those who ate the smallest amount of these foods.

In another study, apple consumption was linked to a lower risk for asthma. When nearly 1,500 adults in the United Kingdom were asked about their eating habits during the previous year, the investigators found that people who ate at least two apples each week had a 22 to 32 percent lower risk of developing asthma than those who ate less of this fruit.

Researchers feel that much of apple's protective effects against heart disease and asthma is related to its high content of flavonoids like quercetin (see page 145 for more information).

Apples are also very high in pectin, a soluble fiber that has been shown to exert a number of beneficial effects. Because it is a gel-forming fiber, pectin can lower cholesterol levels as well as improve the intestinal muscle's ability to push waste through the gastrointestinal tract. One medium (140 gram) unpeeled apple provides 3 grams of fiber, more than 10 percent of the daily fiber intake recommended by experts. Even without its peel, a medium apple provides 2.7 grams of fiber. Adding just one large apple (about 175 grams) to the daily diet has been shown to decrease serum cholesterol by 8 to 11 percent. Eating two large apples a day has lowered cholesterol levels by up to 16 percent.

Apples' insoluble fiber and pectin both help promote bowel regularity, relieving both constipation and diarrhea. In fact, one well-known over-the-counter diarrhea remedy, Kaopectate, actually contains a form of pectin.

HOW TO SELECT AND STORE

As stated above, there are many varieties of apples. So, when it comes to selection, it depends on your palate whether you prefer a sweeter or more tart apple and whether you like to have your apple baked or raw. As a guideline, the Red and Golden Delicious apples are among the sweetest, while the Braeburn and Fuji are only slightly tart. The tartest apples are the Gravenstein, Pippin, and Granny Smith. While these apples may be too tart for some, they retain their texture best during cooking, where the Bramley comes into its own.

In the Northern Hemisphere, apple season begins at the end of summer and runs until early winter. Apples that you see available at other times of the year have been in cold storage or imported from different parts of the world.

Whenever possible, it is strongly encouraged

to buy organic fruit. To certify that it is organic, in the U.K. the fruit will carry a Soil Association label. Nonorganic apples are sprayed with many dangerous chemicals, especially pesticides. Furthermore, nonorganic apples are often waxed to prolong their freshness. However, do not be confused and try to determine if the apple is organic by the waxiness because even organic apples will appear waxy due to their natural coating.

Also, apples should be firm, crisp, and well colored. Apples that are immature and ripened artificially will be less vibrant. Mature apples produce a characteristic snap when you apply fingernail pressure to break the skin. These have more color and enhanced flavor and will store longer. Conversely, overripe apples feel softer when pressure is applied to the skin.

TIPS FOR PREPARING

Wash organically grown apples gently by rinsing them under cool water and patting them dry with a paper towel. Nonorganic apples should be sprayed with a solution of diluted additive-free soap or commercial produce wash and then washed gently under cool running water, then patted dry.

As discussed above, for maximum nutritional benefit, apples should be consumed in their fresh form—either whole or sliced, or as fresh apple juice. In juicing, apples mix very well with other fruit as well as vegetables, because of their sweet but not overpowering flavor. Since there are very small amounts of cyanide in the seeds of apples, many people recommend that you core apples to remove the seeds before eating. This probably is a good idea when eating apples, but the amount of cyanide in the apple seed is below a level that is of concern. If you are making juice in a commercial juicer, it is not necessary, since there is very little liquid in the seed.

To prevent browning when slicing apples for a recipe, simply put the slices in a bowl of cold water with a spoonful of lemon juice added.

QUICK SERVING IDEAS

- Add diced apples to fruit or green salads.
- Lightly sauté slices from one apple with one diced potato and onion.
- Lightly sauté slices from one apple with a few raisins, sprinkle with ground cinnamon, cloves, or ginger, add a few chopped walnuts, then use as a filling for a nutritious omelet.
- For an unusual dessert, skewer apple chunks on cinnamon sticks and bake at 350 degrees F./180 degrees C./gas 4 for 25 minutes.
- Sliced apples (either alone or with other fruit or nuts) and cheese are a favorite European dessert.

SAFETY

As apples are among the top foods containing pesticide residues, we recommend selecting organically grown apples. Also, see "How to Select and Store," above.

If you purchase dried apples, avoid products preserved with sulphur dioxide or sulphites. For more information on the adverse effects of sulphites as a dried-fruit preservative, see page 46.

Apricot

An apricot *(Prunus armenaica)* is a small, round, golden orange fruit with velvety skin and flesh. The apricot is technically classified as a "drupe," a fleshy, one-seeded fruit containing a seed enclosed in a stony pit. It is in the same family as the almond, cherry, peach, and plum. Its flesh is not too juicy and possesses a characteristic muskiness and tartness that is somewhere between those of a peach and a plum. Apricots are often dried, cooked into pastry, and eaten as jam. They are also distilled into brandy and liqueur. Essential oil from the pits is sold commercially as bitter almond oil.

HISTORY

The apricot tree is thought to have originated in China, with records showing that apricots have been consumed there for thousands of years. Alexander the Great is believed to have brought the apricot from China to Greece, and ultimately to Western civilization. In North America, the first apricot tree was delivered to Virginia in 1720. The apricot tree was shown to flourish in the California climate around 1792, and that state is by far the major supplier of apricots in the United States today. Turkey, Italy, the Russian Federation, Spain, Greece, the United States, and France are the leading producers of apricots.

NUTRITIONAL HIGHLIGHTS

Apricots are good sources of potassium, iron, and carotenes. Apricots are also a good source of fiber. A 100 gram serving of apricot (about three apricots) provides 48 calories, 1.4 grams of protein, 0.4 grams of fat, and 11.1 grams of carbohydrate, with 2 grams of fiber and 9.2 grams of natural sugars (sucrose, glucose, and fructose), as well as 0.4 milligrams of iron and 259 milligrams of potassium. The same-sized serving of dried apricot provides 241 calories, 3.4 grams of protein, 0.5 gram of fat, and 62.6 grams of carbohydrate, with 7.3 grams of fiber and 53.4 grams of natural sugars, as well as 2.7 milligrams of iron and 1,162 milligrams of potassium.

HEALTH BENEFITS

For a fruit, apricots are a good source of carotenes such as lycopene and lutein. These carotenes give red, orange, and yellow colors to fruits and vegetables. They are particularly beneficial for preventing macular degeneration, heart disease, and cancer.

HOW TO SELECT AND STORE

The best season for picking apricots is June through to August. Apricots purchased in the U.S. in winter are generally imported from South America. Apricots should be picked when they are still firm because of their high bruisability when soft. A fresh, ripe apricot should be approximately two inches/5 cm in diameter and round and be of a consistent golden-orange hue. An unripe apricot is visibly more yellow and hard, while a soft or mushy apricot is overripe. Apricots should be stored in the refrigerator at 32 to 38 degrees F./0 to 3 degrees C.

Dried apricots are a popular alternative. Unfortunately, dried apricots contain high levels of sulphur dioxide. During the fruit-drying process, sulphur is added to inactivate the enzymes that cause the fruit to spoil. Natural food suppliers carry a healthier alternative to sulphured apricots. These unsulphured apricots are preserved through a blanching process and have a brown color.

TIPS FOR PREPARING

Wash organically grown apricots gently by rinsing them under cool water and patting them dry with a paper towel. If nonorganic, they should be sprayed with a solution of diluted additive-free soap or commercial produce wash and then washed gently under cool running water, then patted dry. Slice them in half and remove the pit.

QUICK SERVING IDEAS

- Eat apricots whole or in fruit salads.
- Add sliced apricots to hot or cold cereal.
- Apricots are a delicious addition to baked goods such as muffins and quick breads.
- The next time you make whole-grain pancakes, add some chopped apricots to the batter.
- Skewer whole or halved fresh apricots, brush with honey, and barbecue on the grill or bake in the oven until brown.
- Add dried, diced apricots to chicken or vegetable stews.

SAFETY

Sulphur-containing compounds such as sulphur dioxide are often added to dried fruits as preservatives to help prevent oxidation and bleaching of colors. These sulphur compounds cause adverse reactions in approximately one in every 100 people and about one in twenty people who suffer from asthma.

Apricots contain moderate amounts of oxalates. Individuals with a history of calcium oxalate-containing kidney stones should limit their consumption of this food. See page 793 for more information.

Avocado

The avocado, also called the alligator pear, is grown from the fast-growing *Persea americana* tree. Despite the dozens of varieties, avocados are divided into three main categories. These are the West Indian, Guatemalan, and Mexican types. West Indian varieties thrive in humid, tropical climates, and Guatemalan types are native to cool, high-altitude tropics and are more hardy. Mexican types are native to dry subtropical plateaus and thrive in a Mediterranean climate. Hybrid types exist among all three forms.

Depending on variety, avocados vary in weight from 8 ounces to 3 pounds/250 grams to 1½ kilograms. When harvested, the flesh is hard, but with time it softens to a buttery texture. The Haas and Fuerte avocados are the most popular varieties in the U.K. The Haas avocado (Guatemalan type) is purple-brown, pebbled, thick-skinned and oval in shape. In contrast, the Mexican Fuerte avocado has a thin, smooth, dark green skin, is pear-shaped, and has less oil content. Its prime season is during December.

HISTORY

Avocados are native to Central and South America and have been cultivated in these regions since 8000 B.C.E. In the mid–seventeenth century, they were introduced to Jamaica and spread through the Asian tropical regions in the mid-1800s. Cultivation in the United States, specifically in Florida and California, began in the early twentieth century. While avocados are now grown in most tropical and subtropical countries, the major commercial producers include the United States (Florida and California), Mexico, the Dominican Republic, Brazil, Colombia, Israel, and Australia. California produces about 80 percent of the U.S. avocado crop.

NUTRITIONAL HIGHLIGHTS

Avocados are an excellent source of monounsaturated fatty acids, as well as potassium, vitamin E, B vitamins, and fiber. In fact, one avocado has the potassium content of two to three bananas. Of course, an avocado also has about three times the calories of a banana. A 100 gram serving is about half of an avocado and provides 160 calories, 2 grams of protein, 14.7 grams of fat, 8.5 grams of carbohydrate, and 6.7 grams of fiber. These fat grams are 9.8 grams of health-promoting monounsaturated fats, 2.8 grams of polyunsaturated fats, and only 2.1 grams of saturated fats. As for minerals, this serving provides 485 milligrams of potassium.

HEALTH BENEFITS

High in monosaturates (unsaturated fatty acids), the unsaturated oil content of avocados is second only to olives among fruits, and sometimes greater. The fat content of an avocado is roughly 20 percent, approximately twenty times that of other fruit. The oils provided by an avocado include oleic acid and linoleic acid, and thereby may help lower cholesterol levels. One study of individuals with moderately high levels of cholesterol who ate a diet high in avocados showed significant decreases in total cholesterol and LDL cholesterol. They also exhibited an 11 percent increase in healthy HDL cholesterol.

HOW TO SELECT AND STORE

Ripe avocados should yield slightly to gentle pressure. Avoid overripe, rancid avocados with brown meat. These will be mushy to the touch.

A firm avocado will ripen in a paper bag or in a fruit basket at room temperature within a few days. As the fruit ripens, the skin will turn darker. Avocados should not be refrigerated until they are ripe. Once ripe, they can be kept refrigerated for up to a week if they have not been sliced. Once sliced or mashed, avocado will keep refrigerated for one day, particularly if the pit is stored in contact with the flesh.

TIPS FOR PREPARING

Use a stainless-steel knife to cut the avocado in half lengthwise. Gently twist the two halves in opposite directions if you find the flesh clinging to the pit. Remove the pit, either with a spoon or by spearing it with the tip of a knife. Place the halves face down, then peel and slice. If the flesh is too soft to be sliced, just slide a spoon along the inside of the skin and scoop it out.

You can prevent the natural darkening of the avocado flesh that occurs with exposure to air by sprinkling it with a little lemon juice or vinegar.

QUICK SERVING IDEAS

- Use chopped avocados as a garnish for black bean soup.
- Add avocado to your favorite creamy tofu dressing recipe to give it an extra richness and beautiful green color.
- Mix chopped avocados, onions, tomatoes, and fresh coriander; lime juice; and seasonings for a rich-tasting guacamole.

- Spread ripe avocados on bread as a healthy replacement for mayonnaise when making a sandwich.
- For an exceptional salad, combine sliced avocado with fennel, oranges, and fresh mint.

SAFETY

Avocados contain enzymes called chitinases that can cause allergic reactions in people with sensitivity to latex. Therefore, individuals with latex sensitivity should avoid touching or eating avocados. The treatment of avocados with ethylene gas to induce ripening can increase the presence of these allergenic enzymes; therefore we recommend selecting organic avocados not treated with ethylene gas, as they have fewer allergy-causing compounds.

Bananas

Bananas are the second leading fruit crop in the world. They abound in hundreds of edible varieties that fall into two distinct species: the sweet banana and the plantain banana. All bananas are elliptically shaped, featuring a firm, creamy flesh inside a thick, inedible peel. While most people think of bananas as having yellow skins, they can also feature red, pink, purple, and black tones when ripe.

Although it looks like a tree, bananas

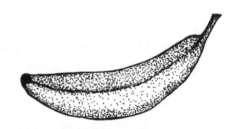

actually grow on a plant. The banana plant grows to 10 to 26 feet/3 to 8 meters in height and belongs to the same family as the lily and the orchid. Bananas grow in clusters of fifty to 150 on the plant, with individual bananas grouped in bunches, known as "hands," of ten to twenty-five bananas.

The most popular type of banana is the large, yellow, smooth-skinned variety of sweet banana familiar to most Europeans and Americans. This banana *(Musa sapienta)* is known as the Manque or Gros Michel (Big Mike). Sweet bananas vary in size and color and are usually eaten raw. The larger, green bananas are known as plantains *(Musa paradisiaca)*. Plantain bananas are prepared similarly to vegetables in that they are usually fried or cooked.

HISTORY

Originating in Malaysia around 4,000 years ago, bananas were introduced to Africa by Arabians during the early part of the Middle Ages and were spread to the Americas by Portuguese explorers during the late fifteenth century; there they thrived, and there the majority of the world's supply is now grown. With the development of refrigeration and rapid transport in the mid-1900s, bananas have become one of the most popular fruits of today. While bananas grow in most tropical and subtropical regions, the main commercial producers are Costa Rica, Mexico, Ecuador, and Brazil as well as Caribbean countries.

NUTRITIONAL HIGHLIGHTS

Bananas are an excellent source of potassium and vitamin B6 and a good source of vitamin C, fiber, riboflavin, magnesium, biotin, and carbohydrates. Since they have a lower water content than most fruit, bananas typically have more calories as well as a higher sugar content. A 100 gram serving is a small (6½-inch/15 cm) banana and provides 89 calories, 1.1 grams of protein, 0.3 grams of fat, and 22.8 grams of carbohydrate, with 2.6 grams of fiber and 12.2 grams of natural sugars (glucose, fructose, and sucrose), 358 milligrams of potassium, 27 milligrams of magnesium, and 5 milligrams of calcium.

HEALTH BENEFITS

Bananas are packed with nutrients, especially potassium. An averaged-sized banana contains 440 milligrams of potassium and only 1 milligram of sodium. Potassium is one of the most important electrolytes in the body, helping to regulate heart function as well as fluid balance—a key factor in regulating blood pressure. The effectiveness of potassium-rich foods, such as bananas, in lowering blood pressure and protecting against heart disease and strokes is well accepted and bolstered by considerable scientific evidence. For example, in one landmark study researchers tracked more than 40,000 American male health professionals over four years to determine the effects of diet on blood pressure. Men who ate diets higher in potassium-rich foods had a substantially reduced risk of stroke.

Bananas are very soothing to the gastrointestinal tract due to their high content of pectin, a soluble fiber that not only lowers cholesterol but normalizes bowel function. In addition, plantain bananas have shown some promise in the treatment of peptic ulcers.

HOW TO SELECT AND STORE

Fresh sweet bananas and plantains are best when they are yellow, with no green showing, and speckled with brown. Sweet bananas and plantains with green tips are not quite ripe, but they will continue to ripen if stored at room temperature, particularly if placed in a plastic bag, as the gases they emit turn around and act on them to stimulate further ripening. After ripening, bananas and plantains may be stored at room temperature for one to two days, when they will continue to ripen and discolor. Ripe bananas and plantains can be stored in the refrigerator, and while the skin will turn dark brown, they will remain fresh for three to five days. Bananas and plantains that are bruised, discolored, or soft have deteriorated and should not be used.

Bananas and plantains can also be frozen and will keep for about two months. Either purée them before freezing or simply remove the peel and wrap the bananas in cling film. To prevent discoloration, add some lemon juice before freezing.

Dried bananas will keep for one to two months, and banana chips will keep for up to three months.

TIPS FOR PREPARING

In addition to being eaten raw, sweet bananas are a wonderful addition to a variety of recipes, including "smoothies," baked goods, and cereals.

Unlike sweet bananas, plantains need to be cooked. Depending on the country and culture, plantains are cooked like any other starchy vegetable. They can be grilled and then mashed into a porridge or, more commonly, roasted or fried. A quick, simple recipe for fried plantains is:

3 ripe plantains (skin should be blackened)
4 tablespoons olive oil

Peel the plantains and cut them into ¼-inch/½ cm slices on the diagonal. In a large, heavy skillet, add the olive oil and heat at a medium level. Sauté the plantains until golden brown and soft (approximately 2 minutes per side).

Yields four to six servings

QUICK SERVING IDEAS

- Purée frozen bananas in a food processor to make a delicious frothy iced dessert.
- Blend bananas and papayas together with a little apple juice, and use as a topping for plain yogurt.
- For a healthy twist on a campfire favorite, cut unpeeled bananas lengthwise midway through the flesh. Spread fruit open and place peanut butter and chopped figs in the opening, wrap tightly in aluminum foil, and grill on the barbecue.
- Add chopped bananas, walnuts, and maple syrup to oatmeal or porridge.

SAFETY

Like avocados, bananas contain enzymes called chitinases that can cause allergic reactions in people with sensitivity to latex. Therefore, individuals with a latex sensitivity should avoid touching or eating bananas. The treatment of bananas with ethylene gas to induce ripening can increase the presence of these allergenic enzymes; therefore we recommend selecting organic bananas not treated with ethylene gas, as they have fewer allergy-causing compounds.

Be sure to purchase unsulphured dried

banana products. See apricot safety on page 256 for more information on the adverse health effects of sulphur used to preserve fruit.

Blueberries

The blueberry *(Vaccinium myrtillus)* is a member of the Ericaceae family, along with many other berries, including huckleberries and bilberries, varieties of blueberry native to North America and Europe, respectively. Blueberries grow in clusters and range in size from that of a small pea to a marble. They are deep in color, ranging from blue to maroon to purple-black, and feature a white-gray waxy "bloom" that covers the berry's surface, serving as a protective coat. The skin surrounds a semitransparent flesh that encases tiny seeds. The difference between the North American blueberry and the European bilberry is that the latter has a purple flesh. Cultivated blueberries are typically mildly sweet, while those that grow wild have a more tart and tangy flavor.

There are approximately thirty different species of blueberries, with different varieties growing in distinctly separate regions. For example, the Highbush variety can be found throughout the eastern seaboard from Maine to Florida, the Lowbush variety throughout the northeastern states and eastern Canada, and the Evergreen variety throughout states in the Pacific Northwest. In the U.K., bilberries can still be picked wild on moors or heathland.

HISTORY

Native to many parts of the world, especially in the Northern Hemisphere, including North America, Europe, and Asia, blueberries have been consumed by man apparently since prehistoric times. Native Americans were particularly fond of blueberries, as they were a key in pemmican, a traditional dish composed of the fruit and dried meat.

The commercial development of blueberries, however, really did not begin until the beginning of the twentieth century, when they were successfully cultivated. There are now hundreds of varieties that exist as a result of both accidental and intentional crossbreeding.

Blueberries continue to grow wild throughout the woody and mountainous regions of the United States and Canada, where they are also grown commercially on farms. In Europe, the fruit is rarely found growing wild, but is also extensively cultivated. Blueberries have only recently been introduced in Australia.

NUTRITIONAL HIGHLIGHTS

Blueberries are an excellent source of flavonoids, especially anthocyanidins. These antioxidant compounds are responsible for the blue, purple, and red pigments. Blueberries are also a very good source of vitamin C, insoluble fiber, and soluble fiber, such as pectin. In addition, they are a good source of manganese, vitamin E, and riboflavin.

A 100 gram serving equals about ⅔ cup and provides 57 calories, 0.7 grams of protein, 0.3 grams of fat, and 14.5 grams of carbohydrate, with 2.4 grams of fiber and only 9.9 grams of natural sugars (fructose and glucose).

HEALTH BENEFITS

The health benefits of blueberries are due mainly to anthocyanidins. These compounds exert exceptional antioxidant activity. In fact, when researchers at Tufts University analyzed sixty fruits and vegetables for their antioxidant capability, blueberries rated the highest.

One of the practical applications of this antioxidant activity may be in the protection against Alzheimer's disease. Researchers have found, in animal studies, that blueberries help protect the brain from oxidative stress and may reduce the effects of age-related conditions, such as Alzheimer's disease. For example, when older rats were given the human equivalent of one cup of blueberries a day, they demonstrated significant improvements in both learning capacity and motor skills, making them mentally equivalent to much younger rats. When the rats' brains were examined, the brain cells of the rats given blueberries were found to communicate more effectively than those of the other older rats that were not given blueberries.

Currently, the most popular medical use of blueberries is in improving vision and protecting against age-related macular degeneration. This use was stimulated by the fact that during World War II, British Royal Air Force pilots consumed bilberry (a variety of European blueberry) preserves before their night missions. Based on folk medicine, the pilots believed that the bilberries would improve their ability to see at night. After the war, numerous studies demonstrated that blueberry extracts do in fact improve nighttime visual acuity and lead to quicker adjustment to darkness and faster restoration of visual acuity after exposure to glare. Clinical studies have shown good results in individuals with sensitivity to bright lights, diabetic retinopathy, and macular degeneration. Additional research also points out that bilberries and blueberries may be protective against the development of cataracts and glaucoma, and quite therapeutic in the treatment of varicose veins, hemorrhoids, and peptic ulcers.

Blueberries were also traditionally a popular remedy for both diarrhea and constipation. In addition to soluble and insoluble fiber, blueberries contain tannins, which act as astringents in the digestive system to firm up a loose stool.

Blueberries also promote urinary tract health because they contain the same compounds found in cranberries that help prevent or eliminate urinary tract infections. In order for bacteria to infect, they must first adhere to the mucosal lining of the urethra and bladder. Components found in cranberry and blueberry juice reduce the ability of E. coli, the bacterium that is the most common cause of urinary tract infections, to adhere.

HOW TO SELECT AND STORE

Choose blueberries that are firm and have a lively, uniform hue colored with a whitish bloom. Avoid berries that appear dull in color or are soft and watery in texture. They should also be free from moisture, since the presence of water will cause the berries to decay. When purchasing frozen blueberries, shake the bag gently to ensure that the berries move freely and are not clumped together. When they are clumped together, it suggests that they may have been previously thawed and refrozen. Blueberries that are cultivated in the United States are now available all year round but are more plentiful from May through October. The British blueberry season runs from mid-July until September. Imported blueberries are available all year round as well.

Ripe blueberries should be stored in a covered container in the refrigerator, where they will keep for about one week, although they will be freshest if consumed within a few days. Always check blueberries before storing and remove any damaged berries to prevent the spread of mould. But don't wash blueberries until right before eating, as washing will remove the bloom that protects the fruit's skin from degradation. If kept out at room temperature for more than one day, blueberries may spoil.

Ripe blueberries can also be frozen, although this will slightly change their texture and flavor. Before freezing, wash, drain, and remove any damaged berries. To better ensure uniform texture upon thawing, spread the berries out on a baking tray, place in the freezer until frozen, then put the berries in a plastic bag for storage in the freezer. Blueberries should last up to one year in the freezer.

TIPS FOR PREPARING

Wash organically grown blueberries by placing them in a colander, then rinse them under cool water. If nonorganic, they should be sprayed with a solution of diluted additive-free soap or commercial produce wash before placing them in the colander. Wash berries just prior to use so as to not prematurely remove the protective bloom that resides on the skin's surface.

When using frozen berries in recipes that do not require cooking, be sure to thaw them prior to using. For cooked recipes, use unthawed berries, since this will ensure maximum flavor; however, you will need to extend the cooking time a few minutes to accommodate for the frozen berries.

You may notice that berries used in baked products may take on a green color. This is a natural reaction of their anthocyanidin pigments and does not make the food item unsafe to eat.

QUICK SERVING IDEAS

- Add ½ cup of fresh or frozen blueberries to your favorite smoothie recipe.
- Fresh or dried blueberries add a colorful and nutritious punch to cold breakfast cereals.
- Layer yogurt and blueberries in wineglasses and top with crystallized ginger.
- Use blueberries as a filling for breakfast crêpes.
- Mix blueberry jam with savory spices to make a spread that is delicious on baked fish or chicken.

SAFETY

Blueberries contain moderate levels of oxalates. Individuals with a history of calcium oxalate-containing kidney stones should limit consumption. See page 793 for more information.

Cantaloupe (Muskmelon)

The cantaloupe (*Cucumis melo reticulatus*), as it is incorrectly referred to, is actually a muskmelon. (In the U.K. the Charentais melon is sometimes referred to as a muskmelon, although this melon has a smoother skin.) The muskmelon or cantaloupe is one of the five most frequently purchased fruits in the United States. In the U.K. the five favourite fruits are apples, oranges, kiwifruit, bananas, and grapefruit, though the city that consumes most melons in Britain is Glasgow.

Along with cucumbers, squash, gourds, and pumpkins, the cantaloupe melon belongs to the Cucurbitaceae family. The cantaloupe is round or oval in shape, grows along the ground with a trailing vine, and has a hollow core that contains its seeds encased in "netting." Cantaloupe flesh has a soft, succulent texture, is yellow to salmon in color, and has a musky aroma that indicates when the melon is ripe.

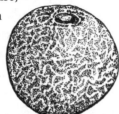

HISTORY

The exact location of origin is uncertain, but the cantaloupe may have originated and been cultivated in India, Persia, or Africa in ancient times. The true cantaloupe is a different species of melon that is grown mostly in France. This European melon was named after a castle's gardens in Italy. The cantaloupe was supposedly named for Cantalupo, a former papal villa near Rome, where the variety was developed. Although the true cantaloupe is not commercially grown in the United States, the muskmelon was introduced to the United States during colonial times, although it was not grown commercially until the late nineteenth century. Today, the United States, Turkey, Iran, and many Central American countries are the major producers of the muskmelon.

NUTRITIONAL HIGHLIGHTS

Cantaloupes are extremely nutrient-dense, as defined by quality of nutrition per calorie. One pound/½ kilogram of cantaloupe is seldom over 150 calories yet provides excellent levels of carotenes, potassium, and other valuable nutrients, especially if the skin is also juiced. In fact, a one-cup serving of cantaloupe contains just 56 calories but provides 129 percent of the daily value of vitamin B6 and 90 percent of the daily value of vitamin C. It is also an excellent source of potassium (417 milligrams per cup, diced) and a good source of dietary fiber, folic acid, niacin (vitamin B3), pantothenic acid (vitamin B5), and thiamine (vitamin B1). For comparison, the standard 100 gram serving equals ⅔ cup of cantaloupe.

HEALTH BENEFITS

Cantaloupe has been shown to contain the compound adenosine, which is currently being used in patients with heart disease to keep the blood thin and relieve angina attacks.

HOW TO SELECT AND STORE

The four major signs of a ripe cantaloupe are:

- No stem but a smooth, shallow basin where the stem was once attached; the stem scar will also be free of mould.
- Thick, coarse, and corky netting or veining over the surface.
- A yellowish buff skin color under the netting.
- A fragrant aroma, which you will be able to detect even if you purchase already cut cantaloupe packaged in a plastic container.

Overripeness is characterized by a pronounced yellowing of the skin, mould, and soft, watery, insipid flesh. Small bruises will do no harm, but large bruised areas should be cut away.

Leaving a firm cantaloupe at room temperature for several days will allow its flesh to become softer and juicier. Once the cantaloupe has reached its peak ripeness, place it in the refrigerator to store. Melon that has been cut should be stored in the refrigerator as well, and it should be wrapped, not only to help retain its nutrient content but also to ensure that the ethylene gas that it emits does not affect the taste or texture of other fruit and vegetables.

TIPS FOR PREPARING

Melons grow resting on the ground, which means their rinds can become contaminated by animal or human waste, or contamination can be transferred from the harvester's or other handler's hands to the melon. Unless the skin is thoroughly cleansed, the knife used to halve a melon can transfer pathogens, such as *Salmonella,* directly onto the flesh. For this reason, all melons should be sprayed with a solution of diluted additive-free soap or commercial produce wash and then scrubbed under cool running water with a vegetable brush. Rinse well and be sure to also wash surfaces that have come into contact with the unwashed melon, such as hands and cutting boards.

After washing, slice the melon into pieces of desired thickness and scoop out the seeds and netting.

QUICK SERVING IDEAS

- Cantaloupe bowls: Halve and seed cantaloupe, sprinkle inside with lime juice, and add your favorite sorbet, cottage cheese, or yogurt.
- Serve cantaloupe in fruit salads. Its flavor combines well with virtually any other fruit, including berries, oranges, pineapple, bananas, and kiwifruit.
- For an appetizer or salad to complement a spring or summer meal, toss chunks of cantaloupe with lemon and watercress, or, for a Mexican flair, try lime, fresh coriander, and sliced jicama.

SAFETY

See "Tips for Preparing," above.

Cantaloupe is among the foods on which pesticide residues have been most frequently found. Individuals wanting to avoid these health risks may want to avoid consumption of cantaloupe unless it is organically grown.

Cantaloupe contains low levels of oxalates. Individuals with a history of calcium oxalate-containing kidney stones should limit their consumption of this fruit. See page 793 for more information.

Cherries

The cherry *(Prunus serotina)* is a small stone fruit, or drupe, that belongs to the same genus of the rose family as apricots, peaches, and plums. There are two types of cherries: sweet and sour.

Among the more than 500 varieties of sweet cherries grown, fifteen are important commercially in the United States, with the undisputed leader being the Bing, a large, round, sweet cherry with purple-red flesh and a burgundy skin so richly dark it appears black when fully ripe. Next in popularity is the Lambert, a smaller, heart-shaped version of the Bing. Other sweet, dark-skinned varieties include the Black Tartarian, Black Republican, Schmidt, and Windsor. Lighter-skinned varieties of sweet cherries include the Rainier, which has yellow rose-blushed skin and is even sweeter than the Bing, and the Napoleon, or Royal Ann, which is typically canned or made into maraschino cherries.

Maraschino cherries actually originated in Yugoslavia and northern Italy, where merchants marinated a local cherry called the Marasca in a liqueur made from the fruit and leaves of the cherry tree. This cherry product was imported to the United States in the 1890s as a delicacy to be used in the country's finest restaurants and hotels. In 1896, U.S. cherry processors began experimenting in an attempt to duplicate the maraschino cherry, using a domestic sweet cherry called the Royal Ann. A combination of almond oil, neroli oil, and vanilla extract was developed to replace the liqueur, and by 1920, the American maraschino cherry supplanted the imported variety in the United States.

Over 270 varieties of sour cherries are also grown in the United States. Sour varieties, which include the Montmorency, Early Richmond, and English Morello, are bright red, smaller, and softer than sweet cherries, and are usually too tart to be eaten fresh but, canned or frozen, make wonderful pie fillings and sauces.

The U.K., by comparison, produces a modest 1,300 tons mostly in the South East where climatic conditions are more favourable. Early varieties include Early Rivers, Merchant, Sasha, followed by Hertford, Van, Stella, and Inga. Main crop varieties are Sunburst, Summit, Lapins, Colney, and Summersun, followed by the late variety Sweetheart. However, consumption of imported cherries doubled in the decade between 1990 and 2000. Most cherries are imported from Spain, Turkey and France, with out-of-season fruit coming from Chile.

HISTORY

Cherries are native to Europe and west Asia. They were named after the ancient Turkish town of Cerasus and date back to at least 300 B.C.E., when they were described by the Greek botanist Theophrastus. Around 70 C.E., Pliny noted that the cherry tree was present in Rome, Germany, England, and France.

Cherries were one of the first fruits the early settlers brought to America in the 1600s. Later, French colonists from Normandy planted cherry pits along the Saint Lawrence River and down into the Great Lakes area, and cherry trees became part of the gardens of French settlers as they established Detroit, Vincennes, and other midwestern settlements.

In the 1840s, Peter Dougherty, a Presbyterian missionary, planted the first cherry orchard in northern Michigan. The area proved to be ideal for growing cherries because Lake Michigan tempers the arctic winds of winter and cools the orchards in summer. Dougherty's cherry trees flourished, so much so that other farmers in the area followed suit.

The first commercial tart cherry orchards in Michigan were planted in 1893 on Ridgewood Farm, near the site of Dougherty's original plantings. By the early 1900s, the tart cherry industry was firmly established, with orchards not only north in the Traverse City area but all along Lake Michigan. Soon cherry production surpassed that of other major crops. The first cherry-processing facility, the Traverse City Canning Company, was built just south of

Traverse City, and the ruby red fruit was shipped to Chicago, Detroit, and Milwaukee.

In the northwestern United States, cherry orchards also flourished. In 1847, Henderson Lewelling planted an orchard in western Oregon, using nursery stock that he had transported by oxcart from Iowa. Lewelling Farms became known for its sweet cherries with orchards beginning commercial production during the 1870s and '80s.

The most famous sweet cherry variety, the Bing, got its name from one of Lewelling's Chinese workmen. Another popular sweet cherry variety, the Lambert, also got its start on Lewelling Farms. The Rainier cherry, a light sweet variety, originated from the crossbreeding of the Bing and Van varieties by Dr. Harold W. Fogle at the Washington State University Research Station in Prosser, Washington. Together, the Bing, Lambert, and Rainier varieties account for more than 95 percent of northwestern sweet cherry production.

The ultimate celebration of cherries is the National Cherry Festival, which is held every year in July in the "Cherry Capital of the World," Traverse City, Michigan. Thousands of visitors come from all over the world to celebrate the harvest and, of course, eat cherries. And, as the cherry tree has long been beloved not only for its succulent fruit but also for the beauty of its blossoms, each year the coming of spring is heralded in Washington, D.C., by the blooming of the ornamental cherry trees.

Cherry trees have played a role in American folklore since George Washington chopped down his father's cherry tree, then could not tell a lie and told his father what he had done.

Today, cherries are grown in most parts of the world but are produced in commercial quantities in just twenty countries. Europe and the Middle East continues to account for the bulk of world production, but the United States is one of the leaders, with an annual sweet cherry crop of 156,730 tons, 85 percent of which comes from Washington, Oregon, and California, and an annual sour cherry crop of 100,000 tons, 77 percent of which is grown in Michigan. Other states with a commercial cherry crop are Utah, Wisconsin, New York, and Pennsylvania.

NUTRITIONAL HIGHLIGHTS

Sour cherries are lower in calories, with 58 calories in 100 grams versus 70 calories in 100 grams of sweet cherries. Sour cherries are also higher in vitamin A, with 1,000 IU per 100 grams, than their sweet counterparts, which contain 110 IU per 100 grams.

In addition to their content of flavonoids, melatonin, and perillyl alcohol, both varieties of cherries contain significant amounts of several nutrients. Sour cherries are an excellent source of vitamins A and C, a very good source of copper, and a good source of manganese. Sweet cherries are a good source of vitamin C and copper.

HEALTH BENEFITS

Cherries, like berries, are rich sources of flavonoids, specifically anthocyanidins and proanthocyanidins, the flavonoid molecules that give this fruit its deep red-blue color. In general, the darker the cherry, whether sweet or sour, the better it is for you because it contains a higher concentration of flavonoids. These flavonoids exert a number of beneficial effects. For example, researchers at Michigan State University investigated the ability of a number of fruits, including cherries, to act as antioxidants and to inhibit cyclooxygenase, an enzyme produced in the body in two forms, called COX-1 and COX-2, each of which has different purposes. COX-1 is made by many different cells to create prostaglandins, hormonelike molecules that are used to send basic "housekeeping" messages to nearby cells, while COX-2 is built only by special cells in response to inflammatory processes and is used to signal pain and inflammation. Most nonsteroidal anti-inflammatory drugs, such as aspirin and ibuprofen, work by blocking both cyclooxygenase enzymes, so no pain messages are sent. Newer drugs such as Vioxx (which has been withdrawn in the U.K.) and Celebrex (which is being reviewed in Europe) work by specifically blocking COX-2, but while these drugs have been linked to serious side effects, cherries have not.

The researchers at Michigan State University found that anthocyanidins from cherries are able to block both COX-1 and COX-2 enzymes. In fact, of all the fruits the investigators tested, cherries had the highest amounts of key anthocyanidins—26.5 milligrams in 100 grams (roughly twenty cherries). The COX-inhibitory activities of cherries' anthocyanidins were even found to be comparable to those of ibuprofen and naproxen. The same group of researchers also discovered that cherries' anthocyanidins possess antioxidant activity superior to vitamin E at equal levels.

In addition to their anthocyanidins, Montmorency tart cherries have been found to contain significant quantities of melatonin, a hormone produced in the pineal gland at the base of the brain that influences the sleep process and is also a very powerful antioxidant. While some other foods, such as bananas, also contain melatonin, the amount is too low to be effective, but, according to studies conducted at the University of Texas, Montmorency cherries contain 0.1 to 0.3 milligrams of melatonin per serving. At this dosage melatonin has been shown to be an effective sleep inducer.

Cherries may also offer significant anti-cancer protection. In research conducted at Michigan State University, two of the anthocyanidins found in cherries—isoquerxitrin and quercetin—have been found to inhibit the growth of colon cancer. Tart cherries also contain perillyl alcohol (POH), a natural compound that appears to be extremely powerful in reducing the incidence of all types of cancer. Recent research suggests that perillyl alcohol shuts down the growth of cancer cells by depriving them of the proteins they need to grow. In studies, perillyl alcohol (POH) has performed favorably in the treatment of advanced carcinomas of the breast, prostate, and ovary, and has also exhibited chemopreventive activity in preclinical breast cancer tests. In animal studies, perillyl alcohol has been shown to induce the regression of 81 percent of small breast cancers and up to 75 percent of advanced breast cancers.

Finally, cherries are particularly useful in the treatment of gout. Gout is a type of arthritis associated with an abnormally high concentration of uric acid in the blood. Uric acid is produced in the liver and enters the bloodstream. Under certain circumstances, the body produces too much uric acid or excretes too little. As uric acid concentrations increase, needlelike crystals of a salt, called monosodium urate, form. In time, these crystals accumulate in the joints, causing the inflammation and pain typical of gout. Cherries' anthocyanidins have been shown to inhibit the activity of xanthine oxidase, the enzyme involved in the production of uric acid. Clinical studies have shown that consuming the equivalent of ½ pound/250 grams of fresh cherries per day is very effective in lowering uric acid levels and preventing attacks of gout.

HOW TO SELECT AND STORE

The cherry season is brief, slightly more than three months long. Bing cherries usually appear at the end of May, peak in June and July, and are available through August, while Lamberts and other sweet, dark cherries arrive in mid-August. Varieties that appear earliest and latest are not as sweet and soft as Bings. Fresh cherries sold after August are either from cold storage or imported from New Zealand or Chile.

Look for cherries kept moist and cool, as warm temperatures quickly cause both flavor and texture to deteriorate. The best sweet cherries are large (an inch/2½ cm or more in diameter) and have bright, glossy, plump-looking skin that is dark-colored for their variety, and fresh-looking green stems. Bings should be a purplish mahogany to an almost black color, and fresh sour cherries should be a bright scarlet color. Sweet cherries should be quite firm, but not hard, while sour varieties should be medium firm. Rock-hard, underripe cherries should be avoided, since cherries do not ripen after picking.

Reject undersized cherries and those that are soft or flabby, have cuts or bruises, or are sticky from leaking juice. Cherries whose stems are darkened or missing should also be passed over.

Darkened stems signal old age or poor storage conditions, and the break in the skin that occurs when the stem is lost allows decay to begin. Brown discoloration and mould growth are also indications of decay. If many of the cherries are old or damaged, shop elsewhere, as a number of spoiled cherries will cause others to decay.

Pack unwashed cherries loosely in plastic bags to minimize bruising or place a single layer in a shallow pan, cover with cling film, and refrigerate. If they are in good condition, fresh cherries will keep for up to one week, but be sure to check them daily and remove any that have begun to spoil.

Frozen cherries, pitted or not, will keep for up to one year. Gently rinse and dry before placing in freezer bags. Seal the bag, leaving just enough of an opening to insert a straw, and suck out as much air as possible before quickly closing the remaining opening. The less air in the bag, the better the cherries will keep. To use, thaw in the bag overnight in the refrigerator or for thirty minutes at room temperature.

TIPS FOR PREPARING

Wash organically grown cherries by placing them in a colander, then rinsing them under cool water. If nonorganic, they should be sprayed with a solution of diluted additive-free soap or commercial produce wash before placing them in the colander. Leave the stems intact if using them whole or in fruit salads; otherwise remove the stems. If you are using cherries in fruit salads or cooking or juicing them, halve them with a paring knife and pry out the pit, or if whole cherries are desired, use a cherry pitter, an inexpensive kitchen tool that works like a hole punch. When adding cherries to fruit salads, add them at the last minute so their color won't stain other ingredients.

Dried cherries can be used as you would use raisins in oatmeal cookies, breads, sauces, desserts, and trail mix. If you wish to rehydrate them, cover with boiling water, juice, or liqueur, and allow to stand for 30 minutes.

Sour cherries are too tart to eat unless gently cooked and sweetened. Sweet cherries can also be cooked and will retain their texture if poached for just a few minutes. Stem and pit the cherries, drop them into a small amount of simmering water, or a combination of water and wine (1 cup liquid to 2 cups cherries), and cook 1 to 3 minutes, until the cherries are slightly softened and heated through. Sour cherries will need a little honey for sweetening. If desired, thicken the liquid with cornflour or arrowroot, and sweeten to taste. Use as a sauce for grilled chicken or a topping for pancakes or waffles.

QUICK SERVING IDEAS

- Enhance the flavor of cooked cherries by adding a few drops of almond extract, a little cinnamon, or some slivers of orange or lemon zest.
- Try cherry rather than strawberry shortcake: Halve a low-fat angel food cake and layer with sliced sweet cherries and vanilla yogurt.
- Top plain or frozen yogurt with pitted cherries and serve as is or blend in your food processor for a sweet, yet healthful smoothie.
- Use either pitted sweet or sour cherries to make chilled cherry soup: Cook the cherries in water and fruit juice or wine (2 cups liquid to 1 cup fruit). Simmer just until fruit is soft, then purée, sweeten with honey to taste, and

chill. Serve topped with a dollop of plain yogurt.

- Make your own chocolate-covered cherries: Wash and thoroughly dry cherries, as the least bit of moisture will result in lumpy chocolate. Melt chocolate in a double boiler, dip in the cherries to cover, and set 1 inch/2½ cm apart on a waxed-paper–covered baking sheet. Refrigerate until the chocolate has hardened.

SAFETY

Be sure to check cherries for any signs of mould or decay when purchasing, refrigerate them promptly, and wash them thoroughly before eating. Cherries are quite susceptible to the growth of *Aspergillus* moulds, which produce a toxin also found in mouldy peanuts, called aflatoxin. Aflatoxin has been found to have a carcinogenic effect in animal studies.

Cranberries

The cranberry, genus *Vaccinium,* grows in the wild in northern Europe, northern Asia, and North America. The North American cranberry (*Vaccinium macrocarpon*) is a member of the family Ericaceae, which is composed of approximately 1,350 species, including rhododendrons and blueberries. Cranberries are low-growing, vining, perennial plants grown in large sandy bogs. Pollination is primarily done by domestic honeybees. The cultivated species grown in the northern United States and southern Canada bears a larger berry than the European cranberry or southern cranberry, which are the wild species native to the eastern United States. The cranberry has often been referred to as the "crane berry" or "bounce berry," since the cranberry's shrub's pale pink blossoms often resemble the head of cranes that haunt the cranberry bogs and the ripe berry can bounce.

HISTORY

The North American cranberry has an extensive and celebrated history. Native Americans used cranberries as food, medicinally, and in ceremonies. They also used the bright berry as a source of red dye, to help stop bleeding via its astringent effects, and as a poultice for wounds. Especially when it was combined with cornmeal (polenta), cranberry was used to counteract blood poisoning.

The Revolutionary War Veteran Henry Hall planted the first commercial cranberry beds in Dennis, Massachusetts, on Cape Cod in 1816. Hall noticed that a wealth of large berries were produced when the tides and wind swept some sand into his bog. Sand helps the cranberries grow by stifling the growth of weeds. The vines produced prolific numbers of different types of berries (some he called "Jumbo"), and by 1820 he was shipping his cranberries to Boston and New York City. The word spread rapidly, and soon many individuals transplanted cranberry vines to their own gardens throughout Massachusetts.

The cranberry industry continued to expand across the United States with the development of the railroad, then eventually crossed the sea to Scandinavia and Great Britain. Cranberries were first introduced to Holland when an American ship carrying barrels of cranberries was shipwrecked on the Dutch coast. The barrels were washed ashore, some berries took root, and cranberries have been cultivated there from then on.

Most of the production of cranberries worldwide can be found in Wisconsin, Massachusetts, New Jersey, Oregon, Washington, and the Canadian provinces of British Columbia and Quebec. The crop grown in the United States produces 154,000 metric tonnes annually, while half of the U.S. crop still comes from Massachusetts. Peak market time runs from October to December.

NUTRITIONAL HIGHLIGHTS

Fresh cranberries are low in calories, with just 46 calories for a cup of whole raw berries or 53 calories for a cup of chopped raw berries (one cup equals a 100 gram serving). They are an excellent source of vitamin C and soluble and insoluble fiber, as well as a good source of manganese and copper. Cranberries are also rich sources of anthocyanidins, antioxidant pigments that give blue, purple, and red pigments to fruits and vegetables.

HEALTH BENEFITS

Native Americans have used cranberry preparations to treat urinary tract infections (UTIs) and other illnesses for centuries. Modern medical research has revealed the chemical and physiological effects cranberries have on the urinary tract and how drinking cranberry juice may help prevent urinary tract infections. For example in a 1994 study published in *The Journal of the American Medical Association (JAMA)*, a placebo-controlled trial of 153 elderly women demonstrated that cranberries help prevent UTIs. A number of other studies conducted since have also corroborated these anecdotal accounts of cranberries' effectiveness in treating and preventing UTIs.

In the above-referenced *JAMA* study, the women given cranberry juice had 42 percent fewer infections than did the control group (those who received a placebo drink that did not contain real cranberry). In this landmark study, the dose of cranberry was 300 milliliters (approximately 1¼ cups), while in later studies, subjects received, each day, 500 milliliters (2 cups) of cranberry juice.

Cranberries contain proanthocyanidins (PACs), which inhibit the fimbrial adhesion of bacteria, including *Escherichia coli,* to the urinary tract epithelium (lining). Adherence and penetration of the bacteria to the mucosal wall is necessary for infection to occur. If the bacteria cannot adhere, they will be washed away with the flow of urine. It is these unique compounds that are pivotal in the prevention of UTI rather than the acidification of the urine, as was previously hypothesized. Furthermore, since 80 to 90 percent of UTIs are caused by *E. coli,* cranberries provide considerable protection.

Another beneficial effect of cranberries is the prevention of kidney stones. In the United States, approximately 75 to 85 percent of kidney stones are made up of calcium salts and similarly in the U.K. the majority are calcium stones. In some studies, cranberries have been shown to decrease the amount of ionized calcium by greater than 50 percent in patients with recurrent kidney stones. Quinic acid, a component of cranberries, is not metabolized by the body and is thereby excreted unchanged in the urine. This increases the acidity of the urine, which then prevents calcium and phosphate ions from forming insoluble stones.

A joint research study by the Cranberry Institute, a trade organization for cranberry growers in the United States and Canada, and the University of Scranton, Pennsylvania, revealed that cranberries are phytochemical phenols that provide five times the antioxidant content of broccoli due to their high concentration of anthocyanidins. These antioxidants have been shown to inhibit the development of atherosclerosis, cancer, and other degenerative diseases. Cranberries were found to have the highest level of these compounds in comparison to nineteen other fruits tested.

It is important to note that the deeper the red color, the higher the concentration of healthy anthocyanidin pigments. The fresh cranberry, compared to the dried, has the highest amount of the antioxidants, while processing, storage, and heating reduce the antioxidant levels. Bottled cranberry drinks and cranberry cocktails that contain added sugars or artificial sweeteners have the lowest level of antioxidants.

HOW TO SELECT AND STORE

Choose cranberries that have a fresh, plump appearance and a deep red luster, and that are quite firm to the touch. Discard any that are soft, discolored, pitted, or shriveled.

Unwashed, fresh cranberries can be stored in the refrigerator for several months. Cranberries may show moisture after removal from the refrigerator, but such dampness does not indicate a lessening in quality, unless the berries are sticky, leathery, or tough or their flesh is discolored.

If frozen, cranberries will keep for several years. To freeze fresh cranberries, spread them out on a baking tray and place in the freezer.

After a couple of hours, transfer the fully frozen berries to a freezer bag, seal, and date. When you are ready to use frozen cranberries, be aware that the berries become quite soft after thawing and should be used immediately to prevent spoilage.

Dried cranberries are available with other dried fruits in many shops.

TIPS FOR PREPARING

Wash organically grown cranberries by placing them in a colander, then rinsing them under cool water. If nonorganic, they should be sprayed with a solution of diluted additive-free soap or commercial produce wash before placing them in the colander.

QUICK SERVING IDEAS

- If you have grown accustomed to the taste of sweetened cranberry juice, here is a healthy alternative to the sugar-filled cranberry drinks available in cans or bottles:

Zesty Cran-Apple Juice

½ cup cranberries
½ lemon
1 handful of grapes
2 apples cut into wedges

Juice the cranberries followed by the lemon, grapes, and apple wedges.

- Because of their extreme tartness, fresh cranberries are best combined with other fruits, such as pears, apples, or oranges, and/or a little honey or maple syrup.
- For a relish: Place 2 cups of fresh or thawed cranberries in your blender along with a cut-up pear, orange, apple, and 1 to 2 handfuls of walnuts or pecans. Blend till chunky but thoroughly mixed. Pour into a large bowl, add 3 to 4 stalks of diced celery, and mix well.
- Instead of dressing your green salad with vinaigrette, just toss it with a little olive oil and add a handful of raw cranberries for color and pizzazz. The cranberries' tartness will replace the usual vinegar or lemon.
- Use dried cranberries as you would raisins. Add some to quick breads or muffins, sprinkle a handful over your hot oatmeal or any cold cereal, or mix them with nuts for a delicious snack.

SAFETY

Cranberries contain low levels of oxalate. Individuals with a history of calcium oxalate-containing kidney stones should limit their consumption of this food. See page 793 for more information.

Dates

Dates grow on the date palm *(Phoenix dactylifera),* a tree similar in appearance to the coconut palm. Mature trees can achieve a height up to 100 feet/30 meters, with the dates growing in clusters that can contain up to 200 dates and weigh up to 25 pounds/11 kilograms. Trees begin to bear fruit at four to five years and may continue fruiting to about eighty years of age, producing annual yields of up to 200 pounds/ 90 kilograms per tree. Sweet, fleshy, and oblong, dates grow to an inch/2½ cm in length and attain a rich red to golden brown color while hanging on the tree.

HISTORY

Called the "Tree of Life," the date palm is said in Muslim legend to have been made from the dust that was left over after the creation of Adam, and it was probably the first cultivated tree in history, having been grown in the Holy Land for at least 8,000 years. Directions for the date palm's husbandry are recorded on sun-baked bricks made in Mesopotamia (Iraq) more than 5,000 years ago, and the date palm is often mentioned in the Bible and in the poetry and proverbs of the East. The date palm was carried to China from Iran about 1,700 years ago, and in the seventeenth century, pioneering Spaniards took date seeds to California.

Today, about three quarters of the world's date crop is grown in the Middle East, the main source of dates in the U.K., but the majority of the United States' supply is produced in date orchards—called "date gardens" in the industry—in California, Arizona, and Texas, where the hot, dry climate and sandy, alkaline soil provide excellent conditions for the date tree's growth.

In the Arab world, dates are often eaten with milk products to boost the protein content, but they are also served alone, fresh or dried, or used in various fruit dishes, baked goods, syrups, candies, ice cream, and salads. In some countries, date pits are roasted, ground, and used as a coffee substitute. Dates have even been fermented and used to make an alcoholic beverage called *arrak,* described by the sixteenth-century traveler Pedro Texeira as "the strongest and most dreadful drink ever invented."

Dates are harvested in late autumn and early winter, but they store quite well, so they are available all year round.

NUTRITIONAL HIGHLIGHTS

Dates are an excellent source of easily digested carbohydrates, with a sugar content that ranges from about 60 percent in soft dates to as high as 70 percent in some dry dates. Glucose or fructose is the sugar found in most varieties, although the Deglet Noor, the most popular date grown in the United States, contains sucrose.

A single pitted date contains only 23 calories, but a cup of chopped pitted dates weighs in at 490 calories. A 100 gram serving equals four Medjool dates or twelve Deglet Noor dates.

Dates are an excellent source of fiber (8 grams per 100 grams); the B vitamins niacin, B6, riboflavin, thiamine, and pantothenic acid; and the minerals copper, potassium, manganese, magnesium, iron, and phosphorus. In addition, they are a good source of folic acid and the trace minerals, zinc and selenium. For each ounce/30 grams, dates provide 260 percent more potassium than oranges and 64 percent more potassium than bananas—but they also contain 60 percent more calories than either of these fruits.

HEALTH BENEFITS

Dates are among the most alkaline of foods (see page 783 for more information) and contain a special type of soluble fiber called beta-D-glucan. Beta-D-glucan fiber has been shown to decrease the body's absorption of cholesterol and to slow or delay absorption of glucose (sugar) in the small intestine, thus helping to keep blood sugar levels even.

Because of its ability to absorb and hold water, beta-D-glucan adds bulk and some softness to the stools, easing both stool movement through the colon and elimination. In addition, this soluble fiber passes through the intestinal tract more slowly than insoluble fiber. By slowing down gastric emptying (the rate at which the stomach digests and empties its contents after a meal), beta-D-glucan increases feelings of satiety and can thus aid in weight loss.

Recent laboratory studies reveal that dates are also surprisingly rich in antioxidant and anti-cancer compounds. Date extract was found to prevent free-radical damage to both fats and protein in a dose-dependent manner—the higher the concentration, the greater the protection against free radicals. And dates' ability to protect against free-radical damage persisted even when the potent cancer-causing chemical benzo(a)pyrene was added to the mixture.

HOW TO SELECT AND STORE

There are three types of dates marketed in the United States:

Soft dates are harvested when still soft and unripe.
Semisoft dates are firmer-fleshed cultivars and are also harvested unripe.
Dried dates are allowed to sun-ripen on the tree.

A semisoft date with firm flesh called Deglet Noor is the most commonly available variety in the United States, accounting for 95 percent of U.S. date production. Other semisoft varieties found in the United States are Medjool and Zahidi. The soft variety most common in the United States is Barhi. The Deglet Noor and Medjool dates are also very popular in the U.K., particularly at Christmas. All of these varieties are sold both fresh and dried, and it's sometimes difficult to tell which is being offered, since fresh dates often appear a bit wrinkled and both types are typically packaged in cellophane or plastic containers. Most often, the dates available in shops are either fresh or partially dried and do not contain any preservatives.

Good-quality soft and semisoft dates are smooth-skinned, glossy, and plump. Slightly wrinkled is fine, but shriveled, cracked, dry, and broken are not. Dried dates should be significantly wrinkled but should not be rock hard. Avoid dates with crystallized sugar on their surface or an off smell that signals spoilage or fermentation. Also, avoid dates with any visible signs of microbial growth.

For the longest shelf life, place soft and semisoft varieties, such as Deglet Noor, in an airtight plastic bag or container to protect them from the odors of other foods, which they will quickly absorb. Store soft and semisoft varieties in the refrigerator, where they will keep for up to eight months. Stored in the same manner at room temperature, they will remain fresh for one month or more.

Dried dates, which are pasteurized to inhibit mould growth, can be kept in the refrigerator for up to one year or in the freezer for up to five years.

TIPS FOR PREPARING

To prepare unpitted dates, simply slice each fruit open and push out the pit. For easier slicing, first firm dates up by separating and placing them on a baking tray in the freezer for about an hour. When chopping dates, snipping them with scissors works as well as or better than cutting them with a knife, but whichever tool you use, be sure to dip the blades into warm water frequently to keep them from gumming up with sugars. If your dried dates have become too dry, a 15-minute soak in some hot water or juice will plump them.

QUICK SERVING IDEAS

- As sweet as candy, dates are a treat all on their own, but this fruit is exceptionally delicious stuffed with an almond, a pecan, or a dab of peanut butter or cottage cheese.
- Use chopped dates instead of other fruit or jam to add flavor, texture, and sweetness to yogurt, any hot or cold cereal, rice dishes, or noodle pudding.
- Substitute chopped dates for raisins in breads, muffins, or cookies.
- Mix chopped dates into your favorite nut butter, and use as a sandwich spread or to stuff celery.
- In North African cuisine, dates are used to add a hint of sweetness to savory lamb stews.
- For a Middle Eastern flair, mix chopped dates into bread crumb stuffings or pilafs.
- Instead of brown sugar, sprinkle finely chopped dates over cooked carrots, parsnips, sweet potatoes, or winter squash.
- Try a Moroccan dish of curried chickpeas, lentils, aubergine, and onion. Top with chopped dates and roasted peanuts, and serve over rice.

SAFETY

Even dates sold as pitted may contain an occasional pit, so check each date before taking a bite. Because of their high sugar content, dates can attract insect pests; be sure to store them in well-sealed containers.

Recent reports from Saudi Arabia indicate that for some individuals, dates are allergenic. Individuals who react to antigens from artemisia, birch, cultivated rye *(Secale cereale),* Timothy grass *(Phleum pratense),* Sydney golden wattle *(Acacia longifolia),* and Bermuda grass *(Cynodon dactylon)* pollens may also react to dates. Although other research has shown that certain date palm cultivars do not produce an allergic reaction, even in individuals with known date allergies, individuals with known allergies to any of the plants noted above may wish to avoid dates.

Figs

Figs grow on the ficus tree *(Ficus carica),* which is a member of the mulberry family. They are unique in that they have an opening, called an "ostiole" or "eye" that is not connected to the tree but that helps the fruit's development, aiding it to communicate with the environment.

Figs have a unique, sweet taste, with a chewy texture to their flesh and skin and a crunchiness to their seeds. Fresh figs are delicate and perishable, so most often figs are dried, either by exposure to sunlight or through an artificial process, creating a sweet and nutritious dried fruit that can be enjoyed throughout the year.

Figs vary dramatically in color and subtly in texture depending upon the variety, of which there are more than 150. Some of the most popular varieties are:

Adriatic: Light green skin and pink-tan flesh; this variety is most often used to make fig bars.

Black Mission: Blackish purple skin and pink flesh.

Kadota (Italian Dottato): Green skin and purplish flesh.

Calimyrna: Greenish yellow skin and amber flesh.

Brown Turkey: Purple skin and red flesh (suitable for cultivation in the U.K.)

White Marseilles: Pale skinned with very pale flesh (suitable for cultivation in the U.K.)

HISTORY

One of the world's first cultivated trees, the fig tree of the family Moraceae, can be traced back to the earliest historical documents, with references in the Bible and other ancient writings. The fig tree, a native of the Middle East and Mediterranean, is thought to have been cultivated in Egypt before being carried to Crete and Greece. Figs were held in such great regard by the Greeks that laws were created to prevent the export of their finest-quality figs. In Roman mythology, the famous characters Romulus and Remus were sheltered by the important fig tree. Already at this time in history, at least twenty-nine varieties of figs were recognized.

Later in history, figs were introduced to other regions in the Mediterranean by ancient conquerors and then brought to the New World by the Spaniards in the sixteenth century. It was not until the late nineteenth century, when the Spanish missionaries established their missions in San Diego, California, that the fig tree was planted there. Unfortunately, due to poor culti-

vation techniques, the figs were inferior in quality to those imported from Europe. It was only in the early twentieth century that California farmers began focusing on proper fig cultivation and processing. As a result, California became one of the greatest cultivators of figs and adds significantly to the world production, along with Turkey, Greece, Spain, and Portugal.

NUTRITIONAL HIGHLIGHTS

Figs are high in natural simple sugars, minerals, and fiber. Figs are fairly rich in potassium, calcium, magnesium, iron, copper, and manganese. A 100 gram serving of dried figs, about eight to ten figs, provides 249 calories, 0.9 grams of fat, 3.3 grams of protein, 63.9 grams of carbohydrate, with 9.8 grams of fiber and 47.9 grams of natural sugars (glucose and fructose), plus 162 milligrams of calcium and 680 milligrams of potassium.

HEALTH BENEFITS

Figs are often recommended to nourish and tone the intestines because they are a very good source of fiber. They are also a good source of potassium, an important consideration in helping to control blood pressure. Figs are among the most highly alkaline foods, making them useful in supporting the proper pH of the body. See page 783 for more information.

Fig leaves have repeatedly been shown to have antidiabetic properties and can actually reduce the amount of insulin needed by persons with diabetes who require insulin injections. In one study, a liquid extract made from fig leaves was simply added to the breakfast of insulin-dependent diabetic subjects to produce this effect.

In addition to their blood-sugar-stabilizing properties, in animal studies fig leaves have been shown to lower levels of triglycerides. And in test-tube studies, fig leaves inhibited the growth of certain types of cancer cells. Researchers have not yet determined exactly which substances in fig leaves are responsible for these health benefits.

HOW TO SELECT AND STORE

The season for California figs is from June to September, with the timing dependent on the variety, while European figs are available throughout the autumn. Figs are quickly perishable and delicate, and are usually best eaten within one to two days after purchase. When choosing figs, select those that are plump and tender, have a rich, deep color, and are free from bruises and not mushy. Ripe figs have a sweet fragrance. When brought home, ripe figs should not be washed until ready to eat. They should be kept covered in the refrigerator on a paper towel-lined plate, where they will remain fresh for approximately two days. If figs are not yet ripe, it is best to keep them at room temperature, away from direct sunlight.

Dried figs will stay fresh for much longer, about several months. When purchasing dried figs, you want to ensure that they are free of mould and soft and have a mild pleasant scent. Dried figs can be kept in a cool, dark place or stored in the refrigerator. Futhermore, they too should be wrapped as to not be overexposed to air, which will make them dry.

TIPS FOR PREPARING

Before eating or cooking figs, wash them under cool water and then gently remove the stem. Figs can be consumed either peeled or unpeeled, depending upon the thickness of the skin, as well as your personal preference.

Since the insides of ripe figs are rather soft and sticky, they are often difficult to chop. Placing them in the freezer for up to one hour will make them a little firmer and easier to handle. In addition, when chopping, dip your knife into hot water several times, as needed, to prevent sticking.

Dried figs can be eaten or used in recipes as they are or simmered for several minutes in water or fruit juice to make them more plump and juicy.

QUICK SERVING IDEAS

- Dried figs can be utilized in baked goods, such as fig bars; jams; and fruit dishes.
- Purée ripe figs and use as a sandwich spread that will complement tofu, chicken, and vegetables.
- Place a sliced fig between two whole-grain biscuits to make a sweet treat that will be as popular with kids as it is with adults.
- When preparing oatmeal or any other whole-grain breakfast porridge, add some dried or fresh figs.
- Poach figs in juice or red wine, and serve with yogurt or frozen desserts.
- Add quartered figs to a salad of fennel, rocket, and shaved Parmesan cheese.
- Fresh figs stuffed with goat cheese and chopped almonds can be served as hors d'oeuvres or dessert.

SAFETY

Figs contain high levels of oxalates. Individuals with a history of calcium oxalate-containing kidney stones should limit their consumption of this food. See page 793 for more information.

Grapefruit

The grapefruit is a large, round citrus fruit related to the orange, lemon, and pomelo (shaddock), but it was named "grapefruit" because it grows in clusters just like grapes. The grapefruit is juicy, tart, and tangy with an underlying sweetness that weaves throughout. Its Latin name, *Citrus paradisi,* signifies its wonderful flavor ("paradise").

Grapefruits usually range in diameter from 4 to 6 inches/10 to 15 cm and come in both seeded and seedless varieties. They are categorized as white, pink, or ruby based upon the color of their flesh and not their skin color.

HISTORY

The grapefruit was first noticed on Barbados in 1750 and is regarded as the result of a natural crossbreeding between the orange and the pomelo or shaddock, a citrus fruit that was brought from Indonesia to Barbados in the seventeenth century. By 1880, the grapefruit had become an important commercial crop in Florida, which is still a major producer of grapefruits in the United States, along with California, Arizona, and Texas. Grapefruits are also commercially produced in Israel, South Africa, and Brazil.

NUTRITIONAL HIGHLIGHTS

Fresh grapefruit is low in calories but is a good source of flavonoids, water-soluble fibers, potassium, vitamin C, and folic acid. Grapefruit also contains phytochemicals, including liminoids, flavonoids, lycopene, and glucarates.

A 100 gram serving is a little less than half the average red or pink grapefruit and provides 42 calories, 0.8 grams of protein, 0.1 grams of fat, and 10.7 grams of carbohydrate, with 1.6 grams of fiber and 6.9 grams of natural sugars (sucrose, glucose, and fructose). For comparison, a whole grapefruit contains 97 calories and 24.5 grams of carbohydrate, with 3.7 grams of fiber and 15.6 grams of natural sugars.

HEALTH BENEFITS

Grapefruit pectin has been extensively studied by researchers led by Dr. James Cerda at the University of Florida since 1973. They have shown that grapefruit pectin possesses similar cholesterol-lowering action to other fruit pectins. The edible portion of the whole fruit contains approximately 3.9 percent, or roughly 7.5 grams, of pectin per grapefruit. Since most of the cholesterol-lowering studies used 15 grams of grapefruit pectin to produce a 10 percent drop in cholesterol levels, this would mean that eating approximately two grapefruits per day would lower the risk for heart disease by 20 percent. Of course, eating other foods rich in pectin and other soluble fibers would have similar effects.

Grapefruit consumption has also been shown to normalize hematocrit levels. Hematocrit refers to the percentage of red blood cells per volume of blood. The normal hematocrit level is 40 to 54 percent for men and 37 to 47 percent for women. Low hematocrit levels usually reflect anemia. High hematocrit levels may reflect severe dehydration or an increased number of red blood cells. A high hematocrit reading is associated with an increased risk for heart disease because it means that the blood is too viscous. Naringin, a flavonoid isolated from grapefruit, has been shown to promote the elimination of old red blood cells by the body. This prompted researchers to evaluate the effect of eating a half to one grapefruit per day on hematocrit levels. As expected, the grapefruit was able to lower high hematocrit levels. However, researchers were surprised to find that it had no effect on normal hematocrit levels and actually increased low hematocrit levels.

This balancing action is totally baffling to most drug scientists but not to experienced herbalists, who have used terms such as alterative, amphiteric, adaptogenic, or tonic to describe this effect. It appears that in addition to performing currently understood actions, many foods, as well as herbs, perform actions that are not at all consistent with modern understanding. For example, many natural compounds in herbs and foods appear to impact body control mechanisms to aid in the normalization of many of the body's processes. When there is an elevation in a certain body function, the herb or food will have a lowering effect, and when there is a decrease in a certain body function, it will have a heightening effect. Grapefruit appears to have this effect on hematocrit levels.

In addition to grapefruit's ability to normalize hematocrit levels, grapefruit, especially those varieties with deep red or pink flesh, is an excellent source of the carotene lycopene, which is an important phytochemical that battles heart disease, cancer, and macular degeneration. Grapefruit is also rich in other cancer-fighting chemicals, such as D-limonene, which inhibits tumor formation by promoting the formation of the detoxifying enzyme glutathione-S-transferase in the liver. This enzyme sparks a reaction in the liver that helps to make toxic compounds more water-soluble for excretion from the body. The pulp of citrus fruits such as grapefruit also contains glucarates, compounds that may help prevent breast cancer by helping the body get rid of excess oestrogen.

HOW TO SELECT AND STORE

Fresh grapefruits of good quality are firm but springy to the touch, well shaped, and heavy for their size.

A good grapefruit doesn't have to be perfect in skin appearance, as discoloration, scratches, or scales do not impact the taste quality. However, if the grapefruit is soft, wilted, or flabby or has green on the skin, it should not be consumed. Other signs of decay include an overly soft spot at the stem end of the fruit and areas that appear water-soaked. These forms of decay usually translate to a flavor that is less vibrant and more bitter than that of a good-quality grapefruit.

Since grapefruits are juicier when they're slightly warm, store them at room temperature if you plan to consume them within one week of purchase. If you will not be using them within this time period or prefer them less juicy or colder, store them in the refrigerator crisper, where they will keep fresh for two to three weeks.

TIPS FOR PREPARING

Since cutting into an unwashed fruit may transfer dirt, bacteria, or allergens that may reside on the skin's surface to the edible flesh, grapefruits should be sprayed with a dilution of additive-free soap or commercial produce wash and then rinsed under cool water before consuming.

Grapefruits are usually eaten fresh by slicing

the fruit horizontally and scooping out sections of the halves with a spoon. To separate the flesh from the membrane, you can cut it with either a sharp knife, a special curved-blade grapefruit knife, or a serrated grapefruit spoon. If there are seeds, you can remove them with a spoon.

Grapefruits can also be eaten like oranges. You can peel them with your hands or with a knife. If using a knife, be careful to cut only through the peel and not into the membrane, especially if you are allergic to citrus peels. The peel can be removed with your hands or with the knife. The membrane can then be separated, as you would do with an orange eaten in this manner.

QUICK SERVING IDEAS

- Eat them whole or in fruit salads, or juice them.
- Instead of your morning glass of orange juice, have a glass of grapefruit juice.
- Grapefruit sections add a tangy spark to green salads.
- Sprinkle grapefruit halves with maple syrup, cinnamon, and nutmeg, and grill.
- Combine diced grapefruit with fresh coriander and chili peppers to make a unique salsa.
- Freeze grapefruit juice in ice cube trays and then purée in a food processor to make a simple and refreshing granita.
- For a salad with a tropical flair, combine chopped grapefruit pieces, cooked prawns, and chopped avocado and serve on a bed of romaine lettuce.

SAFETY

Some people are allergic to citrus peels. When such an allergy is suspected, caution must be employed when eating citrus fruit (see "Tips for Preparing"). But whether you are allergic or not, citrus peels *should not be eaten* in any significant quantity. Citrus peels contain some beneficial oils, but these oils can interfere with some body functions. For example, citrus peels contain a compound known as citral that antagonizes some of the effects of vitamin A.

In addition, grapefruit contains high levels of a flavonoid called naringin that can pose a problem for people taking certain drugs. Naringin reduces the activity of the CYP3A enzymes within the liver. These enzymes are used by your body to break down certain drugs, such as calcium channel blockers (used in the treatment of high blood pressure), cholesterol-lowering statin drugs, sedatives (for example, midazolam), and cyclosporine (an immune suppressant given to people who have received organ transplants). If the drugs are not metabolized, they remain in the body in higher concentrations, thus increasing the risk of unwanted toxic effects. If you are taking a prescription medication, ask your doctor if you should avoid eating grapefruit or drinking grapefruit juice. Some drugs, such as Neoral (oral cyclosporine), already carry a warning. For a complete list of drugs currently known to be affected by grapefruit, see www.drug-interactions.com.

Fortunately for citrus lovers, oranges and tangerines do not contain significant amounts of naringin but have many other important nutrients and flavonoids.

Grapes

Grapes are well-known small round or oval berries that feature a semitranslucent flesh encased by a smooth skin. They are generally sweet in flavor and come in seeded and seedless varieties. Grapes are the leading fruit crop in the world. The three main species are:

- European grapes *(Vitis vinifera):* Varieties include Thompson, seedless and amber-green in color; Emperor, seeded and purple in color; and Champagne/Black Corinth, tiny in size and purple in color. European grapes have skins that adhere closely to their flesh. They are used as table grapes, as raisins, and for making wine. This species accounts for more than 95 percent of the grapes grown in the world.

- North American grapes *(Vitis labrusca* and *Vitis rotundifolia):* Varieties include Concord, blue-black in color and large in size; Delaware, pink-red in color with a tender skin; and Niagara, amber-colored and less sweet than other varieties. North American varieties feature skins that more easily slip away from their flesh. They are available in seedless varieties and are well suited for juicing and use as table grapes, but not for raisins.

- French hybrids: Various species were developed from a crossbreeding of European and North American grapes after the majority of grape varieties in Europe were destroyed by a pest in the nineteenth century. These many varieties are used primarily in the production of wine.

HISTORY

Grapes have been eaten since prehistoric times and cultivated as far back as 5000 B.C.E. In the ancient Greek and Roman civilizations, grapes were revered for their use in wine-making. They were planted in the Rhine Valley in Germany in the second century C.E., at which time more than ninety varieties of grapes were already known.

Spanish explorers introduced the fruit to America approximately 300 years ago during the Spanish mission to New Mexico. Grapes quickly moved to California thanks to its climate and absence of grape-preying insects. In the nineteenth century, almost all of the *vinifera* grape species in France was destroyed by an American-born insect that was accidentally brought to France. Thankfully, agriculturists crossbred some of the American *labrusca* varieties with the *vinifera* and were able to continue cultivation of the grapes in France, which is famous for its grapes and wine.

Researchers today continue to explore the grape's skin and seeds for the health-promoting polyphenolic compounds, called oligomeric proanthocyanidins (OPCs). Italy, France, Spain, the United States, Mexico, and Chile are among the largest commercial producers of grapes.

NUTRITIONAL HIGHLIGHTS

Grapes provide nutritional benefits similar to those of other berries. Their nutritional quality can be enhanced by eating the seeds, which are edible in all varieties. More specifically, grapes are very good sources of manganese and good sources of vitamin B6, thiamine, riboflavin, potassium, and vitamin C. In addition, grapes contain flavonoids and the compound resveratrol. A 100 gram serving is about ⅔ cup and provides 69 calories, 0.7 grams of protein, 0.2 grams of fat, and 18.1 grams of carbohydrate, with 1 gram of fiber and 15.5 grams of natural sugars (glucose and fructose).

HEALTH BENEFITS

Grapes are an excellent source of health-promoting flavonoids. Typically, the stronger the color of the grape, the higher the concentration of flavonoids. Grape seed extracts, which are rich in flavonoids known as procyanidolic oligomers, are widely used in treating varicose veins and other venous disorders. These flavonoids are extremely powerful antioxidants and have also been shown to reverse atherosclerosis. In fact, grapes and products made from grapes, such as wine and grape juice, are thought to explain the "French paradox." The French eat a diet high in saturated fats and cholesterol yet have a lower risk of heart disease than Americans. One clue that may help explain this is their frequent consumption of grapes and red wine, since both red wine and grape juice have been shown to increase the antioxidant capacity of the blood, protect against vascular damage, and prevent blood platelets from clumping together to form potentially serious blood clots.

Another of the key components of grapes is resveratrol. Resveratrol belongs to a group of compounds called phytoalexins that plants produce in self-defense against environmental stressors, such as adverse weather or attack by insects or microorganisms. Resveratrol has been identified in more than seventy species of plants, including mulberries and peanuts, but the flesh of grapes is an especially good source. Resveratrol acts as an antioxidant and has also been shown to reduce the buildup of plaque

in arteries. In addition to possibly reducing the risk for atherosclerosis, animal studies demonstrate some anticancer effects and anti-inflammatory action. Fresh grape skin contains about 5 to 10 milligrams of resveratrol per serving, while red wine concentrations range from 1.5 to 3 milligrams per liter.

HOW TO SELECT AND STORE

Grapes do not ripen after harvesting, so look for grapes that are well colored, plump, firmly attached to the stem, and wrinkle-free. After purchase, grapes should be stored in the refrigerator, where they will maintain their freshness for several days.

While freezing detracts from their flavor, frozen grapes are a wonderful snack that kids really enjoy. To freeze grapes, wash and pat them dry, then arrange them in a single layer on a baking tray and place in the freezer. Once frozen, transfer them to a heavy plastic bag and return them to the freezer, where they will store for up to six months.

TIPS FOR PREPARING

Wash organically grown grapes by running them under cool water. If nonorganic, they should be sprayed with a solution of diluted additive-free soap or commercial produce wash and then rinsed thoroughly under cool running water. After washing, either drain the grapes in a colander or gently pat them dry. If you are not going to consume the whole bunch at one time, use scissors to separate small clusters of grapes from the main stem instead of removing individual grapes. This will help keep the remaining grapes fresh by preventing the stems from drying out.

QUICK SERVING IDEAS

- Eat grapes whole or in fruit salads, or juice them.
- Grapes (best sliced in half) enhance the visual effect and flavor of any fruit or green salad.
- Give your curries a fruity punch by including fresh grapes in the recipe.
- Frozen grapes are delicious as a snack treat.
- Serve stewed and spiced grapes with poached chicken breast for a light and healthy entrée.

SAFETY

Since grapes are among the foods on which pesticide residues have been most frequently found, we recommend choosing organically grown grapes to avoid ingesting pesticide residues.

Concord grapes contain high levels of oxalates and other varieties contain low levels. Individuals with a history of calcium oxalate containing-kidney stones should limit their consumption of this food. See page 793 for more information.

Honeydew Melon

Like cucumbers and squash, honeydew (*Cucurbia melo*) and other melons belong to the Cucurbitaceae family, whose members grow on climbing or trailing vines with round, pointed, or folded leaves and small yellow flowers. Honeydew is a slightly oval melon distinguished by a smooth, creamy white or pale yellow-green rind that ripens to creamy yellow and its extraordinarily sweet and juicy pastel green flesh—although one variety of honeydew has orange flesh and a salmon-colored rind. Ripe honeydews are about 7 inches/18 cm in diameter and 8 inches/20 cm long, and range in weight from 4 to 8 pounds/2 to 3½ kilograms. When fully ripe, the honeydew has the sweetest flesh of all the melons.

HISTORY

Although the origin of the honeydew is obscure, this succulent melon is thought to have originated in Persia and was prized by ancient Egyptians thousands of years ago, appearing in Egyptian hieroglyphics that date back to 2400 B.C.E. Honeydew melons were also cultivated by the Romans and were introduced into Europe during the Roman Empire but did not become well known until the French royal court's love affair with the fruit in the fifteenth century. In fact, the varieties of honeydew we eat today were developed at the end of the nineteenth century from a French strain called the Antibes white melon.

Columbus carried honeydew melon seeds to America, and Spanish explorers settling in what is now California cultivated honeydew melons. Today, most of the honeydew melon produced in the United States is still grown in irrigated fields in California, although it is also cultivated in the southwestern states.

NUTRITIONAL HIGHLIGHTS

Honeydew melons combine the nutritional highlights of their cousins, summer and winter squash. Like summer squash, honeydew is low in calories—60 calories for a cup of diced melon—and high in water content—about 90 percent water. Like cantaloupe, honeydew is an excellent source of vitamin C and a very good source of potassium. One cup (170 grams) of melon provides 56 percent of the daily value of vitamin C along with 12 percent of the daily value of potassium—an amount of potassium comparable to that found in an average-sized banana, but for about half the calories of a banana. Honeydew is also a very good source of the B vitamin thiamine and a good source of several other B vitamins, including niacin, pantothenic acid, and B6, as well as the trace mineral copper.

HEALTH BENEFITS

Honeydew's high water content—90 percent of its weight is water—combined with the amount of potassium comparable to that found in an average-sized banana, make honeydew helpful in maintaining healthy blood pressure levels. Honeydew provides several key nutrients that are particularly helpful for healthy skin, too. For example, both vitamin C and copper are necessary for collagen production and tissue repair.

HOW TO SELECT AND STORE

Honeydews are called "winter melons" because they ripen late in the season and are at their peak during the late summer, autumn, and winter, although they are available all year round. Growers try to pick melons when they are ripe but still firm, so they will be less likely to suffer damage during shipping. Inevitably, this practice results in some melons being picked too early. Melons picked before they are ripe will never reach their full flavor potential because they have virtually no internal reserves of starch before ripening. That means that once they are cut from the vine, they cannot grow sweeter. Although the texture of their flesh will soften as pectic substances in their cell walls become more soluble, their complex taste will not develop. Knowing how to select a melon that has been left on the vine until fully ripe is important.

One good sign of ripeness is a clean break between the melon and the stem, rather than a cut in the stem itself. Check the perimeter of the crater at the stem end. Jagged edges signal that the melon was yanked from the vine before it was ready. Also, the rind of a ripe honeydew will be a pale, creamy yellow, not a greenish white. In addition, the rind of a perfectly ripe honeydew will have a soft, velvety surface with an almost indistinguishable wrinkling, often detectable only by touch. Tiny freckles on the rind's surface are a sign of sweetness, and a ripe honeydew will emit a sweet, almost perfumed odor and will give slightly when pressed at the blossom end with a finger. Another indication of ripeness is a melon that is very heavy for its size.

If you cannot find a ripe melon, choose another fruit instead, as the flesh will lack flavor and sweetness. Also, avoid any that are overly ripe. These will exhibit soft, shriveled, or dark patches; sunken spots; or discolored areas on the rind.

To optimize texture and juiciness, leave uncut melons at room temperature for one to two days to allow pectic substances in the flesh to soften the fruit. Whole, ripe honeydew melons can be stored in the refrigerator for up to five days. Enclose them in plastic bags to protect other produce from the ethylene gas that honeydew gives off. Once cut, honeydew should be sealed in an airtight container or wrapped and stored in the refrigerator, where it will keep for up to three days. Cut melons quickly absorb odors from other foods; plus, their own aroma can transfer to and alter the taste of other foods, so make sure their wrapping is airtight.

TIPS FOR PREPARING

One medium-size, ripe honeydew melon weighs about 2 pounds/1 kilogram and provides 3 cups of chopped fruit. Melons grow resting on the ground, which means their rinds can become contaminated by animal or human waste, or contamination can be transferred from the harvester's or other handler's hands to the melon. Unless the skin is thoroughly cleansed, the knife used to halve a melon can transfer pathogens, such as *Salmonella,* directly onto the flesh. For this reason, all melons should be sprayed with a solution of diluted additive-free soap or commercial produce wash and then scrubbed under cool running water with a vegetable brush. Rinse well, and be sure to also wash surfaces that have come into contact with the unwashed melon, such as hands and cutting boards.

After washing, simply cut the honeydew in half. If you will be storing half of a cut melon, leave its seeds intact. They will keep the melon moist and extend its storage time. Immediately before serving, use a large spoon to scoop out the seeds and stringy flesh.

Honeydew can be cut up in many attractive ways. You can cut it into halves, quarters, wedges, cubes, or, if you have a melon baller, scoop it out in little rounds. One of the easiest ways to eat honeydew is to halve it, scoop out the seeds, and cut it into quarters, then eighths if desired. Slide a knife between the rind and the flesh of each wedge, and then slice the flesh into bite-sized pieces.

For the fullest flavor, serve honeydew barely chilled. To bring out its full fragrance, allow refrigerated melon to stand at room temperature for 15 to 20 minutes before serving. In addition, the contrast in flavors added by a sprinkling of salt, a squeeze of lemon juice, or a little freshly chopped mint will bring out honeydew's succulent sweetness.

QUICK SERVING IDEAS

- Serve honeydew in fruit salads. Its flavor combines well with virtually any other fruit, including other types of melon, berries, oranges, pineapple, bananas, and kiwifruit.
- For an appetizer or salad to complement a spring or summer meal, toss chunks of honeydew with lemon and watercress, or for Mexican flair, try lime, fresh coriander, and sliced jicama.
- To make melon rings, cut the honeydew into thick crosswise slices; then remove the seeds and, if desired, the rind. Place the ring of melon on a plate and fill the center with fruit salad or cottage cheese.
- Use honeydew halves as edible bowls for yogurt or cottage cheese. Quartered honeydew makes an attractive platter for prawns, tuna, or crabmeat salad.
- For a delicious summer brunch or light dessert, combine 1 cup orange juice, ¼ cup finely chopped mint leaves, ½ teaspoon cinnamon, ¼ teaspoon ginger, and 2 teaspoons honey in a large bowl. Add 2 to 3 cups of honeydew melon balls or chunks, and toss lightly. Cover and refrigerate 3 to 4 hours, then let stand for 15 to 20 minutes before serving.

• Make a frosted honeydew frappé: Chill 2 wineglasses by placing them in the freezer an hour beforehand. Blend together 1 cup plain yogurt, 3 cups cold honeydew melon chunks, 2 tablespoons honey, ¼ teaspoon pure vanilla extract, and 3 ice cubes or ¼ cup crushed ice. Process until smooth, pour into the frosted wineglasses, and garnish with sprigs of mint.

SAFETY

See "Tips for Preparing," above.

Since melons are among the foods on which pesticide residues have been most frequently found, we recommend buying organically grown melons.

Kiwifruit

The kiwifruit *(Actinidia chinensis)* is a small, oval fruit that is brown and fuzzy on the outside and inside contains a sherbet green meat surrounding small, jet-black edible seeds. Its flesh is almost creamy in consistency, somewhat between a strawberry and banana, with a very unique, sweet flavor.

HISTORY

Native to China, where it has been consumed for thousands of years, kiwifruit was originally known as *yang tao.* Kiwi trees were taken to New Zealand from China by missionaries in the early twentieth century, and the first commercial plantings occurred several decades later and have flourished.

Prior to 1961, kiwis were known as Chinese gooseberries. In 1961, the Chinese gooseberry made its appearance in the United States. It was at this time that the fruit was given a new name, "kiwi," in honor of the native bird of New Zealand, which has a similar brown, fuzzy coat. Kiwifruit is available worldwide today and is produced in New Zealand, the United States, Italy, Japan, France, Greece, China, Spain, Australia, and Chile.

NUTRITIONAL HIGHLIGHTS

Kiwifruit is an excellent source of vitamin C and a very good source of dietary fiber. It is also a good source of the minerals potassium, magnesium, copper, and phosphorus, as well as the antioxidant vitamins E and A.

A 100 gram serving is about one and a third whole fruit (76 grams per medium kiwi) and provides 61 calories, 1.1 grams of protein, 0.5 grams of fat, and 14.7 grams of carbohydrate, with 3 grams of fiber and 9 grams of natural sugars (fructose and glucose).

HEALTH BENEFITS

Kiwifruit is rich in antioxidants and enzymes. Like other vitamin C-rich foods, kiwis are particularly important in promoting respiratory tract health. In a study of six- and seven-year-old children in northern and central Italy, the more kiwi or citrus fruit these children consumed, the less likely they were to have respiratory-related health problems, including wheezing, shortness of breath, and night coughing.

HOW TO SELECT AND STORE

Kiwifruit is usually available throughout most of the year. Kiwifruit should feel firm but not rock hard. It should give slightly when pressed. If kiwifruit does not yield when you gently apply pressure with your thumb and forefinger, it is not yet ready to be consumed, since it has not reached the peak of its sweetness.

Kiwifruit can be left to ripen for a few days to a week at room temperature, away from exposure to sunlight and heat. Placing the fruit in a paper bag with an apple, banana, or pear will help to speed its ripening process. Ripe kiwifruit can be stored either at room temperature or in the refrigerator. Store it away from other fruits and vegetables that emit ethylene gas, which causes kiwifruit to become overripe quickly.

TIPS FOR PREPARING

Kiwifruit can be peeled with a paring knife and then cut into pieces, or you can cut them in half and scoop the flesh out with a spoon. Organically grown kiwis can also be eaten with the skin on after washing by hand under cool running water. Kiwifruit should not be eaten too long after cutting since it contains enzymes (actinic and bromic acids) that act as food tenderizers, with the ability to further tenderize the kiwifruit itself and make it overly soft. Consequently, if you are adding kiwifruit to fruit salad, you should do so at the last minute so as to prevent the other fruit from becoming too soggy.

QUICK SERVING IDEAS

- Eat kiwifruit whole or in fruit salads, or juice them. Kiwifruit mixes deliciously with most other fruits, especially grapes, apples, and oranges.
- Add kiwifruit to tossed green salads.
- Serve chopped kiwifruit and strawberries, fruits whose flavors are naturally complementary, topped with yogurt.
- Mix chopped kiwifruit, orange, and pineapple together to make a chutney that can be served as an accompaniment to chicken or fish.
- Blend kiwifruit and cantaloupe in a food processor to make a chilled soup. For a creamier consistency, blend yogurt with the fruit mixture.
- Kiwifruit have a wonderful flavor and appearance for use in fruit tarts.

SAFETY

Kiwis contain high levels of oxalates. Individuals with a history of calcium oxalate-containing kidney stones should limit their consumption of them. See page 793 for more information.

Lemon

The lemon (*Citrus limon*) is part of the Rutaceae family. This small, oval fruit is approximately 2 to 3 inches/5 to 7½ cm in diameter. With its bright yellow, pitted outer peel, like that of other citrus fruits, the inner flesh of the lemon is encased in approximately eight to ten segments. The lemon has a characteristic, sour odor with an acidic, tart, astringent taste that is unexpectedly refreshing.

The fruit juice contains mainly sugars and fruit acids, which are principally citric acid. Lemon peel consists of two layers: the outermost layer ("zest"), which contains essential oils (6 percent) that are composed mostly of limonene (90 percent) and citral (5 percent), plus a small amount of citronellal, alpha-terpineol, linalyl, and geranyl acetate. The inner layer contains no essential oil but instead houses a variety of bitter flavone glycosides and coumarin derivatives.

Despite the misconception that lemons are only sour, there is also a sweet variety. The most notable sweet lemon is the Meyer lemon, which is becoming increasingly popular in markets and restaurants. This lemon is relatively easy to grow (indoors) in the U.K. too. It has a much rounder form and a smooth unpitted skin, and takes on a deep yellow to orange color when mature. Meyer lemons have an amazing tangy aroma and are less acidic. The two main sour lemons are the Eureka and Lisbon. The Eureka has few seeds and a more textured skin (there is now a seedless variety of Eureka in the U.K.), while the Lisbon is smoother and seedless.

Lemon trees are much less hardy in their tolerance for cold than orange trees, hence they have been difficult to cultivate. However, the lemon tree flowers continuously and has fruit in all stages of development most of the year. A tree may bear as many as 3,000 lemons annually.

HISTORY

Citrus fruits are native to southern China and Southeast Asia, where they have been cultivated for approximately 4,000 years. In fact, ancient Asian literature includes stories about these fruits. The citron was carried to the Middle East sometime between 400 and 600 B.C.E. Arab traders in Asia carried lemons, citrons, limes, oranges, and shaddocks to eastern Africa and the Middle East between C.E. 100 and 700.

During the Arab occupation of Spain, citrus fruits arrived in southern Europe. From there, they were taken to the New World by Christopher Columbus and Portuguese and Spanish explorers. Lemons became quite well known in Florida and Brazil by the sixteenth century. Superior varieties from Southeast Asia arrived in Europe with Portuguese traders in the sixteenth century. Mandarin oranges from southern China did not arrive in Europe and the New World until the nineteenth century.

The desire for citrus fruits increased greatly after the 1890s when physicians found that people suffering from scurvy (a disease of vitamin C deficiency) could be cured by drinking citrus juice. Lemons were in such demand that people were willing to pay up to $1 per lemon, an astronomical price for that time! Later, scientists discovered that the juice is beneficial because it is the most potent and concentrated source of Vitamin C. Lemons also contain vitamins A, B1, and bioflavonoids, as well as potassium, magnesium, and folic acid.

The United States (California and Florida lead in U.S. production), Italy, Spain, Greece, Israel, and Turkey are the major producers of lemons.

NUTRITIONAL HIGHLIGHTS

Lemons are an excellent source of vitamin C. In addition, they are a good source of vitamin B6, potassium, folic acid, flavonoids, and the important phytochemical limonene. A 100 gram serving is about 2 medium lemons and provides 29 calories, 1.1 grams of protein, 0.3 grams of fat, and 9.3 grams of carbohydrate, with 2.8 grams of fiber and 2.5 grams of natural sugars.

HEALTH BENEFITS

The phytochemical limonene, which is extracted from lemons, is currently being used in clinical trials to dissolve gallstones and is showing extremely promising anticancer activities. The highest content of limonene is found in the white spongy inner parts of the lemon.

HOW TO SELECT AND STORE

When choosing a lemon, one should hold the fruit and determine if it is heavy. The heavier the fruit and the thinner the skin, the more juice it has. A ripe lemon should be firm, with a fine-textured peel with a deep yellow color. Acidity varies with the color of the lemon. A deep yellow lemon is less acidic than a lighter or greenish yellow one. Surface marks usually do not affect the fruit inside, but you should try to avoid buying bruised or dried-out fruit, as well as shriveled or hard-skinned lemons.

Store lemons at room temperature, away from sunlight, and enjoy their cheerful color. They keep without refrigeration for about two weeks. If kept in the refrigerator crisper, it is best to use a plastic bag, where they can remain up to six weeks.

Lemons can also be juiced and stored for later use. First, squeeze the lemons and pour the juice into ice cube trays for freezing. You can then transfer the frozen cubes to a plastic freezer container, where they will keep for up to three months. Lemon zest, which is usually used as a spice, can be dried and stored in a cool place for up to two to three months.

TIPS FOR PREPARING

Lemons in many forms are called for in countless recipes. To produce more lemon juice for a recipe, it is always better for the lemon to be warm (or at least room temperature). If time is a factor, the lemon can be placed in a bowl of warm water or in the microwave for 5 to 10 seconds, or juiced in a juicer or extractor. Rolling the lemon under the palm of your hand on a flat surface will also ensure the extraction of more juice. It is also important to note that before cutting a lemon, it is a good idea to wash the skin of the lemon so that any dirt or bacteria on the skin is not transferred to the fruit's interior. Use caution if you have a citrus allergy.

It is always recommended, if you are using the skin or "zest" of any citrus, to purchase organic fruit. Most conventionally harvested fruits have pesticide residue concentrated on their skin. To obtain the zest of a lemon, first wash and dry the lemon, then use a paring knife or vegetable peeler to remove the colored part of the lemon. The white pith that is under the peel has a very bitter taste and should not be used. The zest can be chopped, diced, candied, or used in whatever fashion called for by the recipe.

QUICK SERVING IDEAS

- Place thinly sliced lemons, peel and all, underneath and around fish before cooking. Baking or grilling will soften the slices so that they can be eaten along with the fish.
- Combine lemon juice with olive or linseed oil, freshly crushed garlic, and pepper to make a light, refreshing salad dressing.
- If you are watching your salt intake (and even if you are not), serve lemon wedges with meals, as the tart lemon juice makes a great salt substitute.

SAFETY

Some people are allergic to citrus peels. When such an allergy is suspected, caution must be employed when eating citrus fruit (see "Tips for Preparing"). But whether you are allergic or not, citrus peels *should not be eaten* in any significant quantity. Citrus peels contain some beneficial oils, but these oils can interfere with some body functions. For example, citrus peels contain a compound known as citral that antagonizes some of the effects of vitamin A.

Lemons contain low levels of oxalates; lemon peel, however, contains high levels of oxalates. Individuals with a history of calcium oxalate-containing kidney stones should limit their consumption of this food. See page 793 for more information.

Since lemons are among the foods on which pesticide residues have been most frequently found, we recommend selecting organically grown lemons.

Lime

The lime *(Citrus aurantifolia)* is a well-known small citrus fruit whose skin and flesh are green in color. It has an oval or round shape with a diameter of 1 to 2 inches/2½ to 5cm and grows on trees that flourish in tropical and subtropical climates.

Limes can either be sour or sweet, with the latter not readily available in the U.S.A. or UK. Sour limes possess a greater sugar and citric acid content than lemons and have an acidic, tart taste, while sweet limes, which lack citric acid content, are sweet in flavor.

There are two general varieties of sour limes available, the Tahitian and the Key. Among Tahitian limes are the egg-shaped Persian and the smaller, seedless Bears. Key limes, famous for the pie bearing their name, are smaller and more acidic than the Tahitian variety.

HISTORY

Limes, originating in Southeast Asia, were carried by Arab traders into Egypt and North Africa around the tenth century. Limes were then taken to Spain by the Moors in the thirteenth century. As with other fruits, it was during the Crusades that limes were spread throughout southern Europe, and they were then brought to the New World with Christopher Columbus in 1493.

The lime is the most susceptible to frost injury of all citrus fruits. It is of no surprise that the lime tree was cultivated successfully in the Caribbean countries, where the weather is hot and humid. It was not until centuries later in the West Indies that British explorers and traders used the Vitamin C-rich lime to prevent scurvy. It was here that they originally earned the nickname "limey."

In the sixteenth century, West Indies limes were introduced into the United States by Spanish explorers to the Florida Keys. This initiated the type of fruit we now know as the Key lime. In the next century, Spanish missionaries tried to take the lime to California. Unfortunately, as stated above, the lime is very susceptible to frost; hence the California climate could not support its growth. This is why today, in the United States, lime growing is confined to the southernmost parts of Florida. The chief commercial producers today are the United States, Mexico, and Brazil.

NUTRITIONAL HIGHLIGHTS

Limes do not differ much in nutritional value from lemons. They are an excellent source of vitamin C and provide good levels of vitamin B6, potassium, folic acid, flavonoids, and the important phytochemical limonene.

HEALTH BENEFITS

Limes contain several distinctive phytochemicals that are high in antioxidant and anticancer properties, including flavonoids and limonene, besides being an excellent source of vitamin C. In particular, research has demonstrated that lime juice can affect cell cycles: specifically, it can modulate the decision a cell makes to divide (mitosis) or die (apoptosis) or even boost the activity of white blood cells.

Furthermore, one of the most intriguing functions of the lime is its antibiotic effect. This was demonstrated in several villages of West Africa during a cholera epidemic. Cholera is a bacterial disease that is caused by the activity of *Vibrio cholerae* in the intestine, which results in severe diarrhea. Researchers found that the inclusion of lime juice in the subjects' main meal (a sauce eaten with rice) was strongly protective against the development of cholera.

HOW TO SELECT AND STORE

Limes should be green in color and heavy for their size. If they have purple or brown spots, it is a sign that they are decaying and may have an undesirable, mouldy taste. Limes are available in the marketplace throughout the year, although they are usually in greater supply from mid-spring through to mid-autumn.

Limes can be kept out at room temperature, where they will stay fresh for up to one week.

Make sure to keep them away from sunlight exposure, since it will cause them to turn yellow and will alter their flavor. Limes can be stored in the refrigerator crisper, wrapped in a loosely sealed plastic bag, where they will stay fresh for about ten to fourteen days. While they can be kept for another several weeks, they will begin to lose their characteristic flavor.

Lime juice and zest can also be stored for later use. Place freshly squeezed lime juice in ice cube trays until frozen, then store the cubes in plastic bags in the freezer, where they will keep for up to three months. Dried lime zest should be stored in a cool, dry place in an airtight glass container, where it will keep for two to three months.

TIPS FOR PREPARING

Limes are prepared in the same manner as lemons (see page 290).

QUICK SERVING IDEAS

- Limes can be used in place of lemons.
- Combine freshly squeezed lime juice, evaporated sugarcane juice (Sucanat), and either plain or sparkling water to make limeade.
- Add an easy-to-prepare zing to dinner by tossing seasoned cooked brown rice with garden peas, chicken pieces, spring onions, pumpkin seeds, lime juice, and lime zest.
- Squeeze some lime juice onto an avocado quarter and eat as is.

SAFETY

Limes contain low levels of oxalates, while lime peel contains high levels of oxalates. Individuals with a history of calcium oxalate-containing kidney stones should limit their consumption of this food. See page 793 for more information.

Limes are generally not an allergic food. However, some people are allergic to citrus peels. When such an allergy is suspected, caution must be employed when eating citrus fruit (see "Tips for Preparing"). But whether you are allergic or not, citrus peels *should not be eaten* in any significant quantity. Citrus peels contain some beneficial oils, but these oils can interfere with some body functions. For example, citrus peels contain a compound known as citral that antagonizes some of the effects of vitamin A. Since limes are among the foods on which pesticide residues have been most frequently found, individuals wanting to avoid health risks associated with pesticides should avoid consumption of lime unless organically grown.

Mangoes

The mango *(Mangifera indica)* is a luscious tropical fruit with a smooth green skin that develops patches of red, yellow, and/or gold as it ripens and orange-yellow flesh that is exceptionally juicy when ripe. The seed of the mango is larger than any other in the fruit kingdom—practically as long and wide as the entire length and width of the fruit. Almost flat, the seed is surrounded first by some fibrous matter, then by plump, fleshy fruit, whose taste is a spicy-sweet mélange of peach and pineapple.

A member of the sumac family (Anacardiaceae), the mango is cousin to pistachios and cashew nuts. Mangoes are one of the leading fruit crops of the world, ranking seventh among the top twenty fruits. In fact, more mangoes are consumed by more people in the world on a regular basis than apples. Mangoes come in more than 1,000 varieties and vary in form from round to kidney-shaped, ranging from diminutive plum-sized to melon-sized fruits weighing up to 4 pounds/2 kilograms. Most commercially grown varieties are about the size and shape of a large avocado: 4 to 5 inches/10 to 12 cm in length and about 8 ounces/250 grams in weight.

The mango tree is a magnificent evergreen that grows up to 100 feet/30 meters tall and produces beautiful, shiny, thick, pointed leaves 8 to 14 inches/20 to 35 cm long. Symmetrical in shape, the mango tree is a beautiful ornamental valued for its cooling shade as well as its fruit.

Mango trees begin to produce fruit four to six years after planting and continue bearing fruit for about forty years. Tiny, delicate pinkish white flowers precede the fruit, which grows in clusters from long stems attached to the main branches. Each mango tree bears an average of 100 mangoes each year.

HISTORY

The wild mango originated in the foothills of the Himalayas in India and Burma, and wild mango trees still grow in India and Southeast Asia today. However, the wild mango, with its tiny size, fibrous texture, and unpleasant turpentine taste, bears little resemblance to the luscious cultivated mangoes we now enjoy. The cultivation of the mango began in Moghul, India, where the fruit is still considered sacred and is thought to have aphrodisiac effects. In the sixteenth century, a special technique employing grafting was developed for propagating the mango.

This technique and variations upon it are still used today because even cultivated mangoes will not develop true from seed but will revert back to their wild ancestry, producing a highly fibrous fruit that tastes like turpentine.

The earliest mention of the mango tree, *Mangifera indica,* which means "the great fruit bearer," is found in Hindu scriptures dating back to 4000 B.C.E. In Tamil, the language of southeastern India, the mango was given its original name, *mancay* or *mangay,* which the Portuguese later changed to *manga.*

Legend relates that the Buddha, delighting in the mango, was given a whole grove of mango trees where he could rest whenever he wished. The mango's association with the Buddha caused the mango tree to be held in awe as capable of granting wishes, and also to be revered in India as a symbol of love. In fact, in the oldest Sanskrit writings, the mango tree is central to a legend of undying love. The king of the land fell in love with and married the beautiful daughter of the sun, Surya Bai, but she was forced to transform herself into a golden lotus to evade persecution by an evil sorceress. When the king then fell in love with the beautiful flower, the sorceress burnt it to ashes. All appeared lost until, with the help of a magnificent mango tree that sprang from the ashes, Surya Bai emerged from a golden ripe mango that had fallen to the ground. The king instantly recognized her as his long-lost wife, and the two were reunited.

Reverence for the mango was extended beyond India when explorers carried the fruit to other tropical countries, including Thailand, Malaysia, Indonesia, and the Philippines, where it was cultivated successfully. As the mango adapted to these new locales, new varieties evolved and were praised with nicknames, such as the "apple of the tropics," the "king of fruits," and the "fruit of the Gods."

The Chinese traveler Hwen Tsang, who visited India during the first half of the seventh century C.E., brought the mango home with him to China. The Chinese were delighted with the beauty of the mango tree as well as its fruit, and the mango soon became a garden favorite. By the end of the seventh century C.E., the mango had journeyed west to Baghdad, where the caliphs used the fruit to make a complex liquor that required six months to a year to ferment fully. Continuing west by camel caravan, the mango traveled from Persia to North Africa, where it arrived about the year 1000 C.E.

Mangoes were first recorded in Europe by Friar Jordanus in 1328, but Europeans did not delight in them as had the inhabitants of countries with tropical climates—a reaction that continues to this day, as the mango remains an infrequently eaten fruit in Europe. However, by the sixteenth century, Portuguese explorers carried the mango to East and West Africa and Brazil, and by the eighteenth century, the fruit had sailed to the West Indies.

In the nineteenth century, the mango continued its travels west, arriving in Florida, Mexico, and Hawaii. Mangoes were grown on the east coast of Florida by 1825, and in 1889 the USDA introduced a special grafted variety from India called Mulgoa or Mulgoba, from which one of today's most popular varieties, the richly sweet and spicy Haden, was developed.

Today, India remains the world's largest producer of mangoes, and the mango is India's main fruit crop, far outnumbering all others.

NUTRITIONAL HIGHLIGHTS

Mangoes are an excellent source of carotenes, vitamin C, and copper, providing 184 percent of the daily value of vitamin A, 61 percent of the daily value of vitamin C, and 20 percent of the daily value of copper in one cup (165 grams) of sliced fruit. They are a very good source of B vitamins, with one cup of sliced mango providing 17 percent of the daily value of vitamin B6, 9 percent of the daily value of thiamine and riboflavin, 7 percent of the daily value of niacin, and 6 percent of the daily value of folic acid. Mangoes are also a good source of vitamin E, potassium, and magnesium. A cup of sliced mango provides 12 percent of the daily value of vitamin E, 7 percent of the daily value of potassium, and 5 percent of the daily value of magnesium.

Raw mangoes are about 82 percent water and a very good source of both soluble and insoluble fiber. A one-cup serving of sliced mango provides 12 percent of the daily value of fiber; more than half is soluble fiber, the type of fiber that latches onto cholesterol and helps to prevent cardiovascular disease.

One cup of chopped mango contains 107 calories. A slice of dried mango provides 32.5 calories.

HEALTH BENEFITS

Mangoes have long been valued as a health-promoting fruit. We now know the health benefits are due to their high concentration of carotenoids, antioxidant nutrients, and various phytochemicals. Research conducted in 2002 by Dr. Sue Percival, an associate professor at the University of Florida's Institute of Food and Agricultural Sciences, confirmed and expanded upon earlier research conducted at the University of Hawaii in 1997. In that study, white blood cells from mice were exposed to cancer-causing substances and then to mango extract. Lab tests showed the mango's ability to stop normal cells from turning into cancer cells. Interestingly, Dr. Percival compared an extract containing mango's carotenes to a water-soluble mango extract in order to test their effectiveness against cancer formation. According to her findings, mango's water-soluble portion was about ten times as effective in preventing cancer cell formation as its carotenes. Compounds in the aqueous portion of the mango include not only water-soluble nutrients, such as vitamin C, but also valuable flavonoid compounds, which appear to contribute to the mango's anticancer effect. Furthermore, there is human evidence that demonstrates that mangoes can help fight cancer. A diet analysis of 64 patients with gallbladder cancer and 101 patients with gallstones showed that mango consumption was correlated with a 60 percent reduction in the risk of gallbladder cancer—the highest reduction in the risk of this cancer found for any fruit or vegetable.

Mangoes also contain a number of enzymes, including one similar to the papain in papayas, that improve digestion. Among them are magneferin, katechol oxidase, and lactase. In fact, in tropical countries where the mango is grown, it is often used as a meat tenderizer since its powerful proteolytic enzymes help break down proteins.

The mango may also offer some protection against infections. The Department of Epidemiology and International Health at the University of Alabama conducted a four-month study of

176 Gambian children in which those who received dried mango were found to have higher blood levels of retinol (vitamin A) than those who were given a placebo. Since vitamin A's nickname is the "anti-infective vitamin," the mango may literally be a lifesaving fruit in developing countries where there is a severe seasonal shortage of carotenoid-rich foods. In other studies indicating the mango's protective effects on overall health, infants in Gambia and India were found to have the best gut integrity and thus the least intestinal disease and diarrhea during the three months when mangoes were in season in each country.

Not surprisingly, the mango was also shown in a study conducted in Mexico to provide protection against giardia, an organism responsible for many cases of what has been dubbed "traveler's diarrhea." Not only was mango found to eliminate giardia, but it did so just as well as tinidazol, a drug commonly used to treat giardia infection. Furthermore, one lab test turned up rather startling results that raised mangoes to the "highest perch." Mango juice was poured into a test tube that contained viruses. Shortly, the viruses were destroyed.

Because of their high iron content, in India mangoes are used as blood builders and are suggested for the treatment of anemia and as a beneficial food for women, especially during pregnancy and menstruation. People who suffer from muscle cramps, stress, and heart problems can benefit from mangoes' high potassium and magnesium content, which also helps those with acidosis. In addition, the mango, one of the most delicious tropical fruits, can be safely enjoyed by persons with diabetes. When plasma glucose and insulin responses to various tropical fruits were compared, the glucose response curve to mango was the lowest of all.

HOW TO SELECT AND STORE

Although mangoes are available in January, those that appear at the market later in the year are typically more flavorful. Mangoes sold in the United States are usually imported from Mexico, Haiti, the Caribbean, and South America. About 10 percent are grown in Florida and are harvested several times throughout the year. From April through September, Mexican mangoes are in good supply. Florida mangoes are plentiful from May through August, with supplies at their peak in June and July. The most popular varieties in the U.K. are the Kent and Keitt, both of which are grown in Florida, South and Central America, and The Gambia.

If possible, choose fruit grown in Florida or Hawaii, as other mangoes are often irradiated or sprayed with chemicals banned in the United States and Europe. Then ask your supermarket produce manager which varieties of mangoes are available. The flesh of the Tommy Atkins, the most common U.S. variety, is a bit blander and more fibrous than that of the Haden, Kent, and Keitt, three of the most flavorful varieties grown in Florida, Mexico, and Central America.

Mango size is related to the variety, not the fruit's quality or ripeness, although the larger the mango, the higher will be the ratio of fruit to seed. A ripe mango will yield slightly to gentle palm pressure and exude an appealing flowery fragrance. Test the fruit with a gentle squeeze. It should be soft but solid. If it feels spongy to the touch, it's definitely overripe and very possibly spoiled. Also avoid mangoes with a loose or shriveled skin, or a fermented or turpentinelike scent. A few black speckles are typical indicators of ripeness, but an abundance of black-speckled skin may signal damaged flesh beneath.

The skin of the mango should be smooth, largely unblemished, and, in most varieties, blushed with an area of yellow-orange or red that will increase in size as the fruit ripens. However, Keitt mango can remain virtually all green with only a slight trace of yellow even when fully ripe, so for this variety, softness and fragrance are the indicators of ripeness.

Mangoes are harvested when they are "mature green" to enable them to travel long distances to market without spoiling. Green, rock-hard mangoes were likely picked too soon and will probably never ripen, but slightly underripe mangoes can be placed along with an apple in a paper bag that has been pierced with a few holes, where they will ripen if left at room temperature for one to three days. Adding an apple creates more natural ethylene gas and decreases ripening time. Since this speeds up the ripening process, be sure to check daily for ripeness. If, however, you've purchased unripe mangoes and don't plan to use them immediately, you can store them for one to two weeks at 55 degrees F./13 degrees C. before setting them out at room temperature or placing them in a paper bag to ripen. Once ripe, mangoes should be put in a plastic bag and stored in the refrigerator, where they will keep for one to three days.

Dried mango slices are also available in most supermarkets as well as health food shops. When purchasing dried mango, look for organic, unsweetened, sulphite-free fruit.

TIPS FOR PREPARING

Mangoes should be sprayed with a solution of diluted additive-free soap or commercial produce wash and then scrubbed under cool running water with a vegetable brush. Since mango peels may be irritating to the skin, you may want to wear rubber gloves when peeling, especially if you will be peeling several mangoes at the same time. Mangoes can also be quite juicy, and their juice is rich in pigment that can permanently stain clothing, so it's a good idea to wear an apron when preparing them, too.

Since its flesh clings tenaciously to the large, flat seed, the mango is not the easiest fruit to prepare, but these peeling and slicing tips will help:

For easiest slicing, cut off both ends of the mango with a sharp, thin-bladed knife, such as a paring knife. Place the fruit on a flat end and cut away the peel from top to bottom along the curvature of the fruit. Then stand the fruit on its wide end and cut vertically, sliding the knife along the seed first on one side, then on the other, creating two near halves of fruit ready for slicing (a little fruit will remain around the seed). Or cut thin slices off the fruit until you reach the seed.

Alternatively, after cutting off both ends of the mango, leave the skin on and make vertical slices to remove each half from the pit. The flesh can then be scooped out with a spoon. If you prefer mango cubes, cut crosshatch lines partway through the flesh with the tip of your knife, being careful not to cut through the skin. Then invert the skin so the flesh pops outward, and slice off the cubes.

In the tropics, people eat mango cubes right off the skin or serve the whole fruit on a fork. To prepare the fruit to be served on a fork, cut an "X" across the skin on the top of the mango, pull the skin away from the fruit in quarters, insert a fork on the unpeeled end, and serve—with an ample supply of napkins. Another common way of eating ripe mangoes in the tropics is to roll the fruit back and forth on a tabletop to soften the pulp, then cut off the tip of the stem end, and suck on the fruit to draw out the pulp.

QUICK SERVING IDEAS

- In their unripe form, mangoes are just as appealing as when fully ripe. For a basic green mango chutney, sauté a large chopped onion in a little oil until clear, then add 1 chopped green mango. Cook over medium heat for a couple of minutes, then add 1 cup vinegar, 1 tablespoon freshly grated ginger, 1 tablespoon finely chopped Serrano or jalapeno chili or ¾ tablespoon red pepper flakes, and ½ cup brown sugar. Mix well and simmer for 10 minutes. Remove from heat, cool to room temperature, and serve or store in covered glass jars in the refrigerator for up to two weeks.

- Try this delicious rice salad: Mix 2 cups chopped green mango, ¾ cup shredded carrot, 4 stalks sliced celery, 2 teaspoons lemon zest, and 2 tablespoons honey into 2 cups cooked brown rice. Cover and refrigerate 2 hours or more before serving.

- Mangoes are a terrific addition to prawn salad, too: Cut 3 ripe mangoes into cubes, 16 large prawns into chunks, and 1 sweet red pepper into thin strips. Toss with a dressing made of ½ cup mayonnaise, 1 teaspoon horseradish, a squeeze of fresh lemon juice, and a tablespoon of honey. Chill for a half hour before serving.

- Mangoes can be sliced, diced, and julienned into fruit salads, and make a delightful, tangy addition to tossed green salads and coleslaw as well. If they are eaten alone, try serving them with a wedge of lemon or lime to bring out their flavor.

- Spice up rice-and-veggie-filled tortillas by topping them with mango salsa. To make the salsa, dice 4 ripe mangos, 4 spring onions, and ¼ cup fresh coriander. Mix together with the juice of 4 limes and add salt and pepper to taste.

- Puréed in the blender with yogurt, mangoes add delectable sweetness to smoothies and creamy dressings for fruit salads.

- Cold soups enjoy a boost in nutrition and a tangy lift in flavor with the addition of fresh mangoes. For an exceptionally delicious cold soup for four, combine 3 cups chopped mango (3 mangoes) with 1 cup milk, 1 cup yogurt, 2 tablespoons honey, and nutmeg and cinnamon to taste. Blend and garnish with mint, edible flowers, or thin slices of lime. For a thick, creamy dessert, just eliminate the milk, or for another wonderfully tangy cold soup, instead of milk and yogurt, use 1 cup orange juice and 1 cup buttermilk.

SAFETY

Mangoes are distant relations of poison oak and poison ivy. Especially when unripe, their peel may be irritating to the skin since it contains a substance that can cause an allergic skin reaction, such as redness and swelling. Even if you have never had a reaction to mangoes before, wearing rubber gloves while preparing them is recommended if you will be preparing several unripe fruits.

Although an infrequent food allergen, mango has been identified as an allergy-provoking food in some individuals with food allergies. In the case of children and other persons with allergies to other foods, introduce mango cautiously and monitor for any allergic reactions. For a description of common signs and symptoms of food allergies, see page 723.

Nectarines: See Peaches and Nectarines.

Olives: See chapter 14.

Oranges

Oranges are round citrus fruits ranging in diameter from about 2 to 3 inches/5 to 7½ cm with finely texturized skins that are, of course, orange in color, just like their pulpy flesh. They are undoubtedly one of the most popular fruits in the world.

Oranges are classified into two general categories—sweet and bitter—with the former being most commonly consumed. Popular varieties of the sweet orange (*Citrus sinensis*) include Valencia, navel, and Jaffa oranges, as well as the blood orange, a hybrid species that is smaller in size, more aromatic in flavor, and has red hues running throughout its flesh. Bitter oranges (*Citrus aurantium*) are used to make jam or marmalade, and their zest serves as the flavoring for liqueurs such as Grand Marnier and Cointreau.

HISTORY

The first known reference to oranges is found in the second book of the traditional text *The Five Classics,* which appeared in China in 500 B.C.E.

Oranges were first cultivated in the Middle East around the nineth century. During the fifteenth century, sweet oranges were introduced to Europe by various explorers and traders during their travels to the Middle East and Asia. However, it was the Spanish explorers who were responsible for transporting the orange to Florida in the sixteenth century. In the eighteenth century, Spanish missionaries brought the fruit to California for cultivation as well.

The modern-day orange was developed from varieties native to southern China and Southeast Asia. In the United States, oranges are the leading fruit crop. Other large world producers of oranges are Mexico, Brazil, Spain, Israel, and China.

NUTRITIONAL HIGHLIGHTS

Oranges are an excellent source of flavonoids and vitamin C—one orange (131 grams) supplies nearly 100 percent of the recommended dietary intake of vitamin C. They are also a very good source of dietary fiber. In addition, they are a good source of B vitamins (including vitamins B1, B2, and B6, folic acid, and pantothenic acid), carotenes, pectin and potassium.

HEALTH BENEFITS

The combination of high vitamin C content and flavonoids make oranges important wherever vitamin C is required to function, especially within the immune system, lens of the eye, adrenal glands, and reproductive organs and in the connective tissues of our body, such as the joints, gums, and ground substance; and in promoting overall good health. One of the most important flavonoids in oranges is hesperidin.

Hesperidin has been shown in animal studies to lower high blood pressure as well as cholesterol, and to have strong anti-inflammatory properties. The concentration of hesperidin is considerably higher in the inner peel and inner white pulp of the orange, rather than in its orange flesh.

The consumption of oranges and orange juice has been shown to protect against cancer and help fight viral infections. The pectin in oranges also possesses properties similar to that of grapefruit pectin in lowering cholesterol levels (see page 279).

Note: Mandarin oranges, tangerines, and satsumas provide similar health benefits as the orange.

HOW TO SELECT AND STORE

Choose oranges that are firm and heavy for their size (this indicates that they are full of juice). Lighter fruit has more skin and drier pulp, which results in less juice. For the juiciest, sweetest fruit, look for oranges with a sweet, clean fragrance. One should avoid oranges that are severely bruised, soft, mouldy, or puffy. Color should not be used as a factor in choosing an orange. Oranges that are green or brown may be as ripe and delicious as those of a solid orange color. Actually, the uniform orange color of nonorganic oranges may be due to the injection of an artificial dye, Citrus Red No. 2 (this additive has no E number, so while it may be found in the U.K., it hasn't been certified by E.U. safety tests).

Like other citrus, oranges can be stored at room temperature for about two weeks or loosely stored in the refrigerator. It is better not to store oranges wrapped, for wrapping leaves the fruit more susceptible to moisture and mould. Also, orange peel can be dried and stored in an airtight container and kept in a dry, cool environment, and orange juice can be squeezed into ice cube trays and frozen for later use.

TIPS FOR PREPARING

Oranges should be sprayed with a solution of diluted additive-free soap or commercial produce wash and then hand washed under cool running water. Oranges can be eaten as a snack—just peel and enjoy. Thin-skinned oranges can easily be peeled with your fingers. For easy peeling of the thicker-skinned varieties, first cut a small section of the peel from the top of the orange. You can then either make four longitudinal cuts from top to bottom and peel away these sections of skin or, starting at the top, peel the orange in a spiral fashion.

If you wish to cut your orange instead, before cutting the orange in half horizontally through the center, wash the skin so that any dirt or bacteria residing on the surface will not be transferred to the fruit. Proceed to cut the sections into halves or thirds, depending upon your personal preference.

Oranges are often called for in recipes in the form of orange juice. As oranges produce more juice when warmer, always juice them when they are at room temperature, or, if you've just taken them out of the refrigerator, place them in a bowl of warm water for several minutes. Rolling the orange under the palm of your hand on a flat surface will also help extract more juice. The juice can then be extracted in a variety of ways. You can use either a juicer or a squeezer or squeeze it by hand. If you happen to have an allergy to any of the constituents in citrus peel, use extra caution when juicing oranges.

If your recipe calls for orange zest, make sure you use an orange that is organically grown, since most conventionally grown oranges have pesticide residues on their skin and may be artificially colored. After washing and drying the orange, use a zester, paring knife, or vegetable peeler to remove the zest, which is the orange part of the peel. Make sure not to remove too much of the peel, as the white pith underneath is bitter and should not be used. The zest can then be chopped finely or diced if necessary.

QUICK SERVING IDEAS

- Eat oranges whole or in fruit salads, or juice them.
- Lightly sauté onions and then deglaze the pan with orange juice. Use this liquid as a marinade and sauce for grilled tofu.
- Blend cooked carrots with orange juice, season with rosemary, and serve as a cold soup.
- Orange segments, fennel, and shaved Parmesan cheese make a delightfully refreshing salad.
- Gently simmer sweet potatoes, winter squash, and orange segments in orange juice. Before serving, sprinkle with walnuts.
- Freeze orange juice in ice cube trays. Once they are mostly frozen, gently blend in a food processor to create a frozen granita dessert.

SAFETY

Oranges are a common food allergen. When such an allergy is suspected, caution must be employed when eating citrus fruit; see "Tips for Preparing" above. For a description of common signs and symptoms of food allergies, see page 723.

Oranges' flesh does not contain oxalates, although the peel contains high levels of oxalates, as do other citrus peels. Individuals with a history of calcium oxalate-containing kidney stones should limit their consumption of them (see page 793 for more information), though citrus peels should never be eaten in any significant quantity. Citrus peels contain some beneficial oils, but these oils can interfere with some body functions. For example, citrus peels contain a compound known as citral that antagonizes some of the effects of vitamin A.

Since oranges are among the foods on which pesticide residues have been most frequently found, we highly recommend selecting organically grown oranges.

Papaya

The papaya *(Carica papaya)* is a spherical or pear-shaped fruit that can be as long as 20 inches/50 cm. Papayas commonly found in the market usually average about 7 inches/18 cm and weigh about 1 pound/½ kilogram. Their flesh is a rich orange color with either yellow or pink hues. Papaya has a wonderfully soft consistency and a sweet, musky taste. Inside the inner cavity of the fruit are round, black seeds encased in a gelatinlike substance. These seeds are edible, though they are quite bitter.

HISTORY

The papaya originated in Central America. In the sixteenth and seventeenth centuries, it quickly became favored by Spanish and

Portuguese explorers, who took papayas from Central America to many other subtropical lands, including India, the Philippines, and parts of Africa. In fact, the papaya was so beloved by the explorers that Christopher Columbus called it "the fruit of the angels."

In the twentieth century, papayas were brought to the United States and have been cultivated in Hawaii, the major U.S. producer since the 1920s. Today, the largest commercial producers of papayas include the United States, Mexico, and Puerto Rico.

NUTRITIONAL HIGHLIGHTS

Papayas are an excellent source of antioxidant nutrients, such as carotenes, vitamin C, and flavonoids. They are also a very good source of folic acid, vitamins E and A, potassium, and dietary fiber. A 100 gram serving is about ⅓ of a medium papaya and provides 39 calories, 0.6 grams of protein, 0.1 grams of fat, and 9.8 grams of carbohydrate, with 1.8 grams of fiber and 5.9 grams of natural sugars.

HEALTH BENEFITS

The fruit, as well as the other parts of the papaya tree, contains papain, an enzyme that helps digest proteins. Papain is more concentrated in the fruit when it is unripe.

In addition to providing protective benefits against cancer, heart disease, and other diseases associated with free-radical damage, papayas are valued for their papain content. This protein-digesting enzyme is used in digestive enzyme dietary supplements and is also used as an ingredient in many meat tenderizers. It is also used in a similar manner as bromelain from pineapple (see page 307) to treat a number of conditions, such as indigestion, chronic diarrhea, hay fever, sports injuries and other causes of trauma, and allergies.

HOW TO SELECT AND STORE

If you want to eat papayas within a day of purchase, choose those that have reddish orange skin and are slightly soft to the touch. Papayas that have patches of yellow color will take a few more days to ripen. Avoid papayas that are totally green or overly hard, as their flesh will not develop its characteristic sweet juicy flavor.

Papayas that are partially yellow should be left at room temperature, where they will ripen in a few days. If you want to speed this process, place them in a paper bag with a banana. Ripe papayas should be stored in the refrigerator and consumed within one to two days to enjoy their maximum flavor.

TIPS FOR PREPARING

Papayas should be sprayed with a solution of diluted additive-free soap or commercial produce wash and then scrubbed under cool running water with a vegetable brush. After washing the fruit, cut it lengthwise and scoop out the seeds. If it is being consumed simply with a spoon, a little lemon or lime juice can be squeezed on top.

To cut papaya into smaller pieces for fruit salad or other recipes, peel it with a paring knife, cut it lengthwise, scoop out the seeds, and then cut it into the desired size and shape. You can also use a melon baller to scoop out the fruit of a halved papaya. If you are adding papaya to a fruit salad, you should do so just before serving, as it tends to cause the other fruits to become very soft.

QUICK SERVING IDEAS

- Eat papayas whole or in fruit salads, or juice them.
- Sprinkle papaya with fresh lime juice and enjoy as is.
- Slice a small papaya lengthwise and fill with fruit salad.
- Mix diced papaya, fresh coriander, jalapeño peppers, and ginger to make a unique salsa that goes great with prawns, scallops, and halibut.
- Combine diced papaya, chopped cooked chicken breast, onions, and cashew nuts with soy mayonnaise to make a chicken salad with a tropical flair.
- In a blender, combine papaya, strawberries, and yogurt for a cold soup treat.
- If you have a papaya that is not too soft, cut it into medium-size cubes. Place the papaya on a skewer with small onions (or other vegetables of your choice) and grill for about ten minutes. Serve as a side dish with a variety of different entrées.

SAFETY

Papaya is not associated with any significant safety issues.

Peaches and Nectarines

The peach *(Prunus persica)* is a round, fuzzy-skinned fruit with a hard pit or stone surrounded by soft, pulpy flesh ranging in diameter from about 2 to 3 inches/5 to 7½ cm. There are two major types of peaches, freestone and clingstone, so named to reflect how easy it is to remove the pit from the fruit. Popular freestone varieties include Elberta, Hale, and in the U.S.

Golden Jubilee. Popular clingstone varieties in the U.S. are the Fortuna, Johnson, and Sims. The nectarine (also *Prunus persica*) is simply a smooth-skinned peach, also available in both freestone and clingstone varieties.

HISTORY

The peach is native to China. It was introduced into the Middle East a few centuries before Christ and eventually was spread by the Romans throughout Europe. Several of its horticultural varieties were brought by the Spanish to North America, where it became naturalized as far north as Pennsylvania by the late seventeenth century.

In the United States, the major peach production centers are California, Texas, Oregon, and the southern Atlantic states. Elsewhere the peach is cultivated in southern Europe, Africa, Japan, Australia, and South America.

NUTRITIONAL HIGHLIGHTS

Peaches and nectarines provide good levels of potassium, carotenes, flavonoids, and natural sugars. A 100 gram serving equals one medium peach or nectarine and provides 49 calories, 0.9 grams of protein, 0.3 grams of fat, and 9.5 grams of carbohydrate, with 1.5 grams of fiber and 8.4 grams of natural sugars (sucrose, glucose, and fructose).

HEALTH BENEFITS

Peaches and nectarines are good sources of carotenes and flavonoids, such as lycopene and lutein, which give red, orange, and yellow colors to fruits and vegetables. These phytochemicals are particularly beneficial in preventing macular degeneration, heart disease, and cancer.

HOW TO SELECT AND STORE

Fresh peaches and nectarines are usually best when in season, June through to August. In the winter in the U.S.A., peaches and nectarines are imported from South America. Ripe peaches or nectarines yield to gentle pressure on the skin. If the fruit is quite hard, it is unripe; if it is quite soft or mushy, it is overmature. Also be sure to check for bruises and other signs of spoilage.

Peaches and nectarines will ripen if kept at room temperature (usually within one or two days). Note that the color indicates the variety of the peach or nectarine more than ripeness, hence it should not be used as a gauge of ripeness. Once ripe, store the peaches and nectarines in the refrigerator, where they will keep for two to three days.

TIPS FOR PREPARING

Peaches and nectarines should be washed by hand under cold running water if organically grown. If nonorganic, they should be soaked or sprayed with a solution of diluted additive-free soap or commercial produce wash and then washed by hand under cool running water. Dry them carefully with a paper towel and eat them whole or slice them in half to remove the pit before eating or slicing.

QUICK SERVING IDEAS

• Eat them whole or in fruit salads.
• Add sliced peaches to hot or cold cereal.
• Peaches are a delicious addition to baked goods, such as muffins and quick breads.
• The next time you make whole-grain pancakes, add some chopped peaches to the batter.
• Skewer whole or halved fresh peaches, brush with honey, and barbecue on the grill or bake in the oven for 2 to 3 minutes.

SAFETY

Since peaches are among the foods most commonly associated with pesticide residues, we encourage you to select organically grown peaches.

Peaches contain moderate amounts of oxalates. Individuals with a history of calcium oxalate-containing kidney stones should limit their consumption of this food. See page 793 for more information.

Pears

The pear *(Pyrus communis)* is a delicious fruit that is related to the apple and the quince. About the size of an apple, pears generally have a characteristic large, round bottom that tapers toward the top. Depending upon the variety, their paper-thin skins can be yellow, green, brown, red, or a combination of two or more of these colors. The white to cream-colored flesh of pears is very juicy and sweet, while their texture is soft and buttery yet slightly grainy. Like apples, pears have a core that features several seeds.

While there are thousands of varieties of pears, each differing in size, shape, color, taste, and storage qualities, the Anjou, Bartlett, Bosc, and Comice pears are those most commonly available in the United States. In the U.K., the National Fruit Collection holds over 500 varieties of pear. Popular varieties include the Comice, Concord and Conference.

HISTORY

The historical record of the pear dates as far back as the Stone Age. The attractive fruit even captured the praise of the Greek poet Homer in the eighth century B.C.E., who referred to pears as a "gift of the gods." Evidently, the Romans agreed, as they proceeded to use grafting techniques to develop more than fifty varieties. Pears were even deemed a luxury item in the court of Louis XIV.

The first pear tree planted in America in 1620 was brought to the New World by the early colonists. And missionaries brought this luscious fruit to California in the 1700s. Today, the world's supply of pears is grown primarily in Italy, the United States, and China.

NUTRITIONAL HIGHLIGHTS

Pears are a very good source of dietary fiber. They are also a good source of vitamin C, copper, vitamins B2 and E, and potassium.

A 100 gram serving equals two-thirds of a medium pear (166 grams) and provides 58 calories, 0.4 grams of protein, 0.1 grams of fat, and 15.4 grams of carbohydrate, with 3.1 grams of fiber and 9.8 grams of natural sugars (fructose and glucose).

HEALTH BENEFITS

Pears are an excellent source of water-soluble fibers, including pectin. In fact, pears are actually higher in pectin than apples. This makes them quite useful in helping to lower cholesterol levels and in toning the intestines.

Pears are often recommended by healthcare practitioners as a hypoallergenic fruit high in fiber that is less likely to produce an adverse response than other fruits. Particularly in the introduction of fruits to infants, pears are often recommended as a safe way to start.

HOW TO SELECT AND STORE

Most pears available are purchased unripe and will require a few days of maturing. As the pear ripens, the skin color changes from green to the color characteristic of the variety: Bosc, Conference and Concord pears turn brown, Anjou and Bartlett pears turn yellow, and Comice pears have a green mottled skin. Fresh pears are best when they yield to pressure as an avocado does.

Unripe pears will ripen if stored at room temperature. If you want to hasten the ripening process, place them in a paper bag, turning them occasionally, and keep them at room temperature. Once ripe, pears should be stored in the refrigerator, where they will remain fresh for a few days. *Note:* Pears should be stored away from strong-smelling foods, whether on the countertop or in the refrigerator, as they tend to absorb odors.

TIPS FOR PREPARING

Wash organically grown pears gently by running cool water over them and patting them dry. Nonorganic pears should be sprayed with a solution of diluted additive-free soap or commercial produce wash before washing.

Since their skin provides some of their fiber and higher levels of nutrients, it is best not to peel the fruit, but to eat the entire pear. You can use an apple corer, cutting from the fruit's base, to remove the core, and then cut as desired. Once cut, pears oxidize quickly and turn a brownish color. You can help to prevent this by applying some lemon, lime, or orange juice to the flesh. For juicing, firm pears are much easier to juice than soft pears.

QUICK SERVING IDEAS

- Combine pears with mustard greens, watercress, leeks, and walnuts for a delicious salad.
- Serve grilled pears and onions on a bed of romaine lettuce dressed with olive oil and fresh rosemary.
- Add chopped pears, grated ginger, and honey to millet porridge for a pungently sweet breakfast treat.
- Core pears, stuff them with raisins and nuts, and poach them in apple juice or wine.
- Puréed stewed pears seasoned with cinnamon make a great dessert.
- Serve pears with goat or blue cheese for a delightful dessert.

SAFETY

Since pears are among the foods on which pesticide residues have been most frequently found, we recommend selecting organically grown pears. Pears are considered a hypoallergenic food, allowing them to be used in allergy elimination diets.

Pineapple

The pineapple (*Ananas comosus*) is a well-known tropical fruit that resembles a large, green pinecone, hence its name. The oval- to cylindrical-shaped fruit has a tough, waxy rind that may be dark green, yellow, orange-yellow, or reddish when the fruit is ripe. The flesh ranges from nearly white to yellow. In size, pineapples measure up to 12 inches/30 cm long and weigh 1 to 10 pounds/½ to 4½ kilograms or more. The edible flesh of the pineapple has a characteristic flavor often described as a mixture of apple, strawberry, and peach all mixed together.

HISTORY

The pineapple is native to South America. When Columbus and other explorers brought pineapples back to Europe, attempts were made to cultivate the sweet, prized fruit until it was realized that the fruit's need for a tropical climate inhibited its ability to flourish in that region. By the end of the sixteenth century, Portuguese and Spanish explorers introduced pineapples into many of their African, Asian, and South Pacific colonies. The United States ranks as one of the world's leading suppliers of pineapples, although pineapples are produced only in Hawaii, to which they were introduced in the eighteenth century. Other countries that grow pineapples commercially include Thailand, the Philippines, China, Brazil, and Mexico.

NUTRITIONAL HIGHLIGHTS

Pineapple is an excellent source of vitamin C and manganese. It is also a very good source of vitamin B1. In addition, it is a good source of vitamin B6, copper, magnesium, and dietary fiber. A 100 gram serving is about ⅔ cup of pineapple and provides 45 calories, 0.6 grams of protein, 0.1 grams of fat, 11.8 grams of carbohydrate, and 8.3 grams of natural sugars (sucrose, fructose, and glucose).

HEALTH BENEFITS

Fresh pineapple is rich in bromelain, which is made up of a group of sulphur-containing proteolytic (protein-digesting) enzymes that not only aid digestion but can effectively reduce inflammation and swelling, as in carpal tunnel syndrome; break down mucus in respiratory conditions, such as pneumonia and bronchitis; and have even been used experimentally as an anticancer agent. A variety of inflammatory agents is inhibited by the action of bromelain. In clinical human trials, bromelain has demonstrated significant anti-inflammatory effects, reducing swelling in inflammatory conditions such as acute sinusitis, sore throat, arthritis, and gout and speeding recovery from injuries and surgery. To maximize bromelain's anti-inflammatory effects, pineapple should be eaten alone between meals or its enzymes will be used up in digesting food.

Pineapple is also an excellent source of the trace mineral manganese, an essential cofactor in a number of enzymes important in energy production and antioxidant defenses. For example, the key antioxidant enzyme superoxide dismutase requires manganese. Just one cup of fresh pineapple supplies 73.1 percent of the daily value of manganese.

HOW TO SELECT AND STORE

A ripe pineapple has a fruity, fragrant aroma, is more yellow than green in color, and is heavy for its size. Avoid selecting pineapple with decayed or mouldy spots, especially at the bottom stem scar.

Pineapple can be left at room temperature for one or two days before serving. While this will not make the fruit any sweeter, it will help it to become softer and more juicy. Yet, as pineapple is very perishable, you should still watch it closely during this period to ensure that it does not spoil. After two days, if you are still not ready to consume it, you should wrap it in a perforated plastic bag and store it in the refrigerator, where it will keep for a maximum of three to five days.

Pineapple that has been cut up should be stored in an airtight container in the refrigerator, where it will keep for up to one week. It will stay fresher and retain more taste and juiciness if you also place some liquid, preferably some juice from the pineapple, in the container. Although pineapple can be frozen, this process greatly affects its flavor.

TIPS FOR PREPARING

Pineapples must be washed thoroughly before cutting. Spray them with a solution of diluted additive-free soap or commercial produce wash and then scrub them under cool running water with a vegetable brush.

After washing, the next first step in preparing a pineapple is always to remove the crown and the base of the fruit with a knife. Then, to peel the pineapple, place it base side down and carefully slice off the skin, carving out any remaining "eyes" with the tip of your knife. Or cut the pineapple into quarters, remove the core if desired, make slices into the quarters, cutting from the flesh toward the rind, and then use your knife to separate the fruit from the rind. Once the rind is removed, cut the pineapple into the desired shape and size.

QUICK SERVING IDEAS

- Eat pineapple (peeled and cut up) on its own or in fruit salads, or juice it. Pineapple is low in calories and makes a fantastic base for low-calorie fruit drinks, especially when mixed with berries.

- Pineapple is a wonderful addition to fruit salads, especially those containing other tropical fruits, such as papaya, kiwi, and papaya.

- Combine diced pineapple with chopped prawns, grated ginger, and a little olive oil. Season to taste and serve on a bed of romaine lettuce.

- Mix diced pineapple, tomatoes, and chili peppers for an easy-to-prepare salsa that is an exceptional complement to fish, such as halibut, tuna, and salmon.

- Drizzle maple syrup on pineapple slices and grill until brown. Serve plain or with yogurt.

- Chopped pineapple, grated fennel, and cashew nuts go well together and are especially delicious as a side dish to chicken.

- Pineapple goes well with virtually all vegetables and meat on the grill. Add some to your next shish kebab.

- Add pineapple to your next homemade pizza. This combination is a favorite with children and adults alike.

SAFETY

Pineapple is not associated with any significant safety issues. It is a hypoallergenic food often used in allergy avoidance diets.

Plantains: See Bananas.

Plums

The plum *(Prunus domestica)* is a relative of the peach, nectarine, and almond. Like these other drupes, plums contain a hard pit or stone surrounded by soft, pulpy flesh and a thin skin. Dried plums are referred to as prunes (see "Prunes").

While more than 200 varieties of plums exist, there are six main categories: Japanese, American, Damson, ornamental, wild, and European/garden. Plums vary in size, shape, and color, depending upon the variety. They may be as small as a cherry or as large as a peach, and although usually round, plums can also be oval or heart-shaped. The skins of plums can be red, purple, blue-black, red, green, yellow, or amber, while their flesh comes in hues of yellow, green, pink, and orange—a virtual rainbow.

HISTORY

Plums are native in China, America, Europe, and the Caucasus Mountains region. Greek writers mention cultivated plums as originally being imported to Greece from Syria. The Romans introduced the fruit into northern Europe. They were also reinforced, in the twelfth century, when the Crusaders brought trees back from their journeys to Syria. In 1864, there were 150 cultivated varieties. They were brought to western and eastern North America by Spanish missionaries and English colonists.

The species that originated in China have been cultivated for thousands of years. The plum was taken to Japan 200 to 400 years ago, and there it thrived. This is the reason it is somewhat falsely called the "Japanese" plum. From Japan, it then moved to many other areas of the world. There are four main types of cultivated, edible plums: European, Japanese, Damsons/Mirabelles, and "cherry plums." Japanese plums are larger and heartier than European plums.

The main producers of commercially grown plums today are the Russian Federation, China, Romania, and the United States.

NUTRITIONAL HIGHLIGHTS

Plums are a very good source of vitamin C. They are also a good source of vitamins B1, B2, and B6, phenolic compounds, and dietary fiber. A 100 gram serving is a little less than 2 plums and provides 46 calories, 0.7 grams of protein, 0.3 grams of fat, and 11.4 grams of carbohydrate, with 1.4 grams of fiber and 9.9 grams of natural sugars (glucose, fructose, and sucrose).

HEALTH BENEFITS

Plums and prunes are often used for their laxative effects. However, prunes are more effective than plums in this capacity (see "Prunes"). Plums are also good sources of neochlorogenic and chlorogenic acid, two related compounds classified as phenols that have well-documented antioxidant and anticancer effects.

HOW TO SELECT AND STORE

With more than 200 varieties of plums, there is a considerable variety in color. Hence, it is important to pick a plum based on the knowledge of its varietal color. Regardless of color, a ripe plum should yield to gentle pressure, especially at the end opposite the stem. Good-quality ripe plums should have a distinctively plummy, sweet fragrance. Although you can buy plums that are firm, in order to have them properly ripen at home, you should avoid those that are markedly

hard because they probably are too immature and will not develop a good taste and texture. Last, avoid plums that have skin damage or discoloration or are mushy.

Plums that are not yet ripe can be left at room temperature. As this fruit tends to mature quickly, check on them within one to two days to ensure that they do not become overripe. Once they are ripe, plums can be stored in the refrigerator, where they will keep for a few days. While plums can be frozen, to ensure maximum taste, remove their pits before placing them in the freezer, where they will keep for up to six months.

TIPS FOR PREPARING

Wash organically grown plums gently by hand under cool running water and pat them dry. Nonorganic plums should be sprayed with a solution of diluted additive-free soap or commercial produce wash and then washed gently under cool running water, then patted dry. Plums are delicious eaten as is. If the plums have been in the refrigerator, allow them to approach room temperature before consuming them as this will help them attain their maximum juiciness and sweetness. If you want to remove the pit, cut the plum in half lengthwise, gently twist the halves in opposite directions, and then carefully take out the pit.

Plums can also be used in a variety of recipes and are usually baked or poached. If you want to remove the skin, this process can be made easier by first blanching the plum in boiling water for 30 seconds. Once you remove the plum from the water, quickly run cold water over it before peeling in order to stop the blanching process and allow for easier handling.

QUICK SERVING IDEAS

- Eat plums whole or in fruit salads, or juice them. Plums are fairly harsh if juiced alone, but they mix very well with pears.
- Make pizza with a twist by grilling sliced plums, goat cheese, walnuts, and sage on top of a whole-wheat (wholemeal) pita bread or pizza crust.
- For a delightful dessert, poach plums in red wine and serve with lemon zest.
- Bake pitted plum halves at 200 degrees F./95 degrees C./gas ¼ until they are wrinkled. Then mix them into a rye bread recipe for a scrumptiously sweet and hardy bread.
- Toss cooked brown rice, diced plums, and spinach in a sesame oil-tamari dressing for a refreshing summer salad.
- Blend stewed plums and combine with yogurt and honey for a wonderful cold soup.

SAFETY

Plums contain moderate levels of oxalate. Individuals with a history of calcium oxalate-containing kidney stones should limit their consumption of this food. See page 793 for more information.

Pomelo: See Grapefruit.

Prunes

A prune is a dried plum, just as a raisin is a dried grape. The most popular varieties, including the Agen and Italian varieties, are made from dried European plums.

HISTORY

The process of drying plums to make prunes originated near the Caspian Sea, in the same region where European plums originated thousands of years ago. With the migration of various cultures and peoples, the prunes spread throughout Europe and consequently traveled to the New World.

Californians, who are the leading producers of prunes worldwide, bolstered the plum-drying process in 1856 after Louis Pellier brought a grafted plum tree from his native France. The principal variety was the Agen, which was extremely well suited to this drying process.

To produce prunes, plums are dehydrated in hot air at 185 to 195 degrees F./85 to 90 degrees C. for approximately eighteen hours. It is after this point that the prune is further processed into juice, purée, or other products.

NUTRITIONAL HIGHLIGHTS

Prunes are a very good source of provitamin A and phenolic compounds. They are also a good source of potassium, thiamine, riboflavin, vitamin B6, boron, and dietary fiber. A 100 gram serving equals about ten to twelve prunes and provides 240 calories, 2.2 grams of protein, 0.4 grams of fat, and 63.9 grams of carbohydrate, with 7.1 grams of fiber and 38.1 grams of natural sugars (glucose and fructose), as well as 732 milligrams of potassium.

HEALTH BENEFITS

A healthy high-energy snack, prunes provide antioxidants, calcium, magnesium, potassium, fiber, iron, and vitamin A that may help reduce the risk of chronic diseases. For example, prunes are notorious for preventing and relieving constipation. The prune provides bulk to stools and decreases transit time. The insoluble fiber in prunes provides food for "good" bacteria in the large intestine. When the "good" bacteria use this insoluble fiber, they produce butyric acid, which is a short-chain fatty acid that is the primary fuel for intestinal cells to maintain a healthy colon. These bacteria also form other short-chain fatty acids, such as acetic and propionic acid, that are used as cellular fuel in the liver and muscles. Additionally, prunes contain a large amount of phenolic compounds (184 milligrams per 100 grams). These compounds, mainly neochlorogenic and chlorogenic acids, act as antioxidants to "bad" LDL cholesterol and thereby may act to protect the heart against disease.

An investigation of the blood of fifty-eight postmenopausal (approximately three to five years postmenopause) women who ate approximately twelve prunes per day for three months revealed the presence of enzymes and growth factors that indicated increased bone formation in their bodies. These markers were not seen in women who did not eat prunes. Furthermore, none of the women in the study suffered any negative gastrointestinal side effects. Last, a single 100 gram serving of prunes fulfills the RDA requirement for boron (2 to 3 milligrams). (There is no RDA for boron in the U.K.) Boron is a trace mineral essential for bone metabolism and is a necessary factor in preventing osteoporosis.

HOW TO SELECT AND STORE

Choose prunes that are blemish-free and have bluish-black skin. They should be moist and somewhat flexible. Packages should be tightly sealed to ensure freshness and minimize moisture loss. Whole prunes with pits are usually less expensive than pitted prunes. Again, as with any dried fruit, it is healthier to choose those without preservatives such as sulphur dioxide. Store prunes in a tightly sealed container to retain moisture in a cool, dry place. They will keep for several months. To maximize freshness, prunes can be stored in the refrigerator for about six months.

TIPS FOR PREPARING

If you have prunes that are extremely dry, soaking them in hot water for a few minutes will help to refresh them. If you are planning on cooking the prunes, soaking them in water or juice beforehand will reduce the cooking time.

QUICK SERVING IDEAS

- Serve stewed prunes with rosemary-scented braised lamb, and enjoy this Middle Eastern-inspired meal.
- Purée stewed prunes. Season them with cinnamon, ground coriander, and honey, and serve with plain yogurt.
- Serve stewed or soaked prunes on top of pancakes and waffles.
- Combine diced, dried prunes with other dried fruits and nuts to make homemade trail mix.
- Prunes make a delicious addition to poultry stuffing.

SAFETY

Prunes contain moderate levels of oxalates. Individuals with a history of calcium oxalate-containing kidney stones should limit their consumption of this food. See page 793 for more information.

Raisins

Raisins are made by dehydrating grapes *(Vitis vinifera)*. The size and shape of small pebbles, raisins have wrinkled skins surrounding chewy flesh that tastes like a burst of sugary sweetness. Raisins are produced via one of three commercially used methods: sun-dried (natural), artificially dried (dipped), and sulphur dioxide-treated (golden) raisins. Among the most popular types of raisins are sultana, Malaga, Monukka, Zante currant, muscat, and Thompson seedless. Although the colors of raisins vary, they are generally a deep brown color.

HISTORY

It's probably safe to say that raisins were discovered by humans the first time they found them accidentally dried out on the vine. But it took several hundreds of years before they determined which of the 8,000 varieties of the grape genus would produce the best raisins.

Historians inform us that the ancient Phoenicians and Armenians took the first steps in perfecting viticulture, the process of grape growing and selection. Between 120 and 900 B.C.E., the Phoenicians started vineyards in Spain and Greece. Concurrently, the Armenians founded vineyards in present-day Turkey, Iran, and Iraq. These growing areas had the perfect climate for making raisins and were conveniently close to Greece and Rome, the first markets for raisins. In ancient Rome, raisins were adorned in places of worship, used as barter currency, and given as prizes for sporting events.

Grapes have flourished in the New World, in Mexico and California, since the nineteenth century. However, it wasn't until 1851 that a profitable muscat raisin was grown near San Diego. As it turned out, San Diego was not ideal for raisin growing. Although it was fortunate to have plenty of sunshine during the summer months, it lacked sufficient water to support large vineyards. Farmers then moved north, searching for a perfect spot to grow their raisins, and discovered the sun of the San Joaquin Valley. The San Joaquin Valley has ample sunshine, a long, hot growing season, and a copious water supply from the Sierra Nevada, which makes it one of the most fertile valleys in the world. As a result, the San Joaquin Valley soon became the center of the California raisin industry.

The other leading world producers of raisins are Australia, Turkey, Greece, Iran, and Chile.

NUTRITIONAL HIGHLIGHTS

Raisins are an excellent source of the trace mineral boron. They are also a very good source of antioxidants and dietary fiber and a good source of vitamins B1 and B6. A 100 gram serving is about ⅔ cup, not packed, and provides 299 calories, 3.1 grams of protein, 0.5 grams of fat, and 79.2 grams of carbohydrate, with 3.7 grams of fiber and 59.2 grams of natural sugars (fructose and glucose), as well as 1.9 grams of iron and 749 milligrams of potassium.

HEALTH BENEFITS

Raisins, like prunes, are often recommended to promote bowel regularity due to their high fiber content. However, a possible new use for raisins is as an alternative to sodium nitrite, a preservative commonly used in bacon, beef jerky, prepared lunch meats, and ham. Sodium nitrite has been found to break down into cancer-causing chemicals known as nitrosamines during digestion. Food science researchers at Oregon State University have shown that ground-up raisins are an excellent substitute for sodium nitrite. In addition to inhibiting bacterial growth, raisins bring multiple nutritional benefits to products traditionally preserved with sodium nitrite because they are high in antioxidants and have lots of fiber.

In blind taste tests, a scientific panel in Oregon State University's Sensory Research Laboratory in Corvallis evaluated raisin jerky, typical commercial-type jerky made with sodium nitrite, and jerky made without any preservatives. The three types of jerky (an ancient way of preserving meat by sun-drying) were evaluated for flavor, texture, chewiness, overall liking, and appearance. Panelists ranked the 10 percent raisin jerky as superior to the sodium nitrite control and the preservative-free jerky in terms of overall liking, flavor, texture, and appearance. The panelists said the sweet and tangy flavor imparted by the raisins was pleasing and that it made the jerky seem less salty.

HOW TO SELECT AND STORE

If possible, purchase raisins that are sold in bulk or in transparent containers so that you can judge their quality, checking to see that they are moist and undamaged. When buying raisins in a sealed, opaque container, make sure that the container is tightly sealed and that the raisins are produced or packaged by a reputable company.

Storing raisins in the refrigerator in an airtight container will extend their freshness and prevent them from becoming dried out. If you purchase raisins in single serving boxes and do not want to transfer them to another container, store the boxes in the refrigerator to extend their shelf life. Raisins stored in this manner can be kept for up to one year.

TIPS FOR PREPARING

Raisins that are fresh and have been stored properly will require no special attention prior to eating them or using them in a recipe. To restore dried-out raisins before adding them to a recipe, place them in a bowl covered with a little hot water for a few minutes; you can even use the nutrient-infused liquid in the recipe. Raisins that are stuck together can be more easily separated by heating them on a baking tray at 275 degrees F./140 degrees C./gas 1 for a few minutes.

QUICK SERVING IDEAS

- Raisins are a great addition to homemade granola or can be sprinkled over any breakfast cereal, hot or cold.
- Soak raisins and other dried fruits in water to soften for an easy-to-make compote that is so versatile it can be served a variety of ways. Some of our favorites include serving the compote on top of grilled chicken or layering it with plain yogurt to make a dessert parfait.
- Raisins go well in most baked goods. Add them to bread, muffins, and cookies.

- Add raisins, almonds, peppers, and onions to brown rice to make a tasty side dish.
- Raisins' sweetness and texture make them a great addition to poultry stuffing.
- Mix raisins with your favorite nuts for a high-energy, protein- and fiber-packed homemade snack or trail mix.

SAFETY

Since grapes, from which raisins are made, are among the foods on which pesticide residues have been most frequently found, we recommend choosing organic, unsulphured varieties.

Raisins contain small amounts of oxalates. Individuals with a history of calcium oxalate-containing kidney stones should limit their consumption of them. See page 793 for more information.

Raspberries

The raspberry (Rubus idaeus) is known as an "aggregate fruit" since it is made up of seed-containing fruits, called "drupelets," arranged around a hollow central cavity. While the most common type of raspberry is red-pink in color, raspberries actually come in a range of colors, including black, purple, orange, yellow, and white. Both loganberries and boysenberries are hybrids of raspberries.

HISTORY

Wild raspberries are native to eastern Asia and the Western Hemisphere and have been consumed as food since prehistoric times. Raspberries began to be cultivated widely in Europe and North America in the nineteenth century, when many new varieties, such as the loganberry and boysenberry, were developed through either accidental or intentional cross-breeding. Currently, the leading commercial producers of raspberries are the Russian Federation, Poland, Yugoslavia, Germany, Chile, and the United States.

NUTRITIONAL HIGHLIGHTS

Raspberries are an excellent source of fiber, manganese, vitamin C, flavonoids, and ellagic acid. They are a very good source of vitamin B2 as well as a good source of other B vitamins, such as folic acid, niacin, pantothenic acid, and vitamin B6. A 100 gram serving is about ¾ cup raspberries and provides 52 calories, 1.2 grams of protein, 0.7 gram of fat, and 11.9 grams of carbohydrate, with 6.5 grams of fiber and only 4.4 grams of natural sugars (fructose and glucose).

HEALTH BENEFITS

Raspberries are an excellent low-calorie, nutrient-dense food. As such, they are an excellent food for individuals with a "sweet tooth" who are attempting to improve their quality of nutrition without increasing the caloric content of their diet. Flavonoids, mainly anthocyanidins, are responsible for the colors of raspberries as well as most of their health benefits. These flavonoids, and others, act as powerful antioxidants. Raspberries are also an excellent source of the cancer-fighting compound ellagic acid (see page 144).

HOW TO SELECT AND STORE

The prime season for raspberries is from mid-summer to early autumn. Plump raspberries that have a rich, deep color and a sweet, berry-like aroma are the most likely to be sweet and succulent. Avoid berries that have a hull attached in the center, which is a sign that they were picked before fully ripening (which makes them more tart), as well as those that are prepackaged too tightly and/or have signs of stains and moisture, for these berries are more likely to be crushed or mouldy.

Raspberries are extremely perishable. Plan on buying small quantities and using them within a day or two. Never wash berries before storing or keep them exposed to sunlight or at room temperature for too long. Remove any crushed berries, because these will mould quickly. Store in the refrigerator. The best storage to prevent crushing and spoilage is to remove them from the original container and store them in a single layer in a shallow glass dish, covered with a damp paper towel. They will keep for one to two days.

Raspberries freeze well. After washing the berries using a low-pressure sink spray if you have one, pat them dry with a paper towel. Spread them on a tray in a single layer and freeze until firm. Then transfer them to a freezer bag or airtight container. They will keep for nine months to one year. Adding a touch of lemon juice to the berries will help maintain their color while frozen. Raspberry purée can also be frozen.

TIPS FOR PREPARING

As raspberries are very delicate, place them in a colander in small amounts, wash them very gently, using the light pressure of a sink sprayer if possible, and then pat them dry. If they are not organically grown, they should be sprayed with a solution of diluted additive-free soap or commercial produce wash before being placed in the colander. They should be washed right before eating or recipe preparation so that they do not become water-soaked and are not left at room temperature for too long. Do not use any berries that are overly soft and mushy unless you will be puréeing them for a sauce or coulis.

QUICK SERVING IDEAS

- Eat raspberries whole, in a bowl as a simple dessert, or in fruit salads, or juice them.
- Add ½ cup raspberries to any protein smoothie recipe. If raspberries are not in season, use unsweetened frozen berries.

SAFETY

Raspberries contain moderate levels of oxalates. Individuals with a history of calcium oxalate-containing kidney stones should limit their consumption of them. See page 793 for more information.

Strawberries

The strawberry (*Fragaria* spp.) is the most popular type of berry fruit in the world. While there are more than 600 varieties of strawberries that differ in flavor, size, and texture, they all have the same characteristic heart shape, red flesh with yellow seeds piercing the surface, small, regal, leafy green caps, and stems that adorn their crowns.

HISTORY

The history of strawberries goes back more than 2,200 years. Native to many parts of the world, hundreds of varieties of strawberries exist due to accident and planned crossbreeding techniques. In 1714, a French engineer commissioned to Chile and Peru to monitor Spanish activities observed that the strawberry native to those regions was much larger than that in Europe. He decided to bring back samples to France to cultivate. Unfortunately, these strawberries did not grow until a natural crossbreeding occurred between this newly transported variety and a North American variety planted nearby. The end result was a large, juicy, sweet hybrid that became extremely popular in Europe.

Like many other fruits, strawberries make their claim in history as a luxury item enjoyed only by royalty. It wasn't until the mid-nineteenth century, when railways were constructed, that a more rapid means of transport developed to ship strawberries longer distances to be enjoyed by increasing numbers of people.

The United States, Canada, France, Italy, Japan, Australia, and New Zealand are among the largest commercial producers of strawberries. In the United States, strawberries have been grown in California since the early 1900s. Today, more than 25,000 acres of strawberries are planted each year in California and the state produces more than 80 percent of the strawberries grown in the United States.

NUTRITIONAL HIGHLIGHTS

Strawberries are an excellent source of vitamins C and K, dietary fiber, and flavonoids. They are also a very good source of manganese, pantothenic acid, vitamin B1, and iodine. Strawberries are also a good source of folic acid, biotin, and vitamin B6. A 100 gram serving is about ⅔ cup strawberries and provides 32 calories, 0.7 grams of protein, 0.3 grams of fat, and 7.7 grams of carbohydrate, with 2 grams of fiber and only 4.7 grams of natural sugars (glucose and fructose).

HEALTH BENEFITS

The health benefits of strawberries are due primarily to their flavonoids. As with other berries, strawberries' anthocyanidins are their most powerful flavonoids. The vibrant red color of strawberries is due to the anthocyanidin known as pelargonidin.

Strawberries' unique flavonoid content makes them a valuable protector against inflammation, cancer, and heart disease. The anti-inflammatory properties of strawberries include the ability of their flavonoids to lessen the activity of the enzyme cyclooxygenase, or COX. Nonsteroidal anti-inflammatory drugs (NSAIDs), such as aspirin and ibuprofen, block pain by blocking this enzyme, which is linked to inflammatory conditions such as rheumatoid arthritis, osteoarthritis, asthma, atherosclerosis, and cancer. Unlike drugs that are COX inhibitors, however, strawberries do not cause intestinal bleeding or heart disease.

Strawberries also have strong anticancer effects. In one study strawberries topped a list of eight foods most linked to lower rates of cancer deaths among a group of 1,271 elderly people in New Jersey. Those eating the most strawberries were one third as likely to develop cancer as those eating few or no strawberries.

HOW TO SELECT AND STORE

Strawberries are usually available all year round, though they are in greatest abundance from spring through to midsummer. Choose berries that are firm, plump, and free of mould, and that have a shiny, deep red color and attached green caps. Since strawberries, once picked, do not ripen further, avoid those that are dull in color or have green or yellow patches, since they are likely to be sour and of inferior quality.

Medium-sized strawberries are often more flavorful than those that are excessively large. If you are buying strawberries prepackaged in a container, make sure that they are not packed too tightly, as this may cause them to become crushed and damaged, and that the container has no sign of stains or moisture, as this is an indication of possible spoilage.

Like all berries, strawberries are very perishable, so great care should be taken in their handling and storage. Make sure not to leave strawberries at room temperature or exposed to sunlight for too long, as this will cause them to spoil. Before storing in the refrigerator, remove any strawberries that are moulded or damaged so that they will not contaminate others. Replace unwashed and unhulled berries in their original container or spread them out on a plate lined with a paper towel, then cover with cling film. Strawberries will keep fresh in the refrigerator for one to two days.

To freeze strawberries, first gently wash them and pat them dry. You can either remove the caps and stems or leave them intact, depending upon what you will do with them once they are thawed. Arrange them in a single layer on a baking tray and place them in the freezer. Once frozen, transfer the berries to a heavy plastic bag and return them to the freezer, where they will keep for up to one year. Adding a bit of lemon juice to the berries will help to preserve their color while frozen. While strawberries can be frozen whole, sliced, or crushed, they will retain more of their vitamin C content if left whole.

TIPS FOR PREPARING

Wash organically grown strawberries by placing them in a colander, then rinsing them with cool water. If nonorganic, they should be sprayed with a solution of diluted additive-free soap or commercial produce wash before placing them in the colander. As strawberries are very delicate, wash them very gently, using the light pressure of a sink sprayer if possible, and then pat them dry. They should be washed right before eating or recipe preparation so that they do not become water-soaked and are not left at room temperature for too long. To remove the stems, caps, and white hull, simply pinch them off with your fingers or use a paring knife.

QUICK SERVING IDEAS

- Eat strawberries whole or in fruit salads, or juice them.
- Add ½ cup fresh strawberries to your favorite protein smoothie. If strawberries are not in season, use unsweetened frozen berries instead.
- Add sliced strawberries to mixed green salads.
- Layer sliced strawberries, whole blueberries, and plain yogurt in a wineglass to make a parfait dessert.
- Mix chopped strawberries with cinnamon, lemon juice, and maple syrup, and serve as a topping for waffles and pancakes.
- Blend strawberries with a little bit of orange juice and use as a refreshing coulis on grilled chicken and prawns.

SAFETY

Strawberries are one of the foods most commonly associated with allergic reactions. For a description of common signs and symptoms of food allergies, see page 723.

Strawberries contain moderate levels of

oxalates. Individuals with a history of calcium oxalate-containing kidney stones should limit their consumption of them. See page 793 for more information.

Since strawberries are among the foods most commonly associated with pesticide residues, we encourage you to select organically grown strawberries.

Tangerines: See Oranges.

Watermelon

The watermelon *(Citrullus lanatus)* ranges in size from a few pounds to upward of 90 pounds/40 kilograms. It is a member of the Cucurbitaceae family, along with cantaloupe, squash, pumpkin, and other plants that grow on vines on the ground. The watermelon most commonly consumed is round, oblong, or spherical in shape and light to dark green in color, with white stripes or mottling. Its flesh is bright red, and it has dark brown or black seeds. The flesh may also be pink, orange, yellow, or white; the seeds can be brown, white, green, or yellow; and a few varieties are actually seedless.

HISTORY

Watermelons are native to the Kalahari Desert of southern Africa. The first recorded watermelon crop was found in Egypt, as it was depicted in hieroglyphics on tomb walls dating back as far as 3000 B.C.E. Being held in such high regard, watermelons were left as food to nourish the dead in the afterlife.

From Egypt, watermelons spread throughout countries along the Mediterranean Sea by way of merchants. They were documented in China in the tenth century, and in the thirteenth century they were introduced to the rest of Europe by the Moors. Ultimately, the watermelon crossed the Atlantic Ocean and made its way to North America with the African slaves. It wasn't until 1615, however, that the word "watermelon" first appeared in the English dictionary.

Presently, the Russian Federation grows much of the commercial supply of watermelon. People there even make a very popular wine of watermelons. The other world watermelon-producing leaders are China, Turkey, Iran, and the United States.

NUTRITIONAL HIGHLIGHTS

Watermelon has an extremely high water content, approximately 92 percent. It is very low in calories, with one cup (154 grams) of watermelon containing only 48 calories, yet is still a very good source of vitamin C, beta-carotene, and lycopene. In fact, one cup of watermelon provides 19.5 percent of the daily value of vitamin C and, through its beta-carotene, 13.9 percent of the daily value of vitamin A. It is also a good source of vitamins B1 and B6, pantothenic acid, biotin, magnesium, potassium, and dietary fiber.

HEALTH BENEFITS

Watermelon, as its name implies, is a good source of pure water and an excellent diuretic. Because it has such a high water content and lower calorie content than many other fruits, it delivers more nutrients per calorie, which is an outstanding health benefit. It is packed with some of the most important antioxidants in nature, including lycopene—the red carotenoid pigment that also gives tomatoes their red color.

HOW TO SELECT AND STORE

People tap on watermelons to determine if they sound hollow and are therefore ripe; however, this practice does not always meet with success. Instead, look for watermelons that have a smooth surface and a cream-colored underbelly. Despite the best precautions, however, it is difficult to judge the quality of a watermelon without cutting it in half. When cut, indicators of a good watermelon include firm, juicy red flesh and dark brown to black seeds. The presence of white streaks in the flesh or white seeds usually indicates immaturity.

Watermelons should be refrigerated in order to best preserve their freshness, taste, and juiciness. If the whole watermelon does not fit in your refrigerator, cut it into pieces (as few as possible), and cover them with cling film to prevent them from becoming dried out and from absorbing the odors of other foods.

TIPS FOR PREPARING

Melons grow resting on the ground, which means their rinds can become contaminated by animal or human waste, or contamination can be transferred from the harvesters' or other handler's hands to the melon. Unless the skin is thoroughly cleansed, the knife used to halve a melon can transfer pathogens, such as *Salmonella,* directly onto the flesh. For this reason, all melons should be sprayed with a solution of diluted additive-free soap or commercial produce wash. Due to its large size, you will probably not be able to rinse a watermelon under water in the sink. Instead, wash it with a wet cloth or paper towel. Be sure also to wash surfaces that have come into contact with the unwashed melon, such as hands and cutting boards.

Depending upon the size you desire, there are many ways to cut a watermelon. The flesh can be sliced, cubed, or scooped into balls. Watermelon is delicious to eat as is, but it also makes a delightful addition to a fruit salad. In addition, jam, sorbet, and juice are some nutritious and delicious things you can make with watermelon. Moreover, while many people are accustomed to eating only the juicy flesh, both the seeds and the rind are also edible.

QUICK SERVING IDEAS

- Watermelon can be eaten on its own, used in fruit salads, or juiced.
- Freeze puréed watermelon in ice cube trays. Once frozen, gently blend in a food processor to create a frozen granita dessert treat.
- In Asian countries, roasted watermelon seeds are either seasoned and eaten as a snack food or ground up into cereal and used to make bread.
- A featured item of southern American cooking, the rind of watermelon can be marinated, pickled, or candied.
- Purée watermelon, cantaloupe, and kiwifruit together. Swirl in a little plain yogurt, and serve as a refreshing cold soup.

SAFETY

Since melons, in general, are among the foods on which pesticide residues have been most frequently found, we recommend buying organically grown melons.

The Healing Power of Grains

Grains are without question the most important food crop in the world, literally the "staff of life" for most people on this planet. Historically, grains have fueled the growth of civilization, and as the earth's population continues to grow, our reliance on grains is greater than ever.

A grain is most often the seed of a member of the grass family and is often referred to as a "cereal" grain. The word "cereal" is derived from Ceres, the Roman goddess of agriculture. Grains were among the first cultivated crops. In fact, archaeological evidence shows that wheat and barley were used more than 10,000 years ago by people living in the Fertile Crescent, a broad crescent-shaped area that curved northward and eastward from what is now the eastern border of Egypt, to the Taurus Mountains of southern Turkey, across to the Zagros Mountains of western Iran, and down to the Persian Gulf. By about 5000 B.C.E., grain farming was also well established along the Nile in Egypt. Since dried grains store well, it is not surprising that their cultivation spread from the Fertile Crescent as people traveled to new lands.

Other areas of the world began grain farming a bit later. By 4000 B.C.E., millet farming was well established along the upper Yellow River in China. At about the same time, rice was being cultivated in Southeast Asia. Rice was originally believed to have been first cultivated in China around 6,000 years ago, but recent archaeological discoveries have found primitive rice seeds and ancient farm tools dating back about 9,000 years.

The cultivation of grains and development of grain foods, such as bread, contributed greatly to the growth of civilization. Without grains it is unlikely that civilization would have developed the way that it has. Several factors promoted the spread of grain cultivation: (1) an increase in population; (2) changes in climate; (3) the domestication of animals; and (4) the development of commerce.

The creation of a consistent food supply

through agriculture led to an increase in the population of early villages. The improved nutrition led to not only increased reproduction but reproduction of healthier people better equipped to deal with the environment. As the population of a village increased, more land was needed for farming, and people were often forced to seek out new areas to farm. Also, as the land changed, so did the natural habitat and culture. This created an increased dependence on farming, which in turn required inhabitants of villages to work together in a cooperative manner. It is noteworthy that every major densely populated ancient civilization throughout the world developed because its people were largely grain farmers.

Climatic events obviously played a major role in the development of grain agriculture, too. Of particular significance was the global warming between 5500 and 3000 B.C.E. that resulted in the melting of much of the polar ice caps and mountain glaciers. The rising sea level would have forced many grain farmers in low-lying areas to migrate to places of higher elevations, while the melting of mountain glaciers allowed some of the grain farmers to migrate northward to central Europe.

Also important to the spread of grain cultivation was the domestication of animals. Animals such as the ox, donkey, and camel were used to help till the soil and carry the harvested grain. This led, in turn, to increased commerce.

The Green Revolution

In ancient times, as the population of a village grew, so did its dependence on grains. Today, as we experience a global population explosion, our dependence upon grains as food is greater than ever. Throughout history, improvements in farming techniques and the development of improved hybrids (crossbreeds) of specific grains have led to better crop yields. However, since there is not much farmland left, there is an ever-growing need for even better utilization of farmland to feed the world's population. The so-called Green Revolution refers to recent breakthroughs in agriculture that have the potential to double or triple the supply of grains and other foods for the world's expanding population and, more immediately, the developing countries of the world. We are in the midst of this Green Revolution.

The "father" of the Green Revolution is considered to be Norman Borlaug, an American agricultural scientist who in 1970 was awarded the Nobel Peace Prize for his breeding of higher-yielding varieties of wheat at the International Maize and Wheat Improvement Center in Mexico. Borlaug's wheat, a hybrid, or offspring, of wheat varieties from the United States, the Russian Federation, Japan, and Mexico, has numerous favorable traits, such as short stature of the wheat stalk, which prevents the wheat from growing too tall and falling or breaking; an increased number of grains per plant; strong resistance to disease; and improved tolerance to the environment.

These same sorts of improvements have been made in rice, most notably by the International Rice Research Institute in the Philippines, which in 1968 released the IR-8 rice strain. This "miracle" rice is a cross between a Chinese semi-dwarf strain and a tall Indonesian strain that yields three times the amount of grain as the older types. Originally the IR-8 strain was a bit chalky, with a strange taste; however, these defects have been overcome and other improvements made by further breeding.

The Green Revolution is not limited to grains, and improvements are continually being made in the production of all crops. However, in terms of satisfying the world's food requirements, grains and legumes are viewed as the greatest prospects. The two foods work well together in many respects. For example, their amino acid patterns complement each other in such a way that the shortcomings of one are compensated for by the other. Specifically, the low lysine content of grains is compensated for by the high lysine content of legumes, while the low methionine and cysteine content of many legumes is compensated for by the higher methionine and cysteine content of grains. Furthermore, certain legumes, such as peanuts and soybeans, convert nitrogen gas from the air to soil nitrogen, making the soil suitable for planting grains. After the grains have depleted the nitrogen, the legumes can once again be planted to renourish the soil with nitrogen. Eventually, the Green Revolution will likely produce grains and legumes that will yield even higher quality protein.

Whole Versus Refined Grains

The following illustration and description of a grain of wheat are representative of all grains, as the anatomy or structure of all grains is basically the same.

The bran is composed of tissues between the outer seed coat and the aleurone, which is the

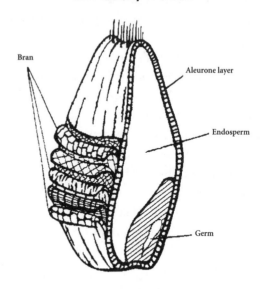

FIGURE 12.1

The Anatomy of Wheat

Bran

Aleurone layer

Endosperm

Germ

granular protein layer in the outermost layer of endosperm. The endosperm, the storage compartment of the grain, is composed primarily of protein and carbohydrates. The germ contains the embryo or sprouting section of the grain.

In the production of flour, the bran, aleurone layer, and germ are typically removed, leaving only the endosperm. This process has both negative and positive effects. The negative effect is that removing the bran and germ results in the loss of many key nutrients (see Table 12.1).

So why are these valuable nutrients removed? It results in increased shelf life. However, while this may be an important benefit in many parts of the world, it is not a significant benefit in the United States or Europe, where the delay from production to market via transportation is not significant. To compensate for the loss of nutrients, white flour is "enriched" with nutrients. Specifically, the following nutrients are added to white flour: iron, thiamine,

TABLE 12.1

Nutrients Lost When the Bran and Germ Are Removed from Wheat

Nutrient	Percentage Lost
Thiamine	97%
Vitamin B6	94%
Niacin	88%
Chromium	87%
Magnesium	80%
Potassium	77%
Zinc	72%
Fiber	70%
Essential fatty acids	70%
Riboflavin	68%
Calcium	60%
Pantothenic acid	57%
Protein	25%

riboflavin, and niacin. The levels of these nutrients in enriched white flour are slightly higher than those found in whole-wheat flour. The addition of other nutrients is optional.

The same type of refining is done with all other whole grains. For example, the overwhelming amount of rice consumed in the world is eaten as white rice. White rice is produced by milling the rice to separate the outer portions of the grain (husk, bran, and aleurone) as well as the germ from the endosperm. After the husk, which is not present in modern wheat, is removed, the rice is sold as "brown rice," or it is milled (polished) at least three more times, removing the bran, aleurone, and germ, to produce white rice. This polishing results in a

significant loss of nutrient. Of particular importance is the loss of thiamine (vitamin B1).

A severe deficiency of thiamine results in a condition known as beriberi. Beriberi is characterized by extreme loss of appetite, congestive heart failure, water retention, psychosis (disorientation, hallucinations, loss of memory, etc.), muscle pain, and other symptoms of disturbed nerve function. Beriberi was relatively common in the general population of Asia, and, globally, in sailors and in prison populations. Prior to the late 1890s, the cause of beriberi was not known. The first clue occurred in 1873, when a Dutch naval doctor observed that European crew members had significantly fewer cases of beriberi than sailors recruited from the East Indies. When the amount of white rice in the diet of the East Indies sailors was decreased, the rate of beriberi was decreased, but it was thought that beriberi was caused by some toxin or infectious agent in the white rice. Kanehiro Takaki, a Japanese naval doctor, was the first to report that beriberi seemed to be a nutritional deficiency based on reducing the incidence of beriberi in Japanese sailors by giving them additional meat, dry milk, and vegetables. The Dutch physician Christaan Eijkman's classic experiments in the 1890s began to clarify the role of diet in the development of beriberi.

Eijkman noticed that when fowl were fed a diet solely consisting of polished white rice, they developed symptoms similar to beriberi. By adding rice polishings, the material removed from whole rice to produce white rice, to the feed, Eijkman was able to cure the fowl of beriberi. His associate later demonstrated that the addition of green peas, green beans, and meat could prevent beriberi in fowl and deduced correctly that there was something in natural foodstuffs that prevented beriberi. In 1911, Funk, working at the Lister Institute in London, isolated from rice polishings what he considered the substance that would cure/prevent beriberi. Funk termed his discovery a "vitamine." What Funk actually isolated, however, turned out to be the antipellagra vitamin, or niacin (vitamin B3). In 1926, pure thiamine, the true anti-beriberi vitamin, was isolated by two Dutch scientists, Barend Jansen and W. F. Donath, working in Java. Today, white rice is often enriched with thiamine and other nutrients lost during milling. However, beriberi is still prevalent in many parts of Asia, where white rice supplies up to 80 percent of the total calories. Beriberi and many other nutrient deficiencies in developing-world countries could be prevented if the people simply ate whole grains.

The story of beriberi and the discovery of thiamine highlights the value of whole grains over polished grains. In addition to many known nutrients, whole grains provide substantially more phytochemicals, and possibly many unknown compounds with health-promoting properties as well. Instead of removing natural nutrients from the grains and then adding back a small portion of their synthetic counterparts, wouldn't it make more sense to eat whole grains?

Whole grains are a major source of complex carbohydrates, dietary fiber, minerals, and B vitamins. The protein content and quality of whole grains are greater than that of refined grains. Diets rich in whole grains have been shown to be protective against the development of chronic degenerative diseases, especially cancer, heart disease, diabetes, and varicose veins; and diseases of the colon, including colon cancer, inflammatory bowel disease, hemorrhoids, and diverticulitis. More specifically, the ability of whole-grain foods to improve insulin sensitivity may be an important mechanism through which whole grains reduce the risk of type 2 diabetes and heart disease. A recent Harvard Medical School study involved having eleven overweight or obese subjects follow a diet that included six to ten servings a day of breakfast cereal, bread, rice, pasta, muffins, cookies, and snacks. For six weeks, subjects received these foods made from whole grains; then, for another six-week period, they ate the same foods, but this time the foods were made from refined grains. After each six-week trial period, subjects consumed a liquid mixed meal, after which their blood samples were taken over a two-hour period.

In contrast to the refined-grain diet, after the whole-grain diet, not only was the subjects' fasting insulin 10 percent lower, but two hours after the meal, their insulin curve was lower, which means that they secreted less insulin. In addition, a test performed the next day found that their rate of glucose infusion was higher, showing that more glucose was being delivered to cells for use as energy.

Preparation and Uses of Whole Grains

Perhaps the healthiest manner in which to enjoy the nutritional benefits of whole grains is simply by boiling or steaming them. This can be done with the help of a double boiler or grain steamer. However, the most common method is to bring the appropriate amount of water (see chart below) to boil in a pot with a fitted lid, add the appropriate amount of whole grain, bring to a boil again, reduce the heat, cover, and simmer for the appropriate amount of time.

Whole grains are excellent foods because they are low in calories, high in fiber, and high in complex carbohydrates. Since cooking whole grains in water results in a tremendous increase in their water content, they are quite satiating due to their high bulk. Whole grains can be used as breakfast cereals, inside dishes or casseroles, or as part of a main entrée.

TABLE 12.2

Guide to Cooking Grains

Grain	Cups of Boiling Water, Juice, or Stock to 1 Cup of Grain	Cooking Time	Yield (Cups)
Amaranth seeds	2½–3	20–25 minutes	2½
Barley, flakes	2	30–40 minutes	2½
Barley, hulled	3	1 hour, 15 minutes	3½
Barley, pearl	3	50–60 minutes	3½
Buckwheat	2	15 minutes	2½
Cornmeal (fine grind)	4–4½	8–10 minutes	2½
Cornmeal (polenta, coarse, grits)	4–4½	20–25 minutes	2½
Millet, hulled	3–4	20–25 minutes	3½
Oats, bran*	2½	5 minutes	2
Oat groats*	3	40–50 minutes	3½
Oats, rolled	2	15 minutes	2½
Oats, steel-cut	2	30 minutes	2½
Quinoa*	2	15–20 minutes	2¾
Rice, brown basmati	2½	35–40 minutes	3
Rice, brown, long-grain	2½	45–55 minutes	3
Rice, brown, quick	1¼	10 minutes	2
Rice, brown, short-grain	2–2½	45–55 minutes	3
Rice, wild	3	50–60 minutes	4
Rye, grains or cracked grain	3–4	1 hour	3
Rye, flakes	2	10–15 minutes	3

* Add to *cold* water, bring to a boil, and simmer.

(continued on next page)

Grain	Cups of Boiling Water, Juice, or Stock to 1 Cup of Grain	Cooking Time	Yield (Cups)
Sorghum	2½	45–55 minutes	3
Spelt, kernels	3	1 hour	2½
Triticale, whole grains	3	1 hour, 45 minutes	2½
Triticale, rolled (flakes) or cracked	2	15 minutes	2½
Wheat, bulgur	2	15 minutes	2½
Wheat, couscous	1	5 minutes	2
Wheat, cracked	2	20–25 minutes	2¼
Wheat, whole grains	3	2 hours	2½

* Add to *cold* water, bring to a boil, and simmer.

The Major Food Grains

While there are more than 8,000 different species of plants that supply grains, only a handful play a significant role in the human diet. The major food grains are corn, oats, rice, and wheat. They are discussed first, followed by brief descriptions of some of the more popular minor food grains.

Corn (Maize)

Covered by a husk and protected by "corn silk," corn grows as rows of kernels. Although corn is typically yellow, there are many variations, including whitish yellow, red, pink, blue, and even black, and these colors may be solid, mottled, or striped. The best corn is fresh, for it retains its juicy flavor. After picking, changes in the fluid content of the corn's starch decrease its moisture content, and it also loses some sweetness. Like many other grains, as it dries, it becomes hard and devoid of water.

There is some confusion over the use of the word "corn." Technically a grain, most of the world refers to corn as "maize," an appellation that reflects its Latin name, *Zea mays*. The confusion comes because many parts of the globe use the term "corn" to reflect the popular grain of that area. For instance, the English refer to wheat as "corn"; what American people call oats, the Irish and Scottish call "corn." In parts of Germany, the German word *Korn* means "rye." For our purposes, we will use the American meaning.

Well-known corn products include grits and polenta. Grits are made from ground corn. This form of corn is less nutritious since the germ and bran of the corn have been removed. This is why grits are commonly found as an enriched product, meaning that some vitamins and minerals are added back in. Cooked cornmeal is known as polenta and is often eaten by itself or used as a substitute for pasta.

HISTORY

The earliest uses of corn date back to approximately 5000 B.C.E. in the areas of today's Central America or possibly Mexico. Native Americans and early colonists alike found corn to be an important staple of their diet and ability to live.

Pellagra, a disease characterized by fatigue, skin rashes, and digestive tract inflammation, is caused by a deficiency of niacin, also known as vitamin B3. People who have a diet that is dominated by corn run the risk of developing pellagra, for the niacin in corn is not readily absorbable. Keenly observing this condition, the Native Americans learned to serve corn with a little limestone that had been burned into ash. Although these ingenious people did not know exactly why this was necessary, they did note that people who ingested this ash with the corn foods were indeed healthier than those who did not. Today we realize that limestone ash, known as potash, helps liberate this important B vitamin so the body can absorb it properly. Although the explorers of the New World marveled at the bounteous rows of corn growing

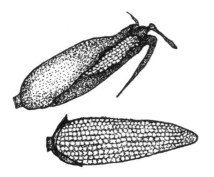

throughout the Americas, they did not pay attention to how the natives prepared this food. As a result, many settlers fell victim to pellagra.

First taken to China in the 1550s, the popularity of corn grew in places where rice could not be well cultivated. As a result, corn became an important factor in the population growth in the 1700s. The American breakfast staple of the cornflake was first introduced around 1907. Today, the largest commercial producers of corn include the United States, China, the Russian Federation, Brazil, and Mexico.

NUTRITIONAL HIGHLIGHTS

Although a healthy food, corn by itself is not nutritionally a complete food. As discussed above, those people subsisting primarily on corn run the risk of developing pellagra, a vitamin B3 (niacin) deficiency. One way to avoid this is to eat it in tortilla form, which contain cornmeal and limestone potash together, to allow the B3 to become available for absorption. Corn is a fine source of vitamin B1 (thiamine). It also is considered a good supplier of vitamin B5 (pantothenic acid), vitamins C, E, folic acid, and the minerals magnesium and phosphorus.

Corn is considered to be low in protein content, as its levels of the amino acids lysine and tryptophan are minimal. However, it is a good source of complex carbohydrate as well as healthful essential fatty acids and fiber.

HEALTH BENEFITS

Various flavonoids and carotenes are responsible for the different colors of different varieties of corn. Among the colors valued by the Native Americans were pink, red, black, and blue, and some also had stripes and spots. The concentration of these healthy phytochemicals is found in the outer layer of the endosperm nutritive tissue in seed plants. Yellow corn, the predominant corn used today, is high in the carotenoid called lutein. Thus, yellow corn food products can protect against heart disease and macular degeneration, a condition of the eye typically seen in older age; 1.5 micrograms of lutein is found in one 100 gram serving of yellow corn.

HOW TO SELECT AND STORE

Since picked corn goes through rapid conversions from sugar to starch, whether from the farmer's market or supermarket, it is best to buy corn that has been stored in a cool environment or refrigerated. Visually inspect the corn husks, and choose those that still look fresh, with minimal drying. You can pull the husk back and down to check the kernels. If they are fresh and well hydrated, they should look turgid and tightly packed. If you pierce a kernel with your fingernail, a milky white liquid should flow out.

As with any food, it is best to buy it as fresh as possible before use. If you have to keep the corn before using, keep it in a tightly sealed plastic bag in the refrigerator. Do not remove the husk until you are ready to cook. After cooking, corn may stay in the refrigerator for up to two days. By using freezer bags, you can also freeze fresh corn for longer-term storage. Simply blanch the whole ears from 7 to 11 minutes (less for smaller corn, more for larger ears). Whole ears can be frozen for up to one year. Alternatively, you can blanch the ears for 5 minutes and then cut off the kernels and freeze just these. These kernels will keep frozen for two or three months.

Other forms of corn, such as cornmeal, grits (such as polenta), and corn flour should be kept refrigerated in airtight containers. There they will stay fresh for up to three months. Frozen products have a six-month freezer life.

TIPS FOR PREPARING

Corn on the cob can be prepared via two different methods, dry or wet. The dry method employs grilling or an oven. With these methods, you must soak the corn in water for a few minutes before cooking. The moisture will help provide steam around the kernels to cook them gently. If using a wet boiling method, dehusk the corn and add it to a pot of cold water. Turn the heat on and take the corn out when the water begins to boil. This will ensure that the corn is not overcooked. Do not add salt to the water.

Corn kernels or niblets can be purchased in cans or frozen; the frozen is preferred. Simply follow the cooking instructions on the label of either form.

Two special preparations of cornmeal that deserve comment are grits and polenta. Grits are a popular breakfast grain in the U.S. made from coarsely ground corn from which the bran and germ have been removed. Therefore, grits provide less nutrition than whole corn. Grits are often enriched, however, with vitamins and minerals lost during processing. Polenta is, simply enough, cooked cornmeal (whole or degerminated). Polenta can be eaten on its own or, better yet, substituted for pasta in recipes. For easy preparation instructions for grits and polenta, see Table 12.2, "Guide to Cooking Grains," on page 325.

QUICK SERVING IDEAS

- Corn on the cob is delicious plain or seasoned with a little organic butter, extra-virgin olive oil or linseed oil, salt and pepper, nutritional yeast, freshly squeezed lemon juice, or practically any other herbs or spices that sound good to you.
- Lightly sauté green chilis, onions, and cooked corn to create a wonderful side dish; you can also serve it cold and use as a filling to spice up your favorite sandwich.
- An ancient Incan cold salad: Combine cooked corn kernels, quinoa, tomatoes, green peppers, and red kidney beans.
- Corn is a great addition to any soup; it increases its robustness as well as its nutritional value. And any bean salad will welcome corn kernels as an addition.
- Cornmeal (or polenta) is an excellent alternative flour for pancakes, crepes, and muffins.
- Creamy corn: Gently heat 1 tablespoon of ghee or organic butter and mix in 4 teaspoons of a flour of your choice. Once it is mixed and blended, add one cup of soy or cow's milk and stir together. Place in a blender and add 1 cup cooked or frozen corn kernels. Blend well, and, if you used frozen kernels, return to the heat to warm.

SAFETY

Corn is one of the most common food allergens. For more information on food allergies, see page 723.

One of the big concerns surrounding food safety in the U.S. right now is the widespread use of genetically modified corn. The insecticidal protein the genetically modified corn was engineered to produce exhibits characteristics of known allergens. Possible health effects of this category of allergen include severe allergies and anaphylactic shock. In addition, the pollen from genetically modified corn has been shown to contaminate naturally occurring corn. More specifically, if a farmer with a one-hectare plot plants a single row with genetically modified seed, it will overtake the natural corn in only seven years. Due to the possible negative health effects of genetically modified corn, we recommend using organic corn, cornmeal, and corn flour.

Corn contains moderate to high amounts of oxalate. Individuals with a history of calcium oxalate-containing kidney stones should limit their consumption of this food. See page 793 for more information.

Oats

In terms of quantity, the oat (*Avena sativa*) is the fourth leading grain produced in the United States, behind corn, wheat, and sorghum (a grass whose seeds are used to make flour and livestock feed). In the U.K., wheat, barley and oats are the most common cereals grown, though oats and barley are used mainly as animal fodder. Oats are an important grain and are famous for their health benefits and have increasingly grown in popularity in the United States.

Although oats are hulled, this process does not strip away their bran and germ, allowing them to remain a concentrated source of their fiber and nutrients. Different types of processing are then used to produce various oat products, which are generally used to make breakfast cereals, baked goods, and stuffing. Common oat products include:

- *Oat groats:* Unflattened kernels good as breakfast cereals or in stuffings.
- *Steel-cut oats:* Produced by running oats through steel blades, which thinly slice them, creating a denser, chewier texture.
- *Old-fashioned oats:* These oats are steamed and then rolled; as a result, they have a flatter shape than do other oats.
- *Quick-cooking oats:* Similar to old-fashioned oats, but after steaming they are cut finely before rolling.
- *Instant oatmeal:* Produced by partially cooking the oats rather than simply steaming them and then rolling them very thin. Often sugar, salt, and other ingredients are added to make the finished product.
- *Oat bran:* The outer layer of the grain that resides under the hull. While oat bran is found in all whole-grain oat products, it may also be purchased as a separate product that can be added to recipes or cooked to make a hot cereal.
- *Oat flour:* A flour made from hulled oats that is used in baking and is often combined with wheat or other gluten-containing flours when making leavened bread.

HISTORY

With their Asian ancestry tracing back to the wild red oat, oats are a relative newcomer to the world grain theater and were the final major cereal grain to be cultivated, in approximately 500 B.C.E. in Europe. Due to their high perishability soon after harvesting, ancient Greeks and Romans saw oats as a type of weed suitable only for horses and barbarians. Interestingly, it was oat-eating barbarians who eventually conquered the Romans.

Oats were originally used as a medicine and later on became a bona fide foodstuff for the Scots, British, Germans, and Scandinavians. The first Scottish settlers brought oats to the New World in the 1600s. Today only 4 to 5 percent of the oats grown commercially are used for human food. The largest cultivators of oats are the United States, Germany, Finland, Poland, and the Russian Federation. Most of the oats grown are used for horse and other livestock feed.

NUTRITIONAL HIGHLIGHTS

Oats are a very good source of the minerals manganese, selenium, and phosphorus. They are also a good source of the minerals magnesium and iron. Oats have more than three times as much magnesium as calcium (177 milligrams versus 54 milligrams per cup of dried oats). In addition, oats are a good source of vitamin B1 and soluble dietary fiber.

HEALTH BENEFITS

Oat bran's dietary fiber is high in beta-glucan, which helps to lower cholesterol by binding bile acids and removing them from the body via the faeces. Since 1963, more than thirty clinical studies have examined the effect of oat bran on serum cholesterol levels. Various oat preparations containing either oat bran or oatmeal have been used, including cereals, muffins, breads, and entrées. The overwhelming majority of these studies demonstrate a very favorable effect on cholesterol levels: In individuals with high cholesterol levels (above 220 milligrams per deciliter/5.7 mmol/l) the consumption of the equivalent of 3 grams of soluble oat fiber per day typically lowers total cholesterol by 8 to 23 percent. This is highly significant, as with each 1 percent drop in serum cholesterol level, there is a 2 percent decrease in the risk of developing heart disease.

Three grams of fiber can be obtained by consuming approximately 1 bowl of ready-to-eat oat bran cereal or oatmeal. Although oatmeal's fiber content (7 percent) is less than that of oat bran (15 to 26 percent), it has been determined that the polyunsaturated fatty acids contribute as much to the cholesterol-lowering effects of oats as does the fiber content. Although oat bran has a higher fiber content, oatmeal is higher in polyunsaturated fatty acids. This makes oat bran and oatmeal quite similar in effectiveness. It is important to note, however, that although individuals with high cholesterol levels will see significant reductions with frequent oat consumption, individuals with normal or low cholesterol levels will see little change.

Studies also show that oat bran has beneficial effects on blood sugar as well. Adults with type 2 diabetes who were given foods high in oat fiber or given oatmeal- or oat bran-rich foods experienced a much lower rise in blood sugar than those who were given white rice or bread.

HOW TO SELECT AND STORE

With a lipid profile of approximately 20 percent saturated fat and 80 percent polyunsaturated and monounsaturated fats, oats have a slightly higher fat content than other grains and can go rancid more quickly. As a result, we suggest to buy small quantities at one time. They are available prepackaged, as well as in bulk. If you purchase already prepared oats, look at the ingredients list to ensure there is no salt, sugar, or other additives. If you buy oats in bulk, make sure that the bins are covered and that the shop has a fast product turnover to ensure maximum freshness. Check the oats' aroma to make sure they are fresh. Fresh oats have a clean, sweet or grassy smell, whereas spoiled oats have a sharper, unpleasant odor. Visually inspect the package or container to be sure there is no moisture in the oats. Oats can be kept for two months if well stored in airtight containers and left in a dark, dry, cool area. Cooked oats are good for two to three days and can be frozen for one month, although the texture may become less favorable.

TIPS FOR PREPARING

Somewhat different cooking methods may be required for making hot oat cereal or porridge (a soft food made by boiling oatmeal, another meal, or legumes in water or milk) from different oat types. No matter what the type, rinsing is not required, and it is best to add the oats to cold water and then heat to a simmer. See Table 12.2, "Guide to Cooking Grains," on page 325 for more oat preparation instruction.

QUICK SERVING IDEAS

- For a hearty breakfast, cook oats and add ½ teaspoon of organic butter, a pinch of salt, sliced dried prunes or fruit of your choice, 1 teaspoon of cinnamon, and raw walnut pieces. Once the oats are in your bowl, finish with 1 tablespoon of linseed meal, and for sweetness add some maple syrup or raw honey.

- Oatmeal is more than just a breakfast food; try adding chopped vegetables, miso, sesame seed butter (tahini), and fresh herbs and spices to make an easy, one-pot meal.
- With or without raisins, oatmeal cookies are a favorite of kids of all ages.
- Add some oat flour or whole oats to your next bread or muffin recipe.
- Oat bran adds healthy fiber to any cold or hot cereal.
- Try oat groats as the foundation of your next turkey, chicken, or quail stuffing.

SAFETY

Oats are not commonly an allergenic food. However, they are classified as a member of the "gluten grains." This grouping of grains has traditionally included wheat, oats, barley, and rye, and it has traditionally been avoided by individuals with wheat-sensitive conditions. While the conclusion that oats should be grouped together with wheat and systematically avoided in a wheat-free diet is not supported by some research studies, most public health organizations continue to place wheat and oats together in the category of "gluten grains" and recommend elimination of oats along with wheat for wheat-sensitive individuals. Celiac disease, also known as "nontropical sprue," is an intestinal disorder caused by an inability to utilize gluten. It is characterized by diarrhea, malabsorption of nutrients, and an abnormal small intestine structure that reverts to normal on removal and avoidance of dietary gluten. Celiac disease is discussed further on page 703.

Oats contain moderate to high amounts of oxalate. Individuals with a history of calcium oxalate-containing kidney stones should limit their consumption of this food. See page 793 for more information.

Rice

A wonderful and versatile grain able to complement practically any food—there are more than 8,000 different types—rice (Oryza sativa) is categorized by size and by the method used to process it. Long-, medium-, and short-grain rices are the main types. Sticky rice is produced by the high-starch short grain, while long grain is generally less heavy and starchy. Medium-grain rice is somewhere in between the two. Milling processes also help define rice, as white rice is the most highly polished rice, with all bran, germ, and nutrients removed. Brown rice, on the other hand, is replete with nutrients, for only the hard, inedible outer hull is removed.

Without question, rice is the most relied-upon grain of sustenance in East Asian countries. In fact, in a number of Asian languages the words for "rice" and "food" are the same. Annually, a typical person in Indonesia, Thailand, Japan, or China consumes anywhere from 200 to 400 pounds/90 to 180 kilograms. In stark contrast, the U.S. per capita consumption of rice is less than 8 pounds/3½ kilograms. Similarly, U.K. consumption is about 10 pounds/4½ kilograms per person a year.

Some of the most popular varieties of rice in the U.S. include:

- Arborio: A round, short-grain, starchy white rice, traditionally used to make the Italian dish risotto.
- Basmati: An aromatic rice that has a nutlike fragrance, delicate flavor, and light texture.

- Sweet rice: Almost translucent when it is cooked, this very sticky short-grain rice is traditionally used to make sushi and mochi.
- Jasmine: A soft-textured, long-grain, aromatic rice that is available in both brown and white varieties.
- Bhutanese red rice: Grown in the Himalayas, this red rice has a nutty, earthy taste.
- Forbidden rice: A black-colored, short-grain rice that turns purple upon cooking; it has a sweet taste and sticky texture.

HISTORY

Rice was first cultivated in China around 7000 B.C.E. Chinese myth tells us rice was a gift to humans from animals: A large flood had wiped out food production. The people, who were afraid they would starve, observed animals with seeds of rice on their mouths. These were planted, and scores of people were saved.

Rice was the secret of Asia for many years. Only later did travelers introduce rice into ancient Greece, and when Alexander the Great brought it to India, rice finally found its way to other corners of the world. Moorish conquerors took rice to Spain in the 700s, and the Crusaders were responsible for bringing rice back to France. Rice was introduced into South America in the seventeenth century by the Spanish during their colonization of the New World. It was taken to West Africa by the end of the 1600s, and slaves introduced rice to South Carolina in the middle 1700s.

Contrary to popular thought, rice does not have to grow in water. The reason rice fields or paddies are flooded is actually to control weeds and insects and to increase productivity. Thailand, Vietnam, and China are the three greatest producers and exporters of rice. The United States is responsible for about only 1 percent of the world's total rice production.

NUTRITIONAL HIGHLIGHTS

Brown rice is by far the most nutritious rice form available. Because of white rice's severe milling and polishing process, it is devoid of practically all vitamins and nutrients. For the last hundred years, great efforts have been made to increase Asians' health by encouraging them to consume unmilled rice. Unfortunately, they prefer white rice to brown, so these efforts have failed. As a result, general malnutrition and beriberi (discussed on page 323) are still too common in many Asian regions. Another plan is to enrich white rice with the lost vitamins and minerals. Due to the expense and practicality of this process, eating brown rice still makes better, and more healthful, sense.

Brown rice is a quality source of vitamins B1, B2, B3, and B6, as well as manganese, iron, selenium, magnesium, phosphorus, and the trace minerals. Additionally, brown rice includes a good supply of protein and gamma-oryzanol, an extract of rice bran oil that has been used to treat digestive, menopausal, and cholesterol problems.

HEALTH BENEFITS

Comparable to whole wheat, brown rice is quite nutritious as far as calories, vitamins, and minerals are concerned. Whole wheat does have a greater protein content (12.6 percent compared to 8.9 percent) and fiber content (12.2 percent compared to 3.5 percent), but in terms of quality, brown rice has better protein as far as essential amino acid quantity is concerned.

Like oat bran (discussed on page 330), rice bran can help treat hypercholesterolemia. In addition to its healthy fiber constituents, rice bran and rice oil have gamma-oryzanol, a compound that not only lowers cholesterol but exerts growth-promoting properties as well. Since brown rice contains rice bran and gamma-oryzanol, it likely possesses a cholesterol-lowering effect.

HOW TO SELECT AND STORE

You can buy rice in packages or as a bulk product. Since its natural oils do spoil over time, check the freshness date on prepackaged rice. When buying in bulk, go to a shop with a high turnover rate and be sure the bins are properly covered. With either bulk or packaged rice, do not buy rice with evidence of moisture.

As the oil in brown rice can turn rancid, keep it in the refrigerator. White rice is fine in a cool, dry place. Brown rice should be stored in an airtight container and can remain in the refrigerator for up to six months. White rice is fine in an airtight container for up to one year. Keep cooked rice in an airtight container to prevent drying, and it will remain fresh for up to four days.

TIPS FOR PREPARING

All grains, save oats, should be rinsed thoroughly under cool running water to remove any dirt or debris. The lighter, fluffy basmati rice should be soaked in a bowl of cool water before cooking. It should be stirred frequently and the water replaced four to five times until it is no longer a milky color. See Table 12.2, "Guide to Cooking Grains," on page 325 for easy preparation instructions.

QUICK SERVING IDEAS

- Cooked rice makes a great dessert. First add milk or soy milk. Then add cinnamon, nutmeg, raisins, and honey for a delicious, easy Asian-style rice pudding.
- Homemade vegetable sushi rolls are easily fashioned by wrapping brown rice and your favorite vegetables in nori sheets.
- Kanji is an easy-to-digest rice dish that is good for cleansing or when you have a flulike cold: Prepare organic vegetable or chicken stock and fill a large pot one half to three-quarters full. Add one to two handfuls of brown rice plus sliced celery, onions, and garlic. Simmer over a low heat. Add shiitake or reishi mushrooms for an immune-boosting effect.
- Try brown rice pasta instead of wheat pasta.
- Use rice leftovers for cold rice salads, which are great for on-the-go lunches. Be creative and add either chicken or tofu, plus your favorite vegetables, nuts, herbs, and spices.
- Rice and beans with the vegetables of your choice are always a filling and healthy meal.
- A rice side dish can be made into anything you like; jazz it up with the toppings of your choice. Some of our favorites include cashews or peanuts, sesame seeds, pineapple pieces, sautéed mushrooms, spring onions, and currants.
- Leftover rice stir-fry: In a large pan, sauté ginger and minced onions in organic extra-virgin olive oil. You can add any leftover meats from the refrigerator. Then add two beaten eggs to the sauté and stir until they are well scrambled. Add the rice and two handfuls of frozen peas. Mix together and let

warm. Take off the heat and season with roasted sesame oil, black pepper, and soy sauce to taste.

SAFETY

Rice is one of the safest foods available. The hypoallergenic (low-allergy) nature of whole-grain, organic brown rice makes it a commonly recommended grain alternative. Rice is also not a food that is commonly contaminated by pesticides.

Brown rice does contain moderate amounts of oxalate, but white rice does not, as the oxalate is contained in the bran of the rice. Individuals with a history of calcium oxalate-containing kidney stones should limit their consumption of brown rice. See page 793 for more information.

Wheat

Wheat *(Triticum aestivum)* is the most important grain in that it provides more nourishment for more people throughout the world than any other food. Greater than one third of the world's population utilizes wheat as a main dietary staple. Wheat is used in a variety of products, but its use as flour for bread and baked goods is the most important. One of the key reasons why wheat is best suited for bread making in comparison to other grains is its high gluten content. Gluten is composed of the two proteins gliadin and glutenin, which are found in many grains but are found in greatest quantity in wheat, followed by rye (a distant second), oats, and barley. Gluten gives wheat flour elasticity and strength and allows breads to "rise." After kneading, gluten traps the carbon dioxide produced by the yeast or other chemical leavening agent, resulting in the expansion, or "rising," of the dough.

HISTORY

Wheat has been the most important grain throughout history. Thought to have originated in southwestern Asia, it has been consumed as a food for more than 10,000 years. First cultivated in the Fertile Crescent and later in Egypt, wheat has been a decisive factor in the development of civilization. In fact, the reverence in which wheat was held is noted in almost every major culture. For example, in Western culture, the Lord's Prayer symbolizes the importance of wheat and bread with the line "Give us this day our daily bread." (For more information about the spread of grain cultivation, see page 320.)

Wheat is not native to the Western Hemisphere and was introduced here only in the late fifteenth century, when Columbus came to the New World. Though wheat was grown in the United States during the early colonial years, it was not until the late nineteenth century that wheat cultivation flourished, owing to the importation of an especially hardy strain of wheat known as Turkey red wheat, which was brought over by Russian immigrants who settled in Kansas.

Wheat accounts for the largest cropland area of any food, with more than 22 percent of all available cropland in the world devoted to growing wheat. The major wheat-producing countries in the world, in order, are the Russian Federation, the United States, China, and India. The leading wheat-producing states in the United States are

Kansas, North Dakota, Oklahoma, Texas, Washington, and Montana. It is also the most common cereal crop grown in the U.K.

NUTRITIONAL HIGHLIGHTS

The story of wheat in the United States unfortunately starts with a raw material that is very nutritious and a final product that in most instances is not. As a standard rule, wheat products such as pasta, noodles, breads, and biscuits use flour that undergoes a process in which 60 percent of the wheat grain is removed. Included in the 60 percent lost are the most nutritious aspects of the wheat: the bran and the germ. As a result, more than half of the B vitamins, folic acid, zinc, copper, phosphorus, calcium, and iron are removed. In the 1940s, the United States instituted laws requiring enrichment as a reaction to the observed health problems of the population. Unfortunately, enrichment does not even replace what has been lost. In the U.K., iron, thiamine, and niacin are, by law, added to white and brown flour (but not wholemeal). This practice began in World War II when food shortages were anticipated.

Unextracted whole wheat (wholemeal), on the other hand, yields a good supply of dietary fiber and manganese. It also contains a healthful portion of vitamins B1, B2, B3, B5, B6, and E and folic acid, as well as calcium, phosphorus, zinc, copper, protein, magnesium, and iron. Wheat germ is the vitamin- and mineral-rich embryo of the wheat kernel that is removed during the refining of whole-wheat (wholemeal) grains into white flour. It is an excellent source of vitamins B1 and B6 and folic acid, as well as the minerals zinc, magnesium, and manganese.

Wheat germ also has a high oil content and therefore is an excellent source of vitamin E.

HEALTH BENEFITS

Wheat's health benefits are maximized when 100 percent whole-wheat (wholemeal) products that include the bran and the germ are used and are virtually nonexistent in products made of bleached white flour. Furthermore, bleached white flour has a higher glycemic index and affects blood sugar levels untowardly. Some of the benefits of unextracted whole wheat (wholemeal) include:

- Reduction of the incidence of colon cancer, a benefit that has not been seen with oat bran or corn.
- Reduction of the risk of breast cancer, as wheat bran has been shown to decrease blood oestrogen, a promoter of breast cancer.
- Promotion of regular bowel function, which can significantly reduce the incidence of diverticular disease.

HOW TO SELECT AND STORE

Found both prepackaged and in bulk, whole-wheat (wholemeal) products are freshest when bought from secure covered bins in a shop with high turnover. Any evidence of moisture is a reason not to purchase. Sealed containers and vacuum packaging often ensure a fresher product as well.

Forms of whole wheat include wheat bran, wheat germ, wheat berries, wheatgrass seeds, whole-wheat couscous, bulgur wheat, cracked wheat, and unbleached whole-wheat (wholemeal) flour. Wheat berries should be stored in an airtight container in a cool, dry, and dark place, where they will keep for up to one month. The optimal way to store other whole-wheat (wholemeal) products, such as flour, couscous, cracked wheat, bulgur, bran, and germ, is in airtight containers in the refrigerator, as the cool temperature will help prevent them from becoming rancid, increasing storage time to three months. Wheat products can also be stored in the freezer for up to six months.

TIPS FOR PREPARING

For any grain except oats, it is best to rinse thoroughly under cool water to remove any dirt and debris. Then see Table 12.2, "Guide to Cooking Grains," on page 326 for easy preparation instructions.

QUICK SERVING IDEAS

- Whole-wheat (wholemeal) bread makes a better sandwich than plain white bread.
- Whole-wheat (wholemeal) flakes, similar to rolled oats, can be prepared as a hot breakfast cereal.
- Sprouted wheat berries (wheatgrass seeds) are a healthy and hearty choice in vegetable and grain salads.
- Try whole-wheat (wholemeal) bread instead of white bread the next time you make French toast.
- Whole-wheat (wholemeal) pitas with tomato sauce, soy cheese, and broccoli make a healthy meal or snack for kids of any age. Whole-wheat (wholemeal) pasta is a heartier, tastier pasta that can stand up to your favorite tomato sauce.

- Whole-wheat (wholemeal) pancakes are easily whipped up by mixing 1½ cups of whole wheat flour, 1 tablespoon of baking powder, 1 tablespoon of honey, 1 organic egg, 1 cup of cow or soy milk, ½ teaspoon of salt, and 2½ tablespoons of rapeseed oil. Mix to a lumpy consistency and ladle out on the griddle in ½-cup amounts. Use real maple syrup with cardamom for an exotic taste.
- Wheat germ works nicely in casseroles, protein shakes, muffins, and pancakes, or used to top cereal, salad or yogurt.

SAFETY

Although whole wheat (wholemeal) can be very nutritious, some individuals do not react well to gluten, a component of wheat, oats, barley, and rye. Celiac disease (nontropical sprue) is a small-intestine disorder whereby reaction to gluten causes severe malabsorptive symptoms, frequent diarrhea, and irregular small intestine luminal structures that can return to normal once the offending gluten products are removed. Celiac disease is discussed further on page 703.

Wheat is a common food allergen, especially in children. Common symptoms associated with an allergic reaction to wheat products include chronic gastrointestinal disturbances; frequent infections, such as ear and bladder infections; enuresis (bed-wetting); asthma and sinusitis symptoms; eczema, skin rash, acne, and hives; bursitis and joint pains; fatigue, headache, and migraine. Also, hyperactivity, depression, and insomnia can be observed.

Since wheat contains moderate to large amounts of oxalate, individuals with a history of calcium oxalate-containing kidney stones should limit their consumption of this food. See page 793 for more information.

The Minor Food Grains

Amaranth

Amaranth is an ancient food of the Aztecs and Mayans of Central America that is currently being "rediscovered." Amaranth, a member of the Amaranthaceae family, is a beautiful broad-leafed bushy plant that reaches a height of 5 to 7 feet/1½ to 2 meters. It has a dramatic flower head composed of a profusion of small deep red or magenta cloverlike flowers—in fact, the name "amaranth" comes from the Greek for "never-fading flower." Once considered a weed, amaranth is now acknowledged as a highly nutritious food; it is grown both as a vegetable for its leaves and as a grain for its seeds.

Each amaranth plant is capable of producing 40,000 to 60,000 tiny, lens-shaped seeds. The seed heads, which look like very full corn tassels, create a striking mass of color—most often a golden to creamy tan, although, like the leaves, the seeds can range in color from buff to dark purple, deep red, green, orange, pink, and white.

Acclaimed as the "miracle grain" of the Aztecs, amaranth is actually not a grain at all but an annual herb that is a close cousin of pigweed (a weed also known as lamb's quarters), the garden plant cockscomb, and the tumbleweeds of the American Southwest. Approximately sixty species of amaranth are grown in North and South America, and all are grown for both leaf and seed rather than specifically as a vegetable for the leaf or as a grain for the seed.

Since amaranth kernels are so tiny, with pinhead-size seeds even smaller than poppy seeds, a pound/half-kilo of amaranth may contain upward of 750,000 seeds. What amaranth seed lacks in size, however, it makes up for in nutritional strength. Amaranth's "supergrain" status, while technically inaccurate, is nutritionally valid. Its seeds are composed of 15 to 18 percent protein, and unlike true grains, which are deficient in the essential amino acids lysine and methionine, the protein provided by amaranth seeds is high in both. When combined with grains such as wheat, rice, or barley, amaranth provides complete, well-absorbed protein.

Amaranth's protein-rich seed has a unique flavor of earthy sweetness reminiscent of beetroot. This makes it an excellent cereal grain. The seeds are also ground into flour to enrich the protein, vitamin, and mineral content of wheat breads, pasta, and other baked goods. Since amaranth does not contain gluten, the protein in wheat responsible for wheat flour's elastic rising dough, as well as its allergenic potential, amaranth cannot be used alone to make bread. However, mixed with maize or rice, which are also gluten-free, this nutritious seed can be used to produce delicious, nonallergenic baked goods.

Amaranth greens' hint of sweetness makes them an interesting addition to salads, although research has shown that the iron contained in the leaves becomes more absorbable when the leaves are cooked.

In addition to being grown as a food, amaranth is used as an ornamental plant. The leaves of ornamental varieties, such as Joseph's coat, are similar in appearance to those of the coleus plant. Plus, since amaranth is resistant to heat and drought and has no major disease problems, this tall, colorful plant is not only one of the most beautiful but one of the easiest to grow.

HISTORY

Originating in what is now Central and South America, amaranth's history began as a staple in the diets of pre-Columbian Aztecs, who believed the plant was endowed with supernatural powers and would give them amazing strength. Because of this belief, amaranth was one of the primary foods eaten by Aztec royalty and was incorporated into Aztec religious rituals, which included human sacrifice. The Aztec women mixed ground amaranth seed with honey and human blood, shaped the reddish paste into figures of bird and snake gods, and baked them for consumption during religious ceremonies. During the Spanish conquest in the early 1500s, the conquistadors were appalled by this practice, which they considered a parody of the Holy Communion host. Reasoning that eliminating amaranth would also eliminate human sacrifice, they burned every crop of amaranth they could find and forbade growing the grain. The punishment for possession of amaranth was severe—having even one seed was punishable by chopping off the hands. As a consequence, amaranth quickly became a "lost" seed, a status that lasted for hundreds of years. Fortunately, amaranth cultivation continued in a few remote areas of the Andes and Mexico; otherwise this wonderful plant might have become extinct and its beauty and health benefits lost to us. Today, amaranth is grown in Mexico, Peru, Nepal, and the United States.

Currently, in the Cuzco area of Peru, amaranth's flowers are used medicinally for toothaches and fevers and, because of their rich purple-red color, cosmetically, both as a food dye for maize and quinoa and as a rouge. In Ecuador, amaranth flowers are boiled, leaching their vibrant color into boiling water that is added to *aquardeinte* rum to create a drink said to purify the blood and help normalize the menstrual cycle.

Amaranth has been grown in the United States since 1975 and is now cultivated in Colorado, Illinois, Nebraska, and other states. Although not yet a mainstream food, amaranth can be found in many natural food stores, and its flour is often added to baked goods.

NUTRITIONAL HIGHLIGHTS

Amaranth seed's primary claim to fame is its unusually high protein content, particularly its content of respectable amounts of lysine and methionine, two essential amino acids that are not frequently found in grains. Just a cup of amaranth seed supplies 60 percent of an adult's daily requirement of protein. The protein provided by amaranth is well absorbed, too. In fact, cooked amaranth seed is 90 percent digestible. In addition, using amaranth in combination with wheat, corn, or brown rice provides a complete protein as high in food value as that of fish, red meat, or poultry.

This tiny but nutritionally mighty seed outperforms whole wheat (wholemeal), not only when it comes to protein but in the categories of fiber and healthy fats, and in a number of minerals and vitamins as well. The fiber content of amaranth is 25 percent higher than that of whole wheat (¼ cup of dry amaranth seeds supplies 31 percent of the daily value of fiber); its iron and calcium content is five times that of

TABLE 12.3

Amaranth: A Clear Nutritional Winner Compared to Whole Wheat: Nutrients in 100 Grams of Amaranth Versus Whole Wheat

	Amount in Amaranth	Percentage of That Found in Hard Red Winter Wheat
Food energy	374 kilocalories	114%
Protein:		
Total protein	14.45 grams	115%
Alanine	0.799 gram	176%
Arginine	1.060 grams	178%
Histidine	0.389 gram	136%
Isoleucine	0.582 gram	127%
Leucine	0.879 gram	103%
Lysine	0.747 gram	223%
Methionine	0.226 gram	112%
Threonine	0.558 gram	153%
Tryptophan	0.181 gram	113%
Valine	0.679 gram	122%
Fiber	15.2 grams	121%
Fats:		
Total lipids (fat)	6.51 grams	423%
Saturated fat	1.662 grams	618%
Monounsaturated fat	1.433 grams	717%
Polyunsaturated fat	2.891 grams	461%
Palmitic acid (16:0)	1.284 grams	549%
Oleic acid (18:1)	1.433 grams	746%
Linoleic acid (18:2/n6)	2.834 grams	472%
Vitamins:		
C	4.2 milligrams	Whole wheat contains none
B2	0.208 milligram	181%
Folic acid	49 micrograms	129%

Minerals:		
Calcium	153 milligrams	528%
Copper	0.78 milligram	179%
Iron	7.59 milligrams	238%
Magnesium	266 milligrams	211%
Potassium	366 milligrams	101%
Zinc	3.18 milligrams	120%
Active compounds:		
Phytosterols	24 milligrams	Whole wheat contains none

whole wheat (¼ cup of cooked amaranth seeds supplies 21 percent of iron's daily value); and it has twice as much magnesium. Amaranth seeds contain twice as much calcium as does milk, providing 7 percent of the daily value of calcium in a mere ¼ cup. Amaranth seeds are also an excellent source of vitamins B2, B3, and B5 and a very good source of vitamin B6 and folic acid. In addition, amaranth seeds are an excellent source of minerals. Aside from their iron and calcium content, cooked amaranth seeds supply 61 percent of the daily value of manganese in a ¼ cup, along with 42 percent of the daily value of both copper and magnesium, 19 percent of the daily value of zinc, and 5 percent of the daily value of potassium. Amaranth seeds are also an excellent source of tocotrienols, a vitamin E fraction with numerous cardiovascular benefits, including cholesterol-lowering activity in humans. Last, unlike whole wheat and other grains, amaranth seeds' abundance of nutritional riches includes significant amounts of phytosterols, which research is beginning to show can play a major role in preventing chronic degenerative disease.

Amaranth's leaves are nutritional stars in their own right. For almost unbelievably fat-free calories, 1 cup of cooked amaranth leaves provides 104 percent of the daily value of vitamin A, along with 72 percent of the daily value of vitamin C. Amaranth leaves are also excellent providers of the B vitamins. In fact, 1 cup of cooked leaves contains 19 percent of the daily value of folic acid, 18 percent of the daily value of B6, 16 percent of the daily value of B2, and 10 percent of the daily value of B3. Amaranth's leaves are an excellent source of minerals, too. A cup of cooked leaves will give you 63 percent of the daily value of manganese, 28 percent of the daily value of calcium, 24 percent of the daily value of potassium, 23 percent of the daily value of copper and magnesium, 17 percent of the daily value of iron, and 15 percent of the daily value of zinc.

HEALTH BENEFITS

Due to its recent introduction to the modern food supply, amaranth tends to be less allergenic than many other grains. Because it's virtually gluten-free, it is also suitable for most people with gluten intolerance. Although it is more expensive than many other common grains, its cost may be justified for allergic individuals.

All amaranth varieties contain tocotrienols (a vitamin E fraction) and squalene (a fatty acid), both of which are known to reduce cholesterol synthesis. Researchers decided to test their effectiveness by looking at what would happen to cholesterol formation in six-week-old female chickens whose diet was supplemented with whole seed, popped and milled amaranth, and amaranth oil, compared to birds given a standard diet. In the birds fed amaranth-containing diets, blood levels of total cholesterol and (bad) LDL cholesterol were lowered by an outstanding 10 to 30 percent and 7 to 70 percent, respectively. Plus, the birds' beneficial HDL cholesterol was not affected by amaranth supplementation.

The scientists think that these very beneficial effects are due to a significant increase in the activity of a liver enzyme called cholesterol 7-alpha-hydroxylase, which is the enzyme responsible for cholesterol breakdown into bile acids. The activity of this enzyme was 10 to 18 percent higher in birds fed amaranth than in birds used as controls. In addition, the activity of another liver enzyme, liver 3-hydroxy-3-methylglutaryl coenzyme A reductase—the rate-limiting enzyme for cholesterol biosynthesis—also dropped by 9 percent in birds fed popped, milled amaranth and its oil. Since amaranth's cholesterol-lowering effects were even greater than can be accounted for by these two mechanisms, the researchers think amaranth must also contain other as yet unidentified, but potent, cholesterol inhibitors in addition to its tocotrienols and squalene.

Amaranth also cut total blood cholesterol levels in two other animal studies. In the first study, researchers fed amaranth seeds to one group of male Wistar strain albino rats (a type of rat specially bred to have high cholesterol), while giving the control group standard rat chow. In the rats given amaranth, the seeds provided the best possible outcome. Potentially harmful LDL and VLDL cholesterol and triglyceride levels measured in the blood dropped significantly lower, while levels of beneficial HDL cholesterol rose.

In the second, later study, researchers looked at the effect of various fats on lipids in the blood and liver of rats. For twenty-eight days, sixty male Buffalo rats were fed one of six diets containing 15 percent fat (provided by lard or sunflower oil), 20 percent protein, and 0.5 percent cholesterol. Amaranth and oat bran were added to the diets to provide a little dietary fiber, but the researchers soon discovered that amaranth significantly decreased total cholesterol levels in the rats' blood (by 10.7 percent in the case of the diet with lard and by 14 percent with sunflower oil) and liver (by 20 percent in the diet with lard and by 23 percent in the sunflower oil diet). Oat bran decreased the level of total cholesterol in the blood even more—by 19 percent in the lard diet and by 22 percent in the sunflower oil diet—and in the liver by 22 percent and 27 percent, respectively. Plus, neither amaranth nor oat bran caused a lowering of the rats' beneficial HDL cholesterol.

In the diets in which amaranth or oat bran was given with sunflower oil, the rats' blood levels of triglycerides also dropped precipitously—by 22 percent! But when amaranth or oat bran was combined with lard, such beneficial effects on triglycerides occurred only in the liver, not in the blood. In the liver, amaranth decreased triglycerides by 10 percent in the lard diet and by 15 percent when given with sunflower oil, while oat bran decreased triglycerides in the liver by 15 percent in the lard diet and 20 percent in the diet with sunflower oil.

Amaranth is also a suitable grain for people with type 2 diabetes. When researchers studied the glycemic index of amaranth, wheat, and rice preparations in persons with non-insulin-dependent diabetes, the amaranth–wheat flour composite diet (25 percent amaranth, 75 percent wheat) was found to have the lowest glycemic index (65.6 percent, followed by the wheat diet (65.7 percent), and then the rice diet (69.2 percent). Surprisingly, an amaranth-wheat flour composite diet in which equal amounts of both grains was used had a higher GI (75.5 percent), as did popped amaranth in milk (97.3 percent). The researchers concluded that, for persons with type 2 diabetes, a 25:75 combination of amaranth and wheat can be considered a low-GI food.

HOW TO SELECT AND STORE

Amaranth flour can be found in prepared cereals and other baked goods, such as crackers, cookies, and breads, and is also available packaged as a whole-grain flour. Because amaranth seeds contain fairly high levels of beneficial polyunsaturated fats, once they have been ground into flour, it is best to store the flour in an airtight freezer bag in the refrigerator or freezer. This will protect the flour's more vulnerable fatty acids from becoming rancid.

Stored in the refrigerator, amaranth flour will keep for two to three months. Stored in the freezer, the flour will keep for up to six months.

Amaranth seeds can be found in most natural food stores sold packaged and, less expensively, in bulk. Air, moisture, and sunlight can cause amaranth seeds to mould and their oils to go rancid. Do not purchase or use amaranth seeds that have a musty or bitter smell, both of which indicate spoilage. Also, look for seeds that are uniform in color. Occasionally, you'll find a few very bitter black seeds mixed in. These are seeds from wild pigweed that have managed to gain a foothold among the cultivated amaranth plants. Don't worry about picking them out; their flavor will not dominate that of the true amaranth seeds.

Stored in a cool, dark, dry place in an airtight container, such as a glass jar, amaranth seeds, which have a hard outer shell, will keep for one year or even longer. If purchased in vacuum-sealed packaging, once the package has been opened, the seeds are best stored in the refrigerator, where they should keep for an additional six to eight months. Cooked amaranth seeds will keep for three days refrigerated, and cooked leaves will keep for one to two days refrigerated.

TIPS FOR PREPARING

Like any seed or green leaf, amaranth should be rinsed thoroughly before use. Seeds are best cleaned by placing them in a bowl, covering them with water, swishing them around with your hand, and then pouring off the water over a fine-meshed sieve. Repeat this process several times. You can wash amaranth leaves as you would any green by rinsing them under cool running water and shaking off excess moisture or placing them in a salad spinner and spinning dry.

Amaranth seed should be cooked before it is eaten because it contains components in its raw form that block the absorption of some nutrients in our digestive system. Lightly cooked, amaranth seeds add protein, flavor, and texture to other whole-grain dishes and stir-fries. The "sticky" texture of lightly cooked amaranth seeds makes a pleasing contrast to the fluffier texture of grains such as rice or quinoa, but take care not to overcook amaranth seeds, as they can become gummy if cooked for more than 10 to 15 minutes. With longer cooking, as, for example, in soups or stews, amaranth seeds make an excellent, nutrient-dense thickening agent.

When cooking amaranth seeds, use a ratio of 2½ to 3 parts water to 1 part grain (see Table 12.2 on page 325). Using less water will make the grain chewier. Using more water will give the grain the texture of mushy cooked cereal. Bring the water to a boil and stir in the grain. Return to a boil, then lower the heat and simmer. Keep covered until all the water is absorbed. Whether boiled or steamed, amaranth will congeal as it cools, much like grits, so enjoy it right away.

If you are relying on amaranth seed as a source of lysine, choose other cooking methods over popping. Of all of the amino acids, lysine is the most sensitive to dry heat, and the amount of lysine in amaranth seed and other sources of this essential amino acid can be significantly reduced by popping. Sprouting, on the other hand, raises the level of some nutrients in amaranth seed, including lysine.

Amaranth flour contains no gluten and must therefore be combined with wheat when a rising loaf of bread is desired. Mix 25 percent amaranth flour with 75 percent wheat or other gluten-containing flour when making yeast breads. Baked goods that do not require gluten, such as biscuits, muffins, pancakes, pasta, and flatbreads, can be made using 100 percent amaranth flour.

Amaranth leaves can be served raw in salads, but research has shown that first blanching and then cooking the mature leaves significantly improves their iron availability while also significantly reducing their oxalic acid content.

QUICK SERVING IDEAS

- Sprout amaranth seeds as you would any seed (see page 408). Enjoy the sprouts on sandwiches, in green and fruit salads, or as a crunchy snack all by themselves.

- For a delicious grain side dish, try lightly cooked amaranth seeds. Add 1 cup seeds to 2½ cups of liquid, such as water, half water and half stock, or apple juice, bring to a boil, lower heat to medium high, and cook until the seeds are tender. Try adding a little chopped fresh turmeric or gingerroot to the pot for even more nutrients and flavor.

- Alternatively, to bring out their nutty aroma, amaranth seeds can be first toasted, then cooked. Toast 1 cup of seeds in a saucepan or wok over medium heat, stirring constantly for 4 minutes, or until they begin to pop. Bring 1 cup of water to a boil over high heat, add the toasted seeds, cover, lower the heat, and simmer for 7 minutes, or until all the liquid has been absorbed. Remove from heat, add any favorite spices, and let steam, covered, for another 5 to 10 minutes. Toss with a little olive or linseed oil and, if desired, sea salt and pepper, and serve.

- Experiment with amaranth by adding ¼ to ½ cup of seeds to your favorite soup recipe. It will expand and thicken, adding a rich, nutty sweetness to your soup.

- For a tasty main dish, stir cooked amaranth seeds in with cooked beans and your favorite spices, then top with grated cheese and bake at 350 degrees F./180 degrees C./gas 4 until heated through and the cheese melts (10 to 15 minutes).

- Amaranth seeds make a hearty breakfast porridge. Add 1 cup of seeds to 3 cups of cooking liquid (water and/or juice), bring to a boil, then lower heat to medium, cover, and cook until the seeds are mushy, about 20 to 25 minutes. If desired, sweeten with a little honey, molasses, or maple syrup; add a handful of raisins, dried fruit, cinnamon, or allspice; and top with a few of your favorite nuts.

- For popped amaranth seeds, heat them in a heavy, dry skillet on medium-high heat, stirring constantly until they pop (5 to 8 minutes). Add to your favorite granola or other dry cereal, or serve topped with milk and strawberries as a protein-rich breakfast cereal or snack.

- Amaranth flour can be used in making breads, muffins, pastry, pasta, and other baked goods. To make your whole-wheat (wholemeal) bread a complete protein, substitute about 25 percent of the wheat flour called for in your favorite bread recipe with amaranth flour. To increase the protein content, when making any yeast or quick bread, for best results, use the same ratio, mixing one part amaranth flour with three to four parts wheat, rice, oat, or other grain flour or cornmeal. When making flatbreads, pancakes, and pastas, 100 percent amaranth flour can be used.

- Amaranth leaves taste much like sweet young spinach and are best served raw in salads when the plant is young and tender. Mature leaves have an earthy sweetness that is best brought out if they are blanched and then steamed, stir-fried, or sautéed as you would any hardy green. One of our favorite ways of preparing amaranth leaves is to quickly blanch and then steam them for 10 minutes, then toss them with a little olive or linseed oil, fresh chopped herbs, and onion or garlic. Serve as a side dish topped with sesame seeds.

SAFETY

Amaranth seeds should always be cooked before they are eaten, since in their raw form, the seeds contain components that prevent the absorption of some nutrients by the human digestive system.

Amaranth contains moderate to large amounts of oxalate. Individuals with a history of calcium oxalate-containing kidney stones should limit their consumption of this food. See page 793 for more information.

Barley

Barley *(Hordeum vulgare)* is reminiscent of the wheat berry, although barley has a lighter color. It is the fourth largest produced cereal globally, behind wheat, rice, and corn. More than 80 percent of the barley produced is used for livestock feed or alcohol manufacture. High in maltose, sprouted barley is the foundation of malt syrup, a much-used sweetener, and also for fermentation to produce a basic component of whiskey, beer, and a number of other beverages.

A versatile glutenous grain, barley has a rich, nutlike flavor and a pleasingly chewy, pastalike consistency.

The forms of barley available in the modern market include hulled barley, pearl barley (an intensely milled whole barley grain), and barley flakes.

HISTORY

As one of the most ancient cultivated grains in the world, barley originated in Ethiopia and Southeast Asia, where it has been cultivated since 8000 B.C.E. It is thought that post-Ice Age climatic changes, plus barley's development of a hardened rachis, which prevented early grain scattering, allowed for better barley cultivation. As one of the first cereals cultivated in the Middle East, barley was used by ancient civilizations as a food for humans and animals, as well as to make alcohol. Actually, the first known recipe for barley wine dates back to 2800 B.C.E. in Babylonia. Barley water has also been used for various medicinal purposes since ancient times.

The ancient Greeks relied on barley to make bread, and athletes attributed much of their strength and physical growth to their barley-containing diets. Roman athletes also honored barley for the strength it gave them. The gladiators were known as *hordearii,* meaning "eaters of barley." Since the heads of barley are heavy and contain numerous seeds, barley was also honored in ancient China as a symbol of male virility. Given the relatively high cost of wheat in

the Middle Ages, many Europeans at that time made bread from a combination of barley and rye. In the 1500s, the Spanish introduced barley to South America. The English and Dutch settlers of the 1600s brought barley to the United States.

Today, the largest commercial producers of barley are Canada, the United States, the Russian Federation, Germany, France, and Spain.

NUTRITIONAL HIGHLIGHTS

Barley provides virtually the same nutritional elements as corn. It is a very good source of fiber and selenium. It is also a good source of the minerals copper, magnesium, and phosphorus, and it contains more than four times as much magnesium as calcium. Unlike corn, however, barley is a good source of niacin (vitamin B3).

HEALTH BENEFITS

The chief health benefit of barley is provided by its fiber components. Like oat bran, barley's dietary fiber is high in beta-glucan, which helps lower cholesterol by binding to bile acids and removing them from the body via the faeces.

HOW TO SELECT AND STORE

Hulled, pearl, and flake forms of barley are available in both bulk and prepackaged forms. For freshness, when buying in bulk, it is always important to ensure that there is no moisture in the food, that the bins are covered, and that your market has a quick turnover. Store in a covered glass container and keep in a cool, dry place. If the weather is particularly warm, barley may be kept in the refrigerator.

TIPS FOR PREPARING

Before cooking hulled or pearl barley, rinse it thoroughly under cool running water to remove any dirt or debris. Then see Table 12.2, "Guide to Cooking Grains," on page 325 for easy preparation instructions.

QUICK SERVING IDEAS

- A lemon twist on a old Roman favorite, barley water: Boil ¼ cup of barley grains in 2 pints/1 litre of water for 5 minutes, then strain and squeeze in the juice of one lemon and 2 teaspoons of honey and drink as a easily digested, healthy drink.
- Barley lends a hearty portion of health to vegetable soups, bean dishes, casseroles, and many other recipes.
- For a change in tastes, mix some barley flour with wheat flour to make breads and muffins that have a uniquely sweet and earthy taste.
- Hot cereals normally made with oatmeal can alternatively be made with cracked or flaked barley.
- Pilaf: Mix cooked barley and garlic-sautéed mushrooms for an eastern European flair.

SAFETY

Barley contains moderate to large amounts of oxalate. Individuals with a history of calcium oxalate-containing kidney stones should limit their consumption of this food. See page 793 for more information.

Buckwheat

The name "buckwheat" comes from the Dutch word *bockweit,* which is indicative of the resemblance to beech tree seeds and the wheatlike character of buckwheat flour. Interestingly, buckwheat is not a cereal grain but a fruit seed from the herbaceous plant buckwheat *(Fagopyrum esculentum).* This plant makes an aromatic flower and subsequently the buckwheat groats, which are small triangle-shaped grain-like seeds covered by a hard shell. When bees collect the nectar of the buckwheat flower, the flavor of the resulting honey is strong and the honey itself is quite dark.

In the United States, the two buckwheat varieties are the common and Tartary types. The color can be anywhere from a tan-pink hue to brown. Buckwheat is also sold as roasted buckwheat, which has an earthy, nutlike taste, or unroasted kasha, which is known for its subtler flavor. Ground unhulled buckwheat yields a nutritious dark flour, while hulled ground groats are lighter and contain fewer nutrients.

Buckwheat contains no gluten and is good for those who need to avoid wheat for allergy purposes.

HISTORY

Buckwheat is a native of Central Asia. Originally, it was cultivated in China and other Eastern countries from the tenth to the thirteenth centuries and subsequently taken to Europe from Asia by the Crusaders. Buckwheat was introduced into the United States by the Dutch during the 1600s. Poles and Russians have used buckwheat as an important main ingredient in their traditional fare for many generations. Other nations to employ commercial buckwheat cultivation include Canada, the United States, and France, the country famous for its buckwheat crêpes.

NUTRITIONAL HIGHLIGHTS

Buckwheat contains two flavonoids with significant health-promoting actions: rutin and quercetin. Buckwheat is also a very good source of magnesium (it has 86 grams of magnesium in a one-cup serving) and has a good supply of manganese, fiber, phosphorus, pantothenic acid, and protein. Finally, the protein in buckwheat is a very-high-quality protein, containing all eight essential amino acids. In this way, buckwheat is quite complementary to other grains and will provide an even more complete protein when combined with them.

HEALTH BENEFITS

The salutary effects of buckwheat are in part due to its rich supply of flavonoids, particularly rutin and quercitin. These flavonoids extend the action of vitamin C and act as antioxidants. They also maintain blood flow, keep platelets from clotting excessively, and protect low-density lipoproteins from free-radical oxidation into potentially harmful cholesterol oxides. Diets that contain buckwheat have also been linked to a lowered risk of developing high cholesterol and high blood pressure. As a result, they can lower heart disease. One Chinese study clearly showed that buckwheat intake was associated with lower total serum cholesterol, lower levels of LDL (the cholesterol linked to cardiovascular disease), and a high ratio of HDL (the health-promoting cholesterol) to total cholesterol. Even though buckwheat lacks bran and germ, it still rates as a very good fiber source.

HOW TO SELECT AND STORE

For freshness, it is always important to ensure there is no moisture in the food, and that bulk buckwheat bins are covered and your market has a quick turnover. Store buckwheat in an airtight container and keep it in a dry, cool place. Buckwheat flour is best kept in the refrigerator in warmer weather. The flour can last for several months, while whole buckwheat will be good for one year.

TIPS FOR PREPARING

The Japanese combine buckwheat flour with wheat flour to make soba noodles. Whole buckwheats are soaked, steamed, dried, and then milled to remove the hulls, to make a product called *soba-mai*, which is used in a similar fashion to rice. People in the United States use buckwheat flour to make buckwheat pancakes, a good alternative for those with a wheat allergy. Buckwheat flour is widely available in the U.K. Russians enjoy kasha, a mashed and cooked buckwheat dish that is popular for breakfast.

Like all grains, before cooking whole buckwheat, rinse it thoroughly under cool running water to remove any dirt or debris. Then see Table 12.2, "Guide to Cooking Grains," on page 325 for easy preparation instructions.

QUICK SERVING IDEAS

- Try the French method of using buckwheat flour to make crêpes that can be filled with sautéed mushrooms, yam purée, or blueberry jam.
- Buckwheat flour combines well with whole-wheat (wholemeal) flour to make delicious breads, muffins, and pancakes.

- For a change of pace from hot oatmeal, make a pot of buckwheat as a delicious hearty breakfast cereal.
- Kasha varnitchkes are made by combining roasted buckwheat with cooked bow-tie noodles, sautéed onions, garlic, and seasonings.
- Cooked buckwheat makes a nutritive addition to soups or stews and yields a more pronounced flavor and deeper texture.
- Add 1 cup of chopped chicken, ½ cup garden peas, ¼ cup pumpkin seeds, ¼ cup sunflower seeds, and ¼ cup spring onions to 1 cup of cooked and cooled buckwheat for a nourishing lunch or dinner salad.

SAFETY

Buckwheat is not a common allergen and is often employed in allergy elimination diets. There is debate as to whether buckwheat can be safely eaten by people who have celiac disease. This intestinal disease is caused by gluten sensitivity, that is, by eating such grains as wheat, oats, or rye, or other foods that contain the protein gluten. Buckwheat is often excluded as well. Although buckwheat is not in the grass family, it does contain prolamines that are similar to the alpha-gliadin of wheat.

Millet

Although millet *(Panicum miliaceum)* is well known as a main ingredient of birdseed, its ramifications for human health are many. The corn-like millet plant grows to about 15 feet/4½ meters tall and can grow in climates inhospitable to wheat and barley. A rounded, tiny bead-shaped grain, millet's color ranges from whitish to gray to yellow and even reddish. This grain alternative contains no gluten and is perfect for gluten-sensitive individuals who still want nutritious foods. Some shops carry the traditional cracked millet couscous, but most shops carry the more common hulled type.

HISTORY

Hailing from prehistoric North Africa, millet is a staple food of many Indians, Africans, Chinese, and Russians. The Egyptians made flat pita bread from millet until they accidentally added one of their brewed beers to it that created a fluffy texture. After this, it is thought that beer was used instead of water to make millet bread. Millet also has a biblical history as an ingredient of unleavened bread and was a key European cultivated grain until the mass cultivation of potatoes and corn. The Asian countries of India and China, along with the African country of Nigeria, together produce more than 90 percent of the global millet production today.

NUTRITIONAL HIGHLIGHTS

The protein content of millet varies from 5 to 20 percent, with an average of 10 to 12 percent. Millet is generally superior to wheat, corn, and rice in terms of protein content. Millet is also a good source of the minerals phosphorus and magnesium, as well as B vitamins such as thiamine, riboflavin, niacin, and B6.

HEALTH BENEFITS

Besides its protein and vitamin content, millet is a hypoallergenic (low-allergy), gluten-free grain. As such, it is a perfect alternative to wheat.

Like many other whole grains, it is a good source of fiber and offers protection against heart disease, diabetes, and cancer.

HOW TO SELECT AND STORE

For freshness, it is always important to ensure there is no moisture in the food, and that for bulk purchasing the bins from which you obtain the millet are covered and your grocer has a high volume and quick turnover. For storage, use an airtight container and keep millet in a dry, cool place, where it can last for several months.

TIPS FOR PREPARING

Like all grains save oats, before cooking hulled millet, it should be rinsed thoroughly under cool running water to remove any dirt or debris. After rinsing, add 1 part millet to 3–4 parts boiling water or organic chicken or vegetable broth. Once the liquid returns to a rolling boil, turn down the heat, cover, and simmer for about 20 minutes. As when cooking rice, this technique will keep the texture of millet fluffy. For a more creamy consistency, stir the millet frequently, adding a little water every now and then as needed. (Also see Table 12.2 on page 325.) To give millet a more nutlike character, roast the grains in a dry skillet over medium heat and stir until they are a golden color. Then add to the boiling water.

QUICK SERVING IDEAS

- Once cooked, millet can be served as a breakfast porridge, to which you can add your favorite fruits and nuts.
- Ground millet is an excellent addition to bread and muffin recipes.
- Add cooked millet to soup to make it more substantial.
- For a wheat-free biscuit, replace wheat flour with millet flour in any biscuit recipe.
- Combine cooked millet with chopped vegetables, bread crumbs, eggs, and seasonings, then form into patties and bake at 350 degrees F./180 degrees C./gas 4 until done.
- Next time you are looking for an alternative to rice or potatoes, serve millet instead.

SAFETY

Millet contains a goitrogen (a substance that interferes with thyroid hormone manufacture) and should not be consumed on a regular basis by people with hypothyroidism.

There is debate as to whether millet can be safely eaten by people who have celiac disease. This intestinal disease is caused by gluten sensitivity when eating such grains as wheat, oats, or rye, or other foods that contain the protein gluten. Millet is often excluded as well. Although millet is not in the grass family, it does contain prolamines that are similar to the alpha-gliadin of wheat.

Quinoa

Although considered a grain, quinoa is technically the seed of a plant that, as its Latin name, *Chenopodium quinoa*, suggests, is related to the beet, chard, and spinach plants. While the most popular variety is transparent yellow, other varieties are orange, pink, red, purple, or black. Quinoa seeds, which are rich in amino acids, are not only very nutritious but also quite tasty.

Cooked quinoa seeds are fluffy and creamy, yet slightly crunchy. They have a delicate and subtly nutty flavor. Rarely seen in today's fresh produce section, the quinoa plant has edible leaves, with a taste not unlike that of its beet, spinach, and chard cousins.

HISTORY

Quinoa is a relative newcomer to North America and the U.K., despite the fact that it has been produced in South America (Peru, Chile, and Bolivia) since 3000 B.C.E. The South American Native Americans enjoyed this plant as a dietary staple, with the Incas honoring quinoa with the title "mother seed." Also known to give strength and stamina, it was called "the gold of the Aztecs."

The Spanish conquistadors all but stamped out the existence of quinoa in an attempt to destroy the South American natives and their culture. With death as a punishment to any offender, cultivation of quinoa was decreed illegal. In the 1980s, however, two people from the state of Colorado became interested in its healthfulness and began to cultivate it there. Since then, the availability of quinoa has increased substantially.

NUTRITIONAL HIGHLIGHTS

A very good source of magnesium and manganese, quinoa contains three times as much magnesium as calcium. It is also a very fine protein source and possesses healthy levels of vitamins B2, vitamin E, and dietary fiber. It is also a good source of the minerals iron, phosphorus, copper, and zinc.

HEALTH BENEFITS

Quinoa is a fantastic wheat- and gluten-free choice, probably the least allergenic of the grains. Like buckwheat, quinoa has an excellent amino acid profile, not only because of its absolute high protein content but also because it contains all the essential amino acids. Quinoa is an excellent protein source for vegans.

HOW TO SELECT AND STORE

For maximum freshness, it is always important to ensure there is no moisture in the quinoa you are purchasing. If you buy in bulk, the bins from which you obtain the quinoa should be covered and your shop should have a high-volume, quick turnover. Store quinoa in an airtight container and keep it in a cool dry place, where it can last for several months. It will keep for longer, approximately three to six months, if stored in the refrigerator. When deciding how much to purchase, remember that quinoa expands to several times its original size during cooking.

TIPS FOR PREPARING

It is best to remove any leftover saponins on the quinoa coat by thoroughly washing the seeds by putting them into a fine-meshed sieve and running cold water over them. Gently rub the seeds with your fingers. At the end, taste a seed: if it is bitter, more washing is required.

For perfectly cooked quinoa, simply add one part grain to two parts liquid in a saucepan. After the mixture is brought to a boil, reduce the heat to a simmer and cover. One cup of quinoa cooked using this method usually takes 15 to 20 minutes to prepare, which is less time than brown rice. The grains become translucent at the end of the cooking process, and the white germ partially detaches from the main body of the grain, appearing like a white spiral tail. To obtain a nuttier flavor, you can dry-roast the quinoa for 5 minutes in a skillet before cooking. (Also see Table 12.2 on page 325.)

QUICK SERVING IDEAS

- Combine 1 to 2 cups cooked, chilled quinoa with one can of organic pinto beans, ¼ cup pumpkin seeds, 3 minced spring onions, and ground coriander. Add extra-virgin olive oil and mustard. Season with salt and pepper to taste and enjoy this south-of-the-border-inspired salad.
- For a breakfast treat, add nuts and fruits to cooked quinoa and serve as a breakfast porridge.
- For a twist on your favorite pasta recipe, try pasta noodles made from quinoa.
- Sprouted quinoa is great in salads and sandwiches, just like alfalfa sprouts.
- Quinoa makes a nice protein-rich addition to your favorite vegetable soups.
- For a varied flavor and texture, quinoa flour can be added to cookie or muffin recipes.

SAFETY

Quinoa contains moderate to large amounts of oxalate. Individuals with a history of calcium oxalate-containing kidney stones should limit their consumption of this food. See page 793 for more information.

Rye

With one of the deepest and heartiest tastes of all the grains, rye *(Secale cereale)* looks like wheat but is longer and more slender. Its color ranges from yellowish brown to grayish green. Rye is available in its whole-grain or cracked-grain form, or as flour or flakes. Since it is laborious to completely separate the germ and bran from the endosperm of rye, rye flour usually keeps more nutrients than its wheat cousin. As the key ingredient in traditional rye and pumpernickel breads, rye is commonly used as a bread grain and is second only to wheat. Since rye's gluten is less elastic and it holds less gas than that of wheat during the leavening process, breads made with rye flour become more compact and dense. Although popular for human consumption, most of the rye grown in the United States is used as livestock feed.

HISTORY

Originally a Central Asian species of wild grass, rye spread among the fields of barley and wheat until it was noticed for its own nutritious qualities. Unlike other grains, this nutritious food has always been a second-class cultivar, somewhat considered a food of the poor. As living standards in the times of the ancient Greeks and Romans and some other European cultures rose, the consumption of rye diminished, though people living in Germany, Scandinavia, and eastern European nations still appreciate rye's taste and nutrition. Maybe as natural health gains a stronger foothold in today's world, so will rye.

Prior to modern farming techniques, because rye grows well in poor soil and moist climates, it was susceptible to the ergot fungus. Ergot grows out of the flowering stalk as a horn-like dark fruit body that looks like a deformed grain. During the Middle Ages, ergot was responsible for frequent epidemics of what was called "holy fire" or "Saint Anthony's fire," a condition characterized by loss of blood flow to the extremities, which results in intense pain and eventually gangrene, along with mental derangement. The compounds responsible for the symptoms are chiefly alkaloids, of which LSD (lysergic acid diethylamide) is a variant. Today, small amounts of ergot compounds are used in the medical treatment of migraines, Parkinson's disease, and shock.

Today, the majority of the world's rye comes from the Russian Federation. Poland, China, Canada, and Denmark grow rye commercially as well.

NUTRITIONAL HIGHLIGHTS

Rye is a very good source of dietary fiber, phosphorus, magnesium, and vitamin B1. It boasts a 4:1 magnesium-to-calcium ratio.

HEALTH BENEFITS

Primarily due to its high fiber content, rye can prevent spikes in diabetics' blood sugar level and reduce the symptoms of people with irritable bowel syndrome. Finnish studies have clearly shown the benefit, by reduction of colon cancer risk, of rye's ability to provide extra soluble and insoluble fiber, as well as its function of encouraging colonic butyric acid production. Butyric acid is a fatty acid needed for the health of the colonocyte. Rye fiber is a rich source of non-cellulose polysaccharides with a high water-binding capacity. By binding water in the intestinal tract, rye breads give the sensation of fullness and help normalize bowel function. Dry rye breads or crackers rich in fiber may be the most useful for this purpose; however, look for products without unnecessary salt and oils.

HOW TO SELECT AND STORE

For maximum freshness, it is always important to ensure there is no moisture in the rye you are purchasing. For bulk items, the bins from which you obtain the rye should be covered and your grocer should have a high volume, quick turnover. Store rye in an airtight container in a dry, cool place, where it can last for several months. As a precaution, when shopping for rye bread, make sure to read the labels since sometimes what is labeled "rye bread" is actually wheat bread colored with caramel coloring.

TIPS FOR PREPARING

Like all grains except oats, rye should be rinsed thoroughly under cool running water to remove any dirt or debris. To cook, add one part whole-grain or cracked-grain rye to three to four parts boiling water, along with a little pinch of salt. Once the liquid has returned to a boil, turn down the heat, cover, and simmer for about 1 hour. For a softer texture and feel, you can soak the rye grains overnight and then cook them for 2 to 3 hours. See Table 12.2, "Guide to Cooking Grains," on page 325 for easy preparation instructions for rye flakes.

- Oatmeal alternative: Use rye flakes instead of oats for a hot breakfast alternative.
- In place of rice, cooked rye grains can be served as a hearty side dish.
- Try rye bread to make your favorite deli-style sandwich.
- Homemade rye granola: Combine rye flakes with raw walnuts, raisins, and other dried fruits. Sprinkle with a little maple syrup and toast in a low-heat oven for a few minutes to make your own delicious, low-sugar granola treat.
- Use rye flour instead of wheat flour to make your best pancake, muffin, and bread recipes yet.

SAFETY

Rye contains gluten and should be avoided by individuals with gluten intolerance.

Sorghum

Sorghum (*Sorghum* spp.) is known as chicken corn, guinea corn, and kafficorn. It is usually grown in hot, dry regions where corn cannot be grown successfully. Sorghum's drought resistance makes it a vitally important crop in areas of the world with very little rainfall, such as parts of Africa and India, where it serves as a primary grain for millions of people.

Like corn, sorghum is a member of the grass family, and in its early growth stages, it looks virtually identical to corn, although its mature appearance is quite different. Four kinds of sorghums are cultivated: grain, grass, sweet, and broomcorn sorghums. As their names suggest, grain sorghums are bred specifically for grain production; grass sorghums are used as silage for animals; sweet sorghums are processed into syrup and sugar; and broomcorn sorghums' stiff branches are used to make brooms.

The grain sorghum stalk retains its similarity to corn, although it typically grows to a height of only four feet/1¼ meters, about half as tall as a cornstalk. The leaves are a brilliant green in spring and summer, then turn light brown in the autumn. Unlike corn, the head of the grain sorghum, which grows out of the center of the stalk, is open and composed of a cluster of hundreds of "berries" that, depending upon the variety, range in color from white to yellow, red, and bronze or even very dark blue to black. The interior of the berries, their endosperm or starch portion, is white or yellow. By harvest time, the berries have matured into hard seeds.

White berry sorghums have long been used in foods for human consumption, while the darker varieties were typically used for animal feed. White berry sorghums were developed in Africa and India, where sorghum has been used to make porridges and flatbreads for thousands of years. Recently, however, new varieties of colorful grain sorghums with high levels of beneficial phytochemicals, such as flavonoids and anthocyanins, have been developed for use in cereals, snack foods, baking, and brewing.

In addition to their array of phytochemical antioxidant compounds, the new varieties of grain sorghum have been bred for their drought resistance, excellent protein availability, and environmental friendliness. Jeff Dahlberg, Ph.D., research director for the National Grain Sorghum Producers, estimates that sorghum uses about one third less water than corn and causes less soil erosion than cotton. When sorghum is planted, soil erosion drops from approximately 15 acres per ton for cotton to approximately 5 acres per ton.

In the United States, sorghum varieties approved for food are identified, tested, and certified by the National Grain Sorghum Producers' "Certified Food Sorghum" programme. Many sorghum varieties produce a mild-tasting meal or flour that blends well with other flours. Boosting nutrition without affecting texture and flavor, sorghum flour can be used as a substitute for up to 50 percent of the wheat flour in baked goods, such as biscuits, breads, and crackers. Sorghum kernels can also be flaked, popped, or puffed and used in flaked cereals, snacks, granola cereals and bars, and other baked goods. In the southern United States, sweet sorghum (called "sorgho") is processed into a flavorful, amber-colored syrup with a sweetness comparable to that of maple syrup but with significant amounts of calcium, potassium, and iron.

HISTORY

Sorghum has been cultivated in Africa and Asia for more than 4,000 years. Although sorghum is the fifth leading grain crop in the world, being exceeded only by wheat, rice, corn, and barley, less than 2 percent of the sorghum grown in the United States is used in foods and alcohol production. The rest, 98 percent, is used as livestock feed. Elsewhere in the world, more than half the sorghum produced is for human consumption. In Asia and Africa, sorghum remains a staple food. The stalks of sweet sorghums are chewed much like sugarcane, while grain sorghums are usually consumed as porridge or flatcakes,

which are made by adding hot water to pounded flour. In Nigeria, immature sorghum is roasted much like sweet corn, and special varieties are popped like popcorn. In India, sorghum grain is ground or cracked, made into dough, and baked as an unleavened bread called rotti. The grain is also parched, boiled whole, and made into alcoholic beverages, including a vitamin B-rich beer made in central Africa and a potent Chinese liquor called *mao-tai.*

In the mid-1700s, Benjamin Franklin introduced the first sorghum seeds to the colonies under the name of "broomcorn." Also called "chicken corn" during colonial times, sorghum was not received enthusiastically until about 100 years later, when grain sorghums and Sudan grass were reintroduced from Africa.

Today, the United States is the world's leading producer of sorghum, growing 20 percent of the world's crop, primarily in the southern Great Plains states.

NUTRITIONAL HIGHLIGHTS

From a nutritional composition standpoint, sorghum is comparable to wheat (without containing gluten) in that it is high-complex-carbohydrate, high-protein grain (½ cup supplies 72 grams of carbohydrate and 11 grams of protein) and also an excellent source of fiber (primarily insoluble fiber), vitamins B3, B1, and B2, and the minerals iron and potassium.

HEALTH BENEFITS

Research now being conducted on new, high-phenol varieties of sorghum is demonstrating that certain varieties of sorghums that are high in tannins also contain high levels of active compounds with anticancer properties.

TABLE 12.5

Levels of Phenols and Fiber in Sorghum and Other Foods (Dry Matter Basis)

Food	Phenols (milligrams per gram)	Tannins (milligrams per gram)	Anthocyanins (abs/g/mL)	Antioxidant Activity (ORAC Value)	Dietary Fiber (%)
Red wheat	3	—	—	31	48
White sorghum	4	—	—	27	41
Brown sorghum	107	175	31	401	45
Black sorghum	22	10	520	114	43
Blueberries	26	20	50	—	—
Berries	1–22	—	—	63–282	—

These sorghums are loaded with phenols, phytochemicals that research shows are able to block the initiation, promotion, and progression of colon, oesophageal, lung, liver, pancreas, and breast cancers. Sorghum contains two major types of phenols, phenolic acids and flavonoids, including tannins and anthocyanins, many of which are potent antioxidants that have also been shown to inhibit cardiovascular disease. In lab tests, these new varieties of sorghum have been found to contain from 4.1 to 20.9 milligrams of phenols per gram.

The anthocyanins, a type of flavonoid found in sorghum but not in most other grains, are powerful antioxidants that research shows exhibit potent free-radical scavenging activity, especially in lung tissue. They also decrease tumor growth; reduce elevated blood cholesterol, and prevent oxidation of LDL (bad) cholesterol and blood cell clumping; enhance the activity of vitamin C; strengthen collagen (the main protein in skin and other tissues, including blood vessel walls); improve peripheral circulation; and help safeguard eyesight, especially in individuals with diabetic retinopathy.

Some sorghum varieties have been found to contain as high or even higher levels of anthocyanins than blueberries, a highly touted source of these protective plant compounds. On a dry-weight basis, blueberries contain 3.4 to 24.2 milligrams per gram of phenols, while some black sorghum varieties boast anthocyanin levels of up to 36.9 milligrams per gram.

In addition to these protective phenols, a number of additional phytochemicals in sorghum cultivars with promising antioxidant/ anticancer activity include gallic, protocat-chuic, p-hydroxybenzoic, vanillic, caffeic, p-coumaric, ferulic, and cinnamic acids.

Scientists used to think that only the free forms of these compounds could provide antioxidant benefits to humans, and since most of them are bound to the bran in sorghum, as well as in other grains, it was thought that they provided only modest benefit. Recently, however, researchers have discovered that enzymes produced by friendly bacteria in the colon can release these beneficial compounds from cereal brans. If the majority of sorghum's phenolic acids are bioavailable, its antioxidant contribution to health may be quite significant.

With its excellent nutritional and phytochemical profile and its absence of gluten, sorghum is a contender in the market for those with celiac disease, autism, food allergy, or other gluten intolerance.

HOW TO SELECT AND STORE

Look for sorghum flour, mixes, cereal, and other baked goods in the gluten-free grains section of your whole-food shop. A variety of products produced from "Certified Food Sorghum" is now becoming available in the U.S.A. but sorghum foods are not too easy to find in the U.K. as yet.

Like any whole-grain flour, flour made from sorghum should be tightly wrapped and refrigerated or frozen until use to protect the germ and prevent rancidity. Crackers made with sorghum flour should be wrapped tightly, stored in a cool place, and used within a few months.

Sorghum grains, like other whole grains, should be stored in a cool, dry area in a sealed glass container, away from air, moisture, and sunlight, which can make the oils go rancid. Kept in this manner, they can be stored for one year or more. As with other stored grains, it's a good idea to write the date of purchase on the container and use packages purchased earliest first.

TIPS FOR PREPARING

Whole-grain sorghum flour will add a delightful nutty flavor to your favorite recipes for biscuits, brownies, quick breads, muffins, pancakes, or cakes. Just replace half of the wheat flour called for by your recipe with sorghum flour.

Since sorghum flour contains no gluten, it cannot be used by itself when baking yeasted products, such as bread. For bread baking, combine sorghum flour half and half with wheat flour. If you are sensitive to gluten but do not have celiac disease, use sorghum half and half with spelt flour.

Sorghum flour also combines well with gluten-free flours, such as that made from rice or from soybeans, mung beans, or chickpeas. Since the taste of sorghum flour is mild while that of the others is more distinctive, you may wish to use three parts sorghum flour to one part of the other flours. For example, if your biscuit recipe calls for 4 cups flour, you could substitute 3 cups sorghum flour, ½ cup chickpea flour, and ½ cup sweet rice flour.

QUICK SERVING IDEAS

- Make a double batch of sorghum flour pancakes. Serve some for Sunday brunch, and wrap and refrigerate the remaining pancakes for use as flatbreads or for sandwiches during the week.
- Substitute sorghum flour for half or all the wheat flour in your favorite recipe for peanut butter or chocolate chip cookies, brownies, or banana nut bread.
- Next time you make oatmeal raisin cookies, instead of mixing the rolled oats with wheat flour, use a combination of half sorghum and half oat flour.

SAFETY

A gluten-free grain, sorghum is considered

hypoallergenic; in addition, its hardiness translates into a reduced need for pesticides in its cultivation, so pesticide residues are unlikely.

Spelt

Spelt *(Triticum spelta)* is a distant elder cousin of modern wheat. It is a grass-derived grain that, unlike other alternative grains, can be used alone to produce loaves of bread, pasta, and other baked goods with a familiar wheatlike taste and texture. Yet spelt differs from wheat in a number of important ways. Modern strains of wheat have been bred for loose husks that are easily dislodged during the threshing or harvesting process, but spelt retains its sturdy protective envelope. When harvested, a grain of spelt, with its tough outer hull surrounding the kernel, looks like a jumbo-sized grain of russet brown rice with a mounded back and a flat, cleaved belly.

Spelt's strong hull protects the grain from pollutants and insects; therefore, spelt is not normally treated with pesticides or other chemicals. It is naturally resistant to insect pests and diseases such as rust, which is a common problem in wheat crops. In addition, since the hull is not removed until just before the grain is milled into flour, spelt's nutrients and freshness are better preserved.

A hardier grain than wheat, spelt can thrive in a wide range of environments that would be inhospitable to wheat. On the downside, spelt's yield per acre is lower than that of wheat, and its processing requires two separate grindings compared to just one for wheat—the first to dehull the grain and the second to mill it. In the early 1900s, these economic disincentives resulted in agribusiness's choice of wheat over spelt.

Spelt aficionados are, however, willing to pay a higher price, not only for the rich flavor of this nutty-tasting grain but also because of its ease of digestion and significantly better nutritional profile compared to wheat. Even though, when ripe, spelt does contain the allergy-provoking protein gluten, the chemical bonds holding it together are more fragile than those found in modern wheat, and thus spelt's gluten is much less likely to cause allergic reactions in wheat-sensitive individuals. Nutritionally, spelt is the clear winner over wheat, which is one reason why a new strain of spelt developed at Ohio State University was given the name Champ. Among its nutritional highlights, 2 ounces/60 grams of spelt flour provide 10 grams of protein replete with eight essential amino acids and 5.27 grams of fiber. In comparison, 2 ounces/60 grams of wheat flour offers 2.74 grams of protein and 1.8 grams of fiber.

Spelt may also be picked unripe, the grain dried while still in the ear, then threshed and harvested. Just like fully ripened spelt grain, unripe spelt is rich in nutrients and, due to a careful drying process, has the same robust flavor. What unripe spelt does not have is any gluten—an important benefit for those whose sensitivity to this protein is so severe that they cannot tolerate even the small amount of easily digested gluten found in ripe spelt. Its lack of gluten renders unripe spelt grain unsuitable for baking, but it is an exceptionally delicious and nutrient-dense hypoallergenic grain for other uses, such as in soups, veggie burgers, or pilafs, or as a flavorful substitute for rice in any dish. Cooking plumps each grain, doubling its volume and transforming it into a barley look-alike, its fiber-rich brown coat yielding to a tender white interior with the savory taste of nuts and wheat.

HISTORY

Spelt's cultivation is thought to have begun sometime during the mid- to late Neolithic (Stone Age), 6000 to 5000 B.C.E., in the Fertile Crescent, an area that spans parts of modern Iraq, Iran, and Jordan, making the grain one of the earliest crops grown in the Western world. Spelt's place of origin is controversial. Archaeobotanists and cereal geneticists have proposed two primary hypotheses: one suggesting a single site of origin in what is now northern Iran; the other claiming two independent but concurrent sites of origin, one in northern Iran and a second in northern Greece.

The majority of evidence indicates that spelt developed when either wild or cultivated emmer, another ancient relative of wheat even older than spelt, was dispersed to regions with an indigenous wild grass species called *Triticum tauschii*. The addition of the genome contributed by this wild grass resulted in spelt, a hardier grain that could flourish in an even wider range of environments.

The evidence that suggests spelt developed at the same time in two geographical regions comes from work done by two British researchers, Terry Brown and Glynis Jones, who analyzed DNA obtained from 3,300-year-old grains found in what was a Bronze Age backwater in northern Greece called Assiros. DNA markers in these ancient grains of wheat suggest that it was spelt, which experts previously did not think had become known in the Mediterranean area until the first century of the Christian era.

This discovery is important since it means that Bronze Age Greeks may have been baking a modern version of bread as early as 3300 B.C.E.—centuries earlier than experts had thought the types of wheat needed to produce bread similar to that made from modern varieties existed. Our modern varieties of wheat with their excellent bread-baking qualities are not naturally occurring; they had to be developed through crossbreeding. Before such grains were developed, wheat's forerunners were consumed as meal or gruel. But the spelt grains analyzed by Brown and Jones could have been stone-ground into flour and used to make a loaf smaller and squatter than that produced with modern wheat, but it would have been a delicious nutty-tasting bread with a close crumb structure.

All the experts now agree that spelt was widely distributed throughout the Balkans, Europe, and Transcaucasia during the Bronze Age (4000 to 1000 B.C.E.), a distribution facilitated by the migration of early civilizations westward. The first reference to spelt is found in an edict of the Roman Emperor Diocletian in 301 C.E. Spelt can also be considered the grain centerpiece of the first politically established welfare system, since it is thought to be the grain that, after food riots in 59 B.C.E., was distributed free to Roman citizens.

That spelt was commonly used in biblical times is indicated by the fact that the grain is included in the list of ingredients in the bread baked by Ezekiel (Ezekiel 4:9): "Take wheat and barley, beans and lentils, millet, and spelt. Put them in a storage jar and use them to make bread for yourself."

Brought by Roman legions to Britain in the first century C.E., spelt remained a prominent grain in medieval Europe, gracing the tables of the aristocracy while most of the population ate rye bread. The twelfth-century naturalist Hildegard von Bingen (Saint Hildegard) sang spelt's praises more than 800 years ago:

The spelt is the best of grains. It is rich and nourishing and milder than other grain. It produces a strong body and healthy blood in those who eat it, and it makes the spirit of man light and cheerful. If someone is ill, boil some spelt, mix it with egg, and this will heal him like a fine ointment. . . . Spelt grain makes body and blood healthy, and the soul content.

Known to the ancient Romans as *farrum,* spelt remains a popular grain in Italy, particularly in Tuscany, Lazio, Umbria, and Abruzzo, the relatively poorer central regions. It is called *farro* by modern Italians and featured in Confarrotio, a favorite wedding soup. Spelt also continues to be a major cereal crop in isolated regions throughout Europe, primarily in Germany and Switzerland, where it is called *dinkle.*

Swiss immigrants, settling in eastern Ohio, are credited with bringing spelt to the United States. With large-scale cultivation beginning in the 1890s, spelt was the primary grain used to produce flour in the United States until about 1920, when wheat's lower processing costs caused its elder's displacement. Grown mostly as animal feed until the 1980s, spelt has recently made significant inroads into the health food market as a nutrient-dense, hypoallergenic alternative to wheat. In fact, a number of spelt products are now available, including spelt pasta, whole-grain and white flours, flaked cereals, breads, biscuits, crackers, cakes, muffins, pancakes, waffles, and mixes for pancakes, muffins, and bread machines. Today the majority of the U.S.'s spelt acreage is in Ohio, where 100,000 to 200,000 acres are grown annually, about ten times as much as produced in any other state. Montana also grows a significant spelt crop, and smaller crops are cultivated in Pennsylvania, Michigan, Indiana, Kansas, and North Dakota as well.

NUTRITIONAL HIGHLIGHTS

Spelt is an excellent source of complex carbohydrates, complete protein, and fiber. It is also a very good source of a number of B vitamins and minerals. In a mere 100 calories, 1 ounce/30 grams of spelt cereal flakes provides 5 grams of protein, along with 3 grams of fiber. Whole spelt grain is slightly lower in protein (3 grams per ounce/30 grams) and calories (90 per ounce/30 grams) but higher in fiber and minerals. Table

TABLE 12.4

Protein Content of Spelt and Whole Wheat in Milligrams per Gram of Fresh Weight

Amino Acids	Spelt	Whole Wheat
Cystine	1.35	1.10
Isoleucine	5.60	4.40
Leucine	9.00	6.00
Methionine	4.00	2.40
Phenylalanine	7.00	5.00
Threonine	5.60	5.50
Lysine	2.75	2.90
Tryptophan	1.80	1.20
Valine	5.80	4.20

Source: www.purityfoods.com.

12.4 provides an average of the differences in protein content between spelt and wheat.

HEALTH BENEFITS

Spelt is an alternative for those allergic to wheat. When ripe, spelt contains gluten, but the gluten found in cereal grains is not all alike. Gluten is made up of two kinds of molecules, glutenin and gliadin, and the amount of each differs in the different grains. The molecular composition of the gluten in spelt is such that its gluten is more fragile than that found in wheat, so it is more easily digested.

In addition, spelt is the only grain that contains a special type of carbohydrate called mucopolysaccharides. Certain mucopolysaccharides, the cyanogenic glucosides, have been found to not only stimulate the immune system but also to help lower cholesterol, and to play a vital role in blood clotting.

Spelt's ease of digestion combined with its high levels of complex carbohydrates and immune-stimulating factors make it a particularly good choice for "carbo-loading" before an athletic event or for replenishment of muscle glycogen stores afterward. Plus, spelt provides at least double the protein and fiber of most common varieties of commercial wheat.

HOW TO SELECT AND STORE

Available all year round, spelt grains (or farro), flour, mixes, pasta, cereal, and baked goods can be found prepackaged from many natural food suppliers. As with wheat, spelt products are available in whole-grain and white (refined) versions.

Like any whole-grain flour, flour made from whole-grain spelt (farro) must be wrapped tightly and refrigerated or frozen until use to protect the germ and prevent rancidity. Whole-grain spelt crackers or pasta should also be wrapped tightly, stored in a cool place or refrigerated, and used within a few months. Once cooked, spelt pasta will keep in an airtight container in the refrigerator for three to five days.

Spelt grains, which may be labeled "Farro," the Italian word for this ancient grain, are divided into three grades: the first and best, grains 6 to 8 millimeters (¼ to ⅓ inch) long; the second, 3 to 5 millimeters (⅛ to ¼ inch) long; and the third, cracked grains broken during processing. Avoid cracked farro. Since its protective outer layer has been breached, it is more likely to have lost nutrients or become rancid. Purchase either the first or second grade of spelt grains and, if the recipe calls for it, crack them at home by whirling them in a blender or electric coffee grinder.

Spelt grains, like other grains, should be stored in a cool, dry area in a sealed glass container, away from air, moisture, and sunlight, which can make the oils go rancid. Kept in this manner, they can be stored for one year or more. As with other stored grains, it's a good idea to write the date of purchase on the container and use packages purchased earliest first.

TIPS FOR PREPARING

Cooking spelt grains requires a little planning, as they must be soaked for at least 8 hours beforehand; but, once soaked, they needn't be cooked right away since they will keep in the refrigerator for a few days. Before soaking, as with any grain, spelt grains should be rinsed well to remove any chaff, grit, or bad grains, which can be identified by their dark color or the fact that they float to the top. For the richest flavor, toast raw spelt grains in a skillet for a few minutes until they pop and crackle, then rinse and soak in water overnight before simmering.

Cook soaked spelt grains in a covered pot. Add enough water or vegetable stock to rise 1 inch/2½ centimeters above the grain. Bring to a boil, then simmer over low heat for 1½ to 2 hours (half this amount of time if cooking cracked spelt). Alternatively, bring 3 cups water to a rolling boil. Stir in 1 cup of spelt grains; lower the heat and simmer for 1 hour. Spelt grains will continue to absorb liquid, puff up, and soften even after they are ready to eat, so if possible, let them rest a while before serving. (Also see Table 12.2 on page 326.)

Spelt flour requires less liquid than other flours. To use spelt flour in a recipe designed for wheat flour, you can either reduce the amount of liquid called for by one quarter or add one quarter more spelt flour than the amount of wheat flour used in the recipe.

While wheat typically requires 10 minutes of initial mixing time (from when water is first added to the flour) when making bread, spelt is ready in just 3½ to 4½ minutes. This is because the gluten found in spelt is much more fragile than that found in wheat, so for a good result, mixing should last no more than 4½ minutes at medium speed. Mix the spelt flour with the liquid just enough to produce a homogeneous dough; you may find that 3½ minutes is enough. Once mixed, treat the dough just as you would wheat dough.

For a lighter bread with more volume, make a sponge dough first. Place half the amount called for of all your recipe's ingredients, including the yeast, in a bowl. Mix just until a dough

forms (about 3 to 3½ minutes), then cover and place in a warm, draft-free spot for later use.

Within 5 hours, you'll have usable sponge dough, but you can let it rest up to 12 hours before finishing your bread. To do so, add the remainder of the ingredients to the sponge dough, mix until well but not overly blended (about 3½ minutes), and proceed as you would with wheat dough.

Creating a sponge dough produces a higher loaf because mixing spelt flour, which is high in complex carbohydrates, with water activates enzymes that convert some of the carbohydrates into simple sugars, which provide an ample source of food for the yeast. The yeast's activity results in bread with a better cell structure, greater loaf volume, and a lighter crust.

If you do not have time to make a sponge dough first, try replacing one quarter or one third of whole-grain spelt flour with white spelt flour. The resulting loaf with be lighter, higher, and only a bit less nutrient-dense.

To cook spelt pasta, boil 2 to 3 quarts/liters of water for each 8 ounces/250 grams of dry pasta and follow the timing directions listed on the package. If you will be using the pasta in a recipe that requires additional cooking, such as lasagna, reduce the cooking time listed in the directions by up to a third. To help prevent the pasta from sticking to the pot or clumping together, add a spoonful of olive oil to the boiling water before adding the pasta. Just before the pasta reaches that perfect state when it is *al dente,* or firm to the bite yet cooked through, the center of each noodle will be a lighter color than the rest. This section will still be slightly under-cooked—but just for another minute or two.

When serving spelt pasta with sauces that

are served hot, such as marinara or spaghetti sauce, simply drain without rinsing, toss, and serve immediately. Rinsing can wash off delicate starches that help to hold the sauce to the noodles.

When using spelt pasta for cold dishes or if you must wait before adding sauce and serving, rinsing with cool running water will help prevent the pasta from sticking together.

If you have time, make double the amount of sauce and pasta, drain and rinse half, place in a casserole, cover with sauce, and refrigerate. A slightly thinner sauce works especially well with elbows and rotini. Just shake the container, and they will fill with sauce.

QUICK SERVING IDEAS

- Use spelt flour and pasta for any dish you would make with wheat. Just be sure to use less liquid and mix for a shorter time as explained above in "Tips for Preparing."
- Precook spelt grains in vegetable stock (or the liquid from chickpeas, beans, or cabbage), let them rest for several hours so they will puff up, and add to minestrone soup. Or add uncooked spelt grains while cooking vegetable broth or your favorite robust soups—just be sure to increase the amount of water since the spelt grains will absorb plenty.
- Spelt's high protein content makes it a good choice for a one-dish main course. Mix cooked spelt grains with chunks of raw vegetables, tofu or cheese, and nuts, then drizzle with olive oil and balsamic vinegar for a summer salad supper. For a hearty winter meal, add pieces of your favorite roasted vegetables, tofu or cheese, and nuts, and serve hot.

- Fold cooked spelt grains into multigrain bread dough, muffin, or pancake batter.
- Serve cooked spelt grains as a hot or cold cereal topped with a splash of milk and sliced strawberries, apples, or your favorite fruit.
- Toss cooked spelt grains with a little butter or oil and serve instead of rice as a side dish.

SAFETY

Although the small amount of fragile gluten found in spelt is much less likely to cause an allergic reaction than the higher amount of sturdy gluten found in modern wheat, individuals allergic or sensitive to gluten may find they also have problems tolerating products made of spelt.

Spelt contains moderate to large amounts of oxalate. Individuals with a history of calcium oxalate-containing kidney stones should limit their consumption of this food. See page 793 for more information.

Triticale

Triticale is a hybrid of wheat and rye. It is not commonly used in the U.K., except in animal feed. It is thought to contain the best of both grains and is attracting much interest due to its higher protein content compared to wheat. Triticale's genetic inheritance from rye enables it to withstand cold temperatures, drought, and acidic soils that would devastate wheat, while its wheat genes donate a high level of disease resistance, a high yield, and a gluten content that, while lower than wheat's, is sufficient to enable triticale to be used alone to bake bread. However, triticale requires fertile, well-watered soil for best growth; yields less grain per acre than wheat; and is susceptible to ergot.

Triticale resembles wheat in size, shape, and color, although triticale produces a grain that is longer and slightly darker in color than wheat and plumper than rye. But each plant produces fewer grains, so its yield per acre has been less than wheat's. Within the last few years, however, new cultivars of triticale have been developed that match wheat's yield in optimal environments and outperform wheat in marginal ones.

Though triticale can be used alone to bake bread, it contains less gluten than wheat and, as a result, produces a squat, heavy loaf. New cultivars are also addressing this deficiency. The key factor in producing light-textured breads is the gluten quality of the flour. The desirable gluten traits in modern bread wheats have been successfully obtained through many years of intensive cultivar development, but little or no effort has been made to encourage similar gluten traits in other grains until recently. In the past ten years, a number of studies have been focused on the gluten quality of not only triticale but the ancient grains einkorn, emmer, and spelt as well. Studies of wheat gluten suggest that specific genes encode for the gluten protein subunits that are responsible for its good bread-making qualities. These same gluten subunits are also found in triticale and the ancient grains, so cereal researchers are working with cultivars in which these gluten subunits are enhanced. These new cultivars of triticale and other grain alternatives to wheat will have not only their own pleasing flavors but the high, light texture now provided only by wheat.

HISTORY

Triticale was developed in 1875, when the Scottish botanist Stephen Wilson married wheat with rye in the hope that their offspring would inherit wheat's high yield and ability to produce a high-rising loaf, along with rye's exceptional hardiness. Unfortunately, the initial seeds produced by this union were sterile, but in 1888, the French botanist Wilhelm Rimpau produced the first fertile wheat-rye hybrid.

During 1918, at the Saratov Experimental Station in Russia, thousands of natural hybrids of wheat and rye spontaneously appeared in a number of wheat fields. For the next sixteen years, G. K. Meister and his colleagues developed these hybrids, which are still grown in Russia and have been exported to many other countries as well.

The name "triticale" first appeared in the scientific literature in 1935 and is attributed to Erich von Tschermak, one of the proponents of the Mendelian law of inheritance, who named the grain for both its parents, wheat (Triticum) and rye (Secale). Also in 1935, the Swedish researcher Arne Müntzing began what became his life's work: the development of triticale. Today, triticale is cultivated on more than 6.4 million acres worldwide, contributing more than 6.5 million metric tons each year to global cereal production. Poland, Germany, China, and France account for nearly 90 percent of world triticale production, but the grain is also produced in significant amounts in the republics of the former Soviet Union, Australia, Argentina, Canada, and the United States..

Although its use for human consumption remains limited, in Europe triticale is used, alone or blended with wheat, to produce local homemade breads. Rolled triticale (triticale "flakes") and triticale wholemeal flour, wholemeal specialty breads, and other health foods are also available in limited amounts.

In the United States, triticale cultivation is steadily increasing, with 500,000 acres now grown annually. Triticale is still primarily used as a feed grain, pasture, and silage crop for animals, but considerable research is ongoing to improve its milling and baking qualities. Triticale cultivars released in recent years have high yields, resistance to lodging (the infestation of pests) and ergot, plump kernels, and an excellent balance of amino acids, plus lysine levels higher than those of other cereal grains. (Lysine is the first limiting amino acid in cereal grains, which means that when the body is trying to make protein, lysine is the first amino acid to be in short supply.)

NUTRITIONAL HIGHLIGHTS

Triticale is similar in nutritional content to wheat. The key difference is that it has an excellent balance of amino acids and is particularly high in lysine, an essential amino acid that is low in most cereal grains.

HEALTH BENEFITS

Triticale provides the same sorts of benefits as other whole grains.

HOW TO SELECT AND STORE

In the U.S., triticale can be purchased as whole or cracked grains or flakes. Triticale flour, cereal, bread, and crackers are available in some health food and whole-food shops. In addition, triticale is often included in prepared mixed-grain hot and cold cereals and muffin mixes.

Like wheat grains, triticale grains should be stored in a cool, dry area in a sealed glass container away from air, moisture, and sunlight, which can make the oils go rancid. Kept in this manner, they can be stored for one year or more. As with other stored grains, it's a good idea to write the date of purchase on the container and use packages purchased earliest first.

Cracked triticale are grains whose outer hulls have been cracked or broken. Since any breach in the grains' outer casings increases the possibility of nutrient loss and oil rancidity, we suggest you make your own cracked triticale immediately before using. Just whirl whole grains in an electric coffee grinder or blender until they are coarsely chopped. Cracked triticale has the advantage of taking much less time to cook.

Triticale flakes, like rolled oats, are grains that have been steamed and flattened. Stored in an airtight container in a cool, dry, dark place, triticale flakes should keep for approximately two months.

Triticale flour, like any whole-grain flour, should be wrapped tightly and refrigerated or frozen until use to protect the germ and prevent rancidity.

TIPS FOR PREPARING

Triticale grains need to be soaked overnight in the refrigerator before cooking. For the best flavor, after soaking overnight, brown triticale grains in a small amount of olive oil before cooking.

Triticale is cooked similarly to rice, although more liquid is needed. Use 1½ cups of water for each ½ cup of triticale grains. Bring the water to a rolling boil, add the grains, lower the heat, and simmer until softened (about 1 hour, 45 minutes). (Also see Table 12.2 on page 326 for easy preparation instructions for rolled [flakes] or cracked triticale.)

Since triticale flour is lower in gluten than wheat flour, if used alone it will produce a heavy, dense loaf. For this reason, triticale is often combined half and half with wheat for bread baking. A 50/50 blend of triticale and wheat flour will produce bread of similar quality to bread made only from wheat.

If using triticale flour alone to make bread, it's a good idea to begin by making a sponge, as this will produce a lighter, softer, well-flavored bread loaf. To make a sponge, place half the amount called for of all your recipe's ingredients, including the yeast, in a bowl. Mix until a dough forms (about 3 to 4 minutes), then cover and place in a warm, draft-free spot. Within 5 hours, your sponge dough will be ready to use, but you can let it rest up to 12 hours before finishing your bread. To do so, add the remainder of the ingredients to the sponge, mix until well but not overly blended (another 3 to 4 minutes), and proceed as you would with wheat. The gluten in triticale is more fragile than that found in wheat, so don't knead the dough too much, as this can damage triticale's delicate gluten.

Creating a sponge produces a higher loaf because mixing flour, which is high in complex carbohydrates, with water activates enzymes that convert some of the carbohydrates into simple sugars, which provide an ample source of food for the yeast. The yeast's activity results in bread with a better cell structure, greater loaf volume, and a lighter crust.

QUICK SERVING IDEAS

- With a flavor similar to that of wheat with a subtle hint of rye, whole triticale grains can be soaked the night before and cooked as a delicious breakfast cereal in about an hour. Top with a little honey and macadamia nut oil. Rolled (flakes) or cracked triticale cooks much more quickly and will be ready in 15 to 20 minutes.
- Substitute triticale for wheat grains or cracked triticale for cracked wheat in any recipe.
- Make tabouleh with triticale instead of bulgur.
- Substitute triticale flakes for rolled oats and make a batch of triticale raisin biscuits.
- Cook whole or cracked triticale grains and use in pilaf-style dishes or casseroles or as a stuffing for poultry or fish.
- Add uncooked triticale grains to soups and stews to thicken them and enrich their flavor.
- Mix cooked whole or cracked triticale grains into veggie burgers, nut loaves, or burgers.

SAFETY

Although the smaller amount of more fragile gluten found in triticale is less likely to cause an allergic reaction than the higher amounts of sturdy gluten found in modern wheat, individuals allergic or sensitive to gluten may find they also have problems tolerating products made from triticale.

Triticale contains moderate amounts of oxalate. Individuals with a history of calcium oxalate-containing kidney stones should limit their consumption of this food. See page 793 for more information.

13

The Healing Power of Legumes (Beans)

Legumes (beans) are among the oldest cultivated plants. In fact, fossil records demonstrate that prehistoric people domesticated and cultivated legumes for food. Today, this extremely large category of vegetables contains more than 13,000 species and is second only to grains in supplying calories and protein to the world's population. Compared to grains, legumes supply about the same number of calories but usually two to four times as much protein.

Legumes are often called the "poor people's meat"; however, they might better be known as the "healthy people's meat." Many legumes, especially soybeans, are demonstrating impressive health benefits. Diets rich in legumes are being used to lower cholesterol levels, improve diabetics' blood glucose control, and reduce the risk of many cancers. Legumes contain many important nutrients and phytochemicals, and when combined with grains, they form a complete protein. According to studies conducted by the U.S. Department of Agriculture, richly colored dried beans offer a high degree of antioxidant protection. In fact, small red kidney beans rated the highest, just ahead of blueberries.

Legumes and Flatulence

One of the problems caused by eating legumes is increased intestinal flatulence (wind) or intestinal discomfort. Most humans pass wind a total of fourteen times per day, for a total of 1 pint. About half of the wind is swallowed air and another 40 percent is carbon dioxide produced by bacteria in the intestines. The remaining 10 percent is a mixture of hydrogen, methane, sulphur compounds, and by-products of bacteria, such as indoles, skatoles, ammonia, and hydrogen sulphide. It is this last fraction that is responsible for the offensive odors.

The flatulence-causing compounds in legumes are primarily oligosaccharides, which are composed of three to five sugar molecules linked together in such a way that the body cannot digest or absorb them. Because the body cannot absorb or digest these oligosaccharides, they pass into the intestines, where bacteria break them down. Gas is produced by the bacteria as they digest the oligosaccharides. Haricot and lima beans are generally the most offensive, while peanuts are the least offensive because of their lower levels of oligosaccharides.

The amount of oligosaccharides in legumes can be significantly reduced by properly cooking or sprouting them. In other words, the amount of flatulence produced by legumes can be dramatically reduced by proper cooking or sprouting. See Table 13.1 for guidance in properly cooking legumes and page 370 for instructions for sprouting them. If, after following these instructions, you still experience increased flatulence when you eat legumes, you may wish to try a commercial enzyme preparation called Beano.

Cooking Legumes

Although most legumes can be purchased precooked in cans, cooking your own offers significant economic, as well as possibly health, benefits. Cooking your own legumes will produce three times the amount compared to canned products.

Dried legumes, with the exception of lentils, are best prepared by first soaking them overnight in an appropriate amount of water (see Table 13.1). This is best done in the refrigerator to prevent fermentation. Soaking will usually cut the cooking time dramatically. If soaking overnight is not possible, here is an alternative method: place the dried legumes in an appropriate amount of water in a pot, for each cup of dried legumes add ¼ teaspoon of bicarbonate of soda, bring to a boil for at least 2 minutes, and then set aside to soak for at least 1 hour. The bicarbonate of soda will soften the legumes and help break down the troublesome oligosaccharides. The bicarbonate of soda will also help reduce the amount of cooking time. Be forewarned, however, that beans cooked using the quick-soak and no-soak methods may split or develop a slightly mushy consistency. For beans that retain an even shape, ideal texture, and tender, creamy bite without mushiness, overnight soaking is optimal. Also, beans that have not been presoaked may need some additional water, about ¼ to ½ cup per cup of beans, to replace the water that evaporates during their longer cooking process.

Before cooking presoaked beans, regardless of soaking method, skim off any skins that have floated to the surface, drain the soaking liquid, and then rinse with clean water. The beans should be brought to a gentle boil and then simmered with a minimum of stirring to keep them firm and unbroken. A pressure cooker or Crock-Pot can also be used for convenience. Regardless of cooking method, do not add any seasonings that are salty or acidic, such as vinegar, wine, tomatoes, or citrus fruits and their juices, until after the beans are cooked, since adding them earlier will make the beans tough and greatly increase the cooking time.

Whenever possible, use the cooking liquid as well as the beans. About 35 percent of the B vitamins and 50 percent of the folic acid leach into the liquid when beans are cooked for 1 hour and 15 minutes.

If you are running short on time, you can

TABLE 13.1

Guide to Cooking Dried Beans

Dried Beans	Cups of Water or Stock to 1 Cup of Beans	Cooking Time (Presoaked)	Cooking Time (Unsoaked)	Yield (Cups)
Adzuki (aduki) beans	4	45–55 minutes	2 hours; if not done, add 20–30 minutes	3
Anasazi beans	2½–3	45–55 minutes	1 hour	2¼
Black beans	4	1–1½ hours	2 hours	2¼
Black-eyed peas	3	30–45 minutes	1 hour	2
Broad (fava) beans skins removed	3	40–50 minutes	1 hour	1⅔
Cannellini (white kidney beans)	3	45 minutes	1 hour	2½
Chickpeas (garbanzo beans)	3–4	2–2½ hours	3 hours	2
Cranberry beans	3	40–45 minutes	1 hour	3
Great Northern beans	3½	1½ hours	2 hours	2⅔
Haricot beans	3	45 minutes–1 hour	1½ hours	2⅔
Kidney beans	3	1 hour	2 hours	2¼
Lentils, brown	2¼	15–20 minutes	45 minutes–1 hour	2¼
Lentils, green	2	15–20 minutes	30–45 minutes	2
Lentils, red	3	Not recommended	20–30 minutes	2–2½
Lima (butter) beans, Christmas	4	1 hour	2 hours	2
Lima (butter) beans, large	4	45 minutes–1 hour	1½–2 hours	2
Lima beans, small	4	50 minutes–1 hour	1½–2 hours	3
Mung beans	2½	1 hour	1½ hours	2
Peas, split, green	4	45 minutes	1 hour	2
Peas, split, yellow	4	1–1½ hours	2 hours	2
Peas, whole	6	1–2 hours	2 hours	2
Pink beans	3	50 minutes–1 hour	1½ hours	2¾
Pinto beans	3	1½ hours	2 hours	2⅔
Soybeans	4	3–4 hours	1½ hours	3

always use canned beans in your recipes. If the beans have been packaged with salt or other additives, simply rinse them after opening the can to remove these unnecessary additions. Canned beans need to be heated only briefly for hot recipes, while they can be used as is for salads or prepared cold dishes.

SPROUTING LEGUMES

Since legumes are actually seeds, they contain the essential factors for the plant to reproduce, which allows them to be sprouted. Sprouting is not only thought to increase the nutritional value for beans, it is thought to improve digestibility as well. Many bean sprouts, such as alfalfa, mung bean, chickpea, and lentil, are available at food shops. Alfalfa sprouts are, by far, the most popular.

Sprouting most legumes at home is quite easy. All you need is a large glass jar or, better yet, a sprouting jar with different types of lids. After rinsing, place the legumes to be sprouted in the jar, covered with water, for 24 hours. You may need to rinse the legumes once or twice and re-cover them with water. After the initial 24 hours, pour out the water, rinse, and allow the moist legumes to sit in an area without direct sunlight. Rinse them twice daily. Once the legumes have sprouted the jar can be placed in more direct sunlight if desired. Most sprouts are ready to eat a day or two after they have sprouted.

Soybeans and Soy Foods

The soybean (*Glycine max*) will be discussed first due to the quantity of information available on its health benefits, many of which apply to other legumes as well. In addition, soybeans are an extremely versatile food and are available in many different forms. No discussion of soy would be complete without mention of the traditional soy foods miso, soy sauce (tamari), tempeh, and tofu (bean curd).

Soybeans

Like other beans, soybeans grow in pods enclosing edible seeds. While we most often think of soybeans as being green, the seeds can also be yellow, brown, or black. The texture of soybeans is so adaptable that they are processed into virtually every imaginable type of food. In the United States and similarly in the U.K., soybeans are usually consumed as a meat substitute in the form of soy hot dogs, hamburgers, lunch meats, and textured vegetable protein, and as soymilk, tofu, and soy protein.

HISTORY

The soybean plant is native to China, where it has been cultivated for well over 13,000 years. The ancient Chinese considered the soybean their most important crop and a necessity for life.

Soybeans were introduced into Japan in the eighth century and, many centuries later, into other regions of Asia, including Thailand, Malaysia, Korea, and Vietnam. Soybeans were brought to the United States in the eighteenth century, but it was not until the early twentieth century, when nutrition pioneers such as George Washington Carver and John Harvey Kellogg began promoting the health benefits of soybeans, that they came to be used for more than animal feed by Americans.

Thanks largely to the United States, which accounts for more than 50 percent of the world's production, the soybean is now the most widely grown and utilized legume, accounting for well over 50 percent of the world's total legume production. In terms of dollar value, the soybean is the United States' most important crop, ranking above corn, wheat, and cotton. Unfortunately, in the United States, despite its use in a variety of food products, the soybean is still used primarily for animal feed (protein meal) and for its oils. However, since the 1970s, there has been a marked increase in both the consumption of traditional soy foods, such as miso, tempeh, and tofu, and the development of so-called second-generation soy foods, which simulate traditional meat and dairy products. Consumers can now find soy milk, soy hot dogs, soy sausage, soy cheese, and soy frozen desserts in their food shops. In fact, excluding soybeans used for animal feed and oil, more than 90 percent of the soybeans consumed in the United States is in the form of soy protein products. These products are made from defatted soybean flakes and range in protein content from 40 to 90 percent.

The increase in soy food consumption in the United States is attributed to a number of factors, including economics, health benefits, and environmental concerns. In terms of cost, soybeans provide a great amount of nutrition per acre. In fact, an acre of soybeans can provide nearly twenty times the amount of protein as the amount of protein an acre used for raising beef provides. We believe the use of and reliance on soy will grow as the world's population continues to expand and its food supply continues to shrink.

NUTRITIONAL HIGHLIGHTS

Soybeans are an excellent source of protein and molybdenum. They are a very good source of iron, calcium, phosphorus, and dietary fiber. In addition, soybeans are a good source of vitamins B1, B2, B6, and E and folic acid.

Soybeans are an especially important protein source, containing 38 percent protein. Soy flour is an even richer source of protein, typically containing 40 to 50 percent protein. Moreover, soy protein concentrates typically contain 70 percent protein, and soy protein isolates typically contain 90 to 95 percent protein. Compared to other legumes, soybeans are also higher in essential fatty acids, with a total fat content of 18 percent, and much lower in carbohydrates, at 31 percent.

Soybeans also contain a number of special health-promoting compounds, including phytosterols, lecithin, isoflavones and other phytoestrogens, and protease inhibitors.

HEALTH BENEFITS

The benefits of soy could fill a large book. It is one of the world's most important foods. The key benefits of soy are its high protein content; essential fatty acids, phytosterols, and lecithin; fiber components; isoflavones; and protease inhibitors. Each of these will be briefly discussed. Please note that these topics are intricately interrelated.

Protein Content

Although the amino acid profile of soy is not perfect as it is a little low in methionine and tryptophan, soy is still regarded as equal to animal foods in protein quality. In addition, when soy is combined with grains high in methionine,

TABLE 13.2

Macronutrient Content of Selected Soy Foods

Food	Calories	Protein (grams)	Carbohydrate (grams)	Fat (grams)
Soybeans, ½ cup, cooked	149	14.3	8.5	7.7
Tempeh, ½ cup	165	15.7	14.1	6.4
Tofu, ½ cup	94	10	2.3	5.9
Soy flour, defatted, ½ cup	81.7	12.8	8.4	0.3
Soy milk, plain, 1 cup	79	6.6	4.3	4.6

such as corn, an extremely high quality protein is made.

Soy protein-based products provide the same order of growth and development in infants and protein nutrition in adults as milk-based formulas. However, the human body appears to handle plant proteins differently from animal proteins. For example, experimental studies in animals and humans have shown that soy protein isolates tend to lower cholesterol levels while protein from animal sources, particularly casein from milk, tends to raise cholesterol levels. In some human studies, soy protein has even been shown to lower total cholesterol levels by 30 percent and to lower LDL, or "bad" cholesterol, levels by as much as 35 to 40 percent.

Researchers have yet to determine exactly how soy protein lowers cholesterol levels, as several factors have been observed that would account for the reduction. However, they do know that the cholesterol-lowering effect of soy protein formulations is more apparent when serum cholesterol levels are high. Human studies have shown that the total and LDL (bad) cholesterol levels are both reduced, as are elevated triglyceride levels. In contrast, consumers should be wary of casein-containing (i.e., milk-based) meal replacement formulas. Casein has been shown not only to increase cholesterol levels but to increase the development of gallstones as well.

Essential Fatty Acids, Phytosterols, and Lecithin

The essential fatty acid content of soybeans further supports its cholesterol-lowering and anticancer effects. Soybeans have a total fat content of approximately 18 percent, of which 85 percent is unsaturated and 15 percent is saturated. The unsaturated portion is composed of linolenic (9 percent of total oil content), linoleic (50 percent), and oleic (26 percent) acids.

Soybeans, as well as most other seeds, nuts, and legumes, also contain compounds known as phytosterols. These plant compounds are structurally similar to cholesterol and steroid hormones. Phytosterols function to inhibit the absorption of cholesterol by blocking absorption sites. The cholesterol-lowering effects of phytosterols are well documented. Phytosterols have also been shown to enhance immune functions, inhibit the Epstein-Barr virus, prevent chemically induced cancers in animals, and exhibit numerous anticancer effects. Soybeans are especially rich in phytosterols, especially beta-sitosterol. A 100 gram serving of soybeans provides approximately 90 milligrams of beta-sitosterol, while unrefined soybean oil provides 315 milligrams per 100 grams. Refined soybean oil provides much less beta-sitosterol, 132 milligrams per 100 grams.

In addition, soybeans are the primary commercial source of lecithin (phosphatidyl-choline), which is a major component of the cellular membranes in humans. Unrefined soy oil contains approximately 3 percent lecithin. During refining, the lecithin is removed as an "impurity" and then sold for use in baked goods, prepared foods, and pharmaceutical preparations. Lecithin is an excellent emulsifier in that it helps oils and water mix. Lecithin also has been shown to produce numerous health benefits. Commercial lecithin preparations containing as much as 90 percent phosphatidyl-choline have demonstrated positive effects in lowering cholesterol levels and improving liver and gallbladder function and various neurological disorders. These effects may be attributed to phosphatidylcholine's important role in maintaining the myelin sheath that surrounds nerve cells, as well as its action as a precursor of the neurotransmitter acetylcholine. Phosphatidyl-choline has been investigated in the treatment of Alzheimer's disease, Parkinson's disease, Tourette's syndrome, and Huntington's disease. The studies have shown both a positive effect and no effect. In addition, at this time it is not known to what degree the lecithin content of soybeans contributes to their beneficial effects.

Fiber

Soybeans contain a mixture of fiber. Approximately 94 percent of the total fiber content is composed of insoluble fiber, and 6 percent is soluble. Of the insoluble fibers, approximately 90 percent are hemicelluloses (see page 74 for a description).

Numerous health effects of soy fiber have been demonstrated in clinical studies. Its effectiveness is largely due to its ability to:

Increase faecal bulk.
Increase faecal water content.
Decrease intestinal transit time.
Reduce blood cholesterol and triglyceride levels.
Improve glucose tolerance.
Increase insulin sensitivity.

These effects of soy fiber make soybeans and other soy fiber-containing foods useful in cases of constipation, diarrhea, high cholesterol levels, and diabetes.

Isoflavones

Soybean consumption is thought to be one of the major reasons for the relatively low rates of breast and colon cancers in Japan and China. Studies in animals have demonstrated that diets composed of as little as 5 percent soybeans can significantly inhibit chemically induced cancers.

Soybeans contain many known, as well as many proposed, anticancer compounds. In addition to fiber and other well-recognized anticancer nutrients, several other potent anticancer agents are found in relatively high concentrations in soybeans. The compounds that have garnered the most attention are the isoflavones. These compounds have been shown to be especially protective against breast and prostate cancers.

The two isoflavones found in soy—daidzein and genistein—act as phytoestrogens, naturally occurring plant compounds that bind to oestrogen receptor sites in human cells, including breast cells. By blocking these receptors, they reduce the effects of oestrogen. This action does not disrupt the normal reproductive and fertility functions of oestrogen but may counteract some of its cancer-causing potential. The isoflavones work not only by occupying oestrogen receptors, but also by other unrelated mechanisms. Researchers have concluded that the anticancer activity of soy isoflavones may not be limited to oestrogen-dependent tumors, as they have also been shown to cause death to cancer cells and inhibit angiogenesis, the formation of new blood vessels needed to fuel cancer cells.

OESTROGEN SENSITIVITY WARNING

Women who have oestrogen-sensitive breast tumors should restrict their soy intake to no more than four servings per week and should avoid soy isoflavone supplements. Studies in test tubes and in animals show that the isoflavone genistein stimulates the growth of oestrogen receptor-positive tumors. However, it inhibits the growth of breast cancer cells that lack oestrogen receptors. Whether these results apply to humans is not yet clear, but until more information is available, it makes sense for women who have oestrogen receptor-positive breast cancer to restrict their soy intake and avoid soy isoflavone supplements.

The amount of soy found to be protective against the development of breast and prostate cancers delivers 25 to 100 milligrams per day of isoflavones. Many soy foods now state the level of isoflavones per serving. As you can see from Table 13.3, you do not need to eat huge amounts of soy foods to meet the recommended levels.

The greatest benefits of soy consumption may occur before and during adolescence in girls. Studies indicate that preadolescent intake of soy enhances the maturation (differentiation) of breast cells. These more mature cells are less susceptible to carcinogens. The anticancer effects of soy intake in premenopausal women appears to be more valuable in preventing the onset of cancer through more favorable oestrogen levels and metabolism. Soy intake has been shown to offer breast cancer protection to postmenopausal women as well.

Although most of the attention has focused on the isoflavone content being responsible for the anticancer effects of soy, new evidence suggests that soy contains other substances that provide even more anticancer benefit. Researchers at the University of Chicago tested soy on laboratory animals with mammary gland tumors. One group of animals received pure soy protein (without isoflavones), another group got pure isoflavones, and a third group got a mix that had both. All three groups had fewer tumors than the untreated animals. Surprisingly, the treatment that worked best was soy *without* isoflavones. Clearly, something else was at work.

Protease Inhibitors

Soybeans, as well as other legumes, nuts, and seeds, contain compounds that inhibit the

TABLE 13.3
Soy Foods and Their Isoflavone Content

Product	Serving Size	Approximate Isoflavone Content (mg)
Cooked soybeans	½ cup	40
Roasted soybeans (soy nuts)	½ cup	40
Tempeh	125 grams	40
Tofu	125 grams	40
Soy protein	½ cup	35
Soy milk	1 cup	40

action of the protein-digesting enzymes (proteases). These compounds are referred to as protease inhibitors, and they are part of the seed's defense against destruction. For example, because of protease inhibitors many seeds, if eaten by birds, are indigestible and are excreted intact so they can still sprout new plants. Does this mean humans cannot digest these foods either? Not necessarily. In humans, there are compensatory mechanisms, such as increased pancreatic enzyme output, that can counteract some of the protease inhibition. In addition, most, but not all, protease inhibitor activity is destroyed by cooking or sprouting.

Raw soybeans, which contain considerable amounts of protease inhibitors, were one of the first dietary factors shown to inhibit the growth of experimental cancers in animals. Numerous studies in animals have confirmed a possible anticancer effect when they are fed soy foods containing protease inhibitors. However, although this anticancer effect may be in part due to protease inhibition, the same degree of

inhibition has been produced by feeding animals soy foods without the protease inhibitors. Furthermore, the anticancer effects of the protease inhibitors may not be a direct effect at all.

Pancreatic enzyme preparations containing proteases, as well as other proteases such as bromelain, have long been used in Europe and by alternative health care practitioners in the United States in the treatment of cancer. There is some clinical evidence that this is quite beneficial. The use of proteases in the treatment of cancer would appear to be in direct opposition to the animal studies demonstrating that protease inhibition does not necessarily inhibit cancers. However, by examining the situation more closely it can be seen that feeding animals (as well as humans) protease inhibitors results in the output of more pancreatic proteases. Although the proteases may be inhibited from digesting the protease inhibitors, other functions of proteases may not be affected. In addition to digesting proteins, pancreatic proteases perform many other valuable functions in the body, including activation of certain immune functions and an increase in the output of the hormone cholecystokinin by the intestines. Increased cholecystokinin levels in the blood result in feelings of satiety and a significant reduction in appetite.

Phytoestrogens

Isoflavones are also known as phytoestrogens, signifying their mild oestrogenic activity. Their weak oestrogenic action is in actuality an antioestrogenic effect, as it prevents the binding of the body's own oestrogen to receptors. This does not disrupt the normal reproductive and fertility functions of oestrogen but may counteract some of its cancer-causing potential.

In a study of postmenopausal women, those women consuming enough soy foods to provide about 200 milligrams of isoflavones demonstrated signs of oestrogenic activity when compared to a control group. Specifically, the women consuming the soy foods demonstrated an increase in the number of superficial cells that line the vagina. Presumably, soy food consumption may offset some of the vaginal drying and irritation in postmenopausal women.

Oestrogens are being widely prescribed for postmenopausal women in an attempt to prevent osteoporosis. This may not be necessary if proper diet and lifestyle measures are followed (see page 760). Furthermore, a diet rich in isoflavones may be a suitable alternative. An intake of approximately 300 milligrams of isoflavones provides the equivalent dosage of about 0.45 milligram of conjugated oestrogens, or one tablet of Premarin, a popular oestrogen used for menopausal symptoms. In addition to the oestrogenic activities, isoflavonoids are demonstrating other beneficial effects in preventing bone loss.

There is also evidence that phytoestrogens may exert a balancing effect when oestrogen levels are high, as is commonly seen in premenstrual syndrome (PMS). The consumption of soy foods is the most economical, and possibly the most beneficial, way to increase the intake of phytoestrogens to relieve the symptoms of PMS.

HOW TO SELECT AND STORE

Dried soybeans are generally available in prepackaged containers, as well as in bulk. For maximum freshness, it is always important to ensure that there is no moisture in the beans you are purchasing and that if you purchase them in bulk, the bins are covered. To maintain fresh stock, your grocer should have a high volume and quick turnover. For storage, use an airtight container and keep your beans in a dry, cool place, where they can last for up to one year. If you buy soybeans at different times, keep them separate, for beans of various ages will require different cooking times. Also, check for insect damage and that the beans are whole and not cracked. If purchasing canned beans, look for those that do not contain extra salt or additives. Once cooked, soybeans can be stored in the refrigerator for up to three days if placed in an airtight container.

Fresh soybeans (edamame) should be deep green in color with firm, unbruised pods. Edamame are now found in the U.K. in natural food shops and Asian markets. They may be in the frozen food section, although some shops offer precooked edamame in their refrigerated display cases too. Many sushi restaurants serve boiled edamame with salt on top. Fresh edamame has a two-day refrigerator life, while frozen edamame will keep for four to five months.

TIPS FOR PREPARING

Prior to washing beans, they should be visually inspected to eliminate any debris, dirt, or damaged beans. One way to do this is to spread them in a single layer over a solid-colored dish. After inspection, rinse the beans by straining them under cool running water. Dried soybeans are best soaked before cooking in order to lessen cooking time and make them easier to digest (see page 369 for instructions).

Soybeans are easily cooked on the stove or more quickly in a pressure cooker. For the stove-top method, take a saucepan and add 3 to 4 cups of fresh water or organic vegetable or chicken stock for each cup of dried beans. The liquid should be about 1 to 2 inches/2½ to 5 cm above the top of the beans. Bring the beans to a boil and then reduce to a simmer, partially covering the pot. If any foam develops, simply skim it off. Soybeans generally take about 3 to 4 hours to become tender using this method. They can also be cooked in a pressure cooker, where they take about 1 hour to prepare (also see Table 13.1 on page 369).

For a more complete protein than either alone, you can mix one part soy with three parts grain, especially corn. By substituting soy flour (40 to 50 percent protein) for an equal amount of wheat flour, you can greatly improve the quality of the protein in baked goods such as breads, rolls, buns, bagels, pancakes, and waffles. If desired, soy protein concentrate (70 percent protein) can be added as well to significantly increase protein levels. Soy protein concentrate can also be used to produce meat analogues and as an extender of minced beef. And soy protein isolate (90 to 95 percent protein) can be used to make a high-protein meal replacement shake or smoothie.

QUICK SERVING IDEAS

- Soybeans can be used in their whole, cooked, or sprouted forms, either on their own or in recipes.
- Soybeans are a great alternative for other beans in soups, stews, and casseroles and can even substitute for meat in stews.
- Soy nuts are great to sprinkle on top of green and grain salads.
- Textured vegetable protein is a vegetarian alternative to meat that is excellent in your favorite chili recipe.
- Mix sprouted soybeans into salads or use as toppings for sandwiches.
- Edamame is simple to prepare and makes a great snack or appetizer. Just add the frozen soybean pods to lightly salted water and boil for approximately 15 minutes so they are still green and somewhat firm. Kids love them.
- Soy milk is great in place of cow's milk both as a beverage and to pour over cereal.

SAFETY

Soybeans are well known as a common allergen. See page 723 for more information.

Those with thyroid problems should limit their consumption of raw or sprouted soybeans. Raw or sprouted soybeans contain goitrogens, which can interfere with thyroid gland activity. Dietary goitrogens are usually of no clinical importance unless they are consumed in large amounts or there is coexisting iodine deficiency. Cooking helps to inactivate the goitrogenic compounds. Cooked soybeans do not pose the same issues.

Soy also contains amounts of oxalate. Individuals with a history of oxalate-containing kidney stones should avoid overconsuming soy. For more information, see Appendix D, page 793.

Women who have or have had oestrogen-sensitive breast tumors should restrict their soy intake to no more than four servings per week and avoid soy isoflavone supplements.

Miso

Miso is a fermented soybean paste that is made by inoculating trays of white rice with a mould, *Aspergillus oryzae,* and leaving it to mould abundantly. A ground preparation of cooked soybeans and salt is then mixed in, and the mass is allowed to ferment for several days more before being ground into a paste the consistency of peanut butter. The entire process may take ten to forty days, depending upon the temperature. Miso is used primarily as a flavoring in soups and on vegetables.

The color, taste, texture, and degree of saltiness of miso depend upon the exact ingredients used and the duration of the fermentation process. Miso ranges in color from white to brown. The lighter varieties are less salty and mellower in flavor, while the darker ones are saltier and have a more intense flavor. Some misos are pasteurized, while others are not.

The different types of miso are:

- Hatcho miso (made from soybeans).
- Kome miso (made from white rice and soybeans, as described above).
- Mugi miso (made from barley and soybeans).
- Soba miso (made from buckwheat and soybeans).
- Genmai miso (made from brown rice and soybeans).
- Natto miso (made from ginger and soybeans).

While "miso" is the Japanese name we are most familiar with in the United States and the U.K., this fermented soybean paste is known as *chiang* in China and *chao do* in Vietnam.

HISTORY

Like almost all soy foods, miso was developed in ancient China and later introduced to the Japanese in the 600s. *Hisio,* miso's precursor, was a mix of fermented soybeans, wheat, salt, alcohol, and a few other ingredients and was used primarily as a seasoning by royal and aristocratic persons. During the 1500s, miso gained credit as a healthful and logical military and survival food due to its storage capabilities and the simplicity of its applications. In the 1960s, the founder of the macrobiotic food diet, George Ohsawa, introduced miso to the European community.

The process of making miso in Asia is tantamount to the level of art used to make fine cheeses or wine and is considered a complex and delicate process. Due to the interest in Asian foods, coupled with the many health-conscious consumers who are interested in macrobiotic foods, miso has become widely available in the United States and U.K. in the last few decades.

NUTRITIONAL HIGHLIGHTS

Miso is a good source of many minerals, including zinc, manganese, phosphorus, iron, and copper. It is also a good source of vitamins B2 and B6. In addition, it is a good source of both protein and dietary fiber.

HEALTH BENEFITS

Miso exerts the same cancer-fighting effects as other soy foods. Experimental studies done specifically with miso have shown it to protect against breast cancer.

Since miso is produced from an organism that makes vitamin B12, it may provide this vitamin to vegetarians. However, it should not be assumed that fermented foods, such as miso and tempeh, are excellent sources of vitamin B12. In addition to a tremendous variation in B12 content, there is some evidence that the form of B12 in these foods is not exactly the form that meets our bodily requirements. Vegetarians should take vitamin B12 supplements.

HOW TO SELECT AND STORE

Miso is generally sold in tightly sealed plastic or glass containers. To check for freshness, look for a sell-by date listed on the container. In addition, check the label to make sure there are no additives, such as MSG (monosodium glutamate).

The type of miso to purchase depends on your personal preferences and intended use. As darker-colored misos are stronger and more pungent in flavor, they are generally better suited to heavy foods. Lighter-colored misos are more delicate and more appropriate for soups, dressings, and light sauces.

Miso should be stored in a tightly sealed container in the refrigerator, where it can keep for up to one year.

TIPS FOR PREPARING

Miso soup is quick and easy to prepare. Heat miso paste and water over low to medium heat. Eat as is or add some traditional fixings, such as shiitake mushrooms, tofu, spring onions, burdock, carrots, or daikon radish.

QUICK SERVING IDEAS

- Miso can be used as an ingredient in marinades for meat, fish, poultry, or game.
- Dried miso soup packets can be carried with you and enjoyed as a hot beverage, just like tea or coffee.

- Combine miso with sesame oil, linseed oil, ginger, and garlic to make an Asian-inspired dressing that can be used on salads or cold grain dishes.

SAFETY

Miso is quite high in salt (sodium chloride). Its use should be restricted by people with high blood pressure or those with salt sensitivity.

Soy Sauce (Tamari)

Soy sauce is made by fermenting soybeans with mould *(Aspergillus oryzae),* then adding wheat and salt. Soy sauce originated in China around 500 B.C.E. and was introduced into Japan in the seventh century. It is a salty brown liquid.

HISTORY

Soy sauce has been used as a condiment in China for close to 2,500 years. In the seventh century, Buddhist monks introduced soy sauce into Japan, where it is known as *shoyu.* The Japanese word *tamari* is derived from the verb *tamaru,* meaning "to accumulate," referring to the fact that tamari was the liquid by-product produced during the fermentation of miso. Japan is the leading producer of soy sauce and has an average annual per capita intake of about 3 gallons/11¼ liters.

NUTRITIONAL HIGHLIGHTS

Soy sauce is a good source of vitamin B3. It is also a good source of certain minerals, including iron, phosphorus, and manganese. It also has free amino acids. Tamari is a source of free amino acids and vitamin B2.

HEALTH BENEFITS

Due to their vitamins and amino acids, soy sauce and tamari do confer some nutritional benefit. One concern is that there may be too much sodium in this food. In truth, you consume less sodium when you use soy sauce because the flavor is more penetrating. Reduced-sodium soy sauces have curbed the sodium in soy sauce even further.

HOW TO SELECT AND STORE

Soy sauce is generally sold in sealed glass bottles, but some shops also sell it in bulk containers. Check the label to make sure that no additives or preservatives have been added, especially MSG. Also, choose low-sodium varieties. For those on a wheat-free diet, wheat-free versions are available. Keep unopened soy sauce in a cool, dry, and dark environment. Keep opened soy sauce refrigerated for up to six months.

TIPS FOR PREPARING

Soy sauce is versatile in that it can be used before cooking as a marinade, during cooking, and added to raw or cooked foods.

QUICK SERVING IDEAS

- Soy sauce can be used as a seasoning when sautéing vegetables.
- A marinade for baked tofu, tempeh, or chicken can be made by combining soy sauce, olive oil, garlic, and ginger.
- Soy sauce can be used instead of table salt and pepper for seasoning foods.
- Sprinkle some soy sauce, sesame seeds, and nori strips on top of brown rice for a Japanese flair.
- Before dry-roasting nuts and seeds, brush them with soy sauce.

SAFETY

Soy sauce is quite high in salt (sodium chloride). Its use should be restricted by people with high blood pressure or those with salt sensitivity. When it is used, reduced-salt varieties should be chosen.

All soy products contain a high amount of oxalate. Individuals with a history of oxalate-containing kidney stones should avoid overconsuming soy products. For more information, see Appendix D, page 793.

Tempeh

Tempeh, an Indonesian specialty, is typically made by cooking and dehulling soybeans, - inoculating them with a culturing agent, such as *Rhizopus oligosporus,* and then incubating the inoculated product overnight until it forms a chunky-textured, solid cake.

HISTORY

Shortly after colonizing Indonesia, the Dutch introduced tempeh and other native foodstuffs into Europe. However, it was not until the twentieth century that tempeh was introduced into the United States. Tempeh is now gaining increased popularity in this country as people look for ways to increase their intake of soybeans and discover tempeh's versatility and unique taste.

NUTRITIONAL HIGHLIGHTS

Tempeh is a very good source of protein, manganese, and phosphorus. It is also a good source of vitamins B2, B6, and B3, as well as the minerals magnesium, copper, and iron. In addition, it is a good source of monounsaturated fats.

HEALTH BENEFITS

As a product of soybeans, tempeh confers the same health benefits as the soybean, including the anticancer effects (see above).

As the organism that makes tempeh also makes vitamin B12, it is thought that tempeh may be a good B12 source for vegetarians and vegans. Unfortunately, evidence shows that the forms of B12 found in fermented foods may not be the best in terms of absorbability into the body. As a result, it is important that vegetarians and vegans supplement their diet with vitamin B12.

HOW TO SELECT AND STORE

Until recently, tempeh could be found only in health food and Asian stores. Now that demand has grown, it is found in more conventional markets, usually in the refrigerator or freezer section. Typical varieties include plain and those that include grains and/or vegetables.

Most tempeh has a thin, whitish cover with a few black or gray spots. If you see any pink, blue, or yellow spots, the tempeh may be overfermented.

Tempeh can remain in the refrigerator for up to ten days. Always wrap the partially used package very well and place back in the refrigerator. Frozen tempeh stays fresh for several months.

TIPS FOR PREPARING

One way to prepare tempeh is to marinate it in olive oil, soy sauce or tamari, garlic, and other spices of your choice for at least 20 minutes and then bake it for 15 to 20 minutes at 350 degrees F./180 degrees C./gas 4.

QUICK SERVING IDEAS

- Tempeh Reuben sandwich: Place grilled tempeh on a slice of whole-grain (wholemeal) bread, layer with sauerkraut, top with regular or soy cheese or "meltable" soy cheese, then grill for a few minutes until the sandwich is hot and toasty. An easy Russian dressing topping is made by combining ketchup and soy mayonnaise. Baked tempeh is a great replacement for luncheon meats in sandwiches and, cut into cubes, makes a wonderful protein-rich addition to salads.
- Tempeh bolognese: Try spaghetti and tempeh sauce. Substitute tempeh for minced beef in your favorite recipe.
- Tempeh chili: Find your best chili recipe and add some extra flavor, texture, and nutrition with some tempeh.
- Place baked tempeh in a food processor with olive oil, pumpkin seeds, ground coriander, and cumin and purée to make a delicious spread.

SAFETY

All soy products contain large amounts of oxalates. Individuals with a history of oxalate-containing kidney stones should avoid overconsuming soy products. For more information, see Appendix D, page 793.

Tofu (Bean Curd)

Tofu, or bean curd, is now a well-known food. After soy sauce, it is the biggest seller among soy foods in the United States.

Tofu is made from soy milk by coagulating the soy proteins with calcium or magnesium salts, often in the form of nigari seaweed. The liquid (whey) is discarded, and the curds are pressed to form a cohesive bond. The degree of pressing produces either soft, regular, or firm tofu.

HISTORY

Like so many soy foods, tofu originated in China. Legend has it that it was discovered about 2,000 years ago, when a Chinese cook accidentally curdled soy milk when he added nigari seaweed.

Introduced into Japan in the eighth century, tofu was originally called *okabe*. Its modern name did not come into use until the 1400s. Although it is a frequently eaten food in Japan, its great popularity came only in the 1600s. In the 1960s, interest in healthy eating brought tofu to Western nations. Since that time, countless research experiments have demonstrated the many benefits that soy and tofu can provide.

NUTRITIONAL HIGHLIGHTS

Tofu is an excellent source of iron and calcium. It is also a very good source of protein, as well as the minerals manganese, selenium, and phosphorus. In addition, tofu is a good source of magnesium, copper, zinc, and vitamin B1.

HEALTH BENEFITS

Tofu is an excellent food from a nutritional and health perspective. It provides the same sort of protection against cancer and heart disease as soybeans. In one study, substituting tofu for cheese demonstrated impressive results in lowering blood cholesterol levels, in both men and women.

HOW TO SELECT AND STORE

Tofu can be found in bulk or individual packages, both of which are refrigerated. Tofu is also sold in sealed containers kept at room temperature, which do not need refrigeration until they are opened. When opened, all tofu needs to be rinsed, covered with water, and kept in a refrigerated container. To keep the tofu fresh for up to one week, the water should be changed every day. If kept in the original package, you can freeze tofu for up to five months. Freezing tofu gives it a more spongy texture. Although not necessary, this texture change is actually desirable for certain uses, such as sautéing.

Some tofu is "calcium-precipitated," meaning that it is manufactured by using calcium to coagulate the soy milk; this type has a higher calcium content. Firm tofus are generally higher in fat content, while the softer tofus (sometimes called silken or silky) are lower.

TIPS FOR PREPARING

Given its neutral taste and range of consistency, tofu has an amazing ability to work with almost all types of flavors and foods. Like a culinary chameleon, tofu can take on and even enhance the flavors of its surroundings. Tofu comes in the firmer, traditional Chinese style and in the smoother, custardlike Japanese type. Extra-firm tofus are best for baking, grilling, and stir-fries, while soft tofu is suitable for sauces, desserts, shakes, and salad dressings. Of course, you can experiment to see how tofu works into your own cooking preferences and preparation style.

QUICK SERVING IDEAS

- Italian tofu dip: Combine tofu, olive oil, garlic, and lemon juice to make a tofu aioli dip. This is great with freshly sliced vegetables.

- Eggless egg salad: Scramble medium or firm tofu with your favorite vegetables and add mustard, paprika, and turmeric to give it a yellow "egglike" coloring. Sauté in a pan with a little olive oil until warm and serve.
- Firm tofu makes a great stir-fry: Add sugar snap peas, minced ginger, cashews, and your favorite vegetables and seasonings.
- Add soft tofu to ½ cup of blueberries, 1 banana, and 1 tablespoon of ground linseed meal and blend in a blender or food processor. This makes great breakfast or parfaitlike dessert.
- Treat firm tofu like a steak: Marinade it in your favorite teriyaki sauce and throw it on the barbecue.

SAFETY

Tofu and all soy products contain large amounts of oxalate. Individuals with a history of oxalate-containing kidney stones should avoid overconsuming soy products. For more information, see Appendix D, page 793.

Tofu is among the foods most commonly associated with food allergies. See page 723 for more information on food allergies.

Other Legumes

Adzuki (Aduki) Beans

Adzuki beans are not only high in protein but easier to digest than most beans. They are small and reddish brown in color, with a soft texture and a strong, nutty-sweet flavor. Surpassed in importance only by soybeans among the Chinese and Japanese, the adzuki bean *(Phaseolus angularis)* first became popular in the United States as a staple food in Zen macrobiotic diets. Similarly, macrobiotic ideas and foods were brought to the U.K. in the late 1960s.

Plant varieties grow to a height of 1 to 2 feet/30 to 60 centimeters, producing leaves and yellow flowers that are followed by a cluster of several smooth, short, cylindrical pods. The pods contain small, dark red oval seeds approximately 5 millimeters in diameter with a distinctive white ridge along the side where the seed attaches to the pod, although some varieties produce green, straw-colored, black-orange, or mottled seeds. Uneven ripening is characteristic of adzuki beans, so the same plant may show mature brown pods along with slightly yellow and even completely green immature pods.

HISTORY

Like the soybean, the adzuki is thought to have originated in China and was introduced to Japan around 1000 C.E. Cultivated ever since, the adzuki is known by a variety of names in Asia, including adsuki, aduki, asuki, azuki, chi dou, feijao, field pea, hong xiao dou, red oriental, and Tiensin red.

Well loved in both Japan and China, adzuki beans are used in ceremonial dishes, serving as a filling for the dumplings traditionally made for the New Year and steamed with sticky rice to tint it a beautiful rosy pink for the Japanese Red-Cooked Rice Festival.

With annual consumption at more than 120,000 metric tons, adzuki beans are one of the largest of Japan's crops, but only recently has this nutty-sweet bean been introduced to America. In the United States, awareness of the adzuki bean is almost entirely due to its prominence in the Zen macrobiotic dietary practices advocated by George Ohsawa. Among natural health food enthusiasts in the United States, the popularity of the Zen macrobiotic diet peaked in the 1960s but dropped off after several deaths were attributed to overzealous adherence to its dietary restrictions. However, many who abandoned the Zen macrobiotic diet continued to enjoy adzuki beans, which they had discovered were delicious, easily digested legumes that could be used in many very tasty dishes.

Currently, in addition to Japan and China, adzuki beans are cultivated in Manchuria, Korea, New Zealand, India, Taiwan, Thailand, and the Philippines. In the United States, adzuki beans are grown in Florida, Minnesota, and California.

NUTRITIONAL HIGHLIGHTS

Adzuki beans are an excellent source of fiber and protein. In addition, they are rich in B vitamins, being an excellent source of folic acid and B3, a very good source of B1, and a good source of B6 and B2. Last, they provide high levels of the trace minerals molybdenum, copper, manganese, and zinc.

HEALTH BENEFITS

In addition to supplying high levels of soluble fiber and protein, adzuki beans are packed full of trace minerals. These trace minerals are utilized by the body as components of enzymes. For example, a ½-cup serving of adzuki beans provides almost 200 percent of the daily recommended intake for molybdenum, which is necessary for the production of an enzyme called sulphite oxidase, one of the most important enzymes in a liver detoxification pathway called sulphoxidation. Poor sulphoxidation is associated with neurodegenerative diseases, such as Parkinson's and Alzheimer's diseases, and with inflammatory conditions, including rheumatoid arthritis, delayed food sensitivity, multiple chemical sensitivities, and diet-responsive autism.

HOW TO SELECT AND STORE

Available all year round, both dried and canned, adzuki beans can be purchased in most Asian markets and natural food shops and supermarkets. Look for shiny beans with a rich reddish brown or brownish purple color.

Store dried adzuki beans in an airtight container or jar. Cooked adzuki beans can be stored in the refrigerator for up to three days or in the freezer for up to six months.

TIPS FOR PREPARING

Adzuki bean sprouts have a wonderful nutty flavor. Sprout them as you would other beans such as mung or soy. See page 370 for easy sprouting instructions.

When still green, young, tender adzuki pods can be harvested and eaten raw like snow peas or cooked like green beans. Like other beans, dried adzuki beans should be sorted and rinsed well to remove any debris and presoaked. See page 368 for presoaking instructions.

Add 3 cups of water to 1 cup of beans and bring to a gentle boil. Boil for 2 minutes, reduce the heat, and simmer, covered, for 30 to 45 minutes, at which point they should be tender but not mushy. One cup of dried beans will yield about 3 cups of cooked beans. If not presoaked, cook 2 hours, then test; if not done, cook an additional 20 to 30 minutes.

Alternatively, pressure-cook ½ cup presoaked beans in 2 cups water for 5 to 7 minutes at high pressure. If you do not have time to presoak the beans, pressure-cook them for 15 to 20 minutes. (For easy cooking instructions, see Table 13.1 on page 369.)

QUICK SERVING IDEAS

- Flavor adzuki beans while cooking: For each ½ cup of beans, add ½ cup sake or dry sherry, three ¼-inch/½ centimeter slices of fresh mashed ginger, and 3 large garlic cloves, peeled and mashed.
- Adzuki beans make a lovely, cool, but protein-rich salad. Toss 1 cup cooked adzuki beans with 1 tablespoon toasted sesame oil, 2 tablespoons tamari soy sauce, 2 tablespoons rice vinegar, 1 teaspoon honey, and ¼ teaspoon wasabi powder. Sprinkle with chopped parsley or watercress and serve with sliced cucumber and spring onion.
- Thai spices, such as coconut milk, ginger, and Panang goong (a spicy red curry paste), are a wonderful complement to adzuki beans' nutty-sweet flavor.
- Jamaican spices also work particularly well with adzuki beans. Try a spring or summer soup made with a cup of cooked adzuki beans, several tablespoons of your favorite fresh garden herbs (parsley, chives, chervil, rosemary, basil), 1 or 2 diced leeks, a generous teaspoon of Jamaican allspice, and several teaspoons of coarsely ground black pepper. Bring to a boil, then simmer for a half hour. Cool slightly, transfer to a blender, and blend until smooth for a rich, sweet, spicy, deep red soup.
- Make winter fried rice with adzuki beans, onion, diced squash or pumpkin, bright green leeks or spring onions, sesame seeds and oil, and soy sauce. Top with crumbled toasted nori.
- Try making your own adzuki bean paste: Pressure-cook a cup of presoaked beans with a strip of soaked, diced kombu (a type of seaweed) and ¼ cup raisins for about 20 minutes. Allow the pressure to come down, add ¼ teaspoon sea salt and a little honey or barley malt to taste, and mash until a thick, smooth paste forms.

SAFETY

Adzuki beans contain purines. Naturally occurring substances found in plants, animals, and humans, purines can be broken down to form uric acid, and excess accumulation of uric acid may contribute to health problems, such as gout and the formation of kidney stones. Individuals who are susceptible to purine-related problems may wish to limit their intake of adzuki beans.

Alfalfa

Most people are surprised to learn that alfalfa *(Medicago sativa)* is a member of the pea family and therefore a legume. A perennial plant, alfalfa has deep roots, trifoliate leaves, bluish purple flowers, and tiny kidney-shaped seeds.

Although alfalfa, which is known as lucerne in many parts of the world, is grown primarily as forage for livestock, the leaves are also dried, ground into a powder, and compressed into tablets for use as a nutritional supplement for humans. Alfalfa seeds, however, are the part of this plant that provide the food with which we're most familiar—alfalfa's threadlike white sprouts with their tiny green tops and mild, sweet flavor.

HISTORY

Most likely planted in southwestern Asia long before recorded history, alfalfa has been grown as forage for livestock longer than any other plant. Taken by the Persians to Greece when they invaded in 490 B.C.E., alfalfa was carried from Greece to Italy in the first century C.E. and from there spread to the rest of Europe. During the early 1500s, Spanish explorers took alfalfa to South America, and in 1736 European colonists introduced it to the United States.

NUTRITIONAL HIGHLIGHTS

One cup of raw alfalfa sprouts contains just 10 calories but supplies a wide array of beneficial phytochemicals, particularly phytoestrogens and saponins. It is also a very good source of vitamins C, B2, and B5 and folic acid, as well as the minerals copper, molybdenum, zinc, manganese, and magnesium.

HEALTH BENEFITS

Alfalfa sprouts, along with soybeans, clover, and linseed, are the most significant dietary sources of phytoestrogens, beneficial compounds that include isoflavones, coumestans, and lignans. A number of studies in humans, animals, and cell culture systems suggest that dietary phytoestrogens play an important role in the prevention of menopausal symptoms, osteoporosis, cancer, and heart disease. Phytoestrogens are thought to work through a number of mechanisms, including:

- Producing oestrogenic and antioestrogenic effects.
- Inducing the return of normal cell differentiation in cancer cells.
- Suppressing angiogenesis, the formation of new blood vessels needed to fuel cancer cells
- Inhibiting proinflammatory cytokines.
- Providing antioxidant activity.

Because phytoestrogens have much lower oestrogenic activity than human oestrogens but do bind to human oestrogen receptors, they can help normalize the effects of oestrogen in the body. When oestrogen levels are too low, phytoestrogens supply some oestrogenic activity, but when oestrogen levels are too high, the same phytoestrogens, by using up available oestrogen receptors, block out powerful human oestrogens, causing an antioestrogenic effect.

Oestrogenic activity is implicated in the majority of breast cancers, and research now suggests that thyroid cancer may also be an oestrogen-dependent disease. A recent population-based case-control study looked at the effects of eating phytoestrogen-rich foods on thyroid cancer incidence. This study of more than 1,600 women in the San Francisco Bay area revealed that those who frequently ate alfalfa sprouts and soy foods had as much as a 65 percent lower risk for thyroid cancer, regardless of whether they were Caucasian, Asian, or pre- or postmenopausal.

In addition to phytoestrogens, alfalfa sprouts are rich in another class of beneficial phytochemicals called saponins. In animal studies, saponins have been shown to lower diet-induced LDL (bad) cholesterol accumulation in the liver without diminishing circulating levels of beneficial HDL cholesterol, thus exerting a protective effect against cardiovascular disease. But alfalfa's beneficial effects on cholesterol cannot all be attributed to its saponins since, in a recent study, when researchers removed the saponins, alfalfa still reduced cholesterol accumulation in the liver. Obviously, alfalfa contains other active components with potentially significant cardiovascular benefit.

The saponins found in alfalfa have also been shown to boost immune function by increasing the activity of natural killer cells, including T lymphocytes and interferon. Alfalfa sprouts also contain L-canavanine, an amino acid analogue that recent studies suggest may be a natural agent effective against leukemia and cancers of the pancreas and colon.

L-canavanine may also offer promise in the treatment of nearsightedness. Yet another animal study, this one using bovine eye muscle, found that L-canavanine produced a relaxing effect on the intraocular muscle that suggests it could possibly be used to help prevent shortsightedness.

When compared to a number of antioxidant-rich vegetables, alfalfa sprouts rank among the leaders of the pack. When tested against two of the most destructive free radicals on a weight basis, alfalfa sprouts were found to have antioxidant activity surpassed only by kale and Brussels sprouts against the hydroxyl radical, and by garlic, kale, spinach, and Brussels sprouts against the peroxyl radical.

HOW TO SELECT AND STORE

Alfalfa sprouts are widely available in the U.S.A. and can be found in most grocery shops, usually in the small, clear plastic containers in which they have been hydroponically grown. Although available in the U.K., the market for alfalfa sprouts is relatively small, though growing. Buy only sprouts that have been kept at refrigerator temperature. Select crisp, clean, moist alfalfa sprouts with the buds attached. Avoid sprouts with any signs of rot, such as yellowing or graying roots, a musty smell, or any dark or slimy spots. Finally, check the sell-by date printed on the package, do a sniff test—fresh spouts have a clean, fresh aroma—and check for clean roots; the stems should be white or cream-colored.

Refrigerate alfalfa sprouts in their container; they will keep for four to five days. Check them daily and remove any that have become discolored or slimy, plus those immediately surrounding them.

If you enjoy alfalfa sprouts, you can always have a fresh supply if you grow your own, which you can easily do in just two to three days. See page 370 for easy sprouting instructions.

TIPS FOR PREPARING

Although alfalfa sprouts are best eaten raw, following good food safety practices is particularly important when preparing alfalfa sprouts (see "Safety," below).

QUICK SERVING IDEAS

- Use alfalfa sprouts as a crunchy layer in sandwiches, as a garnish for any vegetable or fruit salad, or as a substitute for watercress in any recipe.
- A feathery alfalfa sprout bed can be used as a lovely and edible presentation upon which to serve hot or cold foods, such as pasta, bean, crabmeat, or egg salad, or a fillet of fish.
- Fill pita pockets three-quarters full with

grilled vegetables and or hummus, then fill to overflowing with crunchy alfalfa sprouts.

- A grilled veggie burger on sourdough bread topped with a slice of tomato, onion, pickles, and lots of alfalfa sprouts announces that summer has officially arrived!
- Alfalfa sprouts make a crunchy addition to any sandwich. Two favorites: whole-wheat (wholemeal) bread with tuna salad and alfalfa sprouts, or provolone cheese, sliced avocado, and sprouts.
- Top cold summer soups with a dollop of nonfat yogurt and a generous handful of alfalfa sprouts.

SAFETY

Alfalfa sprouts have been linked to outbreaks of foodborne illness caused by the bacteria *Salmonella* and *E. coli*. In 1997 in the U.S.A., contaminated alfalfa sprouts were responsible for four outbreaks, three of which involved *E. coli* 015:H7, a particularly dangerous strain of bacteria. This type of *E. coli* has killed a number of people in outbreaks involving other foods, such as minced beef. In 1998, *Salmonella*-contaminated alfalfa sprouts made sixty people ill in California.

In humans, *Salmonella* can cause salmonellosis, an illness characterized by fever, stomach cramps, and diarrhea that can last as long as seven days. Severe cases may require hospitalization, and rarely, recurring joint pain and arthritis may result.

Mishandling of sprouts during production, packing, or distribution has not been implicated as the source of sprout contamination. It is thought that the seeds from which the sprouts develop may become contaminated by animals in the field or during postharvest storage, and that the use of animal manure in fields of alfalfa intended for nonhuman use may be a problem if the seed is used for sprouting. In addition, the conditions provided by germinating seeds—abundant nutrients, high levels of moisture, and heat generated by the sprouting process—are all conducive to the growth of bacteria.

Because of these outbreaks, in August 1998, the Food and Drug Administration reaffirmed a warning that had been issued by the Centers for Disease Control and Prevention (CDC) in 1997 for high-risk groups to avoid eating raw alfalfa sprouts, and the International Sprout Growers Association (ISGA) began a voluntary quality assurance programme. Sprout growers agreed to follow stringent ISGA-established seed sanitation guidelines and to be certified by third-party independent inspectors. Sprout growers who successfully participate in this ISGA sanitation programme can label their sprouts with an ISGA-certified grower's seal. (Following these problems in the U.S.A., the Food Standards Agency in the U.K. investigated the safety of sprout production in Britain. The report and its conclusions can be found on www.food.gov.uk/multimedia/pdfs/seedsseminarsummary.pdf)

Despite these incidents, the risk of contracting foodborne illness from eating sprouts is far less than that of other common foods. According to the FDA, 93 percent of all bacterial illnesses from human and animal pathogens come from meat, poultry, and dairy products. All alfalfa seeds are now subject to strict scrutiny and purification, and today's sprout industry is in full compliance with the CDC and U.S. Department of Agriculture.

The wisest choice: err on the side of safety. If you belong to one of the groups at high risk for foodborne disease—children, the elderly, and people with a compromised immune system— avoid raw alfalfa sprouts. If you are a healthy adult, follow these tips:

- Buy only sprouts kept at refrigerator temperature and certified with the ISGA grower's seal. Check the sell-by date printed on the container and choose crisp-looking sprouts with the buds attached. Avoid musty-smelling, dark, or slimy-looking sprouts.

- Keep sprouts refrigerated.

- Before and after handling any raw food, wash your hands thoroughly with warm running water and soap for at least 20 seconds.

- Rinse sprouts thoroughly with water before use. Rinsing can help remove surface dirt. Do not use soap or other detergents.

Individuals who have or who are at risk for systemic lupus erythematosus (SLE) might also wish to avoid or limit consumption of alfalfa sprouts. Alfalfa sprouts contain a nonprotein amino acid constituent called L-canavanine that, while protective against prostate and colon cancer, can induce SLE, at least in monkeys. Test-tube studies have also shown that canavanine produces effects in human white blood cells that might induce or worsen SLE.

Black Beans: See Common Beans.

Broad Beans (Fava Beans)

Native to North Africa and the Mediterranean region, the broad or fava bean *(Vicia faba)* was the major bean throughout the Old World prior to the introduction of the common bean. Broad beans resemble lima beans, though they are larger. The broad bean has a very interesting history. It is said that the Greek philosopher and mathematician Pythagoras could have avoided his death at the hands of an angry mob if he had escaped through a field of broad beans. Why didn't Pythagoras run? Historians believe he suffered from favism, a painful blood condition brought on by eating broad beans or by inhaling the pollen of the flowering plant. Evidently, Pythagoras chose the lesser of two evils. Favism is caused by an inborn error of metabolism, a genetic defect, which causes the red blood cells to rupture after consuming broad beans or breathing in the pollen. Favism is thought to affect up to 35 percent of some Mediterranean populations and 10 percent of American blacks. Symptoms of favism include dizziness, nausea, and vomiting, followed by severe anemia. People susceptible to favism should definitely avoid broad beans.

Broad beans provide similar nutritional benefits as common beans. Broad beans are used in a variety of Mediterranean and Chinese dishes.

Butter Beans: See Lima Beans, under Common Beans

Carob

Carob is made from the fruit pod of a large leguminous evergreen tree *(Ceratonia siliqua)* native to the rocky lands surrounding the Mediterranean Sea. The species is ancient, having survived the last ice age, and is adapted to harsh climates and poor soils. Reaching a height of 50 to 55 feet/15 to 16½ meters and a trunk circumference of 33 inches/85 centimeters, the carob tree is richly endowed with shiny green leaves and produces numerous tiny clusters of dark red flowers that become thick, fleshy, sugar-rich pods ranging in length from 3 to 12 inches/7 to 30 centimeters. When developing, carob pods are similar in appearance to broad green beans, but they turn a dark, glossy brown when mature. Although the carob produces no legumes for its first fifteen years, a fully mature tree can remain productive for eighty to 100 years, annually producing 250 to 550 pounds/114 to 250 kilograms of pods. Ancient carob trees in the Mediterranean area are reported to have borne 3,000 pounds/1350 kilograms in a season!

Along with ten to thirteen hard, flat brown seeds that contain a white mucilaginous endosperm most often used to make carob gum, a food stabilizer and thickener, the long, leathery dark brown pods are filled with a sweet, pale brown pulp that can be eaten fresh or dried, roasted, or ground into a powder that can be used like cocoa. Whole pods can be fermented and distilled, creating a drink with the appealing chocolaty flavor of the pulp. When coarsely ground and boiled in water, the pods will also yield a thick syrup. The seeds, after their gum is extracted, can also be ground to produce a flour that is especially useful for individuals with diabetes due to its 40 percent fibre content and absence of starch and sugar. Roasted carob seeds are also used as a coffee substitute in Germany and are sometimes mixed with coffee in Spain.

HISTORY

Native to the eastern Mediterranean, the carob tree has been cultivated for at least 4,000 years for its pods' seeds as well as pulp. The Arabic word for "bean pod," *kharrub,* is the source of not only our word "carob" but "carat," since because of their uniform size, carob seeds were used by the Arabs as the standard measure of weight for gems and precious metals. The plant is also called Saint John's bread or locust bean because carob pods were thought to be the "locusts" eaten with honey by Saint John the Baptist while traveling in the desert (Matthew 3:4). However, biblical scholars now believe he did actually eat migratory locusts.

Mohammed's army ate *kharoub,* and Arab Moors planted the tree in northern Africa and Spain. Spanish conquistadors carried carob to South America and southern California, and the British took the plant to South Africa, India, and Australia. During the nineteenth century, British chemists sold carob pod husks to singers, since chewing them was thought to support the health of the vocal cords by soothing and cleansing the throat. And for centuries carob has been used to treat diarrhea.

Worldwide, about 300,000 tons of carob pods are produced annually, 75 percent of which is grown in the Mediterranean basin in Spain, Italy, Portugal, and Greece. Even in countries surrounding the Mediterranean, although peasants have virtually lived on carob pods in times of famine, the carob pod remains primarily a source of feed for livestock today. In the United States, in addition to carob pods being used as feed for horses, cattle, pigs, goats, and rabbits and the dried ground pulp serving as a substitute for cocoa, carob bean gum is also used in a wide variety of applications, including as an additive in cosmetics, pharmaceutical products, detergents, and commercially processed food products to stabilize and improve the texture of bakery products, milk, cheese, ice cream, confections, frozen desserts, gelatin salads, salad dressings, and meat products.

NUTRITIONAL HIGHLIGHTS

Carob flour is relatively low in calories and high in fiber: 1 cup (100 grams) provides 222 calories and a whopping 40 grams of fiber. Carob is an excellent source of vitamins A, B2, B3, and B6. It is also an excellent source of a number of minerals, including copper, calcium, manganese, potassium, and magnesium. It is also a good source of zinc and selenium.

Although carob powder is somewhat bland compared to chocolate, carob improves upon chocolate in a number of beneficial ways:

- Carob is stimulant-free and requires no additional sweetening, while cocoa contains the potent caffeinelike stimulant theobromine and requires the addition of a sweetener—one reason why carob has only one third the calories of chocolate.

- Another is that carob is virtually fat-free (100 grams—a bit more than 3 ounces—contain less than a gram of fat). In contrast, even low-fat cocoa contains 8 grams of fat per 100 grams, and high-fat cocoa delivers a whopping 23.7 grams of fat, much of it saturated, in 100 grams.

- Both carob and low-fat cocoa powders are low in sodium and high in potassium—a desirable quality for individuals with high blood pressure or congestive heart failure—but cocoas with moderate to high fat content are often quite high in sodium since they are typically processed with an alkali to enable them to dissolve in water.

- Both carob and cocoa contain calcium, but carob provides twice the amount of calcium found in cocoa (290 milligrams in 100 grams of carob versus 123 to 153 milligrams in 100 grams of cocoa). Plus, unlike cocoa, carob contains no oxalic acid, which interferes with calcium absorption.

- Carob pods are also free of phenylethylamines, small nitrogen-containing molecules found in chocolate that, in susceptible individuals, can trigger migraines.

- Also unlike cocoa, carob powder is high in protein and rich in fiber, particularly pectin.

HEALTH BENEFITS

In addition to being a healthy alternative to chocolate, carob provides other benefits. In particular, recent clinical studies have confirmed the use of carob for treating diarrhea. A double-blind clinical study has demonstrated that carob is useful for treating infants with diarrhea, but a less rigorous trial showed it was of little help for adults with traveler's diarrhea.

Carob's beneficial effects are due primarily to its tannins and large sugar molecules. Unlike many tannins, those found in carob are not water-soluble, so they don't bind to proteins and render them unavailable, as many tannins do.

Instead, carob's tannins not only have an astringent or drying effect in the gastrointestinal system but also bind to and inactivate toxins and inhibit the growth of bacteria. Its large sugar molecules make carob pulp gummy and able to absorb water and act as a thickener, helping to bind together watery stools. Taken with plenty of water, 15 grams of carob powder mixed with a little stewed apple or mashed sweet potato provides a palatable, child-safe remedy. Adults should use at least 20 grams of carob powder.

Also, by making food more viscous in the stomach, the dietary fiber and sugars provided by carob may reduce the reflux of acid into the oesophagus, providing relief for sufferers of gastroesophageal reflux disease (GERD).

HOW TO SELECT AND STORE

Carob powder is available at most health food and whole food shops and in the natural food section of many supermarkets. Stored in an airtight opaque container in a cool, dry, dark place as you would cocoa powder, carob powder will keep for up to twelve months.

Carob is also available in drops, bars, biscuits, brownie and cake mixes, and a variety of confections, including frozen desserts. Store as you would store comparable products containing chocolate.

Should whole carob pods be available, choose glossy, dark brown pods, checking carefully for cracks or pits, which could signal infestation, or a musty smell, indicating mould.

TIPS FOR PREPARING

Carob is sweeter than cocoa or unsweetened chocolate, so when substituting carob for chocolate, reduce the amount of sugar or sweetener by 20 percent. Also, since carob has a milder flavor than chocolate, when using carob in a recipe designed for chocolate, consider enhancing the taste by adding spices, such as cinnamon, peppermint, or coffee. In beverages, if no additional spices are used, replace each part of cocoa or chocolate with 1½ to 2 parts carob.

QUICK SERVING IDEAS

- Carob can be used to prepare an incredibly easy but delicious fudge in about 20 minutes. In a large saucepan over medium-low heat, combine 6 cups carob chips with 1½ cups smooth or chunky peanut butter. Add ½ cup soy milk and stir occasionally until completely melted. Add ½ cup raisins, ½ cup diced dates, ½ cup slivered almonds, and ½ cup shredded coconut. Stir until well combined, let cool slightly, and pour into a 9-by-13-inch/20 by 30 centimeter casserole dish lined with baker's parchment or wax paper. Chill until firm. Using the paper lining to help you, remove the fudge and cut into thirty pieces. Store in an airtight container in the refrigerator until served. It will store in the refrigerator for two weeks or in the freezer for two to three months.

- Carob mounds, another healthy, delightful treat made with carob powder and puffed cereal, are also easy and quick to prepare. In a mixing bowl, combine ¼ cup rapeseed oil with ¾ cup carob powder, mixing until smooth. Add ½ cup water, ¼ cup honey, and a generous tablespoon of molasses. Stir well and add 1 cup toasted wheat germ, a pinch of sea salt, ¾ cup lightly toasted sunflower seeds, and 1 teaspoon cinnamon. When this is well blended, mix in 1 cup puffed cereal, such as kashi or rice, and ¼ cup toasted sesame tahini. Roll into 1-inch balls and eat as is or bake at 350 degrees F./180 degrees C./gas 4 for 10 minutes and cool before serving.

- Celebrate the next birthday with a healthy, delicious carob cake with carob icing. To make the cake, mix ½ cup butter with ½ cup honey and ½ cup molasses. Add 1 egg and beat well. Alternating with the addition of ¾ cup hot water, sift 2 cups whole-wheat (wholemeal) flour, ⅓ cup carob powder, 1 teaspoon baking powder, and ½ teaspoon cinnamon into the bowl. When blended, stir in 1 cup chopped walnuts. Pour into a lightly buttered 9-by-9-inch/20-by-20 centimeter tin and bake at 250 degrees F./130 degrees C./gas ½ for about 1 hour, or until the cake easily separates from the sides of the pan. Cool before icing.

- To make carob icing, cream 2 tablespoons butter with ⅔ cup powdered milk and ⅓ cup carob powder. Add ¼ cup honey and 4 tablespoons cream and mix well. Add 1 teaspoon vanilla essence and whip until smooth.

SAFETY

No safety concerns are associated with carob. Allergic reactions are extremely rare, and no drug interactions with carob are currently known.

Chickpeas (Garbanzo Beans)

The Latin name for the chickpea, *Cicer arietinum,* means "small ram," reflecting the unique shape of this legume, which somewhat resembles a ram's head. Chickpeas are also referred to as garbanzo beans, Bengal grams, and Egyptian peas.

Chickpeas have a delicious nutlike taste and a texture that is buttery yet somewhat starchy and pasty. A very versatile legume, they are a common ingredient in many Middle Eastern and Indian dishes, such as hummus, falafel, and curries. Though most people think of chickpeas as being beige in color, some varieties are black, green, red, and brown.

HISTORY

Chickpeas are thought to have originated in what is now Turkey. During the sixteenth century, chickpeas were taken to other subtropical regions of the world by both Spanish and Portuguese explorers.

Although chickpeas are grown in all semidry and subtropical areas of the world, India and Pakistan grow more than 80 percent of the world's supply. Chickpeas have become a major crop in Pakistan and India because they are extremely tolerant of drought and provide excellent protein (when combined with grains) for the large vegetarian populations of these countries. Today, other major commercial producers of chickpeas are Turkey, Ethiopia, and Mexico.

NUTRITIONAL HIGHLIGHTS

Chickpeas are an excellent source of molybdenum. They are a very good source of fiber, folic acid, and manganese. In addition, they are a good source

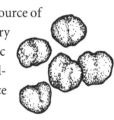

of protein, as well as minerals such as iron, magnesium, copper, and zinc.

HEALTH BENEFITS

A good fiber source, chickpeas can help lower cholesterol and improve blood sugar levels, making them a great food for diabetics and insulin-resistant individuals. Served with high-quality grains, chickpeas are an extremely-low-fat, complete protein food.

Chickpeas also offer a good supply of magnesium and folic acid. Also found in chickpeas is molybdenum, a trace mineral needed for the body's mechanism to detoxify sulphites, a preservative commonly found in wine, luncheon meats, and the fresh salad of most salad bars. Sulphite-sensitive individuals who are deficient in this trace mineral may experience headaches, racing heartbeat, or confusion.

HOW TO SELECT AND STORE

Dried chickpeas are found in both bulk bins and packages. For maximum freshness, it is always important to ensure there is no moisture in the beans you are purchasing, and that for bulk items, the bins from which you obtain your beans are covered. Your shop should have a high volume and quick turnover. Store chickpeas in an airtight container and keep them in a dry, cool place, where they will last for up to one year. If you buy chickpeas at different times, keep them separate, for peas of various ages will require different cooking times. Also, check for insect damage and that the peas are whole and not cracked. If purchasing canned peas, look for those that do not contain extra salt or additives. For chickpea flour, the best recommendation is to buy flour made from milled cooked peas. Milled raw peas tend to create foods that are difficult to digest and produce excess flatulence.

Once cooked, chickpeas can be stored in the refrigerator for up to three days if placed in an airtight container.

TIPS FOR PREPARING

Prior to washing chickpeas, they should be visually inspected to eliminate any debris, dirt, or damaged peas. One way to do this is to first spread them out in a single layer over a solid-colored dish. After inspection, rinse the peas by straining them under cool running water. Dried chickpeas are best soaked before cooking to lessen cooking time and make them easier to digest (see page 368 for instructions).

Chickpeas are easily cooked on the stove, or more quickly in a pressure cooker. For the stovetop method, take a saucepan and add 3 to 4 cups of fresh water or organic vegetable or chicken stock for each cup of dried peas. The liquid should be about 1 to 2 inches/2½ to 5 centimeters above the top of the peas. Bring the peas to a boil and then reduce to a simmer, partially covering the pot. If any foam develops, skim it off. Chickpeas generally take about 2 to 2½ hours to become tender. They can also be cooked in a pressure cooker, where they take about ½ hour to prepare. Chickpeas tend to foam in the pressure cooker. One remedy for this is to add a tablespoon of olive oil to prevent the pressure cooker's vent from being obstructed by the foam. (Also see Table 13.1 on page 369.)

QUICK SERVING IDEAS

- Hummus: Purée 2 cans of drained chickpeas, ⅓ cup extra-virgin olive oil, 4 cloves fresh garlic, 4 tablespoons tahini, fresh lemon juice from one lemon, black pepper, and cumin to make a quick and easy hummus spread. For a smoother, less garlicky hummus, preboil the chickpeas and garlic cloves for 10 minutes, and then strain them before puréeing in the blender. You can add red pepper for a different color and flavor, and you can let the hummus sit in the refrigerator to add texture.
- Chickpeas are a great protein addition to green salads.
- Middle Eastern-inspired pasta: Add chickpeas to penne mixed with olive oil, feta cheese, and fresh oregano.
- Simmer already cooked chickpeas in a sauce of tomato paste, curry spices, and chopped walnuts. You can serve this dahl-style dish with brown rice.
- Chickpeas are a hearty and nutritious addition to any vegetable soup.

SAFETY

Chickpeas can cause a severe allergic reaction in sensitive individuals. They also contain moderate amounts of purines. Since purines can be broken down to form uric acid, and excess accumulation of uric acid may contribute to health problems, such as gout and kidney stones, individuals who are susceptible to purine-related problems may want to limit or avoid intake of chickpeas.

Chickpeas also contain large amounts of oxalate. Individuals with a history of oxalate-containing kidney stones should avoid over-consuming them. For more information, see Appendix D, page 793.

Common Beans

Included in this category are black, haricot, kidney, lima, mung, pinto, and string (French or snap) beans. These are all different varieties of the common bean (note that unless otherwise designated they are variants of *Phaseolus vulgaris*). Common beans are quite versatile, as they can be prepared in a variety of ways.

Black Beans

Black beans are about the size of a pea, oval, and jet black. They have cream-colored flesh; a mild, sweet, earthy taste; and a soft texture. Black beans are widely used throughout Latin America, the Caribbean, and the southern United States.

Haricot Beans

Haricot beans are pea-sized beans that are creamy white in color. They are mild-flavored, dense, and creamy.

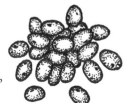

Kidney Beans

Just as its name suggests, the kidney bean is shaped like a kidney. Since these dark red beans hold their shape during cooking and readily absorb surrounding flavors, they are a favorite bean to use in simmered dishes.

Kidney beans that are white in color are known as cannellini beans.

Lima Beans (Butter Beans)

The lima bean *(Phaseolus limensis)* is thought to be named after Lima, Peru, the area where it was first cultivated. Lima beans are most often associated with succotash, a traditional Native American dish that combines this delicious bean with corn. While there are many varieties of lima beans, the ones that are most popular in the United States are the Fordhook, commonly known as the butter bean, and the baby lima bean. Likewise, the most common lima bean in the U.K. is the butter bean. The pod of the lima bean is flat, oblong, and slightly curved, averaging about 3 inches/7 centimeters in length. Within the pod reside two to four flat kidney-shaped seeds, which are what we generally refer to as lima beans. The seeds are most often cream or green in color, although certain varieties have white, red, purple, brown, or black seeds. Lima beans feature a starchy, potatolike taste and a grainy, yet slightly buttery, texture.

Mung Beans

The mung bean *(Phaseolus aureus)* is native to India but has been cultivated in China and Southeast Asia for more than 7,000 years.

Most mung beans are consumed as bean sprouts. Supermarkets often have a ready supply of fresh mung bean sprouts, or you can sprout your own. Mung bean sprouts are most often used in salads, with stir-fried vegetables, and in Asian dishes.

Pinto Beans

Pinto beans have a beige background strewn with reddish brown splashes of color. They are like little painted canvases, hence their name "pinto," which in Spanish means "painted." When cooked, their colored splotches disappear and they become a beautiful pink color, with a delightfully creamy texture.

String Beans (Snap or French Beans)

The string, French or snap bean is different from the other members of the common bean family in that the entire bean, both pod and seed, can be eaten. String beans vary in size, but they usually average 4 inches/10 centimeters in length. They are usually deep emerald green in color and come to a slight point at either end. They contain tiny seeds within their thin pods.

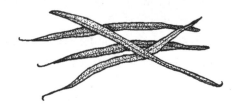

HISTORY

All of the varieties of *Phaseolus vulgaris* originated in Peru more than 7,000 years ago and were spread by migrating bands of Native Americans into Latin and North America. The early European explorers and settlers of the fifteenth, sixteenth, and seventeenth centuries were introduced to these beans by the natives. In fact, the basic recipes for Boston baked beans and succotash were derived from those used by Native Americans. Common beans were then introduced into Europe in the fifteenth century by Spanish explorers returning from their voyages to the New World. They were subsequently spread to Africa and Asia by Spanish and Portuguese traders.

As common beans are a very inexpensive protein source, they have become popular in many cultures throughout the world. Today, the largest commercial producers of dried common beans are India, China, Indonesia, Brazil, and the United States.

NUTRITIONAL HIGHLIGHTS

The key nutritional benefits of common beans are quite similar to those discussed above for soybeans except that they are much lower in fat content—usually only 1 to 2 percent. Their protein content and quality are quite similar, though. Common beans also offer an excellent source of complex carbohydrate and fiber. They are a very good source of folic acid and molybdenum. They are also a good source of phosphorus, iron, protein, magnesium, manganese, and potassium.

HEALTH BENEFITS

The major health benefit of common beans is their rich source of cholesterol-lowering fiber. In addition to lowering cholesterol, the high fiber content of beans prevents blood sugar levels from rising too rapidly after a meal, making these beans an especially good choice for individuals with diabetes, insulin resistance, or hypoglycemia.

Common beans' contribution to heart health lies not just in their fiber but in the significant amounts of antioxidants, folic acid,

vitamin B6, and magnesium they supply. Folic acid and B6 help lower levels of homocysteine, an amino acid that is an intermediate product in an important metabolic process called the methylation cycle. Elevated blood levels of homocysteine are an independent risk factor for heart attack, stroke, and peripheral vascular disease and are found in 20 to 40 percent of patients with heart disease.

According to studies conducted by the U.S. Department of Agriculture, richly colored dried beans offer a high degree of antioxidant protection. In fact, small red kidney beans are rated the highest, just ahead of blueberries.

Beans are also protective against cancer. In one analysis of dietary data collected by validated food frequency questionnaires in 1991 and 1995 from 90,630 women in the Nurses' Health Study II, researchers found a significantly reduced frequency of breast cancer in the women who had a higher intake of common beans or lentils. That was not surprising; what was surprising was that only beans and lentils seemed to offer protection. Intake of tea, onions, apples, string beans, broccoli, green pepper, or blueberries had no protective effect. Eating beans or lentils two or more times per week was associated with a 24 percent reduced risk of breast cancer.

HOW TO SELECT AND STORE

Some beans, such as lima beans (butter beans) and string beans (French or snap beans), are available dried, fresh, or frozen. Obviously, fresh in their pods is preferred. Choose those that are firm, dark green, and glossy; free of blemishes, wrinkling, and yellowing. If lima beans have been shelled, you should inspect them carefully, since they are extremely perishable. Look for those with tender skins that are green or greenish white in color and do not have any signs of mould or decay. If you choose to purchase frozen beans, shake the container to make sure that the beans move freely and do not seem to be clumped together, since the latter suggests that they have been thawed and then refrozen.

Dried black, haricot, kidney, lima (butter), mung, pinto, and string beans are generally available in prepackaged containers as well as in bulk. Just as with any other food that you purchase in the bulk section, make sure the bins are covered and that the shop has a good product turnover rate. Whether purchasing dried beans in bulk or in a prepackaged container, make sure there is no evidence of moisture or insect damage and that the beans are whole and not cracked. Store dried beans in an airtight container in a cool, dry, dark place, where they will keep for up to twelve months.

All of the common beans can be found canned in most markets. Look for those that do not contain extra salt or additives.

Cooked beans will keep fresh in the refrigerator for about three days if placed in a covered container.

TIPS FOR PREPARING

Before washing dried beans, spread them out on a light-colored plate or cooking surface to check for and remove stones and damaged beans. After this process, place the beans in a sieve and rinse them thoroughly under cool running water. It is important to follow the packet instructions regarding the soaking and cooking of kidney beans to ensure that the toxins contained within them are removed.

To shorten their cooking time and make them easier to digest, dried common beans should be presoaked. See page 368 for instructions.

To cook dried common beans, you can either cook them on the stove or use a pressure cooker. For the stovetop method, add 2½ to 4 cups of fresh water or stock for each cup of beans. The liquid should be about 1 to 2 inches/2½ to 5 centimeters above the top of the beans. Bring the beans to a boil and then reduce to a simmer, partially covering the pot. If any foam develops, simply skim it off during the simmering process. (Please see Table 13.1 on page 369 for more specific cooking instructions for each of the common beans.)

QUICK SERVING IDEAS

- Combine cooked kidney beans with black beans and white (haricot) beans to make a colorful three-bean salad. Mix with tomatoes and spring onions, and dress with olive oil, lemon juice, and black pepper.
- Serve cooked beans over a piece of corn bread and top with grated cheese.
- In a food processor or blender, combine cooked beans with garlic, cumin, and chili peppers for a delicious spread that can be used as a crudité dip or sandwich filling.
- Make tacos with a vegetarian twist by using cooked beans in place of minced meat.
- Mix puréed cooked beans with chopped garlic and your favorite fresh herbs. Use this spread as a sandwich filling or a dip for crudités.
- The heartiness of common beans makes them great soup beans, especially when added to a soup that features root vegetables, such as carrots, turnips, beets, and swedes.

- Blend cooked beans and sweet potatoes together. Serve this tasty dish on a plate accompanied by your favorite grain and fresh vegetable.
- Add cooked and cooled beans to a salad of leeks and chard, and top with rosemary vinaigrette.

SAFETY

Common beans can cause severe allergic reactions in sensitive individuals. Common beans also contain moderate amounts of purines. Since purines can be broken down to form uric acid, excess accumulation of purines in the body can lead to excess accumulation of uric acid. As such, individuals who are susceptible to purine-related problems, such as gout and kidney stones, may want to limit or avoid intake of common beans.

Lima beans (butter beans) also contain large amounts of oxalate. Individuals with a history of oxalate-containing kidney stones should avoid overconsuming them. For more information, see Appendix D, page 793.

Haricot Beans: See Common Beans.

Kidney Beans: See Common Beans.

Lentils

Lentils *(Lens culinasis)* grow in pods that contain one to two lentil seeds. There are dozens of lentil varieties, which are classified according to their color. While the most common types of lentils are red, green or brown, they also come in black, yellow, and orange. These round, oval, or heart-shaped beans are small in size, often smaller than the tip of a pencil eraser. They are sold whole or split into halves.

The different types of lentils offer varying consistencies, with the brown and green varieties retaining their shape better after cooking and the others generally becoming soft and mushy. Though the flavor differs slightly among the varieties, they generally feature a hearty, dense, somewhat nutty flavor.

HISTORY

Lentils are one of the most ancient cultivars on Earth; archaeologists have discovered lentil seeds in both Near and Middle Eastern agricultural villages that date back to 6000 B.C.E. Lentils are a biblical food, mentioned in the Genesis story of Jacob and Esau, where Esau trades his future inheritance for a bowl of lentil soup. Lentils were also an ingredient in the bread made during the Babylonian captivity of the Jews. We know that the ancient Egyptians were lentil fans, as lentils have been found in Egyptian tombs. Before the first century C.E. they were introduced into India, a place famous for the spiced lentil dish known as dahl. More than likely, the Egyptians introduced the bean to the Greeks and Romans as well. Interestingly, lentils were used not only as food but also for protecting important cargo. In the first century C.E. 2.8 million pounds/1.3 million kilograms of red lentils were utilized by Egyptians to cushion the famous obelisk that was traveling from their country to where it now stands in front of Saint Peter's Basilica in Vatican City. In more recent times, Catholics have looked to lentils as a staple food to replace meat during Lent. Today, the leading commercial producers of lentils include Turkey, China, India, Syria, and Canada.

NUTRITIONAL HIGHLIGHTS

Lentils do not significantly differ in nutritional content from common beans. They are a good source of protein, folic acid, and dietary fiber. They also contain many trace minerals.

HEALTH BENEFITS

Lentils are an excellent source of cholesterol-lowering fiber. Not only do lentils help lower cholesterol, they are of special benefit in managing blood sugar disorders since their high fiber content prevents blood sugar levels from rising rapidly after a meal.

Interestingly, in one analysis of dietary data collected by validated food frequency questionnaires in 1991 and 1995 from 90,630 women in the Nurses' Health Study II, researchers found a significantly reduced frequency of breast cancer in the women who had a higher intake of beans or lentils. That was not surprising—what was surprising was that only beans and lentils seemed to offer protection. Intake of tea, onions, apples, string beans, broccoli, green pepper, or blueberries had no protective effect. Eating beans or lentils two or more times per week was associated with a 24 percent reduced risk of breast cancer.

HOW TO SELECT AND STORE

Dried lentils are found in both bulk bins and prepackaged containers. For maximum freshness, it is always important to ensure there is no moisture in the lentils you are purchasing, and that for bulk items, the bins from which you obtain them are covered. For fresh stock, your shop should have a high volume and quick turnover. For storage, use an airtight container and keep lentils in a dry, cool place, where they can last for up to half a year. If you buy lentils at different times, keep them separate, for lentils of various ages will require different cooking times. Also, check for insect damage and that the lentils are whole and not cracked. If purchasing canned lentils, look for those that do not contain extra salt or additives. Once cooked, lentils can be stored in the refrigerator for up to three days if placed in an airtight container.

TIPS FOR PREPARING

Lentils are an excellent bean for casseroles, stews, and soups. Prior to washing lentils, they should be visually inspected to eliminate any debris, dirt, or damaged beans. One way to do this is to first spread them out in a single layer on a light-colored dish. After inspection, rinse the lentils in a sieve under cool running water. Unlike larger beans, lentils do not need to be presoaked.

Lentils are easily cooked on the stove or more quickly in a pressure cooker. For the stovetop method, take a saucepan and add 2 to 3 cups of fresh water or organic vegetable or chicken stock for each cup of dried lentils. The liquid should be about 1 to 2 inches/2.5 to 5 centimeters above the top of the beans. Lentils placed in already boiling water will be easier to digest than those brought to a boil with the water. Once the water returns to a boil, reduce to a simmer and cover the pot. Brown lentils take about 45 to 60 minutes to cook, whereas green ones take 30 to 45 minutes, and red lentils are the quickest at 20 to 30 minutes. For firmer lentils to be used in salads, remove from heat 10 minutes earlier than the given cooking time. Dahl or softer lentils should be cooked for 10 to 15 minutes longer. Lentils can also be cooked in a pressure cooker, where they will take less time to prepare (also see Table 13.1 on page 369).

QUICK SERVING IDEAS

- Lentil-stuffed green peppers: Slightly undercook your lentils so they remain firm, and mix with wheat or spelt bread crumbs, spices, and a grated or crumbled cheese, and stuff your pepper. Drizzle with olive oil and bake at 300 degrees F./150 degrees C./gas 2 until the pepper is soft (usually about 45 minutes).
- A cool summer salad idea: Combine 2 cups of cooked lentils, 2 oranges cut into cubes, and 2 chopped sweet peppers to make a delicious cold salad. Season with salt and your favorite herbs and spices.
- For a complete protein meal, toss buckwheat soba noodles with cooked lentils, broccoli florets, and leeks. Add some olive oil mixed with garlic and ginger.
- Quick and easy lentil casserole: Layer cooked millet, cooked lentils, and steamed spinach in a baking dish. Add whole-wheat (wholemeal) bread crumbs, some chopped walnuts, and feta cheese. Bake at 300 degrees F./150 degrees C./gas 2 until thoroughly heated.
- Moroccan lentil soup: Cook your lentils, then add diced vegetables of your choice and season with tamari, ground coriander, cumin, turmeric, and cayenne.

SAFETY

Lentils contain large amounts of oxalate. Individuals with a history of oxalate-containing kidney stones should avoid overconsuming them. For more information, see Appendix D, page 793.

Lima Beans: See Common Beans.

Mung Beans: See Common Beans.

Peas

The pea (*Pisum sativum*) comes in three major types: garden, mangetout (snow), and sugarsnap. Garden peas have rounded pods that are usually slightly curved in shape. They have a smooth texture and vibrant green color. Inside the pods are green rounded pea seeds that are sweet and starchy in taste. Mangetout (snow) peas are flatter than garden peas, and since they are not fully opaque, you can usually see the shadows of the flat pea seeds within. Sugar snap peas, a cross between garden and mangetout, have plump pods with a crisp, snappy texture. The pods of both mangetout and sugarsnap peas are edible, and both have a slightly sweeter and cooler taste than the garden pea.

HISTORY

The exact history of the pea is unknown. The general consensus is that peas originated in the region that spans from the Near or Middle East across to Central Asia. The modern pea varieties were produced by centuries of cultivation and selection for certain desired characteristics in both Europe and Asia. In the nineteenth century, during the early development of the study of genetics, peas played an important role. The monk and botanist Gregor Mendel used peas in his plant-breeding experiments. In the 1970s, sugarsnap peas were developed, the result of a cross between garden peas and mangetout (snow) peas.

Today, almost 80 percent of the world's pea crop is utilized as dried peas rather than as fresh peas. This is the case in the UK, however, in the United States, this is reversed, as 90 percent of the peas are eaten as green peas. Wisconsin, Washington, and Minnesota are the biggest producers of green peas, while the Russian Federation and China are the leading producers of dried peas.

NUTRITIONAL HIGHLIGHTS

All peas are lower in calcium and phosphorus than beans but provide similar levels of protein, carbohydrate, and fat. They are a good source of protein, B vitamins, and a variety of minerals, including phosphorus, manganese, magnesium, potassium, and iron. In addition, dried peas are an excellent source of dietary fiber, and green peas are a good source of vitamin C, vitamin K, and carotenes, while dried peas contain very little of these nutrients.

As dried peas lack water, they are more calorie-dense than fresh peas.

HEALTH BENEFITS

Dried peas provide the same sorts of health benefits as common beans. Green peas provide some additional nutrition (see above) and antioxidants.

HOW TO SELECT AND STORE

Green peas are available in many forms: fresh pods, canned, frozen, and dried. As fresh pods, garden peas are generally available from the spring through to the onset of winter, and mangetout peas can usually be found throughout the year in supermarkets. Snap peas tend to be available only from late spring through to early summer.

Fresh peas should be refrigerated, since heat hastens the conversion of their sugar content into starch. For fresh garden peas, look for those whose pods are firm, velvety, and smooth and have a medium green, alive look. Reject peas whose green color is especially light or dark or those that are yellow, whitish, or mottled with gray. Also, avoid pods that are puffy, water-soaked, or have mildew residue. Pods should contain peas of sufficient number and size so that there is not much empty room in the pod. Avoid pods that rattle when shaken as they may be nearly empty. Although garden peas are typically round, the pods of mangetout peas should look flat. Look for the shape of the peas through the translucent shiny pea pod. Generally, the smaller pods are younger and tend to be sweetner. To find quality, fresh sugarsnap peas, snap one open and see whether it is crisp. These should be bright green in color, firm, and plump.

It is best to eat and enjoy fresh peas on the day you buy them. If this is not possible, it is best to refrigerate them as quickly as possible. Otherwise the sweet sugar will turn to starch rather quickly. Leave peas unwashed and unshelled and stored in the refrigerator in a perforated bag or unsealed container that will allow some air to circulate around the peas. They will keep for several days. Fresh peas can be blanched in boiling water for 1 to 2 minutes and subsequently frozen for up to six months.

TIPS FOR PREPARING

Rinse pea pods briefly, then shell the peas by snapping or cutting off the top and bottom of the pod and removing the tough, undigestible "thread" of the pea pod. If the peas do not have this thread, you can cut the seam of the pod carefully, so as not to damage the tender peas inside. Peas removed from the pod are clean and do not need to be washed.

Rinse mangetout and sugarsnap peas under cool water before using. You can eat mangetout and sugarsnap peas raw, but cooking them will enhance their sweet character. One easy method is to blanch them for ½ to 1 minute (do so briefly to keep them green and fresh-looking), then remove them and plunge them into ice water to stop the cooking.

One traditional pea-cooking method is to use a few wet leaves of roundhead lettuce to line a saucepan and then pour the peas on top. Add some spices and herbs of your choice and cover with a second lettuce layer. Add 2 tablespoons of water, cover the pan, and cook the peas for 15 to 20 minutes over heat.

QUICK SERVING IDEAS

- Peas enhance green salads.
- Blanch sugarsnap peas, sauté them with garlic and shiitake mushrooms, and serve them over brown rice.
- Combine drained peas, chopped apple, and onion in a bowl. Separately combine sour cream or soft tofu, horseradish, and salt and pepper to taste. Add to the salad, mix lightly, and top with freshly squeezed lemon juice.
- Green peas can be mixed with shredded chicken, diced onions, rapeseed-oil mayonnaise, almonds, raisins, and curry powder to make a delicious and colorful chicken salad.
- You can improve on canned split pea soup by adding fresh peas to enhance its flavor, texture, and nutrition.
- Fresh (or freeze-dried) pea pods are a healthy, portable snack food.

SAFETY

Peas contain small amounts of oxalate. Individuals with a history of oxalate-containing kidney stones should avoid overconsuming them. For more information, see Appendix D, page 793.

Pinto Beans: See Common Beans.

String Beans: See Common Beans.

The Healing Power of Nuts, Seeds, and Oils

Nuts and seeds are the vehicles of plant reproduction. Locked inside them is the genetic material for an entire plant. In addition, nuts and seeds provide excellent human nutrition, being especially good sources of essential fatty acids, vitamin E, protein, and minerals. Because of their high oil content, nuts and seeds are often used as sources of oils for use in culinary, medicinal, and cosmetic preparations. In this chapter, we will discuss some of the common nuts, seeds, and vegetable oils.

Nuts, Seeds, and Oils: An Overview

The word "nut" commonly refers to the shell-encased seeds of trees. There are more than 300 types of nuts, and every plant has a seed. However, relatively few nuts and seeds are important food crops.

In the United States, peanuts are by far the leading nut crop, as they account for greater than 70 percent of the yearly nut production. In terms of worldwide production, the coconut is by far the most widely grown and utilized nut crop, followed by the peanut. In fact, coconuts and peanuts account for roughly 94 percent of the world's nut production. One of the main reasons is that coconuts and peanuts provide oils that are among the leading ingredients of cooking oils, margarines, and shortening.

As more people seek healthier food choices, nut and seed consumption is on the rise. Nuts and seeds, like the other plant foods discussed in previous chapters, are rich not only in their nutrient content but also in their phytochemical content. In addition to fiber components, important phytochemicals in nuts and seeds include protease inhibitors, ellagic acid, and other polyphenols. Nuts are also the best source of arginine, an amino acid that plays an important role in wound healing, detoxification reactions, immune functions, and promotion of the secretion of several hormones, including insulin and growth hormone. Recently there has been a considerable amount of scientific investigation regarding arginine's role in the formation of nitric oxide. This compound plays a central role in determining the tone of blood vessels. Specifically, it exerts a relaxing effect on blood vessels, thereby improving blood flow. Normally, the body makes enough arginine, even when the diet is lacking. However, in some instances, the body may not be able to keep up with increased requirements and higher dietary intakes may prove useful. Arginine supplementation has been shown to be beneficial in a number of cardiovascular diseases, including angina pectoris, congestive heart failure, high blood pressure, and peripheral vascular insufficiency (decreased blood flow to the legs or arms). By increasing nitric oxide levels, arginine supplementation improves blood flow, reduces blood clot formation, and improves blood fluidity. The degree of improvement offered by arginine supplementation in angina and other cardiovascular diseases can be quite significant as a result of improved nitric oxide levels. These benefits may also be attainable by eating foods high in arginine, such as nuts.

Because of the high oil content of nuts and seeds, one would suspect that frequent consumption of nuts would increase the rate of obesity. But in a large population study of 26,473 Americans, it was found that the people who consumed the most nuts were less obese. A possible explanation is that consumption of nuts produces satiety. This same study also demonstrated that higher nut consumption was associated with a protective effect against heart attacks (both fatal and nonfatal). Other large studies, including the Nurses' Health Study, the

Iowa Women's Health Study, and the Physicians' Health Study, found that nut consumption is linked to a lower risk of heart disease. Researchers who studied data from the Nurses' Health Study estimated that substituting nuts for an equivalent amount of carbohydrate in an average diet resulted in a 30 percent reduction in heart disease risk. Researchers calculated an even more impressive risk reduction—45 percent—when fat from nuts was substituted for saturated fats (found primarily in meat and dairy products). Other studies have shown nuts to protect against type 2 diabetes. The ability of nut consumption to lower the risk of type 2 diabetes may relate to their ability to improve cell membrane structure and function. As it relates to type 2 diabetes, abnormal cell membrane structure due to eating the wrong types of fats leads to impaired action of insulin. Clinical studies have shown that increasing the intake of monounsaturated fats improves insulin action, and population studies have indicated that frequent consumption of olive oil, nuts, and nut oils protects against the development of type 2 diabetes even in subjects who are obese (a major risk factor for type 2 diabetes).

Oils

Nuts and seeds have long been used as a source of oils for culinary, medicinal, and cosmetic purposes. For culinary purposes, oils can be used in salad dressings and sauces, in baking and in cooking. Some oils offer advantages over others for certain applications. For example, as olive, macadamia nut, coconut, sesame, and rapeseed oil are more stable than other oils, they are preferred for use when exposing foods to heat. In the U.K., olive oil is now the most popular oil, sales having increased by 39 percent between 2000 and 2005. Rapeseed oil is made from rapeseeds that have had a toxic oil, erucic acid, removed. It has gained incredible popularity in a short period of time because it is being promoted for its high level (7 percent) of omega-3 oils. Highly polyunsaturated oils, such as linseed, safflower, soy, and sunflower, are not recommended if they are going to be exposed to heat because the heat changes the chemical structures of the fatty acids and forms free radicals. These oils are best suited for salad dressings.

Still other oils are best avoided altogether, specifically, trans-fatty acids, partially hydrogenated oils, and cottonseed oil. Cottonseed oil may contain toxic residues due to the fact that cotton is so heavily sprayed with pesticides. It also contains gossypol, a substance known to inhibit sperm function. In fact, gossypol is being investigated as the "male birth control pill." Its use as an antifertility agent began after studies demonstrated that men who had used crude cottonseed oil as their cooking oil had low sperm counts followed by total testicular failure.

For medicinal purposes, fish, linseed, evening primrose, borage, and black currant oils are the most popular. Black currant, borage, and evening primrose oil are used because they contain gamma-linolenic acid, an omega-6 fatty acid that eventually acts as a precursor of the favorable prostaglandins of the 1 series (see page 86 for a description of prostaglandin metabolism). However, linseed oil is not only less expensive; it may provide greater benefit due to its high concentration of alpha-linolenic acid, an omega-3 fatty acid (see "Linseeds," page 431). Linseed oil also contains linoleic acid, which is easily converted to gamma-linolenic acid by most people. Fish oils rich in eicosapentaenoic acid(EPA) and other omega-3 oils are also quite popular.

HOW OILS ARE PRODUCED

In the modern oil-pressing factory, the starting material—seed, nut, grain, or legume—is first mechanically cleaned to get it ready for either chemical or mechanical extraction. With chemical extraction, the material is typically rolled into meal, for example, seed meal or cornmeal, and then mixed with a chemical solvent, such as hexane. Once the solvent has separated the oil from the meal, the mixture is exposed to high heat to evaporate the solvent. Although most of the solvent is removed, traces can still be found. The oil that is produced is usually further processed by means of degumming, bleaching, deodorizing, etc., to produce a "refined" oil. A refined oil is one that has had some of the "impurities" removed from it, such as vitamin E, lecithin, chlorophyll, carotenes, aromatic oils, and free fatty acids. Many of these impurities have important health-promoting properties. In the process of refining, the oil is exposed not only to extremely high heat but also to caustic substances, such as phosphoric acid and sodium hydroxide. Because the refined oil has been stripped of most of its natural protection against damage, synthetic antioxidants, such as BHT, are added.

The mechanical method usually differs only in how the oil is initially extracted. The seeds are

TABLE 14.1

Fat Content and Fatty Acid Composition (as Percentage of Total Fat) of Selected Nuts and Seeds

Food	Total Fat (%)	Alpha-Linolenic Acid	Linoleic Acid	Oleic Acid	Saturated Fat*
Almond	54	0	17	78	5
Brazil nut	67	0	24	48	24
Cashew	42	0	6	70	18
Coconut	35	0	3	6	91
Corn	4	0	59	24	17
Hazelnut (filbert)	62	0	16	54	5
Linseed (flaxseed)	33	58	14	19	9
Macadamia nut	72	0	10	71	12
Olive	20	0	8	76	16
Peanut	48	0	29	47	18
Pecan	71	0	20	63	7
Pistachio	54	0	19	65	9
Pumpkin seed	47	15	42	34	9
Rapeseed	30	7	30	54	7
Rice bran	10	0	35	48	17
Sesame seed	49	0	45	42	13
Soy	18	9	50	26	15
Sunflower	47	0	65	23	12
Walnut	60	5	51	28	16

* The saturated fat in nuts is primarily medium-chain fat, rather than the longer-chain saturated fat contained in animal foods.

typically cooked at high temperatures for up to two hours and then mechanically pressed through the expeller. The pressure can be as high as several tons per square inch. This results in the generation of heat, usually around 200 degrees F./93 degrees C. The higher the heat, the greater the oil yield. The oil pressed in this manner can be filtered and sold as "cold-pressed" (no external heat was used during the extraction) or as natural, crude, or unrefined oil. Or the oil can be processed to produce a refined oil. Be aware that even if the oil has undergone refinement, it can still be labeled "cold-pressed" because no external heat was applied during the extraction.

Although far from ideal, the best oils commonly available are the cold-pressed, unrefined oils. However, do not expect these oils to taste as "clean" as the highly processed commercial varieties you may be accustomed to, as the cold-pressed unrefined oils still retain much of their original flavor.

Selecting and Storing Nuts and Seeds

In general, nuts and seeds, due to their high oil content, are best purchased and stored in their shells. The shell is a natural protector against free-radical damage caused by light and air. Make sure the shells are free of splits, cracks, stains, holes, or other surface imperfections. Do not eat or use mouldy nuts or seeds, and also avoid limp, rubbery, dark, or shriveled nutmeats. Store nuts and seeds with shells in a cool, dark, dry environment for up to two to three months. If you must buy shelled nuts or seeds, store them in airtight containers in the refrigerator or freezer (see Table 14.2 for storage times). Crushed nuts, slivered nuts, and nut pieces that you may find for sale are most often rancid. Prepare your own from whole nuts if a recipe calls for these.

Tips for Nut and Seed Preparation

In addition to being eaten as snacks, nuts and seeds can be added to many foods for their unique flavor. And with the aid of a food processor, nut and seed butters can be prepared right at home. Most nuts and seeds have enough natural oils to make nut butter, but occasionally you may need to add some oil. Keep nut butters in airtight containers in the refrigerator, where they will usually keep for three to six months.

You can also prepare your own, healthier version of dry-roasted nuts by laying them out on a baking sheet and then roasting them in an oven at 275 degrees F./140 degrees C./gas 1 for 15 to 20 minutes.

Since nuts and seeds, like grains and legumes, contain the essential factors for the plant to reproduce, they can also be sprouted. Sprouting is thought to not only increase the nutritional value but improve digestibility as well. Sprouting at home is quite easy for most nuts and seeds. All you need is a large glass jar or, better yet, a sprouting jar with different types of lids. After rinsing, place the item to be sprouted in the jar, and cover with water for 24 hours. You may need to rinse the item once or twice and re-cover with water. After the initial 24 hours, pour out the water, rinse, and allow the moist sprouts to sit in an area without direct sunlight. Rinse the sprouts twice daily. Once the item has sprouted (usually in one to three days), it can be placed in more direct sunlight, if desired. Most sprouts will be ready to eat one to two days after they have sprouted.

Safety Issues

There are significant safety issues with nut and seed consumption. As a general rule, nuts are among the foods more commonly associated with allergic reactions. It is estimated that roughly 1 percent of the American population (approximately 3 million people) suffers from tree nut and peanut allergy. One U.K. research team found that about one in 70 children in the U.K. are allergic to peanuts, but it has also been found that about 20 percent of children grow out of their allergy. Overall, 1.3 percent of the

TABLE 14.2

Yield of and Storage Time for Selected Nuts and Seeds

Nut	One Pound/ Half a Kilogram Equals	Can Be Stored in Refrigerator for up to	Can Be Stored in Freezer for up to
Almonds (in shell)	1¼ cups (shelled)	12 months	12 months
Almonds (shelled)	3 cups	9 months	9 months
Brazil nuts (in shell)	3¼ cups	4–6 months	4–6 months
Cashews	3¼ cups	6 months	9 months
Chestnuts (in shell)	2½ cups (shelled)	2–3 weeks	3–4 months
Coconut (dried)	5¾ cups	1 month	6 months
Hazelnuts (in shell)	1½ cups (shelled)	9 months	9 months
Hazelnuts (shelled)	3½ cups	6 months	9 months
Linseeds	2⅔ cups	12 months	12 months
Macadamia nuts	3⅓ cups	6 months	9 months
Peanuts (in shell)	2⅓ cups (shelled)	6 months	9–12 months
Peanuts (shelled)	3 cups	3 months	6 months
Pecans (in shell)	2 cups (shelled)	6 months	12 months
Pecans (shelled)	4 cups	6 months	12 months
Pine nuts (shelled)	4 cups	1 month	6 months
Pistachios (in shell)	2 cups (shelled)	3 months	12 months
Pumpkin seeds	7 cups	6 months	12 months
Sesame seeds (whole)	3⅛ cups (shelled)	12 months	12 months
Sesame seeds (hulled)	3½ cups	6 months	12 months
Sunflower seeds (whole)	3 cups (hulled)	12 months	12 months
Sunflower seeds (hulled)	3½ cups	6 months	12 months
Walnuts (in shell)	2 cups (shelled)	12 months	12 months
Walnuts (shelled)	3½ cups	12 months	12 months

Note: Nuts in their shells can also be stored in a cool, dry place for an average of two to three months. Nut butters can usually be stored in the refrigerator for three to six months after opening.

population is allergic to peanuts (approximately 780,000 people). When people are allergic to nuts, the allergy tends to be severe. One out of four persons allergic to nuts has severe signs and symptoms. Nut allergy can produce:

- A tingling feeling in the lips or mouth.
- Hives.
- Swelling in the throat, causing difficulty in swallowing or breathing.
- Asthma symptoms.
- Vomiting.
- Cramping abdominal pains.
- Diarrhea.
- Faintness and unconsciousness.
- Death due to obstruction to breathing or, more rarely, extremely low blood pressure (anaphylactic shock).

Nut allergies tend to be "fixed"; in other words, children do not outgrow them and life-long avoidance of the allergen is required. People suspecting that they or their child may have a severe nut or peanut allergy should be evaluated by a physician. Possible tests include a diagnostic blood test, called a RAST test, which measures antibodies to specific allergens.

It is especially important to purchase good-quality nuts, especially peanuts and Brazil nuts, as researchers have isolated a number of field and storage fungi on poor-quality nuts. Of particular concern is the fungus *Aspergillus flavus,* which produces a poison called aflatoxin. A known carcinogen, aflatoxin is twenty times more toxic than DDT, and ingestion of this fungus has been linked to mental retardation and lowered intelligence.

To prevent aflatoxin ingestion, the FDA enforces a ruling that 20 parts per billion is the maximum of aflatoxin permitted in all foods and animal foods, including all nuts and nut products. E.U. regulations also restrict aflatoxin levels to 20 parts per billion, but there are concerns that Trading Standards inspectors have found batches with levels of 22 parts per billion in some parts of the U.K. Furthermore, concerns about aflatoxin levels in unshelled Brazil nuts led to E.U. regulations in 2004 limiting the level to 4 parts per billion. To ensure your own safety, when purchasing nuts, do so from a shop where the nuts have been stored in a dry, cool environment (the fungus grows when the temperature is 86 to 96 degrees F./30 to 35 degrees C. and the humidity is high).

Roasting nuts is thought to provide protection against aflatoxin, while also increasing the nuts' digestibility. However, it's best to purchase nuts still in the shell, shell them at home just before using, and roast them at home if so desired.

A less serious safety issue with most nuts and seeds is that they provide a high ratio of arginine to lysine. While arginine does provide significant health benefits, a high arginine-to-lysine ratio is best avoided by individuals susceptible to cold sores or herpes infections, as arginine promotes, while lysine prevents, the activation of the virus.

Finally, another health risk with nut consumption is the fact that the most popular commercial roasting process of nuts is a form of deep-frying, usually in saturated fat such as coconut oil or palm kernel oil. Deep-fried foods have been linked to high levels of LDL (the bad form of cholesterol) and to the thickening of larger artery walls.

Common Nuts and Seeds

Almonds

The almond tree *(Prunus amygdalus)* is a small deciduous tree closely related to the peach, apricot, and cherry. Unlike these other drupes' fruit, the outer fleshy layer of the almond is quite tough and becomes the hull at maturity. The hull must be cracked to free the sweet-tasting nut.

Almonds are off-white in color, covered by a thin, brownish skin and encased in a hard shell. Almonds are classified into two categories: sweet (*Prunus amygdalus* var. *dulcis*) and bitter (*Prunus amygdalus* var. *amara*).

Sweet almonds are the variety that is eaten. They are oval in shape, usually malleable in texture, and wonderfully buttery in taste. They are available in the market either still in their shell or with their shell removed. Shelled almonds are available whole, sliced, or slivered in either their natural form, with their skin, or blanched, with their skin removed.

Bitter almonds are used to make almond oil, which is used as a flavoring agent for foods and liqueurs, such as Amaretto. They are otherwise inedible, as they naturally contain toxic substances, such as hydrocyanic acid. These compounds are removed in the manufacturing of almond oil.

HISTORY

The almond is thought to have originated in western Asia and North Africa. Almonds were a prized ingredient in breads served to Egypt's pharaohs. Explorers ate almonds while traveling the Silk Road between Asia and the Mediterranean. Before long, almond trees flourished in the Mediterranean, especially in Spain and Italy.

The almond has maintained religious, ethnic, and social significance throughout history. For example, the Bible tells the story of Aaron's rod, which blossomed and bore almonds, thus giving the almond the symbolism of divine approval.

The Romans showered newlyweds with almonds as a fertility charm. Today, guests at weddings are often given bags of sugared almonds, representing children, happiness, romance, good health, and fortune. In Sweden, cinnamon-flavored rice pudding with an almond hidden inside is a Christmas custom: find it, and good fortune is yours for a year.

The cultivation of almonds in California, the only U.S. state that produces them, has an interesting history. Almond trees were originally brought to California centuries ago when missions were created by the Spanish, but cultivation of the trees was abandoned when the missions were closed. Almond trees found their way back to California in the nineteenth century via the eastern United States. In 1840, almond trees were brought over from Europe and were first planted in New England. Because the climate on the eastern seaboard did not support their cultivation, the trees were taken to California, where they thrived and continue to do so. Almonds are now second only to grapes in terms of crop acreage in California.

Almonds are now commercially grown in many of the countries that border the Mediterranean Sea, including Spain, Italy, Portugal, and Morocco, as well as in California.

NUTRITIONAL HIGHLIGHTS

Almonds' high fat content (up to 60 percent) translates to a high calorie content. Just 100 grams of almonds provide nearly 600 calories. However, almonds are packed full of nutrition. They are an excellent source of monounsaturated and polyunsaturated oils, protein (20 percent), potassium, magnesium, calcium, iron, zinc, and vitamin E. Almonds are also a good source of important antioxidant flavonoids and of amygdalin (2 to 4 percent), which is better known as laetrile. These components have resulted in the almond's reputation as an anticancer food.

A ⅓-cup serving of shelled almonds contains 280 calories, 24 grams of fat, 9 grams of protein, and 10 grams of carbohydrate.

HEALTH BENEFITS

Like other nuts, almonds appear quite useful in fighting against heart disease. In the most recent study, the effects of roasted, salted almonds and roasted almond butter were compared with that of raw almonds on blood lipid levels. All subjects were given 100 grams of one of three forms of almonds for four weeks. All three forms of almonds significantly lowered "bad" low-density-lipoprotein cholesterol (LDL) from baseline to the completion of the study. Both raw and roasted almonds significantly lowered total cholesterol, whereas the decrease by almond butter did not reach statistical significance. "Good" high-density-lipoprotein cholesterol (HDL) did not significantly change with raw or roasted almonds but slightly increased with almond butter. These results suggest that unblanched almonds—whether raw, dry-roasted, or in roasted butter form—can play an effective role in cholesterol-lowering, plant-based diets.

In addition to their beneficial effects on lowering cholesterol and heart disease, almonds may help fight many cancers. In an animal study of the effect of almonds on colon cancer, animals were exposed to a colon cancer-causing agent and fed almond meal, almond oil, whole almonds, or a control diet containing no almonds. The animals given whole almonds showed fewer signs of colon cancer, including fewer rapidly dividing cells. One reason may be the almond's high fiber content—just ¼ cup of almonds contains 4 grams of fiber.

HOW TO SELECT AND STORE

When selecting any nut, remember that when they are still in their shells, they will have the longest shelf life. If purchasing almonds in shells, look for shells that are not split, mouldy, or stained. Shelled almonds that are stored in an hermetically sealed container will last longer than those that are sold in bulk bins, since they are less exposed to heat, air, and humidity. If purchasing almonds from bulk bins, make sure that the shop has a quick turnover of inventory and that the bulk containers are sealed well in order to ensure maximum freshness. Look for almonds that are uniform in color and not limp or shriveled. In addition, smell the almonds. They should smell sweet and nutty; if their odor is sharp or bitter, they are rancid.

If you want almonds with a roasted flavor and texture, choose those that have been dry-roasted, as they have not been cooked in oil like their roasted counterparts. Even when purchasing dry-roasted almonds, it is important to read the label to be sure that no additional ingredients, such as sugar, corn syrup, or preservatives, have been added.

Since almonds have a high fat content, it is important to store them properly in order to protect them from becoming rancid. Store shelled almonds in a tightly sealed container in a cool, dry place away from exposure to sunlight. Keeping them cold will further protect them from rancidity and prolong their freshness. In the refrigerator, almonds will keep for several months, while in the freezer, they can be kept for up to one year. Shelled almond pieces will go rancid more quickly than whole shelled almonds. Almonds still in the shell have the longest shelf life.

TIPS FOR PREPARING

In addition to being eaten raw, almonds are a wonderful addition to a variety of recipes, from salads to baked goods.

Whole shelled almonds can be chopped by hand or in a food processor. If using a food processor, it is best to pulse on and off a few times, instead of running the blade constantly, as this will help ensure that you end up with chopped almonds rather than almond butter.

If you want to remove the almonds' skins, blanch them for a few minutes until you notice the skin beginning to swell. Drain and then rinse under cold water. Pinch the cooled almonds between your thumb and index finger, and the skin should slide right off the almond meat.

QUICK SERVING IDEAS

- Almonds provide a little crunch to plain yogurt.
- Enhance your next vegetable stir-fry with ½ cup sliced almonds.
- Add two tablespoons of almonds to your morning bowl of oatmeal.
- Utilize a handful of almonds as a quick power snack.
- Make an open-faced sandwich of almond butter and bananas drizzled with a little honey.
- For a delightful side dish, sauté 1½ cups blanched almonds with 2 tablespoons olive oil, 1 teaspoon ground coriander, ½ teaspoon crushed cayenne pepper, and a dash of salt.

SAFETY

See page 408 for more information.

Brazil Nuts

Brazil nuts are the seeds of a giant evergreen tree (*Bertholletia excelsa*) that grows wild in the forests of the Amazon valley in Brazil, Bolivia, and Peru. Reaching a height of 165 feet/50 meters and a trunk width of 6 feet/2 meters, the Brazil nut tree does not begin to produce fruit in significant quantities until it has grown for fifteen to thirty years, but for the rest of its 500-to-800-year life, each year, it will bear 250 to 500 pounds/115 to 230 kilograms of seed pods. The woody, coconutlike pods, inside which the nuts develop in clusters, grow slowly to reach a width of about 6 inches/15 centimeters across, maturing fully in about fifteen months. Each pod houses twenty to twenty-five large, creamy-meated seeds, arranged like segments inside an orange, each of which is protected by its own extremely hard, dark brown, triangular shell.

The Brazil nut is accurately named, since attempts to cultivate the tree outside the Amazon Valley have failed due to the unusual reproductive cycle of these bountiful giants. Even in Brazil, only a few commercial plantations have succeeded. Dependent upon the unique wildlife of their forest habitat, most trees remain in the wild, growing in dense natural stands of fifty to 100 trees, called *castañales* in Brazil and *manchales* in Peru.

Fallen Brazil nut pods are collected carefully, given the fact that the pods, which weigh 4 to 6 pounds/2 to 3 kilograms, often fall more than 100 feet/30 meters (the equivalent of eight storeys), landing with enough force to kill a person. Human harvesters carry shields to protect themselves from falling pods, whose drop velocity causes them to, at times, literally plant themselves on impact.

After the tough fruit capsules are hacked open, the nuts are sold to local factories, where the hard shell surrounding each seed may be left on or removed, and the nuts are dried and graded prior to being packed in vacuum-sealed bags and shipped overseas.

A sweet, rich-tasting nut whose meat is similar in texture to coconut, the Brazil nut is eaten raw as well as roasted and salted and is consumed not just as a protein-rich food, but, in Brazil, used in a special tea for stomachaches. In South America, Brazil nut oil is used for cooking, as lamp fuel, and in moisturizing soaps and hair conditioners. In the Amazon basin, natives burn the husk for fuel, set it smoking to repel mosquitoes and blackflies, and carve it into ashtrays and trinket cases.

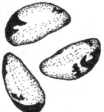

HISTORY

The Brazil nut originated in the Amazon valley, still the only region in which the tree will grow, and remained a food enjoyed only by local Amazon Indians until the end of the fifteenth century, when a troop of Spanish explorers led by the officer Juan Alvárez Maldonado stopped to rest in the middle of a Brazil nut forest near the Madre de Dios River. Told about the nuts by the Cayanpuxes Indians, Maldonado ordered that thousands of what he named *almendras de los Andes* (almonds of the Andes) be collected for rations.

The Spaniards ate the nuts but did not take them back to Spain, and it wasn't until 1633, when trade-savvy Dutch explorers sent their Brazil nuts home, that the giant seeds entered the world market, where they were enthusiastically embraced. In fact, by the second half of the nineteenth century, bowls full of Brazil nuts were a requisite part of the upper classes' lavish celebration of Christmas in Britain.

Most Brazil nuts are still gathered from wild trees; however, attempts to develop plantations continue in various parts of the Amazon. About half the world's Brazil nuts—around 40,000 tons—are still exported from the Brazilian port of Belém, mostly to Britain, France, Germany, and the United States, where Americans consume $17 million worth of the nuts each year, somewhat less than half the $44 million Brazil nut sales provide in annual income to South America.

NUTRITIONAL HIGHLIGHTS

Although just two Brazil nuts provide about 90 calories, the caloric equivalent of an egg, this nut is also a heavyweight when it comes to nutritional value. In addition to being loaded with healthy polyunsaturated fats, Brazil nuts are the richest and most reliable food source of selenium. Just one Brazil nut can provide more than the daily recommended value of this important trace mineral. Brazil nuts are also a very good source of chromium.

One-third cup of shelled Brazil nuts provides 300 calories, 31 grams of fat, 7 grams of protein, and 6 grams of carbohydrate.

HEALTH BENEFITS

In addition to health benefits consistent with other nuts', the Brazil nut gains special attention because of its high selenium content. Selenium has been shown to lower the risk of heart disease and cancer, and also plays a role in reducing allergies and inflammation.

A food's selenium content is determined by the amount of selenium found in the soil in which the food is grown; studies have indicated that nuts grown in the Manaus-Belém region of the Amazon basin are much higher in selenium content than nuts from the Acre-Rondonia region.

HOW TO SELECT AND STORE

Brazil nuts can be found in whole-food shops and some supermarkets all year round. However, in the U.K., the availability of nuts in their shells has been affected by E.U. regulations introduced in 2004 that limited the levels of aflatoxin to 4 parts per billion. Consequently some retailers are no longer stocking unshelled nuts as the legal requirement of "due diligence" has meant that ensuring safe supplies has added significantly to the cost of unshelled Brazils.

Brazil nuts can be purchased raw, both unshelled and shelled. If already shelled, they may be roasted in oil or dry-roasted.

The availability of fresh nuts in the shell—the healthiest choice since the shell protects the nut's delicate fats—is more seasonal than for shelled nuts, with the supply being best soon after the nuts are harvested, in autumn and early winter. When choosing Brazil nuts in the shell, look for clean shells that don't rattle when shaken—a sign they are well filled.

When selecting shelled nuts, choose plump, crisp nutmeats. Avoid nuts that are shriveled (a sign of age and staleness), discolored, or musty-smelling (an indication of mould).

Because Brazil nuts' high polyunsaturated oil content makes them especially susceptible to rancidity, shelled nuts should be stored in an airtight container in the refrigerator or freezer, where they will keep for one to two months. Unshelled Brazil nuts will remain fresh for four to six months if they are kept in a cool, dry place away from humidity and insects.

TIPS FOR PREPARING

One pound/½ kilogram of unshelled Brazil nuts will yield about 1½ cups of nutmeats. Brazil nuts' very hard protective shells are easier to crack after they have been frozen, steamed, or boiled. If steaming or boiling, do so for no more than 3 minutes, then place the nuts under cold running water before cracking them with a nutcracker.

QUICK SERVING IDEAS

- Shelled and coarsely chopped Brazil nuts make a great addition to virtually any pasta dish. Once the pasta is cooked and has been transferred to a serving bowl, lightly toast ½ cup of Brazil nuts for every serving of pasta in a dry skillet over medium-high heat.

Shake the skillet frequently, until the nuts become fragrant—about 2 minutes. Immediately transfer them to the serving bowl full of pasta and toss with olive oil, a little lemon juice and/or lemon zest or balsamic vinegar, chopped parsley, freshly ground pepper, and sea salt.

- Add nutrition and taste by scattering a handful of coarsely chopped Brazil nuts over any tossed green salad.
- Add coarsely chopped Brazil nuts to muffin, cake, or pancake batters.
- Garnish a bowl of granola, fruit salad, vanilla yogurt, or rice pudding with coarsely chopped Brazil nuts.
- For an elegant, easy-to-make-ahead dessert, blend together 1 cup each of chopped Brazil nuts, pecans, raisins, and dates. Add a little orange or lemon rind and just enough honey to provide a sticky consistency. Roll into small balls, refrigerate to harden, and wrap in waxed paper.

SAFETY

See page 408.

Since Brazil nuts can be high in selenium content, their intake should be limited to no more than one to two servings (¼ – ½ cup) a maximum of twice a week.

Brazil nuts contain high amounts of oxalate. Individuals with a history of oxalate-containing kidney stones should avoid overconsuming them. For more information, see Appendix D, page 793.

Cashew Nuts

Cashew nuts are well-known kidney-shaped nuts that are light-colored, delicate in flavor, and slightly spongy in texture. Cashew nuts belong to the same family as the mango and pistachio nut (Anacardiaceae). They are actually seeds that adhere to the bottom of the cashew apple, the fruit of the cashew tree *(Anacardium occidentale)*. Cashew apples are regarded as delicacies in Brazil and the Caribbean.

Cashew nuts in the shell are not available in shops since the interior of their shells contains a caustic resin known as cashew balm. This resin, which is toxic, must be removed before they are fit for consumption. Cashew balm is used in varnishes and insecticides.

HISTORY

The cashew tree is native to the coastal areas of northeastern Brazil. The earliest written reports of cashew are from Brazil, coming from French, Portuguese, and Dutch observers. The French naturalist André Thevet, who visited Brazil in 1558 during the brief period of French settlement, was the first to describe cashew apples and their juice being consumed and that the nuts were roasted in fires and the kernels eaten. He also provided the first drawing of the cashew showing the local people harvesting fruits and squeezing juice from the cashew apple into a large container. In the sixteenth century, Portuguese explorers introduced cashew into other tropical regions, such as India and some African countries, where they are now also cultivated. The cashew tree was a prized resource owing to its precious wood, cashew balm, and cashew apple, but the cashew nut itself did not gain popularity until the beginning of the twentieth century. Today, the leading commercial producers of cashew nuts are India, Brazil, Mozambique, Tanzania, and Nigeria. The cashew ranks second only to the almond among the nine tree nuts of importance in world trade.

NUTRITIONAL HIGHLIGHTS

Cashew nuts are a very good source of monounsaturated fats. They are also a good source of many minerals, including copper, magnesium, potassium, iron, and zinc. In addition, cashew nuts are a good source of biotin and protein. One-third cup of shelled cashews provides 260 calories, 21 grams of protein, and 15 grams of carbohydrate.

HEALTH BENEFITS

The health benefits of cashews center around their excellent nutritional value. Cashew nuts have a lower fat content and a higher protein and carbohydrate content than most other nuts. The fat that they do contain is mostly (65 percent) derived from oleic acid, a monounsaturated oil with known benefits in protecting against heart disease and cancer. Although cashew nuts are lower in vitamin E and calcium than most nuts, they are a good source of protein, magnesium, potassium, iron, and zinc.

HOW TO SELECT AND STORE

Cashew nuts are generally available prepackaged, as well as in bulk. Just as with any other food you may purchase in the bulk section, make sure that the bins are covered and that the shop has good product turnover so as to ensure maximum freshness. Whether you are purchasing cashew nuts in bulk or prepackaged, make sure that there is no evidence of moisture or insect damage and that the nuts are not shriveled. If it is possible to smell the cashew nuts, do so in order to ensure that they are not rancid.

Due to their high content of oleic acid versus polyunsaturated oils, cashew nuts are more stable than most other nuts. Still, they should be stored in an airtight container in the refrigerator, where they will keep for about six months, or in the freezer, where they will keep for about one year. Cashew butter should always be refrigerated once it is opened.

TIPS FOR PREPARING

Cashew nuts can be eaten on their own in raw or roasted form. They can also be added to many fruit and vegetable salads to provide a nutty taste.

QUICK SERVING IDEAS

- Combine cashew nuts with other nuts and dried fruits for a healthy snack.
- Right before taking off the heat, add cashew nuts to sautéed vegetables.
- Cashew nuts with a little bit of maple syrup make a great topping for waffles, pancakes or hot cereals.
- Add cashew nut butter to breakfast soy or rice milk shakes to increase their protein content and give them a creamy, nutty taste.
- In a saucepan over low to medium heat, mix cashew butter with some tamari, cayenne pepper, garlic, ginger, and water to make a wonderful sauce for fish, vegetables, tofu, or rice.

SAFETY

See page 408.

Cashew nuts contain small amounts of oxalate. Individuals with a history of oxalate-containing kidney stones should avoid over-consuming them. For more information, see Appendix D, page 793.

Parts of the cashew contain oleoresins, similar to those in mangoes and pistachios, which have caused allergic reactions. Individuals who are allergic to mangoes or pistachios should therefore avoid cashew nuts as well.

Chestnuts

Enclosed in glossy, soft, mahogany-colored shells, chestnuts are the seeds of the chestnut tree (*Castanea* spp.). A chestnut is about the size of a large walnut, with the shape of an acorn. The tree flowers from late June to July, producing dense white flower clusters, which form the spiny round burs that house its thin-shelled nuts. The chestnuts develop inside their prickly capsules in mid- to late September and are ready for harvest by October. When first picked, chestnuts are starchy, but after a few days, some of the starch turns to sugar, giving these large, chewy nuts their characteristic gentle sweetness.

Virtually always roasted or boiled, cooked chestnuts have the consistency of thick, mashed sweet potatoes; in the United States, they are best known as a treat added to poultry stuffing for festive Thanksgiving and Christmas dinners. During the winter in Europe, boiled chestnuts are often served as a vegetable side dish, and bags full of chestnuts, roasted over hot coals, are sold on street corners, their soft shells easily peeled while the nuts are still warm. Chestnuts are also dried on racks and made into a nutrient-rich flour that is used in a variety of recipes, from soups to breads to desserts. They are also an important food source in parts of China and Japan.

HISTORY

One of the oldest nuts, chestnuts, along with acorns, hazelnuts, and beechnuts, belong to the same family of trees, the Fagaceae, which are represented in Europe, Asia, and the United States because they were already in existence before the continents split apart, some 60 million years ago.

The American chestnut was a spectacular forest tree reaching a height of 100 feet/30 meters and a trunk diameter of 4 to 5 feet/120 to 150 centimeters. Early records indicate that Native Americans gathered chestnuts for food, favoring the sweet, easily shelled chestnuts over the bitter, tannin-filled acorns and the hard-to-shell hickory nuts. The colonists also favored the abundant, easily peeled chestnut, which is estimated to have made up 25 percent of the eastern forest canopies.

Until the nineteenth century, no tree in America's eastern forests was as useful as the chestnut. The nuts were relied upon not only as a source of food for both livestock and humans but as an important cash crop for many Appalachian families. Each autumn, the harvest was so bountiful that, as the holidays approached, trainloads were shipped to New York, Philadelphia, and other big cities, where street vendors sold them fresh-roasted; but enough remained to fill the attics of homes in Appalachia to the rafters with bags full of chestnuts.

This stately, serviceable tree flourished from

southern Maine to Georgia, Alabama, and Mississippi, and as far west as Ohio. So many chestnuts crowded the dry ridgetops of the central Appalachians that in early summer, when their canopies were filled with creamy white flowers, the mountains appeared snowcapped—until the accidental introduction of the chestnut blight fungus, which decimated the species during the first fifty years of the twentieth century. The disease, currently identified as *Cryphonectria parasitica,* was probably imported from Asia. It started near New York City around 1904 and spread rapidly. By 1950, the once-dominant chestnut trees were reduced to a forlorn mass of decomposing trunks and stump sprouts. No cure has been found, and for the last fifty years, most chestnuts consumed in the United States have been imported.

In Europe and Asia, literally hundreds of varieties of the chestnut tree that span the ages of civilization still flourish, but because of plant quarantine restrictions, only a few European and Chinese varieties are currently available in the United States, in addition to what remains of the American chestnut. However, there are three available species from whose combined gene pools American arborists hope to stage a comeback of healthy chestnut forests: the American chestnut *(Castanea dentata),* the European chestnut *(Castanea sativa),* and the Chinese chestnut *(Castanea mollissima).* In the meantime, China, Italy, Japan, and Spain are the principal growers of chestnuts.

NUTRITIONAL HIGHLIGHTS

Chestnuts are the only low-fat nuts, containing just 1 gram of fat and a little less than 70 calo-

ries, primarily from carbohydrates, per 30 grams of dried or roasted nuts. Chestnuts are also a breed apart from other nuts in that they are the only nuts that contain vitamin C. Just 100 grams of chestnuts supply about 45 percent of the RDA of this vital antioxidant nutrient.

Chestnuts radically increase their caloric content once they are boiled. Per 100 grams, raw chestnuts, compared to boiled chestnuts, increase their calorie count from 181 to 297 calories, protein from 1.8 to 4.7 grams, and sugars from 39.4 to 67 grams.

Chestnuts are an excellent source of manganese, molybdenum, and copper and a good source of magnesium. In addition, they are a good source of vitamin C as well as vitamins B1, B2, and B6 and folic acid.

HEALTH BENEFITS

The health benefits of chestnuts center on their nutritional content. However, unlike other nuts, chestnuts are a low-fat variety that does not provide the benefits of a high level of monounsaturated fat.

HOW TO SELECT AND STORE

In season from September through to February, chestnuts are sold fresh and in their shells. Choose firm, plump, heavy nuts whose glossy mahogany shells are free from blemishes.

Because of their high moisture content (chestnuts have a water content of 52 percent, while that of most nuts ranges from 3 to 6 percent), chestnuts should be kept covered and refrigerated lest their moisture provide a favorable climate for the growth of bacteria and moulds. If freshly gathered, however, they should be left to cure at room temperature for a few days to allow some of their starch to be converted into sugar.

Chestnuts in the shell should be stored in a perforated plastic bag in the refrigerator, where they will keep for two to three weeks. To freeze chestnuts, make a small incision in each one, place on a baking tray, and freeze. Then transfer to an airtight container and return to the freezer, where they will keep up to four months.

In gourmet shops and some upmarket supermarkets, prepared chestnuts are available year-round in jars containing a French confection called *marrons glacés*, in which the nuts are peeled and cooked in syrup; in cans, in the form of chestnut purée, which is used for making desserts; and in bags of chestnut flour for baking. Dried chestnuts may also be found in ethnic markets. Due to their low-fat content, properly dried chestnuts store quite well.

TIPS FOR PREPARING

One pound/½ kilogram of fresh unshelled chestnuts will yield 2½ cups of shelled nutmeats. One pound/½ kilogram of shelled, peeled, and cooked chestnuts will yield about 1 cup of purée. Three ounces/85 grams of dried chestnuts equals 1 cup fresh shelled nuts.

Chestnuts can be heated, peeled, and then cooked, or cooked until tender and then peeled. Regardless of which method you choose, first use a paring knife to slash an "X" on the flat side of each nut, being sure to cut all the way through the shell. This will keep the chestnuts from bursting during cooking and make them easier to peel when done.

In Italy, chestnuts are traditionally prepared by dry-roasting them over hot coals. To do so, wrap the precut chestnuts in a sheet of heavy-duty foil, punch a few holes in the foil to allow the air to escape, and place the parcel about 5 inches above the fire, roasting for 30 minutes. Or, place the cut nuts in a fireplace corn popper or chestnut roasting basket and roast for 15 to 20 minutes. Chestnuts are done if tender when pierced with the tip of a knife.

To dry-roast chestnuts in the oven, place the precut nuts in a single layer in a shallow dish or baking tray, cover tightly with foil, and bake at 450 degrees F./230 degrees C./gas 8 for 20 to 25 minutes, shaking the tray several times during cooking. If you prefer your chestnuts lightly browned, remove the foil after the first 15 minutes of roasting time, then continue to roast them, uncovered. However you roast them, be sure to peel chestnuts and remove their thin papery inner shell while they are still warm. To prevent unpeeled nuts from cooling off, remove them from their roasting container one at a time. If they have cooled so much that the shell won't slide off easily, reheat them briefly.

To serve chestnuts as a side dish, blanch them first, then cover and simmer in water or stock until tender, about 20 to 30 minutes, depending upon the size of the nuts. To blanch, bring a medium saucepan of water to the boil, cut the chestnuts with an "X," and drop them into the boiling water. When the shells split and soften, in about 5 minutes, remove the chestnuts and peel them as soon as they are cool enough to handle.

To rehydrate dried chestnuts, cover them with boiling water, bring the water to a boil again, and then simmer until tender—about 1½ hours.

QUICK SERVING IDEAS

- You can serve boiled chestnuts as you would mashed potatoes. Simply put boiled and peeled chestnuts in a food processor and process until mashed.
- Coarsely chop boiled or roasted chestnuts and add to your favorite stuffing recipe.
- Toss roasted, chopped chestnuts with cooked broccoli or Brussels sprouts, olive oil, and balsamic vinaigrette.
- Boil chestnuts and purée them with vanilla and a little maple syrup, if needed. Top with a dollop of whole-milk yogurt or whipped cream for a delicious dessert.
- A rich chestnut-mushroom sauce can be served over polenta, pasta, or grilled vegetables. To make the sauce, blanch 10 to 15 chestnuts, then peel and chop them finely. Pour 2 tablespoons olive oil into a medium skillet or sauté pan, add 1 large, chopped onion, and stir over medium heat until golden. Add ½ pound/250 grams sliced mushrooms, the chopped chestnuts, and ¼ pound/125 grams prosciutto, and sauté for 3 to 5 minutes. Add ½ cup white wine, raise the heat to high for a minute, then add ½ cup vegetable stock and reduce the heat to thicken the sauce. Add 1 bunch of sage leaves, thinly sliced, and season to taste with salt and pepper. Grated Parmesan cheese makes a nice garnish for this hearty sauce.

SAFETY

See page 408.

Chestnuts' high (52 percent) moisture content makes them quite susceptible to mould and bacterial growth. For this reason, chestnuts should be kept covered and refrigerated.

In Massachusetts, the tree most often mistaken for the American chestnut is a much-planted ornamental tree called the horse chestnut *(Aesculus hippocastanum)*. This species displays distinctive conical clusters of flowers 10 inches/25 centimeters long and 3 to 4 inches/7 to 10 centimeters in diameter. The horse chestnut also bears large nuts, but these have a very bitter taste and are considered to be poisonous.

Coconuts

The brown, hairy, egg-shaped coconut sold in the grocery store is actually the seed of the fruit of the coconut palm tree *(Cocos nucifera)*. The tree trunk is about 18 inches/45 centimeters in diameter, with numerous rings marking the places where former leaves have grown, and reaches a height of up to 100 feet/30 meters. At its summit, the tree is crowned with about twenty 10-to-15-foot/3-to-4½-meter-long blade-shaped leaves that droop downward. Amid these leaves, the nuts grow in clusters of ten to twenty or more, each tree typically carrying ten to twelve clusters in varying stages of development. The oval-shaped coconuts, which have a pale green, thick, fibrous outer husk and a dark brown, hard inner shell, grow to about 12 inches/30 centimeters in length when fully mature. Inside their hard outer shells, they are lined with a layer of rich white nutmeat that surrounds a hollow center filled with a thin, slightly sweet fluid referred to as "coconut water" (rather than coconut milk which is made by squeezing grated coconut flesh).

Like most other nuts, the coconut is quite high in fat, but

unlike other nuts, virtually all its fat is saturated. In fact, coconut oil is the most highly saturated of all vegetable oils—a quality that makes this oil extremely stable, which is why it is so often used in sweets, baked goods, shortening, margarines, and deep-fat frying. The richness of coconut oil also makes it useful in soaps, lotions, shampoos, and detergents.

HISTORY

One of the oldest food plants, the coconut palm is thought to have originated somewhere in the Malayan archipelago but was soon dispersed throughout the tropics by man and nature, having been known to survive floating across entire oceans. Its name is recorded in Sanskrit in the Vedas, the oldest (circa 1500 B.C.E.) scriptures of Hinduism, in which the coconut is said to nourish the body, increase strength, and promote beautiful hair and skin. In Ayurvedic medicine, coconut oil infused with herbs has been used medicinally for almost 4,000 years as an effective treatment for skin diseases caused by infestation with parasites, such as scabies and head lice.

Today, about 20 billion coconuts are grown each year, and although the major producers are the Philippines, India, and Indonesia, virtually everywhere the coconut palm grows—in the tropical regions of Latin America and East Africa, as well as Asia, the Pacific Islands, and the Philippines—coconut products serve as a dietary staple. Coconut oil, which we now know contains immune-boosting medium-chain fatty acids, has long been thought to have a special healing power and is an important constituent not only of the cuisines of each of these countries, but also of their traditional medicines—a practice whose appropriateness is underscored by the fact that Thailand, where coconut appears in virtually every dish in the national cuisine, has the lowest cancer rate of the fifty countries surveyed by the National Cancer Institute.

The importance of the coconut throughout the tropics is exemplified by its many uses in the Philippines, where the coconut palm is called the "tree of life." In these islands, virtually all parts of the tree are used medicinally, including its roots, bark, leaves, flowers, and cabbage, as well as the husk, shell, water, endosperm, and oil provided by its fruit, the coconut. Medicinal uses are varied:

- The roots are used for dysentery and other intestinal complaints.

- A poultice made from the bark is used for toothaches and earaches, while ash of the bark is used as a dentifrice, as an antiseptic, and to treat scabies.

- Nourishing and easily digested, the cabbage (actually the buds cut from the top of the tree), called *ubod,* is a cooling diuretic that is often served as a salad vegetable and is also used to make pickles *(achara)* and a native stew called *gulay.*

- The astringent flowers are used in the treatment of dysentery, urinary infection, diabetes, and leprosy, while the unopened flower stalks are distilled to produce a spirit called *arrak.*

- The fibers of the trunk are used as a diuretic, in the treatment of tapeworm, and to soothe an inflamed throat.

- A native medicine made from burning the shell of the coconut in one receptacle while condensing the volatile products that separate out in another is used to treat a number of skin diseases and to relieve toothaches caused by dental caries.

- The milky liquid inside the coconut, called coconut water, is astringent and slightly acidic when fresh but soon loses its astringency. This fluid, which is 95 percent water, holds in solution proteins, sugars, and salts and is used as a diuretic and a treatment for intestinal worms and urinary disorders.

- The sap of the coconut palm, called *tuba* or *toddy,* stimulates peristalsis and acts as a mild laxative.

- Externally, coconut oil is used as a vehicle for liniments in skin medicines, for strengthening the hair, and to make a shampoo in combination with the bark of a native tree, *Entada phaseoloides,* commonly called *gogo,* which is high in saponin and produces a lather that cleanses the scalp very effectively.

The coconut has spawned an export industry that is vitally important to the Philippines, bringing in $1.2 billion annually and providing a livelihood for almost one third of the population. For the islanders, the coconut palm is a source of not merely income but timber; food; fermented and unfermented drink; alcohol; vinegar; thatching material; splints; strips and fiber for making baskets, mats, rope, hats, brushes, brooms, and other articles; fuel; caulking material; eating and cooking utensils; oil for food, cooking, illumination, soap, and ointments; feed for domestic animals; and fertilizer.

NUTRITIONAL HIGHLIGHTS

Like most nuts, coconuts contain significant amounts of fat, but unlike other nuts, which contain mostly long-chain polyunsaturated fatty acids, coconuts provide fat that is almost all in the form of health-promoting medium-chain saturated fats. Fresh, mature coconut meat contains more than 50 percent water and approximately 35 percent coconut oil, 10 percent carbohydrates, and 3.5 percent protein. One cup of the nutmeat provides approximately 500 calories. Fresh coconut milk provides about 600 calories per cup and is composed of 67 percent water, 25 percent coconut oil, 5 percent carbohydrates, and 3 percent protein. Dried or creamed coconut meat provides nearly 900 calories per cup and is composed of 65 percent fat, 23 percent carbohydrate, and 7 percent protein.

Coconuts are an excellent source of manganese, molybdenum, and copper. A 2-by-2-by-5-inch/5-by-5-by-10-centimeter piece provides 0.68 milligrams of manganese (38 percent of the recommended daily intake), 13.28 micrograms of molybdenum (30 percent of the recommended daily intake), and 0.2 milligrams of copper (22 percent of the recommended daily intake). Coconut is also a good source of selenium and zinc, with the same size piece of coconut meat containing 4.54 micrograms of selenium (8 percent of the recommended daily intake) and 0.5 milligrams of zinc (6 percent of the recommended daily intake).

HEALTH BENEFITS

Until the 1950s, coconut oil was commonly used in the food industry in the United States and the U.K. until it was, as we now understand, mistakenly accused of contributing to the development of cardiovascular disease. Coconut oil was implicated in raising cholesterol levels along with the saturated fats found in meats when a researcher in Minnesota fed rats fully hydrogenated coconut oil and saw a dramatic rise in the rats' cholesterol levels. Although Harvard scientists later reviewed this study and concluded that the cholesterol-raising factor was not coconut oil *per se* but the fact that it had been fully hydrogenated and purposely altered to make it completely devoid of any essential fatty acids, coconut oil was labeled as an artery-clogging fat.

In addition to the now well-recognized harmful cardiovascular effects of hydrogenated fats, current research has shown that any diet that causes an essential fatty acid deficiency will also cause a significant increase in blood cholesterol levels when fed to animals. Yet despite the fact that the initial study generated misinformation about coconut oil and other studies in which fresh/raw coconut oil was used showed that natural coconut oil not only does not cause an increase in cholesterol but also increases levels of beneficial HDL cholesterol, coconut oil continues to have a bad and undeserved reputation as an unhealthy saturated fat.

Approximately 50 percent of the significant amount of fatty acids provided by coconut is in the form of a medium-chain (12-carbon) saturated fat called lauric acid, a health-promoting fat whose only other abundant source in nature is human breast milk. In the body, lauric acid is converted into a highly beneficial compound called monolaurin, an antiviral, antibacterial, and antiprotozoal monoglyceride that destroys a wide variety of disease-causing organisms. Studies have demonstrated that monolaurin

eliminates lipid-coated viruses, such as *Cytomegalovirus,* herpes simplex 1, HIV, *Hemophilus influenzae,* measles, *the Vesicular stomatitis* virus, and the Visna virus. Pathogenic bacteria inactivated by monolaurin include *Listeria monocytogenes; Staphylococcus aureus; Streptococcus agalactiae; Staphylococcus epidermidis;* Groups A, F, and G streptococci; Group B gram-positive streptococcus; and *Helicobacter pylori.* In addition, not only does monolaurin inactivate *H. pylori,* but the organism, which has become resistant to a number of antibiotic drugs, appears to be unable to develop resistance to coconut's natural antimicrobials. Lauric acid and its derivative monolaurin also kill or inactivate a number of fungi, yeast, and protozoa, including several species of ringworm, *Candida albicans,* and *Giardia lamblia.*

Besides being 50 percent lauric acid, 6 to 7 percent of the fat in coconut is in the form of another beneficial medium-chain fat called capric acid. Like lauric acid, capric acid is converted in the body to a highly beneficial substance called monocaprin, which has been shown to have antiviral effects against sexually transmitted diseases, including *Chlamydia trachomatis,* herpes simplex 1 and herpes simplex 2, *Neisseria gonorrhoeae,* and HIV.

Many viruses, bacteria, and protozoa are enveloped by a protective membrane composed of lipids (fats). Current research indicates that the medium-chain fatty acids and the monoglycerides produced from them in the body destroy these pathogens by dissolving the lipids and phospholipids in the fatty envelope surrounding them, causing them to disintegrate. Other recent studies suggest that monolaurin also kills bacteria by interfering with signal transduction, thus disrupting the bacteria's ability to interact with the cells they are trying to infect. In addition, lauric acid has been shown to interfere with virus assembly and maturation.

The antiviral properties of the medium-chain fatty acids abundant in coconut have been found to be so potent that they are now being investigated as a treatment for AIDS patients. Studies recently conducted in the Philippines have demonstrated that coconut oil does indeed reduce viral load in AIDS patients. In other studies demonstrating the antiviral potential of coconut against HIV, AIDS patients consumed 20 to 25 grams of lauric acid per day. Approximately 12 grams of lauric acid are provided in 2 tablespoons of coconut oil, 3 tablespoons of creamed coconut, ½ cup of canned whole coconut milk, or ½ cup of dried coconut meat.

Coconut oil also protects against heart disease and promotes weight loss. In one study in which coconut oil was used as part of a high-fat diet, researchers found not only that coconut oil did not increase body fat, but that the coconut oil-enriched diet actually produced a decrease in white fat stores. In another study, when genetically obese mice were given a diet high in either safflower oil or coconut oil and their number of fat cells was measured, those given coconut oil were found to have produced far fewer fat cells than those given safflower oil.

In addition, because coconut's medium-chain fats are easily absorbed and preferentially used as an energy source, their burning actually increases the body's metabolic rate. The result—as long as calories in excess of the body's needs are not consumed—is that more calories are burned, a situation that encourages the burning of the long-chain fatty acids found in other fats

as well. In one study, the thermogenic (fat-burning) effect of a high-calorie diet containing 40 percent fat as medium-chain fatty acids was compared to one containing 40 percent fat as long-chain fatty acids. The thermogenic effect of the medium-chain-fat diet was almost twice that of the long-chain-fat diet—120 calories versus 66 calories—leading the researchers to conclude that the excess energy provided by medium-chain fats was not stored as fat but burned. In a follow-up study, medium-chain fats given over a six-day period increased diet-induced thermogenesis by 50 percent.

HOW TO SELECT AND STORE

Mature coconuts are available in most supermarkets. Store them in a dry, cool area if you purchase them whole to crack open yourself. Once a coconut is opened, its meat should be refrigerated and used within seven to ten days.

A number of prepared coconut products are available in many natural and whole-food markets, including dried coconut meat, creamed coconut (very finely ground dried coconut blended with coconut milk), canned coconut milk (either the fluid found inside the coconut or milk made from the expressed juice of grated coconut), and coconut oil.

- Dried coconut meat is often shredded and may be sweetened, toasted, and/or creamed. Since shredded coconut is often sweetened with sugar and preserved with propylene glycol (a chemical used in antifreeze), we recommend that you read labels carefully to avoid such products or buy whole coconuts and prepare your own shredded coconut with the aid of a food processor. Store shredded coconut in an airtight container in a cool, dry place or a refrigerator, where it will stay fresh for about a month.

- Creamed coconut is found in some super-markets, the refrigerated foods section of Asian and Indian markets and in some whole-food markets and health food shops. Store it in the refrigerator, where it will keep for seven to ten days.

- Canned coconut milk, a good substitute for creamed coconut, can be found in super-markets. Be sure to buy whole, not low-fat, coconut milk (from which much of the ben-eficial medium-chain fat has been removed), and choose a brand that contains no addi-tives. Once opened, canned coconut milk should be used immediately or stored in the refrigerator, where it will keep for seven to ten days.

- Coconut oil of high quality is odorless and tasteless, a white semisolid in cool weather and a creamy-colored oil in hot weather. Choose only food-grade oil and avoid any product that has been hydrogenated. Although coconut oil is quite stable and need not be refrigerated, it is best used within one month after opening.

TIPS FOR PREPARING

Whole green coconuts, called *buko* in the Philip-pines, are harvested when the meat is soft and rubbery. Should you be able to buy these at your market, after removing the husk, poke two holes in the "eyes," the soft spots at the bottom end of the coconut. Place eye side down in a small bowl, allow the liquid to drain out, and save for later use. Then crack open the shell and simply

scoop the meat out with a spoon. Enjoy *buko* on its own or add it along with the coconut liquid to smoothies, soups, curries, or baked goods for flavor.

Mature coconuts are harvested after the shell is quite hard and the meat is firm. To prepare mature coconuts, drain them as described above for *buko*. Their liquid, called coconut water, can be used by itself as a beverage or flavoring agent, or combined with mature coconut meat to pro-duce coconut milk. To remove mature coconut meat, break open the drained coconut by strik-ing it with a hammer or put it in a 350 degree F./180 degrees C./gas 4 oven until the shell cracks open, then use a sharp knife to separate the meat from the shell. Remove the dark outer layer and cut the white coconut meat into small, ¼-inch/½ centimeter chunks. The meat is now ready to be eaten on its own, diced and used in fruit salads or baked goods, ground in a food processor for use in making coconut milk, or shredded and dried to produce homemade dried coconut.

To make coconut milk, place 1 cup of ¼-inch/½ centimeter chunks of coconut meat in a blender or food processor and process until thoroughly broken up. Add 1 cup warm water and process again until fluffy. Line a sieve with cheesecloth, put the processed meat into the sieve, and place it over a glass container. Drain the coconut milk, pressing out all the liquid with the flat back of a large wooden spoon, or with your hands. Freshly made coconut milk should be used immediately or refrigerated and used within two days.

QUICK SERVING IDEAS

- Sprinkle unsweetened, dried shredded coconut over sweet or spicy soups, fruit salads, or tossed greens. Use as a topping for desserts. Add to granola and other cereals, biscuits, cakes, and muffins.

- For a beautiful presentation and tropical taste, garnish any grilled fish with slices of lime and shredded coconut.
- Add blocks of creamed coconut to heated sauces, curries, stocks, soups, and desserts to impart the velvety texture and rich creamy taste of coconut.
- Use coconut milk instead of cow's milk in virtually any recipe. Try coconut milk in smoothies and blender drinks. Substitute coconut milk for cow's milk in your next batch of muffins, pancakes, or chocolate pudding.
- For Haitian flair, add coconut milk and jerk spices to black bean soup.
- Warm up a truly healing bowl of chicken soup by adding coconut milk and freshly ground black pepper.
- The flavor of any creamed soup recipe will be dramatically enhanced by the addition of coconut milk. Try it in tomato soup, clam chowder, or vichyssoise.
- For a tropical variation on bouillabaisse, add coconut milk, lemongrass, and ginger along with canned tomatoes, basil, and lots of freshly ground black pepper to your next fish stew.
- Mix coconut milk with red or green curry paste for a cooking liquid that will add a Thai accent to your next stir-fry.
- Before your next sports competition, try this energizing pasta: Toss cooked and drained pasta with a sauce made from coconut milk combined with 1 to 2 tablespoons of nut butter, such as peanut or almond, a little curry spice, ginger, garlic, and soy sauce.

SAFETY

See page 408.

Products containing hydrogenated coconut oil should be avoided since consumption of hydrogenated coconut oil has been shown to cause a significant increase in blood cholesterol levels, thus increasing the risk of cardiovascular disease.

When purchasing shredded coconut, read labels carefully and avoid products sweetened with sugar and/or preserved with propylene glycol, a chemical used in antifreeze.

Coconut contains small amounts of oxalate. Individuals with a history of oxalate-containing kidney stones should avoid overconsuming this food. For more information, see Appendix D, page 793.

Filberts: See Hazelnuts.

Flaxseeds: See Linseeds.

Hazelnuts (Cobnuts or Filberts)

Hazelnuts and filberts are slightly smaller than acorn-size seeds of two varieties of the same species: the hazelnut (classified as *Corylus americana* or, if beaked, *Corylus cornuta*) is native to the northeastern and midwestern United States, while its larger cousin, the filbert (classified as either *Corylus avellana* or *Corylus maximus,* depending upon its size), is native to Europe and Asia. The European filbert tree, also called the cobnut, can attain a height of 30 feet/10 meters, while the hazelnut grows more like a shrub, reaching a height of 9 to 10 feet/up to 3 meters. Both hazelnuts and filberts do best in moist, temperate climates, producing pale greenish yellow catkins (male flowers) that release their pollen in early winter to fertilize the tiny red-tipped female flowers. The resulting nut clusters ripen in late summer, their fuzzy outer husks opening to allow the hard, glossy brown acorn-shaped seeds they contain to fall to the ground. Although filberts are a little larger than hazelnuts and have a fringed husk, both varieties share the same sweet buttery flavor that has made these nuts a gourmet food, cherished, especially in Europe, in sweets, biscuits, tortes, and liqueurs, such as Frangelica.

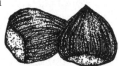

HISTORY

The filbert has been consumed in China for 5,000 years and was also gathered by the ancient Romans. It is believed that its name was adopted either in honor of Saint Philibert, whose feast day occurs on August 22, the beginning of the harvest season, when the fully ripened nuts begin to fall, or because of the nuts' outer husk, which has a fringed appearance described by farmers as having a "full beard," a phrase that evolved into the moniker "filbert."

In the Middle Ages, filberts were thought to possess mystic powers. The wood was fashioned into "divining" rods used to locate valuable mineral ores, and the nuts, considered a symbol of fertility, graced many a marriage feast.

The seventh leading nut crop in the world, with an annual production of 600,000 tons, filberts are grown commercially on a large scale in four countries: Turkey, Italy, Spain, and the United States.

Turkey, where hazelnuts have been cultivated for 2,500 years, produces 350,000 to 600,000 tons per year, approximately 70 percent of the world's hazelnut crop.

NUTRITIONAL HIGHLIGHTS

A 100 gram serving of hazelnuts contains 582 calories, but those calories are nutritionally very well spent. They supply 16 grams of protein (33 percent of the daily recommended value), 13.6 grams of fiber, and 54 grams of fat, almost all of which (82 percent) is healthy monounsaturated or (11 percent) polyunsaturated fat.

Besides their hefty supply of macronutrients, hazelnuts are an excellent source of a number of vitamins and minerals. The same 100 grams provides 89 percent of the recommended daily intake of vitamin E, 53 percent of the recommended daily intake of vitamin B1, 45 percent of the recommended daily intake of vitamin B6, 29 percent of the recommended daily intake of vitamin B3, and 19 percent of the recommended daily intake of vitamin B2, as well as 145 percent of the recommended daily intake of copper, 53 percent of the recommended daily intake of magnesium, 25 percent of the recommended daily intake of zinc, 24 percent of the recommended daily intake of iron, and 14 percent of the recommended daily intake of calcium.

HEALTH BENEFITS

The health benefits of hazelnuts are similar to those of other nuts that provide a high content of monounsaturated fat and arginine. In a recent animal study, the effect of adding hazelnut oil to a diet high in cholesterol was evaluated. Initially, when rabbits were fed a high-cholesterol diet, a number of risk factors for cardiovascular disease increased significantly, including blood levels of oxidized lipids (fats), and levels of LDL (bad) and VLDL (very bad) cholesterol. When the rabbits' high-cholesterol diet was supplemented with hazelnut oil, not only did levels of oxidized lipids, LDL, and VLDL drop, but so did the number of atherosclerotic lesions that had formed in their aortas.

One reason for these very beneficial effects—besides hazelnuts' high levels of mono-unsaturated fats—may be their exceptional concentration of copper, a key component in the intracellular form of an important antioxidant enzyme called superoxide dismutase, which disarms free radicals that would otherwise damage cholesterol and other lipids. Just 30 grams of hazelnuts supplies 41 percent of the daily recommended intake of copper.

HOW TO SELECT AND STORE

Hazelnuts, which are usually packaged whole with their skins removed, can be purchased raw; roasted; finely ground into meal for use as a flour replacement or binding or flavoring agent; or in the form of hazelnut butter or hazelnut paste, which is a sweetened, spreadable, but grainy mixture of ground hazelnuts. Some producers offer hazelnuts already chopped, but unless packaged in an opaque, vacuum-packed container, prechopped nuts should be avoided due to a higher likelihood that their delicate oils may have become rancid.

Store shelled hazelnuts in an airtight bag or container in the freezer, where they will stay fresh and flavorful for one year or more. Hazelnuts placed in an airtight container may also be stored in a refrigerator kept between 32 and 35

degrees F./0 to 1.6 degrees C., where they will remain fresh for six to eight months.

Although hazelnuts will stay fresh much longer if stored in the freezer or refrigerator, they are quite resistant to spoilage. Raw hazelnuts contain 4 to 6 percent moisture, while roasted or baked hazelnuts contain only 2 to 3 percent. Hazelnuts' low moisture content, combined with their high vitamin E level, provides resistance against oxidation and bacteria. If stored in the refrigerator or a cool, dark, dry place in an airtight container, they will keep for up to six months.

TIPS FOR PREPARING

For the best flavor and texture, always allow frozen or refrigerated hazelnuts and filberts to warm to room temperature before using.

Unless already peeled, both hazelnuts and filberts have a bitter brown skin that is best removed before eating. To do so, spread them on a baking tray and bake at 275 degrees F./140 degrees C./gas 1 for 20 to 30 minutes, until the skins begin to flake and the nutmeats turn a pale golden brown. Wrap the warm nuts in a clean terry-cloth towel, allow them to steam for 4 to 5 minutes, then rub vigorously for 1 to 3 minutes to remove the skins.

Alternatively, bring a pot of water to a boil, add 1 teaspoon bicarbonate of soda and the desired amount of nuts, and cook for 45 to 60 seconds. Remove from heat, drain thoroughly, spread out on a clean terry-cloth towel and rub briskly to remove the skins.

One pound/½ kilogram of unshelled hazelnuts or filberts yields 1½ cups nutmeats. If already shelled, one pound/½ kilogram of whole nuts yields 3½ cups.

QUICK SERVING IDEAS

- Top sautéed scallops with a hazelnut vinaigrette: Heat 1 tablespoon of hazelnut oil in a heavy medium saucepan over medium-high heat. Add ¼ cup minced onion, ¼ cup finely chopped roasted hazelnuts, and 1 tablespoon finely minced fresh ginger. Sauté until the onion is translucent, about 4 minutes, remove from the heat, and mix in ¼ cup balsamic vinegar, 1 tablespoon of honey, 3 tablespoons of hazelnut oil, and salt and pepper to taste. Just before pouring over the scallops, stir in 1 tablespoon of fresh minced basil.

- Top a fresh tossed salad of curly endive, radicchio, and watercress with roasted chopped hazelnuts, chopped hard-boiled egg, and crabmeat. Dress the greens first with a tarragon vinaigrette made by combining ¼ cup hazelnut oil, 2 tablespoons white vinegar, 1 tablespoon Dijon mustard, 2 tablespoons finely chopped tarragon, and a pinch each of salt and sugar.

- Make your own toasted seasoned hazelnuts. Melt ⅓ cup butter in a saucepan and add ¼ teaspoon each of salt, Worcestershire sauce, and Tabasco sauce, plus ½ teaspoon garlic powder. Add 4 cups of hazelnuts, stirring until coated. Spread on a baking tray and bake at 275 degrees F./140 degrees C./ gas 1 for 20 to 30 minutes.

- While steaming broccoli or sugarsnap peas until just tender, sauté a couple of tablespoons of chopped hazelnuts in a little butter along with a couple of tablespoons of your favorite fresh herbs, such as basil, tarragon, oregano, sage, or rosemary. Remove the vegetable from the heat, transfer to a bowl, and toss with the herbed hazelnuts.

- Dress up your favorite pasta with an elegant orange hazelnut sauce. Sauté hazelnuts in a little butter for about 5 minutes, add 2 teaspoons grated orange peel (use an organically grown orange if possible), 1 cup orange juice, and ¾ teaspoon salt. Pour the sauce over 4 cups cooked pasta and toss lightly. Garnish with orange slices and parsley.

- Add class to your next tuna salad. Mix water-packed, drained tuna with lime juice, olive oil, salt, pepper, a handful of chopped hazelnuts, and chopped parsley. Line a salad bowl with leaves of Little Gem lettuce. Mound the tuna salad in the center, then surround with slices of avocado and fresh orange segments. Garnish with roasted chopped hazelnuts and serve with a little dressing made with olive oil, lime juice, chopped fresh parsley, salt, and pepper.

- Try a hazelnut risotto. Sauté chopped onion and garlic in a little olive oil over medium-high heat until the onion is translucent. Add 1 cup chopped hazelnuts and 1 cup arborio rice, stirring until coated with oil. Reduce the heat to medium and add vegetable or chicken stock until the rice is just covered. Stir continually until the liquid is absorbed, continuing to add more stock until about 4 cups have been used. When the rice is *al dente,* add ½ cup chopped butternut squash, 1 teaspoon finely diced fresh sage, and ¼ cup shredded cheese, such as Gruyère, provolone, or mozzarella. Cook another 5 to 7 minutes until it is thick and creamy. Transfer to a serving platter and garnish with additional roasted chopped hazelnuts and fresh parsley.

- Serve a hazelnut café au lait as an after-dinner coffee: Heat 2 cups milk and add 2 tablespoons chocolate hazelnut spread. Stir frequently until hot and steaming, but do not bring to a boil. Blend in 2 cups freshly brewed coffee. Divide among two to three serving cups, dust with cinnamon, and serve.

SAFETY

See page 408.

Hazelnuts are a potentially allergenic tree nut. Individuals allergic to other tree nuts, or to birch or alder pollen, have a higher probability of also being allergic to hazelnuts. Symptoms are usually mild and include itching of the mouth and lips, mild gastrointestinal symptoms, swelling of the lips, and difficulty swallowing. Roasting appears to reduce hazelnuts' allergic potential; however, children with asthma who also have food allergies may react to the ingestion of hazelnuts with potentially severe respiratory symptoms. Thus they should avoid hazelnuts altogether.

Hazelnuts also contain large amounts of oxalate. Individuals with a history of oxalate-containing kidney stones should avoid overconsuming them. For more information, see Appendix D, page 793.

Linseeds (Flaxseeds)

Flax *(Linum usitatissimum)*, from which linseeds are derived, is a plant native to the Mediterranean that has been used as a food item for well over 5,000 years. Although whole linseeds contain a toxic glucoside, it is detoxified by heating.

Linseeds are shaped like sesame seeds but are slightly larger and have a hard shell that is smooth and shiny. Their color ranges from deep amber to reddish brown depending upon whether the flax is of the golden or brown variety. The linseed's flavor is warm and earthy with a subtly nutty edge. While whole linseeds feature a soft crunch, they are usually not consumed whole but rather ground, since this allows for the enhancement of their nutrient absorption. Ground linseeds can have a relatively mealy texture with a potential hint of crunch depending upon how fine they are ground.

HISTORY

Flax has been grown since the beginnings of civilization, and people all over the world have celebrated its usefulness throughout the ages. Linseeds originated in Mesopotamia. Historians have documented its use as ancient records show that flax was cultivated in Babylon in about 3000 B.C.E. and burial chambers depict flax cultivation and clothing made of flax fibers. Around 650 B.C.E. Hippocrates wrote about using flax for the relief of abdominal pains. In the same era, Theophrastus recommended the use of flax mucilage as a cough remedy. In the eighth century C.E., Charlemagne considered flax so important for the health of his subjects that he passed laws and regulations requiring its consumption. After this, linseeds became widely appreciated throughout Europe.

It was not until the early colonists arrived in North America that flax was first planted in the United States. In the seventeenth century, flax was first introduced into and planted in Canada, the country that is currently the major producer of this extremely beneficial seed.

NUTRITIONAL HIGHLIGHTS

Linseeds are an excellent source of the omega-3 essential fatty acid alpha-linolenic acid (ALA), as well as phytoestrogens known as lignans. They are a very good source of dietary fiber, magnesium, potassium, and manganese. They are also a good source of the minerals phosphorus, iron, and copper.

HEALTH BENEFITS

The major health benefits of linseeds are derived from their alpha-linolenic acid and lignan content. Linseed oil contains nearly twice the level of omega-3 fatty acids as fish oil, although it contains the shorter-chain alpha-linolenic acid rather than the longer-chain fats, such as eicosapentaenoic acid (EPA) and docosahexaenoic acid (DHA). Alpha-linolenic acid can be converted to these longer-chain omega-3 fatty acids, but the conversion depends upon the presence and activity of an enzyme called delta-6-desaturase, which, in some individuals, is less available or less active than in others. In addition, delta-6-desaturase function is inhibited in those with diabetes and nutrient deficiency, and by the consumption of saturated fat and alcohol.

Although much of the benefit of ALA is via conversion to the longer-chain omega-3 fatty acids, ALA has shown benefits of its own, including reducing the risk of heart disease and cancer. For example, data derived from biopsies of adipose breast tissue at the time of diagnosis from women with breast cancer compared to benign samples indicated that those women with breast cancer had a 64 percent lower alpha-linolenic acid level than those women whose samples were benign. In another study, the higher the level of alpha-linolenic acid in breast tissue, the less likely the cancer was to spread into the lymph nodes of the armpit.

In addition, linseeds and linseed oil are the most abundant sources of plant lignans. These components are fiber compounds that can bind to oestrogen receptors and interfere with the cancer-promoting effects of oestrogen on breast tissue. Lignans also increase the production of a compound known as sex hormone-binding globulin, or SHBG. This protein regulates oestrogen levels by escorting excess oestrogen from the body.

Population studies, as well as experimental studies in humans and animals, have demonstrated that lignans exert significant anticancer effects. In one recent study, researchers followed twenty-eight postmenopausal nuns for a year and tracked blood levels of two cancer-related oestrogens, oestrone sulphate and oestradiol. In addition to their normal diets, the nuns received daily supplements of 0, 5, or 10 grams of ground linseed. Oestrogen levels fell significantly in the women taking ground linseed, but they remained stable in the control group (those taking no linseed). Reducing oestrogen reduces breast cancer risk.

Furthermore, Dr. Paul Gross, director of the breast cancer prevention programme at the Princess Margaret Hospital and the Toronto Hospital, has reported that linseed in the diet may shrink breast cancers. His study involved fifty women who had recently been diagnosed with breast cancer. While waiting for their surgery, the women were divided into two groups. Those in one group were given a daily muffin containing 25 grams (a little less than 2 tablespoons) of ground linseed. The others were prescribed ordinary muffins. After surgery, the investigators found that women who had received the linseed muffins had slower-growing tumors than the others.

LINSEEDS AND PROSTATE CANCER

While alpha-linolenic acid is showing benefit against breast cancer, some studies indicate that ALA may actually increase the risk of prostate cancer. However, in some of these studies, ALA intake was used simply as a marker for meat intake. (In the absence of consuming vegetable sources of ALA, such as linseed or rapeseed oil, the primary dietary source is meat.) It is also possible that deficiencies of zinc or other nutrients involved in the conversion of ALA to EPA are ultimately responsible for the elevations in ALA noted in men with prostate cancer. About 50 percent of all men with prostate cancer are deficient in zinc.

No one has actually looked at the effect of linseed oil on prostate cancer. However, ground linseed appears to be quite helpful not only in preventing prostate cancer, but also in men with existing prostate cancer. In addition to the phytoestrogen effect, linseed lignans bind to male hormone receptors and promote the elimination of testosterone. In a study conducted at the Duke University Medical Center and Durham Veterans Affairs Medical Center involving men with prostate cancer, a low-fat diet (in which fat represented no more than 20 percent of total calories) supplemented with 30 grams (roughly 2 tablespoons) of ground linseed reduced serum testosterone by 15 percent, slowed the growth rate of cancer cells, and increased the death rate of cancer cells after only thirty-four days.

Ground linseeds have also been shown to be helpful in improving blood lipid profiles. In one double-blind trial, thirty-six postmenopausal women were given 40 grams (approximately 3 tablespoons) of either ground linseed or a wheat-based placebo daily for three months. In the women given linseed, blood levels of total cholesterol dropped 6 percent, but no reduction in cholesterol occurred in the women given wheat. In women on the linseed regimen, blood levels of both LDL (bad cholesterol) and HDL (good) cholesterol dropped by 4.7 percent and triglycerides dropped by 12.8 percent, resulting in only a minor reduction in the ratio of "bad" to "good" cholesterol. However, in the women given linseed, blood levels of two cholesterol-carrying molecules, apolipoprotein A-1 and apolipoprotein B, were reduced by 6 percent and 7.5 percent, respectively. Research suggests that these cholesterol-carrying molecules are better indicators of heart disease risk than cholesterol alone.

HOW TO SELECT AND STORE

Linseeds can be purchased either whole or already ground. The two different forms offer distinct benefits. Although ground linseeds may be more convenient, whole linseeds have a longer shelf life.

Whole linseeds are generally available prepackaged, as well as in bulk. We recommend purchasing them in packaged form, preferably refrigerated. Just as with any other food that you may purchase in the bulk section, make sure that the bins are covered and that the store has good product turnover so as to ensure maximum freshness. Whether purchasing linseeds in bulk or prepackaged, make sure that there is no evidence of moisture. If you purchase whole linseeds, store them in an airtight container in a dark, dry, and cool place, where they will keep fresh for several months.

Ground linseeds are usually available both refrigerated and nonrefrigerated. It is highly recommended to purchase ground linseeds that are in a vacuum-sealed package or have been refrigerated since once linseeds are ground, they are much more prone to oxidation and spoilage. Whether you purchase ground linseeds or grind them at home, it is important to keep them in a tightly sealed container in the refrigerator or freezer to prevent them from becoming rancid. Ground linseeds stored in the refrigerator in this manner will keep fresh for six months; in the freezer, for one year.

Linseed oil should definitely be cold-pressed and purchased in opaque bottles that have been kept refrigerated. Linseed oil should have a sweet, nutty flavor. You should never use linseed oil in cooking, but you can add it to foods after they have been cooked.

TIPS FOR PREPARING

Grind linseeds in a coffee or seed grinder in order to enhance their digestibility and therefore their nutritional value. If you are adding ground linseeds to a cooked cereal or grain dish, do so at the end of cooking since the soluble fiber in the linseeds can thicken liquids if left too long.

A typical serving size for ground linseeds is 1 or 2 tablespoons daily.

QUICK SERVING IDEAS

- Sprinkle ground linseeds onto your hot or cold cereal.
- Add ground linseeds to your homemade muffin, biscuit, or bread recipes.
- To pump up the nutritional volume of your breakfast shake, add ground linseeds.
- To give cooked vegetables a nuttier flavor, sprinkle some ground linseeds on top.
- Dredge tofu in ground linseeds before baking.
- Add a tablespoon of linseed oil to your next smoothie.
- Use linseed oil instead of other oils in salad dressings, as an oil for dipping bread, or to drizzle over steamed vegetables, baked potatoes, whole-grain pasta, or brown rice.

SAFETY

See page 408.

Linseeds contain moderate amounts of oxalate. Individuals with a history of oxalate-containing kidney stones should avoid overconsuming linseeds. For more information, see Appendix D, page 793.

Macadamia Nuts

Macadamia nuts, or mac nuts for short, are tasty and crunchy, buttery-flavored nuts that are about the size of a marble when unshelled. Though native to Australia, macadamia nuts are closely associated with Hawaii, and for good reason: Hawaii is the largest exporter of macadamia nuts, providing 95 percent of the world's crop.

Macadamia integrifolia is a fast-growing, regular-shaped, medium-sized tree with heavy, dark green foliage. Leaves develop in whorls of three, paired, or in fours. The leaves are rarely solitary. The leaves are blunt-tipped, oblong, and 1 foot/30 centimeters or more in length, edged with fine teeth. The nuts ripen in the autumn, in both the spring and autumn, or through the year depending upon the climate. The smooth, hard nut shell is encased in a leathery two-valved case that is 1 inch/2½ centimeters in diameter. The case encloses one spherical nut shell or two hemispherical nut shells.

Due to the labor involved in shelling the nuts and the tropical environment required to grow them, they were traditionally more expensive than other nuts. Prices have dropped dramatically in the past twenty years due to new strains with softer shells and increased production. Since the shell is so difficult to crack (much like that of black walnuts), you'll find them always shelled, either raw or roasted, salted or unsalted.

HISTORY

Most people assume the macadamia tree is native to Hawaii; however, it is actually native to the Australian subtropical rainforests of southern Queensland and northern New South Wales. Early British inhabitants learned about the macadamia tree from the native Australian aborigines. The aborigines would congregate on the eastern slopes of the Great Divide Range during the months of autumn and winter (March to June) to feast on the seeds of a tree they called *kindal kindal,* which we now know as the macadamia.

The colonization of Australia by the British began in 1788, but it wasn't until 1875 that the recorded history of the macadamia began. Ferdinand von Müller, royal botanist at Melbourne, and Walter Hill, director of the Botany Garden at Brisbane, were exploring the forest along the Pine River in the Moreton Bay district of Queensland when they discovered a species of tree previously unknown to European and American botanists. This species did not fit into any previously established genera, so in 1858 Müller established a new genus, *Macadamia,* naming it in honor of John Macadam, M.D., secretary of the Philosophical Institute of Victoria.

The macadamia tree was brought to Hawaii in the 1890s, where it has flourished, as it grows best in well-drained soils of moist semitropical climates. While there are now over 20,000 acres that have been planted in the Hawaiian chain, the largest single planting of macadamia trees is on 3,700 acres in Komatipoort, South Africa. Additionally, macadamias are grown commercially in Australia, Malawi, Kenya, South Africa, Israel, Costa Rica, Guatemala, Mexico, Brazil, and many other tropical and subtropical regions, including Florida and California.

NUTRITIONAL HIGHLIGHTS

One of the reasons macadamia nuts have such a wonderful flavor is their high fat content (72 percent). Their protein content, however, is low (8 percent) compared to other nuts'. Macadamia nuts are a good source of magnesium and potassium. They are also a good source of copper, iron, vitamin B3, phosphorus, vitamin B1, zinc, and vitamin E.

One serving (ten to twelve nuts) provides 204 calories, 21.5 grams of fat, 2.2 grams of protein, and 3.9 grams of carbohydrate.

HEALTH BENEFITS

The health benefits of macadamia nuts are similar to those of other nuts that provide a high content of monounsaturated fat and arginine.

Several studies conducted at the University of Hawaii have shown their significant health benefits. For example, the latest study was conducted to assess the cholesterol-lowering potential of macadamia nuts. Seventeen men with elevated cholesterol levels were given macadamia nuts (40 to 90 grams per day), equivalent to 15 percent energy intake, for four weeks. At the end of four weeks, their plasma total cholesterol and LDL cholesterol concentrations had decreased by 3 and 5.3 percent, respectively, and their HDL cholesterol levels had increased by 7.9 percent.

Another study, the Diamond Head Nutrition Research Study, named for the location of Kapiolani Community College campus where study volunteers dined during the one-month investigation, compared three diets: a typical American diet containing 37 percent of calories from fat, a similar diet with the fat calories derived from macadamia nuts, and the American Heart Association's "prudent diet" (30 percent of calories from fat). All meals were prepared and eaten in the college cafeteria. Volunteers—thirty men and women, ages eighteen to fifty-nine—were divided into three groups of ten and assigned one of the three diets for four weeks. Calories were adjusted to maintain constant weight levels; menus contained common local foods. At the end of four weeks, blood lipid analysis indicated that the cholesterol levels of those on the macadamia nut diet were similar to those of the volunteers on the low-fat diet and lower than those of the volunteers on the typical American diet. In addition, the macadamia nut diet produced lower triglyceride levels than either of the other diets.

Macadamia nut oil also provides significant health benefits. While olive oil and rapeseed oil are by far the most popular monounsaturated fats in use, macadamia nut oil is superior to cook with because of its lower level of polyunsaturated fat (3 percent for macadamia nut oil versus 8 percent for olive oil and 23 percent for rapeseed oil). As a result, while olive oil and rapeseed oil can form lipid peroxides at relatively low cooking temperatures, macadamia nut oil is stable at much higher temperatures (over two times more stable than olive oil and four times more stable than rapeseed). Macadamia oil, like olive oil, is also very high in natural antioxidants. In fact, it contains more than four and a half times the amount of vitamin E as olive oil.

HOW TO SELECT AND STORE

Macadamia nuts are most often available in packages or cans after they have been shelled and dried, or in sweets. Vacuum-packed nuts are the best choice for the freshest product. Shelled macadamia nuts have a very high fat content and must be stored carefully to avoid rancidity. The nuts should be light in color; they will darken with age as the inherent oil turns rancid. Refrigerate unopened packages or cans of macadamia nuts for up to six months or freeze for up to one year. Once opened, refrigerate and use within two months.

TIPS FOR PREPARING

To roast your own macadamia nuts: Rinse them well with hot water. Sprinkle salt (optional) over nuts and let drain for about 30 minutes. Spread nuts on a baking tray. Put tray in oven preheated to 350 degrees F./180 degrees C./gas 4 for 10 to 15 minutes. Reduce heat to 250 degrees

F./120–130 degrees C./gas ½ for an additional 35 to 45 minutes, turning the nuts occasionally. Nuts are done when they are golden brown in color. Remove from oven and let cool.

Whole, shelled macadamia nuts can be chopped by hand or in a food processor. If using a food processor, it is best to pulse on and off a few times, instead of running the blade constantly, as this will help ensure that you end up with chopped macadamia nuts rather than macadamia nut butter.

Four ounces/125 grams of shelled macadamia nuts equals 1 cup of nuts. One 5-ounce/160-gram can of shelled nuts yields about 1¼ cups of nuts. One 7-ounce/200-gram jar of shelled nuts yields about 1½ cups of nuts.

QUICK SERVING IDEAS

- Macadamia nuts can be substituted for other nuts, especially almonds, measure for measure in most recipes, and vice versa.
- Chopped macadamia nuts can be used as a filler and flavor enhancer in minced meat, poultry, and seafood dishes.
- Use chopped macadamia nuts in pastry dough or sprinkle on the bottom of pie shells for a delightful change of taste.
- Use macadamia nut oil instead of olive oil when cooking, and in salad dressings.

SAFETY

See page 408. Though macadamia nuts are a potential allergen, they appear to be less allergenic than other nuts.

Olives

Although many consider the olive *(Olea europaea)* to be a vegetable, it is technically a fruit. To confuse matters a bit more, we have included olives in this chapter, for they are a rich source of healthy oil. The Latin word for oil is *olea.*

Most supermarkets sell both green and black olives. In truth, these are the same fruit but sold at different degrees of ripeness, with the least ripe being greener and the most ripe being black. Olives are often cured or pickled by being immersed in oil, water, or brine. They may also be dry-cured or lye-cured. Less ripe green olives are soaked in a lye solution before brining, but black olives can be soaked in brine straight away. Less bitter and more complexly flavored olives have usually been left in their brine for a longer period of time.

Often, pitted green olives are stuffed with a filling. Typical fillings include pimientos, nuts, anchovies, jalapeños, onions, and capers. Black olives are graded into sizes labeled as medium, large, extralarge, jumbo, colossal, and super-colossal. Black olives usually contain more oil than the less ripe green ones.

Healthy olive oil is made from the crushing and then subsequent pressing of olives and is available in a variety of grades. These grades reflect the degree to which it is processed. Please see "How to Select and Store," page 439, for more information on these different grades of olive oil.

HISTORY

An ancient symbol of wisdom and peace, the olive tree has given sustenance, timber, medicine, and fuel to many different civilizations. Olives probably originated in Crete around 3000 to 5000 B.C.E. and were brought to the Americas by Iberian explorers during the 1400s and 1500s. Although a staple in the diet of most Mediterraneans, recent medical research outlining the health benefits of olive oil has increased its demand in other countries such as the United States. Commercially, Italy and Spain are a major olive oil reserve. In the United States, California is a large supplier of this precious fruit and oil.

NUTRITIONAL HIGHLIGHTS

With a total fat content of 15 to 35 percent, olives are a fine candidate to tap into for oil production. Olives and their oil are excellent sources of oleic acid, an omega-9 monounsaturated fatty acid. Olives also contain mixed tocopherols, which is why they are a good source of vitamin E (1.6 milligrams per tablespoon). Olives and their oil also have many unique phenolic and aromatic compounds, including oleuroprein and flavonoids.

HEALTH BENEFITS

In what initially seems to be a paradox, in some parts of the world an excessive fat intake leads to increases in chronic and degenerative conditions such as atherosclerosis, diabetes, colon cancer, asthma, and arthritis, while in other high-fat-intake regions, the risk of developing these conditions is much lower. Why should this be? Well, it seems not to be geographically related. Instead, research is showing that it is the type of fat ingested that is important. Some regions, like the Mediterranean areas, tend to consume the very healthy olive oil and thus their risk of developing these conditions is reduced. Conversely, in places like the United States and the U.K., where people take in high levels of animal fats, the risk is augmented.

How does olive oil make people healthier? Multiple studies conducted around the world are creating a strong body of evidence describing the multiple benefits of olive oil and olive compounds for many difficult diseases.

Scientific investigations reveal that particles of LDL cholesterol (the potentially harmful cholesterol) in the blood that are made up of the monounsaturated fats of olive oil are less likely to become oxidized than other less healthy oils and fats. This is important, for as far as researchers can tell, it is only oxidized cholesterol that adheres to vessel walls and inevitably forms the plaque that can lead to heart attacks or strokes. By ingesting olive oil instead of saturated animal fats, we can prevent the oxidation of cholesterol and help prevent atherosclerosis. Furthermore, when people with high cholesterol levels eliminated the saturated fat from their diet and replaced it with olive oil, total cholesterol levels dropped about 13.4 percent on average, and LDL cholesterol levels dropped 18 percent. Note, however, that these benefits occurred when they used olive oil instead of eating other fats, rather than simply adding olive oil to their normal diet. An important message here is the following: to reap the benefits of olive oil, the unhealthy dietary fats still need to be eliminated from the diet.

Other risk factors of heart disease seem to benefit by the use of olive oil. Investigations with diabetic patients have revealed great benefit. Those patients who ate meals with olive oil gained better blood sugar control, as well as lower levels of triglycerides. These results were better than for those diabetics who ate lower-fat meals without the olive oil. Triglycerides are a compound of fat and sugar that increase risk of heart disease when found in high amounts. Heart disease risk may also be lowered due to high antioxidant levels, which may protect against oxidation of cholesterol in the blood. One double-blinded-placebo-controlled study showed that the extract of olive leaves may decrease blood pressure in those individuals who are hypertensive.

Olives and olive oil may also be important in the prevention and treatment of asthma, arthritis, and cancer. Since healthy oils are important for lowering systemic inflammation, it is not surprising that olive oil intake has been shown to be helpful with arthritis and asthma symptoms as well. Finally, research has shown that women who regularly ingest olive oil also have a smaller risk of breast cancer. One article, published in the *Annals of Oncology,* reported that the oleic acid found in olive oil significantly cut levels of a breast cancer-promoting gene by up to 46 percent.

HOW TO SELECT AND STORE

Picking from green or black, canned or bottled olives really depends on your taste preference as well as what is available in your area. Many prepared olives are also spiced in different ways, many of which reflect the culinary and herbal presence of the geographic area from which they come. Bottled olives, left unopened, can last for two years. Once they are opened, it is best to leave them in a nonmetal container in the refrigerator, where they will last for several weeks.

Oils generally have a tendency to take in any chemicals in their surroundings. As a result, we highly recommend you purchase only organic olive oil. Olive oil is also identified by its grade. And in general, better grades do equate with fresher, tastier oil that confers greater health benefits than the lesser grades. The best grade is "extra-virgin," which refers to the initial unrefined oil garnered from the first crushing of the olive. "Virgin oil" is a name that indicates all first-pressed oil, and "pure olive oil" is virtually any oil that is able to be pressed out of the olive, regardless of the number of pressings. Extra-virgin oil is richer in taste and has up to four times the level of free oleic acids as the other grades. "Cold-pressed" denotes that the crushing of the olive was conducted without any heat. Although this process of eliciting the oil is more difficult, the quality of the oil is even higher, for heat can promote the oil's going rancid. In short, the best-quality oil to look for is organic, cold-pressed, extra-virgin olive oil.

A healthy oil, olive oil is also somewhat subject to going rancid from heat, air, and light. As a result, it is best to choose oil that is sealed in small, dark glass bottles. Unless you will be using a large quantity of oil all at once, it's best to buy it in small bottles, which will ensure that your oil is not excessively exposed to air. Glass containers are best, for metal and plastic containers can leach their own compounds into the oil. Finally, keep oil away from the stove or other heat sources. The best place in which to store it is a cool, dark, dry cabinet.

TIPS FOR PREPARING

Olive oil should be kept in glass containers away from heat and light to preserve freshness.

QUICK SERVING IDEAS

- Italian salad dressing: Mix aged balsamic vinegar, olive oil, a little water, lemon and/or lime juice, and oregano well and pour over salad.
- Fresh olive tapenade: Place pitted kalamata olives and chopped fresh garlic cloves in a blender. Add a touch of olive oil and blend.
- Olive oil is an excellent marinade foundation; try it with beef, chicken, fish, and soy products, such as tofu and tempeh.
- Dipping oil for fresh Italian bread or a French baguette: Mix olive oil, salt, black and red pepper flakes.
- Purée roasted garlic, cooked potatoes, and olive oil together to make great garlic mashed potatoes. Salt and pepper to taste.
- Drizzle olive oil over steamed vegetables before serving. Top with garlic powder and a touch of salt.
- An olive dip: Purée olive oil, garlic, and your favorite beans together in a food processor. Season to taste and serve as a dip or sandwich spread.

SAFETY

Because olives are very bitter in their raw state, they are soaked in a concentrated brine solution that leaves the final olive product a very salty food. As a result, people with high blood pressure and cardiac failure may need to eliminate olives from their diet, though given olive oil's and the olive leaf's probable benefits for these conditions, these products should be fine for people with these conditions. Olives and olive oil are not usually allergenic foods. Neither are they included on the list of twenty foods that most frequently contain pesticide residues. Olives and olive oil are also not known to contain goitrogens, oxalates, or purines.

Peanuts

The peanut is the most popular nut in the United States. (Consumption in the U.K. is a more modest average of 3 grams per person per day, probably because of allergy concerns.) But we have been a bit hoodwinked by the name, for the peanut is actually more "pea" than "nut." It is actually a legume and is a cousin of the pea, as well as the lentil and the chickpea. The peanut plant itself *(Arachis bypogaea)* grows a flower that sends a shoot down into the ground, where it enlarges into tissue that becomes the peanut.

In many nations, peanuts are not just a snack but a food relied on for its nutritional value. Known by a derivative of its African name *(nguba)*, "goober" or "goober pea," its high protein content and nutrients make it a prized nut that is well suited to making oil, flour, butter, and flakes. Although there are many varieties to be found, the most common include the Spanish, Valencia, and Virginia peanuts.

In the United States, approximately 50 percent of peanuts are used for peanut butter, 25 percent are packaged as shelled or unshelled roasted peanuts, and 25 percent are utilized as ingredients in confectionery products.

HISTORY

Known to humankind since at least 1500 B.C.E., it is thought that peanuts originated on the South American slopes of the Andes in Brazil and possibly in Peru, becoming a staple of the native people of South America and Mexico. The Spanish explorers who conquered the New World eventually took these legumes to Africa. There the peanut deeply infiltrated the culture, food, and customs of the African people. When the slave trade began, it was the African people who introduced it to the North American part of the Western Hemisphere.

Two people in the 1800s and one in the 1900s helped bring peanuts to the fore in the U.S.A. George Washington Carver suggested that farmers plant peanuts to replace the post-Civil War cotton fields, which had been ruined by the boll weevil. He also invented more than 300 ways to use this legume. Dr. John Harvey Kellogg invented a version of peanut butter as a protein substitute for his older patients who had compromised dentition and could not chew meat. Although it was probably the Incas who "invented" peanut butter, his new use for it quickly caught on and helped peanut butter become a very well-known food. In the nineteenth century it was P. T. Barnum's traveling circus that familiarized the American people with the famous call "Hot roasted peanuts." As Barnum's circus gained popularity, the notion of eating hot roasted peanuts also became well known.

Every year Americans consume twelve pounds/5½ kilograms of peanuts per person compared to just over 1 kilogram per person in the U.K. The current leading commercial producers of peanuts are Indonesia, India, Nigeria, China, and the United States.

NUTRITIONAL HIGHLIGHTS

Peanuts are composed of half fat, a quarter protein, and the rest carbohydrate. They contain plentiful healthy monosaturated fats. Morover, they yield good levels of biotin, tocopherols, folic acid, vitamins B1 and B3, and the trace minerals magnesium, phosphorus, and manganese.

One-third of a cup of shelled peanuts contains 280 calories, 24 grams of fat, and 11 grams of protein. Two tablespoons of peanut butter provide 190 calories, 7 grams of fat, and 8 grams of protein.

HEALTH BENEFITS

A food high in protein, monosaturated fat, and the antioxidant resveratrol, the peanut is showing itself to be an able protector of the human heart and blood vessels. One study of subjects who consumed a diet that emphasized peanuts, in both nut and butter form, for one month demonstrated that their risk of heart disease dropped by around 21 percent compared to those people who ate typical American/Western fare. A second study, in which the subjects were given two or three servings of peanuts or peanut butter for one month, also found reductions in the "bad" LDL cholesterol with maintenance of "good" HDL cholesterol. Triglycerides, which are another risk factor for heart disease, also dropped. Those who ate peanut foods had results double the benefits of other subjects who had a low-fat diet.

HOW TO SELECT AND STORE

Peanuts are sold as shelled and unshelled roasted nuts, as peanut butter, and as peanut oil. Peanuts are found in both bulk bins and prepackaged containers. For maximum freshness, it is always important to ensure there is no moisture in the peanuts you are purchasing and that for bulk items, the bins from which you obtain your peanuts are covered. For fresh stock, your shop should have a high volume and quick turnover. If possible, try to smell the peanuts, and check for a rancid smell that may mean these particular peanuts are past their prime. For storage, use an airtight container and keep your peanuts in a dry, cool place, where they can keep for up to one year. Also, check for insect damage, and that the nuts are whole and not cracked. Shelled peanuts can keep in the refrigerator for about three months and in the freezer for up to six months. Peanuts should not be chopped if you are going to store them. It is best to chop peanuts only right before eating or using in a recipe, for chopping increases the surface area, thus allowing air to oxidize the oils and encouraging them to turn rancid more quickly. Unshelled peanuts should feel heavy for their size. They should not rattle, since a rattling sound suggests that the peanut kernels have lost moisture, allowing them more space to move around in the shell.

As a matter of heart health, it is recommended that only nonhydrogenated peanut oil be consumed. Although most major peanut butter manufacturers use hydrogenated stabilizing oils to keep the oil and protein from separating, these products are hazardous to the cardiovascular system. A much better choice is to purchase peanut butter that uses only peanuts. Even better is to grind it yourself, and many more health-conscious markets are providing this option. Once opened, freshly ground peanut butter will last up to two months. Unshelled peanuts can be kept in a cool, dry place or in the refrigerator for up to six months. Peanut oil should be purchased in small quantities in dark glass or plastic bottles and stored in a cool, dry environment, where it can keep for up to three months.

TIPS FOR PREPARING

Peanuts can be chopped on a cutting board or in a wooden bowl using a mezzaluna, a curved knife that has a handle sitting atop the blade. Alternatively, they can be chopped in a food processor by adding a handful at a time and pulsing until you have the texture for which you are looking. You can grind further in the food processor for a peanut butter consistency too. Roasting can decrease the heart-healthy profile of the peanut's oil, and it may lose some nutrients. In general, the dry-roasted, unsalted nut is more healthy than the oil-roasted, salted version.

QUICK SERVING IDEAS

- Make a new version of an old campfire favorite: Slice unpeeled bananas lengthwise down the middle. Spread the bananas open wide and place peanut butter and some chopped figs or dates inside. Wrap tightly in aluminium foil and grill on the barbecue.
- George Washington Carver's peanut bisque:

To 3 cups of boiling milk, add half a teaspoon chopped onion, a pinch of salt, and pepper; rub to a smooth paste a tablespoon of flour with water; add half cup of peanut butter; stir in the flour; boil 3 minutes longer; serve with peanut wafers.

- In a food processor, blend together peanut butter, sesame oil, tamari, cayenne pepper, and water. Use as a marinade for baked tofu and tempeh.
- Add peanuts to sautéed vegetables for a protein punch.
- Add a few tablespoons of peanut butter to maple syrup. Heat it until warm, and sprinkle with cardamon. Use this as an alternative pancake topping.
- Use peanut butter loaded onto celery sticks or apple slices for a great lunch bag addition or an afternoon snack.

SAFETY

See page 408.

Aflatoxin is a poison produced by the *Aspergillus flavus* fungus, known to grow well on peanuts. A known carcinogen, it is twenty times more noxious than DDT. It has been related to low intelligence and mental retardation. In fact, one rural Georgia, U.S.A., town had twice the average rate of mental retardation due to a diet high in homegrown peanuts. Because of this link, pregnant women are cautioned to stay away from peanuts and foods containing peanuts during pregnancy.

The FDA and E.U. do have a 20-parts-per-billion maximum limit of aflatoxin in food. Since the *Aspergillus* fungus likes warm and moist environments, you should store your peanuts in a cool, dry place. Roasted peanuts last longer than raw peanuts.

Peanuts also contain large amounts of oxalate. Individuals with a history of oxalate-containing kidney stones should avoid overconsuming them. For more information, see Appendix D, page 793.

Finally, peanuts are a highly allergenic food, with some people at risk for anaphylaxis if they even breathe air containing peanut dust. The rate of severe peanut allergy is increasing, and as a result, peanuts are no longer provided as a snack on airplane flights. It is estimated that approximately 10,000 food-related severe allergic reactions are treated in U.S. emergency departments each year, and 150 to 200 deaths each year are caused by a reaction to peanuts. In the U.K., there are approximately six deaths a year from peanut allergy, which affects about 1.3 percent of the population.

Pecans

Pecans grow on a majestic tree that is a type of hickory *(Carya illindinensis)* native to North America, specifically the Mississippi River valley. Often reaching a height of 150 feet/45 meters with a trunk 7 feet/2 meters in diameter, the pecan tree is widely cultivated commercially in the United States, from Virginia through Georgia to Texas and New Mexico. The pecan tree flowers in April or May, and the nuts ripen through the summer, then drop to the ground, where they are collected from early autumn through to November.

A wild pecan tree takes eleven years to reach full maturity, after which it produces about 200 pounds/90 kilograms of golden brown nuts encased in a thick, hard shell each year. New pecan varieties, developed as a result of research conducted by the U.S. Department of Agriculture, mature in just five to six years. Averaging one inch/2½ centimeters in length, the nuts produced by these cultivated pecan trees are enclosed in a smooth, paper-thin tan shell that is much easier to crack open than the shells of their wild siblings. Each shell contains two pecans, usually plump and oblong in shape, although some varieties are round or pointed. Regardless of their shape, all pecans share the sweet, delicate flavor that makes this nut compatible with virtually any food—a quality that has resulted in pecans being used in a wide array of baked goods, confections, puddings, pies, cereals, stuffings, salads, and meat, fish, and vegetable dishes. Pecans are also enjoyed right out of the shell in their natural raw state or roasted and salted, sweetened, or spiced.

HISTORY

Archaeological evidence reveals that pecans played a major role in the diets of prehistoric American Indians, and fossil remains discovered along most major streams and irrigation canals in Texas and the northern part of Mexico indicate that this area was the birthplace of the pecan. The first historical record of the pecan appears in the diary of a Spanish explorer, Cabaca de Vaca, who was shipwrecked on Galveston Island in the 1540s. He wrote that the Indians so prized the pecan, they gathered in the river valleys each autumn to gather the fallen nuts and, in winter, ground and soaked them in water to make a rich, sustaining, milky drink, as well as a fermented intoxicating beverage called *powcohicora,* from which the word "hickory" is derived.

Hernando de Soto, in his wanderings through the New World, also noted the abundance of this wild nut, and French explorers began mentioning pecans in the early 1700s. A ship's carpenter visiting Natchez with the Sieur d'Iberville in 1704 is credited with the first recorded use of the name *pecane,* a Native American word of Algonquin origin that meant "nuts requiring a rock to crack." The French, who are credited with the creation of the pecan pie, were introduced to the nut by the explorer René-Robert Cavelier, Sieur de La Salle, who, in 1682, visited the site that some twenty years later would become New Orleans, and was given pecans by the Quinipissa and Tangipahoa peoples living nearby.

One of the first known cultivated pecan tree plantings, by Spanish colonists and Franciscans in northern Mexico, appears to have occurred in the late 1600s or early 1700s. By the late 1700s, pecans had reached the English portion of the Atlantic seaboard and in 1775 were planted in George Washington's gardens. Settlers were also planting pecans in community gardens along the Gulf Coast at this time, and Thomas Jefferson had trees sent from Louisiana to his Monticello orchards in 1779.

Also by the late 1770s, French and Spanish colonists settling along the Gulf of Mexico had recognized the economic potential of pecans, and in 1802, the nuts were being exported by the French to the West Indies. Once the pecan was recognized as an item of commerce for the American colonists, the pecan industry was born. New Orleans, located near the mouth of the Mississippi River, was a natural avenue for redistributing pecans to other parts of the United States and the world. As interest in the pecan grew, so did interest in planting orchards in Louisiana, which stimulated the adaptation of propagation techniques specific to the pecan and led to the demand for trees producing superior nuts. The successful use of grafting techniques led to orchards of superior genotypes that were further refined by research conducted by the USDA beginning in 1950. A number of varieties of pecans were developed that produced nuts with thin shells and larger kernels, providing double or triple the yield and making orchards profitable more quickly.

Today, there are more than 1,000 varieties of pecans. Georgia is the leading pecan-producing state with an annual yield of 100,000 tons, 32 percent of the U.S. crop. Although cultivars bred for a paper-thin shell are 70 percent of the U.S. crop, with wild pecans supplying the remaining 30 percent, four fifths of the pecan harvest is sold as shelled nuts.

Pecans have now been introduced into Brazil, Peru, Australia, South Africa, and China, but the United States remains by far the leading producer of this native American nut. According to the USDA, more than 346 million pounds/157 million kilograms of pecans were produced in the United States in 1999—more than 80 percent of the world's pecan crop.

NUTRITIONAL HIGHLIGHTS

The pecan is another delicious nut that owes much of its flavor to its high fat content, which runs about 71 percent, most of it in the form of heart-healthy monounsaturated oleic acid. Although this translates to a high calorie count, the pecan's endowment of macro- and micronutrients justifies its caloric price tag. Each 30 gram (about ¼-cup) serving provides

190 calories, 19.5 grams of fat (46 percent of which is monounsaturated and 27 percent polyunsaturated), 2.6 grams of protein, 3.93 grams of carbohydrate, and 2.72 grams of fiber.

In addition to monounsaturated fat, pecans also contain significant amounts of plant sterols, which have been widely researched for their cholesterol-lowering effects. Pecans can contain as much as 95 milligrams of plant sterols per 100 grams, 90 percent of which is in the form of beta-sitosterol. By competing with cholesterol for absorption from the intestine, beta-sitosterol and other plant sterols have been shown to lower LDL (bad) cholesterol concentrations by 10 to 14 percent. A 30 gram serving of pecans can contain up to 27 milligrams of plant sterols, including as much as 24 milligrams of beta-sitosterol.

Pecans are also an excellent source of vitamin B1 (17 percent of the recommended daily intake per 30 grams) and a good source of vitamin B3 (6 percent of the recommended daily intake), vitamin B6 (5 percent of the recommended daily intake), vitamin B5 (5 percent of the recommended daily intake), and vitamin E (8 percent of the recommended daily intake). In addition, this nut really shines in the mineral department. A 30 gram serving of pecans supplies 71 percent of the recommended daily intake of manganese, 38 percent of the recommended daily intake of copper, 19 percent of the recommended daily intake of molybdenum, 16 percent of the recommended daily intake of zinc, 11 percent of the recommended daily intake of magnesium, 4 percent of the recommended daily intake of iron, 3 percent of the recommended daily intake of potassium and selenium, and 2 percent of the recommended daily intake of calcium.

HEALTH BENEFITS

The health benefits of pecans are similar to those of other nuts that provide a high content of monounsaturated fat and arginine (see page 404). Pecans' concentration of monounsaturated fat and beta-sitosterol are two potential reasons why, in a study recently conducted at New Mexico State University, pecans significantly lowered LDL cholesterol in healthy people with normal lipid levels. Nineteen people completed the study; ten were randomly assigned to the pecan treatment group (seven women and three men ranging in age from thirty-five to fifty-five) and nine to the control group (eight women and one man, ranging in age from twenty-five to forty-nine). Both the pecan treatment group and the control group ate a self-selected diet, the only difference between them being that those in the pecan group consumed pecans daily, while those in the control group avoided all nuts.

Despite the fact that, each day, the subjects in the pecan treatment group consumed about 100 grams of pecans, which delivered 459 calories and 44 grams of fat, their body mass index and weight remained unchanged. Many people avoid nuts, thinking these high-fat foods will lead to weight gain, but this study clearly shows that the healthy fats in pecans do not translate into unhealthy excess fat stores in human beings.

In another study conducted in 2001 at Loma Linda University, adding just a handful of pecans to a traditional low-fat, cholesterol-lowering diet had a dramatic impact on the diet's effectiveness. Study participants—a total of twenty-three men and women between the ages of twenty-five and fifty-five, with normal to mildly elevated cholesterol levels—were randomly placed on either the Step I diet, which is recommended by the American Heart Association as the first line of therapy for individuals with elevated cholesterol levels, or on a pecan-enriched version of the Step I diet. The pecan-enriched diet replaced 20 percent of the Step I diet's calories with pecans, which amounted to about a handful of pecans each day. After staying on their initially assigned diet for four weeks, subjects switched to the other diet.

When the study ended, the data showed that the pecan-enriched diet had lowered study participants' LDL cholesterol levels by 16.5 percent, more than twice as much as the Step I diet, which lowered LDL cholesterol by 6.7 percent from the participants' baseline levels. Similarly, the pecan-enriched diet lowered total cholesterol levels by 11.3 percent, twice as much as the Step I diet, which lowered total cholesterol by 5.2 percent. The pecan-enriched diet also lowered blood triglyceride levels and helped maintain desirable levels of HDL (good) cholesterol compared to the Step I diet. The triglyceride levels of participants on the pecan-enriched diet dropped by 5.7 percent, while in those on the Step I diet, triglyceride levels rose by 4.8 percent.

Once again, in this study, daily consumption of pecans did not affect study participants' weight. Even though the Step I diet contained only 28 percent fat, while the pecan-enriched diet supplied 39.6 percent fat, study participants on the higher-fat pecan diet did not gain weight. One reason may be that pecans add richness, palatability, and satiety to meals and snacks—three factors that can help people stick to a heart-healthy way of eating.

In another study, when researchers at the University of Georgia evaluated samples of pecans from two different years, collected from several states, they found that the vitamin E content of pecans remained abundant and constant, regardless of the year, variety of pecan, or region where it was grown. Pecans contain both the alpha- and gamma-tocopherol forms of vitamin E in levels similar to those of almonds, pistachios, and walnuts, and in higher levels than cashew nuts, macadamia nuts, dry-roasted peanuts, olives, and pine nuts.

HOW TO SELECT AND STORE

Though available all year round, pecans' peak season is the autumn. Due to their high oil content, pecans should preferably be purchased in their shells—although they are also available shelled in vacuum-packed jars, sealed plastic bags, or cans. If choosing shelled pecans, check the sell-by date on the package as, once shelled, pecans turn rancid quickly.

Shelled nutmeats should appear plump and be of similar size and color. Avoid any that are limp, rubbery, dark, or shriveled. Also discard any with a bitter or off taste—a sign that their oil has turned rancid. In addition to their susceptibility to rancidity, shelled pecans will absorb odors, so they should be stored in an airtight container in the refrigerator, where they will keep for up to nine months, or in a moisture-proof Ziplock bag in the freezer, where they will keep for up to two years.

Pecans will mould if not thoroughly dry before storing, even in the freezer, so it's a good idea to place them on a baking tray and bake at 175 degrees F./80 degrees C. for 15 minutes. Then allow them to cool completely to ensure dryness before storing.

When purchasing unshelled pecans, look for clean shells free of stains, splits, cracks, or holes. The best-tasting are heavy for their size and don't rattle when shaken—a sign that the nutmeat is old and dried out. Discard any with a musty scent, as mouldy nuts are unsafe to eat.

Unshelled pecans may be stored in an airtight container in a cool, dry place, where they will keep at room temperature for three to six months. An airtight container will prevent rancidity, and also prevent pecans from absorbing odors and flavors from other foods.

TIPS FOR PREPARING

Two pounds/1 kilogram of unshelled pecans will yield 1 pound/½ kilogram of nutmeats. One pound/½ kilogram of unshelled pecans will yield 2 cups of nutmeats. One pound/½ kilogram of shelled pecans equals 4 cups of pecan halves or 3¼ cups chopped pecans.

Wild pecans are smaller, and their shells are harder to crack than cultivated varieties. Use this method to make shelling all varieties of pecans easier. Place the desired amount of pecans in a pot, cover with water, and bring to a boil. Remove from the heat, cover, and set aside until cool (about 15 to 20 minutes). Drain the pecans, blot dry, and then crack open end to end.

QUICK SERVING IDEAS

- Add a handful of pecans to your favorite banana bread, muffin, corn bread, or pancake recipe.
- Improve on the classic spinach salad by adding pieces of smoked tofu, freshly grated Asiago or Parmesan cheese, and chopped, toasted pecans.
- Try an Asian pasta salad: Dress angel hair pasta with sesame oil and rice vinegar.

Season with chili peppers, green onions, and finely chopped pecans.

- Slice ½-inch/1 centimeter-thick sourdough or French bread rounds, spread with soft goat cheese, and add a sprinkle of minced rosemary or thyme and some finely minced pecans. Grill just until bubbly, and serve with your favorite green salad.
- Stir-fry sweet potato cubes in a stock for 2 to 3 minutes, then add a little olive oil and soy sauce and stir-fry another 2 minutes. Add freshly washed mustard greens. As soon as the greens have wilted, toss in a handful of pecans.
- Make a fresh cranberry-pecan relish: Place a peeled orange, a cored and sliced pear, and 2 cups of fresh cranberries in the blender and blend until just combined. Pour into a bowl and mix in several stalks of chopped celery and a couple of handfuls of toasted pecans.
- Grind pecans into a paste with fresh ginger, olive oil, garlic, and a splash of balsamic vinegar. Slather on tuna steaks and grill until medium rare.
- Season prawns with red pepper, paprika, and salt. Pan-fry in olive oil, spoon over steamed brown rice, and top with toasted pecans.

SAFETY

See page 408.

Pecans contain large amounts of oxalate. Individuals with a history of oxalate-containing kidney stones should avoid overconsuming them. For more information, see Appendix D, page 793.

Pine Nuts

Pine nuts, also called *pignoli, piñons,* and Indian nuts, depending upon the variety, are the seeds of various species of pine trees. Of the more than 100 pine tree species around the world, about a dozen in the Northern Hemisphere yield desirable seeds, the three most prevalent being the *Pinus pinea* (Mediterranean stone pine), *Pinus cembroides* (Mexican nut pine), and *Pinus edulis* (piñon pine of the southwestern United States).

Pine species that produce edible nuts grow in northern Mexico, the southwestern United States, Europe, Asia, North Africa, and South America. Their seeds range in size from the ½-inch/1 centimeter seeds found in Mexican, American, and European pines to the giant 2-inch/5 centimeter seeds of the nut pines of South America. A single pine cone may contain a hundred seeds, but they are lodged securely within the cone, which must be heated to open the scales and loosen the nuts, enabling their removal. After the nuts have been shaken free, the hull protecting each individual nut must be cracked open. This intensive two-step process is the primary reason for pine nuts' high price tag.

If you've already tried pine nuts, you've most likely eaten the seeds of the Mediterranean stone pine, *Pinus pinea,* a tree found from Portugal to Italy to Lebanon that provides the most widely available pine nut. Shaped like torpedoes, these soft, ivory-colored, ½-inch/1 centimeter *pignoli* have a light, delicate flavor with a piney, resinous undertone.

Piñons are similar to *pignoli* in taste and appearance, but the Chinese pine nut, which is shaped like a squat triangle, has a pungent pine flavor so intense that it can overpower some dishes. *Pignoli* are a ubiquitous ingredient in the cuisines of the Mediterranean, Middle East, and North Africa, where they are eaten by the handful as snacks and used in a wide variety of recipes, including classic Italian pesto, while *piñons* have enhanced the traditional dishes of Mexico and native Americans living in the southwestern United States for many centuries.

HISTORY

Not surprisingly, all cultures where nut-bearing species of pines grow have valued their edible seeds since time immemorial. It is thought that the pine nuts from the North American piñon tree were eaten as a staple food some 10,000 years ago, and species are also to be found in Korea, China, Turkey, Pakistan, and Afghanistan, where they have been a traditional food of nomadic tribes.

Piñons were so important a food for Native Americans throughout the region that they were also called Indian nuts and are still harvested in quantity by Native Americans, both for food and for trading.

In the 1500s, Spanish chroniclers traveling among the Hopi and Navajo nations recorded pine nuts being eaten whole, ground for flour and baked, pounded into a buttery paste, used in soup, and either boiled or roasted to make a nourishing porridge. The seeds were cached against the long winters, serving as the mainstay of the Native Americans' diet when weather conditions prevented hunting for fresh meat.

Despite this description of use in America, pine nuts are most often associated with the Mediterranean region, in particular Italy, where they have been used as an ingredient for well over 2,000 years. Evidence found in the ruins of Pompeii, the Italian town destroyed when the volcano Mount Vesuvius erupted in 79 C.E., show that pine nuts were widely used at that time. Some research indicates that the species now grown in Europe, *Pinus pinea,* originated in the Near East and that it was humans who gradually spread it throughout the Mediterranean.

Valued by ancient Greeks and Romans as an aphrodisiac, pine nuts are still a favorite ingredient in Italian cuisine. *Pignoli* are also used in a variety of savory French meat dishes, in *crudités* (raw vegetable salads), and in pastries and baked goods, such as macaroons. In Greece and Turkey, pine nuts, often along with currants, are an integral ingredient in a number of pilaf rice dishes.

In North Africa, pine nuts are a common ingredient in confections; in Tunisia, they are often added to mint tea, the region's ubiquitous equivalent of the American cup of coffee or British cuppa. In India, where they are called *chilgoza,* pine nuts garnish rice dishes and add their sweet richness to desserts, puddings, sauces, and sweetmeats. And, finally, in Korea, they are used in a sustaining breakfast porridge.

Although 3,000 or more metric tonnes of pine nuts are produced annually in Mexico and the southwestern United States, little of this crop enters the nut trade. The majority of pine nuts commercially available in the United States and U.K. are imported from Italy and Spain, the world's top producers.

NUTRITIONAL HIGHLIGHTS

European pine nuts, or *pignoli,* which deliver 24 grams of protein per 100 grams, contain more protein than any other nut or seed. An ounce/30 grams of *pignoli* contains more protein (6.8 grams) and less fat (14 grams), fiber (1.3 grams), and carbohydrate (4 grams) than their American cousins, *piñons,* which provide 3.3 grams of protein, 17 grams of fat, 3 grams of fiber, and 5.5 grams of carbohydrate. The fat provided by both types of nuts is about 50 percent monounsaturated, 40 percent polyunsaturated, and 10 percent saturated.

Pignoli supply 160 calories per 30 grams, while the same amount of *piñons* provides 178 calories. Per 30 grams, *piñons* contain more vitamin B1 (32 percent of the recommended daily intake compared to 21 percent of the recommended daily intake of this nutrient in *pignoli,* although both nuts qualify as an excellent source), while *pignoli* contain more iron (14 percent of the recommended daily intake compared to 5 percent of the recommended daily intake for this mineral in *piñons,* which makes *pignoli* an excellent and *piñons* good source of iron). Both types of pine nuts provide comparable amounts of other vitamins and minerals. Both are an excellent source of vitamins B1 and B3, manganese, copper, magnesium, molybdenum, and zinc and a good source of vitamin B2, vitamin E, and potassium.

A ⅓-cup serving of pine nuts contains 230 calories, 24 grams of fat, 5 grams of protein, and 8 grams of carbohydrate.

HEALTH BENEFITS

The health benefits of *pignoli* are similar to those of other nuts that provide a high content of monounsaturated fat and arginine. In addition, both types of pine nuts deliver a hefty dose of magnesium and potassium, two minerals whose combined effects produce a strong, healthy heartbeat, lowered blood pressure, and improved blood flow. Taken altogether, pine nuts' arginine, monounsaturated fat, and magnesium and potassium content provide powerful effects for counteracting heart disease.

HOW TO SELECT AND STORE

Pignoli are widely available and are sold already shelled. *Piñons* are most likely to be available in the southwestern United States, where they are sold, already shelled, in the produce section of supermarkets and natural food markets. Asian markets are the best places to find Chinese pine nuts.

Because of their high fat content, all varieties of pine nuts are extremely susceptible to rancidity. Purchase pine nuts that are packaged in an airtight container. Be sure to check the sell-by date on the package to ensure freshness.

Store all pine nuts in an airtight container in the refrigerator, where they will keep for up to three months, or in an airtight Ziplock bag in the freezer, where they will keep for up to nine months.

TIPS FOR PREPARING

Toasting pine nuts will intensify their flavor and takes just 2 to 3 minutes on a dry skillet over medium heat or 6 to 8 minutes spread out on a baking tray in an oven preheated to 350 degrees F./180 degrees C./gas 4.

Alternatively, rinse the pine nuts in cold water, drain, sprinkle with salt, put in a covered roasting pan, and steam at 250 to 275 degrees F./130 to 140 degrees C./gas ½ to 1 for 15 to 20 minutes. Remove the cover, and stir until completely dry.

QUICK SERVING IDEAS

- Sauté dried cranberries in a little olive oil until they plump and turn bright red. Add fresh spinach leaves and cook until just wilted. Place in a serving bowl, sprinkle with pine nuts, freshly ground black pepper, and sea salt, and serve.
- The presentation and flavor of creamy tomato or split pea soup are greatly enhanced by topping with a dollop of plain yogurt and a sprinkling of toasted pine nuts.
- Add pine nuts to your favorite quick bread, pancake, waffle, muffin, or cookie recipe.
- Rice cooked with pine nuts, mushrooms, raisins, and onion makes a wonderful stuffing or side dish.
- Try a Mediterranean salad of fresh greens with orange segments and soft goat cheese rolled in pine nuts.
- Drizzle grilled vegetables with balsamic vinegar and a sprinkling of pine nuts.
- For an elegant dessert, place chunks of fresh fruit and berries in a parfait glass and top with generous spoonfuls of yogurt, honey, and pine nuts. Dust with cinnamon or garnish with a fresh mint leaf.

SAFETY

See page 408. Also, asthmalike symptoms have been reported after consumption of pine nuts. Individuals living near a pine forest, who are therefore exposed and possibly sensitized to pine tree pollen, may be more at risk of an allergy to pine nuts. Also, common antigenic (allergy-provoking) proteins have been identified in pine nuts and peanuts, so individuals allergic to peanuts may also want to avoid pine nuts.

Pistachio Nuts

A member of the Anacardiaceae or cashew family, which also includes mangoes, the pistachio is the pea-sized seed of the small tree *Pistacia vera.* Its English name, pistachio, is derived from the Persian word for the tree, *pistah,* which in the conditions provided by Iran (modern-day Persia)—stony, poor soil, high heat, and little or no rainfall—can thrive for centuries, a fact attested to by a number of 200-year-old trees still producing nuts in the Middle East and a 700-year-old tree still living in Iran.

The pistachio tree grows to a height of about 20 feet/6 meters. Some trees are male, others female, and both are needed for reproduction, which, in this case, results in pistachio nuts. The male trees produce the pollen, which is carried on the wind to the female trees, on which the nuts, each enclosed in its own reddish green hull, grow in clusters like grapes. One male tree provides enough pollen for six female trees.

Pistachio trees mature slowly, do not begin to bear fruit until seven to ten years after planting, and take a full twenty years to reach peak production. Even then, like many other nut trees, the pistachio is alternate-year-bearing—producing a large crop one year and very little or nothing at all the next. The trees develop a brownish green flower in early summer, and the nuts ripen in late summer to early autumn.

Encased in a hard, pale beige shell that splits open partially when the bright green seed is mature, pistachios bless us with a rich nutty flavor underscored with a hint of sweetness. The visually appealing green nuts are quite popular in Mediterranean and Middle Eastern cuisines, where their color and flavor enhance both sweet and savory dishes. The introduction of the pistachio tree to California has resulted in a dramatic increase in their popularity in the United States as well. A favorite nut for eating out of hand, pistachios are also used in a wide variety of confections, baked goods, and desserts, in which their lively green hue adds to their appeal. Pistachios are also pressed for their delicious oil, and their pleasing color is used in green food coloring. The green in the pistachio nut is due to its content of chlorophyll, the pigment that makes plants green.

In Turkey, where the pistachios are a little smaller, the nuts are placed in brine with their hulls still on, which gives the shells a pink tint. The first pistachios marketed in the United States were imported from the Middle East in the 1930s and were dyed red. Some nut authorities attribute the practice of dyeing pistachios with red food coloring to an attempt to imitate the appearance of Turkish pistachios. Others claim that the red dye was used to draw consumers' attention to the nuts, while still others assert that the red dye was used to cover imperfections and stains on the shells due to the nuts' poor quality.

Red-dyed pistachios were marketed much more forty to sixty years ago than they are today, but some American-grown pistachios are still dyed red to appeal to consumers who find the color familiar or wouldn't recognize the nuts in their—preferable—natural tan state.

HISTORY

Native to Turkey, Iran, Syria, Lebanon, and the Caucasus Mountains in southern Russia and Afghanistan, the pistachio has been gathered from wild trees in the high desert regions of the Holy Lands since time immemorial and cultivated for at least 3,000 years. Evidence found by archaeologists in a dig site at Jarmo, near northeastern Iraq, indicates that pistachio nuts were a common food as early as 6750 B.C.E.

Pistachios, along with almonds, share the distinction of being the only two nuts mentioned in the Bible. In Genesis 43:11, when Jacob finally sends his sons to Egypt for grain, he tells them to pack a gift of "the best products of the land . . . a little balm, a little honey, some spices and myrrh, some pistachio nuts and almonds."

Pistachio trees flourished in the Hanging Gardens of Babylon during the reign of King Merodach-baladan II, about 700 B.C.E., and the queen of Sheba, who considered them an aphrodisiac, is said to have hoarded the entire Assyrian supply for herself and her court. According to Persian legend, lovers met beneath pistachio trees on moonlit nights in the hope of hearing the ripening nuts crack open—a promise of good fortune. In Syria, pistachios remain to this day an important ingredient at wedding feasts, and guests are often given a small bag of the nuts as a good will parting gift.

During the first century C.E., the pistachio traveled from Syria to Italy, where Apicius, the cook for the Roman emperor Vitellius, singled out the nut in his classical cookbook but refused to share his recipes. Vitellius is said to have commonly finished off his meals by stuffing his mouth full of pistachios.

Hardy travelers that held up well on long journeys, pistachios were carried from Rome throughout the Mediterranean and from Persia to China via the Silk Road. Transported by Arab settlers to southern Spain (Andalusia) and Sicily in the Middle Ages, pistachio trees took well to these regions, producing highly prized nuts that commanded steep prices for their deep green color. Imported into France, pistachios soon became so expensive that only the richest could afford them, but merchants had an ample supply for those able to splurge on the green delicacies. Pistachios finally arrived in England in the sixteenth century; there, however, they were not the gastronomic success they had been in the rest of Europe, and colonists did not take them to the New World.

The United States was first introduced to the pistachio in 1854, when Charles Mason, a seed distributor for experimental plantings, brought some trees to California. Twenty years later, in 1875, a few small pistachio trees imported from France were planted in Sonoma, California. Then, in the 1880s, pistachio nuts were imported from Turkey by American traders, primarily for U.S. citizens of Middle Eastern origin. Fifty years later, introduced in vending machines, the pistachio became a popular snack food, and the birth of the California pistachio industry followed shortly thereafter.

Today, 110,000 acres of pistachios are planted in California, and 98 percent of America's pistachio crop—a record-breaking 302.4 million pounds/137 million kilograms in 2002—is produced in this state.

Currently, pistachios are the eighth leading nut crop in the world, with approximately 220,500 metric tonnes produced annually, principally in Iran and Turkey. In addition to their rapidly increasing production in the United States, pistachios are also cultivated in smaller amounts in India, Syria, Greece, Pakistan, the Far East, and North Africa.

NUTRITIONAL HIGHLIGHTS

Like other nuts, pistachios are high in fat, but the fat they deliver is heart-healthy: 52 percent is monounsaturated and 20 percent is polyunsaturated. Pistachios are also an excellent source of protein and fiber. A single ounce/30 grams of roasted pistachio nuts delivers 13 percent of the recommended daily intake of protein and 12 percent of the recommended daily intake of fiber.

In addition, pistachios are well endowed with B vitamins, being an excellent source of vitamin B6 (37 percent of the recommended daily intake per ounce/30 grams), vitamin B1 (22 percent of the recommended daily intake per ounce/30 grams), and vitamin B3 (12 percent of the recommended daily intake per ounce/30 grams). They're also a very good source of vitamin E (8 percent of the recommended daily intake per ounce/30 grams) and a good source of vitamin B2 (4 percent of the recommended daily intake per ounce/30 grams), folic acid (4 percent of the recommended daily intake per ounce/30 grams), and vitamin B5 (3 percent of the recommended daily intake per ounce/30 grams).

Like many other nuts, pistachios really shine in the mineral department. They're an excellent source of copper (42 percent of the recommended daily intake per ounce/30 grams), manganese (20 percent of the recommended daily intake per ounce/30 grams), and molybdenum (19 percent of the recommended daily intake per ounce/30 grams); a very good source of magnesium (11 percent of the recommended daily intake per ounce/30 grams) and zinc (8 percent of the recommended daily intake per ounce/30 grams); and a good source of selenium (4 percent of the recommended daily intake per ounce/30 grams) and calcium (3 percent of the recommended daily intake per ounce/30 grams).

Furthermore, pistachios are the richest source of potassium of all the nuts—just 1 ounce/30 grams of pistachios deliver as much potassium as an orange, and 2 ounces/60 grams of pistachios provide more potassium than a medium-size banana. But perhaps the greatest nutritional highlight of pistachios is that you can enjoy a lot of them while getting all these nutrients. A 1-ounce/30 gram serving of California pistachios contains an unbelievable forty-seven nuts!

One-third cup of shelled pistachios provides 240 calories, 20 grams of fat, 9 grams of protein, and 6 grams of carbohydrate.

HEALTH BENEFITS

The health benefits of pistachios are similar to those of other nuts that provide a high content of monounsaturated fat and arginine. Additionally, pistachios are a very good source of both magnesium and potassium, two minerals that protect against high blood pressure.

Given their heart-healthy constituents, it's not surprising that two recent clinical research trials have demonstrated that including pistachios regularly in the diet significantly improves lipid profiles in humans with both normal and moderately elevated blood levels of cholesterol. In one study, pistachios were substituted for 20 percent of the daily caloric intake in ten patients with moderately elevated blood cholesterol levels who followed a traditional American diet (35

to 39 percent of their calories from fat). After three weeks, the result was a significant decrease in both total and LDL (bad) cholesterol levels, plus an increase in levels of beneficial HDL cholesterol. In the other study, including 60 to 100 grams of pistachios in a low-fat diet (30 percent calories from fat) produced a 5 to 12 percent lowering of total cholesterol and a 10 to 15 percent drop in LDL cholesterol.

In addition to their healthy fats and sterols, pistachios contain a compound with anti-inflammatory effects. In a 2001 animal study, this compound, oleanolic acid, was found to alleviate dermatitis because of its ability to inhibit the production of the proinflammatory agent leukotriene B$_4$.

Another recent study evaluated the long-held belief in Jordanian folk medicine that pistachios are an effective treatment for jaundice. When intoxicated rats were given a dose of 4 milliliters per kilogram of body weight of a water extract of pistachio, the liver-damaging activity of three enzymes—alkaline phosphatase, alanine aminotransferase, and aspartate aminotransferase—was significantly reduced, along with bilirubin levels. (Bilirubin is a yellowish pigment in bile whose accumulation is a primary symptom of jaundice.) Thus it appears that the practice of using pistachios as a folk remedy for jaundice has merit.

HOW TO SELECT AND STORE

Pistachios are harvested in September, but a good supply and modern storage techniques ensure their availability all year round.

Pistachios can be purchased in the shell or with their shells removed, both raw and roasted. If you are buying pistachios in their shells, choose those with partially open shells that are free of defects. Pistachio shells split open to accommodate the expanding nut kernel. A firmly closed shell indicates that the nut is immature and flavorless. In addition, choose the most colorful nuts; the most flavorful, highest-quality nuts are bright green in color. And avoid salted pistachios and those whose naturally beige shells have been dyed red or whitened.

Since pistachios' split shells expose the nut meats, even those still in the shell should be stored in an airtight container in the refrigerator, where they will keep for up to three months. Placed in heavy-duty freezer bags and frozen, pistachios will keep for up to six months.

Shelled pistachios can also be stored in an airtight container in the refrigerator, where they will keep for up to six weeks, or in the freezer, where they will keep for several months.

If stored pistachios lose their natural crunch, they can quickly be revitalized. Simply place them on a baking tray and heat at 250 degrees F./120 to 130 degrees C./gas ½ for 6 to 9 minutes.

TIPS FOR PREPARING

Because of their characteristic widely split shells, California pistachios are especially easy to open. Two cups of California pistachios can be shelled in about 15 minutes. Unsplit shells contain immature nutmeats and should be discarded; however, slightly split shells are worth opening. The easiest way is to wedge the tip of a half shell from an already-opened pistachio into the split of an unopened one and twist; the shells will pry apart.

One pound/½ kilogram of pistachios in the shell will yield 2 cups of nutmeats. Two cups of pistachios still in their shells will yield 1 cup of nutmeats. One pound/½ kilogram of shelled pistachios equals 3½ cups of nutmeats. One ounce/30 grams of shelled pistachios equals 47 nuts.

If desired, the thin, edible papers surrounding the nut meats can be removed by blanching. To blanch shelled pistachios, cover them with boiling water, let stand for 2 minutes, drain, and cool slightly. The skins will slip right off.

Roasting pistachios at home enables you to prepare them to suit your own taste. A shorter roasting time produces crispness with a minimal roasted flavor, while a longer roasting time develops a stronger roasted flavor. Before roasting, make a salt solution by dissolving 2 to 3 ounces/60 to 85 grams of salt in ½ cup of water. Pour the salt solution into a deep saucepan over high heat. Add 8 to 10 cups of pistachios and stir until all the water has evaporated, leaving a deposit of salt on the nuts. Next, spread the salted pistachios on a baking tray in an oven preheated to 250 degrees F./120 to 130 degrees C./gas ½ and let roast, stirring every 30 minutes, for 1¼ hours for crispness with minimal roasted flavor and for 1¾ hours for a deeper roasted taste.

QUICK SERVING IDEAS

- Try this exceptionally delicious pistachio-artichoke soup. In a soup pot, add 2 cans drained artichoke hearts or 1 package frozen artichoke hearts, 1 peeled and cubed parsnip, 1 small chopped onion, 3 stalks diced celery, 1 thinly sliced leek, 3 tablespoons finely chopped parsley, 1 tablespoon lemon juice, 7 cups vegetable stock, 2 ounces/60 millilitres white wine, and ½ cup finely ground pistachios. Bring to a boil over medium heat, then lower the heat to a simmer and add 1 teaspoon dried marjoram, ¼ teaspoon ground coriander, and salt and freshly ground black pepper to taste. Cover and cook for 1½ hours. Garnish each serving with a dollop of whole-fat yogurt and a sprinkling of roasted pistachios.

- Add raw pistachios to grain dishes at the end of cooking. The color contrast they provide is especially attractive with lighter-colored grains, such as quinoa, millet, rice, and barley.

- One nice pistachio-grain combination is a mix of pistachios and rice with onion, currants or raisins, orange, and cinnamon. Cook 1 cup rice in 2 cups water or vegetable stock to which has been added the juice of one orange along with some zest from the orange skin. Sauté 1 chopped onion in a tablespoon of olive oil, coconut oil, or butter. Add ¼ cup raisins, ½ cup chopped pistachios, and 1 teaspoon cinnamon. Sauté for several minutes, then combine with the cooked rice. To add a festive golden tint to the rice, add ½ teaspoon ground saffron to the sautéed onion along with the other ingredients.

- Ground, raw, unsalted pistachios are an excellent thickener for soups and sauces; just remember, the nuts will affect the color of the dish.

- Make pistachio butter, a delicious topping for baked fish: Blend together ¼ cup of ground pistachios, ½ cup softened butter or olive oil, eight to ten fresh basil leaves or ¼ cup parsley, ¼ cup chopped onion or 1 clove garlic, and a tablespoon of lime juice. Refrigerate until well chilled (make a day or two ahead if desired). When the fish is almost done (after baking about 10 minutes), smear a generous tablespoon on each piece and continue baking for another 5 minutes. Transfer the fish to a serving platter and garnish with chopped pistachios and parsley.

- Try pistachio pasta: Sauté ¼ cup minced onion and 1 clove minced garlic in olive oil over medium heat until the onion is transparent. Add ½ cup chopped pistachios, ¼ cup minced parsley, 1 teaspoon lemon juice, 1 minced basil leaf, and freshly ground black pepper to taste. Cook a couple of minutes, then pour over four cups of cooked pasta and toss. Garnish with pistachios, chopped basil or parsley, and a little grated Parmesan.

- Alternatively, toss pasta with pistachio pesto. To make the pesto, blend together 2 cups fresh basil, 1 cup ground pistachios, 2 to 3 cloves garlic, and ¼ to ½ cup olive oil.

- Try pistachios in your favorite muffin or quick bread recipe. Team the nuts with golden raisins, orange or lemon zest, cardamon, cinnamon, and/or ginger.

- For an unusual, delicious dessert, serve pistachio-stuffed dates, fruit, and cheese. Make ¼-inch/½ centimeter slits in your favorite type of dates and slip in pistachios. Arrange on a large serving dish surrounded by chilled green grapes and slices of your favorite cheese.

SAFETY

See page 408. Also, since the pistachio belongs to the same family as the mango and cashew, parts of the pistachio contain similar oleoresins, which have caused contact dermatitis and have been shown to cause IgE-mediated allergic reactions. Individuals who are allergic to mangoes or cashew nuts should therefore avoid pistachios as well.

Pumpkin Seeds

The pumpkin *(Cucurbita pepo)* was previously described in Chapter 10 (see "Squash, Winter" on page 236). Also known as pepitas, pumpkin seeds are rugby ball-shaped, flat, dark green seeds with some sheathed in a yellow-white husk. There are also varieties of pumpkins which produce seeds without shells. The pumpkin seed has a chewy texture and a subtle, sweet, and nutty flavor. While roasted pumpkin seeds are probably best known for their role as a perennial Halloween-time autumn treat, the seeds of the pumpkin are quite healthful and tasty any time of the year.

HISTORY

Big pumpkins, and their small seeds, were a distinguished food of the Native American Indians. These peoples used the pumpkin seed for both nutrition and making medicine. Pumpkin seeds had a reputation of being able to treat worms. European explorers took these seeds back to the Old World, where they were appreciated for their value and taste. Although used in many cuisines, the Mexicans have especially developed a special taste and purpose for the pumpkin seed. As more scientific research underscores the benefits of the pumpkin seed, its popularity will most certainly increase in years to come. The top producers of pumpkins and pumpkin seeds are the United States, China, Mexico, and India.

NUTRITIONAL HIGHLIGHTS

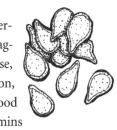

Pumpkin seeds supply minerals such as phosphorus, magnesium, iron, manganese, zinc, and copper. In addition, pumpkin seeds are a good source of vitamin A, vitamins B1, B2, and B3, protein, monounsaturated fats, and phytosterols, particularly beta-sitosterol.

In one-third of a cup of shelled pumpkin seeds there are about 90 calories, 4 grams of fat, 4 grams of protein, and 11 grams of carbohydrate.

HEALTH BENEFITS

Naturopathic doctors have utilized the benefits of pumpkin seeds to treat prostate conditions effectively. The high levels of essential fatty acids, zinc, and phytosterols make them an excellent part of a prostate health regimen, and research supports the notion that these nutrients may benefit prostate enlargement. One of the phytosterols, called beta-sitosterol, helps block conversion of testerone into a metabolite (dihydrotestosterone) that encourages prostate enlargement. Not surprisingly, studies using pumpkin seed oil or beta-sitosterol have demonstrated considerable benefits in improving the symptoms of benign prostate enlargement.

HOW TO SELECT AND STORE

Pumpkin seeds are found both in bulk bins and in prepackaged containers. For maximum freshness, it is always important to ensure there is no moisture in the seeds you are purchasing, and that for bulk items, the bins from which you obtain your seeds are covered. For the freshest stock, your shop should have a high volume and quick turnover. For storage, use an airtight container and keep your pumpkin seeds in the refrigerator, where they can last for up to half a year, although they are best for only the first two months. Also, check for insect damage and that the seeds are whole and not desiccated. Finally, if possible, check for a musty aroma, which may indicate that the seeds have gone rancid.

TIPS FOR PREPARING

For the freshest pumpkin seeds, open a pumpkin and remove the seeds, cleaning the pumpkin flesh off the seeds while they are still moist. Once they are out, you can dry the seeds by leaving them exposed to air for a few days.

If you would like to roast pumpkin seeds, lay the seeds as a single layer on a baking tray and drizzle them lightly with oil and seasonings of your choice. Place them in the oven at 300 degrees F./150 degrees C./gas 2 for about 30 minutes or until golden brown. Shake the pan repeatedly while baking to keep them from burning.

QUICK SERVING IDEAS

- Spicy pumpkin seeds: Follow the above toasting directions. To approximately 3 cups of seeds, you can add 1 teaspoon ground cinnamon, ½ teaspoon ground cloves, ½ teaspoon nutmeg, and salt to taste.
- Pumpkin seeds can be sautéed with carrots, broccoli, and onions and served over your favorite grain.
- Liberally sprinkle pumpkin seeds on top of mixed green salads for an extra healthy crunch.
- For a tasty salad dressing, grind pumpkin seeds with fresh garlic, parsley, and coriander leaves. Mix with olive oil and lemon juice.

- Crushed pumpkin seeds are a healthy addition to any hot or cold cereal dish.
- Pumpkin seeds can be an added treat in your standard oatmeal biscuit recipe.
- Pumpkin seed burger: Try adding pumpkin seeds to your meat or vegetable burger for a seed treat.

SAFETY

Allergy to pumpkin seeds is rare. If an allergic reaction is to occur, it manifests as itching and swelling of oral mucosa, and asthma. Three patients with symptoms after ingestion of roasted pumpkin seeds have been reported; however, all the patients fished for sport and used pressed pumpkin seed flour as bait. The case histories suggest inhalation of the flour to have been the relevant route of sensitization, leading to the allergy.

Sesame Seeds

The sesame plant (*Sesamum indicum*) is cultivated in Central America, India, Sudan, China, and the United States. Surprisingly, this small seed is grown from an annual plant that grows 2 to 4 feet/about 1 meter tall. The plant develops flowers that are tiny, with a pink or white color. The seeds also vary in color, from white to dark brown. The sesame seed itself is encased in a small pod. The Arabian tale of "open sesame" harkens back to the ability of sesame seed pods to burst open when ripe.

Because of their high oil content, sesame seeds are both highly valued and highly susceptible to rancidity. In fact, the seeds are so susceptible that they are harvested by hand. Additionally, the sesame seed is used as food, as oil, and in cosmetic and pharmaceutical preparations.

HISTORY

Thought to be one of the oldest foods, sesame seeds have been grown throughout the world since prehistoric times. The Assyrians claim to hold the earliest records for writing, with ancient stone tablets as evidence. Apparently, on one of the tablets there exists a legend about the Assyrian gods, who drank sesame wine one night, then created the earth the next day.

The sesame seed was thought to have originated in India and was mentioned in many early Hindu traditions. According to these traditions, the sesame seed represents immortality. During the Babylonian era (2100–689 B.C.E.), the Babylonians used sesame oil to make exotic perfumes and medicine. Records also indicate that the Egyptians prescribed the sesame as medicine around 1500 B.C.E. and used the oil as ceremonial purification.

Europeans encountered the sesame seeds when they were imported from India during the first century C.E. In the seventeenth century, the sesame seed was brought to the United States from Africa. Today, the main producers are China, India, and Mexico, where labor is abundant and inexpensive.

NUTRITIONAL HIGHLIGHTS

The sesame seed, one of the smallest seeds, is densely packed with nutrients. The seed is a fantastic source of protein (especially rich in methionine and tryptophan), lignans, fiber, monounsaturated fats, vitamins B1 and B2, minerals such as copper, magnesium, iron, zinc, and calcium, and phytic acid. Sesame seeds are low in carbohydrates and cholesterol-free. One-third cup of shelled sesame seeds yields 280 calories, 8 grams of protein, 23 grams of fat, and 6 grams of carbohydrate.

The fat in sesame seeds is 38 percent monounsaturated and 44 percent polyunsaturated, which equals 82 percent unsaturated fatty acids. The average oil content of the seed is 50 percent. The amino acid profile rivals those of many other vegetarian protein sources, such as soybeans, peanuts, and other legumes.

Natural unhulled sesame seeds are high in calcium. One tablespoon provides 87.8 milligrams, while the hulled type provides only 10.5 milligrams per tablespoon. Some surprising numbers are revealed when comparing the amount of calcium in sesame seeds to that in milk. One cup of natural sesame seeds has 1404.0 milligrams of calcium, while one cup of nonfat milk provides 316.3 milligrams and one cup of whole milk has only 291 milligrams of calcium. However, the 2 to 3 percent oxalic acid in unhulled sesame seeds can interfere with calcium utilization.

HEALTH BENEFITS

Sesame seeds, like other nuts and seeds, contain lignans. The lignan in sesame seeds called sesamin has displayed amazing antioxidant abilities. It has been shown in research that it inhibits the manufacture of cholesterol in the livers of rats as well as reduces cholesterol absorption from the diet. This preliminary research states that sesamin may offer considerable ability to lower total blood cholesterol levels.

The ability of sesame seeds to relieve constipation and to remove worms from the intestinal tract is also well known. These little seeds aid digestion, stimulate blood circulation, and benefit the nervous system. Their high oil content lubricates the intestines and nourishes all the internal viscera. In traditional Chinese medicine, sesame is known to produce *yin* (body fluid) and can promote lactation (for breast-feeding mothers). Sesame oil also makes terrific massage oil because of its excellent emollient and vitamin E properties, and it is thought to aid in chronic skin diseases and burns.

HOW TO SELECT AND STORE

There is a great variety when purchasing sesame seeds. They come dry, cleaned with hulls, white and without hulls, toasted, and made into butter (tahini) or flour. Unhulled sesame seed is more advantageous to purchase because the hulls act as a protective coating to prevent rancidity and keep the oil more stable.

Most of the sesame seeds sold in the United States are hulled. These seeds can be stored in an airtight container in a cool, dry, dark place for one year or in the refrigerator or freezer.

TIPS FOR PREPARING

Sesame seeds are used in a variety of ways and recipes. They can be toasted, baked, or sprinkled. The oil is used in frying or dressings, or tahini can be incorporated into dishes.

QUICK SERVING IDEAS

- Sesame, spinach, and artichoke dip: Blend finely chopped spinach leaves, and artichoke hearts, mint leaves, tahini, lime juice, cumin, salt, and nutritional yeast to an almost smooth purée in a food processor. Transfer to a serving bowl and sprinkle with toasted sesame seeds and a dash of paprika. Serve with toasted pita wedges.
- Peanut butter replacement: Combine sesame seeds with honey, a pinch of carob, a pinch of cinnamon, and a tiny pinch of salt. Place all ingredients in a coffee grinder and blend to a buttery consistency.
- Combine raw or toasted sesame seeds with Asian salad dressings.
- Sesame seed chutney: Blend 1 cup roasted and ground sesame seeds, 1 teaspoon cayenne, and ¼ teaspoon salt until well mixed. Use 1 teaspoon per meal on the side of the plate as a spicy sauce.

SAFETY

See page 408.

Sesame seeds contain moderate amounts of oxalate. Individuals with a history of oxalate-containing kidney stones should avoid overconsuming them. For more information, see Appendix D, page 793.

Sunflower Seeds

While the vibrant, strong sunflower is recognized worldwide for its beauty, it is also an important source of food with its seed-studded center. The Latin name for the sunflower is *Helianthus annuus,* which is derived from the Greek word for "sun," *helios,* as well as *anthos,* the Greek word for "flower." This cheerful flower smiles down upon us, since it can grow to 20 feet/6 meters tall, with the flower diameter being as large as 30 inches/76 centimeters.

The seed-studded center can produce gray-green- or black-shelled seeds with black or white stripes. The seeds have a mild nutty taste with a firm yet tender texture. Oil can be produced from the seeds and is made up of a combination of monounsaturated and polyunsaturated fats, with low saturated fat levels.

Sunflower oil is light in taste and appearance and supplies more Vitamin E than any other vegetable oil.

HISTORY

Sunflowers are native to both North and South America, where indigenous people were the first to cultivate them. Sunflowers have been cultivated for more than 5,000 years by the Native Americans, who used all the parts of the plant for various purposes, such as oil sources and dye pigments. The Spanish explorers took the sunflower back to Europe, from which it extended its beauty to adjoining countries.

Today, sunflower oil is one of the most popular oils in the world. The world's leading commercial producers of sunflower seeds are the Russian Federation, Spain, Argentina, France, China, Peru, and the United States. In the United States, North Dakota, Minnesota, and California are the leading producers.

Considered to be the most "cheerful" flower in the world, the sunflower is a symbol of light, hope, and innocence. The U.S. state of Kansas adopted the sunflower as its state flower, while Russia considers the sunflower its national flower. However, some U.S. farmers inexplicably thought otherwise and considered the sunflower a weed; in fact, in 1972 the state of Iowa officially declared the sunflower a "noxious weed."

NUTRITIONAL HIGHLIGHTS

Sunflower seeds are an abundant source of important nutrients. They are a wonderful source of protein, vitamin E, magnesium, selenium, vitamins B1, B5, and B6, phosphorus, copper, iron, folic acid, and fiber.

A ⅓-cup serving of sunflower seeds provides 24 grams of fat, 11 grams of protein, 270 calories, and 9 grams of carbohydrate.

HEALTH BENEFITS

The health benefits of sunflower seeds are similar to nuts that provide a high content of mono-unsaturated fat and arginine.

Research studies have shown that the important nutrients a sunflower provides are often in insufficient supply in the American diet. Deficient intake of these vital nutrients has been shown to be linked to increased risk of heart attack and stroke, and selenium in particular has anticancer, anti-inflammatory, and anti-allergenic properties as well.

Several folk medicine remedies use sunflower seeds. One remedy that includes sunflower seeds is an old Russian recipe that combined chopped sunflower heads, soap chips, and vodka in a mixture that was sun-aged for a period of nine days. This concoction was then used topically on joints for rheumatism. John Douglas, M.D., a physician at Kaiser-Permanente Medical Center in Los Angeles, recommends raw sunflower seeds for allergy relief and to stop smoking. He recommends the seeds primarily to provide an activity to keep smoker's hands and mouths busy.

HOW TO SELECT AND STORE

Sunflower seeds are available in a variety of forms. For example, they can be roasted, raw, and with or without hulls. The most nutritional gain comes from the fresh, raw, and hulled seed.

Whenever possible, purchase organic sunflower seeds, shelled or unshelled. It is important to make sure they are not broken, dirty, or limp nor appear yellow in color. Sunflower seeds that are limp or yellow are probably rancid. Health food shops are one resource to buy the seeds in bulk. However, many nuts and seeds can now be purchased on the Internet at lower prices.

For best results when temperatures climb above 70 degrees F./18 degrees C., store them in a plastic or glass airtight container and keep them refrigerated year round. They can also be frozen. Sunflower seeds with shells have an extended life and can be kept at room temperature for up to a year in cooler climates. Roasted seeds have a shorter shelf life.

The highest-quality sunflower oil is cold-pressed (this should be clearly stated on the bottle). Once the bottle is opened, store it in the refrigerator to prevent spoilage.

TIPS FOR PREPARING

First and foremost, it is essential to note that albeit beautiful, the sunflower petals themselves are not edible. In fact, they are very poisonous and should not be eaten or used as decorations for food.

It can be a tedious and frustrating task un-shelling sunflower seeds by hand. A more accessible and efficient method is to put a quantity of seeds into a large Ziplock bag and use a rolling pin to break up the shells. Transfer the seeds to a large bowl filled with water and give them a vigorous stir. You'll notice that the kernels sink to the bottom, while the shells float to the surface, where they can be skimmed off.

Toasting sunflower seeds heightens their flavor. To do so, put one or two handfuls of raw sunflower seeds into a dry nonstick skillet. Over high heat, stir them continuously with a wooden spoon until seeds turn light golden brown (2 to 3 minutes) and watch carefully to avoid burning. As soon as they begin to turn color, remove the seeds from heat and place in a dish to cool. Another method is to simply place the raw seeds on a baking tray and bake at 350 degrees F./180 degrees C./gas 4 for approximately 10 to 15 minutes.

QUICK SERVING IDEAS

- Add sunflower seeds to your favorite hot or cold cereal.
- Add sunflower seeds to any rice pilaf dish.
- Healthy sunflower seed pesto: 1 cup hulled raw sunflower seeds, 4 cups coarsely chopped fresh basil leaves, ½ cup olive oil, 1 cup freshly grated Parmesan cheese, and 2 crushed cloves of garlic. In a blender in batches or in a food processor purée the basil with the sunflower seeds, the oil, the Parmesan, and the garlic. Use immediately or if covered and refrigerated it can last for up to two weeks.
- Wasabi sunflower spread: Combine ½ cup sunflower seeds, ½ teaspoon salt, ¼ teaspoon of sugar, ⅓ teaspoon wasabi paste, 1 tablespoon rice vinegar, 3 tablespoons water, and ½ teaspoon tamari in a food processor and process until almost smooth and creamy. Transfer to a small serving bowl and serve with whole-grain bread or raw veggies.
- Linseed dessert balls: Mix together ground linseed, ground sunflower seeds, ground sesame seeds, some carob powder, ground coconut, a pinch of salt, and some honey or maple syrup. Knead the mixture together and form it into balls.

SAFETY

See page 408.

Sunflower seeds contain moderate amounts of oxalate. Individuals with a history of oxalate-containing kidney stones should avoid over-consuming them. For more information, see Appendix D, page 793.

Walnuts

Walnuts are considered to be the oldest tree food known to man. Walnut trees live long (their life span is several times that of humans) and can grow to a height of 150 feet/45 meters. They are a popular tree used to make furniture, as well as a great ornamental tree. Two walnut species are of commercial importance. One is the English walnut *(Juglans regia)*, and the other is the black walnut *(Juglans nigra)*. Most people prefer to eat the English walnut because it is easier to break the shell.

Walnuts are normally 1½ to 2½ inches/4 to 6½ centimeters in diameter and oblong in shape. The external shell is covered by an outer leathery husk, and the inner portion of the shell houses the meat of the nut.

HISTORY

The walnut tree dates back as far as 7000 B.C.E. and has been cultivated ever since. Walnuts have numerous locations of origin. In the early days of Rome, they were considered food for the gods and were named *Juglans regia* in honor of Jupiter. Today, walnuts are commonly called "English" walnuts, in reference to the English merchants whose ships transported the product for trade around the world. The English walnut

originated around the Caspian Sea and in India and was brought to America.

In contrast to the English walnut, the black walnut is native to North America, particularly the central Mississippi valley and Appalachian area. Black walnuts were a staple in the diets and lifestyles of both the Native Americans and the early colonial settlers.

Besides being a food source, walnuts provide shelter and medicine, as well as dyes and lamp oil. The world's leading commercial producers of walnuts are the United States, China, France, Turkey, Romania, and Iran. California alone provides more than half of the world's production.

NUTRITIONAL HIGHLIGHTS

Walnuts are extremely nutrient-dense. They are a wonderful source of antioxidants, vitamin E, minerals such as manganese, copper, phosphorus, and magnesium, and monounsaturated fats. The walnut is one of the few nuts that contain omega-3 fatty acids and alpha-linolenic acid. In fact, walnuts are the main "nonfish" source of alpha-linolenic acid.

Walnuts are also a rich source of protein and dietary fiber and have no dietary cholesterol.

A ⅓-cup serving of shelled walnuts contains 210 calories, 20 grams of fat, 5 grams of protein, and 6 grams of carbohydrate.

HEALTH BENEFITS

The health benefits of walnuts are similar to those of other nuts that provide a high content of monounsaturated fat and arginine (see page 404). In addition, according to the Doctrine of

Signatures, the belief that a food has been signed by the creator and indicates its use, walnuts are considered food for the brain.

Walnuts are an essential component of the Mediterranean diet, and several investigations have been performed into their health benefits. One study in particular compared the effects of the cholesterol-lowering Mediterranean diet to that of a Mediterranean diet that had 35 percent of the calories derived from monounsaturated fats from walnuts. The study found that the forty-nine participants who ate the walnut-enhanced diet had lower levels of total cholesterol, LDL, and lipoprotein a (Lp(a), a form of lipoprotein that is an even more serious risk for heart disease than LDL).

Other research studies have corroborated these beneficial effects of walnuts. For example, a study of thirteen postmenopausal women and five men who ate walnuts also found beneficial results in the ratio of LDL to HDL cholesterol, despite the total cholesterol level remaining the same. In this study, while walnuts were consumed, the subjects' LDL level decreased by more than 30 percent, while the HDL level remained reasonably constant.

Arginine is an essential amino acid present in walnuts. This amino acid is converted into nitric oxide, a chemical that allows the blood vessels to relax, remain smooth, and prevent platelet aggregation. This effect on cholesterol and blood vessels may be the hidden mechanism of the walnut's cardiovascular protective properties.

Walnuts are also rich in antioxidants, in particular ellagic acid. Ellagic acid can impede the metabolic pathways that can usher the way to cancer and heart disease. It does so by protecting healthy cells from free-radical damage, helping to detoxify potential cancer-causing substances, and preventing cancer cells from multiplying.

HOW TO SELECT AND STORE

When shopping for walnuts, one can purchase them shelled or unshelled, purchased in bulk or prepackaged. Unshelled walnuts should feel heavy for their size, not appear rubbery or shriveled. Shelled walnuts should not be cracked, pierced, or stained, for you to be sure they are not mouldy. When purchasing foods from the bulk section, it is key to note that the bins are covered and that your shop has sufficient product turnover to ensure maximum freshness.

It is recommended not to shell walnuts until you are ready to use them. For storing, keep shelled walnuts tightly sealed and refrigerated or store in your freezer for up to one year. Unshelled walnuts will remain fresh for several months when stored in a cool, dry place. However, it is preferable to store them in the refrigerator. It is also important to take special care when storing walnuts with other foods, as they sometimes absorb odors from other foods, such as citrus and fish.

Walnuts are extremely perishable. You will know if walnuts have spoiled by taking a whiff of the nuts; if you smell an odor like paint, the walnuts have turned rancid or have oxidized.

TIPS FOR PREPARING

Walnuts are a delicious addition to savory dishes such as grains, stuffing, salads, and stir-fries. Shelled walnuts can be used straight out of the package. Chopped walnuts are used especially in baking foods such as brownies and cookies, where they are added at the last stage of mixing.

QUICK SERVING IDEAS

- Walnut banana muffins or walnut carrot bread.
- Curried chicken walnut salad: Combine shredded chicken with rapeseed mayonnaise, currants, Major Grey chutney, minced celery, and walnuts. Add curry powder and mix.
- Orecchiette pasta with mushrooms and artichokes: While the pasta is cooking, heat oil in a large skillet. Sauté garlic and peppers in oil for 2 minutes. Stir in mushrooms and cook until tender. Add artichoke hearts and parsley, cook until heated through. Season with salt and pepper. Spoon vegetable mixture over drained pasta and toss. Spoon onto plates and sprinkle with cheese and walnuts.
- Tofu and vegetable hoisin stir-fry with walnuts: Sauté or stir-fry tofu and vegetables. Remove from the heat, add hoisin sauce, and top with chopped walnuts.
- Homemade walnut granola: Mix together approximately ½ cup of honey, 3 to 4 tablespoons of blackstrap molasses, 1 tablespoon of vanilla essence, a dash of salt, and 1 teaspoon each of your favorite spices, such as cinnamon, ginger, and/or nutmeg. Place 6 to 8 cups of rolled oats in a large bowl and toss to coat with the honey–blackstrap molasses mixture. Then spread on a baking tray and bake at 275 degrees F./140 degrees C./gas 1 for 45 minutes. Cool and mix in ½ to 1 cup of chopped walnuts.

SAFETY

See page 408.

Walnuts contain moderate amounts of oxalate. Individuals with a history of oxalate-containing kidney stones should avoid over-consuming them. For more information, see Appendix D, page 793.

The Healing Power of Herbs and Spices

Technically, an herb is a plant that does not have a woody stem. If a plant has a woody stem, it is referred to as a shrub, bush, or tree. The term "herb" is also used to describe a plant or plant part that is used for medicinal purposes. A spice, on the other hand, is technically a plant product that has aromatic properties and is used to season or flavor foods.

Most spices are derived from bark, for example, cinnamon; fruit, for example, red and black pepper; seed, for example, nutmeg; or other parts of herbs, trees, and shrubs. Herbs used in cooking are typically composed of leaves and stems. This makes for an easy way to distinguish herbs from spices. But can herbs be spices and can spices be herbs? Yes. Many herbs are used to flavor foods, thus meeting the definition of a spice, and most spices can be used for medicinal purposes, thus meeting the second definition of an herb.

Absent from this chapter is a discussion of salt (sodium chloride), which we consider a seasoning as it is not an herb or spice. For information on sodium and salt alternatives, see page 738.

Plants as Medicines

Before we discuss the use of herbs and spices in foods, let's first look at their use as medicines. Specifically, let us answer the following question: Are herbs effective medicinal agents, or is their use merely a reflection of folklore, outdated theories, and myth? To the uninformed, herbs are generally thought of as ineffective medicines used prior to the advent of more effective synthetic drugs. To others, herbs are simply sources of compounds to isolate and then market as drugs. But to some, herbs and crude plant extracts are effective medicines to be respected and appreciated.

For many people in the world, herbal medicines are the only therapeutic agents available. It is difficult to assess the extent to which plants are used as medicines throughout the world, but the World Health Organization has estimated that perhaps 80 percent of the world's population relies on traditional therapies for their primary health care needs. Since botanical medicine is the major part of traditional therapies, it can be safely stated that the majority of the world's population relies on plants as medicines.

Unfortunately, most people in the United States and many in the U.K. still know very little of the tremendous value of plants as medicine. However, throughout the world, especially in Europe and Asia, a tremendous renaissance has occurred in the use and appreciation of herbal medicine. Nonetheless, herbal teas and products are a major business in the United States as well, with an estimated annual sales figure of more than $4 billion. In the U.K., while the traditional cup of tea is declining in popularity, sales of herbal teas rose by 50 percent between 2002 and 2004.

This rebirth of herbal medicine, especially in developed countries, is largely based on renewed interest by the public and scientific researchers. During the last twenty to thirty years, there has been an explosion of scientific information concerning plants, crude plant extracts, and various substances from plants as medicinal agents. This research has led to increased marketing and consumption of herbal remedies.

Plants play a major role in modern pharmaceuticals. Many modern drugs were initially derived from plants, and screening for medicinal plant compounds is still an important aspect of research. Generally, the practice was to find compounds that could be used as the base from which to develop a patentable medication.

However, research into the use of herbs as opposed to semisynthetic medications continues to grow.

Cooking with Herbs and Spices

Have you ever heard the expression "Add a little spice to your life"? This little message signifies the belief that herbs and spices add pleasurable taste to foods. It is amazing what herbs and spices can do. For example, potatoes taste fairly bland on their own, but add a little tarragon, dill, or ground red pepper, and you have a whole new experience.

When using herbs, it is far better, for both their health benefits and the flavor they add to foods, to utilize them in their fresh form. To prepare most fresh herbs for use, first remove the stems, then put the leaves in a measuring cup and, with your kitchen shears, mince them to the desired size. Since dried herbs are more concentrated than fresh, you will need to use more of the fresh. If using a recipe that calls for dried herb, simply multiply the amount required by four.

For example, to season enough vegetables for four servings, start with 1 teaspoon of minced fresh or ¼ teaspoon of crushed dried herb. Taste and then add a little more if needed.

If dried herbs and spices are all that's available to you, or if they're your preference, it is worth the time and effort to explore local spice stores or ethnic markets in your area. Often, these stores offer an expansive selection of dried herbs and spices of superior quality and freshness compared to those offered in regular markets. And be sure to choose organically grown whenever possible, since organically grown herbs and spices are much less likely to have been irradiated.

Matching Vegetables and Starches with Herbs and Spices

Some combinations of foods and seasonings are more appealing than others. Here are some pairings that can be used as starting points.

ASPARAGUS
Chives
Lemon balm
Pepper, black
Sage
Tarragon
Thyme

AUBERGINE
Basil
Cinnamon
Dill
Garlic
Marjoram
Mint
Mustard seed
Onions
Oregano
Parsley
Pepper, black
Sage
Thyme

BEANS, RICE, AND OTHER GRAINS
Cumin
Garlic
Horseradish

Mint
Mustard seed
Onions
Oregano
Parsley
Pepper, black
Saffron
Sage
Thyme
Turmeric

BROCCOLI
Basil
Dill
Garlic
Oregano
Pepper, black
Tarragon
Thyme
Turmeric

CABBAGE
Basil
Cayenne (red) pepper
Cumin
Dill
Marjoram
Mustard seed
Pepper, black
Sage

CARROTS
Anise
Basil
Chives
Cinnamon
Cloves
Cumin

Dill

Ginger

Marjoram

Mint

Mustard seed

Nutmeg

Parsley

Pepper, black

Sage

Tarragon

Thyme

Turmeric

CORN

Chives

Pepper, black

Saffron

Sage

Thyme

PEAS

Chives

Pepper, black

Rosemary

Tarragon

Thyme

Turmeric

POTATOES

Basil

Cayenne (red) pepper

Chives

Coriander

Dill

Horseradish

Mustard seed

Oregano

Parsley

Pepper, black

Rosemary

Sage

Tarragon

Thyme

Turmeric

PUMPKIN AND WINTER SQUASH

Basil

Cardamom

Cinnamon

Cloves

Ginger

Marjoram

Nutmeg

Pepper, black

Rosemary

Sage

Turmeric

SPINACH

Anise

Basil

Chives

Cinnamon

Dill

Mustard seed

Pepper, black

Rosemary

Thyme

Turmeric

TOMATOES

Basil

Chives

Coriander

Dill

Garlic

Marjoram
Oregano
Parsley
Pepper, black
Rosemary
Sage
Tarragon
Thyme
Turmeric

Common Culinary Herbs and Spices

There are literally thousands of herbs and spices in use around the world. The following are some of the ones most commonly used.

Anise (Aniseed)

Anise (*Pimpinella anisum*) is a member of the Umbelliferae family along with celery, fennel, dill, and carrots as well as coriander, cumin, and caraway. Although these other spice relatives have a licorice flavor to some extent, anise provides the stronger, true taste of licorice. The oils are distilled from the seeds to impart a strong licorice flavor to sweets, cough syrups, alcoholic beverages, breath mints, etc. The small brown seeds are slightly curved and have a small strand on one end.

HISTORY

Anise is a native of Egypt, the eastern Mediterranean region, and western Asia, but is now grown primarily in Spain and southern Germany. There is written evidence that anise was used in Egypt as early as 1500 B.C.E., making it one of the oldest known spice plants used for both culinary and medicinal purposes. The Romans used anise to aid digestion.

Anise was clearly a valuable item at one time. The Bible, in the book of Matthew, makes mention of anise as being a way to tithe, indicating that it was used as common currency. In 1305, anise was listed by King Edward I as a taxable drug, and merchants bringing it into London paid a toll to help raise money to maintain and repair London Bridge.

HEALTH BENEFITS

Anise provides similar benefits to those of fennel (see page 197) in that it is a rich source of cancer-preventing coumarin compounds, which are the primary components in anise's relatively high concentration of volatile oils. Anise is mildly oestrogenic but much weaker than fennel. Together, the compounds in anise exert a broad range of health benefits, but primarily they help expel wind (carminative effect), relax intestinal spasms (antispasmodic effect), and relieve coughs (antitussive effect). Reportedly, a few seeds taken with water will often cure hiccups.

HOW TO SELECT AND STORE

Anise seed is available dry as whole or ground seed. Whole is preferred, as many of the volatile oils are quickly lost when the seed is ground.

TIPS FOR USE

Anise is used primarily to give its licorice flavor to cakes, biscuits, and ice cream. The seeds can also be used in meat and poultry dishes, breads, pastries, and fruit salads. Ground anise can be sprinkled on seafood appetizers.

QUICK SERVING IDEAS

- Use in small amounts to flavor meat or poultry: ½ teaspoon of anise is generally enough to flavor a dish for four people. Anise can be used whole or ground.
- Rub ground anise under the skin of a chicken before roasting to give the meat a spicy, sophisticated flavor.
- Add 1 teaspoon of ground anise to spiced cake or bread recipes for another level of flavor.
- Ground anise is a unique addition to fruit salads made of primarily berries.

SAFETY

No significant safety concerns are associated with dietary levels of consumption of anise. Please note that anise seed and star anise *(Illicium verum)* are not the same and star anise should not be fed to infants.

Basil

The most common variety of basil is sweet basil *(Ocimum basilicum)*. While the taste of sweet basil is bright and pungent, there are other varieties that differ from this well-known taste, such as lemon basil, anise basil, and cinnamon basil, which all have names indicative of their respective flavor variations. Altogether, there are more than sixty different varieties of basil.

Basil is a bushy annual plant with green leafy stems. Left alone, it can achieve a height of 2 feet/60 centimeters; however, it is rarely allowed to reach this height, for savvy gardeners know that frequent pruning makes the plant bushier, thereby producing more leaves. The basil plant has round leaves that are often pointed. They are green in color, although some varieties feature hints of red or purple. In general, basil looks a little like peppermint, which is not surprising since they belong to the same plant family.

Well known for its unique taste and fragrance, basil is a welcome addition to many foods. One of the best-known uses of basil is as one of the key ingredients of pesto, a mixture of basil, pine nuts, and Parmesan cheese that is one of the famous dishes of Genoa, Italy. In addition to its use as an aromatic herb, the aromatic oil of sweet basil is used in cordials, cosmetics, perfumes, and soaps.

HISTORY

Native to India, Africa, and Asia, basil is now cultivated extensively throughout much of the world after being spread by traders and explorers. In China, the medicinal use of basil can be traced back more than 3,000 years. It is featured prominently in a number of the world's cuisines, including Italian, Thai, Vietnamese, and Laotian.

The name "basil" is derived from the Greek word *basilikon,* meaning "royal," a word indicative of the ancient culture's high respect for this herb. In addition to its regal heritage in Greece, basil has been revered in other cultures. Basil was utilized as a botanical for embalming bodies in ancient Egypt. And in India, it was a cherished sign of hospitality and is still a sacred herb to the Hindus. In Italy, it was considered a symbol of love and it is still. Basil is also referred to as Saint Joseph's wort to pay honor to Joseph, the husband of the mother of Jesus.

HEALTH BENEFITS

Basil has many of the same medicinal effects as other members of the mint family. Specifically, its uses mirror those of peppermint and spearmint, including use as a digestive aid, as a mild sedative, and for the treatment of headaches. The herb is still used in China for spasms of the intestinal tract, kidney ailments, and poor circulation. The volatile oil of basil relaxes the smooth muscle of the intestines and dilates small blood vessels. The volatile oil of a variety of sweet basil has been shown to possess antibacterial as well as anthelmintic (antiworm) activities, which would make it effective in treating intestinal ailments.

Research studies on basil have shown it to contain orientin and vicenin, two water-soluble flavonoids that protect cell structures as well as chromosomes from radiation and free-radical damage. As such, basil provides important anticancer benefits.

HOW TO SELECT AND STORE

Basil can often be found fresh in supermarkets. This is the easiest way to purchase and use basil, as it is much more aromatic when fresh. Look for crisp, vibrant green leaves with no signs of decay. Basil can also be easily grown in pots and can be kept inside for one year, pruned regularly to prevent flowering.

Fresh basil should be lightly rinsed and stored in the refrigerator wrapped in a slightly damp paper towel for up to one week. It may also be frozen, either whole or chopped, in airtight containers. Fresh basil can be also chopped or blended with olive oil and stored in the refrigerator or freezer. Frozen basil is good for three months.

Dried basil can be used if fresh basil is not available. Just as with other dried herbs, when purchasing dried basil, choose organically grown basil if possible, since organically grown herbs are much less likely to have been irradiated. Store dried basil in a tightly sealed glass container in a cool, dark, dry place for maximum shelf life (about six months).

TIPS FOR USE

Basil adds a "clovelike" taste to foods. It can be used alone, although it mixes well with other herbs and spices, such as garlic, thyme, and oregano. However, since the oils in basil are highly volatile, it is best to add the herb near the end of the cooking process, so as to retain its maximum essence and flavor.

Perhaps the best-known use of basil is as an ingredient in pesto. Most pestos contain a lot of Parmesan cheese, which translates into extra saturated fat and sodium. When making your own pesto, go heavy on the basil and garlic and light on the Parmesan. Basil is also a popular ingredient in tomato sauce.

QUICK SERVING IDEAS

- Combine 1 cup fresh chopped basil with 2 to 3 cloves garlic and 2 to 3 tablespoons of olive oil to make a dairy-free version of pesto that can top a variety of dishes, including pasta, salmon, and whole-wheat (wholemeal) bruschetta. Although traditional pestos use chopped *pignoli,* the less expensive walnuts will also suffice.
- To create a refreshing Mediterranean-style iced granita dessert, combine 1 cup chopped fresh basil with ¼ cup lemon juice, 2 to 3

teaspoons xylitol, and 1 cup water, and freeze in ice cube trays. Once frozen, gently blend in a food processor.

- Layer fresh basil leaves over tomato slices and mozzarella cheese to create a traditional, colorful, and delicious Caprese salad.
- Adding basil to stir-fries, especially those that include aubergine, cabbage, chili peppers, tofu, coconut milk, and cashew nuts, will give them a Thai flair.
- Purée 2 tablespoons of basil, 1 tablespoon of olive oil, and ¼ cup onions in a food processor or blender and add to tomato soup.
- Basil can be used to make a spicy tea by infusing ¼ cup chopped basil leaves in 2 cups hot water for 8 minutes, covered.

SAFETY

Basil contains small amounts of oxalate. Individuals with a history of oxalate-containing kidney stones should avoid overconsuming this food. For more information, see Appendix D, page 793.

Cardamom

True cardamom *(Elettaria cardamomum)* is a perennial plant with simple erect stems (or canes) that can reach a height of 10 to 12 feet/3 to 3½ meters. The small, green fruit contains up to eighteen seeds. The seeds are polygonal with flat sides and are used whole or ground as a spice. Cardamom tastes like an airy, gentle ginger with a touch of pine. Cardamom is used prominently in curry powder. It is also used in desserts, especially pastries, and as a fragrance in soaps, detergents, lotions, and perfumes.

HISTORY

Cardamom is native to southern India, Ceylon, and Malaysia, where it still grows wild. Cardamom has been used as a medicine in India and China since records have been kept, making it one of the world's most ancient spices. The ancient Egyptians chewed cardamom seeds as a tooth cleaner; the Greeks and Romans used it as a perfume; it was featured regularly in the "Arabian Nights" for its aphrodisiac qualities; and the ancient Indians regarded it as a cure for obesity. It has been used as a digestive since ancient times. Viking explorers visiting what is now Turkey about 1,000 years ago brought it back to Scandinavia, where it still remains a popular spice.

Cardamom is second only to saffron in terms of price per kilogram. As a result, it is often adulterated or is substituted by inferior cardamom-related plants, such as Siam cardamom, Nepal cardamom, winged Java cardamom, and bastard cardamom. However, only *Elettaria cardamomum* is the true cardamom. Indian cardamom comes in two main varieties: Malabar cardamom and Mysore cardamom. The Mysore variety contains higher levels of cineol and limonene, making it very aromatic.

HEALTH BENEFITS

Its prime uses are similar to those of cinnamon and ginger—as a carminative, digestant, and stimulant. It is also a valuable flavoring agent for herbal medicinal preparations for indigestion and flatulence.

HOW TO SELECT AND STORE

Cardamom can be purchased in the fruits or pods or as whole or ground seeds. It is best to buy them whole and grind them yourself to preserve the volatile oils. The pods are cooked whole and set aside, not to be eaten.

TIPS FOR USE

Although rarely used alone, cardamom enhances the flavor of pumpkins and other squash, sweet potatoes, pastries, and many other foods. Cardamom is often combined with cumin and coriander seed.

QUICK SERVING IDEAS

- When poaching chicken or fish, add a pinch of cardamom to the poaching liquid.
- Add 1 teaspoon ground cardamom to black beans for an interesting side dish, or use them in burritos or nachos to give them a uniquely delicious taste.
- Give a cup of coffee or tea a lift of aromatic flavor by adding ⅛ teaspoon cardamom powder per cup before brewing or steeping.
- Cardamom powder adds depth to pastries and can be mixed into fillings or glazes.
- Cardamom powder can be used to flavor mashed or roasted, diced sweet potatoes.
- A medicinal (perhaps aphrodisiac) cordial can be made by stirring ¼ teaspoon cardamom powder into 1 cup of hot water.

SAFETY

No significant safety concerns are associated with dietary levels of consumption of cardamom.

Cayenne (Red) Pepper and Paprika

Cayenne or red pepper *(Capsicum frutescens)* is the fruit of *Capsicum annuum longum,* a shrubby tropical plant that can grow to a height of up to 3 feet/1 meter. The fruit is technically a berry and is usually ½ to 1 inch/1 to 2 centimeters in diameter and ½ to four inches/1 to 12 centimeters in length. Although cayenne is typically red, other varieties of *Capsicum annuum* can vary in color from purple to orange and yellow. The common name "cayenne" was given to this pepper because of its cultivation in a town that bears its name in French Guiana, on the northeastern coast of South America.

Cayenne and most other *Capsicum* varieties are typically moderately to very spicy. However, paprika is a milder, sweeter-tasting fruit produced by a different variety of *Capsicum annuum.*

HISTORY

Although cayenne pepper is native to Central and South America, it is now cultivated in tropical locations throughout the world and has found its way into the cuisines unique to many warm climates, particularly those of Southeast Asia, China, southern Italy, and Mexico.

It is not surprising that cayenne peppers, as well as other chili peppers, can trace their 7,000-year history to Central and South America, regions whose cuisines are renowned for their hot and spicy flavors. In these regions, cayenne peppers were used first as a decorative item and subsequently as a foodstuff and medicine. The folk remedy uses of cayenne pepper are quite extensive. It was used for asthma, fevers, sore throats and other respiratory tract infections, digestive disturbances, poultices, and cancers. From a nutritional standpoint, cayenne peppers are packed with nutrients, particularly vitamin C and carotene.

During the fifteenth and sixteenth centuries, cayenne and other chili peppers made their global debut. Christopher Columbus encountered these spicy plants while exploring the Caribbean Islands. He brought them back to Europe, where they served as a substitute for black pepper, which, since it had to be imported from Asia at the time, was very expensive. Ferdinand Magellan spread the popularity of cayenne peppers into Africa and Asia during his visits there. For a variety of reasons, the people of these continents quickly incorporated cayenne pepper not only into their culinary life but also into their medicine. While cayenne and chili peppers are actively cultivated on all continents, Spain, China, Turkey, Nigeria, and Mexico are among the largest commercial producers, while the less spicy variety paprika is cultivated extensively in eastern European countries.

HEALTH BENEFITS

The intense heat produced by cayenne pepper is produced by its high concentration of capsaicin. This compound is well recognized in clinical research as an effective pain reliever; as a digestive and antiulcer aid; and for its cardiovascular benefits. In addition, one of the reasons why tropical cultures quickly fell in love with the incredible fruit of this plant is that capsaicin has the ability to lower body temperature, helping to deal with the intense tropical heat. Capsaicin is also the component responsible for cayenne pepper's ability to increase basal metabolic rate and stimulate the burning of fat for energy.

Capsaicin is responsible for the irritating effect of red pepper when it is applied to the skin or ingested via its ability to cause the release of substance P (the "P" stands for "pain") from nerve cells, which in turn results in irritation and pain. However, once substance P is released, capsaicin works to block its reuptake. The net result is that repeated applications of capsaicin deplete substance P from small nerve fibers, thereby eventually blocking the pain sensation. A similar occurrence happens with the ingestion of cayenne pepper in that the more frequently it is consumed, the greater the tolerance.

Capsaicin-containing creams and gels are available as FDA-approved topical treatments for arthritis and pain such as that seen in diabetic neuropathy. They are also licensed for use in the U.K. for the treatment of osteoarthritis. Clinical studies demonstrate that capsaicin products applied topically can produce impressive results in cases of psoriasis, rheumatoid arthritis, and postherpes pain (postherpetic neuralgia). Topical capsaicin preparations have been shown to be an effective treatment for cluster headaches and osteoarthritis pain.

Cayenne pepper exerts beneficial effects internally as well. Perhaps most important are its effects of stimulating and enhancing digestion. A recent *New England Journal of Medicine* study found that daily doses of red pepper significantly reduced symptoms of indigestion in individuals with frequent indigestion (functional dyspepsia). In this placebo-controlled trial, thirty men and women with frequent indigestion were randomly assigned to receive either 2.5 grams of red pepper powder three times a day before meals or a placebo for five weeks. (Individuals who had been diagnosed with gastroesophageal reflux disease [GERD] or irritable bowel syndrome were excluded from the study.) Each day during the trial, the study participants scored and recorded the severity of their symptoms, such as stomach pain, stomach fullness, nausea, and changes in appetite. At the end of the trial, those who had been given red pepper powder were found to have much lower symptom scores (which means they had fewer or less severe symptoms) than those who received the placebo. In the group receiving red pepper, nausea, stomach pain, stomach fullness, and overall symptom scores were 38 percent, 50 percent, 46 percent, and 48 percent lower, respectively, than the scores recorded by the placebo group.

Although people with active peptic ulcer may be bothered by "spicy" foods containing cayenne pepper, spicy foods do not cause ulcers in normal individuals. Furthermore, there is some evidence that supports the idea that spicy foods containing cayenne and turmeric may actually help heal peptic ulcers. Specifically, double-blind studies have shown that red pepper consumption protects against aspirin-induced stomach damage and improves abdominal pain, fullness, and nausea scores in people with nonulcer dyspepsia. Nonetheless, some people definitely seem to be bothered by cayenne pepper ingestion, as it may lower the threshold for heartburn in these people.

Cayenne pepper also exerts a number of beneficial effects on the cardiovascular system. Specifically, it reduces the likelihood of developing atherosclerosis by reducing blood cholesterol and triglyceride levels and platelet aggregation, as well as increasing fibrinolytic activity. Fibrinolytic activity refers to the ability to prevent the formation of blood clots, which can lead to a heart attack, stroke, or pulmonary embolism. People in cultures consuming large amounts of cayenne pepper have much lower rates of these diseases.

Interestingly enough, capsaicin, although hot to the taste, has actually been shown to lower body temperature by stimulating the cooling center of the hypothalamus in the brain. The ingestion of cayenne peppers by cultures native to the tropics appears to offer a way for people living in those areas to get relief from high temperatures.

Finally, several studies have shown that increasing the intake of cayenne pepper may be an effective method of increasing the basal metabolic rate and the burning of fat for energy (lipid oxidation). In the most recent study, after ingesting a standardized dinner on the previous evening, the subjects ate one of the following for breakfast: a high-fat meal, a high-fat meal with red pepper (10 grams), a high-carbohydrate meal, or a high-carbohydrate meal with red pepper (10 grams). The burning of fat for energy was significantly enhanced by the addition of red pepper to either meal, but especially the high-fat meal. Similar results have been noted with garlic and ginger in animal studies. The bottom line from this study and others is that adding red pepper (as well as garlic and ginger) to your diet is a safe, natural way to enhance the burning of fat.

Capsaicin also has a stimulating effect on the mucus membranes of the nose and sinuses. Capsaicin stimulates blood flow through the membranes and causes mucus secretions to become thinner and more liquid. This action makes it beneficial in combating the common cold or sinus infections.

HOW TO SELECT AND STORE

Cayenne peppers are available as whole fresh, whole dried, crushed dried, or ground. Paprika is available dried and ground. Select according to the recipe in which they will be used. If you choose to grind your own, be careful not to inhale any dust that may form, which can be irritating to the lungs.

As with other dried spices, choose organically grown dried cayenne pepper whenever possible, since organically grown herbs are much less likely to have been irradiated.

Cayenne peppers and paprika should be kept in a tightly sealed glass jar, away from direct sunlight, where they will keep for up to one year.

TIPS FOR USE

Cayenne pepper definitely adds a lot of personality to a dish. It is used frequently in Cajun, Creole, Spanish, Mexican, Szechuan, Thai, and East Indian recipes. The heat actually comes from the pith, the membrane on which the seeds grow. The oils from the pith seep down over the seeds, causing them to become hot as well. To decrease the heat of fresh peppers, you can cut them lengthwise and slice out the pith and seeds.

Although chili powder may resemble cayenne pepper, it is actually a combination of several spices, usually cayenne, cumin, turmeric, ginger, and oregano.

Super Chili Powder

2 tablespoons paprika
½ teaspoon ground cayenne
1 tablespoon turmeric
½ teaspoon oregano
⅛ teaspoon cumin

⅛ teaspoon coriander
1 clove garlic, pressed
¼-inch/½-cm slice of ginger, finely minced

Mix all ingredients together. Store in a cool, dry, dark place.

QUICK SERVING IDEAS

- In many cultures that traditionally use cayenne pepper, people keep a container of cayenne pepper or paprika on the table to be added as desired to virtually any food for spicy or sweet pepper flavor.
- To give hot cocoa a Mexican flair, add a dash of cayenne pepper.
- Adding a dash of cayenne pepper spices up the relatively bland taste of canned pinto beans.
- Cayenne pepper and lemon juice make great complements to cooked bitter greens such as collards, kale, and mustard greens. Add cayenne to taste to 2 tablespoons of lemon juice and mix into 3 cups of cooked greens.

SAFETY

After handling cayenne pepper, be careful not to touch your eyes or an open wound, as capsaicin can cause an unpleasant burning sensation. No other safety concerns are associated with cayenne pepper at the usual dietary intake levels.

Chives: See Chapter 10, Onions.

Cinnamon

Cinnamon comes from the inner bark of evergreen trees native to Sri Lanka, southwest India, and Asia. After it is peeled away from the tree, this brown bark curls up into tubes, called "quills," as it dries. In addition to its use as a spice, cinnamon or its oil is used as a flavoring agent in pharmaceutical, personal health, and cosmetic products. Cinnamon is also often used in incense. Cinnamon is available either as cinnamon sticks (in its whole quill form) or as ground-up powder.

Cinnamomum verum, *Cinnamomum zeylanicum* (Ceylon cinnamon), and *Cinnamomum aromaticum* (Chinese cinnamon) are the most popular of the more than 200 varieties of cinnamon. Many consider Ceylon cinnamon to be "true cinnamon," while the Chinese variety is known as "cassia." While both are relatively similar in characteristics, featuring an aromatic, sweet, and warming nature, the flavor of the Ceylon variety is more refined and subtle. In North America, cassia is more popular, probably due to its cheaper price, whereas Ceylon cinnamon is less commonly found and used. In the U.K., Ceylon cinnamon is commonly used along with a blend of Ceylon and cassia.

HISTORY

Cinnamon is one of the oldest spices known. It was used in ancient Egypt not only as a beverage flavoring and medicinal herb, but also as an embalming agent. At one point in ancient history, cinnamon was so highly treasured that it was even considered more precious than gold. Cinnamon also received much attention in ancient China, which is reflected in its mention in one of the earliest books on Chinese botanical medicine, a reference that dates to around 2700 B.C.E. Cinnamon is also mentioned in the Bible, and reportedly, the Roman emperor Nero, in the

first century C.E., burned a year's supply of cinnamon on his wife's funeral pyre as an extravagant gesture meant to signify the depth of his loss.

As the popularity of cinnamon continued to flourish, it became one of the most utilized spices in Medieval Europe. During the Middle Ages, most meals were prepared in a single cauldron; casseroles containing both meat and fruit were common, and cinnamon helped bridge the flavors. Mince pie is a traditional food from this period that still survives today. Due to its great demand during the late Middle Ages, cinnamon became one of the first commodities traded regularly between Europe and the Near East. The demand for cinnamon was enough to launch a number of explorers' enterprises, especially explorations by the Dutch and Portuguese.

In modern times, cassia is mainly produced in China, Vietnam, and Indonesia, while Ceylon cinnamon is produced in Sri Lanka, India, Madagascar, Brazil, and the Caribbean.

HEALTH BENEFITS

Cinnamon has a long history of use in both Eastern and Western cultures as a medicine. Some of its reported uses are in cases of arthritis, asthma, cancer, diarrhea, fever, heart problems, insomnia, menstrual problems, peptic ulcers, psoriasis, and spastic muscles. There are scientific studies to support some of these uses. Some of the confirmed effects of cinnamon are as a sedative for smooth muscle, circulatory stimulant, carminative, digestant, anticonvulsant, diaphoretic, diuretic, antibiotic, and antiulcerative. One recent investigation of sixty people with type 2 diabetes demonstrated that 1 to 6 grams of cinnamon taken daily for forty days reduced fasting blood glucose by 18 to 29 percent, triglycerides by 23 to 30 percent, LDL (bad) cholesterol by 7 to 27 percent, and total cholesterol by 12 to 26 percent. In contrast, there were no clear changes for the subjects who did not take the cinnamon.

Cinnamon's unique healing abilities come from three basic components in the essential oils found in its bark. These oils contain active components called cinnamaldehyde, cinnamyl acetate, and cinnamyl alcohol, plus a wide range of other volatile substances.

Cinnamon is often used in multicomponent Chinese herbal formulas, some of which have been studied for clinical effects. For example, cinnamon combined with Chinese thorough-wax *(Bupleurum falcatum)* and Chinese peony *(Paeonia lactiflora)* was shown to produce satisfactory results in the treatment of epilepsy. Out of 433 patients treated (most of whom were unresponsive to anticonvulsant drugs), 115 were cured and another 79 improved greatly. Improvements were noted not only by clinical symptoms, but also by improvements in brain wave patterns. Other clinical studies have shown cinnamon-containing formulas to be useful in cases of the common cold, influenza, and frostbite. However, it is not really known to what degree the improvements noted are actually due to the cinnamon versus the other components.

HOW TO SELECT AND STORE

Cinnamon is available in either stick or powder form, though most recipes call for the ground powder. You can grind cinnamon sticks into powder on your own at home if you have a spice grinder; otherwise it is quite difficult. Just as with other dried spices, choose organically grown cinnamon when possible, since organically grown spices are much less likely to have been irradiated. Remember, if you want a sweeter, more refined taste, choose the Ceylon variety.

Ground cinnamon as well as sticks should be kept in a tightly sealed glass container in a cool, dark, and dry place. Ground cinnamon will keep for about six months, while cinnamon sticks may stay fresh for as long as one year. The best judge of freshness is your nose.

TIPS FOR USE

Cinnamon is vital to Indian, Moroccan, Indonesian, Middle Eastern, Greek, Chinese, and other cuisines. It is an extremely versatile spice that complements a wide variety of foods and other spices. Cinnamon works well with poultry, in curries, and with fruit, particularly apples and pears.

QUICK SERVING IDEAS

- Here is a great tea to have when you feel a cold coming on. You will need one 1-inch/2½-centimeter slice of fresh ginger, ¼ teaspoon cinnamon, ¼ lemon, and 1 cup hot water. If you own a juice extractor, juice the ginger and lemon and add them, plus the cinnamon, to a cup of hot water. If not, grind the ginger and squeeze the juice from the lemon. Add them, plus the cinnamon, to the cup of hot water.
- Simmer a cinnamon stick with 1 cup soy milk and honey for a delicious warm beverage.

- Enjoy cinnamon toast with a healthy twist: Drizzle linseed oil over whole-wheat (wholemeal) toast and then sprinkle with cinnamon and cane juice.
- When poaching chicken or fish, add 2 cinnamon sticks to the poaching liquid.
- Adding ½ teaspoon ground cinnamon to black beans to be used in burritos or nachos will give them a uniquely delicious taste.
- Sauté small chunks of lamb with 1 tablespoon olive oil, ½ cup cubed aubergine, 2 tablespoons raisins, and 2 cinnamon sticks for a Middle Eastern flavor.
- Add ground cinnamon when preparing curries.

SAFETY

Cinnamon contains moderate amounts of oxalate. Individuals with a history of oxalate-containing kidney stones should avoid overconsuming this food. For more information, see Appendix D, page 793.

Cloves

The clove *(Eugenia aromatica)* is the unopened flower bud of the clove tree. These buds are handpicked when they are pink and then dried until they turn deep brown in color. At approximately ½ inch/12 millimeters long and ⅛ inch/3 millimeters in diameter, and with their tapered stems, they look like small nails. Fittingly, their English name comes from the Latin word *clavus,* meaning "nail."

The flesh of the clove features an oily compound that is essential to their medicinal, nutritional, and gustatory profile. This oil is well protected by a hard outside. Cloves have a warm, sweet, and aromatic taste that evokes the sultry tropical climates where they are grown. Cloves possess a distinctive warm and sweet flavor that is often used to spice up a variety of dishes, especially in the cuisines of Russia, Scandinavia, Greece, India, and China.

HISTORY

Cloves are native to the Moluccas, which is an Indonesian group of volcanic islands formerly known as the Spice Islands. Cloves have been consumed in Asia for more than 2,000 years. Back in 200 B.C.E., Chinese courtiers concerned with offending the emperor would use the clove as a natural breath "mint" in order to freshen their breath. Although in the fourth century Arab traders brought cloves to Europe, this spice did not come into widespread use until the Middle Ages, when it became sought after for its pungent flavor, which served to mask the taste of poorly preserved foods.

Once cultivated almost exclusively in Indonesia, today the leading clove-producing region is Zanzibar in eastern Africa. Additionally, cloves are grown commercially in the West Indies, Brazil, the island of Pemba, Sri Lanka, Madagascar, and India.

HEALTH BENEFITS

Cloves contain significant amounts of an active component called eugenol, which has made them the subject of numerous health studies, including studies showing benefit for the prevention of toxicity from environmental pollutants, such as carbon tetrachloride; prevention of digestive tract cancers; and treatment of joint inflammation.

In the United States, eugenol extracts from

clove have often been used in dentistry in conjunction with root canal therapy, temporary fillings, and general gum pain, since eugenol and other components of cloves, including beta-caryophyllene, combine to make clove a mild anesthetic as well as an antibacterial agent. For these beneficial effects, you'll also find clove oil in some over-the-counter sore throat sprays and mouthwashes.

HOW TO SELECT AND STORE

In the case of cloves, it is best to buy whole cloves instead of clove powder. Since the key components of clove are so volatile, clove powder quickly loses its flavor. To judge the quality of cloves, use your nose. Good-quality cloves will release some of their oil when gently scraped. When buying ground cloves, buy them in small glass containers. Store both whole and ground cloves in a tightly sealed glass container in a cool, dark, dry place. Ground cloves may keep for up to three months, while whole cloves may stay fresh for about a year. In addition to judging by your nose, if you are uncertain as to the freshness of stored cloves, before using place them in a cup of water. Those of good quality will float vertically, while those that are stale will either sink or float horizontally.

As with other dried spices, choose organically grown cloves when possible, since organically grown spices are much less likely to have been irradiated.

TIPS FOR USE

Since cloves have a very intense flavor, especially those that have been ground, care should be taken when deciding how much to use in a recipe so as to not overpower the flavors of the other ingredients.

The easiest way to grind whole cloves into a powder is to use a coffee grinder.

QUICK SERVING IDEAS

- Cloves and apples go very well together. To give a warm, spicy note to apple cider, add ⅛ teaspoon ground cloves and 1 teaspoon ground cinnamon.
- Clove powder livens up coffee; simply add a pinch of clove powder to ground coffee before brewing.
- Add ⅛ teaspoon ground cloves to any stir-fry for a little change of pace.
- Pierce an onion with 5 or 6 whole cloves and add to soups, stocks, or liquids used to poach.
- Clove powder, walnuts, and raisins are flavorful additions to your favorite stuffing recipe.

SAFETY

No significant safety concerns are associated with dietary levels of consumption of cloves.

Coriander (Cilantro)

Coriander *(Coriandrum sativum)* is a bright green annual with slender, erect, hollow stems. Coriander is considered both an herb and a spice, since both its leaves and its seeds are used as a seasoning condiment. Fresh coriander leaves are known in the U.S.A. as cilantro, and they bear a strong likeness to the Italian flat-leaf parsley, both belonging to the Umbelliferae family.

The fruit of the coriander plant contains two seeds. When ripe, these seeds are yellowish brown in color with longitudinal ridges. When these seeds are dried, they are an excellent spice, sporting a fragrant flavor reminiscent of both citrus peel and sage. Coriander seeds are typically available in the whole or ground powder form.

The name coriander comes from the Greek word *koris,* meaning "bug." It is likely named for the offensive buglike smell coriander has when it is unripe.

HISTORY

Coriander is one of the world's ancient spices, as the first known use of coriander was at least 7,000 years ago. Native to the Mediterranean, southern Europe, and the Middle East, coriander was cultivated in ancient Egypt, Greece, and the Roman Empire not only as a spice but also to preserve meats. Coriander was also heavily used as a medicine for thousands of years in these countries as well as in India and China. Like cardamom, cinnamon, and ginger, coriander seeds were used primarily as a carminative, digestant, and stimulant.

Today, the Russian Federation, India, Morocco, and Holland are the main producers of coriander seeds.

Coriander leaves (cilantro) are utilized primarily in traditional dishes of Latin America, India, and China.

HEALTH BENEFITS

Coriander seeds have a health-supporting reputation that is high on the list of the healing spices. The essential oils in the seed make it an effective carminative and digestive aid. In parts of Europe, coriander has traditionally been referred to as an antidiabetic plant. In parts of India, it has traditionally been used for its anti-inflammatory properties. Modern scientific investigations of coriander have focused on its antimicrobial properties, antianxiety action, and cholesterol-lowering effects. These preliminary studies in animals appear to confirm many of its historical uses. For example, its cholesterol-lowering action is the result of coriander stimulating the conversion of cholesterol to bile acids within the liver, an effect that would likely improve digestion of fat.

HOW TO SELECT AND STORE

Fresh coriander (cilantro) should be deep green in color and look vibrantly fresh. The leaves should be free from yellow or brown spots and crisp. Store fresh coriander in the refrigerator wrapped in a damp cloth or paper towel, or keep it in a perforated plastic bag. If the roots are still attached, you can place the roots in a glass of water and cover the leaves with a loosely fitting plastic bag. Whole cilantro will last up to one week, while coriander leaves will last about three days.

Coriander leaves can be frozen, either whole or chopped, in airtight containers. Thaw them just before use to maintain a crisp texture.

Dried coriander seeds are available whole or ground, but whole is preferable. If the recipe calls for ground coriander, simply grind the whole seeds yourself. Coriander leaves and roots, if they can be found, can also be used to make ground coriander. Coriander seeds can be easily ground with a mortar and pestle. You may wish to first soak them in cold water for ten minutes and then drain them, as this process will revive their fragrant aroma.

Just as with other dried spices, choose organically grown dried coriander when possible, since organically grown spices are much less likely to have been irradiated.

Coriander seeds and coriander powder should be kept in a tightly sealed glass container in a cool, dark, dry place. Ground coriander will keep for about four to six months, while the whole seeds will stay fresh for about one year.

TIPS FOR USE

To clean fresh coriander, wash the leaves thoroughly under cool running water. If not organically grown, we recommend soaking the coriander in a mild solution of additive-free soap or use a vegetable wash (see page 51), rinse thoroughly and dry with paper towels or a salad spinner.

Coriander seeds and fresh coriander are used extensively in the cuisines of Asia, China, Latin America, and Spain. The flavor of coriander seed and leaves combines nicely with beetroot, onions, potatoes, and lentils. Fresh coriander is often used to top dishes or is mixed fresh into dishes made from grains, legumes, or meats.

QUICK SERVING IDEAS

- Coriander leaves can be used in place of basil to make coriander pesto.
- Coriander chutney can be made by combining 1 bunch chopped coriander with ½ cup shredded coconut, 2 tablespoons fresh chopped mint, and ½ to 1 diced jalapeño pepper.
- Use coriander seeds in a pepper mill and keep on the dinner table as an alternative to black pepper.
- Add ¼ teaspoon ground coriander and

½ teaspoon cinnamon to decaffeinated black tea for a delicious beverage.
- Lightly sauté 1 bunch fresh spinach, 1 to 2 cloves fresh garlic, and 1 to 2 teaspoons coriander seeds, mix in 1 cup cooked chickpeas, and season with ¼ teaspoon ginger and ½ teaspoon cumin.
- Adding ground coriander to pancake and waffle mixes will give them a Middle Eastern flair.

SAFETY

No significant safety concerns are associated with dietary levels of consumption of coriander.

Cumin

The small cumin seed (*Cuminum cyminum*) possesses a powerful flavor described as being penetrating and peppery with slight citrus overtones. Cumin's unique flavor complexity has made it an integral spice in the cuisines of Mexico, India, and the Middle East.

Cumin seeds are oblong, longitudinally ridged, and yellow-brown in color, and resemble caraway seeds. This similarity is reasonable, since cumin and caraway, like their parsley and dill cousins, belong to the Umbelliferae plant family.

HISTORY

Native to Egypt, cumin has also been cultivated for thousands of years in the Middle East, India, China, and Mediterranean countries, where it has played an important role as a food and medicine and has been a cultural symbol with varied attributes. The Bible includes cumin as a dual treasure, for it is mentioned both as a seasoning for soup and as a legal tender to pay mandatory tithes to the local priest. In ancient Egypt, cumin was also an ingredient used to mummify pharaohs.

Ancient Greek and Roman kitchens highly honored cumin seeds as a culinary seasoning. The rise of cumin's reputation was partially as a result of it being a useful alternative to the more expensive and rare black pepper spice.

During the Middle Ages in Europe, cumin was one of the most common spices used and became recognized as a reminder of love and devotion. Cumin was thought to possess enough power to stop livestock, and possibly a spouse, from wandering away. As a result, guests carried cumin in their pockets when attending wedding ceremonies. When sent off to war, the wives of married soldiers baked cumin bread to be taken by their beloved. Arabic traditions also celebrate a mixture made of ground cumin, pepper, and honey, which was believed to possess aphrodisiac properties.

While maintaining an important role in Indian and Middle Eastern cuisines, the popularity of cumin in Europe declined after the Middle Ages. In recent times, cumin and a number of other culinary herbs have become popular for many diverse uses and cuisines.

HEALTH BENEFITS

Cumin seeds have traditionally been noted to be of benefit to the digestive system, and scientific research is beginning to bear out cumin's age-old reputation. Research in animals has indicated that cumin may stimulate the secretion of pancreatic enzymes, important factors in proper digestion and nutrient assimilation. As with other carminative spices, cumin's digestive

stimulating effects are due to its content of volatile oils.

Cumin seeds may also have anticancer properties. In one study, cumin was shown to protect laboratory animals from developing stomach or liver tumors. This cancer-protective effect may be due to cumin's potent free-radical scavenging abilities, as well as the ability it has shown to enhance the liver's detoxification enzymes.

HOW TO SELECT AND STORE

As with other dried spices, choose organically grown dried cumin whenever possible, since organically grown herbs are much less likely to have been irradiated. Cumin is available both in its whole seed form and ground into a powder. Whenever possible, buy whole cumin seeds instead of cumin powder, since the latter loses its flavor more quickly and the seeds can be easily ground with a mortar and pestle.

Cumin seeds and cumin powder should be kept in a tightly sealed glass containers in a cool, dark, and dry place. Ground cumin will keep for about six months, while the whole seeds will stay fresh for about a year.

TIPS FOR USE

To bring out the fragrance and flavor of cumin, it should be lightly roasted. One method is to roast whole cumin seeds on a tray in an oven at 300 degrees F./150 degrees C./gas 2 for a few minutes or in a skillet on low heat until their aroma gains strength. As the taste of cumin is a great complement to the hearty flavor of legumes, such as lentils, chickpeas, and black beans, add this spice when preparing any recipes with these foods.

QUICK SERVING IDEAS

- Make a cup of warming and soothing cumin tea by lightly boiling 2 teaspoons of seeds in 2 cups water, covered, and then allowing them to steep for 8 to 10 minutes.
- Take 2 cups cooked plain brown rice and give it some zest by adding 2 teaspoons of cumin seeds, ½ cup diced dried apricots, 1 cup almonds, 2 tablespoons olive oil, and ½ teaspoon salt.
- Take 1 cup of vegetables, and season with ½ teaspoon cumin to give them a bit of cumin flair.
- The mixture of equal portions of cumin, black pepper, and honey is considered to be an aphrodisiac in some Middle Eastern countries and is an excellent flavorful addition to vegetable, chicken, and fish dishes.
- For a quick black bean soup, in a quart/1 litre saucepan sauté 1 tablespoon olive oil, 1 cup chopped onions, 1 cup sliced carrots, ½ cup chopped red bell pepper, ¼ cup lime juice, and 1 tablespoon cumin; add a 12-ounce/350-gram can of black beans and 2 cups water and bring to a boil, then simmer for 3 minutes. Garnish each serving with a slice of lime floating in the middle and a sprinkling of finely chopped fresh coriander.

SAFETY

No significant safety concerns are associated with dietary levels of consumption of cumin.

Dill

Dill *(Anethum graveolens)* is a member of the Umbelliferae family, along with carrot, celery, fennel, and parsley. Its name comes from the antique Norse word *dilla,* meaning "to lull." Appropriately, dill was traditionally used to calm the stomach and intestines, and to help sleeplessness. Dill's green leaves are wispy and fernlike and have a soft, sweet taste; both its leaves and seeds are utilized to flavor food. Dried dill seeds are light brown, winged, and oval, with one flat side with two ridges and the other side a convex ridge. Dill seeds are comparable in taste to caraway, with an essence that is aromatic, sweet, and citruslike but also slightly bitter. The leaves and stalks are aromatic and are used fresh or for pickling.

HISTORY

Dill is native to southern Russia, western Africa, and the Mediterranean region, where it has long been popular for its culinary and medicinal properties. Dill was mentioned in both ancient Egyptian writings and the Bible. The ancient Greeks and Romans considered dill a sign of wealth, as it was highly regarded for its many healing properties, and many Greek and Roman soldiers placed burned dill seeds on their wounds to promote healing.

During medieval times, Europe could not grow dill fast enough for love potions, casting spells, and protection against witchcraft. Carrying a bag of dried dill over the heart was considered protection against hexes. In addition, the emperor Charlemagne even made dill available on his banquet tables, so guests who overindulged could benefit from its carminative properties.

Today, dill is a noted herb in the cuisines of Scandinavia, central Europe, North Africa, and the Russian Federation. It is cultivated primarily in Europe and in the United States.

HEALTH BENEFITS

Dill's prime health benefit, similar to that of other aromatic herbs, is as a carminative in the elimination of flatulence and digestive disturbance. Like other aromatic herbs, dill has shown some anticancer and antimicrobial effects. The two major classes of active compounds in dill are the monoterpenes in the volatile oil, including carvone, limonene, and anethofuran, and unique flavonoids. Dill is especially useful in promoting detoxification reactions in the liver to help the liver rid the body of toxic chemicals. Specifically, the monoterpene components of dill have been shown to activate the liver enzyme glutathione-S-transferase. This enzyme helps attach the antioxidant molecule glutathione to toxic molecules that would otherwise do damage in the body. This action makes dill a "chemoprotective" food that can help neutralize particular types of carcinogens, such as the benzopyrenes that are part of cigarette smoke, charcoal grill smoke, and the smoke produced by household waste incinerators.

The flavonoids are thought to assist the volatile components in their carminative and sedative properties.

HOW TO SELECT AND STORE

Fresh dill leaves and seeds are preferred to dried. Dill is also quite easy to grow. The leaves of fresh dill should look feathery and green in color, but dill leaves that are a little wilted are still acceptable, since they usually droop very quickly after being picked.

Fresh dill should always be stored in the refrigerator, either wrapped in a damp paper towel or with its stems placed in a container of water. Since it is very fragile, even if stored properly, dill will stay fresh for only about two days. It can be frozen, either whole or chopped, in airtight containers. Alternatively, you can freeze dill leaves in ice cube trays covered with water or stock that can be added when preparing soups or stews.

Just as with other dried herbs, choose organically grown dill seeds when possible, since organically grown herbs are much less likely to have been irradiated. Dried dill seeds should be stored in a tightly sealed glass container in a cool, dry, dark place, where they will remain fresh for about six months. Dried dill seeds can be used whole or can be ground in a coffee grinder.

TIPS FOR USE

Dill is a familiar flavor thanks largely to the popularity of dill pickles. A versatile herb, dill combines well with fruits and vegetables, as well as fish and poultry. The seeds are slightly stronger than the leaf. Dill, in either its fresh or dried form, should be added toward the end of cooking, since heat can destroy its delicate flavor.

QUICK SERVING IDEAS

- Here is a recipe for a multipurpose dill sauce: Combine 3 tablespoons olive or rapeseed oil, 2 sprigs dill, 1 teaspoon dill seeds, 1 sprig parsley, 1 clove garlic, and the juice and rind of 1 lemon in a blender and blend. This sauce is especially delicious served over potatoes and steamed vegetables.
- Combine ¼ cup chopped dill weed with 1 cup plain yogurt and 1 cup chopped cucumber for a delicious cooling dip.

- Use two to three sprigs dill per piece of fish when cooking, especially salmon and trout, as the flavors complement one another very well.
- Dill seeds were traditionally used as a carminative to soothe the stomach after meals. In order to take advantage of this function, place some seeds in a small dish and place it on the dinner table for all your guests to enjoy.
- Add 2 teaspoons chopped dill to each cup of your favorite egg salad recipe.
- Mix together 2 cups diced potatoes, 1 cup green beans, and 1 cup plain yogurt, then season with 2 teaspoons dill seeds and 1 tablespoon chopped dill weed.

SAFETY

Dill contains small amounts of oxalate. Individuals with a history of oxalate-containing kidney stones should avoid overconsuming this food. For more information, see Appendix D, page 793.

Garlic: See Chapter 10.

Ginger

Ginger is an erect perennial herb that has thick tuberous rhizomes (underground stems and roots). Ginger's botanical name, *Zingiber officinale,* is likely derived from its Sanskrit name, *singabera,* meaning "horn-shaped."

The rhizome is branched with small "arms," usually 2 inches/5 centimeters in circumference. A piece of the rhizome is often called a "hand." It has a pale yellow interior and a skin varying in color from brown to off-white. Jamaican ginger, which is pale buff, is regarded as the best variety. African and Indian ginger is darker-skinned and generally inferior, with the exception of Kenya ginger, and its flesh can be yellow, white, or red in color, depending upon the variety. The brown skin may be thick or thin, depending upon whether the plant was harvested when it was mature or young, respectively. Ginger rhizome has a firm yet striated texture and boasts a taste that is fragrant, pungent, and hot. Interestingly, according to Chinese tradition, dried ginger tends to be hotter energetically than its fresh counterpart.

Ginger is available in various forms:

- *Whole fresh roots.* These provide the freshest taste. The roots are collected and shipped when they are still immature; the outer skin is a light green color.
- *Dried roots.* These are sold either "black" with the root skin left on, or "white" with the skin peeled off. The dried root is available whole or sliced.
- *Powdered ginger.* This is the buff-colored ground spice made from dried root.
- *Preserved or "stem" ginger.* This is made from fresh young roots, peeled and sliced, then cooked in a heavy sugar syrup. The ginger pieces and syrup are canned together. They are soft and pulpy but extremely hot and spicy.
- *Crystallized ginger.* This is also cooked in sugar syrup, then air-dried and rolled in sugar.
- *Pickled ginger.* The root is sliced paper thin and pickled in a vinegar solution. This pickle, known in Japan as

gari, often accompanies sushi to refresh the palate between courses.

HISTORY

Ginger is native to southeastern Asia, India, and China, where it has been a very liberal component of the diet. Ginger is found in ancient Chinese, Indian, and Middle Eastern literature and has long been valued for its aromatic, culinary, and medicinal properties. Ginger has also been important in Chinese medicine for many centuries and is mentioned in the writings of Confucius. The Romans first imported ginger from China almost 2,000 years ago. From that time its popularity in Europe remained focused in the Mediterranean region until the ninth century. Because ginger had to be imported from Asia, it remained a relatively expensive spice. Nevertheless, it was still in great demand. As a result, Spanish explorers introduced ginger to the West Indies, Mexico, and South America in an effort to increase its availability. By the sixteenth century, these areas began exporting the precious herb back to Europe. Subsequently it became so popular in Europe that it was included in every table setting, like salt and pepper. A common article of medieval and Renaissance trade, it was one of the spices used against the plague. In English pubs and taverns in the nineteenth century, bartenders put out small containers of ground ginger for people to sprinkle into their beer—the origin of ginger ale.

In recent times, the top commercial producers of ginger include Jamaica, India, Fiji, Indonesia, and Australia.

HEALTH BENEFITS

Historically, ginger has a long tradition of being very effective in alleviating symptoms of gastrointestinal distress. In herbal medicine, ginger is regarded as an excellent carminative, a substance that promotes the elimination of intestinal wind, and intestinal spasmolytic, a substance that relaxes and soothes the intestinal tract. These properties can be attributed to its volatile component. Modern scientific research has revealed that ginger possesses numerous therapeutic properties, including carminative and intestinal spasmolytic effects, antioxidant effects, an ability to inhibit the formation of inflammatory compounds, and direct anti-inflammatory effects. A combination of ginger, cardamom, cinnamon, and coriander is carminative and stimulating to the digestion.

An indication of ginger's action in eliminating gastrointestinal distress is offered by recent clinical studies with ginger in preventing the symptoms of motion sickness, especially seasickness. In one early study ginger was shown to be far superior to Dramamine, a commonly used over-the-counter and prescription drug for motion sickness. In the study, eighteen male and eighteen female volunteers who had previously indicated an extreme susceptibility to motion sickness were randomly divided into three groups. The first group received a placebo, the second 100 milligrams of dimenhydrinate (Dramamine), and the third 940 milligrams of powdered ginger root 25 minutes before testing. The subjects were then blindfolded, led to a concealed mechanical rotating chair, spun around, and asked to report their feelings of nausea every 15 seconds while they performed mental tasks. The test was stopped when the subject either vomited or asked that it be stopped. Subjects who received ginger remained in the chair an average of 5½ minutes, compared with an average of 3½ minutes for the dimenhydrinate group and 1½ minutes for the placebo group. Once nausea began, however, the sensations of nausea and vomiting progressed at the same rate in all groups.

Gingerroot appears to be equally effective for automobile, airplane, train, or boat trips. It reduces all symptoms associated with motion sickness, including dizziness, nausea, vomiting, and cold sweating. However, unlike dimenhydrinate, which works on the central nervous system, ginger affects the gastrointestinal tract and slows the feedback interaction between the stomach and the nausea center in the brain by absorbing and neutralizing gastrointestinal hormones, toxins, and acids.

Ginger has also been used to treat the nausea and vomiting associated with pregnancy, including hyperemesis gravidarum, the most severe form of pregnancy-related nausea and vomiting. This condition usually requires hospitalization. In a double-blind trial, gingerroot powder at a dose of 250 milligrams four times a day brought about a significant reduction in both the severity of the nausea and the number of attacks of vomiting in nineteen of twenty-seven cases of hyperemesis gravidum during early pregnancy (less than twenty weeks).

Ginger also contains very potent anti-inflammatory compounds called gingerols. These substances are believed to explain why so many people with osteoarthritis or rheumatoid arthritis experience reductions in their pain levels and improvements in their mobility when they consume ginger regularly. Gingerols inhibit the formation of inflammatory cytokines, chemical messengers of the immune system.

To test the ability of ginger to reduce inflammation, a preliminary clinical study was conducted on seven patients with rheumatoid arthritis in whom conventional drugs had provided only temporary or partial relief. One patient took 50 grams per day of lightly cooked ginger, while the remaining six took either 5 grams of fresh ginger or 0.1 to 1 gram of powdered ginger daily. All patients reported substantial improvement, including pain relief, increased joint mobility, and decreased swelling and morning stiffness.

In the follow-up to this study, twenty-eight patients with rheumatoid arthritis, eighteen with osteoarthritis, and ten with muscular discomfort who had been taking powdered ginger for periods ranging from three months to two and a half years were evaluated. Based on clinical observations, the researchers reported that 75 percent of the arthritis patients and 100 percent of the patients with muscular discomfort experienced relief in pain or swelling. The recommended dosage was 500 to 1,000 milligrams per day, but many patients took three to four times this amount. Patients taking the higher dosages also reported quicker and greater relief.

Ginger contains high levels of active substances, so dosages do not have to be high in order to produce beneficial effects. Although most scientific studies have used powdered gingerroot, fresh gingerroot at an equivalent dosage is believed to yield even better results because it contains active enzymes. Most studies utilized 1 gram of powdered gingerroot. This would be equivalent to approximately 10 grams or ⅓ ounce of fresh gingerroot, roughly a ¼-inch/½ centimeter slice.

For nausea, ginger tea made by steeping one

to two ½-inch/1-centimeter slices (one ½-inch/1-centimeter slice equals ⅔ ounce/20 grams) of fresh ginger in a cup of hot water will likely be all you need to settle your stomach. For arthritis, some people have found relief consuming as little as a ¼-inch/½-centimeter slice of fresh ginger cooked in food, although in the studies noted above, patients who consumed more ginger reported quicker and better relief.

HOW TO SELECT AND STORE

Fresh ginger can be purchased in the produce section at most supermarkets. Ginger is generally available in two forms, either young or mature. Mature ginger, the more widely available type, has a tough skin that requires peeling, while young ginger, usually available only in Asian markets, need not be peeled. Fresh ginger can be stored in the refrigerator for up to three weeks if it is left unpeeled.

Whenever possible, choose fresh ginger over dried since it is not only superior in flavor but also contains higher levels of gingerol as well as ginger's active protease, its anti-inflammatory compound. The bronze root should be fresh-looking, firm, smooth and free of mould, with no signs of decay such as soft spots, mildew, or a dry, wrinkled skin.

If fresh ginger is not available, dried ginger is widely available. Just as with other dried spices, when purchasing dried ginger powder, try to select organically grown ginger, since organically grown spices are much less likely to have been irradiated.

Ginger is also available in several other forms, including crystallized, candied, and pickled. It can be found in these forms in Asian markets and natural food stores.

Dried ginger powder should be kept in a tightly sealed glass container in a cool, dark, dry place for no more than six months.

TIPS FOR USE

A paring knife is the best utensil to remove the skin from fresh, mature ginger; gently push it off using the tip of a spoon. The ginger can then be sliced, minced, or julienned. It is important to note that the strength and taste that ginger imparts to a dish depend upon its timely addition during the cooking process. If it is added at the beginning, it will create a subtler taste; however, if you add it near the end, it will be much more pungent.

Ginger is an important spice in cooked dishes but can also be used as a fantastic addition to fresh fruit and vegetable juices, especially pineapple, carrot, and apple. Ginger tea can also be made.

QUICK SERVING IDEAS

- Ginger tea is great to drink when you feel a cold coming on. It is a diaphoretic tea, meaning that it will warm you from the inside and promote perspiration. It's also good when you don't have a cold and just want to warm up and feel good! If you have a juice extractor, juice a 1-inch/2½ centimeter slice of ginger and ¼ lemon and add it to 1 cup of hot water; otherwise you will need to chop the ginger up into fine pieces and let it steep in the hot water. For extra flavor, you may want to add ⅛ teaspoon of nutmeg or cardamom.

- Ginger alternative to lemonade: First add ginger tea to ice, then add xylitol, honey, or some other natural sweetener.

- To jazz up rice side dishes: Sprinkle ½ teaspoon each diced ginger, sesame seeds, and nori strips over the rice.
- Combine ½ teaspoon grated ginger, 2 tablespoons rice vinegar, 1 tablespoon tamari, 4 tablespoons raw sesame oil, and 1 mashed clove of garlic to make a wonderful salad dressing.
- Add 1 teaspoon grated ginger and 2 tablespoons maple syrup to 2 cups puréed sweet potatoes.
- For a more pungent stir-fry, add 1 teaspoon grated fresh ginger to each cup of vegetables while cooking.

SAFETY

Ginger contains moderate amounts of oxalate. Individuals with a history of oxalate-containing kidney stones should avoid overconsuming this food. For more information, see Appendix D, page 793.

Horseradish

Horseradish (*Armoracia rusticana* and *Armoracia lapathifolia*) is a large, long, tapered root with thin, light brown skin, white flesh, and spiky green leaves. Horseradish is a member of the cabbage family and is related to mustard and radish, as well as kale, cauliflower, and Brussels sprouts.

Although the leaves can be used in salads, horseradish is valued primarily for its root's pungent bite. This effect, which develops only when the root is broken and wetted, is the result of the reaction that occurs when a number of chemicals that the plant stores separately are allowed to mix. These chemicals—an enzyme,

myrosinase, and a number of isothiocyanate compounds, including two glucosinolates, sinigrin and 2-phenylethylglucosinolate—react and form the mustardlike oils that enable horseradish to provide such robust enhancement of vegetables, fish, and meat.

The horseradish root is harvested in the spring and autumn and sold in 1,200-pound/550-kilogram pallets to processors, who use it to make one of the world's most popular condiments, both singly and as an ingredient in numerous sauces and dressings. Regardless of the product to be made, horseradish is first grated, then mixed with distilled vinegar, which stops the reaction that forms its isothiocyanates, stabilizing the oils and maintaining their hot, peppery edge. Other spices or ingredients may also be added, but horseradish and vinegar are the *sine qua non* of all prepared horseradish.

HISTORY

Horseradish is an ancient herb native to eastern Europe. Prized for its medicinal and gastronomic qualities for centuries, horseradish was used by the Egyptians in 1500 B.C.E. and still serves as one of the five bitter herbs, along with coriander, horehound, lettuce, and nettle, that Jews are enjoined to eat during the Passover Seder.

Also used by the early Greeks, horseradish is thought to be the plant Pliny called *amoracia* and recommended for its medicinal effects rather than as a food or condiment. According to legend, the Delphic Oracle told Apollo, "The radish is worth its weight in lead, the beet its weight in silver, the horseradish its weight in gold." Like mustard, whose pungent oils it shares, horseradish was used medicinally by both the Greeks and Romans, having been added to smelling salts, chewed to ease toothaches, put into rubs for rheumatic joints and low back pain, and used as an expectorant cough medicine and even as an aphrodisiac.

By 1300 C.E., horseradish had spread to Scandinavia and England, where it was used as a cough expectorant and treatment for food poisoning, scurvy, tuberculosis, and colic. Throughout the Middle Ages, both the root and leaves of horseradish continued to be used medicinally. Then, in 1597, Gerard, who called it *Raphanus rusticanus,* noted that among the Germans, horseradish, crushed with a little vinegar, was used as a condiment for fish and meat. By the early 1600s, the Germans' taste for horseradish with meat had spread to France, where, thinly sliced and mixed with vinegar, horseradish was called *moutarde des Allemands* (German mustard).

By 1640, the culinary use of horseradish had arrived in England among country folk and laborers, but by the end of the 1600s, European chefs had discovered the synergistic bond between horseradish and meat or seafood, with the result that horseradish became *the* accompaniment for an Englishman's beef and oysters. The pungent root was even grown at inns and coach stations, where it was used to make "horseradish ale," a mixture of horseradish, wormwood, and tansy that was sure to revive weary travelers.

In the eighteenth century, horseradish was included in the *Materia Medica* of the London *Pharmacopoeia* under its scientific name *R. rusticanus* and listed with a wide variety of uses, including improving digestion and alleviating the pain associated with chronic rheumatism; as an expectorant and antiscorbutic (a source of vitamin C able to prevent scurvy); and, if taken in large amounts, as an emetic (an agent used to induce vomiting). A horseradish poultice applied to the skin was used to ease sciatica, gout, and facial neuralgias, while an infusion of sliced horseradish in milk served as a cosmetic to clarify and bring color to the skin or, combined with vinegar, to remove freckles. Diluted with water and vinegar and sweetened with glycerin, horseradish juice was said to provide relief for children with whooping cough and, eaten frequently throughout the day, was used to get rid of a persistent cough following influenza.

Brought by early settlers to North America, horseradish was cultivated by the colonists and became so common in the Northeast that it was growing wild near Boston by 1840. When immigrants from central Europe started horseradish farms in the Midwest in the mid-1850s, commercial cultivation in America began.

Today in the United States, each year, approximately 24 million pounds/11 million kilograms of horseradish roots are ground and processed into 6 million gallons/23 million litres of prepared horseradish—more than sufficient, according to the Horseradish Information Council, to generously season enough sandwiches to circle the world twelve times.

HEALTH BENEFITS

Horseradish is an underresearched medicinal food, and unfortunately, little research has been done to either support or refute its historical uses. What is known through scientific investigation is that horseradish definitely helps protect against foodborne illness. Recent research shows that horseradish protects against *Listeria,*

E. coli, Staphylococcus aureus, and other food pathogens. The reason is allylisothiocyanate, one of the pungent chemicals formed when horseradish is cut. This powerful antibacterial ingredient constitutes 60 percent of horseradish oil.

Horseradish is also a cholagogue, an agent that stimulates the release of bile from the gallbladder. Horseradish thus helps to maintain a healthy gallbladder and improve digestion. Increasing bile secretion is a part of digesting dietary fats and oils as well as eliminating cholesterol and waste from the body.

Horseradish also contains an enzyme called horseradish peroxidase (HRP). Commonly used as an assay to check for antibodies indicating infections, to test blood levels of glucose and lactate, and to check hormone levels for possible negative effects caused by chemicals in the environment, HRP may serve another, protective role in the future: treating contaminated soils and wastewater containing amines and phenols.

HOW TO SELECT AND STORE

In the U.S. fresh horseradish is available all year round in most supermarkets, but it's more difficult to find in British chains. Its peak seasons are right after harvest, in autumn and spring. The fresh roots, which can be as long as 20 inches/50 centimeters, are usually sold cut into 2-inch/5-centimeter-long sections with diameters of 1 to 2 inches/2½ to 5 centimeters. Choose firm roots with no soft or green spots, other blemishes, or signs of mould. Also avoid old roots; these will be dry and withered and may even have begun to sprout. Wrapped in a plastic bag and stored in the refrigerator vegetable crisper, fresh horseradish will keep for up to one week. Homemade

prepared horseradish should be stored in a lidded glass jar in the refrigerator, where it will keep for up to six weeks.

Commercially prepared, bottled horseradish is available both white, preserved with vinegar and a small amount of salt, and red, to which beet juice is added. Cream-style prepared horseradish and dehydrated horseradish are also commonly available, in addition to which horseradish is frequently enlisted to add its "heat" to cocktail sauce, specialty mustards, and a variety of other sauces, dips, spreads, relishes, and dressings.

All prepared horseradish is available both coarsely and finely ground. Coarsely ground horseradish is usually more pungent since chewing initiates the formation of additional volatile oils.

Look for white to creamy beige horseradish products. A brownish tinge indicates that the product is old and has lost its potent flavor. Once opened, prepared horseradish should be stored in the refrigerator in a tightly closed glass jar, where it will keep for six months, or in the freezer, where it will remain pungent for several months longer.

TIPS FOR USE

When using fresh horseradish in recipes, it is important to know how it translates to prepared horseradish:

- 1 tablespoon of freshly grated horseradish has the potency of 2 tablespoons of prepared horseradish.
- 1 tablespoon dried horseradish + 1 tablespoon vinegar + 1 tablespoon water + salt to taste = 2 tablespoons prepared horseradish.

It's easy to make your own fresh horseradish sauce, but be forewarned: the powerful pungency of freshly made horseradish makes prepared versions pale in comparison. This is because the volatile oils in horseradish that simultaneously bring a tear to the eye and a flame to the tongue deteriorate rapidly once horseradish is cut or grated and exposed to air. Heat causes these volatile oils to evaporate completely, eliminating both the aromatic and taste effects, which is why true horseradish aficionados prefer their horseradish raw and freshly grated.

Always grate or blend fresh horseradish in a well-ventilated room with an open window; the fumes are quite potent and can actually burn your nose and eyes. For the full flavor experience, simply scrub the roots and peel away the thin brown outer skin before grating. The cores of larger roots may be fibrous and bitter—cut out and discard them. When preparing horseradish for immediate use, the more finely the root is chopped or grated, the more pungent its flavor.

If processing in a blender, wash, peel, and dice the horseradish into small cubes first. Fill the blender no more than halfway, add a small amount of cold water, and grate until the desired consistency is reached. Add 2 to 3 tablespoons of white vinegar or lemon juice and ½ teaspoon of salt for each cup of grated horseradish. For a milder horseradish sauce, add the vinegar immediately. Vinegar halts the enzymatic reaction that produces the volatile oils responsible for horseradish's kick and stabilizes the degree of hotness. Remove the blender lid at arm's length and turn your head away to lessen your exposure to the newly formed volatile oils. Transfer the prepared horseradish to small glass jars, seal tightly, and store in the refrigerator.

If desired, mix horseradish with a little beetroot juice for that bright pink color. To lessen the intensity a bit, mix in a little whole plain yogurt, sour cream, or mayonnaise or, for the traditional Austrian accompaniment to meat, a little apple purée. Also, to retain its maximum bite when serving horseradish with cooked food, add it at the end of the cooking process, after the food has been removed from the heat.

Two final notes: Always serve just the desired amount of horseradish, returning the rest to the refrigerator as soon as possible, as unrefrigerated horseradish will lose its flavor. And always serve horseradish in a glass or ceramic bowl; it will tarnish silver.

QUICK SERVING IDEAS

- Traditionally served at the Passover meal with gefilte fish, this beetroot and horseradish sauce is so delicious you'll want to use it all year round. Coat three to four small beetroot, roasted and diced, with a dressing made of ½ cup olive oil and 3 tablespoons of balsamic vinegar. Add 1 teaspoon coarse salt, ½ teaspoon freshly ground black pepper, 1 cup chopped red onion, ¼ cup sour cream or yogurt, and ⅓ cup freshly grated horseradish. Mix well and enjoy!
- Add an Austrian flair to your next meal of roast beef with homemade apple and horseradish sauce. Grate several Newton or Granny Smith apples and combine with an ounce or two of freshly grated horseradish. Moisten with a couple of ounces of cider vinegar and/or white wine.

- Wake up your Thanksgiving dinner or Christmas turkey with this cranberry horseradish sauce. Bring ¾ cup water to a boil and add ½ cup honey and ½ cup brown sugar, stirring until dissolved. Add a 10-ounce/300-gram package of fresh cranberries, return to a boil, and cook for 10 minutes. Cool slightly and stir in 2 tablespoons freshly grated horseradish and 1 tablespoon Dijon mustard.
- For a sweet, tangy sauce that's an excellent accompaniment to fish or prawns, mix 1 tablespoon freshly grated horseradish and 3 tablespoons Dijon mustard into a cup of orange marmalade. Or try a glaze of apricot preserves, horseradish, and mustard.
- A spoonful of fresh horseradish added to any soup stock adds a lot of surprisingly mild but delicious flavor.
- Enliven your salads by adding a tablespoon of prepared horseradish to ½ cup dressing.
- Mix a spoonful of horseradish with ½ cup plain yogurt, ¼ cup butter, and ½ teaspoon prepared mustard. Use to give corn on the cob, cooked carrots, green beans, peas, or new potatoes a major flavor boost.

SAFETY

Due to its effect of increasing bile flow, horseradish should probably not be consumed in large amounts by individuals with gallbladder stones or obstructions. Otherwise, no other safety concerns are associated with horseradish at normal levels of consumption.

Marjoram: See Oregano.

Mint

The mint family is one of the most useful medicinal and culinary herb families. The reason is the valuable oils produced by the hairlike oil glands on the surfaces of the leaves and stems of these plants. One member of the mint family, basil, has already been described. Other members of the mint family include lemon balm, marjoram, oregano, peppermint, rosemary, sage, savory, spearmint, and thyme.

While there are about twenty-five different species of mints, peppermint (*Mentha piperita*) is actually a natural hybrid cross between *Mentha aquatica* (water mint) and *Mentha spicata* (spearmint). Peppermint has greenish purple lance-shaped leaves, while the rounder leaves of spearmint are more of a grayish green color. Peppermint and spearmint are the most commonly cultivated mints. Both are vivacious, perennial plants growing into 2-to-3-foot/60-to-90-centimeter shrubs.

The taste of both peppermint and spearmint can be described as a cross between pepper and menthol, with peppermint being a bit stronger and spearmint being a little more cool, sweet, and subtle. In addition to peppermint and spearmint, other plants in the *Mentha* genus include apple mint, orange mint, water mint, curly mint, and Corsican mint.

HISTORY

Mint is native to the Mediterranean region, with its origins immortalized in a Greek myth that explains the tale of the nymph Minthe, who attracted the attention of Hades. As a result, Hades' wife, the jealous Persephone, attacked Minthe and was in the process of trampling her to death when Hades turned her into the herb (which was ever sacred to him).

Mint is a symbol of hospitality and wisdom; "the very smell of it reanimates the spirit," Pliny tells us. Ancient Hebrews scattered mint on their synagogue floors so that each footstep would raise its fragrance. Ancient Greeks and Romans rubbed tables with mint before their guests arrived. The Romans took mint and mint sauce to Britain. The Pilgrims brought mint to the United States aboard the *Mayflower*. The Japanese have distilled peppermint oil for several centuries, and the oil is further treated to produce menthol.

Mints are now grown and cultivated virtually all over the world.

HEALTH BENEFITS

Mints exert a wide range of health benefits. Like other aromatic plants, their primary application has been as a carminative and digestant. The oil of the peppermint plant is an excellent example. It has been shown to relieve spasms of the gastrointestinal tract and wind. In fact, an enteric-coated peppermint oil capsule has been shown to be very effective in relieving symptoms of irritable bowel syndrome. (Enteric coating prevents the oil from being released in the stomach.) Peppermint oil relaxes smooth muscle. Once the smooth muscles surrounding the intestine are relaxed, there is less chance of spasm and the indigestion that can accompany it. The menthol contained in peppermint may be a key reason for this bowel-comforting effect.

Peppermint contains a compound known as perillyl alcohol that has been shown to inhibit the growth or formation of cancer. It also contains the substance rosmarinic acid, a powerful antioxidant that blocks the production of allergy-producing leukotrienes. The high content of rosmarinic acid may be the reason extracts of peppermint have been shown to help relieve the nasal symptoms of allergic rhinitis (hay fever).

HOW TO SELECT AND STORE

Many mints are now available fresh in supermarkets. Whenever possible, choose fresh mint over the dried form of the herb, since it is superior in flavor. The leaves of fresh mint should look vibrant and be a rich green color. They also should be free from dark spots or yellowing. If fresh mint is not available in your area, mints are also available as dried leaves or extracts.

To store fresh mint leaves, carefully wrap them in a damp paper towel and place them in a loosely closed plastic bag. Store in the refrigerator, where they should stay fresh for several days. Just as with other herbs, when purchasing dried mint, try to select organically grown mints, since organically grown herbs are much less likely to have been irradiated. Dried mints should be kept in a tightly sealed glass container in a cool, dark, dry place, where they will remain fresh for about nine to twelve months.

TIPS FOR USE

Mints—especially the milder varieties, such as lemon balm and spearmint—mix quite well with many different foods when used fresh and chopped. But perhaps the best-known use for mint is for making soothing tea. For this purpose, dried peppermint is most often selected.

QUICK SERVING IDEAS

- Foods that are enhanced by mints include green salads, marinated vegetables, corn, broccoli, asparagus, and legumes.
- Combine 1 cup chopped fresh mint leaves, the juice of 2 limes, and ⅓ cup fructose or sugar. Add this mixture to 2 quarts/1 litre sparkling water to make a nonalcoholic version of a mojito, the popular Cuban drink.
- To make peppermint tea, add ¼ cup dried peppermint to 4 cups hot water and steep covered for 15 minutes. A cup of fresh mint tea can help to soothe your stomach and your nerves.
- Toss 2 cups of cooked aubergine cubes with ½ cup chopped mint leaves, ½ cup plain yogurt, 1 clove garlic, and ⅛ teaspoon cayenne.
- For a quick and easy salad, combine 1 cup sliced fennel, ¼ sliced red onion, the pieces of 1 peeled orange, and ¼ cup chopped fresh mint leaves.
- Any fruit salad will benefit by adding some fresh mint leaves.
- Add chopped mint leaves to gazpacho or another soup that features tomatoes, as the freshness of the mint nicely complements the sweet acidity of tomatoes.

SAFETY

Allergy to mint is quite rare. Conventionally grown mint is frequently sprayed with pesticides, so choose organically grown mint when possible. Peppermint may be contraindicated in those with gastroesophageal reflux due to its ability to relax the oesophageal sphincter, the ring of muscle that closes the stomach off from the oesophagus.

Mustard Seeds

Mustard greens are discussed in Chapter 10, but as a spice, it is the seeds that are used. Mustard plants are cruciferous vegetables related to broccoli, Brussels sprouts, and cabbage. While there are approximately forty different varieties of mustard plants, there are three principal types used for their seeds: black mustard (*Brassica nigra*), white mustard (*Brassica alba*), and brown mustard (*Brassica juncea*). Black mustard seeds have the strongest flavor, while "white" mustard seeds (which actually have a yellowish color), are the mildest and are the ones used to make American yellow mustard. Brown mustard, which is darker yellow in color, has a pungent, acrid taste and is used in Dijon-style mustards. Mustard seeds are usually found as tiny spheres 2 to 3 millimeters across.

HISTORY

The mustard plant is native to different areas of Europe and Asia, each producing different-colored seeds. The white variety hails from the eastern Mediterranean regions, the brown type comes from the foothills of the Himalayas, and the black seeds originate in the Middle East. Mustard seeds appear in Sanskrit writings dating back to about 3000 B.C.E. In the New Testament the Kingdom of Heaven is compared to a grain of mustard seed.

Most likely, today's popular mustard style is derived from the ancient Greeks and Romans, who originally concocted a paste from ground seeds. The physicians of both these great civilizations, including Hippocrates, the father of Western medicine, used mustard seed medicinally.

Today, the mustard seed is still one of the most popular spices traded around the world. Temperate climates are best suited to mustard cultivation, and Hungary, Great Britain, India, Canada, and the United States are among the top producers in the world.

HEALTH BENEFITS

One of the oldest home remedies is the use of a mustard plaster (a type of poultice) to help to decongest the chest and airways. To make a mustard poultice, mix one part of dry mustard with three parts of flour, then add enough water to make a paste. Spread the paste on thin cotton (an old pillowcase works well) or cheesecloth, fold it, and place it on the chest. Check often, as the mustard can cause blisters if left on too long. After the hot pack, perform postural drainage by lying facedown with the top half of the body off the bed, using the forearms as support. The position should be maintained for five to fifteen minutes, while you try to cough and expectorate into a basin or newspaper on the floor.

Like other cabbage-family vegetables, mustard seeds contain plentiful amounts of phytochemicals called glucosinolates and isothiocyanates. These compounds have been repeatedly studied for their anticancer effects (see page 178 for more information).

HOW TO SELECT AND STORE

Mustard seeds can be purchased as dried whole seeds, dried mustard powder, prepared mustard, and mustard oil.

Just as with other spices, try to select organically grown mustard seeds or powder, since organically grown spices are much less likely to have been irradiated. Mustard powder and mustard seeds should be kept in tightly sealed containers in a cool, dark, dry place, where they will keep for six months for the powder and one year for the seeds. Prepared mustard and mustard oil should both be stored in the refrigerator, where they will keep for up to six months.

TIPS FOR USE

Most popularly, mustard seeds and powder are consumed in the form of the prepared mustard condiment. Mustard seeds and mustard powder can also be used a variety of dishes. Mustard seeds can be used as is or roasted in a skillet over medium heat until they pop. Mustard seeds can be easily ground at home with a mortar and pestle or in a coffee grinder.

While dried mustard powder itself does not exhibit a very strong quality, mixing it with water catalyzes an enzymatic process that greatly enhances its pungency and heat. In order to reduce its sharp flavor, an addition of hot water or an acidic substance such as vinegar will stop the enzymatic process.

A typical mustard condiment is also easily made by boiling 1 cup of apple cider vinegar, 2 tablespoons honey, ⅛ teaspoon turmeric, and ½ teaspoon salt. While hot, pour into a blender, add ½ cup yellow mustard seeds, and immediately blend the mixture thoroughly. When the mixture has achieved a smooth consistency, add 1 tablespoon of olive oil, blend again, and serve.

QUICK SERVING IDEAS

- Dredge chicken breast fillet in prepared mustard and whole mustard seeds and bake.
- Make a delicious cold millet salad by combining 2 cups of the cooked, then cooled, grain with some chopped spring onions, one package of baked tofu cubes, garden peas, and mustard seeds to taste. Dress with lemon juice and olive oil.
- Marinate salmon fillets in a combination of Dijon mustard and white wine. You can also use a marinade like this to keep fish fresher if it is not to be used on the same day it is bought.
- Mix prepared mustard with honey and the seasonings of your choice to make a pungent and sweet dipping sauce.
- Add taste and color to brown, black, white, or wild rice by sprinkling some brown, black, and white mustard seeds on top.
- Add 1 teaspoon of mustard oil to each 1 cup serving of stir-fried vegetables for an extra aromatic kick!

SAFETY

Raw mustard seeds do contain goitrogens, naturally occurring substances in some foods that can interfere with the functioning of the thyroid gland. Individuals with already existing and untreated thyroid problems may want to avoid raw mustard seeds for this reason. However, cooking helps to inactivate these goitrogenic compounds. (See "Cabbage" in Chapter 10 for more information.)

Mustard also contains small amounts of oxalate. Individuals with a history of oxalate-containing kidney stones should avoid over-consuming this food. For more information, see Appendix D, page 793.

Nutmeg

Nutmeg *(Myristica fragans)* is the seed of the apricotlike fruit of a tropical evergreen tree native to the Moluccas, the central Spice Islands of Indonesia. The tree, which can reach a height of sixty-five feet/20 meters, has grayish brown smooth bark and produces pale yellow male and female flowers that scent the air with a spicy aroma. The nutmeg tree yields fruit after eight years of growth, reaches its prime in twenty-five years, and continues to bear fruit for another sixty years or more.

Like apricots, plums, and peaches, the nutmeg contains a hard, oval-shaped shiny brown stone about 1¼ inch/3 centimeters in length and ¾ inch/2 centimeters in diameter. It is the kernel of this seed that is dried and sold whole or ground as the spice nutmeg. When fully ripe, the fruit splits in two, revealing a thin lacy purple-to-crimson-colored aril, or membrane, that envelops the nutmeg seed, separating it from the surrounding pulp. This covering is removed by hand, flattened out, dried, and used as the spice mace. The nutmegs are also dried in the sun, being turned twice daily for six to eight weeks, during which time the nutmeg kernels shrink away from the hard outer seed coat until they rattle when the shell is shaken. A wooden truncheon is then used to crack open the thin shell, and the nutmegs, which now are grayish brown ovals with furrowed surfaces, are removed for enjoyment of their warm, aromatic flavor, which has been described as a combination of cinnamon and pepper.

HISTORY

Nutmeg has a long and fabled history. Nutmeg was one of the spices carried by Muslim traders along routes that have existed between Arabia, India, and the Far East since biblical times. It was introduced to the European markets in the eleventh century by Venetian and Genoese merchants who bought the spice from Arab traders in Constantinople. In the thirteenth century, Marco Polo's dazzling account of the spices of the Far East generated interest in establishing an independent spice trade between Europe and Asia—a desire Columbus was attempting to fulfill when he sailed from Spain in 1492 in the hope of discovering an all-water route to the spice-rich lands of the East. By 1512, Portuguese ships had rounded South Africa and sailed to India and beyond, reaching the famed Spice Islands, which they seized. The Portuguese dominated the spice trade for the rest of the sixteenth century.

By this time, nutmeg, already an immensely popular spice, had become an essential luxury for wealthy Europeans, who carried their nutmegs in tiny silver graters, which they pulled out at mealtimes to season their meat and wine. Always costly, nutmeg rocketed in price when physicians in Elizabethan London asserted that their nutmeg pomanders were the only certain cure for the plague. Overnight, the spice, which had been used for little more than its flavor and its ability to ameliorate flatulence and the common cold, became more sought after than gold.

In the early 1600s, the Dutch and the British drove Portugal from Asian waters, ending the Portuguese monopoly of the lucrative nutmeg and clove trade from the tiny, isolated Banda Islands, part of the Spice Islands. Knowing that these spices did not grow elsewhere, the Dutch established one of the tightest monopolies the world has ever known. Nutmegs were even dipped in lime before shipment in the belief that this made them infertile, so they could not be planted elsewhere.

During the whole of the seventeenth century, nutmeg was in high demand in Europe, and the Dutch East India Company (*Vereenigde Oostindische Compagnie*) could dictate prices at will. This situation finally changed in the eighteenth century, when the French smuggled seedling trees out of the Bandas and planted them on the island of Mauritius in the Indian Ocean, breaking the Dutch monopoly. In the late eighteenth century, a series of transplantings occurred, and in 1843, during the brief period when the British controlled the Spice Islands, they introduced the nutmeg to the West Indian nation of Grenada.

Nutmeg is featured on Grenada's flag, and West Indian nutmeg, more than 40 percent of the world's supply of the spice, is produced in this country. East Indian nutmeg is grown in Indonesia, which exports the spice to Europe and Asia, while Grenada supplies West Indian nutmeg primarily to the United States.

HEALTH BENEFITS

Nutmeg, as both a dried spice and an essential oil, has long been used as a carminative (to lessen wind formation and prevent flatulence). An ointment made with nutmeg butter has also been used as a counterirritant and to treat rheumatism.

These historical uses have been substantiated today. Nutmeg has been found to be an effective antidiarrheal agent, reducing the amount of stool, increasing the period between evacuations, and improving intestinal tone while inhibiting the contractions that would normally be stimulated by irritating agents. In addition, nutmeg's demonstrated sedative effects had no harmful effects on blood pressure.

When expressed, nutmeg yields 24 to 30 percent essential oil. The principal component of this oil, called nutmeg butter or oil of mace, is an active compound called myristicin. In animal studies, myristicin has exhibited "extraordinarily potent hepatoprotective [liver-protective] activity," to quote the authors of one study. These researchers think myristicin works its protective magic by preventing the release of a very inflammatory compound called TNF-alpha from one of the immune system's heavy guns, a type of white cell called a macrophage. High levels of TNF-alpha occur in inflammatory diseases such as rheumatoid arthritis, which may explain the benefit of consuming nutmeg in that condition.

Also, within the last several years, a number of studies have revealed that those Elizabethan physicians who asserted that nutmeg could protect against the plague had some foundation for their claim. In various studies, nutmeg oil has exhibited considerable antibacterial activity against 25 different species of bacteria, including animal and plant pathogens, and food poisoning and spoilage bacteria. Test organisms have included *Listeria monocytogenes*, *Bacillus subtilis*, *Escherichia coli*, and *Saccharomyces cerevisiae*. The results of these studies provide scientific support for the traditional use of nutmeg as a food preservative, disinfectant, and antiseptic.

HOW TO SELECT AND STORE

Formerly, nutmeg was almost always purchased in the form of a whole dried berry and freshly ground with a small grater. Today, nutmeg is most commonly purchased already ground—although once it is ground, the volatile oils responsible for its flavor and taste soon evaporate, so we recommend purchasing whole nutmeg and grating just before use. If you enjoy nutmeg, we highly recommend that you purchase a nutmeg grater, so you can easily get the most flavor from fresh whole nutmeg. If you don't have a nutmeg grater, the finest blade on a larger handheld manual grater will do almost as well. Keep whole fresh nutmegs, as well as ground nutmeg and mace, in a tightly sealed jar or airtight container in a cool, dark, and dry place, where they will keep for one year. Wrap leftover fresh nutmeg tightly in plastic wrap, so its oils do not evaporate.

To test nutmeg, insert a darning needle 1 centimeter into the seed. If the nutmeg is good, a tiny drop of oil will seep out.

Essential oils and oleoresins of nutmeg and mace are available as well. Oil extraction is usually done in the United States. The oils contain just the volatile constituents of the spices, while the oleoresins provide both volatile and nonvolatile components.

Mace is sold in whole pieces called *blades* or ground. Blades are preferable when flecks of spice are undesirable, as, like a bay leaf, they can be removed after they have imparted their flavor. When choosing mace, the color often indicates its origin. Orange-yellow blades are most likely from Grenada, while orange-red blades are probably from Indonesia.

TIPS FOR USE

Add freshly grated nutmeg at the end of the cooking process, since heat, which promotes the evaporation of its essential oils, diminishes its flavor. And when preparing fresh nutmeg for a recipe, keep in mind that

- One whole nutmeg equals 2 to 3 teaspoons of ground nutmeg
- One teaspoon ground mace equals 1 tablespoon of mace blades

Nutmeg, which most Americans associate with holiday eggnog, is also an essential ingredient of the classic white sauce béchamel and a mulling spice, and it can be used to enhance the flavor of baked or stewed fruit, curries, custards, milk- and onion-based sauces, pasta, punches, stewed and braised meats, and cooked vegetables—especially spinach, but also potatoes, pumpkins, squash, sweet potatoes, carrots, broccoli, and cauliflower. Mace is more peppery than nutmeg and works well in creamy sauces and soups.

QUICK SERVING IDEAS

- To make your own mulling spice, combine 3 ounces/85 grams of cinnamon sticks, 6 nutmegs, ⅓ cup chopped dried orange and lemon peel, ¼ cup whole cloves, ¼ cup allspice, and 2 tablespoons finely chopped crystallized ginger in a blender. Blend in bursts until broken into small pieces. Transfer to the center of fourteen square pieces of cheesecloth, wrap and tie with string. To mull wine, use one spice bag per 750 milliliter bottle. In a litre pan over medium-low heat, combine ½ cup water and ⅓ cup sugar until the sugar dissolves. Add the wine and spice bag, reduce the heat to low, and simmer about 20 minutes. To mull cider, use 1 spice bag for 8 cups of apple cider. Bring to a boil in a 3-litre pan, reduce the heat, cover, and simmer for 30 to 35 minutes.
- Stuck in a pumpkin pie rut? Next autumn, try this delicious pumpkin casserole. Combine 2 cups cooked pumpkin with 2 finely chopped apples, 2 cups chopped pineapple, ½ cup broken walnuts, 1 teaspoon cinnamon, ¼ teaspoon cloves, and ½ teaspoon nutmeg. Spoon into a covered casserole dish and bake at 350 degrees F./180 degrees C./gas 4 until soft, about 40 minutes.
- Make your own Jamaican jerk sauce: In a food processor or blender combine ½ cup allspice berries, ½ cup packed brown sugar, 6 to 8 garlic cloves, 4 to 6 Scotch bonnet peppers, 1 tablespoon ground thyme, 2 bunches spring onions, 1 teaspoon cinnamon, ½ teaspoon nutmeg, 2 tablespoons soy sauce, and salt and pepper to taste. Blend, transfer to a sealable jar, and refrigerate; it will keep for several months.
- To make béchamel sauce, sauté 1 tablespoon minced onion in 3 tablespoons olive oil; then add ¼ cup flour, 3 cups milk, ¼ teaspoon ground nutmeg, ¼ teaspoon salt, and white pepper to taste. Cook until thickened while stirring regularly to keep the sauce smooth.

SAFETY

Nutmeg contains myristicin, an essential oil that, ingested in large amounts, is a potent hallucinogen with very unpleasant side effects, including severe headache, cramps, extreme nausea, and, for frequent users, liver toxicity. In his autobiography, Malcom X related using nutmeg in a Boston jail for its hallucinogenic effects. The legendary jazz saxophonist Charlie Parker is also reputed to have availed himself of the spice, which he downed with milk or cola. No need to worry, though—the small amount of nutmeg dusted over eggnog or added to a savory stew, elegant vegetable dish, or festive dessert is much too little to produce anything but delightful sensory effects.

However, several cases of nutmeg poisoning, including one report of fatality thought to be the result of a combined toxic effect between an excessive amount of nutmeg and the drug flunitrazepam, have been published. A good guide is not to consume nutmeg in amounts larger than a tablespoon—an amount more than sufficient to flavor eight stew servings.

In the nutmeg trade, broken nutmegs that have been infested by pests are referred to as "BWP grade" (broken, wormy, and punky). Although BWP-grade nutmegs are legally allowed to be used only for distillation of oil of nutmeg and extraction of nutmeg oleoresin, they are occasionally ground and sold illegally. Since moulds can produce aflatoxin (a highly carcinogenic compound) on BWP nuts, it's safest for consumers to purchase whole nutmegs and grind them as needed or buy ground nutmeg from reputable retailers.

Nutmeg contains small amounts of oxalate. Individuals with a history of oxalate-containing kidney stones should avoid overconsuming this food. For more information, see Appendix D, page 793.

Oregano and Marjoram

Oregano and marjoram are closely related species (*Origanum* spp.) of the mint family. Oregano and marjoram are small shrubs with ¼-inch/½-centimeter-wide oval leaves. Their flavor is earthy and aromatic. Their tastes are quite similar, though oregano is a bit stronger and marjoram is sweeter.

Oregano's botanical name is *Origanum vulgare,* and it is called wild marjoram in many parts of Europe since it is closely related to the herb that we know as sweet marjoram. Its name is derived from the Greek words *oros* (mountain) and *ganos* (joy). Not only was oregano a symbol of happiness, but it also beautified the hillsides on which it grew.

HISTORY

Oregano and marjoram are both native to northern Europe. However, the ancient Greeks and Romans both used the herbs not only for cooking but also for their aromatic properties. In both cultures oregano was regarded as a symbol of joy and happiness. Appropriately, it was a tradition in Greek and Roman marriage ceremonies for the bride and groom to be crowned with laurels of oregano.

Oregano became firmly entrenched in both Mediterranean and French cuisine and has been cultivated for both culinary and medicinal effects in the Mediterranean for thousands of years. Today oregano is cultivated throughout Europe and North America and in other regions of the globe.

HEALTH BENEFITS

Oregano and marjoram provide benefits similar to those of other members of the mint family (see "Mint," page 495). The volatile oil of oregano contains thymol and carvacol, two powerful antimicrobial agents. A clinical study in Mexico compared oregano to tinidazole, a commonly used prescription drug to treat infection by the amoeba *Giardia lamblia.* These researchers found oregano to be more effective against *Giardia* than the commonly used prescription drug. Thymol and carvacrol have also been shown to inhibit the growth of bacteria, including *Pseudomonas aeruginosa* and *Staphylococcus aureus,* two bacteria that are often the cause of impetigo (an infection of the skin).

Oregano also has tremendous antioxidant activity. In one analysis conducted by the U.S. Department of Agriculture, oregano scored the highest in antioxidant activity of any herb or food tested, ranking even higher in antioxidant activity than fruits and vegetables known to be high in antioxidants. Oregano had forty-two times as much antioxidant activity as apples, thirty times as much as potatoes, twelve times as much as oranges, and four times as much as blueberries. The active component was rosmarinic acid, which, as its name suggests, is also found in rosemary as well as other mints.

HOW TO SELECT AND STORE

Whenever possible, choose fresh oregano and marjoram over dried, since they are superior in flavor and health benefits. The leaves of fresh oregano and marjoram should be vibrant green in color and free from dark spots or yellowing. Fresh oregano and marjoram should be wrapped in slightly damp paper towels and stored in the refrigerator, where they will keep for up to seven days. They may also be frozen, either whole or chopped, in airtight containers. They will keep for three months in the freezer. Alternatively, you can freeze the oregano in ice cube trays covered with either water or stock that can be added when preparing soups or stews.

If fresh oregano and marjoram are not available, dried can be used. Just as with other herbs, try to buy that which has been organically grown, since organically grown herbs are much less likely to have been irradiated. Dried oregano and marjoram should be kept in tightly sealed glass containers in a cool, dark, dry place, where they will remain fresh for about six months.

TIPS FOR USE

To clean fresh oregano or marjoram, wash the leaves thoroughly under cool running water. If not organically grown, we recommend spraying them with a mild solution of additive-free soap or use a produce wash; rinse thoroughly and dry with paper towels or a salad spinner.

Oregano and marjoram, in either their fresh or dried form, are best added toward the end of the cooking process, since heat can easily destroy their aromatic oils and delicate flavors.

Oregano is best known as an ingredient of tomato sauce and pizza. It has a hot, peppery flavor that is used in the cuisines of Italy, Greece,

Spain, and Mexico. Marjoram is viewed as a milder oregano. Although either herb adds a delicious flavor to a variety of foods, most often oregano or marjoram will be combined with garlic, onion, thyme, and basil, as these herbs have quite complementary flavors.

QUICK SERVING IDEAS

- Fresh oregano is a great garnish for your next slice of pizza.
- Sautéed mushrooms and onions are brought to new life with marjoram and oregano.
- Adding a few sprigs of fresh oregano or marjoram to a container of olive oil will infuse the oil with the essence of the herb.
- Frittatas and omelets are well complemented by fresh oregano and garlic.
- A sprinkling of chopped oregano is always a welcome addition to homemade garlic bread. Minced garlic can be added on top of the bread, or the garlic can be lightly rubbed on for a milder flavoring.
- Add oregano or marjoram to salad dressings.
- Oregano and marjoram work well with thyme, basil, and garlic to make a great tomato sauce: Sauté 1 chopped onion in 4 tablespoons olive oil with salt and pepper as desired. Add 4 cloves chopped garlic, 1 tablespoon kelp powder, 2 14-ounce/400-gram cans diced tomatoes, 1 medium chopped carrot, and 1 medium stalk of chopped celery. Cook for 1 hour at a gentle simmer. Run the sauce through a food blender and return to the pot. Bring to a simmer and add ½ tablespoon dried basil, 1 teaspoon dried oregano, ½ teaspoon dried marjoram, and ½ teaspoon dried thyme; ½ teaspoon rubbed

sage can be added as well. Cover and simmer for an additional 20 minutes, then serve.

SAFETY

No significant safety concerns are associated with dietary levels of consumption of oregano.

Parsley: See chapter 10.

Pepper (Black)

Black pepper *(Piper nigrum)*, along with salt, is the most widely used seasoning agent in the United States, while in the U.K., sales of salt have fallen over recent years making it the fourth most popular condiment behind pepper, which in 2005 had a market value of £31 million, and, most popular of all, dried and fresh herbs and spices. Pepper accounts for one quarter of the world's spice production, about 124,000 tons a year. The pepper plant produces a black fruit (peppercorn) that is usually ground. Black pepper is the most pungent and flavorful of all types of peppers. Other varieties of peppercorns made from the black pepper plant are green and white. White pepper is produced by removing the outer black skin of the peppercorn and tastes more aromatic, with less bite, than black pepper. Green peppercorns are picked while still unripe and green in color, while white peppercorns are those picked when very ripe and subsequently soaked in brine to remove their dark outer shell, leaving just the white pepper seed. Green peppercorns taste aromatic and have a unique "herb" taste that is lacking in black pepper.

HISTORY

Indigenous to India, the black pepper plant has played a central role in global economic and cultural history and has been a prized spice since ancient times. In ancient Greece, pepper was held in such high regard that it was used not only as a seasoning but also as a currency and sacred offering. In classical times tributes were paid in pepper, and both Attila the Hun and Alaric I the Visigoth demanded pepper as a substantial part of Rome's ransom.

The history of the spice trade could be considered the history of pepper, the "king of spices." During the Middle Ages, pepper was at the center of the European spice trade, with Genoa and Venice dominating the market. The Italian pepper monopoly of overland trade routes was the major factor driving the search for an eastern sea route as well as Columbus's desire to find a western route. This desire led not only to the exploration of many undiscovered lands but also to the development of major merchant cities in Europe and the Middle East.

Pepper became cherished because it served key culinary purposes. Its pungency could spice up otherwise bland foods, and, perhaps more important, it could disguise a food's lack of freshness, an especially important quality in the times before efficient means of preservation. This allowed food to be kept longer, thus conferring a significant economic advantage.

Currently, the major producers of pepper are India and Indonesia.

HEALTH BENEFITS

Pepper was also valued for its medicinal applications for treatment of digestive disorders. Black pepper has diaphoretic, carminative, and diuretic properties. It also stimulates the taste buds in a manner that causes an increase in stomach acid secretion, thereby improving digestion. Black pepper has demonstrated impressive antioxidant and antibacterial properties as well, and the outer layer of the peppercorn has been proven to stimulate the breakdown of fat cells.

Many of the benefits of black pepper are due to the compound piperine. Piperine has been shown to:

- Dramatically increase the absorption of certain nutrients, such as selenium, B vitamins, and beta-carotene.
- Support and assist the body's natural thermogenic activities.
- Support and enhance the liver's detoxification processes.

HOW TO SELECT AND STORE

Black pepper is available whole, cracked, or ground into powder. To ensure the best flavor, buy whole peppercorns and grind them yourself in a mill just before adding to a recipe. In addition to their superior flavor, buying whole peppercorns will help to ensure that you are purchasing unadulterated pepper, since ground pepper is often mixed with other spices. Whole peppercorns should be heavy, compact, and free of any blemishes. And, as with other dried spices, try to purchase organically grown black pepper, since organically grown spices are much less likely to have been irradiated.

Black pepper should be kept in a tightly sealed glass container in a cool, dark, and dry place. Whole peppercorns will keep almost indefinitely, while ground pepper will remain fresh for about three months. Pepper can also be frozen, although this will make its flavor more pronounced.

TIPS FOR USE

Pepper is best ground directly onto food. Since the aromatic oils in black pepper lose their flavor and aroma if heated for too long, it is best to add it near the end of the cooking process. For many palates, the familiar taste of pepper is a welcome addition to any dish.

QUICK SERVING IDEAS

- Rather than a pepper shaker, keep a pepper mill on your dining table to take advantage of the greater intensity and flavor of freshly ground black pepper.
- To make classic peppercorn steak, you need only to coat the meat well with crushed peppercorns before cooking.
- Venison's deeper berrylike meat flavor, whether as a steak or in a stew, is also complemented by black pepper.
- A simple but always appetizing salad dressing recipe: Mix ¼ cup olive oil, the freshly squeezed juice of one or two lemons, and cracked pepper to taste.
- Add whole peppercorns to soups to add to their taste and nutritional profiles.
- While it may sound unusual, the classic pairing of black pepper and vanilla is surprisingly delicious. To experience and enjoy this flavor combination, mix ground black pepper into such vanilla-flavored foods as yogurt, ice milk, cakes, or sauces.

SAFETY

Pepper contains low amounts of oxalate. Individuals with a history of oxalate-containing kidney stones should avoid overconsuming this food. For more information, see Appendix D, page 793.

Rosemary

Rosemary *(Rosmarinus officinalis)* is another member of the mint family, although it has a much different appearance in that it is an evergreen shrub that can grow quite large and has an ash-colored scaly bark and short leaves that look like flat pine tree needles with a deep, sage green color on top and a silver-white color on their underside. The purple flowers are very small. The leaves are the portion of the plant that is most commonly used.

The taste and aroma of the herb rosemary, historically used for strengthening the memory, are unforgettable. Rosemary's name means "dew of the sea," and it has a pinelike flavor that is counterbalanced by a rich pungency, a unique combination that evokes both the deep forest and the open sea. Its memorable flavor makes it an essential herb every place food is prepared.

HISTORY

Originally found in Mediterranean regions, rosemary is now cultivated throughout much of the temperate regions of both Europe and America. Rosemary was a revered culinary herb and natural medicine in both ancient Greece and Rome from 500 B.C.E. Rosemary's popularity came in part from the widespread belief that rosemary stimulated and strengthened the memory, an attribute for which it is still traditionally used. In ancient Greece, to stimulate thought and memory, students would place rosemary sprigs in their hair while studying for exams. Mourners would often throw the fragrant herb into the grave of the deceased as a symbol of remembrance. In Britain, rosemary's ability to strengthen the memory transformed it into a symbol of fidelity, and as such, it played an important role in wedding costumes, decorations, and gifts.

Rosemary oil was first extracted in the fourteenth century and subsequently was used to make Queen of Hungary water, a popular cosmetic of the time. In the sixteenth and seventeenth centuries, rosemary became popular as a digestive aid in apothecaries and other places medicines were sold. As modern research learns more about the beneficial active components in rosemary, we learn that the ancients were correct about many of the beliefs about its beneficial effects on human physiology.

HEALTH BENEFITS

Due to its high essential oil content, rosemary has many effects similar to those of other mints. Rosemary, however, is considered more of a stimulant than other mints. In fact, rosemary oil contains several potent antioxidants, so powerful that an extract of rosemary is being investigated for use as a natural alternative to synthetic antioxidants that are often added to foods as preservatives.

One of the chief antioxidants in rosemary is rosmarinic acid. Studies have shown that this compound can act to reduce inflammatory responses by altering the concentrations of inflammatory messenger molecules, such as leukotriene B_4, making rosemary potentially useful for people with inflammatory conditions, such as rheumatoid arthritis, as well as bronchial asthma and atherosclerosis.

Rosemary also contains substances such as flavonoids and volatile oils that are useful for stimulating the immune system, increasing circulation, and improving digestion. Rosemary has been shown to increase the blood flow to the head and brain, thus improving concentration, too.

HOW TO SELECT AND STORE

Whenever possible, choose fresh rosemary over the dried form of the herb, since it is far superior in flavor. The sprigs of fresh rosemary should be deep sage green in color and free of yellow or dark spots. Fresh rosemary should be stored in the refrigerator either in its original packaging or wrapped in a slightly damp paper towel for up to one week. You can also place the rosemary sprigs in ice cube trays covered with either water or stock that can be added when preparing soups or stews. Frozen rosemary will last for three months.

If fresh rosemary is not available, choose dried. As with other herbs, when purchasing dried rosemary, choose organically grown rosemary, since organically grown herbs are much less likely to have been irradiated. Dried rosemary should be kept in a tightly sealed container in a cool, dark, dry place, where it will remain fresh for about six months.

TIPS FOR USE

Quickly rinse fresh rosemary under cool running water and pat it dry. Most recipes call for rosemary leaves, which can be easily removed from the stem. Alternatively, you can add the whole sprig to season soups, stews, and meat dishes, then remove it before serving.

Rosemary imparts a piny, sweet, somewhat pungent flavor to many foods, particularly roasted meats, soups, and vegetables.

QUICK SERVING IDEAS

- Brush 1 pound/½ kilogram new potatoes with 2 tablespoons olive oil, sprinkle 3 tablespoons fresh rosemary leaves on top, and bake at 350 degrees F./180 degrees C./gas 4 until cooked, approximately 30 minutes.
- Add fresh rosemary to omelets and frittatas for a fresh taste.
- Rosemary is a perfect herbal choice to season fish and lamb dishes.
- Simmer 1 cup milk or soy milk with 1 tablespoon fresh rosemary leaves and honey to make a delicious Italian-inspired beverage.
- Add rosemary to tomato sauces and soups.
- Want something to dip fresh bread in? Purée ¼ cup fresh rosemary leaves with olive oil and use as a dipping sauce. Add a pinch of salt and crushed red or black pepper for extra flavor.
- Making homemade croutons? Toss 2 cups cubed whole-wheat (wholemeal) bread with 2 tablespoons olive oil and 3 tablespoons chopped fresh rosemary leaves, then spread on a baking tray and bake at 225 degrees F./110 degrees C./gas ¼ for 30 minutes.

SAFETY

No significant safety concerns are associated with dietary levels of consumption of rosemary.

Saffron

Saffron is the delicate red stigma (the female part of the flower, which catches pollen) of a small purple crocus *(Crocus sativus)* with grasslike leaves and large, purple, lily-shaped flowers. The saffron crocus, a member of the lily family, generally flowers in the autumn. In a good year, each plant can produce several flowers, each of which contains three bright red stigmas joined to a pale yellow style. To produce saffron, the stigmas must be painstakingly handpicked, leaving behind the yellow stamen (the male part of the flower, which has no flavor or aroma), cut from the white style (which also has no culinary value), and then carefully laid on a sieve and cured over heat until dry to deepen the flavor—a process so labor-intensive that saffron is the most expensive spice in the world. Once cured, saffron stigmas look like pieces of very fine red-orange thread. More than 5,000 flowers must be harvested to yield a single ounce/30 grams of the spice. This translates to 80,000 flowers (240,000 stigmas) to produce a single pound/½ kilogram, which is a primary reason why, by the time saffron reaches retail stores, it sells for $600 to $2,000 a pound!

Even though saffron stigmas are red, their effect is pure alchemy—a mere pinch turns the simplest dish into gold. Saffron's sumptuous color, in addition to its exotic, slightly sweet taste and penetrating aromatic scent, makes the spice essential to a number of classic dishes, including the French fish stew bouillabaisse and the rice dishes risotto milanese, paella Valenciana, and arroz con pollo. Saffron is also used extensively in Indian, Middle Eastern, and North African cuisine, not only for its exquisite flavor but for its ability to add brilliant golden color to food. Fortunately, because of saffron's intense flavor and strong coloring power, just a pinch goes a long way—¼ gram is sufficient for most dishes serving six to eight. An ounce (28.35 grams) of high-quality saffron can be purchased for as little as $36 (£20.60) and, if properly stored, will keep well for several years, so the actual cost of enjoying this gorgeous spice can be as low as $0.04 (£0.02) per serving.

HISTORY

Originating in the Fertile Crescent, the land between the Tigris and Euphrates rivers, the saffron crocus, delighted in for both its beauty as a flower and its vibrant aromatic spice, was carried along the routes of conquerors and traders, its tiny bulbs (called corms) planted wherever they would grow. Ancient Middle Eastern cave paintings demonstrate saffron's early use in art, and the golden spice appears as an aphrodisiac and energizing agent in a Chinese book of medicine dating back to 2600 B.C.E.

The Ebers Papyrus, the most important medical treatise of ancient Egypt, which dates back to 1500 B.C.E., speaks of the medicinal properties of saffron—qualities also noted by Hippocrates and Galen, who attributed to the spice the ability to improve digestion and eliminate flatulence, prevent colic, act as a sedative to calm infants during teething and alleviate their insomnia, and act as an antispasmodic and cough suppressant. Furthermore, in Ayurvedic medicine, saffron has been used for thousands of years in herbal formulations, including medicines to treat menstrual disorders, impotence, headaches, urinary and digestive problems, depression, and overall lack of vitality.

Treasured by the ancient Greeks and Romans, who called the spice *krokos* and *karkom,* respectively, saffron appears in the writings of Homer, who has both Zeus and Jupiter lie down on beds of saffron to increase their amorous intentions. In Rome, patrician men and women adopted the recommendation of Dioscorides, the famous Greek physician, who also praised saffron as an aphrodisiac. Reputed to be so powerful it could corrupt vestal virgins, saffron was used to revitalize revelers at the thermal baths.

Saffron's modern name is a gift of the Arabs, who introduced the cultivation of the *Za'faran* (the Arabic word for "yellow") or saffron crocus to medieval Spain, where it became very popular, especially as a dye. In the thirteenth century, the Crusaders returned from the Holy Land laden with saffron, which in France and England was so costly that a pound/½ kilogram could be traded for the finest horse. The ladies of Henry the VIII's court put gold into their hair with saffron, until the king, fearing a shortage of the spice for his table, forbade the custom. Around this time, the saffron crocus was planted so extensively in Essex that the largest town in the area was named Saffron Walden. The extreme value placed upon saffron can also be seen in the fact that in the fifteenth century, German dealers, caught adulterating the precious spice to increase their profits, were burned at the stake.

Today, in the Middle East, saffron threads are blended with sandalwood in an oil-based perfume called *záfran attar,* which is valued for its properties as a relaxant and used as a natural cure for headaches. A coveted gift item in India, saffron is presented on special occasions, such as engagements and weddings, and given to elders and future in-laws as a sign of respect, and is offered as a sacrifice in many temples.

Currently, saffron is commercially produced in Iran, Greece, Morocco, Kashmir, Spain, and Italy. In terms of both volume and quality, Iran is the most important producer of saffron, and Spain is the largest importer of the spice, much of which is then repacked for export. Germany, Italy, the United States, Switzerland, the United Kingdom, and France also import large amounts of saffron.

HEALTH BENEFITS

Historically, saffron has been used as an aphrodisiac, diaphoretic (to cause sweating), carminative (to prevent wind), and emmenagogue (to bring on menstruation). In Japan, saffron is encapsulated and used as a sleep aid and in the treatment of Parkinson's disease. Modern research suggests the spice may provide protection against cancer, memory loss, heart disease, and inflammation.

Saffron contains a dark orange, water-soluble carotene called crocin, which is responsible for much of saffron's golden color. It has potent antioxidant and anticancer effects, which may help explain saffron's historical use in cancer treatment. Crocin has been found to trigger apoptosis (programmed cell death) in a number of different types of human cancer cells, including liver cancer and leukemia. In addition, in studies conducted in China, saffron has demonstrated anticancer activity against a wide spectrum of cancers, including leukemia, ovarian carcinoma, colon adenocarcinoma, rhabdomyosarcoma, papilloma, squamous cell carcinoma, and soft-tissue sarcoma, and has also been used to protect against coronary heart

disease and hepatitis and to promote healthy immunity.

Researchers in Mexico who have been evaluating saffron extract as a potential cancer-preventive agent have discovered that saffron extract and several of its active components display a dose-dependent ability to inhibit human malignant cells. Plus, not only does the spice inhibit cells that have become cancerous, but it has no such effect on normal cells and actually stimulates their formation and that of lymphocytes (immune cells that help destroy cancer cells). One recent animal study may help explain why. In this trial, one group of Swiss albino mice was given a water extract of saffron for five days, while another group of mice served as controls. The mice were then exposed to genotoxins (agents capable of mutating cellular DNA and inducing cancer). In the mice receiving saffron, the spice provided significant protection, greatly reducing the damage done to cellular membranes and other lipid (fat)-rich molecules, while also increasing the liver enzymes and antioxidants (specifically, reduced glutathione) responsible for removing the carcinogens from the body.

Recent studies have also demonstrated that saffron extract, specifically its crocin, promotes learning and memory retention in experimental animals. On the basis of this early research, scientists are hopeful that saffron may be useful as a treatment for age-related mental impairment.

Saffron has also demonstrated protective effects against heart disease. When twenty human subjects—ten healthy individuals and ten with existing cardiovascular disease—were given 50 milligrams (less than ¼ teaspoon) of saffron dissolved in 100 milliliters (3½ ounces) of milk twice daily, the susceptibility of their cholesterol to damage by free radicals decreased by 57 percent in the healthy subjects and by a whopping 64 percent in those with cardiovascular disease.

Saffron's traditional use in the treatment of both acute and chronic inflammation has recently gained scientific support. In animal studies, whole stigma extracts provided moderate pain relief in acute inflammation and anti-inflammatory effects in chronic inflammation.

Saffron may also ultimately replace some of the synthetic food additives currently in use. For example, instead of FD&C Yellow No. 5/E102—a synthetic food coloring agent that is a very common allergy trigger—saffron's glorious yellow could be an acceptable hypoallergenic choice. Also, when the antioxidant properties of saffron were compared to that of the common food additive butylated hydroxytoluene (BHT), saffron was more effective than BHT in preventing lipid peroxidation, the cause of rancidity.

HOW TO SELECT AND STORE

Saffron is made up of tiny, bright red-orange stigmas or threads; the redder the saffron, the higher its quality. Saffron threads are available both whole and ground into powder. Unless purchased from a reputable and trusted source, whole threads of saffron are the best choice, since when purchasing these, you can check to be sure that the style, which, when dry, curls up against the stigma, has been cut away, leaving only a ⅜-to-½-inch/10-to-12-millimeters piece of all-red stigma. When the saffron has been powdered, it's much more difficult to tell if only stigma was used, plus, in addition to the style, the spice may be adulterated with the stamen or much less expensive spices, such as turmeric.

Determining the quality of saffron requires looking at a photospectometry report. This is a laboratory report that provides an analysis of the quantity of three active chemicals present in saffron: crocin (the chemical responsible for saffron's golden color and many of its beneficial health effects), picrocrocin (the chemical that imparts saffron's flavor expressed as bitterness), and safranal (the constituent on which saffron's aroma depends). The best saffron, which is labeled as Category I, will have a coloring strength (the dye intensity of saffron when immersed in liquid) of at least 190. This is the minimum standard for Category I saffron as set by the International Organization for Standardization (ISO), a body of professionals based in Switzerland who set worldwide commercial quality and labeling standards for various foodstuffs, including spices. Coloring strength, which is dependent on the saffron's crocin level, ranges from 110 to 250+ and should be clearly posted on the container (preferably a tin can), according to the ISO. Coloring strength is the only method used internationally to measure saffron's worth because it directly correlates with saffron's aroma and flavor: the higher the coloring strength, the more intense its flavor and aroma, regardless of whether the spice is in thread or powder form.

The photospectometry report will also list the amount of floral waste in the product. Along with coloring strength, floral waste is a primary criterion used to classify commercial saffron by quality category. Floral waste is composed of pollens, stamens, styles, parts of ovaries, or other parts of the *Crocus sativus* flower—in other words, parts of the saffron flower that contain none of saffron's aromatic, flavoring, or coloring properties. In high-quality saffron, these should not be present in anything but very minute quantities.

High-quality saffron powder, with a high coloring strength and virtually no floral waste, is much more convenient to use than saffron threads. When the threads are crushed into powder, the chemicals responsible for saffron's aroma, flavor, and color are made available immediately. The best powder is then carefully packaged in an airtight tin container to protect the powdered saffron from moisture and light, just as the threads must be to maintain their potency. Saffron powder can be added directly to any recipe, where its deep yellow dye, delicate aroma, and unique flavor will be released immediately.

In order to release the potent chemicals in saffron threads, however, they must be immersed in an alcoholic, acidic, or hot liquid for a minimum of twenty minutes. Depending on their quality, saffron threads can release aroma, flavor, and color for 24 hours or more, but 20 minutes will allow for a generous extraction of saffron's effects.

Before buying either form of saffron, examine the container to see if its coloring strength and crop year are printed anywhere. Do not buy saffron with a coloring strength of less than 190. If the container says "Category I," "Meets ISO Standards," or provides any other "category" name, such as "Mancha Selecto" (the name given to high-quality Spanish saffron) but does not provide a number for its coloring strength, ask whoever is selling the saffron to provide you with coloring strength data. In a food store or supermarket, speak with a manager and ask him or her to provide you with this information

before you buy. The crop year is usually expressed as two years, e.g., 2001/02, indicating that the saffron was harvested in 2001 and exported in 2002. Since saffron stigmas are harvested late in the year and must be cured (dried) and packaged properly to preserve their chemical properties, it is impossible for them to be collected and shipped in the same year.

If information on the saffron's coloring strength level is not available, you can try to evaluate the quality of the spice in two ways. First, look at the color. True powdered saffron, made only from ground stigmas, will be bright red-orange, not any shade of yellow. If you are buying whole stigmas, look for threads whose tips are a slightly lighter orange-red color. This may indicate that the product is not a lower-grade saffron that has been falsely tinted red.

You can determine if a dye has been used to imitate true saffron by immersing a little of the spice in warm water or milk. If the liquid colors immediately, it is simply artificial dye that is quickly leaching out. Genuine saffron must soak in warm liquid for at least 10 to 15 minutes before its deep red-gold color, flavor, and aroma begin to develop. To see the full color, rub real saffron with a spoon after it has soaked for several minutes.

To keep saffron affordable, in addition to checking its coloring strength, buy it by the ounce (30 grams), if possible. Buying high-quality saffron by the gram will be more expensive per serving, while purchasing it by the ounce can bring the price down to just pennies per recipe. If you can afford only a gram, buy Category I saffron in that quantity rather than attempting to substitute another herb or spice in the dish. Because saffron is costly and is packaged in small, easily shoplifted containers, authentic saffron is often kept under lock and key, so you may need to ask the supermarket assistant to get you some. High-quality saffron can also be purchased over the Internet, and doing so may provide you with a better product at a lower price. The best-quality saffron is not necessarily the most costly, since saffron's final price is tied to how much saffron is harvested in a particular country and how many middlemen handle it before it reaches you.

A word of caution: Mexican or American saffron is not true saffron but the red-orange thistles of the safflower plant, which grows wild all over the United States and Mexico. Safflower thistles can produce a light yellow dye but cannot provide the flavor, aroma, or health benefits of true saffron. Those unfamiliar with saffron can, however, mistake these thistles, sold very inexpensively and sometimes labeled "saffron," for the real thing.

Whole saffron threads should be so dry that they are quite brittle. Properly dried stigmas can be crushed into powder between your fingers or, with just a little pressure, between two metal spoons. This is important because not only does the drying process activate the chemical compounds that release saffron's aroma, color, and flavor, but if the stigmas are not cut apart from the styles prior to drying, they will retain moisture that will lessen the saffron's shelf life and quality. Saffron should have a distinct, clean aroma; it should never feel soft or spongy or develop a musty smell.

Both whole and ground saffron should be stored in an airtight opaque container in a cool, dry, and dark place. It is important to note that saffron absorbs other flavors and odors very easily. If you transfer saffron to a new container, make sure that it is clean, dry, and odor-free. High-quality saffron, whether in the form of whole threads or powder, will maintain its potency for several years.

TIPS FOR USE

If using whole saffron, remember that each red stigma is a tiny capsule that encloses the complex chemicals responsible for saffron's aroma, flavor, and golden color. To release these chemicals, saffron threads must be steeped as you would a tea for a minimum of 20 minutes prior to adding to a recipe. The longer the saffron steeps, the stronger its flavor, aroma, and color. The amount of liquid is not important. Use whatever is called for in your recipe, or add just a teaspoon or two of hot water. Then put the threads in the liquid and leave them for a minimum of 20 minutes before you add this "tea" to the recipe.

Do not remove the saffron threads. Presteeped saffron threads will not "boil away" when the saffron "tea" is added at the beginning of the cooking process. They will continue to release aroma, flavor, and color for up to 24 hours, which is why saffron-spiced dishes and breads always taste even stronger as leftovers.

However, saffron preparation differs from making tea in that saffron's chemicals respond to room-temperature alcohol and acids (citrus) as well as hot liquids, so saffron can be infused just as effectively in room-temperature white wine, vodka, rose water, orange blossom water, white vinegar, or citrus juice as in hot water, fat-free stock, or milk. But do not try to steep saffron in an oily cooking liquid—saffron is water-soluble, and the threads will not dissolve well in oils or saturated fats.

Many recipes call for saffron powder. If you've purchased threads, it's easy to grind them into a powder using a mortar and pestle. If the powder must be superfine, add a pinch of granulated sugar. This will create more friction and thus a finer powder. Saffron powder does not require steeping, as the powdering process has already released its essence. If substituting powder for threads, use half the amount. For example, 1 teaspoon of threads will yield ½ teaspoon of powder.

To preserve saffron's delicate flavor and aroma, avoid all but the merest touch of potent spices that might overwhelm it, such as turmeric, hot peppers, or ginger. If used with too heavy a hand, even more subtle herbs and spices can wipe out saffron's subtlety. Saffron itself should be used sparingly, because a delicate touch delivers the best impact. Too much, and the flavor will shift from magical to medicinal. The ideal amount depends on what you are cooking, but most recipes use just a few threads, while those demanding a stronger presence may need up to 1 teaspoon.

When determining how much saffron to use in baking, keep in mind that the saffron flavor will be stronger the second day. Just a pinch (less than ¼ teaspoon) of good-quality saffron powder should suffice for a recipe serving four to six. If you find you prefer a stronger flavor, add a tiny bit more. When using threads, try to envision a teaspoon to begin with and add from there.

QUICK SERVING IDEAS

- A pinch of ground saffron will transform any fish soup or stew into a rich, golden delight, which is why saffron is essential to the French fish and shellfish stew bouillabaisse.

- Saffron also works wonders with rice, as is exemplified by two classic Spanish dishes—paella, an exquisite dish of spicy long-grain rice and seafood or chicken, and arroz con pollo, chicken with rice—as well as the Italian presentation of saffron rice, risotto milanese, moist short-grain rice with bone marrow.

- Complementary foods for saffron are almonds, apples, basil, dairy products (including nonfat versions), fresh coriander, cinnamon, citrus, fish stock, garlic, most grains, pistachios, potatoes, rosemary, thyme, tomatoes, vinegar, and white wine.

- For a delicious twist on your standard omelet, sauté chunks of new potato in olive oil until golden. Whisk together eggs, finely sliced spring onions, chopped tomatoes, and salt. Stir in a pinch of powdered saffron or infused threads that have been allowed to soak for 20 minutes in a few spoonfuls of hot water. Pour into a well-oiled skillet and cook over medium heat until set—about 4 minutes.

- For a wonderful marinade for fish, add saffron threads, garlic, and thyme to vinegar.

- Use saffron to give cakes, pastries, and cookies a buttery golden hue and rich aroma. Add a little lemon zest as well for an even more memorable treat.

- Try biriyanis, fragrant northern Indian rice dishes in which saffron is used in conjunction with peppermint or combined with Indian bay leaves, cinnamon, cloves, green cardamom, star anise, and nutmeg or mace to flavor chicken or mutton, and the finished dish is decorated with pieces of almonds, raisins, or pomegranate seeds.

- Add saffron and cinnamon to whole milk or yogurt and honey for a simple version of the famous Indian yogurt drink lassi.
- Crush a tiny piece of saffron into a glass of champagne or sparkling apple cider and turn the drink into a golden elixir.
- Give cherished visitors a special welcome with the coffee drink prepared for honored guests in Arab countries surrounding the Persian Gulf: coffee spiced with saffron and cardamom. If you prefer tea, white tea prepared with a pinch of saffron is an elegant, soothing, and heart-healthy drink.
- Add a pinch of saffron to a basic plain cake recipe, and sprinkle the mixture with pistachios right before baking. Serve cut into triangular wedges—a Swedish-style festive greeting for family and friends.

SAFETY

Saffron as a spice is generally regarded as safe. Because of its cost, intense flavor, and strong dyeing properties, very little saffron is required for culinary purposes. However, it must be pointed out that in excessively large doses (perhaps as little as 2 tablespoons), it can be narcotic, toxic, and even lethal, causing violent hemorrhages. Generally, saffron is not recommended for use during pregnancy or breast-feeding. Its safety for young children or those with severe liver or kidney disease is not known. If consumed in very large amounts—more than 1 or 2 tablespoons—saffron is toxic, although due to its high price, saffron poisoning is very rare.

In Europe, gathering your own wild saffron is not advised. The plant is much more likely to be the common autumn crocus (*Colchicum autumnale*), one of the most poisonous plants in the European flora.

Sage

The silver-green leaves of the sagebrush make it a popular decorative garden plant, but the sagebrush that grows wild in the United States (*Salvia lyrata*) is much too bitter to eat. Instead, it is garden sage (*Salvia officinalis*) that we add to our recipes. Garden sage belongs to the mint family. The botanical name salvia translates to "savior."

Its leaves are grayish silver green in color and lance-shaped, with prominent veins running throughout. Sage leaves are two to three inches/5 to 7½ centimeters long and ½ inch/1 centimeter wide and have an earthy, aromatic taste that is simultaneously sweet and bitter.

HISTORY

Sage is a native of nations all around the Mediterranean Sea and has been enjoyed in these regions for several thousand years. In medicinal lore, sage has one of the longest histories of use of any herb in cooking and in medicine.

The Greeks and Romans recognized and made the most of the many healing properties of sage. Considering it a sacred plant, the Romans developed a special ritual even just to gather it. Both of these civilizations also took advantage of its utilitarian purpose as a meat preservative, a tradition that continued until the beginning of refrigeration.

Arab physicians of the tenth century believed that it promoted immortality and increased mental acumen. In the fourteenth century, Europeans used it as a safeguard from witchcraft. As a tea, sage was in such high demand in China during the seventeenth century that the Chinese are said to have traded three cases of black tea leaves to the Dutch to procure one case of sage leaves.

The high esteem with which sage is regarded has apparently not faded. Modern-day science is just beginning to confirm the ancient uses of sage as both a medicine and a preservative. It has been shown that sage contains compounds that can keep food preserved and serve as powerful antioxidants. Sage was given the distinguished title of "Herb of the Year" in 2001 by the International Herb Association.

HEALTH BENEFITS

The health benefits of sage are similar to those attributed to other members of the mint family. Sage is perhaps most similar to rosemary (see page 507). The primary medicinal components in sage are volatile oils, flavonoids, and rosmarinic acid.

Some of the distinct effects of sage that have been reported include anhidrotic (prevents perspiration); blood sugar-lowering effects in diabetics; antimicrobial; and drying up the flow of milk during lactation. This latter effect is the reason many herbalists recommend that pregnant and nursing women avoid sage.

HOW TO SELECT AND STORE

Whenever possible, choose fresh sage over the dried form of the herb, since it is superior in flavor. The leaves of fresh sage should be a vibrant silver-green in color and free from dark spots or yellowing. To store fresh sage leaves, carefully wrap them in a damp paper towel and place inside a loosely closed plastic bag. Store in the refrigerator, where they should stay fresh for several days.

If fresh sage is not available, choose dried. A tablespoon of fresh sage equals 1½ teaspoons rubbed or 1 teaspoon powdered sage. Dried sage comes in either whole, rubbed (lightly ground), or powder form. As with other herbs, when purchasing sage, choose organically grown sage when possible, since organically grown herbs are much less likely to have been irradiated. Dried sage should be kept in a tightly sealed glass container in a cool, dark, dry place, where it will remain fresh for about six months.

TIPS FOR USE

The most popular use of sage is in the stuffing of turkey at Christmas, but sage has many other uses as well. Sage can be added to breads, soups, most vegetables, and legumes. Since the flavor of sage is very delicate, it is best to add the herb near the end of the cooking process so that it will retain its maximum essence.

QUICK SERVING IDEAS

- Sage tea is an excellent diaphoretic and can help induce a good sweat if you have a fever.
- Mix 1 cup of cooked haricot beans with 1 tablespoon olive oil, 2 tablespoons fresh, chopped sage, and garlic and serve on baguette slices as an Italian bruschetta.
- Sprinkle some sage on top of your next slice of pizza.

- For stuffing, combine 3 cups cubed bread, ½ cup olive oil, ¼ cup vegetable or chicken stock, ¼ cup water, 1 tablespoon chopped sage leaves, ½ tablespoon chopped thyme, and ¼ teaspoon salt. Stuff the cavity of a chicken or turkey or bake by itself in a covered container for 30 minutes at 350 degrees F./180 degrees C./gas 4.
- Combine 2 tablespoons chopped sage leaves, 2 cups sliced bell peppers, ½ medium sliced cucumber, and ½ sliced sweet onion with 1 cup plain yogurt for an easy-to-prepare, refreshing salad.
- When baking chicken or fish in parchment paper or aluminium foil pouch, place three fresh sage leaves inside for each piece of meat so that the food will absorb the flavors of this delectable herb.

SAFETY

No significant safety concerns are associated with dietary levels of consumption of sage.

Tarragon

Tarragon *(Artemisia dracunculus)* is a sweet, aromatic herb with a slightly peppery flavor reminiscent of fennel, anise, and licorice. The tarragon plant is bushy and grows to a height of up to 3 feet/1 meter. The lance-shaped leaves are light green, 1½ inches/4 centimeters long and ¼ inch/½ centimeter wide. Two varieties of tarragon are cultivated: French and Russian. French tarragon is the type commercially grown to produce the dried spice purchased in supermarkets in the United States and the U.K., while Russian tarragon is the plant more often sold to home gardeners.

A native of southern Europe, French tarragon needs a sunny, warm summer and must be protected from cold and frost or potted and brought indoors for the winter. French tarragon produces tiny greenish white flowers that neither open fully nor produce viable seeds, but its smooth, narrow, dark green leaves, which grow on alternating sides of a round, smooth brown stem, are much sweeter and more flavorful than those of Russian tarragon.

Native to Siberia, Russian tarragon can be propagated from seed and is so hardy that it survives outdoors in Finland. Its leaves, more narrow and spiky and a brighter green than those of French tarragon, are bitter and less flavorful than the French variety. The reason for the disparity is that French tarragon contains up to 3 percent essential oil, while the Russian variety contains much less (approximately 0.1 percent), plus Russian tarragon lacks estragol, the active compound in French tarragon that is responsible for its licorice-like sweetness. Instead, Russian tarragon contains the flavonoids quercetin and patuletin, which give it a harsher, more astringent flavor.

HISTORY

Thought to have originated in Mongolia and Siberia, tarragon was valued by the ancient Romans as a treatment for snakebite, and Pliny the Elder, in his great encyclopaedia of nature and art, *Historia Naturalis,* recommends carrying a branch as a certain way to protect oneself against snake or dragon. Brought to Europe by invading Mongols in the thirteenth century, tarragon was in widespread use in the Middle Ages, when it was placed in shoes before a long trip to prevent tired feet and employed as a breath cleanser and treatment for insomnia. Precisely when and by whom the first aromatically sweet varieties were developed is unknown, but the herb we now know as French tarragon was under cultivation in the fifteenth century, by which time it had become popular in England as a seasoning for vegetables, a sleep-inducing drug, and a breath sweetener. In the sixteenth century, tarragon was one of the plants colonists carried with them, planting it in the first herb gardens grown in America and using infusions as a tea drunk to treat diarrhea, colds, head-aches, and the pains of childbirth.

HEALTH BENEFITS

The traditional medicinal uses of tarragon undoubtedly reflect its high content of active volatile compounds in its essential oil. Modern research has shown that the essential oil con-tains several compounds with potent antifungal activity, including 5-phenyl-1, 3-pentadiyne, capillarin, and methyleugenol. Estragol, a component of French tarragon's essential oil, has also demonstrated antimicrobial activity against *Bacillus subtilis,* a type of bacterium with a close resemblance to the pathogen that causes anthrax.

When evaluated for its ability to disarm free radicals, tarragon was found to have a remark-ably high antioxidant and free-radical scaveng-ing activity, comparable to that of chemicals used commercially in food preservation. The researchers recommended tarragon as a poten-tial source of natural antioxidants for the food industry.

Tarragon has also been used traditionally in herbal treatments for diabetes. When diabetic mice received tarragon as part of their diet for nine days, the animals' desire to overeat and excessive thirst was significantly reduced, plus their loss of needed body weight was lessened—all of which happened without any significant alterations in plasma glucose or insulin concen-trations, suggesting that tarragon's beneficial ac-tions occur independently of any improvement in blood sugar control.

HOW TO SELECT AND STORE

If fresh French tarragon is available at your supermarket, look for sprigs with a firm stem and nice straight leaves without blackening, yel-lowing, or wilting. The fresher the tarragon, the more estragol it will have retained, making for a stronger flavor. Store fresh tarragon in a plastic bag in the refrigerator vegetable crisper or place the stems in a glass of water for up to a week. If placed in an airtight plastic bag and frozen, sprigs of fresh tarragon will keep their flavor for three to five months. There is no need to defrost them before using. Or place the leaves in an ice cube tray, cover with water, and freeze. Add it directly to soups (and sauces that won't be spoiled by the addition of a little water) at the end of the cooking process.

Another way to preserve fresh tarragon's fla-vor is to store the herb in vinegar, which has the added benefit of flavoring the vinegar. Place the sprigs in a glass jar, cover with vinegar, and store in the refrigerator for up to six months. Distilled white vinegar, which has the least flavor of its own, is the best choice if used pri-marily to preserve the herb. Simply rinse the preserved tarragon and pat dry before use in any recipe where fresh tarragon is required.

Tarragon's flavor can also be retained by infusing it in oil. Wash and dry tarragon sprigs, then lightly bruise them to help release their aromatic oils. Place in a clean glass container, cover with warmed olive oil, seal tightly, and leave in a cool, dark, and dry place to infuse for about two weeks. Try a taste; if the flavor is not strong enough, add more tarragon sprigs and let stand another week. When the oil has reached the flavor intensity you prefer, strain out the herbs and store at room temperature for up to two months. The flavor of the tarragon will be more prominent in rapeseed oil, with its very mild flavor, but some rapeseed oil brands are highly unsaturated and perishable and must be refrigerated. Regardless of the oil used, infused oils can be enjoyed in salad dressings and marinades within two months.

Dried tarragon can be used if fresh tarragon is not available. Just as with other dried herbs, when purchasing dried tarragon, choose organically grown if possible, since organically grown herbs are much less likely to have been irradiated. Any discolored or musty-smelling leaves may be mouldy and should be discarded. Should you wish to save homegrown tarragon by drying, be certain the herb is fully dried before placing it in jars for storage to prevent mould.

Dried tarragon should be kept in a tightly sealed glass container in a cool, dark, dry place, where it will remain fresh for about six months.

TIPS FOR USE

When available, fresh French tarragon is a chef's delight. Its spicy sweet flavor perks up a wide variety of dishes but is especially good with fish. A key constituent of the classic French seasoning *fines herbes,* tarragon also gives Béarnaise sauce its characteristic flavor and is used in French cuisine, not only with fish and seafood but in poultry dishes and salad dressings. The sweet, slightly peppery taste of tarragon is also an excellent complement to eggs and a variety of cooked vegetables, such as potatoes, peas, asparagus, carrots, mushrooms, tomatoes, broccoli, and cauliflower.

Although tarragon's sweet anise fragrance will improve many subtly flavored dishes, the herb is not one of the most popular in American cuisine. Perhaps this is because the drying process causes French tarragon to lose much of its flavor. But in the U.K., fresh French tarragon is usually available in the produce section of good supermarkets and it is possible to grow from cuttings. Growing French tarragon from seed is not possible as it reverts to Russian tarragon. Unfortunately, the variety of fresh tarragon most commonly sold to home gardeners is the hardier but much less flavorful Russian tarragon.

The more intense flavor of fresh French tarragon, when available, demands that it be used judiciously. Too much can overwhelm a recipe. You can use the following guide to aid you.

- ½ ounce/15 grams of fresh tarragon leaves equals ½ cup.
- 1 pound/½ kilogram of tarragon leaves equals 16 cups.
- 1 tablespoon of fresh chopped tarragon equals 1 teaspoon dried.

Heat greatly intensifies the flavor of tarragon, whether fresh or dried. If you run out of tarragon, you can substitute chervil or a dash of fennel seed or anise seed; however, the flavor of the recipe will be altered.

QUICK SERVING IDEAS

- Béarnaise sauce is a more flavorful version of Hollandaise sauce made with lemon juice, white wine, egg yolk, and butter. While attempting your own Béarnaise sauce is not for the faint of heart or wrist, the 1½ cups produced by the following recipe will amply reward your taste buds for your efforts.

  In a medium-size, nonreactive saucepan over medium heat, combine 4 finely chopped shallots, 2 tablespoons fresh tarragon leaves, 4 crushed white peppercorns, ¼ cup vinegar, and ⅓ cup white wine. Boil until reduced to about ¼ cup. Strain into the top of a double boiler.

  Fill the bottom of the double boiler about half full with water and bring to a simmer. Place the top of the double boiler over it, checking to see that the water is a bit below the bottom of the upper pot, and whisk in four large egg yolks. Whisk constantly until the mixture begins to thicken, then immediately remove the top of the double boiler from the heat. Turn off the heat, but keep whisking. Add four ice cubes to the water in the bottom of the double boiler to cool it down a bit, then replace the top containing the yolk mixture. Continue to whisk. Heat two sticks (½ cup) unsalted butter in a medium saucepan over medium heat until just melted. Drizzling it very slowly, whisk the melted butter into the egg yolk mixture. If at any time the sauce looks anything but smooth and glossy, lift out the top of the double boiler and continue whisking to cool it down, or whisk in 1 teaspoon of cold water. Still whisking constantly, blend in ¼ teaspoon salt and a pinch of cayenne and serve ⅓ cup over the dish of your choice.

- To make your own *fines herbes,* chop finely and combine 1 tablespoon each of fresh tarragon, chervil, chives, and parsley. Add to the dish at the end of the cooking process, just before serving. Fresh *fines herbes* may also be frozen in airtight containers. Alternatively, you can freeze the combination in ice cube trays covered with either water or stock that can be added when preparing soups or stews. If using dried herbs, combine equal amounts of the four and use one third the amount of the fresh form in recipes. To store, place in an airtight glass jar and store in a cool, dry and dark place for up to four months. Yield: About ¼ cup.

- If you have an herb garden or access to fresh French tarragon, make your own tarragon vinegar. Cut off several stalks on a dry day just before the herb flowers in August. Let dry in the sun for an hour, then use to fill a clean and sterilized, wide-mouthed pint/½ litre bottling jar. Bring 16 ounces/½ litre of your choice of vinegar to near boiling, pour into the jar, seal, and put in a dark and dry place. About two to six weeks later, depending on how strong a tarragon flavor you prefer, strain off the herbed vinegar into another jar and discard the tarragon. Or you can leave the herb in the vinegar until it is used; however, the flavor may deepen. If your first batch is too strong or weak, simply adjust the amount of tarragon put in the jar and the time it stands before use to suit your taste.

- Tarragon-infused oil can also be made in a similar fashion to the vinegar recipe, though the oil should be only warmed, not nearly boiled.

- Toss a salad of cold whitefish, prawns, and scallops with a dressing made from ⅔ cup buttermilk, ½ cup ricotta cheese, 4 tablespoons chopped fresh tarragon, a few drops freshly squeezed lemon juice, and salt and freshly ground pepper to taste.
- Perk up an omelet or scrambled eggs by mixing in a tablespoonful each of fresh tarragon and fresh cream before cooking.
- Dress up fish or seafood with this piquant tarragon rémoulade sauce: In a blender, combine 1 cup mayonnaise with 4 ounces/120 milliliters tarragon vinegar, 2 teaspoons fresh tarragon, 1 chopped spring onion, 2 gherkins, 2 teaspoons fresh parsley, 1 teaspoon capers, 1 anchovy, 1 teaspoon freshly ground pepper, and salt to taste. Blend until smooth. For a mustard rémoulade, blend in 2½ tablespoons Dijon mustard.
- For an easier but still delicious creamy tarragon sauce, melt 1 stick (¼ cup) butter in a medium-size saucepan over medium heat. Add 1 clove finely minced fresh garlic and cook several minutes until golden. Stir in 1 tablespoon of flour and cook several more minutes, until browned. Gradually add 1 cup milk, stirring until the sauce thickens. Mix in ½ cup whole yogurt, 3 teaspoons *fines herbes*, and ½ teaspoon freshly ground black pepper. Serve warm with fish or poultry, or as a topping for steamed new potatoes, asparagus, broccoli, or cauliflower. Stored in an airtight container in the refrigerator, this sauce—the recipe yields about 1½ cups—will keep for up to one week.

SAFETY

Tarragon can be consumed safely in normal amounts. However, the essential oil of tarragon should be used with caution. Based on animal testing, at very high doses, methyl chavicol, an active component in essential oil of tarragon, can cause liver toxicity.

Thyme

Thyme *(Thymus vulgaris)* is a small, evergreen shrub of the mint family that has tiny leaves with a minty, tealike flavor. Thyme leaves are curled and elliptically shaped, ⅛ inch/3 millimeters long and 1/16 inch/1½ millimeters wide. The upper leaf is green-gray in color, with a whitish underside.

Delicate-looking and sporting a penetrating fragrance, thyme is an herb worth investigating if you are not familiar with it. And given that there are approximately sixty different varieties, including French (common) thyme, lemon thyme, orange thyme, and silver thyme, there are many to discover.

HISTORY

A native of the western Mediterranean region, thyme has been drawn on since ancient times for its culinary, aromatic, and medicinal properties. In ancient Greece, thyme was burned as incense for sacred ceremonies as a symbol of courage, fortitude, and admiration. Its association with bravery continued throughout medieval times, as it was a ritual for women to give their knights a scarf that had a sprig of thyme placed over an embroidered bee. The ancient Egyptians found thyme to be an effective embalming agent with which they preserved their deceased pharaohs. Since the sixteenth century, thyme oil has also been used for its antibacterial and cleansing properties, both as a mouthwash and as an antiseptic agent on the skin.

Today, thyme is produced mostly in Asia, southern Europe, the Mediterranean region, and North America.

HEALTH BENEFITS

Thyme has similar benefits as other mints due to its volatile oil content. The volatile oil components of thyme are now known to include carvacol, borneol, geraniol, and, most important, thymol. Thyme oil has been shown to possess antispasmodic, antibacterial, and carminative actions. Applied topically, it is also reported to have strong fungicidal properties. Thyme also contains a variety of flavonoids, including apigenin, naringenin, luteolin, and thymonin. These flavonoids increase thyme's antioxidant capacity and, combined with its status as a very good source of manganese, give it a high standing on the list of antioxidant-rich foods.

One interesting line of research indicates that thyme may help improve brain function. In studies on aging in rats, thymol has been found to protect and significantly increase the percentage of healthy fats found in cell membranes and other cell structures. In particular, the amount of DHA (docosahexaenoic acid, an omega-3 fatty acid) in brain, kidney, and heart cell membranes increased. In other studies looking more closely at changes in the brain cells themselves, researchers found that the maximum benefits of thyme occurred when the food was introduced

very early in the rats' life cycle but was less effective in offsetting the problems in brain cell aging when introduced late in the aging process. The possible human application of this research is using thyme as a method to raise DHA levels in children with attention deficit disorder and possibly improve this condition.

HOW TO SELECT AND STORE

Thyme is available fresh or dried. Whenever possible, choose fresh thyme over the dried form of the herb, since it is superior in flavor and aroma. The leaves of fresh thyme are a vibrant green-gray in color, and they should be free from dark spots or yellowing. Fresh thyme should be kept in the refrigerator wrapped in a slightly damp paper towel, where it will keep for up to seven days.

If fresh thyme is not available, be sure when purchasing dried thyme to choose organically grown thyme, since organically grown herbs are much less likely to have been irradiated. Dried thyme should be kept in a tightly sealed glass container in a cool, dark, dry place, where it will remain fresh for about six months.

TIPS FOR USE

Whether fresh or dried, the timing of thyme can make a difference. It is best added toward the end of the cooking process since heat can easily cause a loss of its volatile oils and thus its delicate flavor.

Thyme mixes nicely with many foods and other herbs. The combination of thyme, garlic, basil, and oregano can be put to good use in marinara tomato sauces for pasta and pizza. Given its versatility, thyme also adds a tasty dimension to most vegetables, beans, grains, soups, casseroles, and other dishes.

QUICK SERVING IDEAS

- Hearty legumes, such as kidney beans, pinto beans, and black beans, taste exceptionally good when seasoned with thyme.
- Grilled or baked fish can have a savory topping by adding thyme and rosemary pesto: Chop enough thyme and rosemary to cover half the surface of the fish. Add chopped pine nuts or walnuts in equal parts to the herbs. Season with salt and pepper. Place on top of the fish and bake.
- Poached fish, whether whitefish or salmon, absorb the taste of thyme quite well. Place at least five sprigs on top of the fish and a few in the water, too, to infuse your fish with thyme's delectable flavor.
- You can infuse your favorite olive oil with a few sprigs of thyme and use as a flavored dipping oil or for cooking.
- Most soups and soup stocks will benefit by the addition of some thyme.

SAFETY

Thyme contains moderate amounts of oxalate. Individuals with a history of oxalate-containing kidney stones should avoid overconsuming this food. For more information, see Appendix D, page 793.

Turmeric

Turmeric (*Curcuma longa*) is a member of the ginger family that is extensively cultivated in India, China, Indonesia, and other tropical countries. In cooking, the rhizome (root) is the part that is utilized. It has a tough brown skin and deep orange flesh, and is similar to ginger with smaller branched arms 1 to 1½ inches/2½ to 4 centimeters around. It is usually cured (boiled, cleaned, and sun-dried), polished, and ground into a powder. Turmeric's flavor is peppery, warm, and bitter, while its fragrance is mild, yet slightly reminiscent of orange and ginger.

Turmeric powder was traditionally referred to as "Indian saffron," as its deep yellow-orange color is reminiscent of saffron's. Turmeric is the major ingredient of curry powder and is also used in prepared mustard as a coloring agent. It is extensively used in a variety of foods for both its color and flavor.

HISTORY

A native of Indonesia and southern India, turmeric has been cultivated and harvested since 3000 B.C.E. Turmeric has played an important role in many traditional cultures throughout the East. It is still used today in rituals of the Hindu religion and as a dye for holy robes. It is also a venerated constituent of the Ayurvedic pharmacopoeia.

Even though Arab traders introduced turmeric into Europe in the thirteenth century, it has become popular in Western cultures only recently. Much of its newfound popularity is owed to the recent scientific study that has characterized its therapeutic abilities. India, Indonesia, China, the Philippines, Taiwan, Haiti, and Jamaica are the leading worldwide producers of turmeric today.

HEALTH BENEFITS

Turmeric has been and still is a key component of both the Chinese and Indian systems of medicine, where it is used as an anti-inflammatory agent and in the treatment of numerous conditions, including flatulence, jaundice, menstrual difficulties, bloody urine, hemorrhage, toothache, bruises, chest pain, and colic. Turmeric poultices are often applied locally to relieve inflammation and pain.

Curcumin, turmeric's yellow pigment, has demonstrated significant anti-inflammatory activity in a variety of experimental models. In fact, in numerous studies, curcumin's anti-inflammatory effects have been shown to be comparable to those of the potent drugs hydrocortisone and phenylbutazone, as well as over-the-counter anti-inflammatory agents, such as ibuprofin (Nurofen). Unlike the drugs, which are associated with significant toxic effects, including ulcer formation, decreased white blood cell count, and intestinal bleeding, curcumin produces no toxicity.

Other clinical studies have further substantiated curcumin's anti-inflammatory effects, including a clinical effect in rheumatoid arthritis. In this study, curcumin was compared to phenylbutazone. The improvements in the duration of morning stiffness, walking time, and joint swelling were comparable in both groups. In a new human model for evaluating anti-inflammatory drugs, 400 milligrams of curcumin was comparable to 100 milligrams of phenylbutazone and 400 milligrams of ibuprofen.

Clinical studies have also substantiated that curcumin exerts very powerful antioxidant effects. Curcumin's antioxidant actions enable it to protect healthy cells from free radicals that can damage cellular DNA and lead to cancer. This action is significantly beneficial to areas of the body such as the lining of the colon, where cell turnover is quite rapid—approximately every three days. Because of their frequent replication, mutations in the DNA of colon cells can result in the formation of cancerous cells much more quickly. Evidence is mounting that aspirin and other nonsteroidal anti-inflammatory drugs (NSAIDs) may prevent colorectal cancer. However, in animal studies, curcumin has been shown to inhibit colon cancer more effectively than aspirin at all stages, from initiation to promotion and progression.

Furthermore, curcumin helps the body to destroy mutated cancer cells, so they cannot spread through the body and cause more harm. In one human study, sixteen chronic smokers were given 1½ grams of turmeric daily, while six nonsmokers served as a control group. At the end of the thirty-day trial, the smokers who had received turmeric had a significant drop in the level of cancer-causing compounds as measured in their urine. Their levels were almost the same as those of the nonsmokers. We suggest that people who smoke, or who are exposed to secondhand smoke, eat foods seasoned with turmeric.

In addition to these preventive actions, curcumin has also been shown to inhibit tumor growth by:

• Inhibiting epidermal growth factor (EGF) receptor sites: EGF stimulates cells to proliferate by connecting to receptors on the cells' surface. About two thirds of all cancers produce an abundance of these receptors, which make them highly sensitive to EGF. By reducing the number of EGF receptors, curcumin decreases the cells' tendency to proliferate.

- Inhibiting angiogenesis: Fibroblast growth factor is a protein that promotes the formation of new blood vessels to feed the growing tumor. Curcumin inhibits production of this growth factor.
- Inhibiting nuclear factor kappa beta (NF-kb): This is a protein that many cancer cells produce to block the signals commanding them to stop proliferating.
- Increasing the expression of the nuclear p53 protein: This protein is essential for apoptosis, the normal process of cell "suicide."
- Inhibiting growth-promoting enzymes.

Some of curcumin's benefits come from its known activity as an antioxidant, but curcumin also:

- Inhibits the formation of cancer-causing nitrosamines.
- Enhances the body's production of cancer-fighting compounds, such as glutathione.
- Promotes the liver's proper detoxification of cancer-causing compounds.
- Prevents overproduction of cyclooxygenase 2 (COX-2), an enzyme that may contribute to the development of tumors.

While more human studies are needed on the use of curcumin in cancer treatment, the experimental and preliminary evidence is quite encouraging. Experimental (test-tube) studies have found that curcumin fights tumors arising from prostate, breast, skin, colon,

stomach, and liver cancers. These benefits have also been seen in a human study involving sixty-two patients who had either ulcerating oral cancer or skin cancer and who had not responded to the standard treatments. Patients received either an ethanol extract of turmeric (for oral cancers) or an ointment containing 0.5 percent curcumin in petroleum jelly. The extract or ointment was applied to the affected area three times daily. After eighteen months, the treatment had effectively reduced the smell of the lesion by 90 percent, the itching and oozing by 70 percent, the pain by 50 percent, and the size of the lesion by 10 percent. These may not seem like spectacular results—but remember, standard treatments had not worked for these patients.

In addition to protecting against cancer, turmeric may be able to help in the prevention of heart disease, as well as degenerative neurological diseases such as Alzheimer's and Parkinson's diseases and multiple sclerosis. Regarding heart disease, turmeric not only helps to lower cholesterol, it also prevents the oxidation of cholesterol. Since oxidized cholesterol is what damages blood vessels and builds up in the plaques that can lead to heart attack or stroke, preventing the oxidation of new cholesterol may help to reduce the progression of atherosclerosis and diabetic heart disease. Regarding its potential as a brain-protective agent, population studies showed that in elderly Indian populations, in whose diet turmeric is a common spice, levels of neurological disease, such as Alzheimer's, were very low. In addition, studies have shown that curcumin slows the progression of Alzheimer's and multiple sclerosis in mice.

HOW TO SELECT AND STORE

Turmeric is available as a ground powder but, like ginger, is available as the fresh rhizome from Asian and Caribbean food shops. Fresh turmeric should be free of dark spots and be crisp. It may be stored in the refrigerator, where it will keep for one month. Alternatively, it can be chopped or sliced and stored in an airtight container for up to three months.

Since the color of turmeric powder varies among varieties, it is not necessarily a criterion of quality. However, try to select organically grown dried turmeric, since organically grown spices are much less likely to have been irradiated. Turmeric powder should be stored in a tightly sealed container in a cool, dark, dry place, where it will keep for up to one year. Curcumin-containing products are available in health food shops.

TIPS FOR USE

Since turmeric's deep yellow and orange color can easily stain, avoid getting it on clothing. To avoid a permanent stain, quickly wash any affected area with soap and plenty of water. Depending upon how much you plan on handling it, it might be a good idea to wear latex gloves when preparing foods with turmeric.

Turmeric is a spice that is heavily relied on in the cuisines of Southeast Asia, India, and Mexico, as it is a primary ingredient in curry and chili powders. Other popular uses for turmeric are for adding color to any grain dish as well as to complement any recipe in which ginger appears.

QUICK SERVING IDEAS

- To make your own curry powder, combine in a grinder 1 tablespoon cumin, 1 tablespoon mustard seed, ½ tablespoon coriander, and 1 teaspoon each fenugreek, fennel, ginger, and turmeric. Store the mixture in a cool, dark, dry place for up to six months.
- Mix 2 cups cooked brown rice, ¼ cup raisins, ¼ cup cashews, and 1 tablespoon olive oil and season with ¼ teaspoon each turmeric, cumin, coriander, and salt.
- Turmeric is a great spice to complement recipes that feature legumes, particularly lentils.
- Add turmeric to egg salad to give it an even bolder yellow color and richer flavor.
- Give salad dressings an orange-yellow hue by adding some turmeric powder to them.

SAFETY

Turmeric is extremely safe and well tolerated, even at higher dosages.

16

The Healing Power of Fish and Shellfish

Fish and shellfish have been important in human nutrition since prehistoric times. Fish farming is also an age-old practice. The ancient Assyrians had fishponds where they bred up to fifty different species of fish, and the Romans also farmed fish in ponds. For thousands of years, the Chinese have farmed fish as well, using their rice fields during the periods when the fields are under water.

Throughout history, fish and shellfish have been a source of economic power. The Vikings traded large amounts of stockfish (salted, dried cod), and Britain's empire was based largely on its control of the oceans as a result of its fishing industry. At one time, the English Parliament even forbade the nation's citizens to eat meat three days a week: Wednesdays, Fridays, and Saturdays. This decree increased the demand for fish and shellfish and, as a result, the demand for fishermen. Many of these fishermen became skilled seamen and a resource for the English navy.

During recent decades, per capita fish consumption has expanded all over the world. Several factors determine the consumption of fish and shellfish, the main ones being a country's own supply of these products, the country's economy, and tradition. One of the major reasons fish and shellfish consumption is increasing in the United States is the desire of many Americans to eat more healthfully.

In 2004, total worldwide seafood production (excluding aquatic plants) was estimated to be nearly 150 million tons, of which 58 million tons came from aquaculture. China was the leading seafood-producing country with 16.5 million tons, followed by Peru (8 million tons), the United States (6 million tons), Japan (5 million tons), and Indonesia (5 million tons).

Nutritional Highlights

Fish and shellfish are nutrient-dense and an excellent source of high-quality protein,

TABLE 16.1
Fish and Shellfish Consumption in the United States per Capita per Year

Year	Fresh and frozen fish* (pounds)	Canned Fish (pounds)	Cured Fish (pounds)	Total (pounds)
1960	5.7	4.0	.58	10.3
1970	6.9	4.4	.44	11.7
1980	7.8	4.3	.32	12.4
1990	9.6	5.1	.30	15.0
2001	10.2	4.2	.30	14.7

* Includes processed fish on a fresh (raw) basis and excludes game fish consumption.

vitamins, and minerals, but it is their content of omega-3 fatty acids that receives the most attention. While virtually all fish and shellfish contain some omega-3 fatty acids, some contain much more than others. The following list provides a general grouping of fish and shellfish based upon their omega-3 fatty acid content.

FISH AND SHELLFISH GROUPED BY THEIR OMEGA-3 FATTY ACID CONTENT

Higher-Level Group (more than 1 gram per 100 gram cooked serving)

Fish

Herring

Mackerel

Salmon

Tuna, bluefin

Whitefish

Medium-Level Group (between 0.5 and 1 gram per 100 gram cooked serving)

Fish	**Shellfish**
Bass, freshwater	Mussels, blue
Bass, striped	Oysters

Smelt

Swordfish

Trout, rainbow

Whiting

Wolffish

Lower-Level Group (½ gram or less per 100 gram cooked serving)

Fish	**Shellfish**
Cod	Clams
Flounder	Crab
Grouper	Lobster
Haddock	Prawns
Halibut	Scallops
Mullet	
Perch	
Pollock	
Pike, northern	
Snapper, red	
Trout, sea	
Tuna, skipjack	
Tuna, yellowfin	

Health Benefits

The beneficial effects of fish and shellfish consumption on human health have been well documented. It is their content of omega-3 fatty acids that is primarily responsible for many of their unique health benefits. All told, based upon more than 2,000 scientific studies, at least sixty different health conditions are either prevented or treatable with a higher intake of omega-3 fatty acids (see Chapter 6 for more information). The best-known condition prevented and treated with omega-3 fatty acids is heart disease.

The idea that eating fish may reduce the risk of heart disease began in the 1970s, when it was noted that among the Eskimos in Arctic Greenland, where high consumption of marine animals was the normal diet, heart disease was very low. Subsequent studies in similar cultures where fish and seafood consumption is high showed the same sort of protection. For example, the inhabitants of the Japanese island of Okinawa, who eat primarily fish, were also observed to have a very low incidence of mortality from heart disease.

In order to better assess the protective effects of fish consumption against heart disease, researchers conducted large studies in which they tracked dietary intake of fish and other seafood over a long period of time. As the results of these studies became available in the mid-1980s and 1990s, they provided even stronger evidence that higher levels of fish consumption were associated with a lower risk of mortality from heart disease. It is now estimated that individuals whose diets include a higher intake of fish, particularly those

---

HOW MUCH FISH SHOULD YOU CONSUME?

Based upon the research that assesses the amount of fish required to offer protection against heart disease, it appears that eating fish twice a week will provide distinct health benefits. This translates into approximately 10 to 12 ounces/275 to 350 grams of fish per week, or roughly an average intake of 200 to 400 milligrams of omega-3 fatty acids per day.

---

high in omega-3 fatty acids, reduce their risk of heart disease by roughly 47 percent compared to those individuals who do not eat fish.

In addition to heart disease, scientists now know that fish consumption can lower the risk of many cancers—particularly breast, prostate, colon, and lung cancer—as well as many chronic diseases, including Alzheimer's disease, asthma, depression, diabetes, high blood pressure, macular degeneration, multiple sclerosis, and rheumatoid arthritis.

How to Select and Store

Available all year round, fish is usually sold already cut into steaks or fillets, both fresh and frozen, with the skin left on to prevent the meat from falling apart during cooking. Fresh fish should be displayed on metal trays or sheets of paper or plastic, and placed on top of clean ice. The flesh should appear freshly cut and should not be sitting in a pool of liquid. The skin should be smooth, moist, and firm, not flaky, and should not feel too slippery or slimy. If the fish is small enough to have been left whole, its

TABLE 16.2

Fat and Cholesterol Comparison Chart (per 100 gram serving)

Food	Calories	Cholesterol (milligrams)	Saturated Fat (grams)
Halibut	140	41	0.4
Cod	105	55	0.2
Mahimahi	109	94	0.2
Salmon	231	85	3.2
Snapper, red	128	47	0.4
Swordfish	155	50	1.4
Tuna, bluefin	184	49	1.6
Tuna, yellowfin	140	58	0.3
Crab, Alaskan king	97	53	0.1
Crab, blue/soft-shell	102	100	0.2
Crab, Dungeness	110	76	0.2
Crab, snow	115	71	0.2
Lobster, Maine	98	72	0.1
Prawns	99	195	0.3
Clam	148	67	0.2
Oyster	137	105	1.5
Scallops	112	153	.2
Beef, top round	207	90	2.0
Chicken, light meat only	173	85	1.3
Egg, one, 50 grams	77	212	1.6
Pork loin	213	85	3.6
Turkey, light meat only	161	68	1.2

eyes should be bright and clear, not cloudy or sunken, and it should be buried in the ice since its skin will protect the flesh from direct contact with the ice. When buying a whole fish, be sure to allow twice as much weight per serving as you would for steaks or fillets.

Rely on your sense of smell to tell you if the fish is fresh. Truly fresh fish will smell like salt water and will not emit a sour, ammonia-like "fishy" smell. Once the fishmonger has wrapped and given you the fish you have chosen, give it a sniff test. If you smell any off-odor, return it. If the fish you are considering has already been wrapped in plastic, it's more difficult to tell, but take a good whiff anyway. If the fish is really not fresh, its sour odor will penetrate the plastic. If you're not sure, ask the fishmonger when it was delivered and wrapped. If uncertain, choose a different fish.

Some fish are flash frozen on the boat right after they are caught, then later thawed out and sold as fresh. Such fish is often of excellent quality, even superior to fresh fish, but should be cooked as soon as possible and not refrozen. If buying frozen fish, avoid fish with whitened, cottonlike patches—a sign of freezer burn—or any package with lots of ice crystals or water stains.

When purchasing any fresh fish, plan your shopping trip so that the fish is your last purchase, and, if at all possible, go directly home, so it can be quickly refrigerated until cooked. In warm weather, or if you cannot go directly home, ask to have the fish packed in ice and/or place it in a picnic cooler in the car to keep it chilled.

When you get home, rinse and rewrap the fish, then place it on paper towels in a clean plastic bag or tightly closed container and set it in the coldest part of your refrigerator. Even better, place the rewrapped fish in a pan of ice and set this on the bottom shelf (the coldest one) in the refrigerator. If keeping the fish until the next day, check once or twice to see that the ice is not melted and replenish if needed. Kept in this fashion, fresh fish can be stored for one to two days. Once cooked, fish should be eaten in one to two days.

If you cannot eat fresh fish within a couple of days, it's best to freeze it. Once frozen and thawed, fish should not be refrozen. Cut the fish, if necessary, into pieces no larger than 2 pounds/1 kilogram. Rinse, pat dry, and wrap tightly in heavy-duty freezer paper or plastic wrap. Wrap again in foil, label with the date, and freeze. If the fish is already frozen and not thawed, just store in its original wrapping. Stored in the coldest part of the freezer, fish will keep for up to six months.

Tips for Preparing

Rinse any fresh or frozen fish briefly in cold water and pat dry before cooking. Always check any fillet for bones. Run your fingers over the fillet and remove any you find with tweezers, then rinse and pat dry.

Frozen fish need not be thawed if extra cooking time is allowed; however, if you wish to thaw frozen fish, place it in the refrigerator overnight. To prevent bacterial contamination, do not thaw at room temperature. For the same reason, if you are marinating fish, do so in the refrigerator.

Follow the same food safety rules you would with raw meat or poultry. Thoroughly wash all surfaces, utensils, and your hands with hot soapy water after preparing raw fish and do not let other food items come in contact with the fish, surfaces on which it was prepared, utensils, or your hands before these have been thoroughly cleaned.

It is important to cook all seafood long enough to destroy any pathogenic organisms. To accomplish this goal, measure the fish at its thickest point (if stuffed, this means after stuffing) and cook for ten minutes per inch/2½ centimeters of thickness, turning the fish (unless it's very thin fillets) halfway through the cooking time. If the fish is frozen, double the cooking time. Add five minutes if cooking the fish in sauce. Properly cooked fish will have firm but still moist flesh. When tested with the tip of a knife, the fish should barely flake, but not fall apart, which indicates that it's overdone.

Fish lends itself to baking, barbecueing, poaching, steaming, or grilling. Baking is a particularly easy way to prepare fish. To bake fish, preheat your oven to 425 degrees F./220 degrees C./gas 7. Lightly oil a shallow baking dish and place the fish in it, skin side down. It is not necessary to add a fat or liquid when baking fish. The fish will remain naturally moist as long as it is not overcooked. Alternatively, poaching fish requires liquid, such as stock or a mixture of wine, vinegar, soy sauce, or other flavored liquids with stock or water. Add just enough cooking liquid to cover the piece of fish and bake as above.

The variety of flavor is as diverse as the different types of fish and shellfish, from the buttery, mild flavor of white fish, such as cod, to the full, rich, complex flavor of most shellfish. Table 16.3 will help you select fish based on both texture and flavor.

Safety

There are several safety concerns regarding fish and shellfish consumption, including the danger of chemical contamination with mercury and pesticide residues, as well as with toxins produced by the fish. There is also bacterial, viral, and parasitic contamination to consider. One of the most common reasons for fish safety warnings is mercury contamination. Mercury is

a problem in many large predator fish, such as shark, swordfish, and some larger species of tuna. These fish accumulate mercury from their prey. Mercury can accumulate in the human body, and too much can cause neurological problems, especially in fetuses and young children. The Food and Drug Administration (FDA), which oversees food safety concerns in the United States, recommends that women of childbearing age eat shark, swordfish, or fresh tuna steaks no more than once per month. The FDA also recommends that all consumers limit their grouper, marlin, and orange consumption to roughly 14 ounces/400 grams per week and consumption of shellfish (as well as canned tuna) to about 2 pounds/1 kilogram per week. In the U.K., the Food Standards Agency also recommends maximum intakes of some fish: adults no more than one portion (140 grams) of swordfish, shark or marlin per week (pregnant women, those trying for a baby, and children should avoid these fish); and four portions of oily fish per week for men, boys and non-child-bearing women; two portions of oily fish for girls and potential child-bearing women, pregnant and breastfeeding women. Babies under six months old should not have fish or shellfish.

Two groups, the Environmental Working Group and the U.S. Public Interest Research Group, have asked the FDA to add Gulf Coast oysters and six more types of fish to the list of fish to restrict during pregnancy: tuna, sea bass, halibut, marlin, pike, and white croaker. They also feel that canned tuna, mahimahi, cod, and pollock should not be eaten more than once a month. According to these two research groups, fish considered safe for pregnant women

TABLE 16.3

Fish and Shellfish Categorized by Flavor and Texture

		Mild Flavor	Moderate Flavor	Full Flavor
Delicate texture	Fish	Cod	Buffalo fish	Bluefish
		Flounder	Butterfish	Mackerel, Atlantic
		Haddock	Cod, black	
		Hake/whiting	Cod, ling	
		Pollock	Croaker, white	
		Skate	Perch, lake	
		Sole	Whitefish	
	Shellfish	Crabmeat		Mussels
				Oysters
Moderate texture	Fish	Rockfish	Mullet	Fish, smoked
		Roughy, orange	Ocean Perch	Herring
		Sheepshead	Shad	Mackerel, king
		Tilapia	Smelt	Mackerel, Spanish
		Pike, walleye	Trout	Salmon, canned
		Tuna, canned	Sardines, canned	
	Shellfish	Crawfish	Conch	
		Lobster	Surimi seafood products	
		Scallops		
		Prawns		
Firm texture	Fish	Bass, sea	Amberjack	Marlin
		Blackfish (Tautog)	Bass, striped	Salmon
		Catfish, ocean	Catfish	Swordfish
		Grouper	Drum	Tuna
		Halibut	Mahimahi	
		Monkfish	Pompano	
		Porgy	Shark	
		Snapper	Sturgeon	
		Tilefish		
	Shellfish	Squid	Octopus	Clams

include wild Pacific salmon, farm-raised trout and catfish, prawns, flounder (summer), mid-Atlantic blue crab, and haddock.

To reduce your chances of eating fish that has been tainted with chemical toxins:

• Limit your intake of freshwater fish (particularly from inland lakes), as they are more likely to be contaminated with pesticides and carcinogens, such as dioxin or PCBs.

• Eat smaller, young fish, as they have had less

time to accumulate toxins in their fat. For example, salmon live only one to two years, compared to halibut, which can live many years and accumulate more toxins.

- Eat open-ocean, deepwater fish more often than freshwater fish, since they are less likely to have been exposed to toxins.

In regard to the safety of the fish people themselves catch in America's lakes, rivers, oceans, and estuaries, we encourage you to visit the National Listing of Fish Advisories (NLFA) website: www.epa.gov/waterscience/fish. This organization, created by the Environmental Protection Agency, provides information on fish consumption advisories issued by the federal government, states, territories, tribes, and local governments.

For information about angling in the U.K., contact the Environment Agency which is responsible for the quality of inland waterways. The website is www.environment-agency.gov.uk/subjects/fish.

In the U.S., most fish consumption advisories involve five primary contaminants: mercury, PCBs, chlordane, dioxins, and DDT. These chemical contaminants persist for long periods in sediments, where bottom-dwelling animals accumulate them and pass them up the food chain to fish. Levels of these contaminants may increase as they move up the food chain, so top predators in a food chain, such as largemouth bass or pike, may have levels a million times as high as that in the water.

Mercury, PCBs, chlordane, dioxins, and DDT were at least partly responsible for 96 percent of all fish consumption advisories in effect in 2002 in the U.S. In 2002, nineteen states issued statewide advisories for mercury in freshwater lakes and/or rivers. Another eleven states issued statewide advisories for mercury in their coastal waters. Thirty-eight states issued PCB advisories and four states added nine new PCB advisories in 2002. The number of dioxin advisories is small compared to the other four major contaminants'. But although its use has been banned since 1975, the number of advisories currently in effect for DDT continues to increase.

Some fish and shellfish are a significant source of purines. Since purines can be broken down to form uric acid, excess accumulation of purines in the body can lead to excess accumulation of uric acid. Gout and the formation of kidney stones from uric acid are two examples of uric acid-related problems that can be caused by excessive intake of purine-containing foods. For this reason, individuals with kidney problems or gout should avoid or limit their intake of fish and shellfish.

Allergic reactions to fish and shellfish are commonly reported in both adults and children. It is generally recommended that people who have had an allergic reaction to one species of fish, or positive skin tests to fish, avoid all fish. The same rule applies to shellfish. Allergic reactions to fish and shellfish can be mild, with just itching skin; moderate, with some difficulty breathing; or severe, causing anaphylaxis. Individuals who are extremely allergic to fish or shellfish should avoid fish and seafood restaurants because of the risk of contamination in the food preparation area of their "nonfish" meal from a counter, spatula, fryer, or grill exposed to fish. In addition, fish protein can become airborne during cooking and cause an allergic reaction. Some individuals have had reactions from simply walking through a fish market or restaurant where fish is cooked.

Fish are not a source of goitrogens. In fact, the iodine in oceanic fish and shellfish prevents iodine-deficiency goiter. Because these foods do contain considerable amounts of iodine, people with a thyroid disorder should discuss fish consumption with their physician.

Fish contain small amounts of oxalate. Individuals with a history of oxalate-containing kidney stones should avoid overconsuming this food. For more information, see Appendix D, page 793.

Common Fish

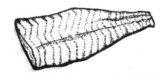

Cod

Cod are saltwater fish that live best in deep, arctic-temperature water in order to grow, reproduce, and survive. It does not seem happenstance that the words "cod" and "cold" are indeed quite similar.

Cod belong to the Gadidae family along with haddock and monkfish (the Latin word *gadus* means "cod"). There are a few varieties of cod that are typically consumed in different parts of the world, such as lingcod, saithe, and zarbo cod. However, North Atlantic cod (*Gadus morhua*) is the best-known type. Cod has a light, almost white color and a noble, buttery taste. It is usually sold as fillets up to 12 inches/30 centimeters long and 4 inches/10 centimeters wide.

HISTORY

Cod has been a dietary staple of seafaring people since the beginning of human history. In addition to being consumed fresh, preservation techniques such as salting, smoking, and drying are used. Historically the early Basque and Nordic colonies preserved cod since the sixth century C.E. This technology allowed cod to be easily transported and stored, and thus it became one of the most commercially important European fishes during the Middle Ages. Salted, dried cod is still quite popular in many nations, including Norway, Portugal, and Brazil.

Interestingly, the coastal town of Cape Cod in Massachusetts was named after the codfish that used to be bountiful in the coastal waters of that area as well as the eastern seaboard of the United States and Canada. Unfortunately, excessive fishing during the past forty to fifty years has greatly decreased the quantity of cod in these waters. In addition to North America, much of the cod available in today's fish markets hails from Iceland, Norway, Greenland, and Newfoundland.

NUTRITIONAL HIGHLIGHTS

Cod is an excellent source of protein, selenium, and vitamin B12. In addition, cod is a very good source of vitamins B6 and D, niacin, and phosphorus. A 100 gram serving has 105 calories, 23 grams of protein, 55 milligrams of cholesterol, and 0.86 grams of fat, with 105 milligrams of EPA and 175 milligrams of DHA, both of which are omega-3 fatty acids.

HEALTH BENEFITS

Fish, particularly cold-water fish such as cod, have been shown to be very beneficial for protecting against heart disease, Alzheimer's disease, and many forms of cancer. For more information, please see page 530.

HOW TO SELECT AND STORE
See page 530.

TIPS FOR PREPARING
See page 532.

QUICK SERVING IDEAS

- Combine 2 fillets of cod, 1 cup stock, 1 medium sautéed onion, and 2 cloves garlic; your favorite vegetables, such as 2 cups chopped leafy greens, 1 diced carrot, and 1 stalk diced celery; and seasonings, such as 1 teaspoon ground fennel or thyme, in a stockpot to make a delicious fish soup.
- Poaching cod is easy: Just cover it with stock and simmer over medium heat until the flesh becomes opaque, usually 7 to 10 minutes.
- Place cod in a baking dish layered with whole-wheat (wholemeal) bread crumbs and steamed spinach. Pour a sauce of olive oil, mustard, lemon juice, and seasonings on top. Bake at 450 degrees F./230 degrees C./gas 8 for about 10 to 15 minutes.
- Serve 4 to 6 chunks of sautéed cod in a large shallow bowl over a thin layer of miso soup. Garnish with chopped spring onions, daikon radish, and shiitake mushrooms.

SAFETY
See page 533.

Halibut

Halibut (*Hippoglossus hippoglossus*) can be found in both the Atlantic and Pacific Oceans, the Atlantic species being larger. A northern seawater fish, halibut is especially plentiful in the northern Pacific Ocean and off the Atlantic coasts of Newfoundland and Greenland. Halibut is big, not only in popularity and nutritional value but also in size. It is one of the largest of all saltwater fishes and weighs from 20 to 500 pounds/9 to 230 kilograms.

Halibut is a lean fish that features finely textured, snow white flesh. It boasts a slightly sweet yet mild flavor.

HISTORY

Halibut has been revered as a sacred fish throughout history and was often served on holidays, especially in medieval Europe. Interestingly, the English derivation of its name is indicative of the sacred status of this large flatfish, as the root word, *hali,* signifies "holy," and *but* signifies "flat."

NUTRITIONAL HIGHLIGHTS

Halibut is an excellent source of protein, potassium, selenium, and vitamin B12. In addition, it is a very good source of vitamin B6, niacin, and phosphorus. A 100 gram serving contains approximately 140 calories, 27 grams of protein, 41 milligrams of cholesterol, and 2.9 grams of fat, with 100 milligrams of EPA and 375 milligrams of DHA omega-3 fatty acids.

HEALTH BENEFITS

Fish, particularly cold-water fish such as halibut, have been shown to be very beneficial for protecting against heart disease, Alzheimer's disease, and many forms of cancer. For more information, please see page 530.

HOW TO SELECT AND STORE

Halibut can be purchased as either steaks or fillets; see page 530 for more information.

TIPS FOR PREPARING

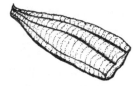

See page 532.

QUICK SERVING IDEAS

- Make fish tacos by wrapping chunks of seared halibut, salsa, and guacamole in a corn tortilla. To sear halibut, cut a 6-inch/15 centimeter piece of fillet into 1-inch/2½-centimeter chunks and place in an oiled pan on medium-high heat. Cook for 1½ minutes on each side.
- Marinate an 8-inch/20-centimeter fillet or medium halibut steak in ½ cup white wine for 1 hour in the refrigerator, dredge in ¾ cup crushed almonds, and bake at 350 degrees F./180 degrees C./gas 4 for 30 minutes.
- Serve cold pieces of baked halibut over a bed of greens. Garnish with tomatoes and orange segments, and top with your favorite dressing.
- Skewer marinated chunks of halibut and your favorite vegetables and bake in the oven or grill on the barbecue for 1 to 2 minutes per side.

SAFETY

See page 533.

Mahimahi

Called mahimahi in Hawaii and dorado in the Florida Keys, Mexico, and Latin America, this large deep-sea food and game fish is widely distributed in temperate and tropical waters around the world but is commercially caught primarily in the Pacific Ocean. Although mahimahi is a member of the Coryphaenidae family, that of the dolphin, and is classified as a common dolphin (*Coryphaena hippurus*), it is not related to the aquatic mammals also called dolphins, which are actually a type of porpoise.

With its iridescent blue-green back, yellow sides, long continuous blue dorsal fin, and steep blunt forehead, mahimahi is one of the most beautiful fish in the ocean. Surface feeders that typically migrate in large schools, mahimahi are gregarious, lively fish that often accompany ships for considerable distances in tropical waters.

The males, called bulls, can grow to a length of more than 5 feet/1½ meters and reach a weight of more than 60 pounds/27 kilograms, although mahimahi typically range in weight from 3 to 45 pounds/1½ to 20 kilograms with 15 pounds/7 kilograms being a common catch. One of the best fighting fish, mahimahi can travel at speeds up to 50 knots and are known for jumping far out of the water when chasing flying fish, their favorite meal.

Mahimahi has firm, pinkish white flesh, and its flavor, which is very similar to that of tuna or swordfish, is sweet, fresh, and mild. When cooked, the meat has a delicate, moist texture and a large flake.

HISTORY

Although found around the world, mahimahi is especially prevalent in the Pacific Ocean around the Hawaiian Islands, where it is the fish often featured, either baked, grilled, or sautéed, at luaus. In the Florida Keys, where this fish is called dorado, it is most readily available freshly caught in the summer months.

NUTRITIONAL HIGHLIGHTS

Mahimahi is an excellent source of protein, potassium, selenium, and vitamin B12. In addition, mahimahi is a very good source of niacin and phosphorus. A 100 gram serving contains approximately 109 calories, 24 grams of protein, 94 milligrams of cholesterol, and 0.9 grams of fat, with 110 milligrams of DHA but only negligible amounts of EPA.

HEALTH BENEFITS

Mahimahi is a lean fish having only 1 gram of fat, of which only ¼ gram is saturated. Therefore, mahimahi is a good fish to include in a diet that is lower in calories and fat intake. Its high DHA content and quality protein make it an excellent "brain" food.

HOW TO SELECT AND STORE

If available in the U.K., mahimahi can be purchased as either steaks or fillets; see page 530 for more information.

TIPS FOR PREPARING

See page 532.

QUICK SERVING IDEAS

- Baked Cajun mahimahi: Sprinkle fish steaks with Cajun seasoning, a dash of cayenne pepper, salt, and freshly ground black pepper. Preheat the oven to 350 degrees F./180 degrees C./gas 4. Heat 1 tablespoon olive or coconut oil in a pan and sear the fish on both sides to brown, then transfer to an oven-safe dish and bake for 4 to 5 minutes. Top with a fruit salsa made of 1 cup of your favorite chopped tropical fruits, such as melon, pineapple, kiwi, and banana, tossed with a tablespoon each of balsamic vinegar and honey or maple syrup.

- Barbecued mango mahimahi: Cut 1½ pounds/700 grams of mahimahi into serving-sized portions (3½ ounces or 100 grams) and place in a glass dish or bowl. Combine ¼ cup olive oil, ½ cup mango juice, and ½ cup finely chopped basil. Pour over the fish, cover, and marinate in the refrigerator for 1 hour. Clean the barbecue surface and coat with olive or coconut oil. When the coals are covered with gray ash, place the mahimahi on the grill about 6 inches/15 centimeters above the coals. Grill 5 to 6 minutes on each side. Be sure to baste before turning.

- Sautéed sweet potato mahimahi: Line up three small bowls. In the first, put ½ cup flour, in the second, ½ cup beaten egg whites, and in the third, 1 medium sweet potato, shredded medium fine. Dredge the fish fillets in flour, then coat with egg white and sweet potato shreds. Sprinkle with salt and pepper and transfer to a large pan coated with olive oil to prevent sticking. Sauté 2 to 3 minutes each side until brown, transfer to a serving platter, and top with pineapple green grape vinaigrette. To make the vinaigrette, sauté ½ cup minced Walla Walla onion or spring onions and 1 tablespoon minced ginger in 2 tablespoons olive oil until the onion turns translucent. Then add 2 tablespoons honey, 1 teaspoon molasses, ¾ cup rice or balsamic vinegar, ½ cup fresh pineapple chunks, and ½ cup chopped seedless grapes. Sauté an additional 5 minutes.

- Macadamia nut-crusted mahimahi: Preheat the oven to 350 degrees F./180 degrees C./gas 4. Combine ¼ cup whole-wheat (wholemeal) bread crumbs, 2 tablespoons finely shredded coconut, ½ cup finely chopped macadamia nuts, 2 teaspoons chopped fresh coriander leaves, ½ teaspoon minced fresh thyme, and ¼ teaspoon jerk seasoning or cayenne pepper. Coat one side of two mahimahi steaks with the macadamia nut mixture. Place fish crusted side up on a baking tray and bake 10 to 12 minutes, then grill 1 to 2 minutes until the crust turns golden brown.

SAFETY

See page 533.

Salmon

Salmon is perhaps the most incredible fish in many ways—both from a nutritional perspective and simply as a marvel of nature. Although born in fresh water, salmon spend a good portion of their lives navigating the open sea, only to swim back hundreds of miles to return to their birthplace in order to spawn. There's a reason why these intelligent, intuitive fish are considered a "brain food."

Salmon varieties are usually classified by the ocean in which they are located. In the Pacific they are considered part of the genus *Oncorhynchus,* and in the Atlantic they belong to the genus *Salmo.* There exist five species of Pacific salmon, including chinook (or king), sockeye (or red), coho (or silver), pink, and chum, and only one Atlantic species. Norwegian salmon, a popular type of salmon often offered on American East Coast restaurant menus, is actually Atlantic salmon that is farm-raised in Norway. In the U.S., much of the salmon available in today's market comes from the waters of Alaska, the Pacific Northwest, eastern Canada, Norway, and Greenland. In the U.K., about 90 percent of fish farms are in Scotland—the main source of salmon in Britain. Wild Alaskan salmon is also available.

Salmon characteristics vary with the species. The colors of these fish range from pink to red to orange. In addition, some salmon are richer and contain more fat than others. Some are considered to be richer in flavor. The chinook and sockeye varieties are fattier than pink and chum, while coho falls somewhere in the middle. Not surprisingly, the Chinook, sockeye, and coho are favorites for steaks and fillets. Pink salmon is usually used primarily for canned food. Chum is generally reserved for processed food production. Chinook salmon are the largest, with a maximum length of 55 inches/140 centimeters and a weight of 80 pounds/36 kilograms. Sockeye is the smallest salmon, growing to only 15 pounds/7 kilograms. Due to the various species parameters, cuts and fillet sizes are variable.

HISTORY

Like other fish, salmon has been enjoyed since time immemorial. In addition to eating fresh fish, techniques such as smoking and salting have been used to preserve salmon. To this day, smoked salmon is enjoyed as traditional fare in the cuisines of the Russian Federation, Britain, and Scandinavia.

NUTRITIONAL HIGHLIGHTS

Salmon is an excellent source of protein, potassium, selenium, and vitamin B12. In addition, salmon is a very good source of niacin and phosphorus. A 100 gram serving contains approximately 231 calories, 25 grams of protein, and 85 milligrams of cholesterol. Wild salmon has more calories than leaner fish, such as mahimahi, because of its fatty acid content. A serving contains 13 grams of fat, with 1,000 milligrams of EPA and 725 milligrams of DHA. Farmed Atlantic salmon has 690 milligrams of EPA and 1,490 milligrams of DHA per serving.

FDA statistics on the nutritional content (protein and fat ratios) of farmed versus wild salmon show that wild salmon have a 20 percent higher protein content and a 20 percent lower fat content than farmed salmon. And while farmed salmon also provide high levels of omega-3 fatty acids, the benefits from these fats are somewhat offset by a higher content of omega-6 fatty acids.

HEALTH BENEFITS

Fish, particularly cold-water fish such as salmon, have been shown to be very beneficial for protecting against heart disease, Alzheimer's disease, and many forms of cancer (see page 530). In terms of health benefits, salmon is one of the most highly valued fish because of its exceptionally high content of omega-3 fatty acids. Wild Alaskan salmon also tends to be one of the cleanest sources of fish, as it typically contains the lowest levels of heavy metals and pesticide residues.

HOW TO SELECT AND STORE

Salmon can be purchased as either steaks or fillets, or smoked; see page 530 for more information.

TIPS FOR PREPARING

See page 532.

QUICK SERVING IDEAS

- Combine leftover cold salmon with greens and vegetables for a delicious salad. Or place between two pieces of whole-wheat (wholemeal) bread, garnish with mustard, and enjoy an easy-to-make yet exceptionally delicious sandwich.

100 grams of fresh fillet of	Total Omega-3 Fats	Total Omega-6 Fats	Ratio of Omega-3 to Omega-6 Fats
Wild coho salmon	0.92 gram	0.06 gram	15.3:1
Farmed coho salmon	1.42 gram	0.46 gram	3.1:1
Wild rainbow trout	0.77 gram	0.33 gram	2.3:1
Farmed rainbow trout	1.00 gram	0.71 gram	1.4:1
Wild channel catfish	0.29 gram	0.24 gram	1.2:1
Farmed channel catfish	0.37 gram	1.56 gram	0.2:1

- For a twist on scrambled eggs, combine eggs with lox (smoked salmon) and onions, a classic New York delicatessen breakfast favorite.
- Combine ½ pound/250 grams silken tofu and ½ pound/250 grams baked or smoked salmon in a blender with 2 tablespoons lemon juice, ½ cup chopped spring onions, and ⅓ cup parsley or dill to create a delicious dip. Season with salt and pepper to taste.
- Serve baked salmon over whole-wheat pasta. Top with a sauce made of 4 tablespoons olive oil, ¼ cup fresh chopped dill weed, ¼ cup lemon peel, ½ cup sliced spring onions, and black pepper to taste.
- For a healthy appetizer, serve smoked salmon on a platter with onions, capers, lemon wedges, and mini rye bread slices.

SAFETY

Fish farms now contribute a large amount of the fish being consumed, including more than 50 percent of salmon in the U.S. In the U.K., it is estimated that only 2 percent of salmon eaten is from the wild, while the Scottish salmon farming industry generates about £500 million per year. However, the bottom line is that wild "free range" fish are superior in many ways to their farm-raised counterparts. Several studies have also shown that farmed salmon accumulate more cancer-causing pesticide residues than wild salmon. However, these studies fail to make a strong case that eating farm-raised fish poses a significant safety concern. To ensure the safety of the food supply, the FDA has studied PCBs and set limits for tolerable levels that are not associated with risks to human health. For fish, the tolerable level of PCBs is millionths of a gram (parts per million, or ppm). At 0.056 part per million, the level of PCBs found in farmed salmon is still 1/35 the unsafe level of 2.0 ppm.

The reason that farm-raised fish have higher levels of pesticides appears to be the type of feed they are given. Farmed fish are given feed pellets that are most often made from fish meal and fish oil—extracted from sardines, anchovies, and other ground-up fish. Pesticides have circulated into the ocean, where they are absorbed by marine life and accumulate in their fat. If the fish oil is not properly distilled to reduce the concentrations of these pesticides, it can lead to much higher concentrations in the salmon feed. One commercial salmon feed analyzed in a Canadian study showed a total pesticide level ten times higher than that of any other feed. The obvious solution is to set limits on allowable pesticide residues in not only farm-raised fish but also the feed that they are given.

There is also concern about some of the synthetic carotenes being used to color farmed salmon. In the wild, salmon absorb carotenes from eating pink krill. On the aqua farm, their rich pink hue is supplied by either synthetic astaxanthin or natural astaxanthin derived from algae or krill. Without the help of supplemental astaxanthin, the flesh of farmed salmon would look similar in color to that of halibut.

While there appears to be no harm with astaxanthin, there does appear to be some risk with using the synthetic carotene canthaxanthin, as this compound was linked to retinal damage in people taking it as a sunless tanning pill. Although no government has banned canthaxanthin from fish feed, most salmon growers are now using astaxanthin instead.

Unfortunately, for consumers, there is no real way to know whether they are getting salmon colored with astaxanthin or canthaxanthin. The FDA does, however, limit the acceptable amount of canthaxanthin to 30 milligrams per pound of salmon, thereby significantly minimizing the safety risk.

Another big concern regarding fish farms is their environmental impact. To address the issue of environmental impact, beginning in the mid-1990s, many salmon farms began using underwater cameras to monitor the salmon as they feed below the surface of the water. By using underwater cameras, the amount of over-feeding and uneaten feed has been reduced considerably, to almost zero.

However, of potentially greater concern is the effect that farmed Atlantic salmon escaping into the wild may have on the gene pool of wild Pacific salmon. Biologists in the U.S. fear that these invaders will outcompete Pacific salmon and trout for food and territory, hastening the demise of the wild fish. An Atlantic salmon takeover could knock nature's balance out of whack and turn a healthy, diverse marine habitat into one dominated by a single invasive species. Similarly, there are concerns in the U.K. about escaped farmed salmon breeding with the dwindling wild stock and weakening the wild salmon's natural resistance to pests, disease and other hardships.

Recently, some large commercial farms have begun seeking U.S. and Canadian approval to alter genes to produce a growth hormone that could shave a year off the usual two and a half to three years it takes to raise a market-size fish. The prospect of genetically modified salmon that can grow six times as fast as normal fish has heightened anxiety that these GMO fish will escape and pose an even greater danger to native species than do the farmed Atlantic salmon.

Please also see page 533 for other safety concerns.

Red Snapper

There are about 185 species of snapper worldwide, all of which belong to the Lutjanidae family of fish. Red snapper *(Lutjanus campechanus)* is a firm, white-meat deep-saltwater fish characterized by a red-and-pink upper body and silvery whitish skin below. Both the flesh and skin of this fish are commonly served as fillets. Red snapper can live up to fifty years and can grow to 3 feet/1 meter in length.

Red snapper has a mild flavor, making it quite easily adapted to a variety of preparation methods. Due to the popularity of snapper around the world, imitator fishes have surfaced to meet the demand. "Pacific red snapper," for example, is not actually red snapper but red rockfish. As a result, it is advisable to buy red snapper only from a verifiable source or a reputable market.

HISTORY

Red snapper comes from deep waters off the United States' Atlantic Coast. It is especially well established in the Gulf of Mexico. Threatened by overfishing, implementation of stricter fishing laws in the late 1980s and 1990s were designed to protect the red snapper in American waters.

NUTRITIONAL HIGHLIGHTS

Red snapper is an excellent source of protein, potassium, selenium, and vitamin B12. In addition, red snapper is a very good source of vitamin B6, niacin, and phosphorus. A 100 gram serving contains approximately 128 calories, 26 grams of protein, 47 milligrams of cholesterol, and 1.72 grams of fat, with 270 milligrams of DHA but only negligible amounts of EPA.

HEALTH BENEFITS

Fish consumption has been shown to be very beneficial for protecting against heart disease, Alzheimer's disease, and many forms of cancer. For more information, please see page 530.

HOW TO SELECT AND STORE

Red snapper can be purchased primarily as fillets; see page 530 for more information.

TIPS FOR PREPARING

See page 532.

QUICK SERVING IDEAS

- Before baking, marinate 2 snapper fillets in ½ cup citrus juice and 2 to 3 tablespoons honey.
- Use snapper in fish tacos.
- Serve 1 fillet baked snapper over 1½ cups whole-wheat pasta and top with your favorite tomato sauce.
- Brush 4 fillets of snapper with olive oil, and dredge in a combination of 1 cup whole-wheat (wholemeal) bread crumbs, 1 cup of your favorite ground nut, and 2 teaspoons ground spices, such as cumin, coriander, and mustard seed for an Indian flair. Bake for 7 minutes at 350 degrees F./180 degrees C./gas 4, then grill for 1 to 2 minutes to crispen the crust.
- Serve leftover or cooled baked or grilled snapper cold over a green summer salad topped with your favorite dressing.

SAFETY

See page 533.

Swordfish

Swordfish is the common name of a food and game fish *(Xiphias gladius)* up to 15 feet/4½ meters long characterized by its distinctive sail-like dorsal fin and the elongation of its upper jaw bones to form a rigid, swordlike blade, which typically constitutes one-third of its body length. Found primarily in tropical waters around the Americas and Hawaiian Islands, swordfish inhabit the Mediterranean Sea and Indian Ocean as well. In the Atlantic Ocean, swordfish range from Nova Scotia to Argentina in the west and from Ireland to South Africa in the east, while in the Pacific they range from Asia to Chile. Also called the broadbill, the swordfish varies in color from a dark metallic purplish cast on its upper back to white on its belly. Fast swimmers easily reaching speeds up to 60 miles/100 kilometers per hour with enormous eyes that enable them to pursue prey at depths of 500 fathoms, swordfish feed principally at night on squid, herring, mackerel, tuna, and other fish, slashing their prey with their swordlike bills since they have no teeth.

The flesh of swordfish is firm, dense, and meatlike, which, combined with its mildly steaklike flavor and moderate fat content, makes this fish an excellent choice for grilling, barbecuing, sautéing, baking, or poaching.

HISTORY

Although most references describe the swordfish as a game fish weighing an average of 200 to 400 pounds/90 to 180 kilograms, the typical weight of swordfish commercially caught in the Atlantic Ocean has steadily declined since the first recorded sale of Atlantic swordfish in 1817. Swordfish caught in 1861 ranged from 400 to 500 pounds/180 to 230 kilograms. By the turn of the twentieth century, the weight had dropped to 300 to 400 pounds/140 to 180 kilograms. In 1961, when long-line fishing largely replaced harpoons as the primary commercial gear used, the average weight dropped to 261 pounds/118 kilograms.

Unlike harpooning, which is limited to catching large fish basking at the surface, long lines catch fish of all sizes and at different depths; these fishing lines stretch for dozens of miles and are baited with hundreds of hooks. As a result, fishermen are able to catch many more fish at a time, including young, immature fish.

Soon after long-line fishing became the standard, so many of the mature swordfish of reproductive age had been caught that the swordfish population began to decline. With heavy fishing, the downward trend accelerated in the late 1980s, and by 1995, the weight of the average swordfish had dropped by almost 70 percent below 1960 levels. As large swordfish have become increasingly rare, the once-thriving harpoon fishery and the recreational fishery for swordfish, both of which targeted the largest fish, have largely disappeared.

Today, the typical weight of commercially caught North Atlantic swordfish is 88 pounds/40 kilograms. Most swordfish—almost two of every three—are now caught before they have a chance to spawn. On average, females do not mature until age five, by which time they weigh about 150 pounds/68 kilograms, while males mature at three years, when they weigh about 72 pounds/33 kilograms. In 1995, 83 percent of the females and 36 percent of the males caught commercially were still immature. Today, swordfish in the North Atlantic are classified as overfished by the federal government and are listed as endangered on the International Union for Conservation of Nature and Natural Resources' Red List of Threatened Species.

Hopefully, swordfish management efforts will soon put a halt to the decline of this magnificent fish, since currently, the Atlantic swordfish population is at a level that is only 50 percent of the maximum sustainable yield (MSY), while a healthy population would be at a level of two times the MSY. Beyond a certain point, the population will have too few adults to sustain itself and, unless fishing pressure is reduced, will continue to spiral downward. Eventually, a point will be reached at which too few adults remain to find one another for spawning, and the population will decline to extinction even if all fishing were to be stopped. The most frightening fact is that no one knows where that point lies.

Maintaining swordfish and other top predators in the Atlantic is critically important to the health of ocean ecosystems that sustain life on Earth. On the ecological bright side, swordfish are prolific egg producers—a large female can produce 30 million eggs each year. Swordfish are capable of rapid recovery if only given the chance, which will necessitate effective conservation by all countries fishing for them.

Like other large ocean-roaming species such as tuna and marlin, swordfish migrate over large distances and are caught by fishermen from the U.S., Spain, Canada, Portugal, and Japan. Spain and the United States dominate the North Atlantic swordfish catch, followed by Canada and Portugal.

In the eastern Pacific, swordfish range from Oregon to Chile, so consumers can help, while still enjoying swordfish, by refraining from purchasing North Atlantic swordfish. Ask your restaurateur or fishmonger where the swordfish on the menu or the shelf comes from. If they don't know, don't buy it. Explain your intent not to buy swordfish from the North Atlantic until adequate recovery measures for these swordfish are in place.

Most of the swordfish taken in the commercial fishery in the north Pacific are four- to five-year-olds, although some as young as one year are occasionally caught as well. As of 1989, scientists still considered Pacific Ocean swordfish stocks to be in good condition and able to withstand increased catches. In the Pacific, the top swordfish-harvesting nations are Japan, Chile, the Philippines, and the United States.

NUTRITIONAL HIGHLIGHTS

Swordfish is an excellent source of protein, selenium, and vitamin B12. In addition, swordfish is a very good source of niacin, potassium, and phosphorus. A 100 gram serving contains approximately 155 calories, 25 grams of protein, 50 milligrams of cholesterol, and 5 grams of fat, with 138 milligrams of EPA and 681 milligrams of DHA, both of which are omega-3 fatty acids.

HEALTH BENEFITS

Fish consumption has been shown to be very beneficial for protecting against heart disease, Alzheimer's disease, and many forms of cancer (see page 530 for more information).

HOW TO SELECT AND STORE

Swordfish can be purchased as steaks. See page 530 for more information.

TIPS FOR PREPARING

See page 532.

QUICK SERVING IDEAS

- Its moderate fat content will help keep swordfish moist when baked. Simply brush a 100 gram serving with a little olive oil, sprinkle with your favorite herbs and a pinch of freshly ground salt and pepper, and bake at 400 to 450 degrees F./200 to 230 degrees C./gas 6 to 8 for 10 to 15 minutes. Serve on a bed of steamed spinach drizzled with fresh lemon juice.

- Its exceptionally firm flesh makes swordfish an excellent choice for kebabs. For a quick delicious summer dinner, try skewering swordfish on rosemary branches, then grilling and serving with vine-ripened tomatoes, onions, and cucumbers. Following are easy directions: Strip the leaves from 6 to 8 mature rosemary branches. Cut 1 pound/½ kilogram of swordfish into 1-inch/2½-centimeter cubes and marinate in the refrigerator for 1 hour in ½ cup olive oil, ¼ cup lemon juice, a clove or two of minced garlic, a teaspoon each of fresh minced rosemary and oregano, and a pinch of salt and pepper. Preheat the grill to medium-high, then skewer the cubes on the rosemary branches, about 5 per branch. Grill until just cooked through, about 3 to 4 minutes each side. Mince some of the remaining rosemary leaves and use to flavor a vinaigrette composed of ½ cup olive oil, ½ cup lemon juice, ½ teaspoon salt, ½ teaspoon honey, and pepper to taste. Use to dress a salad made of 1 medium diced cucumber, 2 halved and sliced Roma tomatoes, ½ sliced red onion, a dozen kalamata olives, and ½ to 1 cup cubed feta cheese.

- Due to both its firm flesh and its moderate fat content, swordfish is an ideal fish to poach. Immerse 2 steaks in a pan of fish stock or a mixture of water and ¼ cup lemon juice or ½ cup white wine. Add several tablespoons of your favorite minced fresh herbs, bring the liquid to a gentle simmer, cover the pan partially, and poach until opaque, about 15 minutes. Or poach in stock seasoned with 1 cup diced tomatoes, 1 cup thinly sliced leeks or onions, 2 cloves minced garlic, 2 to 4 tablespoons lemon juice, 1 tablespoon fresh tarragon and/or thyme, and 2 to 4 tablespoons capers.

- Dip 1-inch/2½-centimeter chunks of swordfish in milk, then dredge in a mixture of 1 cup bread crumbs, ½ cup flour, or cornflour, and sauté in a pan liberally brushed with olive or coconut oil or sprayed with olive oil cooking spray. Cook until browned, turning once. Serve with sautéed onions, sweet peppers, mushrooms, and greens, such as Swiss chard or collards.

- Make your own fish sticks. Dip strips of swordfish in a mixture of milk and egg, then dredge in seasoned bread crumbs. These can

be quickly made by putting herbed croutons in a plastic bag and crushing with a rolling pin. Spray a baking tray with olive oil cooking spray and bake at 400 degrees F./200 degrees C./gas 6 for about 10 minutes.

SAFETY

Sadly, swordfish have been found to contain the highest levels of mercury of any of the larger edible fish. The Food and Drug Administration in the U.S. and the Food Standards Agency in the U.K. recommend that pregnant women, women of childbearing age, and young children avoid eating swordfish, shark, mackerel, and tilefish. These fish often harbor high levels of methylmercury, a potent human neurotoxin. Methylmercury readily crosses the placenta and has the potential to significantly damage the foetal nervous system. For other individuals in good health, swordfish is best consumed no more than once each month.

Several recent studies have confirmed a direct correlation between frequent consumption of swordfish and excessively elevated blood levels of mercury. In a study conducted in San Francisco and published in *Environmental Health Perspectives* in April 2003, involving 123 subjects who consumed thirty different types of fish, frequent consumption of swordfish had the highest correlation with blood mercury levels exceeding the maximum recommended by the U.S. Environmental Protection Agency (EPA) and the National Academy of Sciences.

The mean level for women in this survey was ten times that of mercury levels found in a recent population survey by the U.S. Centers for Disease Control and Prevention. Some children tested were found to have mercury levels greater than forty times the national mean. In another study of sixty-nine subjects conducted at the Harvard Medical School, eleven were found to have blood mercury concentrations greater than 15 micrograms per liter. The EPA and the National Academy of Sciences recommend keeping the whole blood mercury level less than 5 micrograms per liter. Ten of the eleven cases were explained by regular to heavy fish consumption, and six of these ten subjects ate swordfish regularly.

Please see page 533 for other safety concerns.

Tuna

Tuna has a steaklike firmness and density. It boasts the meatiest flavor and texture of any fish. The most popular varieties of tuna are yellowfin *(Thunnus albacares)*, bluefin *(Thunnus thynnus)*, and albacore *(Thunnus alalunga)*. The bluefin and yellowfin are deep red in color, while albacore is a pale pink. Tuna steaks are often found to have a central section of dark brown flesh that has a stronger, more intense flavor. This color indicates the musculature these powerful fish utilize for long-distance swimming. Tuna are found in the warm-water areas of the Pacific, Atlantic, and Indian Oceans, as well as the Mediterranean Sea.

Tuna has become one of the most popular saltwater catches in the world, thanks in part to the commercial success of canned tuna. Although canned tuna can make a tasteful and nutritious meal, many fish lovers will tell you that fresh fish is tastier, and it's even healthier, as the fresh tuna contains more omega-3 fatty acids than its canned counterpart.

HISTORY

Fresh tuna has been enjoyed by seacoast populations throughout recorded history. Smoked and pickled tuna were also popular in more ancient times. Appearing first in 1903, canned tuna is extremely popular throughout the world, and in the United States it is the most widely consumed fish of all (the cod remains the most popular fish in the U.K.). In the United States, annual canned tuna consumption is estimated to be about 50 million cases, or roughly 28 percent of global consumption. It is also the most popular canned fish in the U.K.

The major tuna-producing countries are Mexico, Thailand, the United States, Spain, Italy, Japan, Taiwan, and the Philippines.

NUTRITIONAL HIGHLIGHTS

Tuna is an excellent source of protein, potassium, selenium, and vitamin B12. In addition, tuna is a very good source of niacin and phosphorus. A 100 gram serving of bluefin tuna contains approximately 184 calories, 30 grams of protein, 49 milligrams of cholesterol, and 6 grams of fat, with 363 milligrams of EPA and 1,141 milligrams of DHA, both of which are omega-3 fatty acids. In comparison, the same serving of yellowfin tuna contains approximately 140 calories, 30 grams of protein, 58 milligrams of cholesterol, and 1.2 grams of fat, with 50 milligrams of EPA and 230 milligrams of DHA.

HEALTH BENEFITS

Fish have been shown to be very beneficial for protecting against heart disease, Alzheimer's disease, and many forms of cancer. For more information, please see page 530.

HOW TO SELECT AND STORE

Tuna can be purchased as fillets or steaks; see page 530 for more information.

TIPS FOR PREPARING

See page 532.

QUICK SERVING IDEAS

- Salade niçoise, the classic French dish, features tuna combined with steamed green beans and potatoes. Here are directions for a salade niçoise for eight to ten people. For the vinaigrette: Combine and whisk 3 tablespoons cider vinegar, 1 tablespoon Dijon mustard, 1 cup extra virgin olive oil, 1 medium paper-thin sliced white onion, 2 cloves minced garlic, 3 cups loosely packed flat-leaf parsley leaves, ¾ cup loosely packed mixture of tarragon and fresh chervil leaves, and sea salt and freshly ground black pepper to taste. For the salad: Cook 2 pounds/1 kilogram of tiny new potatoes until just tender, about 15 minutes, and add to ⅓ of the vinaigrette, toss, and set aside. Rub with rapeseed oil and grill 2 pounds/1 kilogram fresh tuna steaks for 5 to 7 minutes on each side, then let cool and remove skin and bones. Drizzle with vinaigrette on both sides and set aside. Steam 1 pound/½ kilogram each trimmed green and yellow beans for 5 to 6 minutes, combine with ½ each red and yellow bell peppers, cut in thin (¼-inch/½ centimeter) strips and enough vinaigrette to coat and arrange them in the center of a serving platter. Top them with 20 anchovy fillets (op-

tional). Place 4 quartered eggs and 6 medium quartered red and yellow tomatoes around the beans and peppers. Drizzle them with 2 to 3 tablespoons of the vinaigrette. Place the potatoes on another platter. Break the tuna apart into large pieces, and arrange the pieces attractively atop the potatoes. Sprinkle with 1 cup niçoise olives. Drizzle with any remaining vinaigrette, and garnish with several sprigs of parsley and chervil.

- There are numerous choices when making tuna salad, as many different ingredients can complement tuna's mild flavor. Some of our favorite tuna salad ingredients include olives, capers, chili peppers, leeks, fennel, and walnuts. A simple combination is 1 cup cooked tuna broken into small chunks, 1 to 2 tablespoons prepared mustard, 1 tablespoon rapeseed-oil-based mayonnaise, 1 tablespoon extra-virgin olive oil, and ¼ cup each diced carrot, celery, and red onion. Combine and season to taste with dill, salt, and pepper.

- Skewer 1½-inch/4 centimeter pieces of tuna fish along with your favorite grilling vegetables, brush lightly with olive oil infused with your favorite herbs, and grill for 1 to 2 minutes per side.

- Enjoy a dinner with the tastes of the Mediterranean: Grill 4 100-gram servings of tuna for 7 to 10 minutes. Serve on a bed of 1 cup combined lightly sautéed peppers, tomatoes, and onions, and top with 3 pitted kalamata olives.

- For an Asian-inspired meal with a fiery flavor, dredge 4 100-gram tuna steaks in a combination of ¼ cup dried wasabi powder, ¼ cup cornflour, and ½ cup sesame seeds before baking at 350 degrees F./180 degrees C./gas 4 for 15 to 20 minutes.

SAFETY

Given the mercury content of tuna, especially larger varieties, you should not consume more than 12 ounces/350 grams of fresh or canned tuna per week. This guideline is particularly important during pregnancy. Please also see page 533 for other safety concerns.

Common Crustaceans

Crustaceans are characterized by having segmented bodies and chitinous exoskeletons. Crustaceans can be divided according to size into two main groups. The larger group includes prawns, lobsters, and crabs. The smaller group includes species that are either microscopic or range up to two inches/5 centimeters in size. Most of the smaller marine crustaceans can be found in plankton and thereby occupy an important position in the marine food chain. The larger crustaceans are often used for human consumption. We will address them in detail here.

Crab

The majority of edible crabs have five pairs of legs, with the front legs being the larger pincers. They can live in both shallow and deep-sea waters, though they are typically found in the intertidal areas up to 10 meters deep because areas with a moderate current and edges of banks provide protection. They prey on a large variety of animals, including clams, fish, other crabs, sea stars, worms, squid, snails, and eggs from fish or crabs.

Since a crab's skeleton is on the outside of its body, the only way for a crab to grow is to shed its old shell. For one to three months after shedding the shell, a crab is soft-shelled. After shedding its shell, a crab will expand its body mass by swallowing water, then form a new shell over this larger mass. Once the new shell is in place, the crab grows to fit the new size. For the first two years of life, a crab sheds its shell several times a year. Once adult-sized (3 years old or more), a crab sheds its shell only about once a year.

Out of the 4,400 varieties of crab, only a few are popular edible varieties in the U.S.: Alaskan king, blue, Dungeness, soft-shell, snow, and stone. In the U.K., the most common edible variety is the brown crab, but shore crabs, spider crabs and velvet swimming crabs are also edible if more fiddly to eat. These vary in size, shape, and the flavor of their meat.

Alaskan King Crab
(*Paralithoides camtschaticus*)

The king of crabs can measure up to 10 feet/3 meters, claw to claw, and weighs an average of 10 to 15 pounds/4½ to 7 kilograms. The delicately flavored meat is snowy white with beautiful bright red edges. King crabs are found

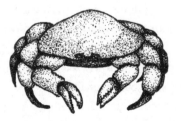

in the Bering Sea and northern Pacific Ocean, with the most abundant harvest in the seas around Alaska, thus lending this crab its name.

Blue Crab (*Callinectes sapidus*)

Named for its blue claws and oval, dark blue-green shell, the blue crab is often found along the Gulf and Atlantic coasts. *Callinectes sapidus* means "beautiful swimmer," and it is indeed a beautiful color. Blue crab is the most prolific species on the East Coast of the United States, ranging from 3½ to 5½ inches/9 to 14 centimeters in size. These crabs turn red when cooked.

Dungeness Crab (*Cancer magister*)

Dungeness crabs are native to the Pacific coast and can be found all the way from Alaska to Mexico. This crab is named for the former small town of Dungeness on the Olympic Peninsula in Washington State, which was the first city to begin commercially harvesting the delicacy, though the Dungeness crab is also a mainstay in the San Francisco area, where it is a featured attraction at the world-famous Fisherman's Wharf. This large crab can range from 1 to 4 pounds/½ to 2 kilograms. Its pink flesh is succulent and sweet. Only males are harvested; female crabs may not be taken as a way to avoid overharvesting.

Snow Crab (*Cancer quanbumi*)

The snow crab, also known as queen crab, measures up to 2 feet/60 centimeters from claw to claw and can weigh as much as 3 pounds/1½ kilograms. Larger snow crabs are harvested in the waters off Alaska, while smaller snow crabs are found in shallow waters.

Soft-Shell Crab (*Callinectes sapidus*)

Soft-shell crabs are simply blue crabs that have shed their shells in order to grow larger ones. Soon after the crab sheds its shell, its skin hardens into a new one. During the few days before the new shell hardens, they are referred to as "soft-shell" crabs.

Stone Crab (*Menippe mercenaria*)

Stone crabs derive their name from their rock-like, oval-shaped shells, of which only the claw meat is eaten. Their large claws, characterized by black tips, have tremendous power and are capable of crushing an oyster shell like a grape. Stone crabs are harvested seven months out of the year, mid-October through to mid-May. Since only the claws are eaten, fishermen twist off one claw from each crab and toss them back to grow new ones. In this manner, they are left with one claw to defend themselves with. Crabs regenerate their claws within eighteen months. The law requires stone crab claws to be boiled for 7 minutes and then either put on ice or frozen. Stone crab claws are usually served cold with dipping sauces. Meat from the claws of the stone crab has a firm texture and a sweet, succulent flavor.

Common Brown Crab (*Cancer pagurus*)

In the U.K., the brown crab is the most commonly consumed type of crab and is available from most fishmongers and good supermarkets. They have large black-tipped pincer claws and a "pie-crust" edge, and most average 6 inches/15 centimeters in their widest part (crabs under 4 inches/12 centimeters should, by law, be thrown back to grow larger). Brown crabs mature between three and five years and can live for twenty years.

Shore Crabs

These crabs are prized in Italy but not commonly eaten in the U.K., either in their "soft-shell" state or normal hard shell. They are easy to catch at the base of sea walls or under jetties.

Spider Crabs

These crabs are spiky and often covered with barnacles and other debris, some scientists think as a camouflage. They are a delicacy in Spain with their sweet, good-textured meat. Most of the U.K. catch goes to Continental Europe, but spider crabs can be bought from some fishmongers or off the boats at fishing ports.

Velvet Swimming Crabs

These purplish, velvet-covered crabs turn bright orange when cooked and have good-flavored meat. They can be found in some U.K. fishmongers, but most of the catch is exported to the south of France for Provençal fish soup.

HISTORY

Crabs are among the oldest species on Earth. The horseshoe crab dates back over 200 million years and is literally a living fossil. Not surprisingly, crabs have been consumed by humans since man first walked the earth.

NUTRITIONAL HIGHLIGHTS

The meat of these varieties of crab is low in fat, high in protein, and a moderate source of omega-3 fatty acids. A 100 gram serving contains an average of 100 calories and 20 grams of protein.

Like other crustaceans, crabmeat does contain cholesterol (king has 53 milligrams per serving, snow has 71 milligrams, Dungeness has

76 milligrams, and blue has 100 milligrams), but it is very low in fat (3 grams per serving) and even lower in saturated fat (1 gram per serving). While not quite as high in omega-3s as salmon, crabmeat contains about 300 to 400 milligrams of omega-3 fatty acids per serving.

HEALTH BENEFITS

Because of its high content of omega-3 fatty acids, the meat of these varieties of crab provides the same sort of benefits as fish. For more information, see page 530.

HOW TO SELECT AND STORE

When Alaskan king, stone, and snow crabs are caught at sea, they are cooked and blast frozen; therefore, they are most often purchased already cooked. Dungeness and blue crabs are often available previously cooked and either displayed on ice or frozen. Soft-shell crabs should be purchased from April to September. If available alive, they should be alert and brandish their pincers when poked. Crabs should have a fresh saltwater aroma; avoid those that smell of ammonia, sour or extremely fishy. Typically, a good crab feels heavy for its size. The yield of meat from a healthy crab will be about one third of its total weight. Normally, the larger the crab, the better the yield and the easier it is to clean.

Crab or crabmeat is available all year round in some form, including live, raw, frozen, cooked, and canned. Live crabs should be refrigerated and used on the day of purchase. Thawed, cooked crab should be used within the same day of purchase. Vacuum-packed crab can be stored in the refrigerator up to one month and used within four days of opening, or stored in the freezer for up to six months. Canned crab is good for six months. To freeze fresh crabmeat, cook the crabs and remove the meat. Pack into airtight containers and cover with a light brine (4 teaspoons of salt to 1 liter of water), leaving ½ inch/1 cm headspace in the container. Frozen crab can be stored up to one month.

TIPS FOR PREPARING

For Alaskan king and snow crabs, reheating is all that is usually required. First thaw the crabs in the refrigerator for 12 to 24 hours. If you're in a big hurry, the crabs can be rinsed under cold running water for 45 to 60 minutes. To determine if the crabs are thawed, try bending the legs at their joints. Once thawed, the crabs can be prepared for cooking. Steaming for 6 to 7 minutes is preferred to maintain moistness. Usually the meat can be accessed by cracking the shell with a nutcracker.

Stone crab claws are usually served cold with a dipping sauce (follow thawing instructions above). Again, a nutcracker is usually all that is required, though some people enjoy getting at the meat with a mallet.

Dungeness and blue crabs or British brown and spider crabs, if they are live, will have to be steamed in a large pot. Place one crab in at least 2 inches/5 centimeters of boiling water and close the lid. The crab won't be happy, but the steam acts fast. Once the pot is boiling again, add the next crab, and so on. Let the pot boil for 20 minutes after the last is put in for crabs up to 1½ kilograms (add another 5 minutes per extra 500 grams). The smaller shore and velvet swimming crabs need only 5 to 8 minutes in boiling water.

Before cooking soft-shell crabs, they need to be cleaned by first turning the crab upside down. With scissors, lift up the "apron" from the abdomen of the crab, and cut it off where it joins the body. Turn the crabs right side up and lift each flap where the shell comes to a point; pull or scrape off the spongy gills and remove the brain sac from behind the eyes.

Most people remove only the dark meat from the main shell and the white meat from the claws. However, the white meat found in the smaller legs and the body carapace is quite delicious, far sweeter than the claw meat, though it is more difficult to remove. The only inedible parts are the gills (dead men's fingers), which are finger-shaped and very gray in color, and located immediately behind the head. Contrary to popular belief, they are not poisonous. To remove the gills from the main body, at the back of the shell, force the handle end of a fork in between the top and bottom. Twist the fork handle and pop off the shell. Pull the gills off the body and wipe or rinse away any remaining green or brown residue.

QUICK SERVING IDEAS

- The quickest and easiest way to enjoy any crab is to eat it in a simple fashion—steamed, with a little clarified butter or olive oil.
- One of the more popular ways to eat Dungeness and blue crab is in the form of crab cakes. Here is an easy recipe:

  In a large bowl whisk together 1 large egg, 3 tablespoons mayonnaise, 1½ teaspoons of English-style dry mustard, ¼ cup chopped, drained pimiento, 3 tablespoons parsley, 1 teaspoon Worcestershire sauce, 2 dashes Tabasco, ¼ teaspoon pepper, and ¼ teaspoon salt. Add 1 pound/½ kilogram crabmeat and ¼ cup of finely crushed salted crackers, and toss the mixture gently. Spread another ½ cup finely crushed crackers on a plate, and gently form the crab mixture with a ⅓-cup measure into eight ¾-inch/2-centimeter-thick patties, coating the top and bottom of each patty carefully with the crackers. Transfer the crab cakes to a sheet of greaseproof paper as they are formed. In a large skillet heat 2 tablespoons vegetable oil and 1 tablespoon unsalted butter over moderately high heat until the foam subsides, and sauté the crab cakes, in batches if necessary, for 1 to 2 minutes on each side, or until they are golden. Transfer them to a heated platter after they are cooked. Serve the crab cakes with the lemon wedges.

• Soft-shell crab can be prepared by combining 1½ cups low-fat milk and 4 small, cleaned soft-shell crabs in a shallow bowl large enough to hold the crabs in a single layer, and letting them soak for 1 hour. Drain and discard the milk. Combine ¾ cup flour, salt, and pepper and lightly dredge each crab in the flour. Heat ¼ cup rapeseed or olive oil (not extra-virgin) over medium-high heat and sauté the crabs in batches until golden, about 4 minutes per side. Garnish with 2 tablespoons chopped flat-leaf parsley.

SAFETY

As with meat and fish, crustaceans must be handled, stored, and cooked properly to prevent foodborne illness. Never buy uncooked dead crab as the meat starts to deteriorate rapidly after death.

As with fish and other shellfish, allergic reactions to crustaceans are commonly reported in both adults and children. It is generally recommended that individuals who have had an allergic reaction to one species of crustacean avoid all other species. Allergic reactions to crustaceans can be severe and are often a cause of anaphylaxis. See page 723 for more information on food allergy.

Lobster

Lobsters include large crustaceans from two groups, one with a pair of large claws and the other without. In the United States and Canada, the most popular lobster is a clawed variety, the Maine or Atlantic lobster (*Homarus americanus*). With its five pairs of legs, including two large foreclaws, and its curling tail, the clawed lobster typically resembles its land counterpart, the scorpion. Also popular are the spiny or rock lobsters native to the Florida and California coasts. These lobsters do not have claws. The lobster found around Britain's coast, the *Homarus gammarus*, is dark blue with a yellow underbelly and claws, one larger than the other.

Often called the "king of shellfish," the Maine or Atlantic lobster's body, tail, and claws are hard-shelled. Live lobsters range in color from brownish rust to greenish brown; but all lobster shells turn bright orangey red when cooked. The white flesh is pleasantly firm and dense with a rich, savory flavor.

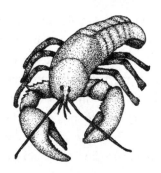

Lobsters grow by molting, or shedding their shells. After a molt (typically in summer), the lobster is soft-shelled and filled with the seawater it has absorbed in the process. Up to two months pass before the absorbed seawater is replaced by new lobster meat. As the shell hardens in the cold waters of the North Atlantic, the meat's texture and taste improve, and the lobster acquires a denser, fuller feel.

The lobsters collected on the shores of New England during colonial times were often much larger than we are used to seeing today. While the average market size for a lobster is now 1 to 2 pounds/½ to 1 kilogram, in earlier days lobsters often weighed in at as much as 40 pounds/18 kilograms. The world record was caught in 1977 in Nova Scotia, Canada, weighing in at 44 pounds, 6 ounces (just over 20 kilograms), and measuring nearly 4 feet/1¼ meters long. Considering it takes five to seven years for a lobster to reach the weight of 1 pound/½ kilogram, the best estimate is that it would take a lobster sixty to seventy years to reach 40 pounds.

HISTORY

While Maine or Atlantic lobsters are now considered a luxury food, they were so plentiful at one time that Native Americans used them to fertilize their fields and to bait their hooks for fishing. In colonial times, lobsters were considered "poor people's food." They were harvested from tidal pools and served to children, prisoners, and indentured servants, who exchanged their passage to America for seven years of service to their sponsors. In Massachusetts, some of the servants finally rebelled and had it put into their contracts that they would not be forced to eat lobster more than three times a week.

Until the early 1800s, lobsters were gathered by hand along the shoreline—they would often be piled up as high as two feet/60 centimeters thick. Lobstering as a trap fishery came into existence in Maine around 1850. Today Maine is the largest lobster-producing state in the United States. Though the number of lobstermen has increased dramatically, the amount of lobsters caught has remained relatively steady through the years. In 1892, 2,600 people in the Maine lobster fishery caught 7,983 metric tonnes; in 1992, approximately 6,000 Maine lobstermen landed 10,600 metric tonnes of lobster. The amount of lobsters harvested in 2002 in Maine exceeded 16,000 metric tonnes. Lobsters are harvested that are between 3½ and 5 inches/9 to 12 centimeters carapace length, the distance from the eye to the beginning of the tail.

The United States and Canada are the world's largest lobster-producing countries. Together, these two countries account for 37 percent of the total production. Other major producers are the United Kingdom, Australia, Cuba, Ireland, and France.

NUTRITIONAL HIGHLIGHTS

Lobster is an excellent source of protein, copper, selenium, and vitamin B12. In addition, it is a very good source of phosphorus. A 100 gram serving contains approximately 98 calories, 21 grams of protein, and 72 milligrams of cholesterol.

Atlantic lobster is one of the leanest protein sources available. It contains less saturated fat, calories, and cholesterol than beef, pork, and even the light meat of chicken. In fact, lobster contains 15 percent less dietary cholesterol than chicken. Given its low fat content, only 0.6

grams per serving, the omega-3 fatty acid content of lobster is not as rich as that of fish, but a serving contains 100 milligrams of omega-3 fatty acids, of which 53 milligrams is EPA.

HEALTH BENEFITS

Lobster has been shown to be very beneficial for protecting against heart disease, Alzheimer's disease, and many forms of cancer. For more information, please see page 530.

HOW TO SELECT AND STORE

In general, larger lobsters are sold into the fresh/live market, where they command premium prices, while smaller lobsters are cooked and either frozen whole or shelled for their meat.

Live lobsters should be active, and their tails should curl, not dangle, beneath them. After buying a live lobster, store it in the refrigerator covered with a damp cloth as soon as possible and cook within six to twelve hours. Do not let it sit out at room temperature for more than half an hour, and never put a live lobster in fresh water for storage purposes. Denizens of the ocean, lobsters will die in fresh water.

Cooked lobster should be refrigerated and consumed within two days. Cooked lobster can be easily frozen, too. To freeze cooked lobster, prepare a brine made of 1 tablespoon of salt to 1 cup of water. Remove the meat from the shell and place it in a container or sealable bag with brine to cover and freeze. Frozen lobster should be eaten within one month.

When purchased in the supermarket, frozen lobster tails packed in special vacuum packs can have an extended shelf life of twenty-four months. Vacuum packs are also available in different meat combinations: whole pieces, chopped, and salad meat; tails; and claws.

TIPS FOR PREPARING

Boiled and served whole with clarified butter is the most popular way to enjoy lobster, but there is virtually no limit to the uses that can be made of this meat. Served hot, it adds an unmistakable taste of luxury to casseroles, stir-fries, stuffings, sauces, bisques, omelets, soufflés, quiches, crêpes, and many other dishes. Cold, it is elegant in salads, hors d'oeuvres, and the famous "down East" lobster roll.

The empty shells can be used in bisques or for lobster au gratin; the tomalley (liver) provides extraordinary flavor for spreads, butters, sauces, or dips; the coral (unfertilized eggs) presents an unusually colorful garnish for hors d'oeuvres or salads; and the claws make an extravagant statement atop a salad.

The traditional method of boiling lobsters is as follows:

1. Fill a large pot one half to two thirds full of water, enough to cover two 1¼- or 1½-pound/½ to ¾ kilogram lobsters. Add 1 teaspoon salt, 1 bay leaf, and 1 tablespoon fresh lemon juice. Cover and bring to a full boil.

2. Melt 1 stick (½ cup) butter in a separate saucepan and set aside.

3. Grasp the first lobster firmly at the middle of the back and place it headfirst into the boiling water. For safety reasons, leave on the bands or pegs securing its claws. Repeat with the second lobster.

4. Cover the pot and bring back to a boil, being sure to regulate the heat to prevent the

water from boiling over. Cook for no more than 12 to 15 minutes or the meat will become tough.

5. When the antennae pull out easily and the lobsters are bright red, they are done. Plunge cooked lobsters into cold water for 1 minute to stop the cooking process.

6. Serve with clarified butter (or olive oil) and lemon wedges.

7. To collect the meat for other dishes, working over a large bowl to catch juices, cut off lobster tails and claws. Crack tail and claw shells and remove lobster meat. Coarsely chop lobster meat; cover and chill.

QUICK SERVING IDEAS

- For a special treat, try barbecued lobster. Preheat the barbecue to medium. Boil the lobster in a large pot of boiling water for 2 minutes. Pat dry. From below the head, cut the lobster in two lengthways and remove and discard the small pouch close to the head. Baste generously with a mixture of lemon juice and melted butter or oil. Season to taste, but do not salt. Place the lobster flesh side down on the grill, calculating about 7 minutes grilling time per pound/½ kilogram.

- Here's an easy and delicious recipe for lobster salad: In a large bowl, mix together ½ pound/250 grams chopped lobster meat, 1 sliced yellow pepper, 1 sliced stalk celery, ½ sliced red onion, 1 to 2 tablespoons rapeseed mayonnaise, and black pepper to taste until evenly combined. Chill for 2 hours before serving.

- Lobster bisque is one of the most popular lobster dishes. Bring a large pot of water to boil. Prepare the lobster meat from two 1-pound/½-kilogram live lobsters as instructed above. Reserve 2 cups cooking liquid and juices from lobster in a large bowl. Coarsely chop lobster shells and bodies and sauté in 2 tablespoons olive oil until shells begin to brown, about 8 minutes. Add 1 sliced onion, 1 sliced large celery stalk, 1 sliced small carrot, 1 garlic head cut in half crosswise, 1 sliced tomato, 2 tablespoons chopped fresh tarragon, 2 tablespoons chopped fresh thyme, 2 bay leaves, and ¼ teaspoon ground black pepper. Mix in ½ cup brandy and ½ cup dry sherry and boil until almost all liquid has evaporated, about 4 minutes. Add 4 cups fish stock or bottled clam juice, plus the reserved 2 cups lobster cooking liquid and lobster juices, and simmer 1 hour. Strain soup through sieve set over large saucepan, pressing firmly on solids. Whisk ¼ cup tomato paste into soup. Simmer until soup is reduced to 3 cups, about 15 minutes. Add ½ cup whipping cream (low-fat milk is an option) to soup and simmer 5 minutes. Dissolve 2 teaspoons cornflour in 1 tablespoon water, add to soup, and boil until slightly thickened, about 2 minutes. Just before serving, mix lobster meat into soup and stir to heat through.

SAFETY

See page 533 for more information.

Prawns (shrimp)

Prawns (or shrimp) are second only to canned tuna as the most popular seafood in the United States. They are equally popular in the U.K., where approximately 65 million kilograms are consumed per year. The firm, translucent flesh of raw prawns sports a variable color palette that can be pink, gray, brownish, or yellow, depending on the variety. Upon cooking, the flesh of these crustaceans typically becomes opaque and a cream or pinkish color.

At 3 to 4 inches/7½ to 10 centimeters in length and reddish pink in color, the deepwater shrimp, also referred to as the pink shrimp, is the most commonly available type in the United States. Giant tiger prawns are also becoming popular in the United States. These large prawns, measuring 6 to 12 inches/15 to 30 centimeters in length, are one of the most widely consumed types in many regions of Asia. Globally, 300 different species of prawn are harvested worldwide. Of these species, thousands of edible varieties are available.

HISTORY

The word "shrimp" hails from the Middle English *shrimpe,* meaning "pygmy" or "crustacean." Although Chinese prawn markets were commented on in the 1300s by Marco Polo, harvesting is first known to have taken place in the seventeenth century, in Lousiana. Prawns are found throughout almost the entire world. While many countries farm-raise prawns, much of the world's supply comes from the coastal waters of the United States, South and Central America, Japan, Thailand, and Taiwan. The United States alone harvests more than 650 million pounds/295 million kilograms a year, more than any other country. Nonetheless, nearly 500,000 tons of prawns are imported into the United States each year, making it the number one seafood import.

NUTRITIONAL HIGHLIGHTS

Prawns are an excellent source of protein, selenium, and vitamin B12. In addition, prawns are a very good source of iron and phosphorous. A 100 gram serving—about 12 large boiled prawns—contains approximately 99 calories, 21 grams of protein, 195 grams of cholesterol, and 1 gram of fat, with 171 milligrams of EPA and 144 milligrams of DHA. Since prawns do have a high cholesterol content, many people tend to avoid eating this seafood delicacy. Scientific evidence does not seem to justify this, as research studying prawn intake does not show it to significantly increase LDL (bad) cholesterol levels, while the same research shows it to produce a modest increase in HDL (good) cholesterol levels.

In one clinical study, researchers analyzed the effect of a diet that contained 300 grams of prawns per day to another where subjects ate 2 large eggs per day. Results indicated that the prawn diet did raise LDL (bad cholesterol) levels by 7 percent but also raised HDL (good cholesterol) levels by 12 percent. In contrast, the egg diet raised LDL levels by 10 percent and HDL by 7 percent. This shows us that the prawn diet actually lowered ratios of total cholesterol to HDL and lowered ratios of LDL to HDL cholesterol more than the egg diet did. Additionally,

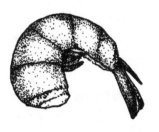

for people who ate the prawn diet, levels of triglycerides decreased by 13 percent.

HEALTH BENEFITS

Prawns, like fish and other shellfish, have been shown to be very beneficial for protecting against heart disease, Alzheimer's disease, and many forms of cancer. For more information, please see page 530.

HOW TO SELECT AND STORE

As with any seafood, it is best to purchase prawns from a shop that has a good reputation for having a fresh supply. When you will be preparing the prawns should influence your decision as to whether you should buy fresh or frozen prawns, as frozen prawns can be kept for several weeks, whereas fresh prawns keep for one to two days. Fresh prawns should have firm bodies that are still attached to their shells, be free of black spots, and not appear yellow or gritty. Smell is a good indicator of freshness; good-quality prawns have a slightly saltwater smell. After purchasing prawns, return them to a refrigerator as soon as possible, preferably in a baking dish filled with ice on the bottom shelf of the refrigerator. Replenish ice one or two times per day. See page 530 for more information.

TIPS FOR PREPARING

Depending upon the recipe, prawns can be cooked either shelled or unshelled. To remove the shell yourself, rinse the prawns under cool water in a colander, then pull off the head and legs, and then, holding the tail, peel the shell off the body. If shelling frozen prawns, it is easier to remove the shell if they are still slightly frozen. To defrost prawns, place them in a bowl of cold water or in the refrigerator. Do not thaw the prawns at room temperature or in a microwave, since this can lead to a loss of moisture and nutrients. To remove the prawn's intestines before cooking or eating, make a shallow incision along the back of the prawn and pull out the dark vein that runs throughout.

Prawns cook quickly. Depending on their size, they will cook within 1 to 2 minutes for small prawns to 10 minutes for large Asian prawns. Prawns, like lobster, are a very versatile food and are amenable to every cooking technique.

QUICK SERVING IDEAS

- Combine 1 pound/½ kilogram chopped cooked prawns with 1 cup diced papaya, ½ cup chopped spring onions, 1 to 2 diced chili peppers, ½ cup cashew nuts, and 2 tablespoons olive oil. Season to taste and serve this aromatic prawn dish over steamed brown rice or as a salad on a bed of romaine lettuce.
- Traditional appetizer plates serve cold cooked prawns with salsa dip or prawn cocktail sauce.
- Lightly sauté prawns in olive oil, garlic, and seasonings to make a quick and easy prawn dish that can be served with rice.
- Skewer prawns and your favorite grilling vegetables, brush lightly with olive oil, and barbecue.

SAFETY

Please see page 533.

Common Mollusks

The mollusk family of shellfish includes clams, mussels, oysters, and scallops since all are bivalves, meaning marine species that have two shells of equal size that protect a soft body.

Mollusks have a long and venerable history, having been around since prehistoric times. When Linnaeus was formulating his system of binomial nomenclature, the mollusks were grouped along with most invertebrates under *vermes,* or worms. The name Mollusca, which derives from the Latin *mollis,* meaning "soft," was first used in 1798 by the great French zoologist Georges Cuvier to refer to cephalopods, such as squids and cuttlefish, but was later extended to include other organisms, including snails and bivalves.

Safety

One of the big concerns about mollusk consumption is safety. The National Academy of Sciences in the U.S. has issued a federal report on seafood safety that warns, "The major risk of acute disease is associated with the consumption of raw shellfish, particularly bivalve mollusks." The reason mollusks are particularly risky is that they live by filtering 15 to 20 gallons/57 to 76 liters of water per day. If the water they inhabit is polluted, they end up concentrating any pathogen, such as the coliform bacteria that get into fresh and salt water from untreated sewage. Some shellfish can store toxins in their bodies for up to two years.

Many of the mollusks can be collected in the wild. Always check on the status of the waters with your local marine fishery government agency (the Environment Agency in the U.K.) before harvesting your own. Also, purchase mollusks only from reputable markets. The U.K. shellfish industry is regulated by strict controls under the E.U. Bivalve Shellfish Hygiene Directive. In the U.S. ask to see the tag certifying that the mollusks were harvested from state-certified-as-clean waters. In many states, the National Shellfish Sanitation Program monitors the harvesting of clams and other bivalves. Pre-packaged clams should bear a sticker from the state agency, as well.

Although harvesting has been limited to areas certified as clean, such certification cannot provide complete assurance of safety when a mere handful of agents are charged with overseeing more than 10 million acres of approved shellfish beds along the Atlantic, Pacific, and Gulf coasts. Thus, eating raw mollusks, even when they are from an area certified as clean, carries health risks, including gastrointestinal infection (diarrhea, nausea, and abdominal cramps) and infection with shellfish-borne viruses, such as hepatitis A. These illnesses pose significant risk to the very young or old, as well as individuals whose health is compromised, such as those with cancer, diabetes, cardiovascular disease, or any disease that impairs immunity, such as hepatitis C or AIDS.

Another concern is paralytic shellfish poisoning, or PSP. Normally associated with red tide, PSP can be present even in clear waters. Caused by a marine biotoxin ingested by shellfish, including clams, PSP can cause symptoms that include nausea, vomiting, diarrhea, abdominal pain, and tingling or burning lips, gums, tongue, face, neck, arms, legs, and toes.

Should you experience any of these symptoms, immediately seek emergency medical assistance as no specific antidote exists. In the E.U., member states must run programmes to monitor algal toxin levels in all commercial fishing areas. Fisheries can be closed if necessary.

Your risk of contracting PSP can be further reduced by eating only the light, white portions and not any of the dark areas, such as the tip of the siphon, or digestive organs, of mollusks. Remove these portions before cooking and wash the remainder thoroughly.

Steamed mollusks are typically cooked just until they open, which takes only a minute or two, not nearly enough time to raise the temperature in the mollusk to a level hot enough to kill bacteria and inactivate any virus that may be present. To protect your health, enjoy your mollusks on the well-done side, steaming them for a minimum of 15 minutes.

Please see page 533 for more information.

Clams

Most clams are only a few inches long, but the biggest of the 15,000 different species of clams worldwide, *Tridacna gigas,* the giant clam of the South Pacific's coral reefs, grows up to five feet/1½ meters long and can weigh upward of 550 pounds/250 kilograms!

Virtually all clam meat is creamy white, but their shells come in many colors, including shades of brown, red-brown, yellow, and cream. The shells are attached by a muscular hinge (the clam's adductor muscle), which the clam uses to close its shells tightly when threatened. Clams also have a foot, which they use to burrow into the sand, and a double-tubed siphon that operates somewhat like a snorkel, one tube drawing in the water from which they extract oxygen and filter plankton (the tiny organisms clams eat), and the second expelling water and waste products from the digestive tract. The siphon projects from the end opposite the foot and may be united in a single column referred to as the neck.

Clams may be hard- or soft-shelled. Hard-shell clams close completely, but soft-shelled clams, which have a long, rubbery siphon that extends beyond the edge of their shells, cannot. The edible parts of the clam are the siphon, through which the clam takes in water; the foot, which the clam uses to propel itself over the sand; and the muscles that open and close the shell. Regardless, the flesh is sweet, being somewhat chewy in the smaller clams and more so in the largest.

In the U.S., clams are harvested along the Atlantic, Pacific, and Gulf coasts, with each location providing slightly different varieties of basic clam species. We'll discuss the most popular varieties.

Of East Coast hard-shell clams, *Mercenaria campechiensis* are the northern variety; *Mercenaria mercenaria,* the southern type, are called quahogs, the Native American word for "clam." Abundant from the Gulf of Saint Lawrence to the Gulf of Mexico, these mollusks, which have brown, vaguely heart-shaped shells and creamy, slightly salty flesh, come in three sizes. The eastern surf clam, *Spisula solidissima,* with a shell diameter of 3 to 6 inches/7½ to 15 centimeters, is the largest. Comparatively tough, it is often used for bait or cut up and cooked in chowder, which is why it is often also called the chowder clam. Next in size, ranging from 2½ to 3 inches/6 to 7½ centimeters, are the cherrystones. The smallest members of the species, which are also the most tender and sweet, are the littlenecks, measuring 2 to 2½ inches/5 to 6 centimeters across.

The steamer clam *(Mya arenaria)*, the most common species of soft-shell clam on both of North America's coasts, has an off-white thin, brittle round shell, which doesn't close entirely because this clam's long siphon extends out from its body. When disturbed, steamer clams eject a spurt of water and withdraw to safer depths in the sand. Commonly about 3 inches/7½ centimeters in length (although they can grow twice as long), steamer clams, as the name suggests, are usually steamed, but are also good shucked and sautéed or deep-fried. They have a moderately sweet flavor and moderately chewy texture.

The Atlantic razor clam *(Enis)* has a soft shell that looks like a folded old-fashioned straight-edge razor. It can be found from Labrador to Florida. Prized for its flavor, this clam can attain a length of 10 inches/25 centimeters.

The Pacific Northwest is famed for its geoduck (pronounced gooey-duck), a large soft-shell clam found from Alaska to the state of Washington that can reach a weight of as much as 12 pounds/5½ kilograms. Typically a 6-inch/15-centimeter-long clam with a neck that can extend about 1½ feet/45 centimeters and a weight of 2 to 4 pounds/1 to 2 kilograms, the geoduck *(Panopea abrupta)* has sweet, soft flesh and is often shucked and sautéed, but also makes an excellent chowder.

The Pacific Ocean also provides soft-shell razor clams *(Siliqua patula)*, which range from Alaska to California; hard-shell varieties, including the small sweet butter clams or littlenecks found in Puget Sound; and several surf clams, including mud clams and white sand clams. From mid-California southward along the California coast, a delicious hard-shell clam called the pismo *(Tivela stultorum)* is now protected by law from excessive harvesting. One of the largest of the California clams, the pismo can grow up to 7 inches/18 centimeters, although legal clamming size is 4½ inches/12 centimeters.

Around the British Isles there are about twenty species of clam, all of which are edible though some are easier to find than others. Carpet shell clams are the ones most likely to be sold in fishmongers, although they can easily be collected from beaches too. The pink tellin clams are tiny, but the American quahog—a species that has found its way into British waters—is almost as large as a scallop. Razor clams also abound, though they are not easy to collect. Good fishmongers may stock them.

HISTORY

Found in intertidal areas throughout the world, clams have been eaten since time immemorial. In addition to being relied upon as a source of food, clams provided the material for a type of currency used by the American Indians, who removed the purple lining from clamshells to make wampum—beads strung and used for barter, ornamental, and ceremonial purposes.

NUTRITIONAL HIGHLIGHTS

Clams are an excellent source of low-calorie, low-fat, complete protein. Clams are also an outstanding source of vitamin B12, providing 1,319 percent of the RDA. In addition, clams are an excellent source of other B vitamins, iron, selenium, manganese, copper, zinc, and potassium. One-half cup of cooked, drained clams provides 20.44 grams of protein for a mere 118 calories and about 1.5 grams of fat, most of which is unsaturated, including 250 milligrams of omega-3 fatty acids. Clams are not high in cholesterol. This misconception was the result of older, less accurate methods of food analysis that identified certain fats in shellfish that are similar to cholesterol as true cholesterol. Newer, more sophisticated analytical methods indicate that the cholesterol content of most shellfish is just 50 to 70 milligrams per 100 gram serving—less than that of cooked skinless chicken or turkey breast.

HEALTH BENEFITS

Consuming clams as a primary source of protein markedly reduces levels of cholesterol in both the blood and the liver—at least in mice. In a recent study, when male mice on high-cholesterol diets were given little-neck clams, their serum and hepatic (liver) cholesterol levels dropped significantly—a reduction not seen in control animals given casein (a protein found in dairy products) instead.

Earlier studies on humans have produced similar results. In one study, eighteen men with normal cholesterol levels were given diets in which shellfish—one of which was clams—were used to replace animal foods normally in their diet. When the men ate clams or oysters and prepared these foods with less than half the amount of fat found in the animal foods they normally ate, their total cholesterol, VLDL (very bad) cholesterol, and LDL cholesterol dropped, while diets using squid and prawns did not

produce these beneficial effects on blood lipids (see page 558 for more information on the effects of prawns on blood lipids).

HOW TO SELECT AND STORE

Clams are typically harvested—dug from the sand at low tide or scooped from beds in deeper waters—and sold locally, so the clams available for purchase on the East Coast will be Atlantic clams, while Pacific varieties are sold in the West. On the East Coast and in the Pacific Northwest, clams are available all year round, while in California, the season runs from November to April. In the U.K., clams can be collected all year round, although traditionally they were not collected between May and September, possibly because this is the breeding season and the clams are in poorer condition.

Clams are sold fresh, in the shell or shucked and packed in their own juices. Clams in their shells should smell briny but fresh. The shells should be hard (except for soft-shell clams'), moist, and appear bright and clean. Hard-shell clams should be so tightly closed that you cannot pull them apart or, if open, should close tightly when the shell is tapped. Soft-shell clams' protruding necks should retract when lightly touched. Do not purchase clams whose shells are cracked or remain open; these are likely dead and are unfit to eat.

Live clams are highly perishable and highly susceptible to bacterial contamination once they die or get too warm, so they must be kept alive until ready to be cooked and eaten. Store live clams in a cold (32 to 35 degrees F./0 to 1½ degrees C.) refrigerator in an open container, covered with a moist cloth or paper towels. Kept in this manner, live clams should remain fresh for two to three days. Do not put live clams in an airtight container or submerge them in fresh water; either will kill them. Check daily for any open shells—a sign the clam has died—and remove these clams promptly so they do not contaminate the rest. Live clams can also be frozen in the shell and kept up to three months. To do so, place the live clams in moisture vapor-resistant bags, press out excess air, and freeze.

If shucked, clams should look plump, be submerged in their own clear liquor, and smell fresh with absolutely no fishy or ammonia odor. Shucked clams are also available canned or already frozen. Shucked clams should be stored in a tightly sealed container immersed in their own liquor. Kept in the refrigerator, they will remain fresh for up to three days. Shucked clams can also be frozen. Clean and wash the meat thoroughly, then drain and pack in freezer containers, leaving ½ inch/1 centimeter headspace. Use within three months. When ready, thaw frozen clams in the refrigerator for 6 hours.

TIPS FOR PREPARING

To shuck hard-shell clams: Discard any clams with broken or gaping shells—these have died and are unsafe to eat. Scrub the outside of each clam with a stiff bristle brush. Then, to purge the grit all clams accumulate, place them in a gallon of cold water to which has been added ¼ cup cornmeal (polenta) and ⅛ cup salt for each liter of clams. Let them soak for 2 to 3 hours, which also lightens the meat color. Rinse well and then cover with cold water for 5 minutes. Discard any clams found floating after either of these procedures. Under cold running water, scrub the remaining clams again with a

stiff brush, scraping off any encrustations with a sturdy knife. Wearing work gloves to protect your hands and using a clam knife—a sturdier version of a paring knife with a rounded tip— hold the clam, rounded side up with the shell's hinge toward your wrist, firmly in your palm. Work the knife blade between the shell halves on the broad side opposite the hinge, twisting the blade when it is well inside to pry apart the shells. Cut the muscles on either side of the hinge, and then slide the knife along the inside of the top and bottom shells to cut the interior muscles, freeing the clam. If you don't have a clam knife, try a short screwdriver or beer can opener. To shuck soft-shell clams: Since the shells are softer, a paring knife can be used. Be sure to pull off the dark membrane covering the edible "neck" of the clam.

All clams should be cooked gently over low heat to prevent toughening. Clams in their shells can be cooked on a barbecue until the shells open or steamed to open before continuing to cook them by another method. You can steam clams in the shell by placing them in a pot with a couple of inches of boiling liquid—water seasoned with wine or stock—then cover and steam over high heat for 6 to 8 minutes. Discard any that have not opened.

Fresh or frozen clams are best for sauces, soups, and stews. Canned clams, which have been cooked, are already soft, so, if using them in a soup or stew, add them at the last minute so they retain their texture.

QUICK SERVING IDEAS

- For an easier way to enjoy clams, simply scrub the clams and set them on a barbecue 4 to 6 inches/10 to 15 centimeters above the coals. After several minutes, when the clams begin to pop open, turn them over and continue to cook until they open wide, about another 3 to 4 minutes. Hold them over a pan of melted butter so the juices drain in, pluck out the meat with a fork, dip in the butter, and enjoy.

- Have an easy indoor clambake: Place clams still in their shells at the bottom of a tall stockpot, then cover with layers of small new potatoes, shucked pieces of corn on the cob, quartered onions, several sprigs of fresh thyme, and last of all, fresh spinach (a reasonable and more edible stand-in for seaweed). Pour in a little stock, clam juice, lemon juice, and/or white wine. Sprinkle with salt and pepper to taste, top with a "tester" potato, and let steam until fully cooked—about 30 to 40 minutes or when the potato pierces easily with a fork.

- Serve clams baked on the half shell. Preheat the oven to 450 degrees F./230 degrees C./gas 8. In several tablespoons of butter, sauté a clove of garlic along with a couple of tablespoons of finely chopped green pepper. Add ¼ cup seasoned bread crumbs and additional butter to make a moist, cohesive mixture. Open 2 dozen cleaned cherrystone clams and discard the top shell. Place the clams in a shallow baking dish and top each with a teaspoon of the bread crumb mix, a little lemon juice, and a sprinkle of Parmesan cheese. Bake for 10 minutes.

- Make homemade clam sauce for linguine. Mince one medium onion and one clove of garlic and sauté in olive oil. Add a 13-ounce/370-gram can of minced clams in their juice, a 6-ounce/175-gram can of tomato paste, 1 cup water, 2 tablespoons lemon juice, fresh chopped parsley, and ¼ teaspoon each of rosemary and thyme. Simmer uncovered for 15 to 20 minutes.

- New England-style clam chowder can be made by adding a can of minced clams with their liquor and some diced potato and celery to a couple of cups of milk, then seasoning with a tablespoon of butter, a spoonful of chopped onion or onion flakes, chopped parsley, salt, and pepper. A Manhattan-style clam chowder can be made similarly. Just add minced clams, clam juice, a splash of lemon juice, and up to a cup of water to your favorite basic marinara sauce. Heat and serve topped with a spoonful of Parmesan cheese.

SAFETY

Please see page 560 for safety concerns.

Oysters

Oysters have rough, fluted shells enclosing a creamy flesh with a delicate briny flavor. Oysters grow wild in estuaries, sounds, and bays, flourishing in conditions varying from brackish water to very salty lagoons. A member of the mollusk family, which also includes clams, mussels, and scallops, the oyster is a bivalve—a marine species whose soft body is protected by two shells of roughly equal size.

The oysters we eat belong to two genera,

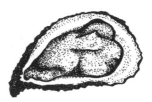

Ostrea and *Crassostrea,* which differ both in appearance—*Ostrea* have round, scalloplike shells, while *Crassostrea*'s shells are long and asymmetrical—and in their reproductive habits.

Within each genus, there are two major species of oysters, whose common names are typically derived from their geographical location: *Crassostrea virginica,* the eastern or Atlantic oyster, whose small, relatively smooth shells average 2 to 4 inches/5 to 10 centimeters in length, is found in cold coastal waters from the Canadian Maritimes to the Mexican border and from the North Atlantic to the Gulf of Mexico. This mild-tasting oyster, which provides most of the American oyster supply, is known by a variety of common/locale names, including Apalachicola, Bluepoint, Chincoteague, Cotuit, Lynnhaven, Malpeque, Pemaquid, and Wellfleet.

Crassostrea gigas, the Pacific or Japanese oyster, is a briny delicacy that ranges in size from the tiny 1½-inch/4 centimeter Kumamoto to the common Pacific oyster, which can grow to more than 8 inches/20 centimeters long and 5 inches/12 centimeters wide, so it's usually cut up for stews or fried rather than served on the half shell. Introduced to the northwestern coast of the United States from Japan in the 1920s, locally grown Pacific oysters go by names such as Yakima Bay, Golden Mantle, and Penn Cove.

Ostrea lurida, the Olympic oyster, is the only oyster native to the West Coast, specifically Seattle's Puget Sound. A tiny variety about 1½ inches/4 centimeters across, the Olympic oyster is related to the European flat oyster. Other so-called Pacific oysters cultivated on the West Coast were originally eastern transplants and are graded and sold by size rather than name.

Ostrea edulis, the European flat oyster, is found in the coastal waters surrounding the British Isles and the Continent. One special French oyster hails from a specific part of Brittany. Considered a real delicacy, this oyster, which the Bretons call the *bélon,* fetches upward of $80 per dozen (€22.50 for half a dozen). In America, *bélons* are farm-grown and sold as Westcott European flat oysters. Other French varieties include the green-tinged *marennes* and oysters the French call *portugaises,* although this variety, which used to be abundant in Europe, is now extinct. Today's French *portugaises* are actually close relatives of the Eastern and Pacific oysters found in the United States. Other European varieties, born and bred in the British Isles, include Ireland's Galway and England's Colchester, Helford, and Whitstable oysters.

Where taste is concerned, in oysters, it's truly about "location, location, location." Oysters are filter feeders, which means they "breathe" water in and out, filtering algae and other treats through their gills for food, so their flavor varies from bland to quite salty depending on their growing environment. The salinity, mineral content, water temperature, and chlorophyll content of the local plankton all affect an oyster's flavor. Generally, raw oysters from the coldest waters are considered tastier than their warmer-bred brethren; however, some southern oyster advocates would firmly disagree. Once cooked, the difference in flavor between northern- and southern-grown oysters is negligible. Prized by epicures, who usually prefer the plump moist morsels raw or barely cooked, oysters are also delicious—and safer to consume— steamed, baked, or grilled, although they must be cooked gently or they'll quickly toughen.

HISTORY

One of the oldest living species, oysters have been around for more than 200 million years. Among the few animals people of the world eat raw and live, oysters have a long history of nourishing the human race and have been a prized food since the pre-Christian era. To the ancient Greeks, oysters were the food of love. Aristotle wrote about oysters in 320 B.C.E., and it's no mistake that Aphrodite, the Grecian goddess from whose name we derive the word "aphrodisiac," rose from the sea on an oyster shell and gave birth to Eros.

The Romans so loved the tasty bivalves that they were imported to Rome from all over the empire. Collected at the order of the Emperor Vitellius, who was reputed to have eaten them day and night, oysters were gathered from the shores of the English Channel by thousands of slaves, packed in seaweed and ice, and carried back to Rome. So popular was the oyster that the Romans learned to cultivate them and even made a monetary unit, the *denarius,* equal in value to one oyster. Oysters were also adored by the ancient Chinese, who figured out how to raise them in ponds.

Popular even in the Middle Ages as an aphrodisiac, oysters were featured in a cookbook written circa 1390. Several hundred years later, in the seventeenth century, oysters were the most frequently mentioned (sixty-eight times) seafood in the diary of Samuel Pepys (1660–1669). Like many other shellfish in Pepys's day, oysters were cheap and plentiful, brought to London from Whitstable, a town on the north Kent shore famous for its oysters since Roman times, and also imported from France. Even today, Whitstable oysters still enjoy an enormous reputation for their succulence and this small town is a fashionable destination for shellfish lovers.

In the eighteenth century, Henry Fielding, in one of the most provocative descriptions of food in literature, introduced his hero Tom Jones to the delights of love over a succulent serving of oysters for two, and the infamous Casanova, a sixty-oyster-a-day kind of guy, called them "a spur to the spirit and to love." Oysters have also appeared in the works of some of the best writers in the English language, including William Shakespeare, Lewis Carroll, Jonathan Swift, and Ernest Hemingway.

In North America, the great piles of oyster shells along many different areas of the shoreline attest to the voracious appetite for oysters shared by Native Americans on both coasts. On the East Coast, however, the early colonial settlers may have outdone even the local tribes. The colonists consumed oysters by the gross (144 at a time!), rather than by the dozen, with per capita consumption said to have been 10 bushels per year. Today, a dozen oysters is considered a standard serving in Europe, while a mere half dozen is the usual portion in the United States. Despite this smaller portion size, Americans alone consume more than 100 million pounds/45 million kilograms of oysters per year.

Although coastal development and its attendant pollution have nearly stripped North America's waters of their natural oyster beds, national seeding programmes have been created to restore the original bounty, and commercial oyster farmers, cultivating oysters from seed, provide a good supply of these delectable bivalves all year round. Unlike fish farming, a relatively new phenomenon, oyster farming dates back more than 2,000 years to ancient Rome. Cultivated oysters take about three years to travel from their spawning grounds to the table and, in North America, range from 1½ to 6 inches/4 to 15 centimeters long—at most, just half as large as the foot-long giants found by early European explorers. Today, the leading oyster-producing countries are the United States, Australia, New Zealand, and Canada.

NUTRITIONAL HIGHLIGHTS

Oysters provide the highest concentration of zinc of any food, more than 33 milligrams per serving, and are also an exceptionally good source of vitamin B12 and the trace minerals copper, iron, and selenium. A 100 gram serving contains approximately 137 calories, 14 grams of protein, 105 milligrams of cholesterol, and 4.9 grams of fat, with 536 milligrams of EPA and 584 milligrams of DHA, both of which are omega-3 fatty acids.

HEALTH BENEFITS

One of the storied historical uses of oysters is as an aphrodisiac. This effect, if in fact true, could be due to oysters' high zinc content. Zinc is essential to the proper action of testosterone and is a key nutrient in sperm production.

HOW TO SELECT AND STORE

The old warning—to eat oysters only in months spelled with the letter "R"—was due in part to the fact that before refrigeration, oysters would spoil quickly. Even today, however, the best seasons for eating oysters are autumn, winter, and early spring. When oysters spawn, which they do from May to August (although oysters in the

Gulf of Mexico spawn all year round due to its warmer waters), they lose their lean, firm texture and dusky shellfish flavor and become fatty, watery, and soft. Therefore, if you must eat raw oysters in the summer, choose those imported from colder waters.

Oysters are sold live, both in their shells and shucked, then cooked or smoked and packed in jars and cans. When purchasing live oysters, keep in mind that the smaller an oyster is for its species, the younger and more tender it will be. Also, reject oysters whose shells are broken, do not snap shut when tapped, or are not already tightly closed.

Oysters are highly perishable and highly susceptible to bacterial contamination once they die or if they get too warm, so they must be kept alive until ready to be cooked and eaten. Live oysters should be refrigerated. Handle them carefully and avoid dropping them. If an oyster's shell is chipped, the ensuing loss of liquor will dramatically reduce its shelf life. To properly store in the refrigerator, place the larger shells down on a platter or baking tray and cover with a damp cloth or paper towel. They should keep for up to three days. Do not put live oysters in an airtight container or submerge them in fresh water; either will kill them. Check daily for any open shells and give them the "tap test." If they don't close, it is a sign the oyster has died. Remove and dispose of these oysters promptly, so they do not contaminate the rest. Live oysters can also be frozen in the shell and kept up for to three months. To do so, place the live oysters in moisture vapor-resistant bags, press out the excess air, and freeze.

Fresh shucked oysters should be submerged in their own clear liquor, should be plump, uniform in size, and a pale creamy white in color, and should smell like clean salt water, with no ammonia or "fishy" scent. Shucked oysters should be refrigerated in an airtight container covered in their own liquor. If additional liquor is needed to cover them fully, make some by dissolving ½ teaspoon salt in 1 cup water. Kept in this manner in the refrigerator, they will remain fresh for up to two days but are best eaten on the day they are purchased. Shucked oysters can also be frozen. Clean and wash the meat thoroughly, then drain and pack in freezer containers, leaving ½ inch/1 centimeter headspace. Use within three months. When ready to use, simply thaw the frozen oysters in the refrigerator for 6 hours.

TIPS FOR PREPARING

To shuck oysters: Discard any with broken or gaping shells—these have died and are unsafe to eat. Scrub the outside of each oyster with a stiff-bristle brush. Then, to purge the grit all oysters accumulate, place them in a gallon of cold water to which has been added ¼ cup cornmeal (polenta) and ⅛ cup salt for each liter of oysters. Let them soak for 2 to 3 hours, which also lightens the color of the meat. Rinse well, then cover with cold water for 5 minutes. Discard any oysters found floating after either of these procedures. Finally, with a stiff brush, scrub the oysters once more under cold running water before opening.

Oysters placed in the freezer for 10 to 20 minutes before opening will open more easily.

Wearing work gloves to protect your hands and using an oyster knife—a short, very strong blade with a guard to protect your fingers—hold the oyster, with its deeper-cupped shell down

and the hinge toward you, firmly in your palm or place it on a firm surface on top of a folded cloth. Work the knife blade between the shell halves into the small opening near the hinge and twist until the hinge gives. Holding the oyster over a bowl to catch its liquor, slide the knife along the top shell to sever the hinge muscle, and remove the top shell. Pick out any pieces of grit or broken shell or hold the oyster and bottom shell under running water. Then slide the knife along the inside of the cupped shell, freeing the oyster meat.

If you don't have an oyster knife, try using a short screwdriver or beer can opener to pry open the oyster.

Before using the oyster liquor, strain it to remove any pieces of shell that may have broken off and fallen in.

If oysters are to be used in a cooked dish, they can easily be opened by steaming. Times vary with size and shell thickness, so watch carefully and remove them as soon as they start to open. Steam oysters in the shell by placing scrubbed live oysters flat side up in a pot in a couple of inches of water, stock, or water seasoned with sherry or wine. Bring to a boil, and then reduce the heat, cover, and steam until the shells open in about 6 to 8 minutes. Discard any that have not opened. Serve in bowls with stock. To steam shucked oysters, use a collapsible steaming rack and steam for 2 minutes. When poaching oysters, remove them from the heat as soon as their flesh is opaque and their edges curl.

Fresh or frozen oysters are best for soups and stews. Canned oysters, which have been cooked, are already soft, so if you are using these in a soup or stew, add them at the last minute so they retain their texture and do not toughen.

QUICK SERVING IDEAS

- Cook oysters in their shells on the barbecue about 6 inches/15 centimeters above the coals until the shells pop open, about 3 minutes. Then bake on the half shell topped with a teaspoon of sauce or stuffing—combine 1 cup bread crumbs, ½ cup shredded, cooked spinach, and 2 tablespoons butter for the classic oyster dish Oysters Rockefeller.
- For a classic American Thanksgiving treat, add 1 cup cooked quartered oysters to the stuffing.
- Barbecue shucked oysters with a few slices of tomatoes and fennel on each. Or, in the center of a 12-inch/30-centimeter square of foil, place a wedge of ripe summer tomato, ¼ cup fennel, and ½ cup oysters. Season with ¼ cup chopped parsley, a few dashes of crushed red pepper, a thread of saffron on each oyster, and a drizzle of olive oil. Add salt and pepper to taste, seal foil tightly around contents, and barbecue for 18 minutes.
- Try pan-fried oysters Sicilian style: Heat 2 tablespoons olive oil in a frying pan. Dust fresh shucked oysters in whole-wheat (wholemeal) flour, then place carefully in the pan; cook for 5 minutes, flipping once. Slip onto a plate and serve with fresh lemon wedges and a drizzle of extra-virgin olive oil.

SAFETY

Please see page 560 for safety concerns.

Scallops

Scallops are mollusks that feature shells that are beautifully and convexly ridged, or scalloped. The fleshy part of the scallop that is generally consumed is the "nut," the white muscle that serves to open and close the two shells. It has a soft texture and a subtle flavor that can be mild or retain a more saltwater taste, depending upon the variety. The "coral," the reproductive glands, is also edible, although it is not widely consumed in North America.

Though there are several hundred different scallop species, the most widely available types of scallops in the United States include the Atlantic deep-sea scallop (*Aequipecten irradians concentricus*) and the bay scallop (*Argopecten irradians*). The flesh of the Atlantic scallop is large, usually about 1½ inches/3 centimeters in diameter, while the bay scallop is tiny, averaging about ½ inch/1 centimeter in diameter. In Europe, the most popular type is the great or Coquille St.-Jacques scallop (*Pecten maximus*).

Scallops make their home in many waters throughout the entire world. The great scallop is well established in the Mediterranean Sea, while the Atlantic and bay scallop are found in concentrations along the U.S. eastern seaboard.

HISTORY

The scallop gained notoriety during medieval times. Religious pilgrims visiting the shrine of Saint James in Santiago de Compostela, Spain, utilized empty scallop shells for a dual purpose: eating and begging. The scallop and its shell speedily came to symbolize this magnificent shrine. In honor of this holy place, scallop shells became known as the shell of Saint James, now best known by their French name of "Coquilles St.-Jacques." As this treasured shell gained notoriety, many people began using shells to decorate their doorways, and the scallop shell form began to appear in family coats of arms.

NUTRITIONAL HIGHLIGHTS

Like other mollusks, scallops are a nutrient-dense food. They have a very high protein content and virtually no fat. They are also a good source of vitamins B6, B12, and E, magnesium, and potassium. A 100 gram serving contains approximately 112 calories, 23 grams of protein, 153 milligrams of cholesterol, and 1.4 grams of fat, with 166 milligrams of EPA and 200 milligrams of DHA, both of which are omega-3 fatty acids.

HEALTH BENEFITS

Scallops, similarly to fish, offer significant health benefits, including protection against heart disease, and many forms of cancer. For more information, see page 530.

HOW TO SELECT AND STORE

Since scallops are extremely perishable, they are usually shelled, washed, and frozen, or else packed in ice, as soon as they are caught. Fresh scallops should have flesh that is white and firm, with no evidence of browning. Smell is a good indicator of freshness when selecting them. They should be odorless or have a slightly sweet scent. Since a slightly "off" smell cannot be detected through plastic, if you have the option, purchase displayed scallops as opposed to those that are packaged. Once the fishmonger wraps

and hands you the scallops that you have selected, smell them through the paper wrapping and return them if they do not smell fresh. After purchasing scallops, make sure to return them to a refrigerator as soon as possible. If the scallops are going to accompany you during a day full of errands, keep a cooler in the car where you can place the scallops to make sure they stay cold and do not spoil.

The temperature of most refrigerators is slightly warmer than ideal for storing scallops. Therefore, to ensure maximum freshness and quality, it is important to use special storage methods to create the optimal temperature. One of the easiest ways to do this is to place well-wrapped scallops in a baking dish filled with ice. The baking dish and scallops should then be placed on the bottom shelf of the refrigerator, which is the coolest area. Check the ice once or twice during the day and replenish if necessary. Scallops can be refrigerated for up to two days.

You can extend the shelf life of scallops by freezing them. If you are planning on freezing scallops, make sure to ask the fishmonger whether they are fresh or defrosted (if it is not clearly marked), since you will need to cook previously frozen scallops before refreezing. To freeze scallops, wrap them well in plastic and place them in the coldest part of the freezer, where they will keep for about three months. If you plan to buy scallops that are already frozen, be sure that they are solid and shiny and that the inside of their packaging is free of frost. To defrost frozen scallops, place them in milk (or water) that has been boiled and removed from the heat, where they will defrost in 1 to 3 minutes. Alternatively, they can be placed in the refrigerator to defrost for 6 to 8 hours.

TIPS FOR PREPARING

Smaller scallops can be cooked whole; larger ones can either be cooked whole or sliced into smaller pieces. Scallops are usually added at the end of cooking sauces and stews or quickly seared, since exposure to too much heat will cause them to become tough and fibrous.

QUICK SERVING IDEAS

- Serve 6 seared sea scallops with a salsa made of 1 cup diced papaya, ¼ cup fresh coriander, 1 diced jalapeño pepper, 1 teaspoon grated ginger, 1 tablespoon lemon juice, 2 tablespoons olive oil, and a pinch of salt.
- Marinate scallops in 2 cups water, ½ cup tamari, 2 cloves mashed garlic, and ½ inch/1 centimetre sliced peeled ginger for 4 hours. Skewer marinated scallops, sliced leeks, and cherry tomatoes, and cook under the grill or on the barbecue.
- Braise 8 sea scallops with 4 tablespoons white wine and reduce to 2 tablespoons. Serve the scallops on a bed of lightly sautéed spinach and thinly sliced garlic. Sprinkle 2 tablespoons lemon juice and ½ cup cashews on top.
- Place cold, cooked scallops on a bed of whole-wheat pasta. Top with a chunky tomato sauce that features olives, green peppers, and courgette.
- Combine grilled scallops with lightly sautéed shiitake mushrooms. Serve on a bed of chopped romaine lettuce and Swiss chard, and top with the dressing of your choice.

SAFETY

Please see page 560 for safety concerns.

The Healing Power of Milk and Other Dairy Products

The U.S. dairy industry tells us that everybody needs milk through an enormous annual advertising budget. The U.S. Department of Agriculture and various other agencies of the U.S. government seem to echo this sentiment. The result is that Americans have an enormous love affair with milk. The average person living in the United States consumes more than 600 pounds/270 kilograms of dairy products every year, including about 420 pounds /190 kilograms of fluid milk and cream, 70 pounds/32 kilograms of various milk-based fats and oils, 30 pounds/14 kilograms of cheese, and 17 pounds/8 kilograms of ice cream. In all, U.S. dairy farmers produce 163 billion pounds/74 billion kilograms of milk and milk products a year.

In the U.K., the Food Standards Agency also recommends milk and dairy products as good sources of proteins, vitamins and calcium. The U.K. produces 14 billion liters of milk per year, half of which is sold as milk. Each person consumes an average of 112 kilograms of milk, 10 kilograms of cheese, 3½ kilograms of butter, 1 kilogram of yogurt, 8 liters of ice cream. The U.K. also consumes 16½ million liters of fermented dairy drinks.

Does milk do a body good? Perhaps, but certainly not to the extent that one might think based on the marketing claims of the dairy industry. Rather, moderation seems warranted. Many people are lactose-intolerant or allergic to milk, and growing evidence suggests that unlimited dairy consumption may be linked to various other health conditions, including some forms of cancer, heart disease, asthma, diabetes, and obesity. Milk and cheese are often loaded with fat and cholesterol, which at elevated levels can lead to obesity, heart disease, diabetes, and some forms of cancer. Milk products may also be contaminated with pesticides, dioxins, and drug residues, and concern is growing about the use of hormones in cows to boost milk production. These contaminants can lead to cancer and asthma.

In addition, good evidence exists that milk consumption actually *increases* the risk of osteoporosis, the very disease that the dairy industry uses as a selling point in its ads. While numerous clinical studies have demonstrated that calcium supplementation can help prevent bone loss, despite what the dairy industry claims, the data are inconclusive regarding any link between a high dietary calcium intake from milk and prevention of osteoporosis and bone fractures. One of the first clues that milk consumption may not be beneficial for bone health is data showing that countries with the highest dairy intake have the highest rate of hip fractures per capita. In analyzing data from the Nurses' Health Study, a study involving 77,761 women, researchers found no evidence that a higher intake of milk actually reduced fracture incidence. In fact, women who drank two or more glasses of milk per day had a 45 percent increased risk for hip fracture compared to women consuming one glass or less per week. In other words, the more milk a woman consumed, the more likely she was to experience a hip fracture. However, this negative effect may turn out to be due to the vitamin A added to the milk—at higher levels, vitamin A, but not beta-carotene—interferes with bone formation. Interestingly, the rate of osteoporosis worldwide is much higher in countries where milk intake is highest.

But there are health benefits to consuming dairy products in moderation. Dairy foods are good sources of protein. Fermented dairy products that contain live beneficial microorganisms are especially healthful and contribute to a longer, healthier life. Milk and milk products from goats and sheep tend to be lower in fat and cholesterol than milk from cows.

Cow's Milk

Cow's milk, whether poured over breakfast cereal, used to dip biscuits in, or enjoyed on its own, has become a staple of the American diet. Many different types of milk and dairy products are available.

Types of Milk

Whole milk contains not less than 3.25 percent milk fat and 8.25 percent nonfat solids. The addition of vitamins A and D is optional. If vitamin A is added, it must be present at a level of not less than 2,000 International Units (IU) per quart. If vitamin D is added, it must be present at a level of 400 IU per quart.

Reduced fat/low-fat/semi-skimmed milk contains 0.5 percent, 1.5 percent, or 2 percent milk fat and not less than 8.25 percent nonfat solids. Two percent reduced-fat milk contains 2 percent milkfat. One percent low-fat milk, also called "light" milk, contains 1 percent milk fat. In the U.K., semiskimmed milk has 1.7 percent fat and 1 percent low-fat milk is also available. Reduced-fat/low-fat milks must contain 2,000 IU of vitamin A per liter. The addition of vitamin D is optional. If added, vitamin D must be present at a level of 400 IU per quart. (In the U.K., vitamin and calcium fortification is optional.) Flavoring ingredients may also be added.

Fat-free milk, also called skimmed or nonfat milk, contains less than 0.5 percent milk fat and not less than 8.25 percent nonfat solids. Vitamin A must be added at a level of 2,000 IU per quart. The addition of vitamin D is optional but must be present at a level of 400 IU per quart if added. (In the U.K., vitamin and calcium fortification is optional.) Flavoring ingredients may also be added.

Reduced-lactose milk is prepared at a processing plant by adding the enzyme lactase to pasteurized milk and storing it for twenty-four hours. When the appropriate level of reduction has been reached, the milk is pasteurized again to stop the activity of the lactase enzyme. A milk labeled "lactose-reduced" must contain at least 70 percent less lactose than regular milk. Milk that has 99.9 percent of its lactose hydrolyzed may be labeled "lactose-free." In addition to lactose-reduced and lactose-free milks (2 percent fat, 1 percent fat, and nonfat), other lactose-reduced dairy products are on the market. In general, reduced-lactose milks and other reduced-lactose dairy products taste sweeter than traditional counterparts. Reduced-lactose milk is not easy to find in the U.K., but one product, "Lactolite", is available. Contact www.lactolite.co.uk.

Organic milk comes from cows fed and raised without the use of pesticides, synthetic fertilizers, antibiotics, or hormones.

Other Milk Products

Acidophilus cultured milk is pasteurized or ultra-pasteurized milk, usually reduced-fat or non-fat, cultured with *Lactobacillus acidophilus*. Reduced-fat acidophilus milk (2 percent or 1.5 percent milk fat) must have at least a 25 percent reduction in total fat compared to the regular product. Low-fat acidophilus cultured milk can have no more than 3 grams of total fat per serving, whereas nonfat acidophilus cultured milk must contain less than 0.5 gram fat per serving.

Acidophilus milk is not easily distinguished from regular milk.

Cultured buttermilk is produced by culturing whole, low-fat, or nonfat (skimmed) milk with appropriate characterizing bacteria, such as *Streptococcus lactis* or *Lactococcus lactis*. The product may be labeled "cultured buttermilk," "cultured reduced-fat buttermilk," or "cultured skim (nonfat or fat-free) buttermilk," depending on the level of milk fat in the finished product. Buttermilk is pale yellow and somewhat thicker than regular milk, with a pleasantly mild sour aroma.

Sour cream or *cultured sour cream* results from the culturing of pasteurized cream with *Streptococcus lactis* until the acidity is at least 0.5 percent (0.6 percent in the U.K.), calculated as lactic acid. Rennet extract also may be added in small quantities to produce a thicker-bodied product. Cultured sour cream must contain not less than 18 percent milk fat (unless nutritive sweeteners are added, in which case not less than 14.4 percent milk fat must be present). In the U.K., the usual fat content is 12 to 30 percent depending on the product. Sour cream is white, thick enough to be spooned out of a container, and has a sharp, sour flavor.

Acidified sour cream results from the souring of pasteurized cream with safe and suitable acidifiers, with or without the addition of lactic acid-producing bacteria. Federal standards of identity regarding milk fat concentration are the same as for cultured sour cream. Acidified reduced-fat sour cream must have at least a 25 percent reduction in total fat compared to the regular product. Acidified sour cream looks and tastes similar to cultured sour cream with variation based on the type of acidifier used.

Sour half-and-half (single) or *cultured sour half-and-half (single cream)* results from the addition of lactic acid-producing bacteria to single cream. Sour single cream contains not less than 18 percent milk fat. The product may or may not contain lactic acid-producing bacteria. Reduced-fat single cream must have at least 25 percent less fat per serving than the regular product. These milk products are similar to buttermilk and the thickness increases with higher fat content.

Acidified sour half-and-half (single cream) results from the souring of single cream with safe and suitable acidifiers, with or without the addition of lactic acid-producing bacteria. Federal standards (milk fat content) for this product are the same as those for sour single cream. Acidified sour single cream is similar to buttermilk.

Concentrated milks are made by the partial removal of water from fluid milk. These products are pasteurized and may be homogenized and/or fortified with vitamin D. According to federal definitions, the milk fat and total milk solids content of concentrated milks must not be less than 7.5 percent and 25.5 percent, respectively. Variations of concentrated milks include evaporated and sweetened condensed milks. Either concentrated milks are sterilized or their osmotic pressure is increased so that no microorganisms survive.

Evaporated milk is made by removing about 60 percent of milk's water, homogenizing, standardizing to the required percentages of components, adding vitamins (vitamin D up to 25 IU per ounce; vitamin A is optional), and stabilizing. Evaporated milk is a heat-sterilized product with an extended shelf life and is available in cans. The product must contain not less than 6.5 percent milk fat, not less than 16.5 percent nonfat milk solids, and not less than 23 percent total milk solids. Because of its yellowish color and cooked flavor, evaporated milk is generally limited to use in baking. Reduced-fat and nonfat versions of evaporated milk are available. Evaporated nonfat milk contains not less than 0.5 percent milk fat and 20 percent total milk solids.

Sweetened condensed milk results from the removal of about 60 percent of the water from a mixture of milk (whole and nonfat pasteurized, homogenized milks) and safe and suitable nutritive carbohydrate sweeteners, such as sucrose, at levels of about 40 to 45 percent of the condensed milk, to prevent spoilage. This product contains not less than 8 percent milk fat and not less than 28 percent total milk solids. Reduced-fat and nonfat versions of sweetened condensed milk are available. Sweetened condensed nonfat milk must contain not less than 0.5 percent milk fat and not less than 24 percent total milk solids.

Dry Milk Products

Nonfat dry milk is made by removing water from pasteurized skimmed (nonfat or fat-free) milk. The product must contain 5 percent or less by weight of moisture and no more than 1.5 percent by weight of milk fat unless otherwise indicated. A number of tailor-made nonfat dry milks (as well as other dry milks), including lactose-reduced, low-sodium, and "instant" (i.e., disperses immediately in cold water), are available.

Nonfat dry milk fortified with vitamins A and D is the same as above, except it is fortified so that it has 2,000 IU of vitamin A and 400 IU of vitamin D per quart when reconstituted.

Dry whole milk contains all of the components of whole milk, but in a concentrated form. Dry whole milk is typically made from pasteurized whole milk from which water has been removed by spray or, sometimes, roller drying. On a dry-weight basis, dry whole milk must contain not less than 26 percent or more than 40 percent milk fat and not more than 5 percent moisture on a nonfat milk solids basis. The addition of vitamin A and/or D is optional.

Dry milk products generally resemble their fresh counterparts when reconstituted.

Cream Products

Half-and-half (single cream) is a mixture of milk and cream containing not less than 10.5 percent milk fat but less than 18 percent milk fat. It is pasteurized or ultrapasteurized and may be homogenized. It is similar to milk in color, with a richer flavor and slightly thicker texture.

Light cream, also called single cream, coffee cream or table cream, contains not less than 18 percent milk fat but less than 30 percent milk fat. It is pasteurized or ultrapasteurized and may be homogenized. It is similar to milk in color, with a richer flavor and slightly thicker texture, but not as much as half-and-half.

Light whipping cream (also called whipping cream) is cream that contains not less than 30 percent and no more than 36 percent milk fat. Whipping cream is generally ultrapasteurized to extend its shelf life and may be homogenized. Light whipping cream looks and tastes similar to light cream until whipped, when it becomes semisolid and light.

Heavy cream (double cream) or *heavy whipping cream* must contain a minimum of 36 percent milk fat. The product is pasteurized or ultrapasteurized and may be homogenized. Heavy cream is similar to milk in color, with a richer flavor and a thicker texture than the other cream products. When whipped, it makes a heavier semisolid with a richer flavor than light whipping cream.

Butter, according to USDA standards, is a concentrated source of milk fat made from milk or cream or both that contains a minimum of 80 percent fat along with some water and nonfat milk solids (casein, lactose, and minerals). Butter is made by churning pasteurized cream using batch-process (35 to 45 percent fat cream) or continuous (42 to 44 percent fat cream) churns. Butter may be salted or unsalted. Lightly salted butter is also referred to as "sweet cream butter" and unsalted butter as "sweet butter." Lightly salted butter and unsalted are made from pasteurized sweet cream to which no starter has been added. Ripened cream or lactic butter, such as Lurpak, is made using starter-ripened cream, or cream that has a bacterial culture added to start fermentation. Natural coloring agents, such as annatto and carotene, may be added to give butter a golden yellow color. Otherwise, fresh butter may be almost white.

Clarified butter, or ghee, can be obtained by melting butter and separating the nonfat ingredients (water, proteins, and carbohydrates) in the upper layer of foam and the whitish bottom layer from the yellowish middle layer of fat (clarified butter). Compared to regular butter, clarified butter can be heated to a higher temperature without burning and has a longer storage life. However, clarified butter lacks the characteristic buttery flavor of butter. The color of clarified butter is golden yellow, and it has a nutty flavor.

Light or reduced-fat butter typically contains nonfat milk, water, and/or gelatin and is 40 percent (or less) milk fat. Reduced-fat butter should not be substituted for regular butter in baking or frying due to its high moisture content and its lighter, less rich flavor.

Ice Cream and Frozen Desserts

Ice cream is a frozen food made from a mixture of milk, cream, and nonfat milk combined with sweetening agents, flavorings, fruits, nuts, stabilizers, emulsifiers, and other ingredients. Federal standards require that ice cream contain a minimum of 10 percent milk fat and 20 percent total milk solids by weight. French ice cream or frozen custard is an ice cream product containing at least 1.4 percent egg yolk solids.

In the U.K., 80 percent of ice cream sales comprise ice cream made with no milk fat, but it must be made with a minimum 5 percent fat and not less than 2½ percent milk protein. A product described as "dairy ice cream" must contain 5 percent milk fat.

Reduced-fat, low-fat, light, and fat-free ice creams are varieties of ice cream products reduced in fat that have entered the marketplace. Reduced-fat ice cream contains 25 percent less fat than the original product. Low-fat ice cream contains 3 grams or less of fat per serving. Light ice cream is reduced in fat by at least 50 percent or more, and fat-free ice cream contains less than 0.5 grams of fat. In the U.K. more low-fat ice cream products are now available, ranging from 2.6 to under 1 percent fat.

Sherbet contains not less than 1 percent or more than 2 percent milk fat and 2 to 5 percent total milk solids along with fruit or other flavors. This product contains more sugar than ice cream.

HISTORY

The earliest record suggesting the use of animals' milk as food was unearthed in a temple in the Euphrates Valley near Babylon, where an archaeologist found a wall painting believed to be about 5,000 years old depicting the practice of drinking milk. However, the practice undoubtedly predates this occurrence to at least 6000 to 8000 B.C.E. In ancient Egypt, consumption of milk was a sign of wealth and status. Milk was also recorded as a popular beverage in the Bible and ancient Hindu texts.

By 400 C.E., sheep and cow's milk began to become a staple in the diet throughout Europe, but it really was not until the 1300s that cow's milk became the most popular form. Cows were brought to America by the Jamestown colonists in 1611 and by the Pilgrims to Plymouth Colony in 1624.

The major commercial development for milk occurred in the later part of the nineteenth century with the widespread adoption of pasteurization, Louis Pasteur's process for destroying bacteria, moulds, spores, and other microorganisms by exposing milk and other food to a high temperature. Prior to pasteurization, many diseases were transmitted through raw milk to children and adults alike. When milk is pasteurized, it is heated to a high enough temperature to kill certain (but not all) bacteria and to disable certain enzymes, minimizing the effect on taste as much as possible. Milk can be pasteurized by heating to 145 degrees F. (62.8

degrees C.) for thirty minutes or 163 degrees F. (72.8 degrees C.) for fifteen seconds. Refrigeration keeps the bacteria from growing further.

Homogenization was developed in the twentieth century and is the process of breaking up the fat globules in cream to such a small size that they remain suspended evenly in the milk rather than separating out and floating to the surface. If you take a gallon of fresh milk straight from a cow and allow it to sit in the refrigerator, all of the cream will separate, leaving you with skimmed milk and a layer of cream on top. Homogenization specifically involves pumping milk, under pressure, through very small openings, thus breaking the fat into minute globules that are immediately surrounded by a film of protein that prevents them from reuniting.

The history of milk production in the United States is particularly significant. In 1856, Gail Borden received a patent on producing condensed milk followed by the building of the first condensery in Burrville, Connecticut. In 1884, another major advancement occurred when Dr. Hervey D. Thatcher, of Potsdam, New York, invented the milk bottle. Other important dates in American milk history:

1895: Commercial pasteurizing machines are introduced.
1908: Chicago passes the first compulsory pasteurization law applying to all milk except that from tuberculin-tested cows.
1911: The automatic rotary bottle filler and capper are perfected.

BOVINE GROWTH HORMONE

Bovine growth hormone (BGH) is a normal product of the pituitary gland of cows. It greatly increases milk production by stimulating the production of another hormone called insulinlike growth factor 1, or IGF-1 for short. IGF-1 directly stimulates milk production.

In 1990, Monsanto scientists developed recombinant bovine growth hormone (rBGH), also known as recombinant bovine somatotropin (rBST). Cows injected with rBGH every two weeks produce 10 to 20 percent more milk than untreated cows. The U.S. Food and Drug Administration (FDA) in late 1993 approved rBGH use in cows and declared the milk from rBGH-treated cows to be safe. However, this approval and declaration have been extremely controversial, as there are many unresolved safety issues. While Europe, Japan, and Canada have banned the use of rBGH, according to Monsanto, more than a quarter of U.S. milk cows are now in herds given rBGH. Complicating the matter is that the vast majority of the country's 1,500 dairy companies mix rBGH milk with non-rBGH milk during processing to such an extent that an estimated 80 to 90 percent of the U.S. dairy supply is now contaminated. Furthermore, while the focus has been on the effects of rBGH in milk, about 40 percent of the beef used to make hamburgers comes from "old" dairy cows.

For U.S. consumers, it is very difficult to know if the milk they are consuming is free of rBGH. Monsanto has filed lawsuits opposing the labeling of milk produced by drug-treated cows and has gone one step further by

(continued on next page)

enlisting the help of the FDA to also oppose labeling of products that are free of rBGH. While the FDA says there is "no significant difference" between milk from rBGH-treated cows and milk from cows not treated, and thus a label saying "rBGH-free" would imply a difference that did not exist, this position may not be entirely true. The FDA's position on labeling was developed under the direction of Michael R. Taylor, a lawyer who joined the FDA in 1991 after almost a decade as a partner in the law firm that Monsanto hired to gain FDA approval of rBGH, and also to bring Monsanto's lawsuits against milk producers who labeled their products as rBGH-free.

So what are the concerns about rBGH? Well, there are many that are currently known and many, we suspect, that are currently unknown, as there have been no long-term safety studies on humans. It is currently known that:

- *rBGH increases the risk of about twenty different health conditions in cows, including mastitis (25 percent increase in risk), infertility (18 percent increase in risk), and lameness (50 percent increase in risk).*
- *rBGH milk is more likely to be contaminated by pus from mastitis induced by rBGH and antibiotics used to treat the mastitis.*
- *rBGH milk is supercharged with high levels of a natural growth factor (IGF-1), excess levels of which have been suggested to increase the risk of breast, colon, and prostate cancers.*

Our view is that even if there were no health concerns associated with the use of rBGH, its use might not be a good thing for economic reasons. The government already subsidizes the milk industry by buying approximately $2 billion of milk surpluses each year. Furthermore, the Congressional Office of Technology Assessment predicted in 1995 that widespread use of rBGH could put 30 percent of all dairy farmers out of business. It is clear that we do not need more milk production. Greater milk production will only suppress the price of milk enough to make dairy farming unprofitable for most small dairy farmers.

Organic milk, on the other hand, is rBGH-free, as required by organic standards. Therefore, even if labeling for rBGH-containing products is not available, you can be confident that if a dairy product is organic, it is also rBGH-free. The E.U. banned rBGH (or BST) on the grounds of animal welfare, effective from January 2000.

1914: Tank trucks are first used for transporting milk.

1919: Homogenized milk is sold successfully in Torrington, Connecticut.

1932: A practical method of increasing the vitamin D level in milk is developed.

1932: The first plastic-coated paper milk cartons are introduced commercially.

1933: Fluid milk is included in army rations.

1938: The first farm bulk tanks for milk begin to replace milk cans.

1946: The vacuum pasteurization method is perfected.

1948: Ultra-high-temperature pasteurization is introduced.

1964: The plastic milk container is introduced commercially.

1974: Nutritional labeling of fluid milk products begins.

1975: Metric measurement equivalent is introduced.

1980: The American Dairy Association

TABLE 17.1

Milk Production by Selected Countries (millions of tons)

	2002	2003	2004
World	593.6	600.1	611.5
15 European Union nations	126.7	126.8	125.5
India	84.6	87.0	91.3
United States	77.1	77.2	77.5
Russian Federation	33.5	33.3	31.9
Pakistan	27.7	28.4	29.1
Brazil	22.8	23.5	24.4
China	14.0	17.5	21.0
New Zealand	13.9	14.4	15.0
Ukraine	14.1	13.6	13.6
Poland	11.8	11.9	11.9
Mexico	9.6	9.9	10.0
Australia	11.3	10.3	10.0
Argentina	8.5	7.9	9.5

From: United States Department of Agriculture, Foreign Agricultural Service. www.fas.usda.com

TABLE 17.2

Nutritional Components of a 1-Cup (8-Ounce/250 milliliters) Serving of Milk

	Calories	Protein (grams)	Fat (grams)	Carbohydrate (grams)
Whole milk	146	8.0	7.9	11.5
2 percent milk	122	8.0	4.8	11.5
1 percent milk	102	8.0	2.4	11.5
Fat-free milk	83	8.0	0.2	11.5

TABLE 17.3

Nutritional Components of a 100 gram Serving of Milk

	Calories	Protein (grams)	Fat (grams)	Carbohydrate (grams)
Whole milk	60	3.3	3.25	4.9
2 percent milk	50	3.3	2.0	4.9
1 percent milk	42	3.3	1.0	4.9
Fat-free milk	34	3.3	0.08	4.9

launches the national introduction of the "REAL"® Seal dairy symbol.

1981: UHT (ultra-high-temperature) milks gain national recognition.

1983: The National Dairy Promotion and Research Board is created.

1988: Lower-fat dairy products gain widespread acceptance. Low-fat and skimmed milk sales combined exceed whole-milk sales for the first time.

1993: A mandatory animal drug residue testing programme is established.

1994: rBST, or recombinant bovine somatotropin, is approved for commercial use in the United States as a safe and effective means of increasing cows' milk production.

1994: The Nutrition Labeling and Education Act requires mandatory nutrition labeling.

1994: The National Fluid Milk Processor Promotion Board launches the "Milk, what a surprise!" ad campaign.

1995: Americans' milk consumption rises for the first time in twenty-five years.

NUTRITIONAL HIGHLIGHTS

The basic composition of milk is 87.4 percent water and 12.6 percent milk solids. In whole milk, the solids portion is made up of 3.7 percent fat and 8.9 percent nonfat milk solids. The nonfat milk solids contain protein (3.4 percent), lactose (4.8 percent), and minerals (0.7 percent). Milk is also a rich source of many important vitamins.

Milk Fat

Milk fat is composed primarily of triglycerides (97 to 98 percent); phospholipids (0.2 to 1 percent); free sterols such as cholesterol and squalene; traces of free fatty acids; and the fat-soluble vitamins A, D, E, and K. Milk fat is extremely complex, as more than 400 different fatty acids and fatty acid derivatives are found in milk, including a relatively high proportion of short-chain and medium-chain saturated fatty acids. Milk fat contains about 7 percent short-chain fatty acids (C4 to C8), 15 to 20 percent medium-chain fatty acids (C10 to C14), and 73 to 78 percent long-chain fatty acids (C16 and higher). The composition of milk fat varies according to such factors as the breed of the cow and composition of the feed. The fatty acids in milk fat are approximately 65 percent saturated, 32 percent monounsaturated, and 3 percent polyunsaturated, with minor amounts of other types of fatty acids.

Milk is a good source of conjugated linoleic acid (CLA), especially if it is from pasture-fed cows. Other interesting milk fat components being investigated for their potential health benefits include sphingomyelin, butyric acid, and myristic acid.

Protein

Cow's milk is an excellent source of high-quality protein. The basic composition of cow's milk protein is about 80 percent casein and 20 percent whey protein. The two proteins have different physical characteristics. Casein is generally defined as the protein precipitated at pH 4.6, a property used in the manufacturing of cheese. Whey protein is separated out in the manufacture of cheese and consists predominantly of beta-lactoglobulin and alpha-lactalbumin. Alpha-lactalbumin has a high content of the amino acid tryptophan. The action beta-lactoglobulin possesses is still speculative. Other whey proteins present in smaller amounts are serum albumin, immunoglobulins (e.g., IgA, IgG, and IgM), protease peptones, lactoferrin, and transferrin.

Carbohydrates

The principal carbohydrate in milk is lactose, a natural disaccharide consisting of one galactose and one glucose unit. Lactose accounts for about 54 percent of the total nonfat solids content of whole milk and about 30 percent of its calories. Minor quantities of glucose, galactose, and oligosaccharides are also present in milk.

Water-Soluble Vitamins, Minerals, and Other Components

Milk contains a very good supply of most B vitamins and minerals. While it is easy to think of milk as supplying only calcium, it actually provides very good levels of virtually every other mineral, including trace minerals.

PASTURE-FED VERSUS GRAIN-FED COWS

Roughly 85 to 95 percent of the cows in the United States are now being raised in confinement in feedlots, not on pasture. The only grass they eat comes in the form of hay, and the ground that they stand on is a blend of dirt and manure. Most dairy cows are fed grain because grain-fed cows produce three times as much milk as those grazing on green grass.

However, while cows fed grain produce a higher quantity of milk, it is definitely lower in quality than that produced by grass-fed cows. For example, milk from a pastured cow can contain five times as much CLA as that from a grain-fed animal. Milk from pastured cows also contains an ideal ratio of the essential fatty acids linoleic acid (the essential omega-6 fatty acid) and alpha-linolenic acid (the essential omega-3 fatty acid). As you can see in the figure, when a cow is raised on pasture, her milk has an ideal ratio of omega-6 to omega-3 fatty acids. Take away one third of the grass and replace it with grain, and the omega-3 fatty acid content of the milk goes down while the omega-6 fatty acid content goes up, upsetting an essential balance. Replace two thirds of the pasture with a grain-based diet (illustrated by the two bars on the far right) and the milk will have a very top-heavy ratio of omega-6 to omega-3 fatty acids, a ratio that has been linked with an increased risk of a wide variety of conditions, including obesity, diabetes, depression, and cancer. Much of the milk bought in U.S. supermarkets has an even more lopsided ratio because the cows producing it get no pasture whatsoever.

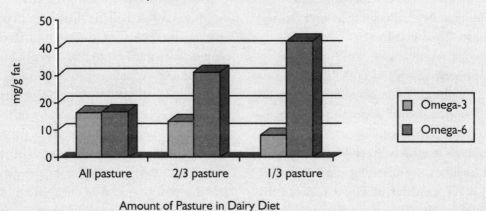

100 percent Pasture Creates Ideal EFA Ration

Milk from pastured cows offers additional health benefits, as it is much higher in beta-carotene, vitamin A, vitamin E, and other vitamins.

Unfortunately, the label on a milk carton won't tell you whether the cows were fed grass or grain. Even an organic label is no guarantee that the cows grazed on pasture. At the present time, there are at least two large organic dairies that make a point of raising their cows on pasture: Organic Valley and Natural by Nature.

HEALTH BENEFITS

Cow's milk has long been valued for its health benefits by many cultures. These benefits revolve around its high nutritional content, yet in addition to being a rich source of protein and many nutrients, milk contains a large number of unique health-promoting ingredients. In addition, fermented milks and yogurts containing health-promoting bacteria offer significant health benefits (discussed below). Dairy foods provide the ideal food system for the delivery of these beneficial bacteria to the human gut, given the suitable environment that milk (and certain dairy products including yogurt and cheese) provides to promote growth and/or support viability of these cultures.

Compounds in milk that have been shown to be beneficial to human health include a range of protein fragments (peptides) produced by digestion of milk's main proteins that are very bioactive. These include:

Caseinophosphopeptides (CPPs), which possess the ability to bind and to solubilize minerals such as calcium and thereby increase their absorption.

Antihypertensive milk peptides, which block angiotensin-converting enzyme (ACE), a key regulator of blood pressure that causes blood vessels to constrict and the kidneys to retain sodium and water.

Lactoferrin, an iron-binding protein that is often cited for its immune-enhancing and antiviral effects.

Glycomacropeptide, which has been shown to slow gastric emptying in animals and is now being promoted as an appetite suppressant in the United States.

Milk fat also contains a number of bioactive components, including conjugated linoleic acid (CLA), sphingomyelin, and butyric acid. Although milk contains saturated fatty acids and trans-fatty acids, which are associated with atherosclerosis and coronary heart disease, it also contains monounsaturated and essential fatty acids, which are negatively associated with these diseases. A twenty-five-year study of 5,700 Scottish men found that the heart disease death rates among men drinking more than two-thirds of a cup of milk each day were 8 percent lower than among those who drank less. Deaths from cancer and strokes were also 10 percent lower among the regular milk drinkers. It appears that the other components of milk counteract the adverse effects of the saturated fat content.

Conjugated linoleic acid (CLA) has been shown to possess activities that prevent cancer and the formation of cholesterol-containing plaques that contribute to heart disease; activate the immune system; enhance the effects of insulin; and promote lean body mass (have an antiobesity effect). For example, when French researchers compared CLA levels in the breast tissue of 360 women, they found that the women with the most CLA in their tissue (and thus the most CLA in their diets) had a 74 percent lower risk of breast cancer than the women with the least CLA.

Milk is also a very good source of myristic acid, a very important fatty acid that the body uses to stabilize many different proteins, including proteins used in the immune system and to fight tumors.

Like CLA, sphingomyelin is a milk fat component that has shown anticancer effects. In

MILK AND TYPE I DIABETES

Type I diabetes develops as the result of an autoimmune process where the insulin-producing cells of the pancreas are destroyed by the body's own immune system. What triggers this destruction can vary from one case to another. In some cases, it looks as if the immune system develops antibodies to dietary protein that cross-react with antigens on or within the beta cells of the pancreas. In humans, the two proteins that have been most often incriminated are those found in milk (bovine serum albumin as well as bovine insulin) and wheat (gluten).

Numerous population-based studies have shown that breast-feeding offers considerable protection against the development of type I diabetes as well as many other diseases. This protective effect against type I diabetes is probably related to two factors: the important role that breast milk plays in the formation of a healthy gut-associated immune system and the delaying of introduction of cow's milk or infant formulas containing cow's milk proteins to the infant. In case-controlled studies, people with type I diabetes were more likely to have been breast-fed for less than three months and to have been exposed to cow's milk or solid foods before four months of age. A critical review and analysis of all relevant studies indicates that early cow's milk exposure may increase the risk about one and a half times. While the risk of diabetes associated with exposure to cow's milk was first thought to relate only to intake during infancy, additional studies showed that ingestion at any age may increase the risk of type I diabetes.

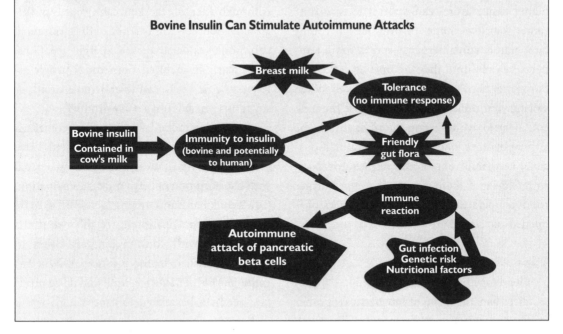

Bovine Insulin Can Stimulate Autoimmune Attacks

one study in mice, sphingomyelin from milk reduced the incidence of colon tumors by 57 percent. Butyric acid, another fatty acid in milk, has also been shown to inhibit the growth of a range of cancer cells, especially colon cancer.

HOW TO SELECT AND STORE

To help ensure you are getting fresh, unspoiled milk, it is always best to check the sell-by date before you buy milk. Also, be sure to smell the top of the container to make sure that the milk doesn't smell of spoilage. In some supermarkets or transportation settings, the milk may experience an extended period of time outside refrigeration, thus moving its freshness date forward from that stamped on the container. Select milk from the coldest part of the refrigerator case, which is often the lower section and/or at the back.

Although some milk in Europe and now in the United States is sold at room temperature in sealed containers, most typical supermarket-refrigerated milk should be refrigerated since higher temperatures can cause it to turn sour rather quickly. Some of the newer room-temperature containers may stay at room temperature only until they are opened. After this point, they need to be refrigerated as well. When storing your milk, always seal or close the milk container to avoid having the milk absorb the aromas of other foods in the refrigerator. If possible, keep milk out of the refrigerator door, since storing it there exposes it to the warmer room temperature each time the refrigerator is opened and closed.

QUICK SERVING IDEAS

- Blend together 1 to 2 cups of milk, 1 frozen sliced banana, ½ cup of blueberries (or other favorite fruits), and 1 teaspoon of cinnamon for a delicious shake.
- Add 1 cup of milk and some raisins, cinnamon and nutmeg to a pot of cooked brown rice to make rice pudding.

- A relaxing evening drink is warmed milk, stirred over low heat. Some Ayurvedic (Indian medicine) practitioners recommend adding a pinch of nutmeg to the milk and drinking it 1 hour before bed to ensure a good night's sleep.
- Make hot chocolate by combining milk, unsweetened cocoa powder, and honey in a saucepan over low heat. Stir frequently to avoid burning on the bottom. Also watch closely, for milk can heat up and boil out over the pot.
- Milk has been enjoyed for generations over a favorite bowl of hot or cold cereal in the morning.

SAFETY

Although allergic reactions can occur to virtually any food, cow's milk is one of the foods most commonly associated with allergic reactions, particularly in children. Sometimes people allergic to cow's milk can tolerate goat's milk or soy milk (which is not a dairy product).

In addition to food allergy, many people lack the enzyme lactase, needed to digest lactose (see page 70). Another adverse reaction associated with consumption of cow's milk is constipation. Cow's milk consumption was determined to be the cause of constipation in roughly two thirds of children with constipation, according to studies published in the prestigious *New England Journal of Medicine*. Milk and dairy products seem to be related to type 1 and type 2 diabetes (see box on page 585). Presumably, the same significance regarding constipation and diabetes holds true for adults.

Finally, milk intake does not appear to change the risk of fracture due to osteoporosis.

Because of this, milk should not be the only source of calcium in the diet. To avoid cows treated with recombinant bovine growth hormone (rBGH), buy organic dairy products.

Cheese

Cheese, a concentrated dairy food made from milk, is defined as the fresh or matured product obtained by draining the whey (moisture or serum of original milk) after the coagulation of casein, the major milk protein. The basic art of cheese making has changed little over the course of its history. Milk is coagulated to produce curd by the separate or combined action of lactic acid (produced by the breakdown of lactose by selected microorganisms) and coagulating enzymes. Whey is subsequently removed from the curd, and the latter is further treated to produce the many varieties of cheese.

Different ingredients and processes employed during the making and aging of cheese result in a wide variety of available cheeses, each with its own distinct texture and flavor profile. More than 2,000 varieties of cheese are produced around the world, and more than 200 types are made in the United States. In the U.K., there are over 700 types of cheese, including the ten main varieties.

Natural cheese is a general classification for cheese that is made directly from milk. In fresh, unripened cheese, the curd, separated from the whey, can be used immediately; whereas in matured or ripened cheese, the curd is further treated by the addition of selected strains of bacteria, mould, yeast, or a combination of these ripening agents. The bacteria, mould, and yeast continue to ripen the cheese over time, changing the cheese's flavor and texture as it ages.

Because natural cheese is a living system, its functional and physical properties change over time. When choosing natural cheese as an ingredient, it's important to understand how a cheese will perform in a finished product based on its age and storage conditions.

Pasteurized processed cheese, and cheese spread are made by blending one or more different kinds of natural cheese into a homogeneous mass. Through the addition of other optional ingredients such as salt and emulsifier, the appearance, texture, and flavor of the cheese mass are modified. These cheeses are available in a variety of color intensities and flavors tailored to a variety of food-processing applications.

Cheese powders, or dehydrated cheeses, are prepared using a single cheese variety or a blend of various cheeses. Products may be all cheese or a blend of cheese with other dairy ingredients (whey, nonfat dry milk, etc.), food ingredients, and/or color. Some typical applications for cheese powders include prepared dry mixes, sauces, and dips.

The amount and variety of cheese and cheese products consumed and manufactured in the United States have increased tremendously in recent years. Americans consumed nearly 2.5 times as much cheese in 1997 as they did in 1970. In fact, since 1970, per capita consumption of cheese has increased yearly. Today, more than one third of all cow's milk produced each year in the United States is used to make cheese. In the U.K., about 20 percent of milk produced is used for cheese making.

Types of Natural Cheeses

While all cheeses are made from the same raw ingredient—the milk of an animal such as a cow, sheep, or goat—the more than 2,000 different varieties of cheese throughout the world each feature their own unique taste and texture. Here are some of the more popular varieties:

Cheddar, originating in Somerset and still Britain's most popular cheese, makes up the largest share of American-type cheeses produced in the United States. The distinctive processing step is the matting or cheddaring of the curd particles into a cohesive state.

Colby is manufactured similarly to cheddar up to the point of draining off the whey. The curds of Colby cheese receive no cheddaring or milling. Instead, the curds are kept separate. Colby cheese has a softer body (higher moisture content), lower salt content, and more open texture than Cheddar cheese but has a mild flavor resembling that of young Cheddar cheese.

Swiss cheese is characterized by the holes or "eyes" that develop during early stages of ripening. This cheese is one of the more difficult types of cheese to manufacture, involving several complicated procedures. During the principal ripening period, propionic acid is released from the bacterium *Propionibacterium shermanii* and related organisms. The propionic acid contributes to the characteristic sweet flavor, and carbon dioxide collects to form holes or "eyes."

Edam and Gouda have tiny shiny holes or eyes. Gouda generally contains more fat and is softer in texture than Edam. They are also manufactured similarly to cheddar cheese. However, the curd develops little acidity, and it is not cheddared.

Parmesan is the most widely known variety of *grana* (hard grating) cheese and the most important cheese in northern Italy. This salty, sharp-flavored grating cheese is also manufactured in the United States.

Romano is a sharply piquant Italian grating cheese resembling Parmesan and other *grana* cheeses. It is usually made from sheep's milk.

Provolone is representative of the *pasta filata* or stretched-curd cheeses. In these stringy-textured cheeses, the curd is cooked to a relatively high temperature and is pulled and moulded into various shapes while hot. The name provolone is derived from the Neapolitan word *prova,* meaning "ball-shaped."

Mozzarella is a soft *pasta filata* cheese made in a way resembling provolone. Available forms of mozzarella cheese include part-skimmed mozzarella, low-moisture mozzarella, and low-moisture, part-skimmed mozzarella. String cheese derived from mozzarella is also popular.

Blue cheese is characterized by visible blue-green veins of mould throughout the interior and by a sharp, piquant flavor. There are several blue-veined varieties of cheese known by various names. However, they differ appreciably only when the milk source varies. Cheeses in this family include Roquefort, which is made only in the Roquefort area of France from sheep's milk, and its various cow's milk counterparts, known as bleu cheese in other areas of France, blue in the United States; other region-specific varieties are Stilton in England, and Gorgonzola in Italy. In the preparation of blue cheese, whole milk, usually homogenized, may be inoculated with mould spores of *Penicillium roqueforti* or a similar mould that will result in blue-green mottling of the cheese. The mould produces a water-soluble enzyme that liberates free fatty acids. The mould spores then convert the fatty acids to ketones, which are largely responsible for the flavor of the finished cheese.

Limburger has a very strong and characteristic odor and flavor. It is produced by exposing a culture of salt-tolerant yeasts and a culture of *Bacterium linens* to the surface of the cheese. Within a few days, the yeasts establish conditions favorable for the growth of bacteria on the surface of the cheese. *Bacterium linens* produces a brownish red surface growth and is essential to the development of Limburger's characteristic strong flavor and aroma and soft, waxy body. After two to three weeks of ripening, the cheese is wrapped in parchment, waxed paper, and foil and stored at 50 degrees F./10 degrees C. for one to two months. When fully ripe, Limburger cheese must be marketed immediately, as it becomes overripe rapidly, which results in an excessively strong flavor. It is not commonly available in the U.K. but some specialist delicatessens stock it.

Camembert is another surface-ripened cheese that has a creamy, semiliquid interior consistency due to the activity of *Penicillium camemberti.*

Brie is also surface-ripened and is similar to Camembert. Differences exist, however, in the manufacturing details, the internal ripening, and the characteristic flavor and aroma. Like Camembert, Brie ripens rapidly, is perishable, and must be consumed soon after ripening.

Cottage cheese is a lactic acid-precipitated type of cheese not subjected to prolonged ripening. Fresh pasteurized nonfat milk, concentrated nonfat milk, or reconstituted nonfat dry milk may be used. Coagulation is initiated by lactic acid, formed by active lactic acid starters.

Cream cheese is a soft, unripened lactic acid-coagulated type of cheese, which is made in a manner similar to that described for cottage cheese. The coagulated mass is stirred and drained by centrifugal procedures.

Whey cheeses are obtained by concentrating whey (the watery liquid remaining after the curd is formed in cheese making) and by coagulating the whey protein with heat and acid, with or without the addition of milk and milk fat. *Ricotta cheese* is a well-known type of whey cheese, although it is now frequently manufactured from whole or low-fat milk.

Reduced-fat cheeses are produced by the same basic principles used to make traditional cheeses, with subtle changes depending on the degree of fat reduction. The lower the fat content of cheese, the more challenging the cheese-making process. Because of the high moisture content of low-fat cheeses, extended aging may not be possible. These cheeses therefore are often available in only mild forms. Reduced-fat cheeses generally have a shorter shelf life than full-fat cheeses. To qualify as low-fat, a cheese must contain no more than 3 grams of fat per serving. To be called "reduced-fat," the cheese must contain at least 25 percent less fat than its traditional counterpart. Fat-free cheese must contain less than 0.5 grams of fat per reference amount and per labeled serving size.

HISTORY

The practice of making cheese is thought to be an age-old process, dating probably before 8000 B.C.E. Like many discoveries in the distant past, it seems that the ability to produce cheese was unearthed by happenstance: a traveler in the Middle East placed his milk ration in a container that was actually the stomach of a freshly killed sheep. After traveling across the desert for a few hours, he noticed that the contents of his container had turned into a hard, curdlike substance. Unknown to our surprised traveler, the enzymes in the sheep stomach and the heat of the desert sun had catalyzed an enzymatic process that curdled the milk into the first cheese.

Since this early time, cheese has become a much-appreciated food in many cultures. For the ancient Romans, it was so important that if someone was fortunate enough, he would create a separate room in his home for cheese to be made and matured in. During these times, the art of cheese making was greatly advanced, with certain varieties, such as Parmesan and pecorino, being developed by the Romans, and as such, cheese became a staple food at emperors' feasts.

In the Middle Ages, monks became the experts of the cheese-making world. In fact, many of the cheeses developed during that time still carry the name of their monastic origins, including Limburger, Munster and Pont l'Évêque. Even though cheese fell out of popularity during the Renaissance, as it was perceived to be unhealthy, the nineteenth century saw a renewal in the interest of cheese with the development of larger-scale production techniques.

One might say that some countries can be distinguished by their brand of cheese, as many cheeses are closely associated with their country of origin—and countrymen are often quite proud of their respective cheese. For example, England is well known for its Cheddar and Stilton. From Norway comes Jarlsberg. Italy is proud of its Parmesan. And even the relatively new United States (specifically Wisconsin) has its Colby cheese, which is well known around the globe.

In the United States, cheese making was confined to on-farm locations until 1851, when the first small Cheddar cheese factory opened in Rome, New York. About 1900, the following five developments in cheese technology contributed to the rapid growth of commercial cheese making:

- The use of acidity measurements, which led to better control in cheese production.
- The introduction of bacterial cultures as "starters".
- The pasteurization of milk used in cheese making, which destroys harmful microorganisms.
- Refrigerated ripening.
- The development of processed cheese.

By using controlled scientific methods, cheese makers in the United States have successfully manufactured virtually all foreign types of cheeses, including Swiss, Camembert, Limburger, blue, Parmesan, and mozzarella. In addition, distinctive original varieties, such as brick, Colby, Monterey, and others, have been created in the United States.

NUTRITIONAL HIGHLIGHTS

Cheese contains a high concentration of essential nutrients, in particular high-quality protein and calcium, as well as other nutrients such as phosphorus, zinc, vitamin A, riboflavin, and vitamin B12.

TABLE 17.4
Cheeses: Fat Content per 100 gram Serving

Cheese	Calories	Fat (grams)	Protein (grams)
Blue	353	28.7	21.4
Brie	334	27.7	20.8
Camembert	300	24.3	19.8
Cheddar/Colby*	173	7.0	24.4
Cottage cheese, 1%*	72	1.0	12.4
Cream cheese*	231	17.6	10.6
Edam/Gouda	357	27.8	25.0
Limburger	327	27.3	20.1
Mozzarella*	302	20.0	26.0
Parmesan, hard	392	25.8	35.8
Provolone	351	26.6	25.6
Romano	387	26.9	31.8
Swiss*	179	5.1	28.4

*Lowfat

HEALTH BENEFITS

Cheese provides many of the same nutritional benefits and health benefits attributed to milk. An additional benefit of cheese is that it usually contains beneficial bacteria. For example, Emmental Swiss cheese contains *Propionibacterium freudenreichii,* a member of the propionic acid-producing bacteria family. This substance, propionic acid, nourishes the cells of the colon and has shown metabolic activity, including lowering blood cholesterol levels, improving blood sugar control, preventing the overgrowth of the yeast *Candida albicans,* and enhancing calcium absorption. Furthermore, it produces a growth factor that dramatically stimulates the growth of *Lactobacillus* and *Bifidobacterium* species, two important health-promoting bacteria (discussed below in "Yogurt").

Cheese has been shown to help protect against dental caries (cavities). Dental caries result from the breakdown of tooth enamel (i.e., demineralization) by acids produced during the fermentation of sugars and starches by plaque bacteria. The critical pH for demineralization is in the range of 5.2 to 5.7. Human dental plaque acidity studies, which measure a food's cavity-causing potential, demonstrate that aged cheeses such as Cheddar, Swiss, blue, Monterey Jack, mozzarella, Brie, and Gouda prevent plaque pH from falling to a level conducive to the development of caries. Population-based studies also support a beneficial effect of cheese on dental health, as cavities are fewer in areas where cheese consumption is higher.

Because cheese is not usually fortified with vitamin A, it may be a better choice than milk to help delay or minimize age-related bone loss and reduce the risk of osteoporosis.

HOW TO SELECT AND STORE

There are different purchase qualities to look for, depending upon the cheese type. Soft cheeses should be uniform in color throughout, and the cheese should fill out the crust casing, which itself should be free of cracks and not too dry. Semifirm cheese should not be too crumbly or dry, with the color being relatively uniform. Hard cheeses should be uniform in color and have a firm, uncracked rind that is not too dry or pasty. Blue cheeses should not be too dry or too crumbly and should feature veining that is evenly distributed.

If your supermarket has a cheese department, speak with the person who specializes in cheese. She or he can help you choose the best-quality cheese as well as introduce you to different cheeses that you may not have yet tried, which can help you to expand your repertoire and more greatly appreciate this wonderful food.

All cheeses, regardless of variety, should be well wrapped and kept in the warmest section of the refrigerator. (The refrigerator door is often one of the warmest spots.) As storage life is related to the moisture content of the cheese, the softer the cheese, the less time it will keep fresh. In general, firm and semifirm cheeses will keep for two weeks, while soft, blue, and grated cheeses will keep for about one week.

TIPS FOR PREPARING

If you need a grating cheese, choose cheese that has a firm texture, such as a Parmesan cheese, since it is the only kind suitable for grating. Typically, it is easier to grate if it is still cold, rather than if it has equilibrated to room temperature.

Since the flavor of cheese is more intense when it is a bit warmer, it can be removed from refrigeration at least thirty minutes before using. Some cheeses, such as Brie, are very good when warmed in the oven or, like halumi cheese, can be heated in a skillet and served hot.

QUICK SERVING IDEAS

- Enjoy a classic Italian salad—sliced onions and tomatoes topped with mozzarella or Parmesan cheese. Don't forget to drizzle it with olive oil. In fact, freshly grated cheese makes a nice addition to any green salad.
- For a favorite party food, wrap a piece of Brie in premade phyllo dough (filo pastry) and bake at about 350 degrees F./180 degrees C./gas 4 until the dough turns darker brown. Then top with marmalade, dried cranberries, and pine nuts and/or walnuts.
- For a quick, healthy "pizza," lightly toast a whole-wheat pita. Top it with tomato sauce and your favorite vegetables, then with sliced mozzarella, and cook under the grill until the cheese melts.
- Combine sliced fennel and orange pieces. You can add a teaspoon of balsamic vinegar and then top with grated Parmesan cheese.
- Cheese makes a delightful pairing with fruits such as apples, pears, grapes, and melons. Serve with wine as an appetizer or as a cheese plate dessert.

• Feta cheese combines nicely with chilled cooked lentils, minced red onion, and diced green pepper for a delicious cold salad.

SAFETY

Even though many people find milk and cheeses hard to digest, there are variations among these foods. Although a cup of cow's milk contains approximately 10 to 12 grams of lactose, the bacteria and fermenting process that accompany cheese production tends to decrease lactose levels in the final cheese product. In general, soft cheeses contain more lactose than hard cheeses. Aged cheeses, such as Cheddar and Swiss, contain little or no lactose. While a cup of soft cheese may be nearly identical to a cup of cow's milk in terms of lactose content, 1 ounce/30 grams of hard cheese typically contains much less (6 to 12 grams versus 0 to 3 grams, respectively). The more a hard cheese ages, the lower the lactose content. As a result, many people with lactose intolerance can eat modest amounts of these harder cheeses without suffering intestinal distress.

Cheese and other dairy products are among the foods most commonly associated with allergic reactions, particularly in children. Aged cheeses are also associated with tension and migraine headaches.

Yogurt

Once eaten only by certain populations, yogurt is now an established fermented dairy product. Yogurt is made by adding bacterial cultures to milk. These cultures carry on the conversion of the milk's lactose sugar into lactic acid. This clever process gives yogurt its unique tart and

---

KEFIR VERSUS YOGURT

Kefir is another cultured milk product. Traditional-style kefir has a tart, refreshing taste and is usually effervescent, owing to the presence of carbon dioxide, which is an end product of the fermentation process.

Kefir contains different types of beneficial bacteria than yogurt does. Yogurt contains transient beneficial bacteria that keep the digestive system clean and provide food for the friendly bacteria that reside there. But kefir bacteria can actually colonize the intestinal tract, a feat that yogurt does not seem to accomplish. Some of the major strains of friendly bacteria found in kefir include Lactobacillus caucasus, Acetobacter *species, and* Streptococcus. *Unlike yogurt, kefir also contains beneficial yeasts, such as* Saccharomyces kefir *and* Torula kefir, *which help control and eliminate destructive pathogenic yeasts in the body.*

---

sour flavor and unique puddinglike texture. The texture is the reasons the Turks gave it the name *yoghurmak,* meaning "to thicken." The lactic acid bacteria that are traditionally used to make yogurt—*Lactobacillus bulgaricus, Lactobacillus acidophilus, Bifidobacterium lactis,* and *Streptococcus thermophilus*—are also responsible for many of yogurt's health benefits.

Yogurt can be purchased in a variety of flavors, including vanilla, fruit flavors such as strawberry, peach, or blueberry, and even chocolate. Plain yogurt, however, is the simplest, lowest in sugar, and most wholesome and versatile. Soy yogurt has recently become available; it is made from soy milk and also has the benefit of healthy bacterial cultures.

HISTORY

Although it is not known when and where yogurt was first created and produced, fermented dairy products have probably been consumed ever since the beginning of the domestication of cows, a practice man has performed for thousands of years. The legend often told about yogurt is that it was born on the slopes of Mount Elbrus in the Caucasus Mountains, between the Black and Caspian Seas. On the hot southern slopes a pitcher of milk belonging to a Turkish nomad was contaminated by a mixture of organisms that thrived in the warm (104 to 113 degrees F./40 to 45 degrees C.) milk. The result was what the Turks call *yogurut*. The name *yogurut* was supposedly introduced in the eighth century and was changed in the eleventh century to the current version, "yogurt."

An early historical account of yogurt is found in the history of Genghis Khan. In thirteenth-century Central Asia, Genghis's armies were allegedly sustained by this healthful food. This is most likely true, for yogurt and other fermented dairy products have long been a staple in the diets of people living in Central Asia, Russia, and the eastern European countries. Surprisingly, the acknowledgment of yogurt's special health benefits did not occur in western Europe and North America until the twentieth century, when research investigating the health-promoting effects of yogurt was conducted by Dr. Elie Metchnikoff. His research, focused on the health benefits of lactic acid-producing bacteria, led to the development of his belief that the long life of certain peoples, such as the Bulgarians, was related to their high consumption of yogurt and fermented dairy products.

Yogurt continues to play a leading role in a host of cuisines, including Turkish, Greek, Indian, and Middle Eastern, as well as eastern European and Asian.

NUTRITIONAL HIGHLIGHTS

Like other milk products, yogurt is a very good source of protein, calcium, phosphorus, riboflavin, and vitamin B12. It is also a good source of pantothenic acid, biotin, selenium, zinc, and potassium. A 100 gram serving of low-fat yogurt provides 63 calories, 5.3 grams of protein, 6 milligrams of cholesterol, 1.6 grams of fat, and 7 grams of carbohydrate, mostly as lactose. Frozen yogurt provides 127 calories, 3 grams of protein, 13 milligrams of cholesterol, 3.6 grams of fat, and 21.6 grams of carbohydrate, mostly as sugars.

HEALTH BENEFITS

Interest in the health benefits of cultured (fermented) dairy foods dates back to the early 1900s, when Elie Metchnikoff, in his book *The Prolongation of Life,* associated intake of large quantities of Bulgarian fermented milk with a long life. Today, researchers are investigating the therapeutic role of probiotic bacteria (i.e., beneficial bacterial cultures such as *Lactobacillus* and *Bifidobacterium*) in dairy foods. The following are some of the potential health benefits associated with intake of cultured dairy foods.

Improved Tolerance of Milk

A number of studies have demonstrated that intake of yogurt enhances lactose digestion in individuals with low intestinal levels of lactase, the enzyme necessary to digest lactose. The lower lactose content of some cultured dairy foods compared to milk's may contribute to the beneficial effect of these foods for individuals who have difficulty digesting lactose. The beneficial effect may also be explained by the ability of the starter cultures used in the manufacture of yogurt with live, active cultures to produce the enzyme lactase, which digests the lactose in yogurt.

Improved Intestinal Health

Yogurt containing live active cultures has been demonstrated to help maintain the normal intestinal microflora balance and suppress harmful bacteria in the intestine. Yogurt can aid in the treatment and prevention of antibiotic-associated diarrhea, traveler's diarrhea, and acute diarrhea in children.

Lactobacillus acidophilus has been shown to protect against stomach ulcers by suppressing the growth of *Helicobacter pylori,* a known ulcer-causing bacterium.

Lowering of Blood Cholesterol Levels

The blood cholesterol-lowering effect of fermented milk was demonstrated more than thirty years ago during studies conducted with Masai tribesmen in Africa. While some more recent studies support a cholesterol-lowering effect of cultured dairy foods, the data are conflicting. Different strains of lactic bacteria in cultured dairy foods appear to have different effects on blood cholesterol levels. In a study of older adults, intake of about 1 cup of yogurt with live cultures per day for one year prevented an increase in blood total and low-density lipoprotein (LDL) cholesterol levels.

Anticancer and Immune-Enhancing Effects

Several studies have suggested that the consumption of high levels of cultured milk products, such as yogurt and buttermilk, may reduce the risk of colon cancer. The anticancer effects of these foods extend well beyond the colon, however. Various probiotic species have demonstrated immune-enhancing and antitumor effects, but they also play a critical role in the detoxification of many cancer-causing substances, including hormones, meat carcinogens, and environmental toxins.

One of the key ways in which the body gets rid of "bad" substances, such as excess oestrogen and fat-soluble toxins, is by attaching them to a molecule called glucuronic acid and then excreting this complex in the bile. However, the bond between the "bad" molecule and its escort can be broken by glucuronidase, an enzyme secreted by bacteria. Excess glucuronidase activity means more of the "bad" molecules are present in the body. This, in turn, is associated with an increased cancer risk, particularly the risk of oestrogen-dependent breast cancer. Glucuronidase activity is higher in people who eat a diet high in fat and low in fiber. The level of glucuronidase activity may be one of the key underlying factors explaining why certain dietary factors cause breast cancer and why other dietary factors are preventive. The activity of harmful bacterial enzymes can be reduced by making sure the digestive system maintains the proper balance of bacterial flora, especially the health-promoting lactic acid bacteria found in yogurt.

As for yogurt's ability to boost immune function, researchers in New Zealand recruited thirty healthy elderly volunteers ranging in age from sixty-three to eighty-four years for a three-stage dietary supplementation trial lasting nine weeks. For the first three weeks, study participants were given a glass of low-fat milk twice a day to establish a base-control diet. For the next three weeks, they were given milk to which *Bifidobacterium lactis* had been added in either a standard dose (5×10^{10} organisms per day) or a low dose (5×10^{9} organisms per day). For the final three weeks, study subjects once again received low-fat milk with no added *Bifidobacterium lactis*.

After each three-week period, the researchers evaluated the numbers of study participants' various white blood cells and their tumor cell-killing activity. After the three-week period when they received *Bifidobacterium lactis*, significant increases were seen in the proportions of total, helper, and activated T lymphocytes and natural killer cells in the subjects' blood. Plus, their immune cells' ability to phagocytize, or engulf and destroy, invaders and the tumor cell-killing ability of their natural killer cells also increased.

Most encouraging was that the greatest improvements in immunity were seen in those subjects who had had poor immune responses before receiving *Bifidobacterium lactis*. In general, both the low and standard doses of probiotic produced similar effectiveness.

HOW TO SELECT AND STORE

Some yogurt manufacturers pasteurize their yogurt products, while others do not. Although the aim of pasteurization is to kill any harmful bacteria, it also kills the beneficial lactic acid bacteria in the yogurt, substantially reducing its health benefits. Therefore, to fully enjoy the benefits of yogurt, look for those that feature "live active cultures" or "living yogurt cultures" on the label. Most yogurts currently sold in the U.K. are "live"—i.e. they have live bacteria when sold up to their sell-by date. In the U.S., yogurts with live active cultures can be identified by the National Yogurt Association's "Live and Active Culture" seal. In order to meet the NYA criteria, live and active culture yogurt must satisfy all of these requirements:

- The product must be fermented with both *L. bulgaricus* and *S. thermophilus*.
- For refrigerated yogurt, the total viable count at the time of manufacture must be 10^{8} CFU (colony forming units) per gram. In the case of frozen yogurt, the total viable count at the time of manufacture must be 10^{7} CFU per gram.
- The cultures must still be active at the end of the stated shelf life, as determined by the activity test described in the "Sampling and Analytical Procedures."
- In the case of frozen yogurt, the product shall have a total titratable acidity expressed as lactic acid of at least 0.3 percent at all times.

Be sure to check the expiration date on the side of the yogurt container to make sure that it is still fresh. Avoid yogurts that have artificial colors, flavorings, or sweeteners. While fruit-filled yogurt can be a delicious treat, be aware that often these yogurt products contain excess sugar.

Look for yogurt made of organic milk. It is becoming more widely available in an array of sizes, flavors, and varieties.

Store yogurt in the refrigerator in its original

container. If unopened, it will stay fresh for about one week past the expiration date.

QUICK SERVING IDEAS

- Sauté cubes of aubergine and then stir in some plain yogurt. Add chopped mint leaves, garlic, and cayenne.
- You can't go wrong making a raita: Add chopped cucumber and dill weed to plain yogurt. Eat this delicious, cooling salad as is or use as an accompaniment to grilled chicken, lamb, or curry dishes.
- Breakfast with an Eastern twist: Top waffles or pancakes with a dollop (or two) of plain yogurt and then sprinkle on your favorite nuts and fruits.
- Yogurt parfaits are a healthful, visual, and gustatory treat. In a large wineglass, alternate layers of yogurt and your favorite fruits.
- Yogurt is a wonderful foundation for salad dressings. Simply place plain yogurt in the blender with enough water to achieve the desired consistency. Add to this your favorite herbs and spices.
- Mix cold cereal or granola and fresh blueberries with yogurt for a twist on the traditional cereal-and-milk breakfast.
- Try using regular or soy yogurt instead of milk for your breakfast smoothie.

SAFETY

The same issues of safety that apply to milk apply to yogurt, although to a lesser extent due to yogurt's ability to lessen allergic reactions to milk and improve lactose tolerance.

To avoid products from cows treated with recombinant bovine growth hormone (rBGH), buy organic dairy products.

Goat's Milk

In the United States and the U.K., goat's milk is thought of as an alternative to cow's milk, but in most areas of the world, the opposite is true: on a global level, more people drink goat's milk than cow's milk.

Most people in the U.S. and U.K. assume that goat's milk has the same potent musky taste for which goat cheese is notorious. The truth is that good-quality goat's milk has a delicious, slightly sweet, and sometimes slightly salty taste.

HISTORY

Goats have played a role in food culture since time immemorial; ancient cave paintings illustrate the hunting of goats. Since goat herding is thought to have evolved around 8,000 B.C.E. in the mountains of Iran, goats are considered to be one of the oldest domesticated animals.

Goat's milk and cheese were revered in ancient Egypt, with some pharaohs supposedly having these foods placed alongside the other treasures in their burial chambers. Goat's milk was also frequently consumed by the ancient Greeks and Romans. Greek mythology tells us the story of the infant god Zeus, who was raised on the milk-filled teats of the goat-nymph Amalthaea. The Chinese believed goat's milk to be an excellent food to maintain general health, and it was was employed to treat conditions of the throat and windpipe. In 1970, the U.N. Food and Agriculture Organization published *Observations on the Goat,* a book that provided many useful insights into the history and benefits of goat's milk. In more recent times, European goat's milk producers such as France and the Netherlands have focused on making goat cheeses.

NUTRITIONAL HIGHLIGHTS

Goat's milk has many of the same nutritional characteristics as cow's milk (see above). It is a very good source of protein, phosphorus, calcium, riboflavin and biotin. It is also a good source of pantothenic acid and vitamin D. A 100 gram serving of goat's milk provides 69 calories, 3.6 grams of protein, 11 grams of cholesterol, 4.1 grams of fat as saturated and monounsaturated forms, and 4.5 grams of carbohydrate as sugars. A 100 gram serving of goat's milk cheese provides 364 calories, 21.6 grams of protein, 79 grams of cholesterol, 29.8 grams of fat of which 20.6 grams are saturated, and 2.5 grams of carbohydrate.

HEALTH BENEFITS

Perhaps the greatest benefit of goat's milk is that some people who cannot tolerate cow's milk are able to drink goat's milk without any problems. Allergy to cow's milk has been found in many people with conditions such as recurrent ear infections, asthma, eczema, and even rheumatoid arthritis. Replacing cow's milk with goat's milk may help to reduce some of the symptoms of these conditions.

Goat's milk can sometimes even be used as a replacement for cow's milk for children who have difficulties with dairy products. Unfortunately, goat's milk is lacking in several nutrients that are necessary for growing infants, so parents interested in trying goat's milk instead of a cow's milk-based formula for their infants should ask their pediatrician or other qualified health care practitioners for recipes and ways of adding these important and vital nutrients. For older children and adults, however, goat's milk can be an excellent calcium-rich alternative to cow's milk, for in addition to calcium, it contains many of the same nutrients found in cow's milk.

HOW TO SELECT AND STORE

To help ensure you are getting fresh, unspoiled goat's milk, it is always best to check the sell-by date before you buy your milk. Also, be sure to smell the top of the container to make sure that the milk isn't spoiled. In some supermarkets or transportation settings, this milk may spend an extended period of time outside refrigeration, thus moving its freshness date forward from that stamped on the container. Select your goat's milk from the coldest part of the refrigerator case, which is often the lower sections and/or at the back.

Goat's milk can sour quickly if not refrigerated. Also, do not store goat's milk in the refrigerator door, since this exposes it to the warmer room temperature each time the refrigerator is opened and closed. Always seal or close the container to avoid the goat's milk's absorbing the aromas of other foods in the refrigerator.

QUICK SERVING IDEAS

- Try goat's milk as an excellent change from regular cow's milk.
- Yogurt made from goat's milk makes an excellent base for tasty dips. Simply mix in your favorite herbs and spices and serve with crudités.

- Lightly sauté figs in olive oil and serve with goat cheese slices for a delicious appetizer dish.
- Crumble some goat cheese on a salad with romaine lettuce, pears, and pumpkin seeds.
- Crumbled goat cheese is a wonderful and rich topping, great for lentil or split pea soup.
- Add a slice of goat cheese to have more taste and extra protein in any vegetable sandwich.
- Mix oatmeal with fresh herbs such as thyme, rosemary, and sage and top with goat's milk or goat's milk yogurt.
- Soft, spreadable goat cheese is a fine accompaniment to crusty whole-grain (wholemeal) bread or crackers and fruit.

- Instead of mozzarella, try a pizza with goat cheese, sun-dried tomato, and sautéed mushrooms.
- The classic Greek cucumber salad is made with tomato, onion, kalamata olives, and chunks of feta—a type of goat's milk cheese—and dressed with olive oil and vinegar.

SAFETY

Although goat's milk is not typically an allergenic food, like cow's milk it contains the milk sugar lactose and can produce adverse reactions in lactose-intolerant individuals. Goat's milk is minimally lower in lactose than cow's milk (with 4.1 percent milk solids and 4.7 percent, respectively).

The Healing Power of Meat, Poultry, and Eggs

Meat and poultry are the edible muscle, fat, and organs of animals. Meat usually comes from grass-eating mammals but may also come from reptiles and amphibians. Poultry is the meat of birds. Because of their high protein content, many different animals and birds are eaten around the world, but in the United States and U.K., the meats most commonly eaten are beef, pork, and lamb, with chicken and turkey weighing in as poultry favorites. As culinary horizons expand, people are also trying out less common sources of meat, such as alligator and ostrich, and interest is also turning to game animals, such as venison and quail.

While moderate consumption of meat and animal products may be health-promoting, there is no question that overconsumption of these foods is spurring a global epidemic of lifestyle diseases, such as heart attacks, strokes, and cancers, as well as creating new pressures on land and water resources, contributing to water pollution, and exacerbating global warming.

World meat production has surged nearly six-fold since 1950, and per capita meat production stands at 36 kilograms, more than double the 1950 level. Per capita consumption of milk, cheese, yogurt, ice cream, and eggs has also climbed to all-time highs.

Since meat production is an inefficient use of natural resources compared to high-protein crops, in a world where an estimated one in every six people goes hungry each day, the politics of meat consumption are increasingly heated. Currently, in the United States alone approximately 70 percent of the grain grown goes to feed livestock and poultry. In the U.K. almost 50 percent of cereal crops are used for animal food. Each kilo of meat represents several kilos of grain, either corn or wheat, that could be consumed directly by humans. If the 670 million tons of the world's grain used for feed were reduced by just 10 percent, this would free up 67 million tons of grain, enough to sustain 225 million people, or keep up with world

TABLE 18.1

Meat Consumption Around the World (kilograms per person per year)

Country	Beef	Pork	Poultry	Lamb	Total
United States	44	31	48	1	123
Germany	16	54	15	1	86
Italy	26	35	19	2	82
Argentina	58	—	21	1	80
United Kingdom	16	25	27	6	74
Brazil	36	9	24	—	70
New Zealand	37	—	—	29	66
Mexico	21	10	20	2	53
China	5	35	11	2	53
Russian Federation	19	13	13	1	46
South Africa	17	—	24	4	44
Japan	12	17	12	1	40
Egypt	8	—	6	1	16
India	1	—	1	1	3
Indonesia	—	—	2	—	2
All industrial nations	21	25	24	2	72
All developing nations	5	11	7	1	24

population growth for the next three years. In addition, if each American reduced his or her meat consumption by only 5 percent, roughly equivalent to eating one dish less of meat each week, 7.5 million tons of grain would be saved, enough to feed 25 million people—roughly the number estimated to go hungry in the United States each day.

Over the past two centuries, but especially in the last fifty years, vast ecosystems have been altered, and massive resources have been devoted to supporting livestock populations. The

ecological impact of world meat production includes forest destruction for ranching in Central and South America, suppression of native predators and competitors in the United States, and the introduction of invasive forage species virtually everywhere commercial ranching exists. In addition, the massive quantities of waste produced by livestock and poultry threaten rivers, lakes, and other waterways. In the United States, the waste generated by livestock is 130 times that produced by humans. Consider this: one 50,000-acre pig farm in Utah produces more waste than the entire city of Los Angeles. Such livestock waste is implicated in waterway pollution, toxic algal blooms, and massive fish kills throughout the country.

A lot of attention has been given to the depletion of the ozone layer. What many people do not realize is that according to the EPA, the world's livestock herds are the largest single source of emissions of methane, a potent greenhouse gas contributing to ozone depletion and climate change.

We hope that these concerns about livestock farms will encourage you to eat a moderate amount of the foods described in this chapter. If you choose to eat meat, we encourage you to:

- Limit your intake to no more than 3 to 4 ounces/100 to 125 grams daily—about the size of a deck of playing cards. And choose the leanest cuts available, keeping in mind that the USDA allows the meat and dairy industry to label fat content by weight rather than by percentage of calories. Fat labelling in the U.K. is confusing: U.K. law doesn't specify maximum fat content for mince unless it is described specifically as "lean minced meat", in which case it must have a maximum of 7 percent fat. But "minced meat—lean" describes the product in a different way and the law doesn't apply! The Food Standards Agency recently did a survey on minced meat and found some "extra lean" products had more fat than "standard" mince, or more fat than stated on the package. Sausages are equally confusing/misleading. A standard 3-to-4-ounce/100-to-125 gram serving size of meat provides a good amount of protein.

- Avoid consuming well-done, chargrilled, and fat-laden meats, which are associated with the development of heart disease and cancer.

- Don't eat cured meats, such as bacon and hot dogs, especially if you are pregnant or a child under age twelve. The chemicals used to cure meats are associated with the development of cancer.

- Buy only Certified Organic meat, eggs, and poultry to avoid unnecessary and potentially harmful consumption of agricultural chemicals, hormones, and antibiotics that are concentrated in conventionally raised meat, eggs, and poultry.

Beef

Beef comes from the domestic cow, *Bos taurus*, and is the most frequently consumed meat in the United States (in the U.K. it is poultry). There is a large variety of beef cattle breeds, but the Hereford and Angus are the most common in the U.S., and Limousin and Charolais in the U.K. Beef is available in a wide variety of cuts that can fulfill many different recipe needs. Although the word "beef" is used to describe the meat from this one animal, the truth is that there are many different textures, tastes, and characteristics found from one cut to another. Even within the same cut, various types of beef (for example, Angus from the United States versus Kobe beef from Japan) vary. Generally speaking, the fat content is higher in the underbelly of the cow. Here we find brisket, spareribs, ribs, and rib eye (brisket, hindquarter flank and skirt in the U.K.). As these are fattier, many people believe

FIGURE 18.1
Cuts of Beef

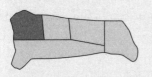

Chuck: *The chuck section comes from the shoulder and neck of the beef, and it yields some of the most flavorful and economical cuts of meat. The downside is that these cuts tend to be tough and fatty, and they have more than their fair share of bone and gristle. It's usually best to cook them slowly in a liquid; therefore, they are usually large cuts such as a pot roast.*

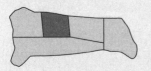

Rib: *Meat from the rib section tends to be tender and well marbled, with fat that makes steaks and roasts juicy and flavorful. Rib steaks and roasts are sometimes called prime rib. It's best not to marinate rib cuts because of their high fat content.*

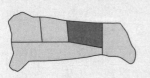

Loin: *The loin yields the most tender and expensive cuts of beef—but not necessarily the most flavorful. The choicest portion is the tenderloin, which is an exquisitely tender and lean smaller cut that includes filet mignon and Chateaubriand cuts. The top loin and sirloin aren't as tender, but they're a bit more flavorful and larger cuts. Cuts from the loin require very little work to taste great. Indeed, steak lovers consider it almost a sacrilege to marinate them or to cook them beyond medium rare, both of which take away the tenderness of these cuts.*

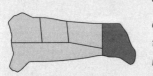

Topside, top rump and silverside: *These are terms for the rear end of the carcass. Those muscles are well exercised, so these cuts tend to be a bit tougher, and they are the leanest cuts of beef. Hindquarter cuts do well if they're cooked with moist heat, and many of them can also be roasted, as long as they're not overcooked. Cuts from the hindquarter vary in size.*

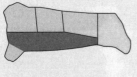

Breast and flank: *The breast and flank yield an assortment of cuts. Smaller cuts from this area include skirt steak and short ribs, while larger cuts include flank steak, hanger steak, and brisket.*

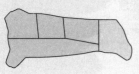

Miscellaneous cuts: *This category includes cuts taken from different parts of the carcass, including minced beef, stew meat, and soup bones as well as organs, including liver, kidney, heart, and tongue. They vary in fat content and tenderness depending on the part they come from.*

these are also the tastiest part. Fat content is decreased in the back leg of the animal, for the cow uses this muscular part for locomotion. This area is called the round in the U.S. and is made up of bottom round, top round, and eye of round. In the U.K., this area is known as the hindquarter comprising leg, thick flank, topside, top rump and silverside cuts. Beef is generally a deep red with streaks of white fat within and sometimes around the cut. High-fat cuts usually appear to have more white streaks, which are referred to as marbling. Marbling generally occurs more when the muscle is used less, a phenomenon that also occurs in humans who are not well exercised.

TABLE 18.2

Roasted Lean Cuts of Beef in Increasing Order of Fat Content per 100 gram Serving

Cut	Calories	Fat, Total/ Saturated (grams)	Protein (grams)	Cholesterol (milligrams)	Omega-3 (grams)
Eye round roast*	163	4.0/1.4	29.6	54	0
Topside steak*	209	4.6/1.6	36.0	90	0.04
Chuck steak†	114	4.7/1.6	18.9	54	0
Silverside roast*	164	4.9/1.7	28.4	61	0.01
Top sirloin steak†	212	4.9/1.9	29.3	73	0.06
Sirloin tip roast‡	188	5.0/1.8	26.8	93	0.04
95 percent lean minced beef	193	5.0/2.4	29.2	89	0.05
Brisket, flat half*	289	5.1/1.9	28.8	76	0.20
Shin‡	263	5.4/1.9	30.7	80	0.14
Chuck shoulder roast‡	129	5.7/1.8	19.5	59	0.03
Chuck roast†	297	5.7/2.2	29.8	95	0.19
Sirloin (strip) steak*	201	6.0/2.3	29.2	79	0.02
Ribeye steak†	182	6.4/2.4	29.9	61	0.02
Sirloin roast†	188	7.1/2.5	26.8	93	0.04
Fillet steak*	200	7.2/2.7	29.0	79	0.02
T-bone steak‡	202	8.2/3.0	27.0	57	0.03

* Trimmed to ⅛ inch/¼ centimeter fat.

† All fat trimmed.

‡ Trimmed to ¼ inch/½ centimeter fat.

HISTORY

Cows have been venerated in many civilizations throughout history. As cows are a source of life and sustenance, many cultures, including some Native American tribes, made it a point to thank the gods and the animals as part of their killing and eating rituals. In some parts of India and Africa, cows have been elevated to the level of sacred. In traditional Chinese medicine terms, meat has been essential to build energy and healthy blood.

In more Westernized cultures, the ability to afford beef has been indicative of a person's affluence and good fortune. Interestingly, beef is a relative newcomer to the United States, for before the 1500s there was no known beef in the Western Hemisphere. The Spanish settlers were the first to bring cows to the hemisphere, taking them along to Central and South America. Later, colonists brought the livestock to North America.

NUTRITIONAL HIGHLIGHTS

Beef is an excellent source of protein and vitamin B12 and a very good source of zinc and selenium. In addition, beef is a good source of riboflavin, vitamin B6, niacin, iron, and phosphorus. Calf's liver, in particular, deserves special mention because of its tremendous storehouse of nutrients, especially B vitamins. A lean cut of beef is defined in the U.S. as having less than 10 grams of total fat, 4.5 grams or less of saturated fat, and less than 95 milligrams of cholesterol per 100 gram serving.

HEALTH BENEFITS

While studies have linked red meat consumption to heart disease and cancer, it is important to point out that most studies do not separate out quality, focusing instead only on the amount of meat consumed. While overconsumption of meat, especially high-fat, char-grilled, or well-done cuts, is not healthful, lean cuts of organic, grass-fed beef, eaten in moderation, are an excellent source of many nutrients (see section on page 606 about types of feed). Lean beef is an excellent source of protein, providing 64.1 percent of the daily value for protein in just 4 ounces/125 grams. In addition to being a very good source of protein, lean, organic beef is an excellent source of vitamin B12 and a good source of vitamin B6, two key vitamins for proper cellular function. And, contrary to popular belief, lean red meat has no greater effect on blood cholesterol levels than an equivalent amount of lean chicken or turkey.

It may not be simply that red meat intake alone is associated with cancer. What may eventually be shown is that the manner in which the meat is prepared determines whether it is carcinogenic. For example, researchers from the University of South Carolina gave questionnaires to 273 women who were diagnosed with breast cancer between 1992 and 1994, as well as 657 women who were cancer-free. They found that women who routinely ate three meats—hamburger, beefsteak, and bacon—very well done had a 462 percent greater chance of developing breast cancer. The risk for very well-done versus rare or medium was 50 to 70 percent greater for hamburger and bacon and 220 percent greater for beefsteak. These results coupled with other evidence suggest that avoiding well-done meats can dramatically reduce the risk of developing breast cancer.

TYPES OF ANIMAL FEED

Although meat is considered to contain some fats (called omega-6 fats) that are proinflammatory and may increase the risk of health issues such as cardiovascular disease and autoimmune conditions, as we learn more about fats in the diet, scientific research is beginning to show that animals raised on a plant-based, grassy diet tend to have fats that are much healthier for the human body (omega-3 fats). Grass-fed meat also has higher concentrations of conjugated linoleic acids, which are fatty acids known to decrease cancer risk and may help people maintain a healthy weight.

It seems that the health benefits found in the fat of animals greatly diminish when they are fed animal by-products, grain, and/or cornmeal, all of which are the typical feeds used for modern industrial livestock. In one study on bison, it was observed that grass-fed bison had significantly higher omega-3 to omega-6 ratios than their grain-fed counterparts. In a parallel manner, cold-water fish such as salmon, whose omega-3 fat profile was generally considered healthy, are displaying more unhealthy omega-6 dominant fatty acid profiles when they are farmed and given feeds that are unnatural to their habitat. Similar effects are being seen with eggs, lamb, chickens, and other meats.

Since some of these terms are confusing, we are going to define them:

- Grain-fed: Refers to feeds made of grain products such as wheat, corn, oats, barley, and soybeans. Commercially raised animals are given processed grains (usually bioengineered corn) sprayed with pesticides and antibiotics to prevent infection and stimulate growth. These animals convert much of the starch in these grains into saturated fat, and the ingested pesticides are stored in their fat tissue, flesh, milk, and other products, such as eggs.

  As a result, this type of feed creates a less healthy, dominant omega-6 fat profile in the animal meat, which is less healthy for human consumption. Although supposedly restricted because of the increased threat of mad cow disease, in the U.S. grain feed may also still contain meat by-products such as ground bone, tendon, and central nervous system.
- Organic grain-fed: The grain products the animals eat are grown without pesticides or chemicals, and should also be hormone- and antibiotic-free.
- Grass-fed: In general, these animals are given foods more natural to their habitat: grasses and plant foods. Grass-fed animals typically have a healthier fatty acid profile, which translates into a less inflammatory effect on the humans who eat them versus grain-fed animals. Grass feed is generally more healthful than grain feed. Grass-fed animals are sometimes, but not always, free-range (see below).
- Organic grass-fed: The plant food these animals feed on is grown without pesticides or chemicals on the plants themselves or the soil.
- Free-range: Free-range animals may be fed grain or be allowed to roam the land eating grasses and plant food. Free-range animals are generally healthier, for they are allowed to move their bodies more than animals kept in tight quarters. Also, they do not experience the chronic exposure to sick animals and faeces that non-free-range animals do. Some animals are more free range than others, meaning that some are given a limited area in which to roam, while others may have more unlimited access to land. Free-range animals may also be given supplemental grasses or grains. These feeds may or may not be organic.

When barbecued or grilled at high temperatures, meat forms many potent carcinogens, including heterocyclic amines (toxic forms of amino acids) and toxic lipid peroxides (especially those from alpha-linolenic acid). These toxic compounds damage cell membranes as well as the DNA within cells, setting the stage for the development of cancer.

HOW TO SELECT AND STORE

Unquestionably the healthiest and most environmentally sound choice is to buy organic grass-fed, free-range beef. Beyond this, beef selection should revolve around the sell-by date and visual inspection of the meat to make sure it is fresh. If you spend time at your supermarket or butchers looking at the various meats, you will begin to get a sense of what very fresh cuts look like. Typically, they should look "alive," with a bright red or sometimes even purple color. Brownness indicates that there has been overexposure to air and oxygen and that the meat is in the process of spoiling. Additionally, what fat is present should have a white look—any yellowing is also indicative of lost freshness.

Type of Meat (raw)	Maximum Storage Time
Refrigerated minced beef	1–2 days
Refrigerated steaks and sliced beef cuts	2–3 days
Refrigerated roasts	3–4 days
Frozen minced beef	2–3 months
Frozen steaks and sliced beef cuts	2–3 months
Frozen roasts	6 months

If you are looking for a healthy, everyday meal, it is probably best to choose the less fatty back leg portion of the animal. If you are cooking a special meal and want a tastier (and fatty) cut, look for underbelly cuts such as flank steak and brisket (see above). No matter which cut you choose, try to have the cuts taken from a larger piece, for this ensures that the maximum amount of surface area is not exposed to air. Any fully cooked meats can be safely stored in the refrigerator for two to three days. If you cannot cook and serve the meat immediately, it is best to refrigerate the raw meat as soon as possible in its original packaging to decrease handling and exposure to air. Larger single pieces of meat will stay fresher longer. Thinner-sliced meat and minced meat have a much larger surface area exposed to air, so these should be stored for less time. If fresh, meats can tightly wrapped with freezer paper or aluminium foil and frozen immediately. See the chart on this page for specific maximum storage times.

TIPS FOR PREPARING

It is important to handle beef and all animal flesh in a manner consistent with minimizing spoilage and contamination with germs.

When in the supermarket, try to purchase raw meat last. After choosing meat, place an extra plastic bag around it in order to avoid spreading any drippings and blood, which might contaminate your hands or other items purchased. If the meat will be away from refrigeration for any length of time, it is best to pack it in ice until you can store it in your refrigerator or freezer.

Once home, always place the meat in the refrigerator or freezer. Never leave it sitting out at room temperature. If you need to thaw frozen meat, it is best to allow twenty-four hours for it to thaw in the refrigerator. If you are in a hurry, you can thaw the meat in cold water by leaving it in the original package and changing the cold water every half hour. When preparing meals that include meat, be sure to wash all surfaces, utensils, clothing, and body parts that come into contact with the meat very well. Do not serve cooked foods on the same dishes that have held raw food, unless they are thoroughly washed. Use hot soapy water to wash surfaces and utensils that touch your food, and you can use a mild bleach solution to wash down countertops and cutting boards (1 teaspoon of chlorine bleach to 1 liter of water will suffice).

When preparing any meat, trim any excess fat, usually present as a strip on one side of steaks. It is not necessary to wash raw meat before cooking it. Any bacteria that might be present on the surface will be destroyed by cooking.

Meat can also be made tenderer by pounding it with a mallet made for the purpose. Place the beef between two pieces of cling film, then pound with the mallet, using glancing blows to prevent tearing the meat. Pound about ten times on each side of a steak, then let it rest for twenty minutes prior to cooking. Marinating meats can enhance their flavor but should be done only in the refrigerator. Since used marinade contains blood and bacteria, if you wish to serve marinade with the meal, make a little extra previous to marinating that will not be required for marinating the meat itself.

Cooking should always be thorough. Never partially cook or brown meat and then store it in the refrigerator, for this can encourage widespread growth of bacteria. Since internal temperature is the only true reliable indicator of whether the meat is fully cooked (and harmful bacteria are completely killed), buy a meat thermometer if you do not have one, and place the tip in the deepest portion of that particular piece of meat.

Cook to a minimum internal temperature of 130 to 135 degrees F./54 to 57 degrees C. for medium-rare and 140 to 150 degrees F./60 to 65 degrees C. for medium-cooked, whole cuts of meat. However, a roast can be removed from the oven when its internal temperature has reached 135 to 140 degrees F./57 to 60 degrees C. and allowed to stand for 15 minutes before carving. During this time, the internal temperature will rise to 150 to 155 degrees F./65 to 68 degrees C., but the meat will still be juicy and the center will remain just slightly pink.

The cooking time needed for meat depends upon the size and thickness of the cut, whether the bone remains or it is boneless, and the method of cooking. Note that lean cuts of beef cook more quickly than cuts with a higher fat content and toughen easily if overcooked. Therefore, use shorter cooking times, especially at high heat. Lower-temperature cooking is the best way to control the resultant texture of your dish as well as prevent lipid peroxide and nitrosamine formation.

QUICK SERVING IDEAS

- An Asian-style beef dish: Sauté 1 pound/ ½ kilogram thin slices of cube steak with 1 medium or large sliced onion, 2 cloves minced garlic, ½ cup fresh basil, 1 stalk chopped lemongrass, and 1 to 2 chili peppers (depending on how spicy you prefer it).

BSE OR MAD COW DISEASE

"Mad cow disease" is the common name of bovine spongiform encephalopathy (BSE), a transmissible, slowly progressive, degenerative, fatal disease affecting the central nervous system of adult cattle. The transmissible agent in BSE is a modified form of a normal cell surface component known as a prion protein. Unlike infectious organisms, prions are resistant to common treatments, such as heat and digestive secretions. Eating the meat of an animal with BSE may lead to a disease similar to BSE in humans called variant Creutzfeldt-Jakob disease, or vCJD. According to the USDA, as of December 1, 2003, a total of 153 cases of vCJD had been reported in the world: 143 in the United Kingdom, 6 in France, and 1 each in Canada, Ireland, Italy, and the United States.

BSE was first reported among cattle in the United Kingdom in 1986 and has been a major concern ever since. The outbreak in the United Kingdom may have started from the feeding of scrapie-contaminated sheep meat-and-bone meal to cattle. Scrapie is a disease of sheep that is related to BSE in cattle. In addition, there is strong evidence that the outbreak in cattle was amplified in the United Kingdom by feeding rendered bovine meat-and-bone meal to young calves. As a result of BSE in the U.K., the use of MBM (meat-and-bone meal) in animal feeds for cattle and other farm livestock is now illegal in Britain.

BSE has now been reported in cattle throughout Europe, and a third case was reported in Canada in January 2005. In the United States, a single case was reported in December 2003, and wild game, such as deer and elk, have been affected with a similar disease known as chronic wasting disease (CWD). The reason American cattle have been spared may be due to the active surveillance and import measures taken by the Food and Drug Administration and the U.S. Department of Agriculture.

The USDA has restricted the importation of live ruminants, such as cows and sheep, and food products from these animals from BSE countries since 1989, and from all European countries since 1997 after a second case in the United Kingdom in 1996 and a third in 2001 that spread to other countries in the European Union. In addition, the FDA prohibits the use of most mammalian protein, particularly meat, bone meal, and nerve tissue such as brain and spinal cord, in the manufacture of animal feeds given to ruminants because this kind of feeding practice is believed to have initiated and amplified the outbreak of BSE in the United Kingdom.

To reduce the risk of ingesting beef with BSE, we recommend taking the following steps:

- *Buy beef only from a trusted source, and know the country of origin. As of 2004, in the U.S. supermarkets were required to post this information. Ask how the cattle were raised, where they originated from, and how they were fed. Since BSE, supermarket chains in the U.K. should be able to trace all meat back to the source farm.*
- *Consider using organic grass-fed beef rather than industrial beef in order to minimize your exposure to animal by-products through livestock feed. In most supermarkets the beef is usually industrial beef. Most industrial cattle have gone through calf feeding, background feeding, and feedlots where possible use of animal by-products could occur.*
- *Purchase beef from smaller USDA-inspected abattoirs, where cattle are individually slaughtered at a rate slow enough to allow the inspector to observe the cow prior to and during slaughter. Currently more than 95 percent*

(continued on next page)

of the beef in the United States is processed at the rate of 400-plus cows per hour by unskilled labor. If you are not sure, ask the meat department manager of the supermarket you frequent or your butcher. Since the mid-1980s in the U.K., the number of abattoirs has declined by 1,000 to just over 300. Small and medium-sized abattoirs in particular have closed, largely as a consequence of E.U. regulations stipulating that, in addition to Meat Hygiene Service Inspectors, a vet is present during the slaughter of animals. This increased costs significantly in smaller abattoirs where animals tend to be processed more slowly. Purchasing meat from small local abattoirs helps to safeguard the environment and the animals' welfare by not subjecting them to long, stressful journeys, and makes tracing meat easier. The importance of traceability was made clear in the 2001 outbreak of foot-and-mouth disease which spread as a consequence of difficulties in tracing the source of the disease and distance the infected animals traveled between farm and abattoir.

- *Consume minced beef made from whole muscle tissue rather than from beef trimmings, which are often combined from many animals. Beef trimmings can include brain, spinal cord, and central nervous system tissue, where the prions that cause BSE are concentrated.*
- *See the USDA website at www.usda.gov, where you can click on Agriculture, then on Animal Production, then on Bovine Spongiform Encephalopathy (BSE). You can also search the USDA site for "bovine spongiform encephalopathy" for information not readily apparent on the BSE page.*

- For an Italian bolognese sauce: Sauté garlic in olive oil, then add minced beef and sear until the meat turns a dark brown. Add the meat to tomato sauce and cook. Then serve over pasta.
- Skewer 1 pound/½ kilogram of 1-inch/2½-centimetre cubes of beef from a lean cut with your favorite vegetables, such as pearl onions, small potatoes, bell peppers, and cherry tomatoes. Brush them with a little olive oil or vinaigrette and grill.
- Thinly slice tenderloin and cook in a skillet. Place inside a toasted fresh baguette, and add sautéed onions, peppers, and garlic.
- To make the classic steak dish steak au poivre, you need only to coat the meat well with crushed peppercorns before cooking.

SAFETY

See "Tips for Preparing" on the proper handling and storage of beef.

Beef contains purines. Since purines can be broken down to form uric acid, individuals with gout should avoid beef or limit their consumption of it. See page 728 for more information.

Since beef contains small amounts of oxalates, individuals prone to calcium oxalate kidney stones should limit their consumption of beef. See page 793 for more information.

Beef is also a rich source of arginine, an amino acid necessary for replication of certain viruses, including the herpes simplex virus. People who have regular outbreaks of herpes should limit or avoid consumption of beef.

Chicken

Chicken *(Gallus gallus)* is a very popular food, as it can be prepared a multitude of ways. From traditional roast chicken to barbecued chicken to tandoori chicken to homemade chicken soup, chicken is appreciated by people of all ages as well as by diverse cultural culinary traditions.

Chicken consumption is increasing as people look for ways to reduce the fat in their diets. The entire bird is consumed, often roasted whole or cut into parts. Dark meat parts include the back, legs, thighs, and wings. The white meat, the leanest part of the chicken, is the chicken breast, which has less than half the fat of a trimmed T-bone steak. Chicken fat is also less saturated than beef fat. However, eating the chicken with the skin on doubles the amount of fat and saturated fat in the dish. For this reason, chicken is best skinned before cooking.

HISTORY

It is believed that chickens are originally from Southeast Asia, probably the area of Thailand. With domestication of chickens for the last 4,000 years, poultry has been a staple item throughout much of history. From Thailand, chickens were taken to China; from there they were introduced into India, western Asia, and finally into the African continent.

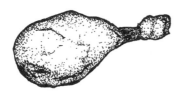

The early colonists brought chickens from Europe to the United States. In the 1800s, better refrigeration methods allowed for more widespread chicken production. Although President Herbert Hoover promised Depression-era Americans "a chicken in every pot," it was only after World War II that poultry production expanded into today's fowl popularity. Most chicken is currently produced by the United States, Brazil, the Russian Federation, Mexico, Japan, and China.

NUTRITIONAL HIGHLIGHTS

Chicken is a very good source of protein, niacin, selenium, and vitamin B6. It is also a good source of pantothenic acid and phosphorus.

HEALTH BENEFITS

Chicken is a versatile source of protein that is low in fat and easy to prepare. Probably the best-known use of chicken is in chicken soup, particularly for colds. In fact, chicken soup has been shown to affect some aspects of the immune system, resulting in relief of some symptoms of the common cold. According to traditional Chinese medicine, chicken in moderate amounts is a good food for building energy as well as supporting the digestive function.

HOW TO SELECT AND STORE

The healthiest and most humane approach is to purchase free-range, organically fed chickens. For a full description of what this means and the differences among free-range, grass-fed, and grain-fed animals, please see the box "Types of Animal Feed" on page 606.

Beyond this, your chicken selection should revolve around the sell-by date and visual

TABLE 18.3
Cuts of Chicken in Increasing Order of Fat Content per 100 gram Serving (Roasted, No Skin)

Cut	Calories	Fat Total/Saturated (grams)	Protein (grams)	Cholesterol	Omega-3 (grams)
Breast	165	3.6/1.0	31.0	85	0.05
Drumstick	172	5.7/1.5	28.3	93	0.11
Thigh	191	8.4/2.3	27.0	94	0.14
Back	239	13.2/3.6	28.2	90	0.21

inspection of the chicken meat to make sure it is fresh. If you spend time at your supermarket or butchers looking at the various meats, you will begin to get a sense of what very fresh chicken looks like. Typically, it should look "alive," and the meat should give a bit when gently pressed. Furthermore, it should not smell "fowl" or have a strong odor. The color of the skin may vary depending on its feed and type, but it should be somewhat translucent and not mottled.

If you are purchasing chicken already cut into pieces, what you should purchase depends on your needs. If you are looking for a healthy everyday meal, it is probably best to choose the less fatty white meat. Whole chicken is generally a better choice freshness-wise, for this ensures that the maximum amount of surface area is not exposed to air. Whole chickens tend to be a better choice economically as well. Frozen chickens should be fully frozen and without visible freezer burn or frozen liquid inside that may signify meat that has thawed and been refrozen.

Carefully wrapped chicken that will not leak may safely be stored in the refrigerator for two to three days. If you cannot cook and serve the meat immediately, it is best to refrigerate the raw chicken as soon as possible by taking it from its original package, washing it in cold water, patting it dry, then wrapping it tightly in aluminium foil or freezer paper. One year is the limit on storing frozen chicken.

TIPS FOR PREPARING

Unlike beef, chicken needs to be washed thoroughly by rinsing under cool water before preparing. Also, if a recipe calls for stuffing a chicken, do not stuff it until just prior to roasting to prevent bacterial growth in the stuffing. Chicken should be cooked until a meat thermometer registers 170 to 175 degrees F./77 to 79 degrees C. when inserted into the thickest part of the meat, not touching gristle or bone. If roasting a whole bird, a meat thermometer is usually inserted into the breast. Another sign that a roasted bird is done is the presence of clear juices on the thigh after being stuck deeply with a fork. Usually, roasting a 4-pound/2-kilogram chicken will take 1 hour; if it is larger, plan on 1 hour of cooking for the first 4 pounds/2 kilograms, plus 8 minutes more for each additional pound/½ kilogram. Let the chicken rest on a platter for 15 minutes before carving. For other safety guidelines in handling, thawing, marinating, and cooking chicken, see page 607.

QUICK SERVING IDEAS

Any cut of chicken can be used in the following recipes based on your own taste preferences. White meat is lighter in flavor and lower in fat than dark meat. Therefore we recommend white meat for regular chicken consumption.

- Chicken salad can be prepared numerous ways and can be served for lunch or dinner. One of our favorite recipes is to combine 1 pound/½ kilogram cubed cooked chicken with 1 cup low-fat plain yogurt, ½ cup garden peas, 1 medium sliced leek, ½ cup sliced almonds, and ¼ cup raisins. Season to taste with dulse flakes and pepper.
- For a quick meal with an Asian flair, lightly sauté 2 chicken breasts sliced ½ inch/1 centimetre thick with 3 to 4 cups of your favorite vegetables. Add 2 tablespoons tamari, 2 tablespoons lightly crushed sesame seeds, 1 inch/2½ centimeters peeled and diced ginger, 1 to 2 cloves sliced garlic, 1 teaspoon rice vinegar, and 1 teaspoon honey.
- Making homemade chicken soup is easy. Just add 1 pound/½ kilogram chopped chicken, 1 medium chopped onion, 1 medium diced carrot, 1 diced celery stalk, 2 tablespoons olive oil, 1 teaspoon thyme, 1 teaspoon sage, 1 tablespoon dulse flakes, and ½ teaspoon pepper to 1½ to 2 liters of water. Cover, bring to a boil, and simmer for 45 minutes. Remove from heat and refrigerate overnight.
- Barbecued chicken is a perennial favorite, which is not surprising as it is easy to prepare and delicious. Simply marinate the chicken in your favorite barbecue marinade or brush the chicken with barbecue sauce right before placing on the barbecue or baking in the oven.

- Try a Mexican dish: Wrap leftover chicken pieces in a whole-wheat or corn tortilla, then sprinkle with chopped tomatoes and onions, top with shredded soy or regular cheese, and grill, making yourself a healthy burrito.
- Mix shredded leftover chicken meat with mayonnaise, minced celery and carrots, raisins, Major Grey chutney, and curry powder for an Indian-inspired chicken salad.

SAFETY

The major safety issue surrounding chicken is contamination with *Campylobacter, Salmonella,* or *Shigella,* bacteria that are common causes of foodborne infection. Chickens are also often given antibiotics to deal with poor sanitation and to stimulate growth. This widespread practice is creating problems, as research shows that the number of bacteria that are resistant to antibiotics is increasing. The FDA's Center for Veterinary Medicine has even stated that these drugs should be banned to avoid the development of further resistance and of humans being sickened by resistant bacteria.

Unfortunately, chicken is also a primary culprit in many food-allergenic reactions and sensitivities, particularly in children. See page 723 for a list of signs and symptoms associated with food allergies.

Chicken contain purines. Individuals with gout should avoid or limit their intake of chicken. See page 728 for more information.

Chicken contains low amounts of oxalates, and individuals with a history of kidney stones should limit their consumption of this food. See page 793 for more information.

Chicken is also a rich source of arginine, an amino acid necessary for replication of some viruses, including the herpes simplex virus. People who have regular outbreaks of herpes should limit or avoid consumption of chicken.

Lamb

The word "lamb" comes from the German word *Lambiz,* and the word itself refers to the meat from young sheep *(Ovis aries)* under one year of age. Given that lamb is generally a lower-fat red meat, it is unfortunate that people in the United States tend to eat much less lamb than those in other nations. In the U.K., the average consumption of lamb per person per year is 6.1 kilograms—about 360,000 tonnes, more than a third of which comes from New Zealand. Mutton is, by contrast, not popularly consumed. At the butcher, you can ask for various cuts, including the leg, shank or loin, rack, and shoulder. Minced lamb is also available and can be used to make sauces, burgers, meatballs, or meat loaf, like its beef, chicken, and turkey counterparts.

HISTORY

Domesticated for human use in the Middle East and Asia more than 10,000 years ago, lamb became a popular food, as well as the source of the wool and parchment industry, in many areas of the world. The ancient Romans actually took the first sheep into Britain. The Spanish conquistador Hernando Cortés brought the first sheep into the Western Hemisphere during early exploration expeditions with the Spanish army.

In mythology and established world religions, lamb has been a strong symbol. In the fifth pillar of Islam, it is required by all who make a pilgrimage to sacrifice a lamb. The Old Testament describes lamb as a symbol of sacrifice. In the New Testament, many experts believe lamb was served during the Last Supper, and Jesus has been referred to by Christians as "the Lamb of God." Fittingly, lamb has become a traditional Easter entrée. Although the United States is still relatively young in its lamb interest, many world cuisines have lamb as a centerpiece, including those of Turkey, New Zealand, Australia, Middle Eastern countries, and Greece.

NUTRITIONAL HIGHLIGHTS

Lamb is an excellent source of vitamin B12 and protein as well as a very good source of selenium, niacin, and zinc. In addition, it is a good source of phosphorus and riboflavin.

HEALTH BENEFITS

Lamb offers health benefits similar to those of beef and should be considered a red meat. In traditional Chinese medicine, lamb is a food considered to warm the body.

HOW TO SELECT AND STORE

As with other meats, we strongly recommend choosing organic varieties of lamb. While USDA inspection of lamb is mandatory, grading is voluntary; therefore not all lamb is labeled with a grade. Those that are carry the titles Prime, Choice, and Select (no such system exists in the U.K.). Prime and Choice are the most tender and flavorful but also have a higher fat content. Although lamb is generally tender, you can ensure taste and quality in your lamb choice by buying lamb with pink, firm flesh and white marbling. Flesh that is soft, deeper in color, and

TABLE 18.4

Lean Cuts of Domestic Lamb in Order of Fat Content per 100 gram Serving, Trimmed to ⅛ inch/¼ centimeter fat

Cut	Calories	Fat Total/Saturated (grams)	Protein (grams)	Cholesterol	Omega-3 (grams)
Leg shank	217	11.4/4.6	26.7	90	0.14
Foreshank	243	13.5/5.6	28.4	106	0.19
Shoulder	269	19.1/7.8	22.7	91	0.32
Minced	293	19.7/8.1	24.8	97	0.26
Loin	290	21.1/9.1	23.3	93	0.37
Rib	341	27.5/11.7	21.8	96	0.40

has fat with a yellow tinge may be past its freshness point. In past times, lamb was labeled "Spring" to let the consumer know that it was a fresh lamb brought to market in the spring or summer. Today, lamb is available during the whole year. So the "spring" label does not denote any greater freshness advantage.

Like all fresh meats, the expiration date for purchase and use should be double-checked. Like other perishable red meat, lamb should be stored cold or frozen and can be kept in the store packaging if it has not been compromised. Minced lamb has a refrigerated shelf life of two days, while lamb chops and roasts may be stored in a cold part of the refrigerator for three to five days. To freeze it, it is best to wrap it snugly in aluminium foil or freezer paper. Minced lamb will keep for three to four months, while roasts and chops will remain fresh for six to nine months.

TIPS FOR PREPARING

Please see page 607 for tips on preparing lamb for cooking.

QUICK SERVING IDEAS

• Place bite-size pieces of lamb on a skewer with your favorite vegetables and make lamb shish kebabs. Grill for 3 to 5 minutes on each side or bake for 15 to 20 minutes at 350 degrees F./180 degrees C./gas 4.

• Lamburgers: Make, season, and cook as you would a regular beef hamburger.

• Braise 1 pound/½ kilogram lamb loin pieces in a covered skillet with ½ cup red wine, 2 to 4 cloves mashed garlic, and 1 tablespoon fresh rosemary for 5 minutes on each side.

• The hearty flavor of lamb makes it an excellent choice for a stew. A basic stew recipe includes 1 pound/½ kilogram of stew meat, such as lamb, 1 medium chopped onion, 1 medium chopped carrot, and 1 medium stalk chopped celery combined with 3 to 4 cups stock, ½ cup red wine, 1 tablespoon fresh thyme, ½ teaspoon salt, and pepper to taste. Simmer gently, covered, for 1½ to 2 hours. The flavor will be best if served the next day.

• For a healthy twist on a traditional food pairing, serve lamb with a mint yogurt sauce made from 1 cup plain yogurt, ⅓ cup chopped fresh mint leaves, 1 clove mashed garlic, ⅛ teaspoon cayenne pepper, and ¼ teaspoon salt.

SAFETY

Please see page 607 for safety guidelines in handling, thawing, marinating, and cooking lamb. One advantage of lamb over beef is that it is significantly less allergenic; thus it is often used as a meat source in allergy elimination diets.

Lamb contains purines. Individuals with kidney problems or gout should avoid or limit their intake of lamb. See page 728 for more information.

Since lamb contains low amounts of oxalates, individuals with a history of calcium oxalate kidney stones should limit consumption of lamb. See page 793 for more information.

Lamb is also a rich source of arginine, an amino acid necessary for replication of some viruses, including the herpes simplex virus. People who have regular outbreaks of herpes should limit or avoid consumption of lamb.

Pork

Pork is the flesh of the domestic pig *(Sus scrofa).* It is sold in a variety of fresh and cured meat products, such as pork chops, ham, bacon, sausage, spareribs, and hot dogs. While still high-fat fare, today's pork is significantly leaner than it was twenty years ago due to improvements in the way pigs are bred, raised, and fed. Compared to 1983, fresh pork now averages 31 percent lower in fat, 29 percent lower in saturated fat, 10 percent lower in cholesterol, and 14 percent lower in calories. In fact, the leanest cuts of pork have a fat content comparable to that of the leanest cuts of beef, plus the fat found in pork is less saturated than beef fat.

Only a third of the pork butchered each year is sold fresh; the remaining two thirds is cured, smoked, or otherwise processed. In the U.K., 21 percent of pork consumed was fresh or frozen, the remaining 79 percent being used for processed meats such as bacon, sausage and ham. Before refrigeration, curing pork was a necessity to retard spoilage; today, although most cured pork products must still be kept refrigerated, curing is used primarily to add flavor. Salt, sugar, and sodium nitrite—a chemical that has been linked to the development of stomach cancer—are the main ingredients used to cure pork, but other chemicals, including various flavorings, sodium erythorbate (which shortens curing time), and sodium phosphate (which retains moisture), may also be added. Because not only salt but other sodium-containing chemicals are used to cure pork, the resulting products are typically very high in sodium, although some cured pork products with less sodium are now available.

Like beef, pork is initially divided into wholesale cuts whose names refer to the body parts from which they come: loin (upper back), leg, shoulder, and side (belly). Retail cuts of pork—the ones found in the meat section of the supermarket—are subdivisions of these four wholesale cuts.

Loin

The cuts with the least fat come from the flavorful loin section. Cuts taken from the center loin are not only the lowest in fat but the most tender, and thus, the most expensive. Tenderloin, with only 26 percent of its calories coming from fat, is the leanest of all pork cuts.

Leg

The back leg section is the source of fresh and smoked hams. Hams are either brine (wet)-cured or dry-cured and may also be smoked. Most hams are brine-cured, which involves injecting or soaking the meat with a solution of water, salt, sugar, and sodium nitrite, then smoking it.

Country-cured hams are typically dry-cured in salt, then smoked over fragrant hardwoods and aged at least six months. A mould usually forms during the aging process that must be scraped off and washed away before cooking.

Prosciutto, a golden pink, thinly sliced Italian ham, is dry-cured but not smoked. Eaten uncooked, prosciutto is usually added to dishes as a final touch or served as an appetizer with melon or figs. Westphalian ham is made from pigs fed with acorns in the Westphalia Forest of Germany. After curing, the meat is smoked slowly over a mixture of beech wood and juniper wood, producing a very dark brown, dense ham with a light smoky flavor. Black Forest ham is similar.

Hams are sold with the shank bone still in (bone in), with the shank bone removed but the leg bone in (semiboneless), rolled and packed into a casing with the bones removed (boneless), and as pieces that have been fully cooked and vacuum-sealed (canned).

In the U.S., hams are also categorized according to the percentage of protein or fat contained:

- "Ham" means the product contains no added water and is at least 20.5 percent protein.
- "Ham with natural juices" signifies a minimum of 18.5 percent protein.
- "Ham—added water" must be at least 17 percent protein.
- "Ham and water" may contain any percentage of water but must list the percentage of water on the label.
- "Lean ham" must contain no more than 10 percent fat by weight.
- "Extra-lean ham" must contain no more than 5 percent fat by weight.

Shoulder

The shoulder is cut primarily into roasts, including one called a "picnic ham," which is not a true ham since it comes from the upper part of the foreleg. A less expensive substitute for regular ham, picnic ham is sold both fresh and smoked; however, it usually contains about 24 percent fat. The shoulder is also cut into chunks for grilling or kebabs.

Side

The side cut provides two pork favorites, both of which are cured: bacon and spareribs. Since both are extremely fatty (40 to 45 percent fat for bacon, 24 to 30 percent fat for spareribs), they should be enjoyed infrequently.

HISTORY

Pigs have been domesticated and used as a source of food by people around the world since 7000 B.C.E. In wooded areas surrounding villages, pigs could be turned loose to grow fat on nuts and roots. On farms, pigs could be fed the remains of the grain used for brewing, the whey left after cheese making, scraps from the kitchen, or any spoiling fruit or vegetable. No matter what they ate, pigs converted it into food for people, and many of the foods produced from the flesh of pigs have become culinary staples. Two examples are the pork pies still beloved in England and the barbecue that, in the United States, has become an icon of the South.

The pork pie has been an English tradition since at least 1390, when the first recipe for pork pie was recorded by the cooks at the court of Richard II. The traditional pork pie is thought to have originated from the Roman technique of sealing meat in a flour-and-oil paste to prevent the juices from seeping away while cooking. In the royal and noble households of medieval England, the humble pork pie was transferred to a moulded container for a more elegant presentation at table—an upgraded appearance it has retained to this day.

In 1493, Christopher Columbus loaded pigs among the other provisions put on board his ship, crossed the Atlantic, and introduced them to the Americas. By the time the colonists arrived, pigs, a low-maintenance animal that could be put out to root in the forest and caught when needed, were an omnipresent food staple.

In the South, wild pig catching and slaughtering became a neighborhood activity, with everyone invited to share in the work and the largesse. Every part of the pig was utilized: the meat either eaten immediately or cured for later consumption, the bones saved for stock and flavoring, and the ears and organs transformed into an assortment of delicacies. Such gatherings were the birthplace of the traditional southern barbecue, which was already well established by the end of the colonial period but

rose to great heights in the fifty years before the Civil War, when plantation owners regularly held large barbecues that lasted for days and were the social events of the year.

Although pigs are now raised in virtually every state in the United States, Iowa farmers raise 26 to 28 percent of the pigs that become U.S. pork, making the state number one in pork production.

NUTRITIONAL HIGHLIGHTS

Pork is an excellent source of protein. A 100 gram serving of fresh pork tenderloin, grilled, provides 185 calories, 30 grams of protein (63 percent of the daily value), and 6.3 grams of fat (9 percent of the RDA), just 2.2 grams of which (11 percent of the RDA) are saturated. Generally, commercially raised pork contains no omega-3 fatty acids.

In addition to its protein content, a 100-gram serving of pork tenderloin is an excellent source of several B vitamins, especially thiamine (of which pork is the leading food source, providing 89 percent of the RDA), niacin (82 percent of the RDA), vitamin B12 (41 percent of the RDA), riboflavin (35 percent of the RDA), and pantothenic acid (18 percent of the RDA). A mineral-rich meat, a 100-gram serving of pork tenderloin is also an excellent source of selenium (providing 93 percent of the RDA) and zinc (37 percent of the RDA); a very good source of potassium (13 percent of the RDA) and magnesium (12 percent of the RDA); and a good source of iron (8 percent of the RDA) and copper (7 percent of the RDA).

A 100-gram serving of extra-lean cooked pork ham contains 145 calories and provides 21 grams of protein and only 5 grams of fat, less than 2 grams of which are saturated. Unfortunately, ham, which is cured, is quite high in sodium, serving up 1,126 milligrams in 100 grams.

HEALTH BENEFITS

Pork is a versatile source of protein that is easy to prepare, and some cuts are low in fat, including the tenderloin and extra-lean ham. However, many cuts, such as those from the side and other forms of ham, are high in fat.

HOW TO SELECT AND STORE

Choose cured pork products that are nitrate- and nitrite-free. These sorts of products are gaining in availability. However, keep in mind that pork products that have been cured with sodium nitrate have a much longer storage life than fresh.

Fresh Pork

Fresh pork tenderloin should be deep red, while leg and shoulder cuts should be pink or pinkish gray in color. Choose cuts with the external fat trimmed to no more than ⅛ inch/¼ centimeter; the remaining fat should be creamy white. Bones, if present, should be red and spongy at the ends. The whiter the bone ends, the older the animal when it was slaughtered and the tougher the meat will be.

Pork roasts should be rosy pink. A darker red indicates acidic meat that, while juicy and delicious, will not keep well and must be eaten immediately.

Purchase fresh pork no more than two to three days before you plan to cook it. Since pork contains much more unsaturated fat than beef, it turns rancid more quickly. Stored in its original store wrapper in the coldest part of the refrigerator, it will stay fresh for three days.

Once cooked, pork should still be refrigerated and will keep for four to five days, or it can be frozen and kept for one month. To freeze, wrap the meat well in plastic, foil, or butcher paper and store at 18 degrees F./−7 degrees C. Once thawed, do not refreeze.

Ham

Read the label carefully when choosing cured hams. It will list the ingredients used; the protein, fat, and sodium content; and directions for storage and cooking.

Cured hams can range from 6 to 24 pounds/3 to 11 kilograms, depending upon the cut and whether the bone remains in or not. If the ham is in a clear plastic wrapping, look for one that is firm and plump, with rosy pink, fine-grained meat. If the ham is canned, you must rely on the reputation of the producer.

Canned hams that require refrigeration, even before opening, generally have a better flavor and texture than those that can be stored at room temperature until opened. This is because the very high heat required to process shelf-stable meat negatively affects the product's flavor, aroma, texture, and nutritional value. Also, be aware that higher-quality meat is typically reserved for the more expensive products.

Canned and dry-cured hams will keep for up to six months if stored in the refrigerator unopened. Once opened, wrap leftovers tightly and use within one week or freeze for up to one month.

Vacuum-packed, brine-cured hams should be stored in the refrigerator, where they will keep for about one week, or they can be frozen for up to three months. Once opened, wrap leftovers tightly in their original wrapping or aluminium foil and use within one week.

Some country-style hams can be stored in a cool place for one to two months; check the label for storage length and instructions. Also, keep in mind that longer storage equals more evaporation, which will shrink and toughen country ham. Once cut, country ham must be refrigerated and should be used within four to five days, or leftovers can be frozen for up to one month.

Bacon

Unopened vacuum-packed bacon should be marked with a sell-by date. If unopened, it will keep for one week past this date, and it can be frozen before this date, keeping for three months. Once opened, if tightly wrapped, it should keep about one week. Slab bacon, if tightly wrapped and refrigerated, will keep for several weeks. Lean bacon will keep up to one week if in large pieces, three to four days if sliced.

TIPS FOR PREPARING

Fresh Pork

- Please see page 607 for safety guidelines for handling, thawing, marinating, and cooking fresh pork. To roast fresh pork, place all cuts to be roasted fat side up in a baking pan and insert a meat thermometer. When done, the internal temperature of the meat should reach 170 degrees F./77 degrees C.

Cured Ham

- Fully cooked hams need not be heated before serving, but uncooked and partially cooked hams must be cooked. Check the label to determine which type you have.
- To remove excessive salt, rinse the ham, then soak it, refrigerated, for up to 24 hours before cooking.
- To bake uncooked ham, remove any skin, trim fat to ¼ inch/½ centimeter, and allow the ham to stand at room temperature for 1½ to 2 hours. Preheat oven to 325 degrees

	TABLE 18.5	
	Cooking Temperatures and Times for Cuts of Pork	
Cut	Temperature (degrees F./degrees C./ gas mark)	Time (minutes per pound/ ½ kilogram)
Tenderloin	425/220/gas 7	20–30
Boneless loin	325–350/170–180/gas 3–4	20–30
Bone-in loin	325–350/170–180/gas 3–4	20–25
Crown roast	325–350/170–180/gas 3–4	20–25
Fresh leg cuts	325–350/170–180/gas 3–4	38–45
Shoulder with blade	325–350/170–180/gas 3–4	40–45

F./170 degrees C./gas 3. Place ham on a rack in a shallow roasting pan, fat side up, insert a meat thermometer into the thickest portion, and bake until the thermometer reads 160 degrees F./71 degrees C. Let rest 15 to 20 minutes before carving. Ready-to-eat and canned hams should be treated like uncooked ham but need to be cooked only until the internal temperature reaches 130 degrees F./54 degrees C., about 8 to 10 minutes per pound/½ kilogram.

- If the bone has been left in, wrap tightly and refrigerate for later use, within three to four days, to flavor soups and stews.

Country-Cured Ham

- A day or two before serving, place the ham in a very large oval kettle. If necessary, saw off the hock to fit the ham in. If salt crystals are visible, the ham will be excessively salty. Remove some of the salt by covering the meat with cool water, leaving it at room temperature and, over the next 24 hours, changing the water three to four times. If no salt is visible, it is still necessary to let the meat soak for 24 hours, but the soaking water need be changed only once or twice.

- After 24 hours of soaking, remove the ham from the pot and scrub well under running tepid water to remove any mould and pepper. Wash the ham again thoroughly in tepid water before placing it on a rack in the same large kettle. Add cool water to cover, place a cover on the kettle, and bring to a boil over high heat. Remove the cover and skim the froth from the surface. Replace the cover, adjust the heat to a slow simmer, and cook 25 to 30 minutes per pound/½ kilogram, or until a

fork can be easily inserted and the bone feels loose. Allow the ham to cool in the cooking liquid while you preheat the oven to 350 degrees F./180 degrees C./gas 4.

- Remove the ham from the kettle, peel off the rind, and trim the fat to ½ inch/1 centimeter. Use a sharp knife to score the meat in a crisscross pattern, stud with cloves, and pat on a thick glaze (bread crumbs liberally mixed with brown sugar is the traditional glaze for Smithfield hams). Transfer the ham, glazed side up, to a rack in a shallow roasting pan and bake at 350 degrees F./180 degrees C./gas 4, uncovered, 45 minutes or until the glaze is well caramelized. Place the ham on a serving platter and let cool at least 20 minutes before serving. In the South, country hams are typically served at room temperature or chilled, rather than hot. Carve into paper-thin slices.

QUICK SERVING IDEAS

- To braise a pork roast, place it in a heavy pot over medium-high heat. Add a little oil, cooking liquid, and seasonings and bring the heat to a simmer. Cover and place in a slow (300 to 325 degrees F./150 to 170 degrees C./gas 2 to 3) oven until the meat is tender enough that a fork can be easily inserted— about 3½ to 4 hours.

- Tenderloin is the best cut for barbecuing. Rub the outside with oil, pepper, and seasonings. Place on the barbecue over hot coals and cook about 2½ minutes on each side. Brush with barbecue sauce or other glaze and cook an additional 2 minutes on each side. When fully cooked, the meat will be pinkish white and should reach an internal temperature of 160 degrees F./71 degrees C.

> ### THE MANY COLORS OF PORK
>
> *Fresh pork turns almost white when cooked, but cured ham retains its rosy hue because the myoglobin in the meat reacts with the nitrites and nitrates used in curing to form nitrosomyoglobin, a compound that stays red at high temperatures.*
>
> *On cut ham, a glistening, greenish, or rainbow iridescent appearance is not necessarily an indication of spoilage. The nitrates and nitrates used to cure pork that cause the meat to remain a rosy red, even when fully cooked, can also trigger a chemical reaction that produces pigment changes in pork when exposed to light and air.*

- Add a Cajun flair to pork chops by seasoning with a mixture of ½ teaspoon cayenne pepper, 1 teaspoon fine ground black pepper, 2 teaspoons garlic powder, 2 teaspoons thyme, and 1 tablespoon paprika before grilling.
- Slit four thick (at least ¾ inch/1½ centimeters) pork chops in the center and stuff with a sautéed mixture of 1 medium peeled and diced Granny Smith apple, 1 medium diced onion, 1 stalk diced celery, and ¼ cup finely chopped nuts, such as walnuts, pecans, or pine nuts. Close the opening with a toothpick and brown the chops in a skillet in a little olive oil. Add about ¼ cup apple juice, a sprinkle of celery seed, and freshly ground black pepper. Cover and braise for 15 to 20 minutes.
- Make your own sweet-and-sour pork: Slice 1 pound/½ kilogram fresh pork loin into ¼-inch/½ centimeter strips and stir-fry with 1 cup pineapple chunks; 1 sliced sweet pepper; 1 medium sliced onion; 1 inch/2½ centimeters peeled, grated fresh ginger; 2 cloves sliced garlic; 1 tablespoon vegetable oil; and 2 tablespoons soy sauce. Top with cashews and serve over brown rice.
- Rosemary grilled pork tenderloin is quick and easy: Rub the meat with oil, then salt, pepper, onion powder, and rosemary. Insert a meat thermometer, place on the barbecue above hot coals, and cook on all sides for a total of about 5 minutes. When done, the meat will be pinkish white, and the internal temperature should be 160 degrees F./71 degrees C.
- If you have a covered barbecue, barbecuing even larger roasts is simple. Preheat the barbecue, oil the meat, rub in your favorite spices, insert a meat thermometer, and place the roast inside, away from direct heat. Cook for about 45 minutes or until the internal temperature reaches 160 degrees F./71 degrees C.

SAFETY

The major safety concern with pork products is trichinosis, a parasitic disease caused by microscopic live worms called trichinae. These parasites live and reproduce in the intestines, and their larvae can migrate into the bloodstream and travel to the muscles, causing pain, fever, muscle deterioration, and even death. Human trichinosis infection after consuming pork products was once very common but today is relatively rare because of:

- Legislation prohibiting the feeding of raw meat swill to pigs.
- Commercial and home freezing of pork (freezing at a temperature of −10 degrees F./

–23 degrees C. for several weeks will kill trichinae in pork).

- Government standards, which require that cooked pork reach an internal temperature of 160 degrees F./71 degrees C. (cooking to an internal temperature of 137 degrees F./58 degrees C. kills trichinae).
- Public awareness of the danger of eating raw or undercooked pork products.

Although U.S. consumers can trust that pork products produced by responsible meat processors are free of trichinae (and trichinosis hasn't existed in the U.K. since 1979), it's still best to err on the safe side by adopting the following precautions:

- Cook pork products until the juices run clear, or to an internal temperature of 160 degrees F./71 degrees C.
- Do not microwave uncooked or partially cooked pork. Microwaving is not an adequate method of cooking pork, since microwaving meat does not consistently kill infective worms.
- Freeze pork less than 6 inches/15 centimeters thick for twenty days at 5 degrees F./–15 degrees C. to kill any worms.
- If you prepare your own minced meats, always be sure to clean the meat mincer thoroughly.
- Trichinae are not found in Europe, allowing the production and consumption of prosciutto, an Italian delicacy of thinly sliced raw pork, which can now be imported into the United States. Some country-cured hams have been advertised as "American prosciutto," claiming that they can be eaten raw. To prevent possible infection with trichinae, avoid such products.

Pork is not considered a commonly allergenic food, although gallbladder attacks have been associated with pork allergy.

Pork contains purines. Since purines can be broken down to form uric acid, individuals with gout should avoid or limit their intake of pork. See page 728 for more information.

Since pork contains low amounts of oxalates, individuals prone to calcium oxalate-containing kidney stones should limit their consumption of pork. See Appendix D, page 793, for more information.

Pork is also a rich source of arginine, an amino acid necessary for replication of some viruses, including the herpes simplex virus. People who have regular outbreaks of herpes should limit or avoid consumption of pork.

Turkey

Turkey *(Meleagris gallopavo)* is increasing in its popularity beyond its association with the holidays of Thanksgiving (in the U.S.) and Christmas, due to its increased availability and the desire by many to eat leaner sources of protein. Like its supermarket chicken predecessor, turkey parts such as breasts, tenderloins, cutlets, and minced turkey are now widely available. Since parts are quicker to prepare, it is now more practical for many people to enjoy turkey more regularly.

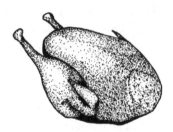

HISTORY

Native to both Mexico and the United States, this native American food was introduced to Europeans when Christopher Columbus returned from the New World with these beautiful gobbling fowl. By the mid- to late 1500s, the French, English, and Italians were domesticating turkeys for commoners' tables, after the bird originally was found only at the table of royalty.

The history of the United States is forever entwined with the turkey, in the form of the famed Pilgrim Thanksgiving dinner. Benjamin Franklin's affection for the turkey was so strong that he was reportedly quite disgruntled to learn that the eagle had been chosen as the national bird.

Although people of many nations enjoy the turkey, the greatest turkey consumers per capita include the United States, Italy, France, the Netherlands, Canada, Israel, and the United Kingdom.

NUTRITIONAL HIGHLIGHTS

Turkey is a very good source of protein, providing 65 percent of the daily value in one 4-ounce/125-gram portion. Along with protein, turkey is a very good source of selenium, niacin, and vitamin B6 and a good source of zinc and vitamin B12. Almost all of the fat in turkey is found in the skin, and the dark meat is higher in fat than the light meat. The skinless white meat is an excellent high-protein, low-fat food.

HEALTH BENEFITS

Turkey is particularly high in the amino acid tryptophan, a building block of the brain compound serotonin. Since serotonin is an inducer of sleep, consumption of turkey may help improve sleep quality. The meat's high level of tryptophan may also explain why some people want to take a nap after their Christmas or Thanksgiving meal.

Other health benefits center around its excellent nutritional profile, especially as a lean source of high-quality protein.

TABLE 18.6
Cuts of Turkey in Order of Fat Content per 100 gram Serving,
No Skin and Roasted

Cut	Calories	Fat Total/Saturated (grams)	Protein (grams)	Cholesterol	Omega-3 (grams)
Breast	135	0.7/0.24	30.1	83	0.01
Drumstick/leg	159	3.8/1.3	29.2	119	0.06
Thigh (with skin)	157	8.5/2.7	18.8	62	0.14
Back	170	5.6/1.9	28.0	95	0.09

HOW TO SELECT AND STORE

If possible, purchase turkey that has been organically raised or that is free-range, since these methods of raising turkey are both more humane and produce turkeys that are tastier and better for your health. Organically grown turkeys have been fed an organically grown diet and have been raised without the use of hormones or antibiotics. Free-range turkeys are allowed access to the outdoors, as opposed to being kept in buildings where large numbers of turkeys are confined with little space to move (see the box "Types of Animal Feed" on page 606).

Always check the date the bird was packaged, as well as the sell-by date, to ensure freshness. When visually inspecting a whole turkey, look for ones that are firm but pliable when touched and plump, with a rounded breast. Whether purchasing a whole turkey or turkey parts, the meat should not smell "fowl" or have any strong odor associated with it. Turkey skin should look white and without mottling or blemishes. Do not buy turkey with visible bruising or cuts. Frozen turkeys should feel rock solid, with no freezer burn or visible frozen liquids that may indicate unwanted freeze-thaw cycles.

Turkey is best stored in the bottom and back of your refrigerator to keep it as cold as possible and away from the warmth of the opening refrigerator door. Turkey can be stored in the refrigerator in its original packaging unless you have purchased a whole turkey with giblets (internal organs). Giblets keep best stored in another container, with your turkey rewrapped and resealed tightly so as to not allow it to leak its liquids into your refrigerator. Raw turkey can remain in the refrigerator for one to two days, while cooked turkey can stay three to four days. Frozen turkeys can keep for up to six months.

TIPS FOR PREPARING

For safety guidelines in handling, thawing, marinating, and cooking turkey, see page 607. Turkey should be rinsed thoroughly under cool water before preparing.

QUICK SERVING IDEAS

- On a bed of 2 cups chopped romaine lettuce, serve ½ cup diced cooked turkey, ½ cup cooked cubed sweet potatoes, 2 tablespoons dried cranberries, and 2 tablespoons walnuts tossed with a light vinaigrette for a salad that recalls the flavors of Thanksgiving.
- Minced turkey makes excellent turkey burgers and turkey meat loaf, or it can be used in a red tomato sauce to create a turkey bolognese pasta dish.
- Try a turkey burrito: Place already cooked turkey pieces on a corn tortilla, then sprinkle with shredded regular or soy cheese and add diced tomatoes and onions. Grill for a few minutes until hot and enjoy.
- Leftover Christmas/Thanksgiving sandwich: Toast a sliced French baguette, add turkey meat and top with cranberry sauce, turkey gravy, and a little salt and pepper for a post-Christmas/Thanksgiving luncheon delight.
- Mix shredded leftover turkey meat with rapeseed mayonnaise, minced celery and carrots, raisins, Major Grey chutney, and curry powder for an Indian-inspired turkey salad.

SAFETY

Turkey is not commonly an allergenic food; however, gallbladder attacks have been attributed to turkey allergy. Turkey contains purines. Since purines can be broken down to form uric acid, individuals with gout should avoid or limit intake of turkey. See page 728 for more information.

Since turkey contains small amounts of oxalates, individuals prone to calcium oxalate-containing kidney stones should limit their consumption of turkey. See page 793 for more information.

Turkey also is a moderate source of arginine, an amino acid necessary for replication of some viruses, including the herpes simplex virus. People who have regular outbreaks of herpes should limit or avoid consumption of turkey.

Check labels carefully if you use turkey cold cuts. Food processors may combine the dark meat with organ meats, such as the heart and gizzards, which makes the product higher in fat.

Venison

Deer are a plentiful animal all around the world and are present on every continent with the exception of Antarctica. Native species exist everywhere, with the exception of Australia, where several varieties were introduced by the British. Venison refers to the meat that comes from deer, such as mule *(Odocoileus hemionus)*, red *(Cervus elaphus)*, white-tailed *(Odocoileus virginianus)*, and many other varieties (red, roe, fallow, sika and muntjak in the U.K.) that are either wild or farm-raised. With its very pliable and tender texture, deer meat flavor is diet-dependent. Many people describe venison as having a flavorful deep woodsy or gamey taste not unlike that of a berry-flavored fine red wine.

HISTORY

The hunting and consumption of deer predate that of other domesticated animals. Europeans in the Stone Ages relied on domesticated deer before learning to consume other animals, such as cattle and sheep. Many cultures and families throughout the world rely on deer hunting for food and/or sport. People in Korea, China, and Taiwan have used deer not only for food but to make products from the antlers and other body parts. Traditional Chinese medicine has used the antlers, tail, and other deer parts for thousands of years. Recently, farm-raised deer meat is also becoming more popular. The United States and New Zealand are the leading countries currently domesticating the deer.

NUTRITIONAL HIGHLIGHTS

Venison is an excellent source of both protein and vitamin B12. It is also a very good source of riboflavin, vitamin B6, niacin, iron, and phosphorus. In addition, venison is a good source of the minerals selenium, zinc, and copper.

Venison is a nutrient-dense meat that is an excellent source of protein that is very low in fat, especially saturated fat. A 100 gram serving of venison loin, lean only, supplies 150 calories, 30.2 grams of protein, 79 milligrams of cholesterol, and 2.4 grams of fat (0.9 grams saturated). Wild venison has a high omega-3 fatty acid level similar to that of range-fed beef.

HEALTH BENEFITS

Venison is a versatile, low-fat, high-protein meat that is flavorful in the way that other red meat, such as beef, is but is a healthier alternative.

HOW TO SELECT AND STORE

First, always take a look at the "sell-by" date to ensure freshness. Wild, free-range, and organically grass-fed animals are the healthiest choices (see the box "Types of Animal Feed" on page 606). Venison is tastiest when brought to market at a younger age. Younger deer generally has darker, more finely grained meat and a more purely white fat.

TIPS FOR PREPARING

For safety guidelines in handling, thawing, marinating, and cooking venison, see page 607. Venison does not need to be rinsed before handling.

QUICK SERVING IDEAS

- Venison jerky is easy to make: Cut 2 pounds/1 kilogram venison steaks into ¼-inch/½-centimeter-thick slices, and marinate overnight in 1 liter water, 1 tablespoon salt, 1 teaspoon ground pepper, 4 cloves mashed garlic, and ¼ cup sugar. Arrange on an aerated roasting rack, and bake at 150 degrees F./65 degrees C. for 6 hours.
- Minced venison is an excellent healthier replacement for beef when making meat loaf, meat sauce and burger recipes which call for minced beef.
- A winter stew: Take some venison steak pieces, and combine with root vegetables, spices, and broth to make a warming, hearty stew. See page 615 for an easy stew recipe in which venison stew meat can be used.
- Cubes of venison steak are easily skewered with your favorite vegetables. Brush with olive oil and grill in the oven or on the barbecue.

SAFETY

For safety information on venison, see page 607.

Venison is a source of purines. Individuals with kidney problems or gout should avoid or limit their intake of venison. See page 728 for more information.

Venison contains low amounts of oxalates; individuals with a history of calcium oxalate-containing kidney stones should limit their consumption of venison. See page 793 for more information.

Venison is also a rich source of arginine, an amino acid necessary for replication of some viruses, including the herpes simplex virus. People who have regular outbreaks of herpes should limit or avoid consumption of venison.

Eggs

An egg holds all the nutrition a developing young chicken *(Gallus gallus)* needs. Eggshells' colors are breed-dependent, most of them being white or brown, with some speckled. Inside this beautiful example of nature's engineering are the white and the yolk, which contains various fats, some vitamins and nutrients, cholesterol, and lecithin. Eggs are an important and influential ingredient in cooking, as their particular chemical makeup is literally the glue of many important baking reactions, including foaming, coagulation, emulsification, and the ability to brown.

Because of the many ways eggs can be cooked, they can become virtually any texture from soft and creamy to firm and formed.

HISTORY

Since the domestication of the chicken more than 4,000 years ago in the region of what is now Thailand, people have been enjoying and nourishing themselves with the egg. As a longtime symbol of fertility and rebirth, the egg has taken its place in religious as well as culinary history. In Christianity, the symbol of the decorated egg has become synonymous with Easter. Easter occurs in the spring, traditionally the time when hens begin laying many eggs. The eggshell-painting tradition has been popular in many countries, including Greece, China, Egypt, and Persia. Even today the Fabergé eggs, originally decorated as Easter tributes for the Russian royalty, are a museum favorite.

NUTRITIONAL HIGHLIGHTS

Eggs are an excellent source of vitamin K and a very good source of the B vitamins, including biotin, thiamine, and vitamin B12. They are also a very good source of selenium, vitamin D, and protein. One serving (1 large egg) contains 78 calories, 6.3 grams of protein, 212 milligrams of cholesterol, and 5.3 grams of fat (1.6 grams saturated). For comparison to the serving sizes of other foods we have discussed, two large eggs equal a 100 gram serving and contain 155 calories, 12.6 grams of protein, 424 milligrams of cholesterol, and 10.6 grams of fat (3.3 grams saturated).

Some eggs contain omega-3 fatty acids, de-

pending on what the chickens have been fed. The omega-3 content varies, and these eggs are usually labeled as containing omega-3 fatty acids. Otherwise, commercially produced eggs contain virtually no omega-3 fatty acids.

HEALTH BENEFITS

Eggs are a very good source of low-cost, high-quality protein. Since eggs are high in cholesterol and public health advocates have long recommended that cholesterol consumption be limited to no more than 300 milligrams per day, people with high cholesterol levels have been recommended to avoid eggs. However, several recent studies suggest that instead of contributing to heart disease, eggs actually lower the risk. These results highlight the exceptional nutritional profile of eggs and the fact that saturated fat in the diet, not dietary cholesterol, is what influences blood cholesterol levels most.

A statistical analysis of 224 dietary studies carried out over the past twenty-five years that had investigated the relationship between diet and blood cholesterol levels in over 8,000 subjects clearly demonstrated that saturated fat is more significant in raising blood cholesterol levels than dietary cholesterol. In addition, in a study published in *The Journal of the American Medical Association,* it was shown that people who reported eating four eggs per week had a significantly lower mean serum cholesterol concentration than those who reported eating one egg per week (193 milligrams per deciliter versus 197 milligrams per deciliter). The daily nutrient intake of people consuming eggs was significantly greater than that of non-egg eaters for all nutrients studied, except dietary fiber and vitamin B6. The bottom line from all of the existing research is that most people can eat 1 to 2 eggs a day without measurable changes in their blood cholesterol levels.

Eggs are rich in several nutrients that promote heart health. For example, they are a rich source of betaine. Researchers from the Netherlands found that betaine can reduce levels of homocysteine, a metabolite of the amino acids methionine and cysteine. Homocysteine can damage the blood vessel walls. Not surprisingly, elevated homocysteine levels are linked to increased risk for heart disease as well as other chronic diseases, including neural tube defects, osteoporosis, Alzheimer's disease, and cancer. Like folic acid, betaine plays a role in converting homocysteine to nondamaging forms. Folic acid is the primary agent in the conversion of homocysteine in all cells, while betaine's methylation activity is confined mainly to the liver. In one study in a group of healthy volunteers, just two weeks of betaine supplementation resulted in approximately a 50 percent reduction in their homocysteine levels. In patients with homocystinuria (a condition characterized by excessively high levels of homocysteine), betaine was even more beneficial. In these patients, betaine supplementation was found to lower total plasma homocysteine concentrations by up to 75 percent.

Eggs are also a rich source of choline, a key component of many fat-containing structures in cell membranes, providing flexibility and structural integrity. Two fat-like molecules in the brain, phosphatidylcholine and sphingomyelin, account for an unusually high percentage of the brain's total mass, so choline is particularly important for brain function and health. Choline is also involved in homocysteine metabolism and is also the key component of acetylcholine—one of the brain's key neurotransmitters. One large egg provides 300 micrograms of free choline (all in the yolk) and also contains 315 milligrams of phosphatidylcholine.

During pregnancy and breast-feeding, an adequate supply of choline is particularly important, since choline is essential for normal brain development. In an experiment with rats, newborn rats that received choline supplements, either in utero or during the second week of life, showed improved brain functioning and greater memory capabilities not just as young rats, but throughout their entire lives. Researchers think these effects are probably due to choline's beneficial effect on the development of the memory center (hippocampus) in the brain.

In traditional Chinese medicine, eggs are recommended to strengthen one's blood and energy by enhancing digestive and kidney function.

HOW TO SELECT AND STORE

Choose eggs from free-range or organically raised chickens, the difference being that organically raised chickens may not receive any antibiotics and any supplemental feed is organically grown (see the box "Types of Animal Feed" on page 606). In turn, commercially raised chickens are given processed grains (usually bioengineered corn) sprayed with pesticides and antibiotics to prevent infection and stimulate growth. The chickens convert much of the starch in these grains into saturated fat, and ingested pesticides are stored in fat. This pesticide-laden fat ends up in the yolk of the eggs these chickens produce. Widespread antibiotic use in chickens has lead to the development of harmful, antibiotic-resistant bacteria. In contrast, free-range and organic eggs are produced by range-fed chickens, whose feed is primarily naturally occurring seeds and insects. Since these chickens are free of crowded conditions, antibiotic use is essentially unnecessary. Sometimes free-range and organic chickens are fed linseed or special meal enriched with DHA (docosahexaenoic acid), which increases the omega-3 content of their eggs.

According to the USDA, eggs are graded according to freshness, with a grade of AA, A, or B. AA is considered the best. Sizes range from extra large to small, with the largest eggs having more protein, nutrients, and fats. In the U.K., approximately 85 percent of eggs are produced in accordance with the Lion Quality Code of Practice, which determines freshness and size along with safety standards. Very large eggs are more than 73 grams, large eggs are 63 to 73 grams, medium eggs are 53 to 63 grams and small eggs are under 53 grams. Eggs should always be visually inspected at the store before buying. It is best to lift the eggs out of the carton and check for cracks and dried egg liquid on the box to ensure that there are no broken ones. Eggs from local farms can also be a good choice. While supermarket eggs in the U.S. are generally washed and cleaned for bacteria, farm eggs may not be, so it is best to ask your farmer if he or she washes the eggs before selling. In the E.U., class A eggs (those found in shops and supermarkets) are not permitted to be washed.

Although in certain cooler climates and cultures eggs are not refrigerated, they are best stored in the refrigerator, where they may remain for up to one month. Eggs that have a higher omega-3 fatty acid content are best eaten as fresh as possible to keep these oils fresh. Since the eggshell is somewhat porous, it helps to keep the eggs in their carton to reduce their absorption of odors and compounds from other foods in the refrigerator. The eggs are best stored point down, so as to keep the most beneficial placement of the air chamber and yolk. Try not to store eggs in the door, as variations in temperature caused by opening and closing of the door can contribute to spoilage.

TIPS FOR PREPARING

To reduce the possibility of contamination of your recipe by a spoiled egg, break each egg separately into a small bowl and visually inspect it before combining with the other ingredients.

Some experts suggest that poaching, hard-boiling, or soft-boiling an egg is the most healthy method of preparing an egg, for this heats the egg at lower temperatures (boiling is at 212 degrees F./100 degrees C., versus frying, which can attain temperatures up to 400 degrees F./200 degrees C. or more). Furthermore, these methods keep the fats in the yolks from being oxidized before and during the cooking process. For anyone frequently eating eggs, poached or soft- or hard-boiled is recommended.

QUICK SERVING IDEAS

• To hard-boil eggs, place them in a saucepan and cover with water. Bring to a boil for 8 minutes. Remove from heat and let sit covered in the hot water for 8 minutes. If you turn the eggs over after removing from heat, the yolk will be centered in the white.

- For a delicious egg salad, mix 4 chopped-up hard-boiled eggs with 2 to 3 tablespoons tofu mayonnaise, 1 medium chopped leek, 1 medium grated carrot, ¼ cup chopped fresh dill, and salt and pepper to taste.
- For a healthy southwestern-influenced breakfast, add 1 to 2 diced fresh jalapeño peppers (remove seeds and pith) to 4 scrambled eggs. Divide in two portions and serve each with ½ cup black beans and 2 steamed corn tortillas. Top with a small dollop of nonfat, organic sour cream and 1 to 2 tablespoons chopped fresh coriander leaves.
- To make a classic breakfast treat, French toast, dredge 8 slices of your favorite whole-grain (wholemeal) bread in 4 eggs beaten with ⅓ cup milk and 1 teaspoon vanilla. Place each slice on a griddle and top with cinnamon before flipping after 2 to 3 minutes.
- Use eggs to bind other ingredients together into a savory dish. For example, combine 3 large, lightly beaten eggs, 1½ cups low-fat milk, 2 teaspoons olive oil, and ½ teaspoon each salt and pepper. Pour the mixture over 2 cups of your favorite chopped vegetables in a whole-grain (wholemeal) pastry case or a small baking dish lined with 1 to 2 sliced medium parboiled potatoes. Bake at 375 degrees F./190 degrees C./gas 5 for 30 minutes.

SAFETY

With regard to eggs, the main concern is risk of *Salmonella* food poisoning. Once thought to be an issue only with cracked eggs, these chicken intestinal bacteria have been found in eggs with uncompromised shells as well. Although washing the egg may be of use, the best protection is cooking your eggs at high enough temperatures for a long enough period of time. Eggs that are soft-cooked, raw, or sunny side up have a greater risk of causing salmonellosis and if cooked in a dish, such as a casserole, should be heated to at least 160 degrees F./71 degrees C. Poached, scrambled, and hard-boiled carry a much lower risk. Similar to precautions when working with chicken, dishes, cutlery, and utensils need cleaning in warm soapy water. Surfaces in contact with raw egg matter should be washed and then sanitized with a chlorine bleach solution (this can be made by mixing 1 teaspoon chlorine bleach in 1 liter of water). Hand washing is essential after egg handling.

Eggs contain purines. For this reason, individuals with kidney problems or gout should avoid or limit intake of eggs (see page 728 for more information).

Eggs contain low levels of oxalate. Individuals with a history of oxalate-containing kidney stones should avoid overconsuming eggs. For more information, see Appendix D, page 793.

Eggs are also a modest source of arginine, an amino acid necessary for replication of some viruses, including the herpes simplex virus. People who have regular outbreaks of herpes should limit or avoid consumption of eggs.

Another safety concern regarding eggs is that they are a common food allergen, particularly among children. See page 723 for a list of common symptoms associated with an allergic reaction to food.

19

The Healing Power of Miscellaneous Foods

A number of foods that possess healing benefits do not fit into the other categories, so we have put them together here. These foods include blackstrap molasses, brewer's yeast, chocolate (yes, chocolate!), honey and other bee products, maple syrup, mushrooms, sea vegetables, and tea.

Blackstrap Molasses

The truth of the phrase "slow as molasses" becomes apparent when you consider molasses's thick, viscous, syrupy texture. Featuring a robust bittersweet flavor, blackstrap molasses helps create the distinctive taste of baked beans and gingerbread. Blackstrap molasses, as its name suggests, is very dark brown, almost black, in hue.

Molasses is the syrupy dark liquid that comes from processing raw sugar into its more refined form. Blackstrap molasses is one type, which is produced in the third cycle of boiling the sugar syrup. Once the sugar's sucrose has been crystallized, the syrup becomes more concentrated.

HISTORY

Dating back to the earliest American colonies, blackstrap molasses was brought into the United States from the beautiful sugar-filled islands of the Caribbean. Given its less expensive price tag than the more refined table sugar's, molasses was the most used sweetener of the time.

Two historical events have been defining moments in the timeline of the human–molasses relationship. In 1733, the British attempted to tax early colonists to dissuade them from entering business relationships with West Indian people not under the king's control. The molasses tax was an incendiary spark in the embers that became the Revolutionary War. In 1919, a fatal molasses accident occurred when a 2 million gallon storage container broke and unleashed a 35-mile/56 kilometers-per-hour,

10-meter-wide tidal wave that killed twenty-one Bostonians. Molasses' popularity has increased, especially in recent years, as the interest in natural health has grown. Molasses production now takes place primarily in Brazil, India, Thailand, the Philippines, Taiwan, and the United States.

NUTRITIONAL HIGHLIGHTS

Blackstrap molasses is an excellent source of iron. It is also a very good source of vitamin B6 as well as many minerals, including calcium, copper, manganese, potassium, and magnesium. In addition, it is a good source of selenium and pantothenic acid. A 100 gram or 5-tablespoon serving of blackstrap molasses provides 235 calories primarily from the 61 grams of carbohydrate. There is no fat or protein in molasses.

HEALTH BENEFITS

Unlike most other sweeteners, molasses is high in minerals and thus provides a number of health benefits. Because it is minimally processed, molasses retains a number of trace minerals (see "Nutritional Highlights" above). White sugar and corn syrup are highly refined compounds, completely devoid of any nutrients except glucose. Similarly, artificial sweeteners are suspect, as research has observed sensitivities in susceptible individuals, and there is a suspicion that they may contribute to certain serious chronic illnesses.

HOW TO SELECT AND STORE

It is recommended to buy organic, unsulphured blackstrap molasses and store it in an airtight container, either in a cool area or in the refrigerator. An opened container has a six-month shelf life, while unopened jars can last up to one year.

TIPS FOR PREPARING

Heating blackstrap molasses by placing the container in hot (not boiling) water can help reduce its viscosity, allowing it to be poured or scooped out more effectively.

QUICK SERVING IDEAS

- To make baked beans with the traditionally robust flavor, combine 2 cups cooked brown (borlotti) beans with a small amount of water, 1 medium chopped onion, 2 tablespoons blackstrap molasses, 2 tablespoons rapeseed or olive oil, and 1 teaspoon mustard powder. Place the mixture into a 1½-liter crock with a lid and bake at 300 degrees F./150 degrees C./gas 2 for 1 to 1½ hours.

- Combine 2 tablespoons blackstrap molasses with 2 teaspoons cinnamon and 1 tablespoon rapeseed oil and use as a glaze for 2 cups baked sweet potatoes.

- Blackstrap molasses imparts a wonderfully distinctive flavor to gingerbread cakes. Mix 3¼ cups whole-grain flour, such as wheat or barley, 2½ teaspoons bicarbonate of soda, 1½ teaspoons ground cinnamon, and ¼ teaspoon salt. In a second bowl, mix 1 cup blackstrap molasses, 2 tablespoons freshly grated ginger, ½ cup cane sugar, ¼ cup nonfat sour cream, 2 large eggs, and 2 teaspoons vanilla extract. Then whisk in ¾ cup boiling water and rapeseed oil, then the dry ingredients. Pour into a loaf pan and bake at 350 degrees F./180 degrees C. gas 4 for 45 minutes.

- Basting chicken or turkey with blackstrap molasses will give it a rich color and taste.

When roasting a bird, thin 2 tablespoons blackstrap molasses with 1 tablespoon rapeseed oil. Baste the bird liberally before roasting in the oven.

- Mix 1 tablespoon blackstrap molasses with 1 tablespoon olive oil, 2 tablespoons tamari, 2 teaspoons rice vinegar, and ¼ teaspoon cayenne pepper to use as a marinade for preparing baked tofu or tempeh, or as a barbecue sauce for grilled fish.

SAFETY

No safety concerns are associated with blackstrap molasses. Since conventional products concentrate the agricultural chemicals used in their production, organic blackstrap molasses is recommended.

Brewer's Yeast

Yeasts are single-cell organisms that convert their food, through a process called fermentation, into alcohol and carbon dioxide—a trait that in the case of brewer's yeast *(Saccharomyces cerevisiae)* has endeared it to the brewers of beer and ale, the two alcoholic beverages for which this yeast, whose species name is derived from the Latin word for "beer," *cerevisia,* works best. While varieties of yeast abound, very few species provide significant benefit to humans. Within the small group of human-friendly yeast organisms, *S. cerevisiae* is perhaps the most beneficial of all, since both brewer's and baker's yeast are strains of this species.

Brewer's yeast can be made in one of two ways. When recovered as a by-product of beer making, brewer's yeast is typically grown on grain, usually barley, and has a bitter, unpalatable taste. When bred as a food supplement, brewer's yeast is often grown on sugar beets (which absorb nutrients from the soil faster than any other crop) and in the presence of vitamin B12 and trace minerals, such as chromium, selenium, copper, iron, and zinc. This process creates an exceptionally nutrient-dense food with a slightly sweet, nutty flavor. Brewer's yeast, when cultivated specifically for use as a food supplement, is dried at a higher temperature than baking yeast, killing the live enzymes and producing a nonleavening yeast that will not ferment.

Regardless of strain, all species of *S. cerevisiae* divide about twenty times before they die, which means that each yeast cell gives rise to millions of offspring. To accomplish this feat, these yeasts require many of the same vitamins and amino acids needed by humans. Since yeasts are typically grown on foods that lack certain nutrients, the yeasts must manufacture their own amino acids and vitamins, becoming, in the process, a much more complete food for any human who consumes them.

HISTORY

Saccharomyces cerevisiae has been an extremely useful yeast for humans for many millennia. Thousands of years ago, naturally occurring yeasts managed to land on some flour or drinks with results so pleasant that eventually people learned how to cultivate the yeasts and select the strains that would work best on various food sources common in their region.

Via fermentation, yeast significantly enhances the nutritional value of foods, such as breads and beers. In some societies, cloudy-looking beers are a major contribution to daily nutritional needs, because the cloudy sediment is composed of yeast cells that contain essential B vitamins, minerals, and amino acids. In fact, during the Middle Ages, it was common practice to feed infants with the sediment from cloudy beer to keep them healthy.

But while yeast's beneficial effects on health were recognized early, the identification of the nutritional factors responsible did not take place until the early twentieth century, when B vitamins were discovered. A number of these vitamins—including biotin, niacin (vitamin B3), pantothenic acid (vitamin B5), and thiamine (vitamin B1)—were first extracted and analyzed from yeast.

Since *S. cerevisiae* is unicellular and very small, large numbers of the yeast can be grown in culture in a very small space, just like bacteria. But *S. cerevisiae* is a eukaryote, an organism whose cells have a nucleus, like human cells, so genetic studies with this yeast provide information that is more directly applicable to human genetics. *S. cerevisiae* was the first eukaryote to have its entire genome sequenced and has been used in genetic studies for many decades.

Like all yeasts, *S. cerevisiae* reproduces rapidly and abundantly, making it the perfect organism for the study of cellular division. In fact, in 2001, Leland Hartwell, a researcher at the Fred Hutchinson Cancer Research Center in Seattle, won the Nobel Prize in Medicine for his pioneering work on the genes responsible for cell division in *S. cerevisiae*. The genes he discovered and characterized, using the yeast as a model organism, have led to some important discoveries in fighting cancer in humans.

NUTRITIONAL HIGHLIGHTS

The nutritional quality of brewer's yeast depends on the host on which the yeast was grown and can therefore vary significantly from one supplier to another. The only way to know precisely what you're getting is to read the label carefully.

In general, brewer's yeast is an excellent source of high-quality protein comparable in value to soy protein. Approximately 40 percent of the weight of dried brewer's yeast consists of protein that includes all the essential amino acids. Plus, like soybeans, brewer's yeast is rich in lysine, which makes both of these foods excellent supplements to cereals, whose proteins are generally low in lysine. A tablespoon of nutritional brewer's yeast can provide 8 grams of protein for a mere 58 calories.

Depending upon the way in which it is grown, in addition to its high-quality protein, brewer's yeast can also be a good to excellent source of a number of important trace minerals, including chromium, selenium, copper, iron, zinc, potassium, and magnesium. For example, while the brewer's yeast that is a by-product of beer making may contain 1 or 2 parts per million (ppm) selenium, commercial "high-selenium" brewer's yeasts may contain as much as 2,000 ppm selenium, 75 percent of which is organically bound. Nutritional brewer's yeast typically provides at least 32 micrograms of selenium in a tablespoon, 57.5 percent of the daily recommended value of this trace mineral, along with around 95 micrograms of chromium.

In addition, brewer's yeast is an ideal supplement for vegetarians because, when grown in the presence of vitamin B12, this nutritional yeast provides excellent amounts of all the B vitamins. A tablespoon of nutritional brewer's yeast may provide more than 100 percent of the RDA of vitamin B12 and pantothenic acid, more than 80 percent of the daily recommended value of thiamine and riboflavin, 50 percent of the RDA of niacin, more than 40 percent of the RDA of vitamin B6, and 30 percent of the RDA of folate—all for less than 60 calories! This is particularly important for vegans, who eat no meat, fish, poultry, eggs, or dairy products, the only other sources of vitamin B12.

HEALTH BENEFITS

Nutritional brewer's yeast has been shown to keep homocysteine levels low; lower triglycerides and raise HDL levels while reducing LDL levels; help control blood sugar; protect against liver cancer; and help clear up acne. By serving as an excellent source of all the B vitamins, brewer's yeast keeps homocysteine levels low. A good deal of research has shown a very strong association between elevated blood levels of homocysteine—an amino acid that is an intermediate product created during an essential cellular process called methylation—and cardiovascular disease and some forms of cancer.

Brewer's yeast also helps lower triglycerides and raise levels of HDL (good) cholesterol while reducing LDL (bad) cholesterol. In one study, a group of eleven men with normal cholesterol levels and sixteen men with elevated cholesterol were given 20 grams (⅔ ounce) daily of a high-chromium brewer's yeast. After eight weeks, not only was HDL cholesterol increased in both groups by 5 to 6 milligrams per deciliter, but in 84 percent of the men, the total cholesterol/HDL ratio improved significantly.

When a second group of nineteen subjects with high cholesterol levels was given just 10 grams of high-chromium brewer's yeast daily for eight weeks, total cholesterol levels also decreased significantly, but by a lesser amount than in the first group of subjects, who had received 20 grams per day. In the second group, levels of beneficial HDL cholesterol were increased by 4 milligrams per deciliter, while the ratio of total cholesterol to HDL was decreased significantly in 79 percent of these subjects.

Recent test-tube studies suggest that the ability of brewer's yeast to lower cholesterol is due not simply to chromium but to the fact that in brewer's yeast, niacin is also present. In one study, the ability of rat liver cells to produce cholesterol was inhibited whether the rats had been fed high-chromium or low-chromium yeast. When researchers isolated the substance responsible for the inhibition of cholesterol synthesis (which, like statin drugs, occurs at the step where acetyl-CoA is converted into mevalonate), it was found to be nicotinamide riboside, a biologically active derivative of niacin produced during the digestion of brewer's yeast.

Similarly, the chromium in brewer's yeast is particularly helpful since it is present in an organic form that is combined with nicotinic acid (niacin) and biologically active peptides to produce glucose tolerance factor (GTF). As part of glucose tolerance factor, chromium helps insulin bind to its proper receptors on the cell membrane, thus improving the transport of blood sugar across cell membranes and into cells, where it can be burned for energy.

In addition to individuals with diabetes,

many older people have a lower tissue chromium content, a decreased ability to absorb chromium (which some studies suggest may be due to suboptimal dietary levels of niacin), or a higher incidence of impaired glucose tolerance. In one study, twenty-four men with an average age of seventy-eight, eight of whom were mild non-insulin-dependent diabetics, were divided into two groups, one of which was given 9 grams of chromium-rich brewer's yeast, while the control group received chromium-poor torula yeast. Not only did glucose tolerance improve and insulin output decrease markedly in the men given chromium-enriched brewer's yeast, but levels of cholesterol and triglycerides also fell significantly in this group. Men whose cholesterol levels were highest (greater than 7.7 mmol/liter, 300 milligrams per deciliter in U.S.) experienced the biggest decrease. In the control group, no significant changes occurred in glucose tolerance, insulin output, or cholesterol and triglycerides levels.

In another study of individuals with type 2 (non-insulin-dependent) diabetes, seventy-eight subjects were divided randomly into two groups and given chromium-enriched brewer's yeast, then a placebo, and finally a chromium supplement over three successive eight-week periods. At the beginning and end of each eight-week stage, the subjects were weighed, their diet and drug dosage were recorded, and blood and urine samples were collected. Both the chromium-enriched brewer's yeast and the chromium supplement caused a significant decrease in fasting and after-meal levels of glucose and triglycerides, and a drop in the average drug dosage, with some patients no longer even requiring insulin. A higher percentage of the subjects responded positively to brewer's yeast enriched with chromium, and its beneficial effects on blood sugar, triglycerides, and HDL cholesterol continued in some patients even during the eight-week period when they were on placebo.

Brewer's yeast can also be an excellent source of selenium. Plus, the selenium in brewer's yeast is almost all in the form of selenomethionine, an organic form in which selenium is complexed with a molecule of the amino acid methionine and that studies have demonstrated is more bioavailable than nonorganic forms of this trace mineral.

Selenium is a necessary component of the enzyme glutathione peroxidase, which is essential for protecting the liver from the free radicals created during the detoxification process. In addition, this selenium-activated enzyme protects cell membranes against oxidative damage, which can lead to the premature aging of cells throughout the body.

In a study conducted in China, high-selenium yeast provided significant protection against primary liver cancer. In this study, 4,075 individuals (226 with a very high risk for liver cancer, plus 3,849 of their close relatives) were randomly divided into two groups, one of which was given common brewer's yeast, while the second received selenium-enriched brewer's yeast. After two years, the incidence of liver cancer in the group that had been taking selenium-enriched brewer's yeast was less than half the incidence of liver cancer in the group taking common brewer's yeast. Even more important, after four years, in the group receiving selenium-enriched yeast, none of the individuals initially considered at highest risk had developed liver cancer, while a significant number of those at high risk who were taking common brewer's yeast did.

Brewer's yeast also has been shown to be an effective treatment for acne. In a double-blind study, 130 patients with various forms of acne were given either nutritional brewer's yeast or a placebo over a five-month period. In more than 80 percent of the patients given brewer's yeast, the acne was either completely healed or considerably improved, while the corresponding figure among those receiving placebo was only 26 percent.

HOW TO SELECT AND STORE

Brewer's yeast comes in powdered form (the most potent form), in flakes, and in tablets (good if you don't enjoy the taste).

Check the label of the brand you are considering purchasing, as the nutrients in different brands vary considerably. Some brands contain not only excellent-quality protein but good to high levels of the B vitamins, including folate, niacin, pantothenic acid, riboflavin, thiamine, and vitamins B6 and B12, plus minerals, including calcium, potassium, magnesium, copper, iron, zinc, manganese, selenium, and chromium.

Store brewer's yeast in an airtight opaque container in a cool, dark and dry pantry, where it should keep for six to eight months; or in the refrigerator, where it will keep for at least three years.

TIPS FOR PREPARING

If you're not used to it, a hefty serving of brewer's yeast may trigger diarrhea or nausea. To accustom your system to this beneficial food

supplement, start out with a small amount—about ¼ teaspoon—and double the amount taken every other day until you reach the typical dose of 1 to 3 tablespoons per day.

QUICK SERVING IDEAS

- Sprinkle a tablespoon of brewer's yeast over cold cereals or hot oatmeal.
- Mix it into soups, stews, casseroles, or sauces. The flavor of nutritional brewer's yeast goes especially well in split pea soup or in any dish made with tomato sauce.
- Add a tablespoonful of brewer's yeast to baked goods.
- Put a tablespoon of brewer's yeast in your morning smoothie.
- Sprinkle a spoonful of brewer's yeast over cottage cheese or yogurt.
- Mix a small amount of brewer's yeast into salad dressings.
- Our favorite way of eating brewer's yeast? Toss 4 cups air-popped popcorn with 3 tablespoons melted organic butter, then sprinkle generously with 2 to 4 tablespoons brewer's yeast and toss again.

SAFETY

The high purine content of brewer's yeast makes it unsuitable for people with gout, kidney disease, or arthritis. About 20 percent of the crude protein nitrogen in yeast is in the form of purines. If consumed in large amounts—more than 3 tablespoons of nutritional yeast daily—these purines can cause problems in anyone, since a high intake can result in elevated blood levels of uric acid. When blood levels of uric acid are high, it tends to crystallize and precipitate in joints, where it can cause gout or arthritis. In addition, high levels of uric acid in the bloodstream stress the kidneys.

Since the chromium–niacin combination found in chromium-enriched brewer's yeast may affect blood glucose and insulin levels, people with diabetes or hypoglycemia should consult their doctors before supplementing their diets with these forms of brewer's yeast.

Some people may be allergic to brewer's yeast. In a study using an elimination diet to treat sixty migraine patients, brewer's yeast was found to be one of the foods likely to contribute to the initiation of a migraine.

Brewer's yeast is not related to *Candida albicans,* the typical culprit in vaginal yeast infections in women.

The nutritional and chemical profile of brewer's yeast depends on the medium on which it was grown. Therefore, purchase organic brewer's yeast when possible.

Chocolate

Chocolate is produced from the beans of the cacao tree, named *Theobroma cacao* by Linnaeus. There are three main varieties of cacao trees. The most common, Forastero, gives us nearly 90 percent of the world's cacao crop. The beans of the Criollo, the rarest and most prized variety, are sought after by the world's best chocolate makers for their rich aroma and delicacy. The Trinitario variety is a cross between Criollo and Forastero.

Despite experiments in crossbreeding to make these three types of cacao trees more productive and pest-resistant, so far the cacao remains a rather delicate and strictly tropical tree, thriving only in geographical areas within 20 degrees (about 600 miles/960 kilometers) north and south of the equator. Only in these regions does the cacao tree find the necessary hot, stable climate (temperatures never below 68 degrees F./20 degrees C.), humidity (rainfall between 70 and 90 inches/175 to 225 centimeters a year), damp soil, protection from the wind, and heavy shade it requires, especially in its first two to four years of growth.

Making matters more difficult is that only 3 to 10 percent of cacao trees mature to develop full fruit. The fruit, the source of the world's chocolate and cocoa, appears in the form of green or sometimes maroon pods on the trunk of the tree and its main branches. Shaped a bit like tiny rugby balls, the pods ripen to a golden color or sometimes develop a scarlet hue with multicolored flecks. The Criollo produces a soft, thin-skinned pod, with a light color and a unique, pleasant aroma. The fruit of the Forastero is a thick-walled pod with a pungent aroma, and that of the Trinitario has characteristics that vary between the two but generally possesses a rich, aromatic flavor. The trees cross-pollinate readily, and in the Western Hemisphere, plantations composed of just one species of cacao are uncommon. Even single trees with all the characteristics of a specific type are rare.

When fully mature, cultivated trees attain a height of 15 to 25 feet/4½ to 7½ meters, while wild trees may reach a stately 60 feet/18 meters or more. Individual trees are known to have reached an age of more than 200 years, but no one has determined the real life span of the species. After twenty-five years, the fruit production, and thus economic usefulness, of a tree comes to an end, so older cultivated cacao trees are often replaced with younger ones.

Harvesting Cacao Pods

Once mature, each cacao tree, planted in the shade of a larger tree, will produce 5 pounds/2¼ kilograms of chocolate per year—or about fifteen to thirty pods since, once dried, the beans from an average pod weigh less than 2 ounces/60 grams, and approximately 400 are required to make 1 pound/½ kilogram of chocolate. Anywhere from twenty to fifty cream-colored beans are scooped from a typical pod, and the husk and inner membrane discarded.

Exposure to the air quickly changes the color of the beans from cream to lavender or purple, but they are far from what we would recognize as chocolate and lack its characteristic fragrance. At this point, the cocoa beans are put into boxes or thrown into heaps and covered with burlap. The layer of pulp that surrounds each bean starts to heat up and ferment—a simple "yeasting" process that converts the sugars in the beans to acids, primarily lactic and acetic acid. Fermentation, which takes from three to nine days and generates temperatures as high as 125 degrees F./52 degrees C., kills the germ of the bean, removes the beans' bitter taste, and activates enzymes that form the precursors of the compounds that will produce chocolate's luscious flavor when the beans are roasted. The result is a bean ready for drying.

During drying, the beans lose more than half their weight and nearly all their moisture, reaching a moisture content of no more than 7 percent. Once dried, the beans are loaded into 130-to-200-pound/60-to-90-kilogram sacks and sent to shipping centers, where they are inspected by buyers. To sample the quality of a crop, buyers cut open a number of beans to check that they are uniformly dark brown rather than purple at the center, which indicates incomplete fermentation. If the beans meet with approval, the grower is paid at the current market price, which depends not only on the abundance of the worldwide crop and the quality of farmers' crops in a number of countries, but on a number of economic conditions around the world. The chocolate industry has set up cocoa exchanges, similar to stock exchanges, in principal cities such as New York, London, Hamburg, and Amsterdam, where the prices are set.

Creating Chocolate

The art of creating chocolate from cacao beans differs slightly from plant to plant, but all chocolatiers follow the same general pattern. First, all manufacturers carefully catalogue each shipment of beans according to the particular type and its origin. Later, this allows them to maintain exact control over the flavor by selecting a variety of beans for roasting. The finest chocolatiers may combine up to twelve different varieties of beans from all over the world. After being sorted by hand, since each variety of bean is roasted separately, the beans are carefully stored in an isolated area, so the sensitive cacao does not absorb any strong odors.

The first step in the actual manufacturing process is cleaning. The cacao beans are sent through a cleaning machine that removes dried cacao pulp, pieces of pod, and any other extraneous material still present. Once thoroughly cleaned, the beans are weighed and then blended according to the chocolatier's particular specifications—often a well-guarded formula based on long years of experience in the art and science of chocolate making.

To bring out their characteristic chocolate aroma, the beans are roasted in large rotary cylinders. Depending upon the variety of the beans and the desired end result, roasting can last from 30 minutes to 2 hours at temperatures of 250 degrees F./120 degrees C. or higher. As the beans are turned over and over, their moisture content drops even further, and they develop the rich brown color and characteristic aroma of chocolate.

After roasting, the beans are quickly cooled and their thin, now brittle outer shells are removed, usually with the help of a giant winnowing machine called a "cracker and fanner" that passes the beans between serrated cones, separating the nibs—the kernels of the chocolate bean, which are the basic product used for chocolate production—into large and small grains while a fan blows away the thin, light shells. Next, the nibs, which are about 53 percent cocoa butter, are transferred to a machine called a *mélangeur,* whose granite runners, which revolve on a steel or stone bed, mash the nibs into a thick paste. The frictional heat generated by this process liquefies the cocoa butter, forming what is commercially called *chocolate liquor,* which in this case means liquid, not alcohol. Poured into molds and allowed to solidify, the chocolate liquor hardens into cakes of unsweetened or bitter chocolate.

At this point, the manufacturing process diverges, one path leading to chocolate and the other to cocoa. The chocolate liquor whose destiny is to become a cup of cocoa is pumped into giant hydraulic presses weighing up to 25 tons, and pressure is applied to express the cocoa but-ter, a yellow liquid that is drained away through metallic screens, collected, and used in the manufacture of chocolate. Cocoa butter is unique among vegetable fats in that it is solid at normal room temperature and melts slightly below body temperature, at 89 to 93 degrees F./ 32 to 34 degrees C. In addition, cocoa butter's ability to resist oxidation and rancidity translates into an exceptionally long shelf life. Under normal storage conditions, cocoa butter will keep for years without spoiling.

The pressed cake that remains after the cocoa butter's removal is then cooled, pulverized, sifted into cocoa powder, and, if its residual cocoa butter content is 10 percent or more, packaged for sale to supermarkets or put into bulk for use as a flavoring by dairies, bakeries, and confectionery manufacturers. In the U.K. cocoa powder is defined as having not less than 20 percent cocoa butter. If it is to be used as "breakfast cocoa," a less common type, it must contain at least 22 percent cocoa butter. If Dutch cocoa is to be made, the cocoa is treated with an alkali, which causes it to develop a slightly less sharp taste and gives it the characteristic lighter color of Dutch cocoa.

While cocoa is made by removing most of the cocoa butter, all types of chocolate—whether dark, bittersweet, or milk—are made by adding it. In addition to enhancing the flavor, cocoa butter makes chocolate rich and creamy. Sweet and semisweet chocolate, a combination of unsweetened chocolate, sugar, cocoa butter, and often a little vanilla, are made by combining the ingredients and melting them in a large mixing machine to produce a mass with the consistency of dough. Milk chocolate is made essentially the same way, except that less unsweetened chocolate is used and milk is added.

Regardless of the ingredients used, the resulting chocolate mass is further ground by being sent through a series of heavy rollers, which refine the mixture to a smooth paste ready for "conching." In conching, a flavor development process that takes its name from the shell-like shape of the containers originally used, the chocolate is kneaded in machines equipped with heavy rollers that plough back and forth through the chocolate mass for anywhere from a few hours to several days. Under regulated speeds, these rollers produce different degrees of agitation and aeration that develop and modify the chocolate flavors.

In some manufacturing setups, an emulsifying operation either takes the place of conching or supplements it. Often the emulsifier lecithin is added, and if so, about 5 percent less of the expensive cocoa butter is needed. Carried out by a machine that works like an eggbeater, breaking up the sugar crystals and other particles in the chocolate mixture, this process gives the chocolate a fine, velvety smoothness.

After it has been conched and emulsified, the well-blended liquid chocolate is tempered for several hours. In tempering, the chocolate liquor is heated and then cooled in several stages, a process that stabilizes the cocoa butter crystals, so they become more uniform in size, and gives the chocolate its bright luster and a sharp snap when broken. Finally, the chocolate is poured into molds ranging in size from those that form the standard 1.4-ounce/40 gram individual bars for consumers to the 10-pound/4½ kilogram blocks used by confectionery manufacturers.

Once in the mold, the chocolate is sent to the cooling chamber, where cooling proceeds at a fixed rate that keeps the chocolate's flavor intact. The bars are then removed from the molds and passed along to wrapping machines to be packed for shipment. In addition to being shipped as bars, chocolate is also frequently shipped as a liquid to sweet, biscuit, and ice cream manufacturers.

Besides the equipment already described, the chocolate industry employs a number of fascinating machines that shape and package chocolate into its array of available forms. Shaping machines perform at amazing speeds, spurting jets of chocolate that solidify into special shapes at a rate of several hundred a minute, while other machines wrap and package the solidified products at speeds impossible for human hands.

One machine worth mentioning is the enrober. Employed in the creation of assorted chocolates, the enrober receives lines of assorted centers—nuts, nougats, fruit, cream fillings, etc.—and drenches them in a waterfall of liquid chocolate. Other confectionery machines achieve the same end by creating a hollow, molded shell of chocolate that is then filled with a soft or liquid center before its bottom is sealed with chocolate.

While all this is going on, so are numerous tests that double-check the viscosity of the chocolate, its cocoa butter content, acidity, fineness, purity, and, of course, its taste, which can vary from having nuances of fruit to a bitterness similar to that of coffee, often with both flavors combined.

In the United States, all chocolate manufacturers must meet the standards set forth by the Food and Drug Administration, which govern manufacturing formulas to the extent of specifying the minimum content of chocolate liquor and milk, and which flavorings and other ingredients may be used. Secrets abound, however, where methods of manufacturing are concerned, and no master chef ever guarded his favorite recipes more zealously than chocolate manufacturers guard their secret formulas for key manufacturing operations, such as blending the beans, the time intervals used in conching, and the temperatures used to temper the final product.

But the secrets of chocolate manufacturers' work are certainly appreciated in the United States, where per capita chocolate consumption runs about 12 pounds/5½ kilograms per year, or about ½ ounce/15 grams of chocolate per person per day. For Valentine's Day in 1997, Americans purchased more than $709 million worth of chocolate. In 2000, they gave their sweethearts more than 35 million heart-shaped boxes of chocolate, close to $1 billion worth.

Sound like a lot? It's not even close to the Swiss, whose annual per capita consumption of chocolate is 22 pounds/10 kilograms, while the British, Germans, and Belgians, at about 20 pounds/9 kilograms per capita, aren't far behind.

HISTORY

The exact origin of the cacao tree is disputed. Some claim the cacao was born in the Amazon basin of Brazil, others say its birthplace was the Orinoco Valley of Venezuela, while still others contend the cacao is native to Central America. While the exact origin remains disputed, it is clear that the Olmec, Mayas, and Aztecs all enjoyed the cocoa bean for at least 5,000 years before it made its way to Europe.

Symbols of life and fertility in the Mayan civilization, cocoa pods were carved into stone palaces and temples as early as 300 C.E. By 600 C.E., Mayan territory had expanded from the Yucatán Peninsula north to the Pacific Coast of Guatemala. In the Yucatán, Mayans were cultivating the earliest known cocoa plantation, and the cocoa pod, which was often represented in religious rituals, was referred to as "the gods' food."

By the sixth century C.E., the Maya, who called the cocoa tree *cacahuaquchtl,* were already using its seeds to make a cold, very spicy, bitter drink they called *xocoatl,* meaning "bitter water." Since sugar was unknown, various other foods, such as hot chili peppers and cornmeal, were used to flavor this thick, cold, potent brew, which they considered a health elixir.

By 1200 C.E., the Mayan culture had been conquered by that of the Aztecs, a civilization that attributed the creation of the cocoa tree to their god Quetzalcoatl, who, descending from Heaven on a beam of the morning star, brought with him a cocoa seedling stolen from Paradise. To the Aztecs, cocoa beans were so valuable they were used as currency and only those wealthy enough to have money to drink used the beans to make *xocolatl,* which they pronounced *shoco-latle,* a drink thought to confer wisdom and power.

The Aztecs also believed that *xocolatl* had nourishing, fortifying, and even aphrodisiac qualities. The Aztec emperor Montezuma is said to have considered the drink much more valuable than the golden goblets in which it was served, throwing them away after only one use. If addiction to chocolate is possible, Montezuma was probably the first to succumb. He liked *xocolatl* so much, he purportedly drank fifty goblets of it every day!

Columbus was the first European to come in contact with cacao. On August 15, 1502, during his fourth and last voyage to the Americas, Columbus and his crew encountered a large dugout canoe near an island off the coast of what is now Honduras. The largest native vessel the Spaniards had seen, the canoe was "as long as a galley" and filled with local goods for trade, including cacao beans. In typical European conqueror style, Columbus and his crew seized the vessel and retained its skipper as his guide.

Later, when Columbus's son Ferdinand wrote about the encounter, he was struck by the value the Native Americans placed on cacao beans, saying, "They seemed to hold these almonds [the cacao beans] at a great price; for when they were brought on board ship together with their goods, I observed that when any of these almonds fell, they all stooped to pick it up, as if an eye had fallen." What Ferdinand didn't know was that cocoa beans were the local currency. In fact, in some parts of Central America, cacao beans were used as currency until as recently as the last century.

The cacao bean was first introduced to Europe when Columbus returned in triumph from the New World and laid before the court of King Ferdinand a treasure trove of strange and wonderful things, one of which was a pile of dark brown beans that appeared most unpromising. Not until 1513, when the conquistador Hernando de Oviedo y Valdez, who went to America as a member of Pedrarius de Avila's expedition, reported that ten cocoa beans bought the services of a prostitute, four cocoa beans got you a rabbit for dinner, and that he had purchased a slave for 100 cocoa beans, were its monetary possibilities even considered by the Spanish.

In 1519, when the great Spanish explorer Hernando Cortés led an expedition into the depths of Mexico, they were welcomed by Emperor Montezuma as "white Gods, risen from the sea," and served *xocolatl*, a bitter-tasting, frothy cold drink made of ground cacao beans mixed usually with water, but sometimes with wine, and seasoned with chili peppers. Cortés is said to have toasted Montezuma with a golden goblet full of the Aztecs' favorite libation before betraying and murdering the proud emperor. Although he was not enthusiastic about the taste of the beverage, finding it too bitter, Cortés wrote to King Carlos I of Spain, calling *xocolatl* a "drink that builds up resistance and fights fatigue."

After discovering that Emperor Montezuma, a devout "chocoholic," had drunk nothing but *xocolatl*, especially before visiting his harem, since he believed it to be a powerful aphrodisiac, Cortés planted a cacao plantation to grow the seeds for Spain. In 1528, he returned to his native land with three chests full of cacao beans and the tools needed to make the drink, which he continued to dislike personally—at least until the Aztecs' recipe was greatly improved upon by the Spanish cooks, who replaced the chili peppers with sugar and added cinnamon and vanilla.

Quickly adopted by the court of King Charles V, the new chocolate drink, served in deep, straight-sided cups for breakfast, was made from cacao beans that were heavily spiced, sweetened, and boiled in wine. For the next hundred years, the Spanish kept the origin of chocolate a secret while developing cocoa plantations in their equatorial colonies around the world and building up quite a profitable trade in the popular new beverage.

In 1544, however, when Dominican friars took a delegation of Mayans to meet the Spanish monarch, Philip, the Spanish monks who had been consigned to process the cacao beans leaked the secret, and it wasn't long before chocolate found its way into the golden cups of all the European monarchs, who began planting cacao plantations wherever an area of fertile soil and the right climate could be found.

Obviously, the word hadn't spread everywhere, because in 1579, after capturing a Spanish ship loaded with cacao beans, British buccaneers set it on fire, thinking the beans were sheep dung, and, in 1587, destroyed the cacao cargo of yet another Spanish ship, assuming it was worthless.

In 1615, Anne of Austria, daughter of the Spanish monarch Philip III, brought the beverage with her as part of her dowry when she wed the French monarch, Louis XIII. So delighted was the French court with chocolate that in 1643, when the Spanish princess Maria Teresa was betrothed to Louis XIV of France, her engagement gift to her future husband was an ornate chest filled with chocolate. Louis XIV, who was said still to be making love to his wife twice a day at age seventy-two, enjoyed chocolate so much that he appointed Sieur David Illou to develop it for manufacture and sale, beginning a chocolate craze that took Paris by storm and soon spread throughout France.

With its reputation as an aphrodisiac flourishing in the French courts, French art and literature were soon filled with erotic imagery inspired by chocolate. The Marquis de Sade mixed chocolate's sensuous qualities with its ability to disguise poisons, while Casanova reputedly used chocolate and champagne to seduce the ladies. In the court of Louis XV, Madame de Pompadour combined her chocolate with ambergris to stimulate her desire for the king, but to no avail; even replete with chocolate, she remained cold to him. Madame du Barry, a nymphomaniac with the opposite problem, gave her lovers chocolate in the hope they would be able to keep up with her.

The drinking of chocolate soon spread across the Channel to Great Britain, where, in London in 1657, a Frenchman opened the first of the many famous London chocolate houses, which quickly became the "in" places where London's elite met to savor the new brew. In 1711, Emperor Charles VI brought his court—and chocolate—from Madrid to Vienna, and by 1720, Italian chocolatiers from Florence and Venice, now well versed in the art of making chocolate, were welcomed into Germany and Switzerland.

As other countries challenged Spain's monopoly on cacao, chocolate became more widely available. Soon the French, English, and Dutch were cultivating cacao in their colonies in the Caribbean and, later, elsewhere in the world. More cacao and the appearance of a perfected steam engine in 1730, which mechanized the cocoa-grinding process, hastened the development of chocolate's mass production. Prices dropped, and soon the masses in Europe and the Americas were enjoying chocolate. For many people, however, the expanded production of cacao in the New World meant slavery and privation since cacao production relied heavily on the forced labor of Native Americans and imported African slaves.

In 1765, the first chocolate factory in the United States, founded by Dr. James Baker in

Dorchester, Massachusetts, appeared in pre-Revolutionary New England, although the first wholly machine-made chocolate was produced in Barcelona, Spain, in 1780. In 1792, the Josty brothers from Grisons, Switzerland, opened a confectionery shop in Germany and were so successful selling chocolate that they opened a chocolate factory in Berlin. Shortly afterward, in 1819, François-Louis Cailler, who had learned the secrets of the chocolate trade in Italy, founded the first chocolate factory in Switzerland in a former mill near Vevey.

As cacao became more commonly available, people began experimenting with new ways of using it. Chocolate began to appear in cakes, pastries, and sorbets, but it wasn't until 1828 that "modern chocolate" was born. In this year, the Dutch chocolate maker Conrad J. van Houten patented the cocoa press, an inexpensive method for pressing the fat from roasted cacao beans. The center of the bean, the nib, contains an average of 54 percent cocoa butter. The machine van Houten developed—a hydraulic press—reduced the nib's cocoa butter content by nearly half, creating a pressed cake that could be pulverized into a fine powder known as cocoa.

Van Houten, a Dutchman, treated the powder with alkaline salts (potassium or sodium carbonates), so it would mix more easily with water, a process known today as "dutching." The final product, Dutch cocoa, was not only much less rich and more soluble, making the creation of chocolate drinks much easier, but also could be combined with sugar and then remixed with cocoa butter to create a solid form of chocolate—a feat first accomplished in 1830 when the British chocolatiers J. S. Fry and Sons, building on van Houten's success, developed the world's first bar of chocolate.

Cadbury Brothers chocolate made its international debut in 1851, at the famous International Exposition orchestrated by Queen Victoria's husband, Prince Albert, and held at Bingley Hall in Birmingham, England; milk chocolate appeared in 1875, developed after eight years of experimentation by Daniel Peter, a Swiss chocolate manufacturer who had the idea of using powdered milk (invented by the Swiss chemist Henri Nestlé in 1867) to make a new kind of chocolate.

In 1879, Rodolphe Lindt of Berne, Switzerland, invented "conching," a means of heating and rolling chocolate to refine it that transformed chocolate into *fondant,* today's creamy velvety chocolate that melts in your mouth. And in 1888, Milton Snavely Hershey opened his first chocolate factory in Lancaster, Pennsylvania, where he developed the Hershey bar, a name that became synonymous with chocolate in the United States.

By 1900, the Swiss had overtaken Spain as the leading producers of chocolate, while the Germans consumed the most per capita, followed by the United States, France, and Great Britain. In 1913, Jules Séchaud of Montrèux, Switzerland, introduced the process for filling chocolates. By this time, chocolate was such big business that in 1923, the Chocolate Manufacturers Association of the United States was organized, followed shortly, in 1925, by the New York Cocoa Exchange, so buyers and sellers could get together for international transactions.

In 1938, just before the outbreak of World War II, the importance of chocolate was recognized by the U.S. government, which allocated precious shipping space for the importation of cocoa beans, knowing chocolate would boost the troops' morale. Today, U.S. Army D rations include three 4-ounce/125-gram bars of chocolate, which is even taken into space as part of the food supplies of U.S. astronauts.

Most cacao beans now come from small farms in West Africa and Brazil, but the tree is also cultivated in other areas of South America close to the equator, in Mexico, the Caribbean, Southeast Asia, the South Pacific, Hawaii, and the islands of Samoa and New Guinea.

NUTRITIONAL HIGHLIGHTS

The primary components of chocolate are sugar and fat, in roughly equal amounts. According to U.S. government standards, true chocolate must derive its fat solely from cocoa butter, unless it's milk chocolate, in which case 80 percent of the fat must be from cocoa butter and 20 percent from milk. Chocolate is rich in plant sterols and many types of flavonoids. A 100 gram serving of milk chocolate provides 535 calories, 7.7 grams of protein, 23 grams of cholesterol, 29.7 grams of fat (14.2 grams saturated), 59.5 grams of carbohydrate (51.5 grams of sugar), and 13.4 milligrams of flavonoids. The same serving of semisweet chocolate provides 479 calories, 4.2 grams of protein, 30 grams of fat (17.8 grams saturated), 63.1 grams of carbohydrate (54.5 grams of sugar), and 53 milligrams of flavonoids. The same serving of unsweetened chocolate provides 501 calories, 12.9 grams of protein, no cholesterol, 52.3 grams of fat (32.4 grams saturated), 29.8 grams of carbohydrate (0.9 grams of sugar), and 135 milligrams of sitosterols.

HEALTH BENEFITS

At the center of chocolate's health benefits are flavonoids. These plant pigments are responsible for many of the health benefits of many fruits and medicinal plants, but chocolate may be a much more sensually pleasing vehicle. In addition, there is evidence that not only is chocolate rich in flavonoids, but that factors in chocolate somehow dramatically increase the absorption of these compounds. The key flavonoids are proanthocyanidins (also called procyanidins) similar to those found in grape seed extracts, apples, berries, and pine bark extract. Chocolate is very well endowed with these compounds. In fact, procyanidins constitute from 12 percent to as much as 48 percent of the dry weight of the cocoa bean. Cocoa powder can contain as much as 10 percent flavonoids on a dry-weight basis.

One of the key areas of research into the benefits of chocolate consumption is its effect on cardiovascular disease. A growing amount of recent research suggests that:

- Unlike the saturated fats found in meat and dairy products, the saturated fats found in chocolate do not elevate cholesterol levels.
- Cocoa butter contains small amounts of the plant sterols sitosterol and stigmasterol, which may help inhibit the absorption of dietary cholesterol.
- Chocolate can be a rich source of flavonoid antioxidants, which are especially important in protecting against damage to cholesterol and the lining of the arteries.
- Chocolate flavonoids prevent the excessive clumping together of blood platelets that can cause blood clots.

TABLE 19.1

**Flavonoid Content (as Flavonols and Procyanidins) and
Antioxidant Capacity of Chocolate and Other Foods and Beverages**

	Flavanols and Procyanidins (milligrams)	ORAC (mmol Trolox equivalents*)
Dark semisweet chocolate, 3 ounces (100 grams)	170	40.0
Milk chocolate, 3 ounces (100 grams)	70	6.7
Hot chocolate,† 1 cup	35	3.4
Apples, 1 medium	106	0.2
Red wine, ½ ounce/15 milliliters	22	0.7
Brewed black tea, 2 bags	40	1.6

* Antioxidant activity is reported as oxygen radical absorbance capacity (ORAC) (water-soluble vitamin E) and expressed as mmol Trolox equivalents.

† The flavonol content of unsweetened powdered cocoa is actually double that of dark chocolate, but when it is made into a cup of hot chocolate, the cocoa is diluted with water or milk and sugar, so its flavonoid total per serving drops to half that found in milk chocolate.

• Chocolate can provide significant amounts of arginine, an amino acid that is required in the production of nitric oxide. Nitric oxide causes blood vessels to dilate, which helps regulate blood flow, inflammation, and blood pressure.

Although chocolate is primarily sugar and fat, it does not appear to adversely affect cholesterol levels (as long as total fat and calorie intake is held constant), based on recent studies. For example, in one study participants experienced no rise in cholesterol levels despite the fact that they were eating 10 ounces/300 grams of chocolate per day. In another study, twenty-three healthy volunteers were placed on two diets in succession: a typical American diet or the same diet plus about four tablespoons of cocoa powder and ½ ounce/15 grams of dark chocolate daily for four weeks. While on the chocolate diet, not only did the volunteers experience 8 percent less oxidative damage of their LDL (bad) cholesterol, but their levels of HDL (good) cholesterol actually increased by 4 percent compared to when they were on the chocolate-free diet.

Chocolate also contains small amounts of the plant sterols sitosterol and stigmasterol. These sterols, which compete with cholesterol for absorption from the gut, can contribute to improved blood lipid profiles by inhibiting the uptake of dietary cholesterol. Although the amounts of plant sterols present in cocoa butter are so small their impact is likely to be small as well, these sterols are still yet one more component of chocolate with potential cardiovascular benefit.

Chocolate flavonoids also work like a very low dose of aspirin to prevent blood platelets from aggregating. When blood platelets are too sticky, they tend to clump together and form a blood clot. A blood clot can become dislodged, leading to a heart attack, stroke, or pulmonary embolism. In one study, the effect of a flavonoid-rich cocoa drink containing 25 grams (a little less than an ounce) of semisweet chocolate compared to an 81 milligram dose of aspirin (i.e., a baby aspirin) showed that the two were similar in their effects on preventing platelets from clumping together or clotting. However, aspirin's effects are longer-lasting than those produced by chocolate flavonoids, so unlike aspirin, which can be taken once daily, a dose of flavonoid-rich chocolate would need to be consumed every six to eight hours.

HOW TO SELECT AND STORE

Chocolate is available in many different forms, but the FDA has a classification system based upon the percentage of key ingredients in chocolate products (no such percentage classification exists in Europe and cocoa content varies widely between manufacturers, although the E.U. defines dark chocolate as having a minimum 35 percent cocoa solids and milk chocolate a minimum of 25 percent):

- *Unsweetened or baking chocolate:* In the U.S., this is the most basic chocolate product. It is simply the hardened chocolate liquor made from the cacao beans' ground nibs. Also called bitter chocolate, it must contain between 50 and 58 percent cocoa butter. Baking chocolate is usually sold in 1-ounce/30-gram squares. It is not the same as the "substitute" chocolate traditionally called "baking chocolate" in the U.K.
- *Semisweet chocolate:* Called bittersweet chocolate in Europe, semisweet chocolate must contain at least 35 percent chocolate liquor, but it also contains sugar, added cocoa butter, vanilla, and other flavorings, and may contain lecithin as an emulsifier. The most popular choice for cooking, semisweet chocolate is available in chips, bars, squares, and sweets. Bittersweet or bitter chocolate in Europe refers to any strong chocolate and a good-quality product should have 55 to 70 percent cocoa solids.
- *Sweet chocolate:* A dark chocolate containing at least 15 percent chocolate liquor, flavorings, and more sugar than semisweet chocolate.
- *Mexican chocolate:* A grainier-textured chocolate than other forms, this sweet chocolate is flavored with cinnamon, almonds, and vanilla. Found in some supermarkets and specialty shops, Mexican chocolate is sold in squares.

CHOCOLATE: AN APHRODISIAC, LOVE POTION, AND ANTIDEPRESSANT?

Chocolate has long been associated with love, and scientists have finally discovered a possible chemical connection. Chocolate contains phenylethylamine (PEA), a neurotransmitter that is released by neurons at moments of emotional euphoria, including feelings of love. It may be that one of the reasons that chocolate is by far the most common cause of food addiction is that people are actually getting minute quantities of PEA from chocolate. What is curious, however, is why we don't have similar affection for a number of foods—such as salami, pickled herring, and Cheddar cheese—that actually contain significantly more PEA than a comparable serving of chocolate.

One explanation may be controversial findings suggesting that chocolate contains pharmacologically active substances with the same effect on the brain as marijuana. In marijuana, the pharmacologically active substance is THC (tetrahydrocannabinol). Brain cells have receptors for THC. A receptor is a structure on the surface of the cell's outer membrane that will lock onto certain molecules, allowing them to transmit a signal through the cell wall, triggering a reaction inside the cell. In the case of THC, the reaction would make someone feel "high."

THC is not found in chocolate, but another neurotransmitter called anandamide is. Like THC, anandamide is naturally produced in the brain and binds to the same receptors, which may help explain why, while eating chocolate will not make you high, it's likely to engender some pleasant feelings or at least make you feel more relaxed and less anxious. Like other neurotransmitters, anandamide is broken down quickly after it's produced, but other chemicals in chocolate inhibit the natural breakdown of anandamide, allowing it to remain in the brain longer, making us feel good when we eat chocolate.

- *Milk chocolate:* Semisweet or sweet chocolate to which dry milk has been added, milk chocolate must contain a minimum of 10 percent chocolate liquor and 12 percent milk solids, along with sugar, cocoa butter, vanilla, and/or other flavorings. Milk chocolate is sold as bars and sweets.
- *Cocoa powder:* Dried, powdered chocolate liquor that contains 10 to 22 percent cocoa butter (20 percent minimum in the U.K.) is classified as cocoa powder.
- *Dutch-process cocoa powder:* Lighter in color and mellower in flavor than regular cocoa powder, Dutch-process cocoa powder (also called European-style cocoa) is treated with alkali to neutralize cocoa's natural acidity and make it more soluble.
- *Liquid chocolate:* This is a mixture of unsweetened cocoa powder and vegetable oil. Developed for convenience in baking since it does not require melting, liquid chocolate comes in 1-ounce/30 gram packages. It cannot, however, duplicate the flavor or texture of melted unsweetened chocolate since it contains much less cocoa butter.
- *Couverture:* A very glossy, dark coating chocolate that contains a minimum of 32 percent cocoa butter defines couverture.
- *White chocolate:* A mixture of sugar, cocoa butter, milk solids, lecithin, and vanilla produces white chocolate. Since it contains no chocolate liquor, it provides none of the beneficial flavonoids found in other chocolates.

In order to provide the most healthful choices of chocolate products, we offer the following suggestions:

- For the biggest flavonoid bang for your caloric buck, choose high-quality semisweet, dark chocolate with the highest cocoa content that suites your palate.
- Avoid chocolate sweets and treats made with hydrogenated fats or refined flour, neither of which promotes health.
- Also pass on products labeled "artificial chocolate" or "chocolate-flavored." These imitations are not even close to the real thing in flavor, texture, or health benefits.
- Since the chocolate's beneficial polyphenols have been removed from white chocolate, we cannot recommend it as a healthful food.

Chocolate can pick up odors from other foods, so never store it near onions, garlic, or strong spices. All types of chocolate should be stored in an airtight plastic bag or other airtight container in a cool, dry place (60 to 70 degrees F./15 to 21 degrees C.), or in the refrigerator or freezer. Dark chocolate is so rich in potent polyphenol antioxidants that protect it from oxidation that it will keep, under ideal conditions, for as long as ten years. Milk chocolate, which contains milk solids, will keep, unrefrigerated, for about nine months. Refrigerated or frozen, it will remain fresh for at least a year.

White chocolate, since it contains none of chocolate's antioxidant polyphenols, will remain fresh, unrefrigerated, for about six months. Stored in the refrigerator or freezer, it should keep for nine months to one year. If storing chocolate in the refrigerator or freezer, let its full flavor return by allowing it to warm to room temperature before serving.

In the summer or in a warm climate, chocolate is best refrigerated since warm temperatures can cause it to "bloom" with surface streaks and blotches that are the result of the cocoa butter rising to the surface. Damp, cold conditions can sometimes produce tiny gray sugar crystals on the surface of chocolate. Neither condition means the chocolate has spoiled, although its flavor and texture may be slightly affected.

In both dark and milk chocolate, the amount of polyphenols present will vary depending upon how the cacao beans were processed. To minimize the losses of these valuable constituents, cocoa processors and chocolate manufacturers are beginning to take precautions. Mars recently developed a proprietary method for processing cocoa beans called CocoaPro that preserves polyphenols by changing the way the beans are selected, fermented, and dried, as well as how they're processed and formulated. Some Mars chocolate bars already feature the CocoaPro label, and it's highly likely that other chocolate manufacturers will develop similar polyphenol-retaining procedures and labels that inform consumers that their products retain more of these beneficial compounds.

TIPS FOR PREPARING

All forms of chocolate scorch easily, which completely ruins the flavor. To prevent this, always melt chocolate slowly over low heat. Perhaps the safest way to melt chocolate is in the top half of a double boiler over simmering water. When a little more than half the chocolate is melted, remove the top pot from the heat and stir until all is melted and completely smooth.

It's also a good idea to rub a little butter over the inside of the pan you will be using to melt the chocolate or spray the pan with rapeseed oil cooking spray. Not only will this help prevent the chocolate from scorching, but it will slide right out when melted. If you have a little one waiting to help "clean" the pot, you may want to skip this and just be extra careful when melting.

Don't substitute milk chocolate for dark chocolate when cooking. Because of milk's sensitivity to heat, milk chocolate will not perform comparably. When melted, unsweetened chocolate is runny, but semisweet, sweet, and white chocolate can be fully melted yet will retain their shape until stirred. Chocolate chips melt more quickly than squares. Don't wait to check until you think these forms of chocolate are melted, or the chocolate may be singed.

Chocolate can be melted with liquid—at least ¼ cup for every 6 ounces/170 grams of chocolate—but once melted, even a *single* drop of moisture will cause the soft, glossy mass to clump and harden ("seize" in the terminology of chocolatiers). If this happens, all is not lost. Immediately stir in 1 tablespoon of a mild vegetable oil, such as rapeseed, for each 6 ounces/170 grams of chocolate, then melt the mixture again over low heat, stirring until fully smooth.

The following measurements may come in handy:

- One 12-ounce/350-gram package of chocolate chips = 2 cups.
- 1 ounce/30 grams unsweetened chocolate = 3 tablespoons unsweetened cocoa + 1 tablespoon butter.
- 1 ounce/30 grams semisweet chocolate = ½ ounce/15 grams unsweetened chocolate + 1 tablespoon granulated sugar.

If substituting Dutch-process cocoa powder for regular cocoa in a recipe, omit any bicarbonate of soda, since it also acts as an alkalizer.

When making hot cocoa, heat the milk gently. The temperature of heated milk should never exceed 170 degrees F./77 degrees C. Overheating milk destroys its flavor and texture. Whisking hot cocoa for about 30 seconds before serving will result in an appealing foamy topping and enhance the flavor of the cocoa.

QUICK SERVING IDEAS

- Enhance the flavor of prepared cocoa mixes for a single serving by:
  - Adding freshly grated cinnamon to the bottom of the cup before pouring in the cocoa and hot milk or water.
  - Adding a drop of vanilla to the hot water or milk along with the cocoa.
  - Adding a dash of nutmeg or a drop of peppermint extract to the cocoa before adding water.
  - Adding 1 tablespoon of your favorite liqueur immediately before serving.
- For chocolate fondue, in a small saucepan over low heat, melt 8 ounces/250 grams semisweet chocolate chips and 1 cup whipping cream, stirring until smooth. Remove from the heat and stir in 1 teaspoon vanilla and a couple of teaspoons sherry, brandy, or your favorite liqueur. Serve with a bowl of organic, unsweetened, shredded coconut and a plate of whole berries, chunks of pineapple, banana, melon, peaches, or any

fruit you choose. Dip the fruit into the chocolate, then sprinkle with shredded coconut.

- Transform refried black beans into something special by adding a little homemade mole sauce: Sauté 1 medium chopped onion, 2 cloves diced garlic, 1 to 2 fresh, seeded chilies, and ¼ cup ground pumpkin or sesame seeds until the onion is translucent. Then add 1 ounce/30 grams of Mexican chocolate (or dark chocolate) and cook over low heat until melted, stirring so that all ingredients are well combined. If you don't have pumpkin or sesame seeds, use ground almonds. If you don't have Mexican chocolate, substitute 1 ounce/30 grams semisweet chocolate, ½ teaspoon ground cinnamon, and, if you haven't already used ground almonds, 1 drop almond extract. Mix the mole into 12 ounces/350 grams of refried black beans.

- Whip up this incredibly rich, dairy-free chocolate mousse: Melt a 10-ounce/300-gram package of semisweet chocolate chips in the top of a double boiler until the chips are soft but still retain their shape. Remove from the heat and let rest while you purée two 12-ounce/350-gram packages of silken tofu in a food processor until they are the consistency of pudding. Add 1 teaspoon of honey or your favorite liqueur and mix the melted chocolate into the tofu until well blended. Pour into parfait glasses and chill until set (about 1 hour). Garnish with a chocolate leaf, chocolate shavings, or grated chocolate and some fresh raspberries. For a chocolate "cream" pie, pour into a prepared chocolate cookie pastry case instead.

SAFETY

Chocolate can produce a stimulant effect and lead to feelings of nervousness and anxiety in some people. It is also a common food allergen. Chocolate, along with red wines and aged cheeses, has been linked with nervous tension, as well as migraine headaches. All of these foods contain compounds known as vasoactive amines that can dilate brain vessels, triggering headaches in susceptible individuals.

Since chocolate contains oxalic acid, a compound that can bind to calcium in the urinary tract to form kidney stones, dark chocolate should be avoided by individuals prone to kidney stones. According to a study conducted in Brazil, while consumption of dark chocolate caused a 20 percent increase in urinary oxalate excretion, no such increase was observed in the group receiving milk chocolate, suggesting that as long as enough calcium is also present, it will bind to oxalates in the gut, preventing the formation of kidney stones.

Chocolate is a food high in arginine, an amino acid required by the herpes virus to replicate. Chocolate and other arginine-rich foods should be avoided by those with active and frequently recurring herpes infections.

Chocolate does not contain goitrogens or purines.

Honey and Other Bee Products

Honey can be found in its standard amber state but may also be red, brown, and even nearly black. Made by bees in an elegantly natural process, honey is designed for bees' nourishment. Incredibly, each bee makes on average only about $\frac{1}{12}$ of a teaspoon of honey in its entire lifetime. Considering the tons of honey produced each year, that is a lot of bees at work! The honeybee (Latin name *Apis*) first travels several miles to collect nectar from local flowers into its mouth. Enzymes in the bee saliva then create a chemical reaction that turns this nectar into honey, which is deposited into the walls of the hive. Incredibly rapid movement of the bees' wings aerates the honey, which decreases its water content and makes it ready to eat. Textures and flavor are dependent on which flowers the honeybees choose. Typical choices include heather, alfalfa, clover, and the acacia flower. Less common but well-known flowers that confer their own special taste characteristics on the honey include thyme and lavender.

In addition to honey, bees produce bee pollen, propolis, and royal jelly. These products concentrate many phytochemicals with powerful health-promoting activity. Yet, for the most part, these foods have been underappreciated and underutilized in North America.

- *Bee pollen* comes from the male germ cell of flowering plants. As the honeybee travels from flower to flower, it fertilizes the female germ cells with some of the male germ cells it picks up. Honeybees make possible the reproduction of more than 80 percent of the world's grains, fruits, vegetables, and legumes. The remaining male pollen is collected and brought to the hive, where the bees add enzymes and nectar to the pollen. Bee pollen is comprised of tiny, golden yellow to dark brown granules that have a delicate flavor and aroma that varies according to the plant pollen it was made from and is used as a nutritive tonic as well as to desensitize seasonal allergies.

- *Propolis* is the resinous substance collected by bees from the leaf buds and barks of trees, especially poplar and conifer trees. The bees utilize the propolis along with beeswax to construct the hive. Propolis has antibiotic activities that help the hive block out viruses, bacteria, and other organisms. Propolis is yellow to brown, waxy, and bitter-flavored and is used as an antimicrobial.

- *Royal jelly* is a thick, milky substance produced by worker bees to feed the queen bee. The worker bees mix honey and bee pollen with enzymes in the glands of their throats to produce royal jelly. Royal jelly is believed to be a useful nutritional supplement because of the queen bee's superior size, strength, stamina, and longevity compared to other bees. It is used as a nutritive tonic.

HISTORY

Referred to in ancient Sumerian, Vedic, Egyptian, and biblical writings, honey has been employed since ancient times for both nutrition and healing medicine. For centuries honey has been a multipurpose food, used to give homage to the gods and to help embalm the dead, as well as for medical and cosmetic purposes. Some evidence suggests that despite the risk of bee sting, collection of honey has occurred since 7000 B.C.E., and since at least 700 B.C.E., beekeeping for the production of honey (apiculture) has been used. To the surprise of the Spanish conquistadors, the natives of Central and South America were already keeping bees for the purpose of collecting honey when they arrived. Honey was considered a food of the rich for many years. More recently, honey has decreased in popularity as refined sugar, which is cheaper and sweeter, has replaced the sweet, viscous liquid in ordinary households all over the world.

NUTRITIONAL HIGHLIGHTS

Honey is a source of riboflavin and vitamin B6. It also provides iron and manganese. A 100 gram serving of honey provides 304 calories, mostly as 82.4 grams of carbohydrate, almost all of which is sugar, 0.3 gram of protein, and no fat. However, honey is more likely to be consumed by the tablespoon (15 grams), which provides 64 calories, 17.3 grams of carbohydrate, and 0.1 gram of protein.

Bee pollen is often referred to as "nature's most perfect food" because it is a complete protein (typically containing 10 to 35 percent total protein) in that it contains all eight essential amino acids. Bee pollen also provides B vitamins, vitamin C, carotenes, minerals, DNA and RNA, numerous flavonoid molecules, and plant hormones. Propolis and royal jelly have similar nutritional qualities as pollen but have considerably higher levels of different biologically active compounds. A 100 gram serving provides 313 calories, 25 grams of carbohydrate, 25 grams of protein, and 12.5 grams of fat. A tablespoon provides 25 calories, 2 grams of protein, 2 grams of carbohydrate, and 1 gram of fat.

HEALTH BENEFITS

The health benefits of a particular honey depend on its processing as well as the quality of the flowers the bees utilize when collecting the pollen. Raw honey is honey that has not been pasteurized, clarified, or filtered, and this form typically retains more of the healthful phytochemicals lost to the standard processing of honey. Propolis is a product of tree sap mixed with bee secretions that is used by bees to protect against bacteria, viruses, and fungi. Propolis is unfortunately lost in honey processing, thus greatly reducing the level of phytochemicals known to protect against the germs; recent research suggests that these may also prevent certain types of cancer. Also important, healthy, organic flowering plants will provide the raw nectar that will confer a higher-quality nutrient profile to the honey produced.

Within the propolis are well-researched phytochemicals that have cancer-preventing and antitumor properties. These substances include caffeic acid, methyl caffeate, phenylethyl caffeate, and phenylethyl dimethylcaffeate. Researchers have discovered that these substances in propolis prevent colon cancer in animals by shutting down the activity of two enzymes, phosphatidylinositol-specific phospholipase C and lipoxygenase, that are involved in the production of cancer-causing compounds.

The following sections address the health benefits of honey in its raw form; see page 658 for information on bee pollen, propolis, and royal jelly.

Antioxidant Effects

Honey, particularly darker honey, such as buckwheat honey, is a rich source of phenolic compounds, such as flavonoids, that exert significant antioxidant activity. A recent human trial showed that daily consumption of honey actually improves blood antioxidant levels and helps prevent lipid peroxidation. Lipid peroxidation, the damaging of lipids (such as cholesterol) by free radicals, is central to the initiation and progression of atherosclerosis. Honey's ability to prevent lipid peroxidation may translate into a protective effect against atherosclerosis, since oxidized cholesterol is a well-known risk factor for this cardiovascular disease. In one human trial, twenty-five men aged eighteen to sixty-eight years drank a mixture equivalent to about 4 tablespoons of honey in a glass of water every day for a period of five weeks. The honey, which had antioxidant levels similar to those in apples, bananas, oranges, and strawberries, was shown to significantly improve blood antioxidant levels in all the subjects.

Earlier studies conducted by Dr. Nicki Engeseth, of the University of Illinois at Urbana-Champaign, Illinois, determined the antioxidant capacity of buckwheat, Hawaiian Christmas berry, tupelo, soybean, clover, fireweed, and acacia honeys. Using the test that is the gold standard for such research—the oxygen radical absorbance capacity (ORAC) assay—Engeseth found that the darkest-colored honeys, such as buckwheat honey, have the highest ORAC values, which are related to the amount of phenolic compounds they contain. The human trial, also led by Engeseth, showed that the higher a honey's ORAC activity, the better able it was to inhibit lipoprotein (cholesterol) oxidation. Engeseth's research suggests that honey could be used as a healthy alternative to sugar and serve as a source of dietary antioxidants in many products.

Energy-Enhancing Effects

Honey is an excellent source of readily available carbohydrate, a chief source of quick energy. In the time of the ancient Olympics, athletes were reported to eat special foods, such as honey and dried figs, to enhance their sports performance. Recently, one group of researchers investigated the use of honey as an performance aid in athletes. The study involved a group of thirty-nine weight-trained athletes, both male and female. Subjects underwent an intensive weight-lifting workout and then immediately consumed a protein supplement blended with sugar, maltodextrin, or honey as the carbohydrate source. The honey group maintained optimal blood sugar levels throughout the two hours following the workout. In addition, muscle recuperation and glycogen restoration (carbohydrates stored in muscle) was favorable in those individuals consuming the honey-protein combination.

Sustaining favorable blood sugar concentrations after endurance training by ingesting carbohydrates before, during, and after training is important for maintaining muscle glycogen stores (glycogen is the form in which sugar is stored in muscle as ready-to-use fuel), so that muscle recuperation is more efficient and the athlete is ready to perform again at his or her highest level the next day. So for now, honey appears to be a suitable source of carbohydrate that can help athletes perform at their best, but it does not appear to be a superior choice compared to other carbohydrates.

Wound-Healing Properties

The wound-healing properties of honey may be its most promising medicinal quality. Honey has been used topically as an antiseptic therapeutic agent for the treatment of ulcers, burns, and wounds for centuries. One study in India compared the wound-healing effects of honey to a conventional treatment (silver sulphadiazene) in 104 first-degree burn patients. After one week of treatment, 91 percent of honey-treated burns were infection-free compared with only 7 percent receiving the conventional treatment. At the conclusion of the study, a greater percentage of patients' burns were healed more readily in the honey-treated group. Another study examined the wound-healing benefits of honey applied topically to patients following cesarean section and hysterectomy surgeries. Compared to the group receiving the standard solution of iodine and alcohol, the honey-treated group was infection-free in fewer days, healed more cleanly, and had reduced hospital stays.

Several mechanisms have been proposed to explain the wound-healing benefits that are observed when honey is applied topically. Because honey is composed mainly of glucose and fructose, two sugars that strongly attract water, honey absorbs water in the wound, drying it out so that the growth of bacteria and fungi is inhibited. Secondly, raw honey contains an enzyme called glucose oxidase that, when combined with water, produces hydrogen peroxide, a mild antiseptic.

In addition to the glucose oxidase enzyme found in honey, which may help in the healing process, honey also contains antioxidants and flavonoids that may function as antibacterial agents. One antioxidant in particular, pinocembrin, which is unique to honey, is currently being studied for its antibacterial properties. One laboratory study of unpasteurized honey samples indicated the majority had antibacterial action against *Staphylococcus aureus,* a common bacterium found readily in our environment that can cause infections, especially in open wounds. Other reports indicate honey is effective at inhibiting *Escherichia coli* and *Candida albicans.* Darker honeys, specifically honey from buckwheat flowers, sage, and tupelo, contain a greater amount of antioxidants than other honeys, and raw, unprocessed honey contains the widest variety of health-supportive substances.

Anticancer Benefits

Propolis contains well-researched phytochemicals that have numerous cancer-preventing and antitumor properties. These substances include caffeic acid, methyl caffeate, phenylethyl caffeate, and phenylethyl dimethylcaffeate. Researchers have discovered that these substances prevent colon cancer in animals by shutting down the activity of two enzymes, phosphatidylinositol-specific phospholipase C and lipoxygenase, that are involved in the production of cancer-causing compounds.

HOW TO SELECT AND STORE

Honey is usually found pasteurized, although more health-conscious consumers can find the raw version as well (see "Health Benefits" above). Pasteurized honey is generally translucent; honeys that are "creamy" are usually produced by mixing crystallized honey into the liquid honey mixture. Darker honey is usually of a stronger flavor. Flavors also depend on the flower nectars from which the honey is produced, so it is fun to try honey made from various sources to experience the gustatory nuances in this delicious food.

High sugar and acid content helps this liquid

BEE POLLEN, PROPOLIS, AND ROYAL JELLY

While honey has some major health benefits, it is a source of significant amounts of simple sugars; if you are look-ing for the health benefits without so much sugar, it is best to choose another bee product. These products and their primary uses are:

Product	Effective for
Bee pollen	Allergies
	Antioxidant support
	Energy enhancement
	Menopausal symptoms
	Support for chemotherapy and radiation therapy
Propolis	Common cold
	Gastrointestinal infections
	Immune enhancement
	Topical anti-inflammatory
	Upper respiratory tract infections
Royal jelly	Elevated cholesterol levels
	Energy enhancement

Bee Pollen

Little research has been done on bee pollen—probably because there is little financial reward to justify such an in-vestment—but the research that does exist is impressive. For example, studies in animals show that bee pollen can promote growth and development, protect against free-radical and oxidative damage, and protect against the effects of harmful radiation as well as toxic exposure to chemical solvents.

Bee pollen extract has also been shown to produce significant improvement in menopausal symptoms, includ-ing headache, urinary incontinence, dry vagina, and decreasing vitality, in double-blind studies. The improvements were achieved even though the pollen extract produces no oestrogenic effect, an important consideration for women who cannot take oestrogens of any kind.

Propolis

Propolis has inherent antibiotic activity to help the hive block out viruses, bacteria, and other organisms. It seems these same effects can help humans block out organisms as well, since propolis has shown considerable antimi-crobial activity in test-tube studies. Propolis also stimulates the body's immune system, according to preliminary human studies. Test-tube and animal studies have shown that propolis exerts some antioxidant, liver-protecting, anti-inflammatory, and anticancer properties, too.

(continued on next page)

One of the key uses of propolis may turn out to be offering protection against and shortening the duration of the common cold. A preliminary human study reported that propolis extract reduced upper respiratory infections in children. In a double-blind study of fifty patients with the common cold, the group taking propolis extract became symptom-free far more quickly than the placebo group did.

Another possible application of propolis is in the treatment of inflammatory bowel diseases (IBDs), such as Crohn's disease and ulcerative colitis. In June 2001, Ralph Golan, M.D., the author of Optimal Wellness, *described an interesting case of ulcerative colitis that responded to propolis therapy in an article in the* Townsend Letter for Doctors. *Dr. Golan feels that the antimicrobial and anti-inflammatory properties of propolis are put to good use in the treatment of IBD.*

The antimicrobial properties of propolis may also help protect against parasitic infections in the gastrointestinal tract. One preliminary study of children and adults with giardiasis (a common intestinal parasite infection) showed a 52 percent rate of successful parasite elimination in children and a 60 percent rate in adults in those given propolis extract (amount not stated). However, these results are not as impressive as those achieved with conventional drugs used against giardiasis, so propolis should not be used alone for this condition without first consulting a physician about available medical treatment.

Royal Jelly

There has been reasonable scientific investigation of royal jelly's cholesterol-lowering effect. Specifically, ten human studies have been published, seven of which were double-blind. Of these seven double-blind studies, only three studies utilized an oral preparation. An injectable form was used in the other four. Results of a detailed analysis of the double-blind studies indicate that with oral preparations, despite shortcomings in the design of the studies and lack of standardization of the commercial preparations used, royal jelly can produce decreases in total cholesterol levels of about 14 percent in patients with moderate to severe elevations in blood cholesterol levels (initial values ranging from 210 to 325 milligrams per deciliter/5.4 to 8.4 mmol/l). Even better results may be noted when using higher-quality royal jelly products.

remain quite fresh for long periods of time. Honey does easily absorb moisture from air, and honey stored in an airtight container will keep practically indefinitely. Since cold promotes viscosity and changes honey's flavor and taste, it is best not to store honey in cold conditions.

Bee pollen, propolis, and royal jelly are most often available in the refrigerated sections in health food stores in opaque containers to maintain optimal freshness. Fresh royal jelly is more difficult to find in the U.K., but there are some suppliers on the Internet. These foods should be stored in the refrigerator. Bee pollen and propolis will keep for up to one year, while royal jelly will keep up to six months.

TIPS FOR PREPARING AND USING

Honey may crystallize, but you can easily remedy this by heating the jar in hot water for 15 to 20 minutes. Honey heated in the microwave might have an altered taste, as its hydroxymethylfurfural content can change through exposure to microwave radiation. Honey can replace sugar, where ½ to ¾ cup of honey is equivalent to one cup of sugar. Honey is a bit sweeter, so you can use less. In addition, since honey adds liquid content to your recipe, remember to decrease the liquid by a quarter cup for each cup of honey used. Finally, since honey browns well, reducing baking temperature by 25 degrees F./4 degrees C. will avoid overbrowning.

QUICK SERVING IDEAS

- Honey is a fine replacement for white cane sugar as a sweetener in your coffee or tea.
- A healthy light snack is to slice an apple, drizzle it with honey, and sprinkle it with ½ teaspoon of cinnamon.
- Buy plain yogurt and add honey for a natural sweetener that is not too sugary.
- Children of all ages have always enjoyed sandwich bread with a combination of peanut or almond butter, plus bananas and honey.
- In a saucepan over low heat, combine 2 cups soy milk, 2 tablespoons honey, and 2 tablespoons unsweetened cocoa to make a deliciously nutritious hot cocoa.
- Enjoy the pleasure of homemade honey-roasted nuts. Drizzle a little honey onto nuts, such as almonds and walnuts, and roast in a low-temperature oven until hot.
- To give baked sweet potatoes even more of a sweet taste, pour a little bit of honey on top.
- Add a nutritious punch to your protein smoothie by adding 1 teaspoon or more bee pollen or royal jelly.

SAFETY

Because honey can contain spores of *Clostridium botulinum*—the causative agent of botulism, an infection in infants—children less than twelve months old should not be fed honey. Due to their more mature digestive tract, honey is safe for children one year of age and older.

Allergic reaction is the most common side effect from bee products. If you know you are allergic to honey, bee pollen, or conifer and poplar trees, do not use bee products. Allergic reactions can range from very mild, such as mild gastrointestinal upset, to more severe reactions, including asthma, anaphylaxis (shock), intestinal bleeding, and even death in people who are extremely allergic to bee products.

Honey contains small amounts of oxalates. Individuals with a history of calcium oxalate-containing kidney stones should limit their consumption of this food. See page 793 for more information.

Maple Syrup

Maple syrup is derived from various maple trees, such as the sugar maple *(Acer saccharum),* red maple *(Acer rubrum),* or black maple *(Acer nigrum).* In the process of making maple syrup, the bark of the maple is tapped, allowing the syrup to flow out. This nearly clear, almost tasteless liquid is subsequently boiled, which concentrates the sugar and creates the flavor and often deep color of the syrup.

HISTORY

The Native Americans of North America were likely the discovers of maple syrup. These indigenous people used it as a medicine as well as a food. Using tomahawks, they made short incisions and employed birch bark to help corral and collect the flow. The heating process necessary was accomplished by placing hot stones in the sap, or by allowing the nighttime to freeze the sap and then removing the frozen water layer when the sun came back up the next morning. The early American colonists were fascinated by this process and quickly came to appreciate the wonderful taste of maple syrup. The colonists employed iron bits and boiling in metal kettles to update the process the natives had begun.

Although maple syrup was an important sweetener in early colonial times, extravagant tariffs gave sugar from the West Indies an economic edge, and as a result maple syrup was less desired. Today, maple syrup production is only 20 percent of what it was in the early 1900s. Trees that produce true maple syrup are located only in certain North American areas. Thus the largest producer of maple syrup in the world is Quebec, Canada. Other main producers include the state of Vermont and New York State.

NUTRITIONAL HIGHLIGHTS

Maple syrup is a very good source of the trace mineral manganese. It is also a good source of zinc. A 100 gram serving provides 261 calories, mostly as the 67.1 grams of carbohydrate. It contains 59.5 grams of sugar, mostly glucose. There is no protein and only 0.2 gram of fat. A tablespoon (15 grams) provides 52 calories, 13.4 grams of carbohydrate, 11.9 grams of sugar, no protein, and 0.04 grams of fat.

HEALTH BENEFITS

Maple syrup is a very good source of manganese, an essential cofactor in a number of enzymes important in energy production and antioxidant defenses. For example, the key oxidative enzyme superoxide dismutase, which disarms free radicals produced within the mitochondria (the energy production factories within our cells), requires manganese. One ounce/30 grams (2 tablespoons) of maple syrup supplies 37.7 percent of the daily value of this very important trace mineral. Maple syrup also has a good supply of zinc, which can help decrease progression of atherosclerosis, help with skin problems such as acne, support a healthy prostate, and keep the immune system healthier.

HOW TO SELECT AND STORE

Maple syrup can be purchased in small individual containers or in bulk. Syrup quality varies by color, taste, and consistency. Maple syrup is labeled with a grade based upon an official U.S. Department of Agriculture (USDA) grading system with three basic types of Grade A, including Light Amber, Medium Amber, and Dark Amber. A lighter color indicates a more subtle flavor and thinner texture. Maple syrup is also available in a Grade B version, which has a stronger taste. Grade B is typically reserved for cooking and use in processed foods. Canadian maple syrup has different designations for these grades: AA No 1 Extra Light (Light Amber); A No 1 Light (Medium Amber); B No 1 Medium (Dark Amber); C No 2 Amber and D No 3 Dark (B grades). Pure maple syrup is distinguished in its labeling from maple-flavored syrups. Many commercial-brand syrups contain little or no actual maple syrup. Although pure maple syrup is generally more expensive, its unique, rich flavor makes it well worth the price differential.

You can store maple syrup in a cool, dry, and dark place providing it is unopened. Once opened, the maple syrup should be kept in the refrigerator, where it will keep for three to six months. Maple syrup can be stored in the freezer, where it can keep for one year. If you see mould in the syrup or on the surface, it is time to dispose of it.

TIPS FOR PREPARING

Maple syrup, used in place of table sugar as a sweetener, gives tea and coffee a richer flavor and aroma.

QUICK SERVING IDEAS

- Pour some maple syrup on oatmeal, and top with cinnamon, cardamom, walnuts, and raisins.
- Spoon some plain yogurt on pound cake and drizzle maple syrup on top.
- Maple syrup and cinnamon topping are an excellent addition to puréed, cooked sweet potatoes.
- Combine ¼ cup maple syrup with ½ cup orange juice and ¼ cup tamari, and marinate 1 pound/½ kilogram tofu or tempeh cut into ½-inch/1-centimeter slices for 2 hours or overnight. Bake at 325 degrees F./170 degrees C./gas 3 for 30 to 40 minutes.
- Spread almond or peanut butter on a piece of sprouted whole-wheat toast, and top with sliced bananas. Finally, drizzle maple syrup on top for a sweet, sticky treat.

SAFETY

No safety concerns are associated with maple syrup. Maple syrup is not a common allergenic food and does not contain goitrogens or purines. Since maple syrup contains small amounts of oxalates, which can bind to calcium in the urinary tract to form kidney stones, it should be limited or avoided by individuals prone to kidney stones.

Maple syrup is usually tapped from wild trees. However, only organically certified maple syrup is guaranteed to be free of agricultural chemicals.

Mushrooms (Button)

Button mushrooms generally look like tiny umbrellas, having a dense parasol-like cap attached to a stem that can be short and thick or thin and slightly curvy. There are three different types of button mushrooms—white mushrooms, crimini (brown button) mushrooms, and portobello (brown open) mushrooms—all of which share the same scientific name, *Agaricus bisporus*. The white mushroom, the most common type, is the cream-colored mushroom that often adorns salads and is usually one to three inches/2½ to 7½ centimeters across. It has a mild earthy flavor with a meaty texture. The crimini mushroom, which looks just like the button but is coffee-colored, features a more distinctive and stronger flavor. The portobello mushroom, whose large size, up to 8 inches/20 centimeters across, and meaty flavor make it a wonderful vegetarian entrée, is actually an overgrown crimini mushroom.

Button mushrooms are grown on straw-based compost in a controlled environment that is kept warm, moist, and dark, as well as free of other fungi that may parasitize the mushrooms.

HISTORY

Eaten by the earliest hunter-gatherers, button mushrooms have been a healthy food source since the prehistoric era. Ancient Egyptians believed mushrooms to possess keys to immortality, and thus decrees were imposed allowing only the pharaohs access to these. A common person was not allowed to eat or touch this prized fungus. Ancient Romans sometimes called the mushroom a food of the gods, or *cibus diorum.* Following these times, common thought in many nations throughout the world hailed mushrooms as conferring superhuman power. In the 1600s, mushrooms began to be actively cultivated near the Paris city limits. Even today, miles of underground Parisian tunnels and caves host dark, moist areas in which delectable French mushrooms are grown. Button mushroom cultivation in the United States commenced in the late 1800s. Today, people in many countries enjoy and cultivate button mushrooms. In the Northern Hemisphere, the state of Pennsylvania is now a leader in producing these fungi.

NUTRITIONAL HIGHLIGHTS

White button mushrooms are an excellent source of many minerals, including selenium, copper, potassium, and zinc, and phytochemicals. They are also an excellent source of B vitamins, including thiamine, riboflavin, pantothenic acid, and niacin. In addition to possessing all of the nutritional highlights of white button mushrooms, Crimini mushrooms and portobellos are very good sources of vitamins B6 and B12.

A 100 gram serving of button mushrooms provides 22 calories, 3.1 grams of protein, 0.3 grams of fat, and 3.2 grams of carbohydrate with 1.2 grams of fiber and no cholesterol.

HEALTH BENEFITS

For the past thirty or more years, phytochemicals found in mushrooms have been the object of anticancer research. Most of this research has centered on their polysaccharide and beta-glucan components. While most of this research has focused on shiitake, maitake, and reishi mushrooms, even the three common mushrooms have been shown to contain polysaccharide and beta-glucan components and anticancer properties. For more information on the anticancer aspects of mushroom phytochemicals, see the discussion under "Maitake" on page 665.

HOW TO SELECT AND STORE

With both fresh and dried button mushrooms available throughout the year, try to buy fresh mushrooms when you find them to be firm, plump, and clean. Avoid mushrooms that are wet, slimy, or wrinkled. Darkening is a sign of a mushroom's age, so choose those mushrooms that are lightest in color. In general, fresh button mushrooms should be white, while the crimini and portobello can be tan. Storage of mushrooms is best when they are placed in a loosely closed paper bag. If you are concerned with them drying prematurely, you can wrap them in a slightly damp cloth or place on a glass dish and then cover with a moistened cloth. These methods will help retain freshness for several days. Prepacked mushrooms can be stored in the refrigerator for up to one week in their original container. If you choose dried mushrooms, these should be stored in a tightly sealed container in either the refrigerator or freezer. This way they can stay fresh for six months to one year. Cooked mushrooms can be refrigerated for three to four days.

TIPS FOR PREPARING

Mushrooms are best cleaned using very little or no water. A damp cloth, damp paper towel, or mushroom brush is best to avoid the mushroom's tendency of soaking in water, which will result in a soggy dish. Sometimes fresh mushrooms get dry if left out too long. In this case, a soak in water for 30 minutes should return them to their more fresh selves. Dried packaged mushrooms often have instructions for preparation. Generally, smaller pieces can be rehydrated by soaking, covered, in hot water or stock for 30 minutes. If the dried mushrooms are used in a baked dish that contains a fair amount of cooking liquid, the mushrooms can often be mixed right into the dish. If your recipe calls for whole mushrooms, slice and discard about ¼ to ½ inch/½ to 1 centimeter of the often spongy bottom of the stem. To prepare a caps-only dish, gently break the stem off with your fingers. You can save the stems for a soup or use them diced in a stuffing side dish.

QUICK SERVING IDEAS

- Sautéed mushrooms and onions are fine additions to a red tomato sauce and make a great side dish to meat dishes.
- Skewer a few mushrooms with some vegetables, then coat lightly with olive oil and grill for approximately 10 minutes.

- After removing the stems from mushrooms, stuff them with diced vegetables, bread crumbs, and soft cheese.

SAFETY

See page 667 for more information.

Mushrooms (Shiitake, Maitake, and Reishi)

Although numerous types of mushrooms provide wonderful tastes, textures, and healthful properties, these three mushroom superstars have been recently receiving widespread attention due to their health benefits and, as a result, are increasingly available:

- Shiitake *(Lentinus edodes):* These have fleshy, brown, slightly convex caps that range in diameter from about 2 to 4 inches/5 to 10 centimeters. Shiitakes are cultivated on logs in the United States and in many East Asian countries for their meaty, robust flavor and texture.

- Maitake *(Grifola frondosa):* Cultivated on tree stumps, these mushrooms grow in a formation of clustered brownish 1-to-2-inch/2½-to-5-centimeter fronds forming a fan shape. Commonly known as "Hen of the Woods," maitakes have a mild, slightly aromatic flavor.

- Reishi *(Ganoderma lucidum):* These usually have an antler or rounded fan shape, with the most popular type of reishi being red in color, although that is just one of the six colors in which they grow. These mushrooms are cultivated on dead trees and are very woody. Therefore, they generally are not eaten but cooked and removed from dishes.

HISTORY

Shiitake, reishi, and maitake mushrooms have been objects of gathering and eating since prehistoric times. Prized in Asia for their therapeutic value, they have played an essential role in Asian medicinal traditions and are noted in some of the early botanical medicine texts written thousands of years ago. In addition to China, Japan, Korea, and Taiwan, these mushrooms are produced in a number of other countries, including the United States. As the scientific evidence mounts regarding the health benefits of these fungi, they are becoming more and more popular as a food in the United States and other countries.

NUTRITIONAL HIGHLIGHTS

Shiitake, maitake, and reishi mushrooms are typically excellent sources of selenium and polysaccharides and very good sources of iron. They are also good sources of protein, dietary fiber, and vitamin C.

HEALTH BENEFITS

Although the chemical profiles of all three mushrooms are quite complex, the health benefits of these mushrooms are due primarily to their polysaccharide components, such as lentinan (from shiitake) and beta-glucans (from maitake).

Shiitake

The shiitake mushroom is a symbol of longevity in Asia because of its health-promoting properties, and has been used medicinally by the Chinese for more than 6,000 years. Recent studies have traced shiitakes' legendary benefits to an active compound contained in these mush-

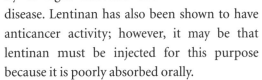

rooms called lentinan. Among lentinan's healing benefits is an ability to power up the immune system, strengthening its ability to fight infection and disease. Lentinan has also been shown to have anticancer activity; however, it may be that lentinan must be injected for this purpose because it is poorly absorbed orally.

The shiitake mushroom has also been shown to lower cholesterol levels. In this action, a compound known as eritadenine is responsible.

Maitake

The maitake mushroom has also been used as a food to help promote wellness and vitality. Recent scientific research has focused on its immune-enhancing and anticancer properties. Modern research on maitake began in the late 1970s in Japan under the direction of Dr. Hiroaki Nanba, who was researching the immune-enhancing properties of mushrooms when he came to the conclusion that maitake extracts demonstrated more pronounced anti-tumor activity in animal tests than other mushroom extracts. Dr. Nanba also found that maitake extracts were quite effective when given orally. In contrast, the other mushrooms Dr. Nanba was studying, such as shiitake, were effective only when injected into the bloodstream.

The primary compounds responsible for maitake's immune-enhancing effects are beta-D-glucans. Numerous experimental studies in test tubes and animals have shown the beta-glucan fraction of maitake activates white blood cells. The beta-glucan components of maitake actually bind to receptors on the outer membranes of macrophages and other white blood cells, including natural killer (NK) cells and cytotoxic T cells. These immune cells are very important in protecting against and fighting cancer because they can attack tumor cells directly.

Just like a key in a lock, the binding of the maitake components literally flips white blood cells on and triggers a chain reaction leading to increased immune activity. In addition to increasing the ability of the macrophages to engulf and destroy cancer cells, microbes, and other foreign cells, the binding stimulates the production of important signaling proteins of the immune system, such as interleukin-1, interleukin-2, and lymphokines. These immune activators ramp up defenses by activating immune cells.

Maitake beta-glucans also stimulate the production of white blood cells within the bone marrow—the major area for white blood cell production. Reduced bone marrow production means lowered white cell counts and an increased risk of infection and cancer. This beneficial effect of the beta-glucan is put to good use in cancer patients undergoing radiation therapy or chemotherapy. Maitake researchers have identified four primary mechanisms by which maitake fights cancer:

- It protects healthy cells from becoming cancerous.
- It enhances the immune system's ability to seek out and destroy cancer cells.
- It helps cancer cells regain control of cell division and programmed cell death (apoptosis).

- It helps prevent the spreading (metastasis) of cancer.

Maitake beta-glucan fractions are perfectly suited as an addition to conventional cancer therapies. In addition to exerting some direct benefits of its own, maitake helps reduce the side effects of conventional chemotherapy and radiation, such as nausea, weight loss, fatigue, and immune suppression, while at the same time enhancing the effectiveness of these treatments.

Reishi

Reishi is the premier longevity herb in classical Chinese medicine and is the medicinal mushroom/herb most often used as a general health tonic. Preliminary clinical studies have shown it to be helpful in boosting the immune system and in the treatment of viral infections, including hepatitis B. Unlike shiitake and maitake, the beneficial effects of reishi appear to be primarily due to its triterpene fraction rather than its polysaccharides.

HOW TO SELECT AND STORE

Shiitake mushrooms are typically more commonly found than reishi or maitake. If your supermarket does not carry these, look for the nearest Asian food shop and try to find them there. With both fresh and dried mushrooms available throughout the year, try to buy fresh mushrooms when you find them firm, plump, and clean. Avoid mushrooms that are wet, slimy, or wrinkled. Reishi mushrooms are usually available in the dried form and may hold a brown to dark reddish orange, waxlike top with firm gills underneath. When dried, maitakes have thin brown strands with a uniform color. Look for fresh shiitakes with a light brownish gray top with splits in the surface. These should have a single color.

Fresh shiitakes and maitakes are best stored loosely in a paper bag kept in the refrigerator, where they can remain for about one week. Dried mushrooms can be kept in airtight containers, and refrigerated or frozen will keep for six months to one year. Cooked mushrooms will last three or four days. Reishi mushrooms decocted or used to make stocks are usually discarded after cooking.

TIPS FOR PREPARING
See page 664.

QUICK SERVING IDEAS
- Shiitake mushrooms are traditionally added to miso soup.
- A healthy sautéed side dish starts with sautéing garlic in extra-virgin olive oil; add sliced mushrooms, quickly sauté, and remove from heat.
- When preparing hamburgers or lamb burgers, mix lightly sautéed mushrooms in with the minced meat before cooking.
- To give vegetable stock an extra depth, add specialty mushrooms such as shiitake or reishi.
- For a quick and easy pasta dish, lightly sauté shiitake mushrooms with blanched sugar-snap peas and tofu. Season to taste and serve over buckwheat soba noodles (or your favorite type of pasta).

SAFETY
These mushrooms have an excellent record of safety but have been known to induce temporary diarrhea and abdominal bloating when used in high dosages (above 15 to 20 grams per day).

Allergic reactions, mainly skin rashes, have also been reported.

Mushrooms are a significant source of purines. Since purines can be broken down to form uric acid, excess accumulation of purines in the body can lead to excess accumulation of uric acid. Gout and the formation of kidney stones from uric acid are two examples of uric acid-related problems that can be caused by excessive intake of purine-containing foods. For this reason, individuals with kidney problems or gout should avoid or limit their intake of mushrooms.

Mushrooms, particularly button mushrooms, may be treated with various chemicals while grown to prevent contamination with bacteria or other fungi. Choose organically grown varieties when possible.

Mushrooms contain moderate amounts of oxalates. Individuals with a history of calcium oxalate-containing kidney stones should limit their consumption of this food. See page 793 for more information.

Sea Vegetables

Sea vegetables, often called seaweed, enhance our diets, from both a culinary and nutritional perspective. Generally found on coral reefs or rocky areas, sea vegetables grow in marine salt waters and some freshwater lakes and seas. Interestingly, it is not well known that sea vegetables are neither plants nor animals—they are

TABLE 19.2

Nutritional Content of Various Seaweeds per 100 gram serving

	Calories	Protein	Fat	Carbohydrate as Fiber	Calcium (milligrams)
Arame	20–60, depending on protein content	5–15 percent dry weight for brown seaweeds	1–5 percent dry weight*	30–35 percent dry weight for soluble, 4.5–5.5 percent dry weight for insoluble	1,000
Wakame					1,300
Kelp					1,093
Kombu					800
Hijiki					1,400
Dulse	80–120, depending on protein content	20–30 percent dry weight for red seaweeds	1–5 percent dry weight†	17.9 percent dry weight for soluble, 6.8 percent dry weight for insoluble	296
Nori					1,000

* Contains some omega-3 fatty acids as alpha-linolenic acid.

† Contains some omega-3 fatty acids as EPA and DHA.

actually a form of alga. As green algae, they do need exposure to sunlight for growth.

Sea vegetables are broadly grouped into three main types: brown, red, and green. However, scores of sea vegetables exist, and each is unique, having a distinct shape, taste, and texture. While many types are not ingested, the following are some of the most popular edible types:

Brown Seaweeds

• Arame *(Eisenia arborea)* is a lacy, wiry sea vegetable that is sweeter and milder in taste than many others.

• Hijiki *(Hizikia fusiformis)* has a green to brown color when found in the wild. After it is collected, it is boiled and dried, making it look like small strands of black wiry pasta. It has a strong flavor.

• Kelp *(Laminaria* spp.) is light brown to dark green in color and is often available in flake form.

• Kombu *(Laminaria japonica)* is a specific species of kelp that is very dark in color and generally sold in strips or sheets. It is often used as a flavoring for soups and beans.

• Wakame *(Undaria pinnatifida)* is similar to kombu and is most commonly used to make Japanese miso soup.

Red Seaweeds

• Nori is a Japanese term used to refer to edible varieties of seaweed in the various species of the red alga *Porphyra,* including most notably *P. yezoensis* and *P. tenera.* Nori also refers to food products created from sea vegetables. Finished products are made by a shredding and rack-drying process that resembles paper making. The dried sheets are dark purple-black in color and turn phosphorescent green when toasted. Nori is famous for its use in making sushi rolls.

- Dulse *(Palmaria palmata)* has a soft, chewy texture and a reddish brown color. It is available as large dried pieces or ground into flakes that can be sprinkled on food.

HISTORY

Studies indicate that sea vegetables have been eaten since at least 8000 B.C.E. by cultures in the Japanese region. The ancient Chinese considered the sea vegetable a delicacy to be given to guests of honor and royalty. Outside Asia, many nations and cultures surrounded by water have learned about and taken advantage of sea vegetables. Probably the most famous example of this in the British Isles is the Welsh delicacy laver bread.

Kombu has historically been the most-consumed seaweed in Japan. The earliest written record of kombu appeared in 797 B.C.E. as being a gift and tax from the Tohoku region of Japan. A way to cultivate kombu was not discovered until the early 1900s, after which it became cheap and readily available everywhere. Presently, Japan is the largest producer and exporter of sea vegetables. This may explain why many of these precious foods are called by their Japanese names.

NUTRITIONAL HIGHLIGHTS

Sea vegetables offer the broadest range of minerals of any food, containing virtually all the minerals found in the ocean—the same minerals that are found in human blood. Sea vegetables are an excellent source of calcium,

iodine (up to 1,500 to 8,000 parts per million dry weight for brown seaweeds), and sodium, a very good source of folic acid and magnesium, and a good source of iron, potassium, riboflavin, and pantothenic acid. In addition, sea vegetables contain good amounts of lignans, plant compounds with cancer-protective properties, and fucans, which can reduce the body's inflammatory response.

HEALTH BENEFITS

A rich iodine source, sea vegetables can play a role in supporting thyroid function, as iodine is a needed precursor to make thyroid hormones. These sea plants may also help prevent cancer via inhibiting the growth of vessels that feed tumor cells and via their lignans, which can block the hormonal signaling of oestrogen-dependent cancers. Fucan substances in these plants can decrease inflammation processes in the body. Therapeutic levels of folic acid and magnesium also retain excellent protection for the heart and cardiovascular system, while magnesium and the lignans can be an excellent help to women experiencing menopausal symptoms. Finally, pantothenic acid and riboflavin are B vitamins very useful to help someone who has too much stress and anxiety, both of which may deplete these nutrients.

HOW TO SELECT AND STORE

The freshest sea vegetables are sold in airtight packaging. As they are sold in a number of forms (sheets, flakes, and powders), you can choose which form will work for your recipes for a particular meal. A tightly closed container can keep them fresh for several months. Dried sea vegetables do not require refrigeration or freezing and, once cooked, have a refrigerated life of three to four days.

TIPS FOR PREPARING

Sea vegetables come in their dried form and rehydrate into long pieces four to five times their dried sizes. Large, dried pieces can be cut into strips prior to cooking. Sea vegetables can also be rehydrated by soaking in cool water for 30 minutes or until soft and either cooked or used raw.

QUICK SERVING IDEAS

- Nori sheets are the type to use to wrap your own sushi. Vegetarian rolls can be made using sliced avocado, thinly sliced cucumber, and daikon radish. But virtually any vegetable you like can be incorporated.
- Sliced nori or kelp and dulse flakes make a good mineralized sprinkle for any salad or seasoning for foods.
- Sea vegetables can be ground into powder and used in place of salt.
- Combine ¼ cup soaked hijiki, 1 cup soaked arame, 1 cup shredded carrots, and 1 tablespoon ginger with 2 tablespoons olive oil, 1 teaspoon toasted sesame oil, 2 tablespoons tamari, and 2 teaspoons rice vinegar.
- When cooking beans, put 3 to 6 inches/7½ to 15 centimeters of dried kombu in the cooking water for each cup of dried beans. It will not only expedite the cooking process but will improve the beans' digestibility by reducing the chemicals that can cause flatulence.
- Add 2 tablespoons soaked sea vegetables to your next bowl of miso soup.

SAFETY

The Food Standards Agency in the U.K. advises people not to eat a type of seaweed called hijiki because they have found high levels of arsenic in some samples. Hijiki is also sold for use in soups and salads and some vegetarian and vegan dishes where seaweed is an ingredient. Other seaweeds tested (e.g., arame, kombu, nori and wakame) did not contain arsenic.

Tea

Both green and black tea are derived from the same plant, *Camellia sinensis,* a 3-foot/1-meter shrub that is shade grown, producing leaves that are 1 to 5 centimeters long. Four times as much black tea is produced and consumed as green tea each year, but green tea is healthier for you because it contains compounds called polyphenols that have high levels of therapeutic activity, including anticancer activity.

The difference between green and black teas results from the manufacturing process. To produce black tea, the leaves are allowed to oxidize. During oxidation, enzymes present in the tea convert polyphenols into substances with much less biological activity. In contrast, green tea is produced by lightly steaming the fresh-cut leaf. Steaming prevents the enzymes from converting polyphenols, so oxidation does not take place and the polyphenols remain intact. Oolong tea is partially oxidized.

White tea is still green tea, but the new, unopened buds are picked and steamed or dried. The resulting tea is pale yellow and low in caffeine and tastes mild and slightly sweeter than green tea.

HISTORY

The use of tea as a beverage is nearly 5,000 years old. Legend has it that it was discovered in 2737 B.C.E. by a Chinese emperor when some tea leaves accidentally blew into a pot of boiling water. From that time, tea consumption spread throughout the Chinese culture, reaching into every corner of the society.

The first tea seeds were brought to Japan by the Buddhist priest Yeisei (1215–1141 B.C.E.), who had seen the value of tea in China in enhancing religious meditation. Tea was elevated to an art form in Japan, resulting in the creation of the Japanese tea ceremony and tea houses.

As European explorers began to visit the Orient, information concerning tea began to filter back to Europe. The first European to write firsthand information about tea was the Portuguese Jesuit father Jasper de Cruz, in 1560. Subsequently, the Portuguese developed a trade route by which they shipped their tea to Lisbon and then Dutch ships transported it to France, Holland, and the Baltic countries.

Great Britain was the last of the three great seafaring nations to break into the Chinese and East Indian trade routes. The first samples of tea reached England between 1652 and 1654. Tea proved popular enough to replace ale as the national drink. It took some time, but eventually tea mania swept across England as it had earlier spread throughout France and Holland. Tea importation rose from 40,000 pounds/ 18,000 kilograms in 1699 to an annual average of 240,000 pounds/110,000 kilograms by 1708. Tea was drunk at all levels of society.

English and Dutch colonists brought tea to North America in the 1600s. It was especially a favorite of colonial women, a factor Britain was to base a major political decision on later. The tea trade was centered in Boston, New York, and Philadelphia, future centers of American rebellion. As tea was heavily taxed, even at this early date, contraband tea was smuggled into the colonies by independent-minded American merchants from ports far away, and herbal teas were adopted from the Indians.

Tea was at the center of the American Revolution. In the 1760s, Britain had imposed on colonists in America a higher tax on newspapers (which it considered far too outspoken in the colonies), tavern licenses (too much free speech there), legal documents, marriage licenses, and docking papers. The colonists rebelled against taxes imposed upon them without their consent and that were so repressive. The initial rebellion, however, led to even heavier taxes levied by Parliament in retaliation. Among these heavier taxes was, in June 1767, the tea tax, which would become the watershed of America's desire for freedom.

The colonists rebelled and openly purchased other imported tea, largely Dutch in origin. In further retaliation, Britain granted British tea companies the right to bypass colonial merchants and sell tea directly to the colonists. In plotting this strategy, Britain was counting on the well-known passion among American women for tea. It was a major miscalculation. Throughout the colonies, women pledged publicly at meetings and in newspapers not to drink British-sold tea until their rights (and those of their merchant husbands) were restored.

By December 16, 1773, events had deteriorated enough that the men of Boston, dressed as Indians (the original justification of Britain for increased taxation had been the expense of the

French and Indian War), threw hundreds of pounds of tea into the harbor. This became known as the Boston Tea Party. Such leading citizens as Samuel Adams and John Hancock took part. Britain had had enough. In retaliation, the port of Boston was closed and the city occupied by royal troops. The colonial leaders met, and independence from Britain was declared.

America began direct trade with China soon after the Revolution was over in 1789, and throughout the 1800s, the British experimented with growing tea outside of China. Many of these experiments failed due to bad soil selection and incorrect planting techniques. Through each failure, however, the technology was perfected. Finally, after years of trial and error and fortunes made and lost, the British tea plantations in India and other parts of Asia flourished. The great British tea marketing companies were founded and production was mechanized as the world industrialized in the late 1880s.

One of the greatest inventions in tea history occurred in 1904, at the Saint Louis World's Fair. Exhibitors from around the world brought their products to America's first World's Fair. One such merchant was Richard Blechynden, a tea plantation owner. Originally, he had planned to give away free samples of hot tea to fair visitors. But when a heat wave hit, no one was interested. To save his investment of time and travel, he dumped a load of ice into the brewed tea and served the first "iced tea." It was the hit of the fair.

Four years later, Thomas Sullivan, a tea merchant of New York, developed the concept of "bagged tea." He carefully wrapped each sample delivered to restaurants for their consideration. He recognized a natural marketing opportunity when he realized that the restaurants were brewing the samples in the bags to avoid the mess of tea leaves in the kitchens. Thus the tea bag was born.

Tea is produced primarily in East Asia, with China, India, and Japan being the world's leading producers. Other producers include Sri Lanka, Taiwan, Kenya, and Vietnam.

NUTRITIONAL HIGHLIGHTS

Both green and black tea contain relatively high amounts of vitamins C, D, and K and riboflavin, as well as good amounts of the minerals calcium, magnesium, iron, zinc, sodium, nickel, and fluoride. However, it is the polyphenols of green tea that are responsible for its health benefits.

A six-ounce/170-milliliter cup of tea contains only 1 calorie as carbohydrate, with no protein or fat.

HEALTH BENEFITS

Green tea provides significantly more health benefits than black tea due to its higher content of free polyphenols. The major polyphenols in green tea are flavonoids, the most active of which is epigallocatechin gallate. In addition to serving as antioxidants, green tea polyphenols may increase the activity of antioxidant enzymes in the small intestine, liver, and lungs. A number of experiments conducted in test-tube and animal cancer models have shown that green tea polyphenols inhibit cancer by blocking the formation of cancer-causing compounds, such as nitrosamines, suppressing the activation of carcinogens, and detoxifying or trapping cancer-causing agents. The forms of cancer that appear to be best prevented by green tea are cancers of the gastrointestinal tract, including cancers of the stomach, small intestine, pancreas, and colon; lung cancer; oestrogen-related cancers, including most breast cancers; and prostate cancer. Although important in fighting all of these cancers, green tea is especially important in preventing breast and prostate cancer.

In contrast to green tea's protective effects, population studies seem to indicate that black tea consumption may increase the risk of certain cancers, including cancer of the rectum, gallbladder, and endometrium.

HOW TO SELECT AND STORE

More than 150 cultivars, or types, of *Camellia sinensis* appear in the commercial marketplace. Not surprisingly, there are many different grades of tea, which are determined by the quality of the leaf: whole leaves are the highest grade, followed by broken or small leaf tea comprised of smaller or slightly torn leaves. Fannings are smaller leaf fragments; next in quality comes tea dust, the leftovers of processing. Tea grading is not universal, with the same tea potentially getting different grades in different countries.

Most consumers in the United States and the U.K. purchase tea in the form of either loose tea or tea bags.

As previously stressed, green tea is more beneficial than black tea. There are seven main forms of green tea:

- *Sencha* is the most popular of Japan's green teas. There are numerous grades of sencha, which vary drastically in both price and quality. Sencha is grown on open plantations, and, after plucking, the leaves are first steamed and then shaped. It is the steaming that makes the leaves more pliable for twist-ing and shaping. Twisting and shaping are done both by hand and machine. Premier teas are usually shaped by hand, and lower-grade teas are machine rolled and shaped. After being dried, the leaves are sorted according to size and shape, and then finishing tools remove any remaining stalks and debris. Sencha produces a clear yellowish green liquor with a sweet, grassy, but slightly astringent flavor. Lesser-quality sencha tea is called bancha.

- *Dragon well (Long Jing)* is considered the ultimate green tea from China. The name comes from a legendary well in the West Lake region of China where the tea is produced. The color is bright green, and the flavor is quite brisk. Be prepared to pay more than usual for this quality tea.

- *Macha* is the kind of tea used in traditional Japanese tea ceremonies. It's ground up very fine, and the tea is whisked when prepared. The flavor is light and sweet. Macha works well added to desserts, too.

- *Young hyson* contains the smallest leaves picked in the spring before the monsoon rains begin. The name means "bright spring." The leaves are dried without bruising or fermenting and retain their bright green color. When properly brewed, young hyson has a yellow-gold color and a light, grassy flavor.

- *Hyson* contains the larger leaves picked in the spring before the monsoon rains. When brewed properly, this tea has a more full-bodied flavor and slightly darker color than young hyson. Higher in caffeine than young hyson, it is excellent in the morning and for afternoon tea.

- *Pinhead gunpowder (Zhucha)* is picked in the early spring before the monsoons. The smaller leaves are rolled between the fingers of the picker before being dropped into the basket. It is dried before it begins to ferment. A light gold color when brewed properly, it has a light, airy flavor with a slightly "minty" aftertaste.

- *Gunpowder* is sometimes called "temple of Heaven." These spring leaves are harvested before the monsoons. The larger leaves are most commonly used. The hearty, full-bodied flavor of this tea is its source of fame. It is best in the morning or afternoon as an invigorator.

We encourage you to sample a variety of brands and types of green tea before settling on the types you like best. But while selecting tea is important, more important is how you store it. Tea will degrade if exposed to heat, moisture, or light, so it is important to store it properly. While properly sealed and stored tea can maintain its quality for up to one year, we encourage using it up much sooner. To preserve tea, always place loose tea in a bottle or canister with a tight seal and in a cupboard away from light, heat, and moisture. Also consider transferring tea bags contained in flimsy cardboard boxes and wrapped in paper to canisters or plastic bags.

TIPS FOR PREPARING

While the brewing and drinking of tea is an art and all over the world there are tea ceremonies celebrated with reverence, in the United States and the U.K., most consumers simply steep their tea bags in hot water for an unspecified time. Nonetheless, the following are guidelines for brewing a proper pot of tea:

- Rinse an empty teapot.
- Fill the teapot with freshly drawn hot tap water. If the quality of your tap water is poor, try using filtered or bottled spring water.
- For green tea, the water should be heated to just below boiling. For all other teas, bring the water to a boil.
- To draw out the best flavor of the tea, the water must contain oxygen, which is reduced if the water is left boiling too long or is boiled more than once.
- Empty the hot water from your teapot and add 2¼ grams, or one rounded teaspoon, of tea leaves, or one tea bag, for each cup (5.5 ounces/160 milliliters) of water.
- Or, for maximum flavor, place the tea directly into the bottom of the pot or use a basket infuser. (Tea balls, while convenient, often yield poorer-tasting tea as they are often too small to allow all of the leaves to fully unravel. If you do use a tea ball, be sure to use one that is sufficiently large.) Pour the freshly boiled water over the leaves in the teapot.
- Steep the tea for 3 to 5 minutes. Tea will become bitter if brewed for longer than 5 to 6 minutes.
- When brewing tea, time with a timer, not with your eyes. It is a common mistake to brew the tea until it looks a particular color or shade. The color of tea is a poor indicator of its taste.
- Serve the tea. If you used a tea bag, basket infuser, or tea ball, remove it promptly when the brewing time has expired. If you placed

TABLE 19.3
Caffeine Content of Tea and
Other Caffeinated Beverages

Espresso (2 ounces/60 milliliters)	60–90 milligrams
Drip coffee (6 ounces/170 milliliters)	60–180 milligrams
Black tea (6 ounces/170 milliliters)	25–110 milligrams
Oolong tea (6 ounces/170 milliliters)	12–55 milligrams
Green tea (6 ounces/170 milliliters)	8–16 milligrams

the tea directly in the pot, pour the tea into cups through a strainer to catch the leaves. In this case, if you do not wish to serve your tea immediately, pour the tea through a strainer into another preheated teapot.

- Your tea is now ready. Add milk or lemon and/or honey to taste.
- Once made, tea should be consumed within one day and will keep, refrigerated, for up to three days.

QUICK SERVING IDEAS

- For iced green tea, pour 1 cup of boiling water over 2 green tea bags, and let steep for 3 to 5 minutes. Remove and squeeze out the tea bags. Add ice and enjoy. Make a larger quantity using more tea bags and water, and refrigerate the rest to drink throughout the day.
- For a hot tea punch, brew 5 bags of green tea in 6 cups of boiled water along with 2 cinnamon sticks and 8 whole cloves. Add 1½ cups orange juice and ⅓ cup fresh lemon juice. Serve hot, reheating if necessary.

SAFETY

Some green teas contain caffeine. Drinking green tea or taking caffeine-containing green tea extracts may be overstimulating, leading to such symptoms as nervousness, anxiety, insomnia, and irritability. Fortunately, decaffeinated green teas and decaffeinated green tea extracts are now widely available.

Green tea can interfere with the blood thinner warfarin (Coumadin). This drug blocks blood clotting in part by interfering with the actions of vitamin K. Since green tea is a significant source of vitamin K, it may reduce the effectiveness of warfarin. However, warfarin can effectively be used even if you drink green tea, as long as the quantities you drink remain constant from day to day. The standard blood tests done when you are taking warfarin will show any effects from the extra vitamin K contained in green tea, and your doctor can simply adjust the warfarin dose to compensate.

Virtually all forms of tea contain high levels of oxalate. Individuals with a history of calcium oxalate-containing kidney stones should limit their consumption of this food. See page 793 for more information.

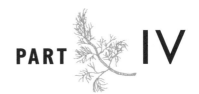

PART IV

Food Prescriptions for Specific Diseases

Promoting Health and Healing with Food

The doctor of the future will give no medicine, but will interest his patient in the care of the human frame, in diet and in the cause and prevention of disease.

—THOMAS EDISON

Were Edison's words prophetic? We believe so. In fact, the doctor of the future may very well be the naturopathic physician of today. Naturopathic doctors are trained in the use of many natural therapies, but nutrition is the foundation of all of them.

There is an ever-growing body of knowledge on the use of foods and nutrients in preventing as well as treating disease. Many common medical conditions respond quite well to diet therapy. They respond because good nutrition addresses the underlying cause of the illness rather than simply covering up the symptoms.

Have you ever heard the expression "You are what you eat"? Is there any truth to this statement? What determines the composition of your body? Your genes certainly play an important role, but the way in which they are actually expressed, your phenotype, is largely determined by the foods you eat. Whether you are in a state of poor health or simply desire better

health, improving the quality of the foods you regularly consume is a must.

Simply following the recommendations given for designing a healthy diet using the guidelines in chapter 2 has the potential to be quite therapeutic for most common illnesses. However, many medical conditions can be further benefited by more specific recommendations. The purpose of this section is to provide those recommendations.

These recommendations are not designed to substitute for proper medical treatment. In all cases involving a physical or mental complaint, ailment, or therapy, please consult a physician. Proper medical care and advice can significantly improve the quality and duration of your life. Readers are strongly urged to develop a good relationship with a physician knowledgeable in the art and science of natural and preventive medicine, such as naturopathic physicians.

Following are food prescriptions to help combat various diseases and conditions.

Acne

Acne is a common skin disorder that occurs in two forms: superficial *(acne vulgaris)*—affecting the hair follicles and oil-secreting glands of the skin and manifesting as blackheads, whiteheads, and inflammation—and cystic *(acne conglobata)*—a more severe form, with deep cyst formation and subsequent scarring. In both forms, the lesions occur predominantly on the face and, to a lesser extent, on the back, chest, and shoulders. These areas of the skin have more sebaceous glands that produce sebum, a mixture of oils and waxes that lubricates the skin and prevents the loss of water.

Signs and Symptoms

Acne is associated with the presence of blackheads, pimples, nodules (tender collections of pus deep in the skin that discharge to the skin's surface), and cysts (deep nodules that fail to discharge contents to the surface).

Causes

Acne is most common at puberty due to increased levels of the male sex hormone testosterone. Although men have higher levels of testosterone than women, during puberty there is an increase of testosterone in both sexes, making girls in this age group just as susceptible to acne. Testosterone causes the sebaceous glands to enlarge and produce more sebum. In addition, the cells that line the skin pore produce more keratin, a waxy protein. The combination of increased secretion of sebum and keratin can lead to blockage of the pore and the formation of a blackhead. With the blockage of the pore, bacteria are allowed to overgrow and release enzymes that break down sebum and promote inflammation. This process can lead to the formation of a whitehead or pimple. If there is no passageway to discharge the contents to the surface of the skin, it can lead to a cyst or boil (a deep nodule full of white blood cells and fluid).

Food Prescriptions

In addition to a healthy diet, a few specific food prescriptions are in order. All refined carbohydrates and fried foods must be eliminated, and foods containing trans-fatty acids (margarine, shortening, and other synthetically hydrogenated vegetable oils) or oxidized fatty acids (fried oils) should be avoided, as these foods may aggravate acne. Consumption of milk and milk products should also be limited or eliminated due to their potential hormone content.

Specific nutrients have been shown to exert a positive effect in treating acne. They include zinc, vitamin A, selenium, vitamin E, and chromium (from brewer's yeast).

Zinc, in particular, is vitally important in the treatment of acne. As discussed in the section on zinc, this important mineral plays a role in the action of many hormones as well as in wound healing, the immune response, and tissue regeneration. As it relates to acne, too little zinc seems to enhance the effect of testosterone on increasing sebum and keratin secretion and makes it difficult for the skin to heal quickly.

Zinc supplementation in the treatment of

acne has been the subject of much controversy and many double-blind studies. However, the inconsistency of the results may be due to differences in absorption of the various zinc salts used. For example, studies using effervescent zinc sulphate show effectiveness similar to that of the antibiotic tetracycline (with fewer side effects from chronic use) while those using plain zinc sulphate have shown less beneficial results. The majority of patients required twelve weeks of supplementation before good results were achieved, although some showed dramatic improvement immediately. Zinc levels are lower in thirteen- and fourteen-year-old males than in any other age group, so it is particularly important for this group to supplement, and the best way to do that is through natural food sources. Foods rich in zinc include most nuts, whole grains, and legumes.

Also important are dietary antioxidants, as male acne patients have significantly decreased levels of antioxidant enzymes. This normalizes when vitamin E and selenium are supplemented in the diet. What's more, the acne of both men and women improves with this treatment. This improvement is probably due to inhibition of lipid peroxide formation and suggests the use of other antioxidants. In addition to regular daily consumption of ¼ to ½ cup of raw nuts and seeds, supplementing the diet with selenium (100 to 200 micrograms per day) and vitamin E (200 to 400 IU per day) appears indicated.

Brewer's yeast may also be of benefit in healing acne. In one double-blind study, in more than 80 percent of the patients given brewer's yeast, the acne was either completely healed or considerably improved after five months of use, while the corresponding figure among those receiving a placebo was only 26 percent. This improvement was thought to be due to the high content of chromium within the brewer's yeast, though other nutrients may also have been responsible.

The widespread belief that chocolate *per se* causes or aggravates acne is apparently not true. In two studies, one conducted at the Pennsylvania School of Medicine and the other at the U.S. Naval Academy, eating chocolate did not produce any significant changes in the acne conditions of study participants. Nonetheless, we recommend that individuals with acne choose dark chocolate since it is has the highest levels of anti-inflammatory phenols and that they avoid sweet chocolate products (too much sugar!) and those that contain trans-fatty acids. Milk chocolate should also be avoided due to the high hormone content of most commercially available milk.

Other Recommendations

Here are six additional recommendations that should help to clear up acne:

1. Avoid medications that contain bromides or iodides.
2. Avoid exposure to oils and greases.
3. Avoid the use of greasy creams or cosmetics.
4. Thoroughly cleanse the face daily with sulphur-containing soap or a suitable alternative, such as calendula soap.
5. Extract blackheads every two to three days, and have cystic lesions incised and drained by a physician every two weeks.
6. Topical treatment with tea tree oil has produced results equal to those of benzoyl peroxide, but with fewer side effects.

AIDS and HIV Infection

Acquired immunodeficiency syndrome (AIDS) is characterized by a profound defect in immune function. The primary cause of AIDS is infection with the human immunodeficiency virus (HIV). Diagnosis of HIV is made by a positive blood test for HIV antigen and antibodies. Diagnosis of AIDS depends on meeting certain criteria, such as positive HIV test plus a total helper lymphocyte (an important white blood cell) count (CD4 count) of less than 200 cells per microliter, or a percentage of helper cells to total lymphocytes (CD8 count) of less than 14 percent.

Signs and Symptoms

The spectrum of HIV infection ranges from a person with a positive test for HIV without any signs of immune deficiency to a person with full-blown AIDS. The onset of AIDS can be either sudden, with the development of fever, sweats, malaise, fatigability, joint and muscle pain, headaches, sore throat, diarrhea, generalized swelling of lymph glands, and/or rash on the trunk; or it can be more insidious, presenting as unexplained progressive fatigue, weight loss, fever, diarrhea, and/or generalized swelling of the lymph glands. Anyone experiencing symptoms suggestive of AIDS or HIV infection should consult a physician.

Causes

HIV is now regarded as the causative agent in AIDS. Primary risk factors for developing AIDS and HIV infection include sexual contact with an HIV-infected person, intravenous drug use involving needle sharing with an HIV-infected person, and being born to a mother who has HIV.

Food Prescriptions

The immune system requires a constant supply of nutrients to function properly. Unfortunately, AIDS patients have many obstacles to overcome in order to supply their immune system with the nutrition it needs. Chief among these obstacles are gastrointestinal tract infections and the wasting (muscle breakdown) caused by the progressing infection. These factors make it difficult to absorb and utilizes nutrients properly. In short, it is easier to institute nutritional therapies early on than after AIDS has developed.

It is often recommended that the diet of HIV-positive persons and AIDS patients be rich in whole, natural foods, such as fruits, vegetables, grains, beans, seeds, and nuts; low in fats and refined sugars; and contain adequate, but not excessive, amounts of protein. For people with AIDS, the protein requirement is at least 2 grams per kilogram (2.2 pounds) of body weight. Supplementing the diet with whey protein (high in the amino acid glutamine) and nutritional antioxidants, such as vitamins C and E plus zinc and selenium, appears particularly useful in cases of AIDS, in terms of both addressing the wasting syndrome of AIDS and healing the gastrointestinal tract. HIV infection causes a significant increase in free-radical production that causes oxidative damage, particularly in the immune system. High-quality, undenatured whey protein supplementation to reach the recommended protein requirement is particularly recommended for people who show signs of weight loss or the wasting syndrome (progressive weight loss and weakness, often associated with fever and diarrhea). Undenatured whey protein provides specific proteins, such as immunoglobulins, that stimulate immunity in the digestive tract. Whey protein is also easily digestible, providing a highly available source of amino acids for weight gain.

Other Recommendations

Further discussion of HIV and AIDS is beyond the scope of this text. For additional recommendations, please see your naturopathic physician or consult the *Encyclopaedia of Natural Medicine.*

Alcoholism

Alcoholism has been defined by the World Health Organization as "alcohol consumption by an individual that exceeds the limits accepted by the culture or injures health or social relationships." Current estimates indicate that more than 18 million people in the United States (roughly 10 percent of the adult population) are alcoholics, making alcoholism one of the most serious health problems today. According to Alcoholics Anonymous, one person in thirteen is alcohol-dependent in the U.K.

Signs and Symptoms

Psychological and social signs of excess alcohol consumption include depression, loss of friends,

arrest for driving while intoxicated, excessive drinking, drinking before breakfast, frequent accidents, and unexplained work absences. Physical signs of excess alcohol consumption include alcohol odor on the breath, flushed face, tremor, and unexplained bruises.

Causes

Alcoholism is a multifactorial condition influenced by genetic, physiological, psychological, and social factors, all of which are of equal importance. Increased risk occurs in families with an alcoholic parent. Tolerance occurs with regular consumption and can lead to physiological and psychological addiction. In addition, alcohol consumption not only is socially accepted but is a popular activity, reinforcing other risk factors for alcoholism.

Food Prescriptions

While many of the nutritional problems of alcoholics relate directly to the effects of alcohol, a major contributing factor is that alcoholics tend not to eat because they substitute alcohol for food. As a result, the alcoholic has to deal with not only secondary nutritional deficiencies caused by excessive alcohol consumption but also primary nutritional deficiencies due to inadequate intake.

It is important for alcoholics to avoid refined sugars and caffeine, as they stress blood sugar control mechanisms and may increase the craving for alcohol. In one study, excluding caffeine, junk food, dairy products, and peanut butter was compared to a control diet for six months. Eighty-one percent of the subjects on the treatment diet remained sober, compared to less than 40 percent on the control diet.

B vitamins are extremely critical in the nutritional support for alcoholism. Alcoholics are almost always deficient in at least one of the B vitamins. In fact, a thiamine (vitamin B1) deficiency is both the most common and the most serious of the B-vitamin deficiencies in the alcoholic. In addition, evidence indicates that a thiamine deficiency results in greater intake of alcohol, suggesting that thiamine deficiency is a predisposing factor for alcoholism. Excellent food sources of thiamine include asparagus, mushrooms, peanuts, pork, soybeans, sunflower seeds, and yeast. Good sources are whole wheat and nuts.

Other Recommendations

A high-potency multiple vitamin and mineral formula (zinc is especially important) or a B-vitamin complex is the best first-step nutritional supplement. A good dosage of thiamine is 50 to 100 milligrams daily.

Alzheimer's Disease

Alzheimer's disease (AD) is a degenerative brain disorder that manifests as a progressive deterioration of memory and mental function, a state of mind commonly referred to as dementia. In the United States, 5 percent of the population over age sixty-five suffers from severe dementia, while another 10 percent suffers from mild to moderate dementia. With increasing age, there is a rise in frequency. For example, in people over age eighty, the frequency rate for dementia is over 25 percent. In the U.K., approximately 5 percent of people over sixty-five will suffer some form of Alzheimer's and 20 percent of people over eighty.

Signs and Symptoms

Progressive mental deterioration, loss of memory and cognitive functions, and an inability to carry out activities of daily life are the characteristic symptoms of AD.

Causes

Alzheimer's disease is characterized by distinctive changes in the brain. In particular, there is a reduced level of acetylcholine, a key neurotransmitter in the brain that is especially important for memory. The primary feature is the formation of what are referred to as neurofibrillary tangles and plaques. Simplistically speaking, these neurofibrillary tangles and plaques are "scars," composed of deposits of various proteins and cellular debris. The result is massive loss of brain cells, especially in key areas of the brain that control mental function.

Although genetic factors probably play a significant role in determining who is going to develop AD, like most chronic degenerative diseases, environmental factors are important. Increased oxidative damage, traumatic injury to the head, chronic exposure to aluminium and/or silicon, and exposure to toxins from environmental sources have all been implicated as causative factors.

Considerable attention has been given to the aluminium concentration in the neurofibrillary tangle. Whether the aluminium concentration develops in response to AD or initiates the lesions has not yet been determined, but significant evidence shows that it contributes, possibly very significantly, to the disease. At this point, it certainly seems appropriate to avoid all known sources of aluminium, including antacids and antiperspirants that contain aluminium; aluminium pots and pans; aluminium foil as food wrapping; and nondairy creamers.

Food Prescriptions

Studies have shown that elderly people's mental function is directly related to nutritional status. High nutritional status equals higher mental function. Given the frequency of nutrient deficiency in the elderly population, it is likely that many cases of impaired mental function may have a nutritional cause. In particular, folic acid and vitamin B12 deficiency are found much more often in patients with dementias of all types.

Also, there is considerable evidence that lack of omega-3 fatty acids (especially DHA from fish oils) and oxidative damage play major roles in the development and progression of AD. Since diets rich in fish oils and antioxidants, such as vitamins C and E, prevent AD, it makes sense to eat at least two servings of fish and other seafood per week, as well as a multitude of green leafy vegetables; highly-colored vegetables rich in carotenes, such as carrots, yams, and squash; and flavonoid-rich fruits, such as citrus and berries, particularly blueberries, cherries, and strawberries. Also, the spice turmeric (the chief component of curry) contains curcumin, a compound currently being investigated for its effects in prevention of AD.

Finally, poor detoxification of harmful chemicals is associated with neurodegenerative diseases such as AD. In particular, research indicates that people with AD have impaired sulphoxidation, a process the liver uses to bind sulphur to a toxin to promote its removal from the body. If this process of sulphoxidation is hindered, the body has impaired ability to clear toxins that damage nerve cells, such as cyanides and heavy metals.

Other Recommendations

Significant improvements in mental function and mood in patients with the early stages of AD have been reported with the daily supplementation of ginkgo biloba extract, 40 to 80 milligrams of the extract standardized to 24 percent ginkgo flavonglycosides, three times a day, and acetyl-L-carnitine, 500 to 1,000 milligrams, three times a day, for at least three months. However, less noticeable improvements have been noted in patients with more advanced stages of AD.

Anemia

Anemia is a condition in which the blood is deficient in red blood cells or the hemoglobin (iron-containing) portion of red blood cells. The primary function of red blood cells is to transport oxygen from the lungs to the tissues of the body in exchange for carbon dioxide. The symptoms of anemia, such as extreme fatigue, reflect a lack of oxygen being delivered to tissues and a buildup of carbon dioxide.

Signs and Symptoms

Anemia can lead to pallor, weakness, and a tendency to become fatigued easily. Laboratory results may indicate a low blood volume, low total red blood cell level, or abnormal red blood cell size or shape.

Causes

Anemia can be due to excessive blood loss, excessive red blood cell destruction due to abnormal red blood cell shape, as in sickle-cell anemia, or, most commonly, deficient red blood cell production as a result of nutritional deficiencies. Although deficiency of any of several vitamins and minerals can produce anemia, the most common causes are deficiencies of iron, vitamin B12, or folic acid.

Iron deficiency is the most common cause of anemia; however, anemia is the last stage of an iron-deficient state. Studies in several developed countries, including the United States, have found evidence of iron deficiency in 30 to 50 percent of the population. The groups at highest risk for iron deficiency are infants under two years of age, teenage girls, pregnant women, and the elderly. In the U.K., while the average man consumes enough iron, an average 25 percent of women have a low intake (50 percent of fifteen-to eighteen-year-olds; 42 percent of nineteen- to twenty-four-year olds; 41 percent of twenty-five- to thirty-four-year-olds). Iron deficiency may be due to an increased iron requirement, decreased dietary intake, diminished iron absorption or utilization, blood loss, or a combination of factors.

The diagnosis of iron deficiency can best be made by measuring serum ferritin, the iron storage protein. This is by far the most sensitive test for iron deficiency. Other measures of iron stores, such as serum iron, total iron-binding capacity, and red blood cell (RBC) hemoglobin, are less sensitive but are often performed on a routine basis. Long-term iron deficiency is characterized by low RBC levels, low hematocrit (volume of red blood cells), small RBCs, and low serum ferritin levels.

Vitamin B12-deficiency anemia is most often due to a defect in absorption and not to a dietary lack of B12. In order for vitamin B12 to be absorbed, it must be liberated from food by hydrochloric acid and bond to a substance known as intrinsic factor within the small intestine. Lack of intrinsic factor results in a condition known as pernicious anemia. The defect is rare before the age of thirty-five and it is more common in individuals of Scandinavian, English, and Irish descent. It is much less common in southern Europeans, Orientals, and blacks. Pernicious anemia is frequently associated with iron deficiency as well.

A dietary lack of vitamin B12 is most often associated with a strict vegetarian or vegan diet. Since body stores of vitamin B12 may remain normal for three to six years, deficiency of vitamin B12 is usually not apparent until after many years of vegetarianism. Fermented foods, such as soy sauce, miso, and tempeh, may contain some vitamin B12, but strict vegetarians and vegans should supplement their diet with additional B12.

Folic acid deficiency can occur with the use of some medications or a genetic defect in the body's ability to activate folic acid. Some medications, such as anticonvulsants and birth control pills, increase the use of folic acid, and other medications, such as methotrexate, block normal use of folic acid. Folic acid deficiency appears similar to vitamin B12 deficiency in blood tests and should be distinguished.

Dietary Factors

Calf's liver is often recommended for nutrition-related anemia, as it is rich not only in iron but also in all B vitamins, including vitamin B12 and folic acid. Brewer's yeast can also be an excellent source of iron and B vitamins. However, green leafy vegetables are of great benefit to individuals with any kind of anemia. These vegetables contain natural fat-soluble chlorophyll as well as other important nutrients, including iron and folic acid. The fat-soluble chlorophyll molecule is similar to the hemoglobin molecule and is efficiently absorbed from the gastrointestinal tract, providing all of the structural elements for hemoglobin.

Foods rich in iron, in addition to calf liver, green leafy vegetables, and brewer's yeast, include: dried beans; blackstrap molasses; lean beef, pork, and venison; dried apricots, raisins, and other dried fruits; almonds; mangoes; and shellfish. Vitamin C supplementation has been shown to greatly enhance the absorption of dietary iron. In fact, vitamin C is regarded as the most potent enhancer of iron absorption, and vitamin C alone will often increase body iron stores. Five hundred milligrams with each meal is a suitable dose for this effect.

Several foods and beverages contain substances that inhibit iron absorption, including coffee, tea, egg yolk, and foods high in phytates, such as Brazil nuts and wheat bran. Antacids and overuse of calcium supplements also decrease iron absorption. These items should be restricted for individuals with iron deficiency.

Other Recommendations

In the treatment of nutrition-related anemias, it is critical to supplement with the corresponding nutrient to address the deficiency, such as iron, vitamin B12, or folic acid. Iron-deficiency anemia can be treated with 50 milligrams of iron citrate in a liver-based supplement, three times per day. In an individual with pernicious anemia or a vegetarian with vitamin B12 deficiency, the standard approach involves injecting vitamin B12 at a dose of 1 microgram daily for one week, followed by a daily oral dose of 1,000 micrograms (1 milligram), preferably as a sublingual tablet or liquid. Folic acid can be taken as a 400 microgram supplement twice a day, on an empty stomach.

Anxiety

Anxiety is an unpleasant emotional state ranging from mild unease to intense fear. Anxiety differs from fear in that while fear is a rational response to a real danger, anxiety usually lacks a clear or realistic cause. Though some anxiety is normal and in fact healthy, higher levels of anxiety are not only uncomfortable, they can lead to significant health problems.

Signs and Symptoms

Anxiety is often accompanied by a variety of physical symptoms. The most common symptoms relate to the chest, such as heart palpitations (awareness of a more forceful or faster heartbeat), throbbing or stabbing pains, a feeling of tightness and inability to take in enough air, and a tendency to sigh or hyperventilate. In addition, tension in the back and neck muscles often leads to headaches, back pains, and muscle spasms. Other symptoms can include excessive sweating, dry mouth, dizziness, digestive disturbances, and the constant need to urinate or defecate.

Anxious individuals usually have a constant feeling that something bad is going to happen. They may fear that they have a chronic or dangerous illness—a belief that is reinforced by the symptoms of anxiety. Inability to relax may lead to difficulty in getting to sleep and to constant waking through the night.

Causes

Anxiety can be the result of both physical and psychological factors. For example, extreme stress can definitely trigger anxiety, but so can certain stimulants, such as caffeine. Anxiety can also be triggered by elevations in blood lactic acid level. Lactic acid is the final product in the breakdown of blood sugar (glucose) when there is a lack of oxygen.

Food Prescriptions

There are at least seven nutritional factors that may be responsible for triggering anxiety by raising blood lactic acid levels: caffeine, sugar, deficiency of B vitamins, deficiency of calcium or magnesium, alcohol, and food allergies. Simply avoiding caffeine, sugar, alcohol, and any foods that trigger allergies, along with boosting B vitamins, calcium, and magnesium, can go a long way in relieving anxiety. In fact, cutting out caffeine alone often results in the complete elimination of symptoms. The diet should be rich in foods that have higher levels of B vitamins, such as leafy vegetables, whole grains, and legumes. Foods high in calcium and magnesium include sea vegetables, sesame, milk, and dairy products as well as leafy green vegetables.

Other Recommendations

Stress reduction and relaxation exercises are often recommended for those suffering from anxiety. Some of the popular techniques are meditation, prayer, progressive relaxation, self-hypnosis, and biofeedback. The usual recommendation is to set aside at least five to ten minutes each day for the performance of a relaxation technique.

Arthritis: See Gout, Osteoarthritis, or Rheumatoid Arthritis.

Asthma

Asthma is an allergic disorder characterized by spasms of the bronchi (the airway tubes), swelling of the mucous lining of the lungs, and

> **WARNING:** An acute asthma attack can be a medical emergency. If you are suffering from an acute attack, consult your physician or nearest hospital immediately.

excessive production of a thick, viscous mucus. The major concern with asthma is that it can lead to respiratory failure—the inability to breathe.

Signs and Symptoms

Chronic asthma is associated with recurrent attacks of shortness of breath, cough, wheezing, and excessive production of mucus. Typically, the asthma patient will show laboratory signs of allergy, including increased levels of eosinophils in the blood, increased serum IgE levels, and positive food and/or inhalant allergy tests.

Causes

Asthma has typically been divided into two major categories: extrinsic and intrinsic. *Extrinsic,* or *atopic, asthma* is generally considered an allergic condition, with a characteristic increase in levels of serum IgE—the allergic antibody. Hay fever is also associated with an increase in IgE, but the symptoms affect the eyes and nose more than the bronchi and lungs. *Intrinsic asthma* is associated with a bronchial reaction that is due not to allergy but rather to such factors as toxic chemicals, cold air, exercise, infection, and emotional upset. Both extrinsic and intrinsic factors trigger the release of chemicals, such as histamine, that mediate (produce or control) inflammation from mast cells—specialized white blood cells that reside in various body tissues, including the lining of the respiratory passages.

The rate of asthma in the United States and the U.K. is rising rapidly, especially among children. Reasons often given to explain the rise in asthma include increased stress on the immune system due to greater chemical pollution in the air, water, and food; earlier weaning and earlier introduction of solid foods to infants; food additives; and genetic manipulation of plants, resulting in food components with greater allergenic tendencies.

Food Prescriptions

Many studies have indicated that food allergies play an important role in asthma. Adverse reactions to food may be immediate or delayed. Double-blind food challenges in children have shown that immediate-onset sensitivities are usually due to, in decreasing order of frequency, eggs, fish, shellfish, nuts, and peanuts; while foods most commonly associated with delayed-onset reactions include, in decreasing order of frequency, milk, chocolate, wheat, citrus, and food colorings. Although lemons and limes are not common allergens, all citrus can be associated with food allergy in asthma. Elimination diets have been successful in treating asthma, particularly in infants and children (see "Food Allergy").

Vitally important in the control of asthma is the elimination of food additives. Tartrazine (FD&C Yellow No. 5 or E102), benzoates, sulphur dioxide, and, in particular, sulphites, have been reported to cause asthma attacks in susceptible individuals. Tartrazine is found in most processed foods and can even be found in vitamin preparations and anti-asthma prescription drugs (e.g., theophylline). And it is estimated that 2 to 3 milligrams of sulphites are consumed each day by the average U.S. citizen, while an additional 5 to 10 milligrams are ingested by wine and beer drinkers.

Switching to a vegetarian diet may also be of benefit, as a long-term trial of a vegan diet (elimination of all animal products) provided significant improvement in asthma symptoms in 92 percent of the twenty-five treated patients who completed the study (nine dropped out). The researchers also found a reduction in the tendency to develop infections. It is important to recognize, however, that while 71 percent of the patients responded within four months, one year of therapy was required before the 92 percent level was reached.

The diet excluded all meat, fish, eggs, and dairy products. Drinking water was limited to spring water (chlorinated tap water was specifically prohibited), and coffee, ordinary tea, chocolate, sugar, and salt were excluded. Herbs and spices were allowed, and water and herbal teas were allowed, up to 1½ liters per day. Vegetables used freely were lettuce, carrots, beets, onions, celery, cabbage, cauliflower, broccoli, nettles, cucumber, radishes, Jerusalem artichokes, and all beans, except soybeans and green peas. Potatoes were allowed in restricted amounts. A number of fruits were also used freely: blueberries, cloudberries, raspberries, strawberries, black currants, gooseberries, plums, and pears. Apples and citrus fruits were not allowed, and grains were either very restricted or eliminated.

The beneficial effects of this dietary regime are probably related to: (1) elimination of common food allergens, (2) altered fatty acid metabolism, and (3) higher intake of dietary antioxidants. The compounds that contribute to the allergic and inflammatory reactions in asthma are derived primarily from arachidonic acid, a fatty acid found exclusively in animal products. In contrast, consumption of foods rich in omega-3 fatty acids decreases allergic and inflammatory reactions. Even though fish was avoided in this particular study, cold-water fish is a good source of omega-3 fatty acids. Using olive oil instead of foods high in animal fats, such as butter, also prevents a buildup of arachidonic acid. In addition, several of the foods consumed (e.g., onions, garlic, and berries) have exerted anti-asthmatic effects in experimental studies. Onions are particularly beneficial.

Diets high in antioxidants have also been shown to improve asthma. Vitamin C and other antioxidants are thought to provide important defenses, since oxidizing agents can both stimulate constriction of the bronchi and increase allergic reactions to other agents. Both treated and untreated asthmatic patients have been shown to have significantly lower levels of ascorbic acid in serum and white blood cells. Vitamin C inhibits induced bronchial constriction in both normal and asthmatic subjects. Vitamin C appears to normalize fatty acid metabolism and reduce histamine production. Carotenes (especially lycopene), vitamin E, and selenium are also important. Vitamin C is found in peppers, berries, citrus fruit, kiwis, and green vegetables from the cabbage family. These green, yellow, and orange fruits and vegetables are also high in carotenoids. And wheat germ oil, nuts and seeds, and grains are high in vitamin E.

Other Recommendations

Asthma can be a serious medical emergency. Proper medical care is essential. In severe cases, the best treatment is a combined approach using natural measures to reduce the allergic threshold and prevent acute attacks, along with proper drug treatment of acute attacks.

Studies have shown that being overweight increases the risk of asthma. Fortunately, losing weight has been shown to lead to significant decreases in episodes of shortness of breath, increases in overall breathing capacity, and decreases in the need for medication to control symptoms.

Atherosclerosis

Atherosclerosis is the process of the hardening of an artery due to the buildup of cholesterol-containing plaque. Atherosclerosis is responsible for coronary artery disease, the leading cause of death in America and the U.K., and many cases of stroke. Altogether, atherosclerosis is responsible for at least 43 percent of all deaths in the United States. In the U.K., 39 percent of deaths were a result of circulatory diseases including stroke and coronary heart disease.

Signs and Symptoms

Atherosclerosis is often referred to as the "silent killer" because the first symptom or sign in many cases is a fatal heart attack or stroke. However, most people with significant atherosclerosis have a history of elevated cholesterol levels and may also experience angina.

Causes

The initial step in the development of atherosclerosis is damage to the lining of an artery.

This damage is usually the result of free radicals (highly reactive toxic chemicals most often produced by body processes). Once the artery lining has been damaged, the site of injury attracts monocytes (large white blood cells) and platelets (small blood cells involved in the formation of blood clots), which adhere to the damaged area, where they release growth factors that stimulate plaque formation and the accumulation of fat and cholesterol deposits.

Reducing premature death from heart disease and strokes involves reducing—and, when possible, eliminating—the following major risk factors:

- Smoking.
- Elevated blood cholesterol levels.
- High blood pressure.
- Diabetes.
- Physical inactivity.
- Obesity.

Food Prescriptions

The guidelines detailed in Chapter 2 are especially important in fighting against atherosclerosis. Specifically, the key dietary recommendations to reduce the risk of atherosclerosis are as follows.

- Reduce the amount of saturated fat, trans-fatty acids, cholesterol, and total fat in the diet by eating fewer animal products and more plant foods.

- Increase your intake of omega-3 oils by eating linseed oil, walnuts, and small amounts of cold-water fish. There is considerable evidence that people who consume a diet rich in omega-3 oils from either fish or vegetable sources have a significantly reduced risk of developing atherosclerosis. Atherosclerosis is associated with a deficiency in omega-3 oils.

- Increase your intake of heart-healthy monounsaturated fats by eating more nuts and seeds, including almonds, Brazil nuts, coconut, hazelnuts, macadamia nuts, pecans, pine nuts, pistachios, and sesame and sunflower seeds, and using a monounsaturated oil, such as olive or rapeseed oil, for cooking purposes.

- Eat five or more servings daily of a combination of vegetables and fruits, especially green, orange, and yellow vegetables; dark-colored berries; and citrus fruits. Antioxidant compounds in these plant foods, such as carotenes, flavonoids, selenium, vitamin E, and vitamin C, are important in protecting against the development of atherosclerosis. These foods are also rich in B vitamins, which can help lower homocysteine levels.

- Increase your intake of fiber. A diet high in fiber has been shown to be protective against atherosclerosis. Dietary fiber, particularly the soluble fiber found in legumes, fruits, and vegetables, is effective in lowering cholesterol levels.

- Limit your intake of refined carbohydrates (sugar and refined grains). Sugar and other refined carbohydrates are a significant factor in the development of atherosclerosis. Sugar consumption elevates levels of the hormone insulin. Elevated insulin levels, in turn, are associated with increased cholesterol,

triglycerides, blood pressure, and risk of death from cardiovascular disease.

Other Recommendations

We recommend using a high-quality fish oil supplement as an alternative to eating large amounts of cold-water fish to avoid the common contaminants found in fish, such as mercury, PCBs, and dioxins. Look for products that are designated "pharmaceutical grade," and take approximately 400 to 600 milligrams of omega-3 fatty acids daily. It is estimated that the use of fish oil supplements may reduce overall cardiovascular mortality by as much as 45 percent.

Bronchitis and Pneumonia

Bronchitis is an infection or irritation of the bronchi—the passageways from the windpipe (trachea) to the lungs. Pneumonia, by contrast, is an infection or irritation of the lungs themselves. Both of these conditions are much more common in the winter, as they usually follow an upper respiratory tract infection (cold).

Signs and Symptoms

Bronchitis usually manifests with bouts of coughing, shaking, chills, fever, and chest pain that are usually preceded by an upper respiratory tract infection (cold). In addition to the symptoms of bronchitis, pneumonia shows classic signs of lung involvement, including shallow breathing, coughing, and abnormal breath sounds, and a chest X-ray shows infiltration of fluid and lymph into the lungs.

Causes

Bronchitis and pneumonia can be caused by a variety of viruses and bacteria. In healthy individuals, pneumonia and bronchitis most often follow an insult to the immune system. Viral infection, especially influenza or the common cold; cigarette smoke and other noxious fumes; loss of consciousness, which depresses the gag reflex, allowing the breathing in (aspiration) of fluids; cancer; or hospitalization, which increases exposure to organisms that can cause pneumonia, are all risk factors for bronchitis and pneumonia.

Food Prescriptions

Optimal immune function requires a healthy diet that (1) is rich in whole, natural foods, such as fruits, vegetables, grains, beans, seeds, and nuts; (2) is low in fats and refined sugars; and (3) contains adequate, but not excessive, amounts of protein. In particular, studies have shown that higher fruit and vegetable consumption reduces the risk of developing chronic bronchitis and pneumonia. Pineapple, because it contains the protein-digesting enzyme bromelain, is one fruit that may help more specifically in the treatment of bronchitis and pneumonia. Clinical studies with bromelain have shown it to be quite helpful in these conditions because it helps to break down thick mucus and exerts some mild antibiotic effects as well.

Garlic also has a long history of use as an infection fighter. In fact, it has been referred to as "Russian penicillin" to denote its antibacterial properties. Unfortunately, the antimicrobial activity is due to allicin, the primary pungent principle. Raw garlic is thus required to take advantage of this antibiotic action. Crush one medium clove of garlic and let it sit for 10 to 15 minutes, then mix with a tablespoon of honey to make it more palatable. Eat one to two cloves daily.

Food allergies may be an underlying factor in cases of chronic bronchitis. In particular, cow's milk allergy has been associated with bronchitis in children. If you suffer from chronic bronchitis, you may want to try eliminating cow's milk from your diet.

Other Recommendations

One of the main treatment goals in cases of bronchitis and pneumonia is to help the lungs and air passages get rid of excessive mucus. You can aid this process by performing postural drainage by lying facedown with the top half of your body off the bed and, using your forearms for support, trying to cough and expectorate into a basin or newspaper on the floor. The position should be maintained for 5 to 15 minutes.

Cancer (Nutritional Support for Cancer Patients)

No other disease strikes as much fear deep within our souls as cancer. The reason? Almost all of us have witnessed firsthand the ravaging effect that cancer, as well as chemotherapy and radiation, has had on a loved one. U.S. cancer statistics present us with some sobering facts. Each year:

- More than 1,250,000 new cases of invasive cancer will be diagnosed (275,000 in the U.K. in 2002).
- An additional 1,500,000 new cases of noninvasive cancer will be diagnosed.
- More than 500,000 people will die from cancer (160,000+ in the U.K. in 2000).
- Cancer causes one in five of all deaths (26 percent of all deaths in the U.K.).
- Cancer will affect one out of every three people alive today.
- Fifty percent of those diagnosed with cancer will die of their disease.
- The economic toll of cancer will be greater than $110 billion (the NHS spent £2.1 billion in the U.K. in 2004).

Cancer develops when there is damage to the genetic code of the cell—the DNA—that results in the cells growing and reproducing out of control. Most of the time when DNA becomes damaged, the cell is able to repair it or the cell simply dies. In cancer, the damaged DNA is not repaired and the cell does not die. Instead, it replicates out of control. Although some people are born with damaged DNA, the initial damage to the DNA is most often caused by free radicals, highly reactive molecules that can destroy cellular components including DNA, membranes, and proteins. So if you want to reduce your risk of cancer, it's important to:

- Reduce free-radical formation in your body.
- Limit your exposure to dietary and environmental sources of free radicals (especially cigarette smoke).
- Increase your intake of foods rich in antioxidants.

It is also important to support the immune system. Cells of the immune system circulate throughout the body not only to protect us against invading organisms, but also to seek out and destroy cancer cells. Impaired immune function greatly increases the risk of cancer.

Cancer is definitely a multifactorial disease in that a myriad of genetic, lifestyle, psychological, environmental, and dietary factors have been shown to either increase or decrease the risk of cancer. Cancer Research U.K. reports that half of all cancers diagnosed in the U.K. could be prevented by changes to lifestyle. Obviously, the goal in prevention is simply to reduce the controllable factors that are linked to causing cancer (e.g., we can quit smoking, but we can't change our DNA or biological parents) while at the same time increasing the dietary factors that prevent cancer. Keep in mind that even the American Cancer Society acknowledges that roughly 85 percent of all cancers are related to diet, lifestyle, and environmental factors.

The Encyclopaedia of Healing Foods provides a compendium of foods and dietary strategies for the prevention of cancer. Our goal for the entry here is to stress the importance of high-quality nutrition and offer some suggestions for dealing with some of the nutritional challenges seen in cancer patients. The bottom line is that cancer patients who have higher nutritional sta-

TABLE 20.1

American Cancer Society Recommendations for the Early Detection of Cancer

Site	Recommendation
General	A cancer-related checkup is recommended every three years for people aged twenty to forty and every year for people aged forty or older. This exam should include health counseling and, depending on a person's age and sex, might include examinations for cancers of the thyroid, oral cavity, skin, lymph nodes, testes or ovaries, as well as for some nonmalignant diseases.
Breasts	Women forty and older should have an annual mammogram and an annual clinical breast examination (CBE) by a health care professional. They also should perform monthly breast self-examination. The CBE should be conducted close to the scheduled mammogram. Women aged twenty to thirty-nine should have a CBE by a health care professional every three years and should perform monthly breast self-examination.
Colon and rectum	Beginning at age fifty, men and women should follow one of the examination schedules below: • A faecal occult blood test every year and a flexible sigmoidoscopy every five years. • A colonoscopy every ten years. • A double-contrast barium enema every five to ten years. A digital rectal exam should be done at the same time as the sigmoidoscopy, colonoscopy, or double-contrast barium enema. People who have a family history of colon cancer should talk with a doctor about a more frequent testing schedule.
Prostate	The ACS recommends that both the prostate-specific antigen (PSA) blood test and the digital rectal examination be offered annually, beginning at age fifty, to men who have a life expectancy of at least ten years and to younger men who are at high risk. Men in high-risk groups, such as those with a strong familial predisposition (i.e., two or more affected first-degree relatives) and blacks, may begin at a younger age (i.e., forty-five years).
Uterus	*Cervix:* All women who are or have been sexually active or who are eighteen and older should have an annual Pap (smear) test and pelvic examination. After three or more consecutive satisfactory examinations with normal findings, the Pap test may be performed less frequently. Discuss the matter with your physician. *Endometrium:* Women with a family history of cancer of the uterus should have a sample of endometrial tissue examined when menopause begins.

Source: Modified from information from the American Cancer Society, Inc.

tus are not only more likely to fight off infections and tolerate therapy and its side effects, they also have better odds of actually winning the battle. Our book *How to Prevent and Treat Cancer with Natural Medicine* provides a comprehensive approach to the topic.

It is important to stress that one key strategy in reducing the risk of dying from cancer is getting a regular checkup by your doctor to look for cancer. Regular checkups are important for everyone, but especially important for people who have certain risk factors, such as a family history of certain cancers, a history of cigarette smoking, or exposure to environmental toxins. The earlier a cancer is discovered, the more likely it is that treatment will be successful.

Signs and Symptoms

Nausea and vomiting are among the most troubling complications of cancer. If nothing is done to control nausea and vomiting, patients may develop anorexia (loss of appetite). When they stop eating a healthy balanced diet, patients may gradually lose a large amount of weight. This wasting away, called cachexia, is a sign that the body has started to use up all of its energy reserves. After it burns all the energy stored in fat cells, it begins using the muscle cells. Rapid weight loss is one of the most serious signs of trouble for a cancer patient.

Causes

The problems of nausea and vomiting, anorexia, and cachexia are sometimes the results of the cancer itself, but often they are an adverse effect of chemotherapy or radiation. Cachexia can also occur in people who are eating enough but whose bodies are so ravaged by disease that they cannot properly absorb the nutrients. In some cases, tumors produce large amounts of cell proteins called cytokines that act on the body by revving up the metabolism, thus burning more energy, accelerating tissue breakdown, and speeding up the wasting process of cachexia. By some estimates, approximately 40 percent of cancer fatalities result not from the disease itself but from malnutrition.

Food Prescriptions

The nutritional support for cancer is a spectrum; for someone with a minor cancer with good energy levels, appetite, and nutritional status, following the guidelines given in chapter 2 may be all that is necessary to provide them optimal nutrition. However, at the other end of the spectrum, people with advanced cancers or those going through chemotherapy will usually be challenged with such things as low energy levels, loss of appetite, and nausea (and possibly even vomiting). For these individuals, the following dietary suggestions can help improve nutritional status:

- Eat small, frequent meals (every one to two hours), rather than larger meals less often.
- Stay well hydrated and drink 18 to 24 ounces/500 to 700 milliliters of fresh vegetable juice daily. It can be taken with food, or, better yet, take a midmorning "juice break."
- Drink a high-protein smoothie once or twice daily (discussed below). Smoothies can take the place of breakfast and as a midafternoon snack.
- Try ginger—nature's nausea and vomiting remedy—as a tea or juice (use fresh ginger) or in rice.
- Use extra seasonings, spices, and flavorings to improve food's taste appeal, but avoid flavorings that are very sweet or very bitter.
- Eat soft, moist foods such as smoothies,

bananas, brown rice, yams, etc.; avoid hard, dry foods such as cereals, crackers, and hard sweets.

- Take small bites and chew completely.
- Be sure to get 6,000 to 9,000 milligrams of EPA and DHA daily from a pharmaceutical-grade fish oil product.

In patients with anorexia or cachexia, it may be necessary to suspend healthy eating habits and focus on eating the things that appeal to them. That is fine for the short term, but we cannot stress enough the importance of high-quality nutrition to fight cancer effectively. Sometimes it just may not be possible for cancer patients to get the nutrition and fluids they need through eating and drinking. They may need additional measures, such as enteral nutrition (feeding via a tube directly into the stomach) or parenteral nutrition (infusion through a vein). These methods are helpful when:

- Upper gastrointestinal blockage prevents eating or drinking.
- Side effects of treatment (for example, burns or irritation to the throat resulting from radiation therapy to the oesophagus) limit eating or drinking.
- Anorexia or other problems such as severe depression, confusion, or disorientation keep a patient from eating or drinking sufficiently.
- Pain makes it difficult to chew or swallow.
- Surgery has involved removal of part of the gastrointestinal tract.
- The patient has difficulty maintaining adequate body weight and muscle mass.

HIGH-PROTEIN SMOOTHIES

Cancer patients often need to increase their intake of protein, especially if they are showing signs of cachexia or are on chemotherapy. Protein is especially important for many of the functions necessary for recovery. It helps maintain muscle mass, nourishes the lining of the gastrointestinal tract, boosts blood counts, heals tissues, and boosts the immune system to help fight cancer and prevent infections. On the other hand, inadequate protein intake slows recovery from illness and decreases resistance to infection. Undergoing conventional cancer therapy may require as much as 50 percent more protein than usual.

Smoothies are an ideal—and delicious—way for people with cancer to consume lots of high-quality protein. The highest-quality protein powder comes from whey, a natural by-product of the cheese-making process. Whey is called a complete protein because it contains all essential and nonessential amino acids. (Amino acids are smaller chunks of protein that are assembled during digestion to make the thousands of different kinds of protein your body needs.) Whey protein, when processed properly, also has the highest biological value (BV) of all proteins. BV is a measure that indicates how much of the protein you eat is actually absorbed, retained, and used in the body (as opposed to the amount that passes out of the body unused). One reason the BV of whey protein is so high is that it has the highest concentrations of glutamine (an amino acid) and branched-chain amino acids (BCAAs) found in nature. Glutamine and branched-chain amino acids are critical to cellular health and protein synthesis.

Glutamine, the most abundant amino acid in the body, is involved in more metabolic processes than any other amino acid. Glutamine is especially important as a source of fuel for white blood cells and for cells that divide rapidly, such as those that line the intestine. It has become an important component of intravenous feeding mixes in hospitals, since double-blind studies have shown that it dramatically increases survival in critically ill subjects. Glutamine also prevents mouth ulcers (stomatitis) and suppression of the immune system in cancer patients receiving chemotherapy. Supplementation with glutamine has been shown to heal peptic ulcers, enhance energy levels, boost immune function, and fight infections.

We recommend that patients obtain their glutamine by taking daily doses of 20 to 30 grams of whey protein concentrate twice a day. We believe that acquiring glutamine from whey protein provides additional benefit over simply taking glutamine. Whey protein is more beneficial because it contains other compounds (called fractions and peptides) that are known to improve immune function and boost glutathione concentrations. If for some reason (e.g., allergy) you cannot take whey protein, you can take glutamine supplements, 3 to 5 grams one to three times daily (dosage determined by size and severity of need). If you have trouble keeping your weight up, we recommend using one of the whey-based weight gain products in the marketplace.

Whey protein can be found in premeasured individual serving packets and bulk canisters and is available in many different flavors—chocolate, vanilla, strawberry, piña colada, orange, and others—from many different manufacturers. For many of the products, just mixing the whey protein with 8 to 12 ounces/240 to 340 milliliters of water, juice, nonfat milk, or soy milk and a few ice cubes is all that is needed to make a delicious shake. You can also add some frozen or fresh fruit, ½ to 1 cup, to make it even more nutritious and higher in calories. Not only is the protein quality of these powders higher, but these smoothies are much easier and more palatable for the cancer patient to consume than fish, chicken, or meat.

SOY IN CANCER TREATMENT

Increasing the intake of soy foods also appears to be helpful in most cancers. The possible exception is in women who have oestrogen-sensitive breast tumors. While studies in test tubes and in animals show that the isoflavone genistein stimulates the growth of oestrogen-receptor-positive tumors, it inhibits the growth of breast cancer cells that lack oestrogen receptors as well as most other cancer cells. It appears that for most cancers, especially prostate and lung cancer, increasing the consumption of soy foods offers significant benefits. Soy foods include tofu, tempeh, and miso, and "second-generation" soy foods that simulate traditional meat and dairy products, such as soy milk, soy hot dogs, soy sausage, soy cheese, and soy frozen desserts.

Soy isoflavonoids prevent the formation of new blood vessels, thus preventing tumors from obtaining a blood supply necessary for continued growth as well as preventing tumor cells from dividing and growing by inhibiting enzymes involved in cell replication.

We encourage cancer patients to consume at least one serving of soy (or 50 to 90 milligrams of soy isoflavones) per day unless you have a history of oestrogen-positive breast cancer, in which case we encourage you to limit soy consumption to no more than three or four servings per week. Remember that you can use soy milk as the basis of whey protein smoothies.

Other Recommendations

For people with cancer, especially those undergoing chemotherapy, it's absolutely essential to maintain good hydration. Without adequate water your body cannot detoxify the drugs and remove them from the system. The buildup of these toxins will lead to further symptoms and discomfort. Fluid is needed to remove the metabolic by-products of the fight against cancer, including the debris from dead cells.

Inadequate water intake can cause a range of medical complications, including bladder infections, excess calcium buildup, electrolyte disturbances, fatigue, muscle spasms, and irregular heartbeat. The risk of dehydration is higher if chemotherapy causes vomiting and diarrhea. Here are some tips for maintaining good hydration:

- Prepare herbal iced tea and keep a glass at your side throughout the day. If you sip just 4 to 6 ounces/125–180 milliliters every hour, you'll reach your daily quota for fluids.
- Avoid caffeine and alcohol. These act as diuretics, which means they draw water from your cells and cause you to urinate more fluid than you are consuming.
- Eat more soups, stews, and other "watery" foods. These are often easier to digest. They're also easy to reheat when you are tired, and they increase your total water intake with each serving.

- Freeze lollipops made with weak fruit juice and water or seltzer and suck on them when your mouth is sore.
- Drink most of your fluids between meals to leave more room to take in nutritious food when you eat.
- Avoid drinking large amounts of fluids all at once, since that can cause nausea and perhaps aggravate the dehydration. Instead sip several ounces, wait about 15 minutes, and sip some more.
- Eat more fresh fruits, especially juicy ones. Watermelon is a particularly good choice.
- Choose sorbets and ices for dessert.
- If you are extremely tired, keep an ice chest by your chair or bedside to make it easier to reach fluids throughout the day.

SUGGESTIONS FOR DEALING WITH DEHYDRATION

Electrolytes (such as potassium, calcium, and sodium) are chemicals your cells need to function. Dehydration can cause an electrolyte imbalance. If you are dehydrated due to vomiting or diarrhea, it is important to drink fluids that replenish electrolytes. You can make your own electrolyte drink by combining 1 liter of water, 4 tablespoons of honey, 1 teaspoon of salt, and 1 teaspoon of bicarbonate of soda. For milder dehydration, fruit juices and teas are adequate (and taste better).

For severe dehydration, intravenous fluid replacement may be necessary. This can be done at your doctor's surgery or with the assistance of a visiting home nurse. Replacement of fluids can often lead to an immediate return of well-being and reduction of nausea. Be sure to notify your doctor if you are unable to drink fluids, if you have severe diarrhea or vomiting, or if you experience a rapid weight loss within several days. Other signs of dehydration include dry lips, dark urine, and becoming dizzy or light-headed upon standing up.

Again, for more information on natural approaches to cancer, consult *How to Prevent and Treat Cancer with Natural Medicine.*

Candidiasis, Chronic

Chronic candidiasis, or chronic yeast infection, is a complex medical syndrome attributed to an overgrowth in the gastrointestinal tract of the usually benign yeast (or fungus) *Candida albicans.*

Signs and Symptoms

Fatigue, allergies, immune system malfunction, depression, chemical sensitivities, and digestive disturbances are just some of the symptoms patients with chronic yeast infection have been reported to experience. Laboratory techniques, such as stool cultures for *Candida,* and measurement of antibody levels to *Candida* or *Candida* antigens in the blood, can help confirm the diagnosis.

Causes

Prolonged use of antibiotics is believed to be the most important factor in the development of chronic candidiasis. Antibiotics suppress the immune system and the normal intestinal bacteria that prevent yeast overgrowth, strongly promoting the proliferation of *Candida.* Other

factors predisposing to *Candida* overgrowth include: decreased digestive secretions; use of other immunosuppressive drugs, such as corticosteroids; increased oestrogen exposure, such as oestrogen dominance or birth control pill use; and impaired immunity.

Food Prescriptions

A number of dietary factors appear to promote the overgrowth of *Candida;* therefore, a special diet must be employed in the treatment of candidiasis. The diet should be free of refined sugar, including sucrose, fructose, commercial fruit juices, honey, and maple syrup, since *Candida* thrives in a high-sugar state. Milk and milk products should be avoided due to their high content of lactose (milk sugar) and trace levels of antibiotics. Refined-flour products should be avoided and replaced with whole grains eaten in moderation.

All known allergens should also be eliminated, since allergies can weaken the immune system and provide a more hospitable environment for the yeast.

Foods that can be eaten freely include all vegetables and protein sources (legumes, fish, poultry, and meat). One 1-cup serving of the following low-sugar fruit may be eaten per day as well: apples, blueberries, cherries, other berries, and pears.

A special food for the *Candida* sufferer is garlic. Garlic has demonstrated significant antifungal activity against a wide range of fungi. Garlic is especially active against *C. albicans,* being more potent than nystatin, gentian violet, and six other reputed antifungal agents.

Other Recommendations

There are seven important steps in successfully controlling *Candida albicans:*

1. Eliminate the use of antibiotics, steroids, other immune-suppressing drugs, and birth control pills (unless there is absolute medical necessity).

2. Follow the *Candida* control diet under "Food Prescriptions" above.

3. Enhance digestion with the use of digestive aids, if necessary. One simple method is to sip 8 ounces/240 milliliters of water with 1 to 2 tablespoons fresh lemon juice or 5 to 15 drops bitter herbs, such as equal amounts of artemisia and gentian, 15 minutes before meals. If digestion is particularly weak, digestive enzymes can be taken with each meal.

4. Enhance immune function through high-quality nutrition and, if necessary, herbal supplements such as astragalus, Siberian ginseng, and medicinal mushrooms, including shiitake, maitake, and reishi mushrooms.

5. Enhance liver function by eating a high-fiber, low-fat diet.

6. Use nutritional and herbal supplements that help control against yeast overgrowth and promote a healthy bacterial flora, such as oregano oil, thyme oil, lauric acid, *Lactobacillus acidophilus,* and *Bifidobacteria.*

7. Eliminate *Candida* toxins by using a water-soluble fiber source, such as guar gum, psyllium seed, or pectin, which can bind to toxins in the gut and promote their excretion.

Carpal Tunnel Syndrome

Carpal tunnel syndrome (CTS) is a common, painful disorder caused by compression of the median nerve, which passes between the bones and ligaments of the wrist.

Signs and Symptoms

Compression of the median nerve in the wrist causes weakness; pain when gripping; and burning, tingling, or aching that may radiate to the forearm and shoulder. Symptoms may be occasional or constant.

Causes

CTS is most frequently caused by repetitive minor injury. This injury occurs most commonly in people who perform repetitive, strenuous work with their hands (e.g., carpenters) but may also occur in people who do light work (e.g., typists and keyboard operators). It may follow more serious injuries of the wrist, too. CTS can also be caused by anything that produces inflammation or swelling of the tissues of the wrist, such as rheumatoid arthritis, diabetes, and hypothyroidism.

Food Prescriptions

The increased frequency of CTS since 1950 parallels the increased presence of compounds that interfere with vitamin B6 in the body. Particularly incriminating is tartrazine (FD&C Yellow No. 5 or E102). Tartrazine is added to almost every packaged food. In the United States, the average daily per capita consumption of certified dyes is 15 milligrams, of which 85% is tartrazine. Eliminating tartrazine from the diet and increasing vitamin B6 intake through diet or supplementation may help CTS. Foods rich in vitamin B6 include brewer's yeast, sunflower seeds, soybeans, walnuts, lentils and other legumes, brown rice, and bananas.

During flare-ups, fresh pineapple juice, along with fresh ginger, may help due to their anti-inflammatory activity.

Other Recommendations

Curcumin is perhaps nature's most potent anti-inflammatory agent. Curcumin is derived from turmeric and may be useful in decreasing inflammation of the median nerve, particularly when combined with bromelain. These preparations should be taken on an empty stomach. Vitamin B6 has been used with some success in the treatment of CTS at a dose of 50 to 100 milligrams one to two times per day for at least twelve weeks.

Cataracts

Cataracts are white, opaque blemishes on the normally transparent lens of the eye. They occur as a result of free-radical or oxidative damage to the protein structure of the lens, similar to the damage that occurs to the protein of egg whites when eggs are heated. Cataracts are the leading cause of impaired vision and blindness in the world.

Signs and Symptoms

Clouding or opacity in the crystalline lens of the eye occurs in a progressive manner, causing a gradual loss of vision.

Causes

Aging-related (or "senile") cataracts form when the normal protective mechanisms of the eye are unable to prevent free-radical damage. The lens, like many other tissues of the body, depends on adequate levels and activities of antioxidant nutrients and enzymes for its normal protective mechanisms. When it is either overwhelmed by the demand for or deficient in the supply of antioxidant nutrient and enzymes, cataracts form. For example, exposure to cigarette smoke or sunlight increases the risk of cataracts by creating an increased need for antioxidant nutrients and enzymes in the lens of the eye.

Food Prescriptions

Individuals with higher dietary intakes of antioxidant nutrients, particularly vitamins C and E, selenium, and carotenes, have a much lower risk of developing cataracts. To increase your intake of these nutrients, include an assortment of high-antioxidant-containing foods, such as leafy greens, yams, carrots, broccoli, and other highly colored vegetables; fresh fruits, particularly citrus fruits and dark-colored berries; and wheat germ oil for vitamin E. It is also important to avoid salt, saturated fried foods, rancid foods, and other sources of free radicals, which are linked to cataract formation.

Particularly important in the prevention of cataracts may be raising glutathione levels. Glutathione is found in very high concentrations in the lens of the eye, where it plays a vital role in maintaining a healthy lens. Specifically, glutathione functions as an antioxidant, maintains the structure of the lens proteins, acts in various enzyme systems, and participates in amino acid and mineral transport. Glutathione levels are diminished in virtually all forms of cataracts. To raise glutathione levels, eat plenty of fresh raw fruits and vegetables, as the glutathione content in these foods is substantially higher than in their cooked counterparts.

Other Recommendations

In addition to eating a diet rich in antioxidants by focusing on fresh fruits and vegetables, when cataracts are already apparent, it appears to be worthwhile to supplement the diet with additional antioxidant nutrients. You can try taking vitamin C, 1 gram, three times daily; vitamin E, 600 IU per day; and selenium, 400 micrograms per day.

Celiac Disease

Celiac disease, also known as nontropical sprue, gluten-sensitive enteropathy, or celiac sprue, is characterized by malabsorption of nutrients and an abnormal small intestine structure, which reverts to normal on removal of dietary gluten. The protein gluten and its derivative gliadin are found primarily in wheat, oats, barley, rye, spelt, kamut, and triticale grains.

Signs and Symptoms

Symptoms of celiac disease most commonly appear during the first three years of life, after cereals are introduced into the diet. A second peak incidence occurs during the third decade. Symptoms generally involve loose stools or diarrhea, often with fat drops in the toilet showing malabsorption. Other signs of malabsorption include inability to gain weight or weight loss, as well as failure to thrive. However, often, especially in adults, the symptoms of celiac disease can be insidious and nonspecific. Celiac disease is being diagnosed more commonly than was once the case, due to increased detection of those with low-grade celiac disease.

Causes

In celiac disease, the body creates an immune reaction against the lining of the small intestine. This autoimmune reaction is triggered primarily by gluten. In addition to sensitivity to gluten, the early introduction of cow's milk is believed to be a major causative factor of celiac disease. Research has clearly indicated that breast-feeding and delayed administration of cow's milk and cereal grains, are primary preventive steps that can greatly reduce the risk of developing the disease.

Celiac disease also appears to have a genetic cause. The frequency of individuals with the genetic trait for celiac disease is much higher in northern and central Europe and the northwest Indian subcontinent. Wheat cultivation in these areas is a relatively recent development (1000 B.C.E.). The prevalence of celiac disease is much higher in these areas than in other parts of the world, for example, 1:300 in southwest Ireland compared with 1:2,500 in the United States. In the U.K., until recently it was thought that the prevalence of celiac disease was 1:1,500 but since the introduction of more sensitive tests it is now estimated that as many as one in 300 people may suffer from the disease.

Dietary Considerations

Cereal grains belong to the Gramineae family. The closer a grain's taxonomic (classification) relationship to wheat, the grain with the highest gluten content, the greater its ability to activate celiac disease. Gluten is composed of gliadins and glutenins. Only the gliadin portion has been demonstrated to activate celiac disease. In the gluten-containing grains, the proteins that appear to activate the disease are termed secalins, hordeins, and avenins individually, and prolamines collectively. Rice and corn, two grains that do not appear to activate celiac disease, contain very little gliadin.

Once the diagnosis of celiac disease has been established, a gluten-free diet is indicated. This diet does not contain any wheat, rye, barley, triticale, spelt, kamut, or oats. Buckwheat and millet are often excluded as well. Although buckwheat is not in the grass family and millet appears to be more closely related to rice and corn, they do contain prolamines that are similar to the alpha-gliadin of wheat.

After a gluten-free diet is started, improvement will be apparent within a few days or weeks. Generally, 30 percent of people with celiac disease respond within three days, another 50 percent within one month, and 10 percent within another month. However, 10 percent of individuals respond only after twenty-four to thirty-six months of avoiding gluten.

Maintenance of a strictly gluten-free diet is quite difficult in the United States, due to the wide distribution of gliadin in processed foods. Individuals with celiac disease must be encouraged to read labels carefully in order to avoid hidden sources of gliadin, such as gluten-containing grains found in some brands of soy sauce—tamari is wheat-free, while shoyu contains wheat; modified food starch; ice cream; soups; and alcohol, such as beer, wine, vodka, whiskey, and malt. Many gluten-free products are available in natural food stores and online catalogs. In the U.K. in recent years, the main supermarket chains have introduced special "gluten-free" lines such as flour, bread, pasta, cakes and Yorkshire puddings. Labeling on foods has also been improved so it is easier to find gluten-free products. A guide, *The Gluten-Free Food and Drink Directory*, is published (and updated monthly) by the Coeliac Society. It lists all types of commonly available food and drink and their gluten status. Certain staple foods are also available on prescription from the NHS.

The absence of gluten in sorghum (which is not common in the U.K.), combined with its excellent nutritional and phytochemical profile, make this grain a contender in the market for those with celiac sprue disease. Other beneficial grains for replacement of gluten-containing grains include amaranth, quinoa, and a variety of rices, such as brown, red, black, and wild.

Other Recommendations

The protein-digesting enzyme in papaya, papain, has been shown to be able to digest wheat gluten and render it harmless in celiac disease subjects. Taking a papain supplement (500–1,000 milligrams) with meals may allow some individuals to tolerate small amounts of gluten.

There are also some excellent resources for more information on celiac disease and gluten-free recipes:

Gluten Intolerance Group
15110 10th Avenue SW, Suite A
Seattle, WA 98166-1820
Web site: www.gluten.net

Celiac Sprue Association
P.O. Box 31700
Omaha, NE 68131-0700
Web site: www.csaceliacs.org

Celiac Disease Foundation
13251 Ventura Boulevard, Suite 1
Studio City, CA 91604
Web site: www.celiac.org

Coeliac UK
Suites A–D
Octagon Court
High Wycombe
Buckinghamshire HP11 2HS
www.coeliac.co.uk

Cervical Dysplasia

Cervical dysplasia is the appearance of abnormal cells on the surface of the cervix. These abnormal cells are detected by a Pap smear, a sample of cells collected from the surface of the cervix. Cervical dysplasia is generally regarded as a precancerous lesion; in other words, it is not a cancerous state, but if untreated it could lead to cancer of the cervix.

Signs and Symptoms

Cervical dysplasia does not have any symptoms. It is discovered by a Pap smear. It is the presence of abnormal but not yet cancerous cells. Cervical dysplasia, if untreated, can progress to cervical cancer, which also is asymptomatic until the late stages.

Causes

Recently, attention has focused on the role of the human papillomavirus (HPV) as the major cause of cervical dysplasia. The risk factors for becoming infected with HPV and developing cervical dysplasia include early age at first intercourse; multiple sexual partners or a sexual encounter with someone who has had multiple partners; herpes simplex type 2; smoking; oral contraceptive pill use; and many nutritional factors, such as deficiency of vitamin A and folic acid.

Food Prescriptions

A high fat intake has been associated with increased risk of cervical cancer, while a diet rich in fruits and vegetables offers significant protection against carcinogenesis, probably due to its higher content of fiber, beta-carotenes, and vitamin C. If you have HPV, cervical dysplasia or risk factors for developing cervical dysplasia, we recommend eating five or more servings daily of a combination of vegetables and fruits, especially green, orange, and yellow vegetables; berries; and citrus fruits. Folic acid is an important nutrient to get through eating whole grains, legumes, and leafy green vegetables.

Particularly helpful in fighting HPV and cervical dysplasia are members of the cabbage family of vegetables, including broccoli, Brussels sprouts, cabbages (green, red, Napa, bok choy), collards, kale, mustard greens, radish, rocket and turnip greens. In addition to increasing antioxidant defense mechanisms and improving the body's ability to detoxify and eliminate harmful chemicals and hormones, components in cabbage-family vegetables exert direct activity against HPV, cervical dysplasia, and cervical cancer. Specifically, one of the key phytochemicals in cabbage, indole-3-carbinole (I3C), has been shown to be effective in reversing cervical cancer at dosages of 200 to 400 milligrams per day.

Other Recommendations

Avoid cigarettes, as smoking is a major risk factor for cervical dysplasia and cervical cancer. In fact, the incidence of cervical dysplasia in smokers is two to three times greater than that in nonsmokers. Smoking depresses immune functions, allowing HPV to promote abnormal cellular development; it depletes body stores of vitamin C; and cervical cells may concentrate carcinogenic compounds from inhaled smoke.

Cholesterol, Elevated

Cholesterol is a fatty substance in the body that serves several vital roles. It is a building block for various hormones and bile acids; and it plays a major role in stabilizing cell membranes. While proper cholesterol levels are important to good health, the evidence overwhelmingly demonstrates that elevated blood cholesterol levels greatly increase the risk of death due to heart disease. (See also "Atherosclerosis.")

Cholesterol is transported in the blood by lipoproteins. The major categories of lipoproteins are very-low-density lipoprotein (VLDL), low-density lipoprotein (LDL), and high-density lipoprotein (HDL). VLDL and LDL are responsible for transporting fats (primarily triglycerides and cholesterol) from the liver to body cells, and elevation of either VLDL or LDL is associated with an increased risk of developing atherosclerosis, the primary cause of heart attack and stroke. In contrast, HDL is responsible for returning fats to the liver, and elevations of HDL are associated with a low risk of heart attack.

Currently, experts recommend that your total blood cholesterol level should be less than 200 milligrams per deciliter (5.18 mmol/liter) from a fasting blood sample. (See the British Heart Foundation website, www.bhf.org.uk, for further information.) The HDL level should be greater than 40 milligrams per deciliter (1.04 mmol/liter). The LDL level limit is based on your current health history and risk factors:

• Less than 100 milligrams per deciliter (2.59 mmol/liter) for people who have coronary heart disease. These people have had a myocardial infarction, angina, or a revascularization procedure, such as a coronary bypass surgery. The same limit applies to people who have not had one of these cardiac events but have atherosclerosis outside of the heart, such as carotid artery or other peripheral arterial disease, diabetes, or an elevated ten-year risk estimate, as determined by a physician.

- Less than 130 milligrams per deciliter (3.37 mmol/liter) for people who do not have coronary heart disease or equivalent risk for it but have two or more risk factors. Risk factors include age, lack of physical activity, smoking, and being overweight.

- Less than 160 milligrams per deciliter (4.14 mmol/liter) for people who have no or one risk factor for coronary heart disease.

For every 1 percent drop in LDL levels, there's a 2 percent drop in the risk of heart attack. By the same token, for every 1 percent increase in HDL, the risk of heart attack drops by 3 to 4 percent.

The ratio of your total cholesterol to HDL and the ratio of LDL to HDL are clues that indicate whether cholesterol is being deposited into tissues or is being broken down and excreted. The ratio of total cholesterol to HDL should be no higher than 4.2:1, and the LDL to HDL ratio should be no higher than 2.5:1.

Another important lipoprotein to be aware of is a form of LDL called lipoprotein (a), or Lp(a). This form of LDL has an additional molecule of an adhesive protein called apolipoprotein. That protein makes the molecule much more likely to stick to the artery walls and cause damage. New research suggests that high Lp(a) levels constitute a separate risk factor for heart attack. For example, it appears that high Lp(a) levels are ten times as likely to cause heart disease as high LDL levels. Lp(a) levels lower than 20 milligrams per deciliter (0.52 mmol/liter) are associated with low risk of heart disease; levels from 20 to 40 milligrams per deciliter (0.52 to 1.04 mmol/liter) pose a moderate risk; and levels higher than 40 milligrams per deciliter (1.04 mmol/liter) are considered extremely risky.

Signs and Symptoms

Elevated blood cholesterol is usually without symptoms. However, elevated cholesterol leads to atherosclerosis in the arteries of the heart, called coronary heart disease, and elsewhere, called peripheral vascular disease. Development of atherosclerosis is associated with angina, diabetes, high blood pressure, and myocardial infarction (heart attack).

Causes

Elevated cholesterol levels are usually due to an increased manufacture of cholesterol within the liver rather than an increased dietary intake of cholesterol. However, elevated cholesterol levels are also reflective of dietary and lifestyle factors, such as high saturated fat intake and lack of physical exercise. Elevated cholesterol can also be due to genetic factors.

Food Prescriptions

See "Atherosclerosis," page 691.

There are many ways to approach lowering cholesterol, including decreasing absorption, increasing excretion, and decreasing production. Preventing oxidation of cholesterol also reduces the propensity for cholesterol to contribute to atherosclerosis. Many of the foods discussed below perform one or more of these actions. Also, many foods have shown a cholesterol-lowering effect, but the mechanism of how this occurs has yet to be understood. For people with normal cholesterol levels, many of these foods do not affect their cholesterol levels. For each of these foods, further details can be found under their description in Part III.

Fiber generally helps to lower cholesterol by binding to bile acids and removing them from the body via the faeces. Fiber comes primarily from whole grains, fruits, vegetables, and legumes. Eat a variety of whole grains, particularly oats and barley, which are rich in the special cholesterol-lowering soluble fiber beta-D-glucan. Bran from whole grains, such as barley, oat, rice, and wheat bran, can also be eaten.

Although oatmeal's fiber content (7 percent) is less than that of oat bran (15 to 26 percent), it has been determined that the polyunsaturated fatty acids contribute as much to the cholesterol-lowering effects of oats as the fiber content. This makes oat bran and oatmeal quite similar in effectiveness.

In addition to the fiber components, other grain components help to lower cholesterol. Rice bran contains gamma-oryzanol, a compound that only lowers cholesterol. Amaranth contains tocotrienols (a vitamin E fraction) and squalene (a fatty acid), both of which are known to reduce cholesterol synthesis. Also, diets rich in buckwheat have been linked to lowered risk of developing high cholesterol due to buckwheat's content of hesperidin, a beneficial flavonoid. Anthocyanin flavonoids are found in sorghum (this is not common in the U.K.) but not in most other grains and are powerful antioxidants that research shows exhibit potent free radical-scavenging activity.

Eat a variety of fruits for their antioxidant effects (see "Flavonoids," page 145) and soluble fiber. Pectin is a soluble fiber that can help lower cholesterol levels through decreasing both absorption and synthesis of cholesterol and is found in apples, bananas, grapefruit, oranges, and pears. Whole fruit contains more pectin than fruit juice. Two pieces of these fruits per day contain enough pectin to reduce the risk of heart disease by 20 percent. Dates also contain the soluble fiber beta-D-glucan.

Prunes contain large amounts of phenolic compounds, which inhibit free-radical damage to LDL cholesterol. Olives and olive oil also contain antioxidants, including oleuroprein and flavonoids, that act to protect against damage to LDL cholesterol. In contrast, deep-fried foods have been linked to high levels of damaged LDL and to thickening of larger-artery walls.

When attempting to lower cholesterol through diet, it is important to eat a variety of cholesterol-lowering vegetables, including celery, beetroot, aubergine, garlic and onion, peppers, and root vegetables. In addition, dandelion root and Jerusalem artichoke contain the fiber inulin, which improves production of antioxidant enzymes while decreasing total cholesterol and triglyceride levels and raising concentrations of beneficial HDL cholesterol.

Peppers, especially chilis, contain substances that have been shown to prevent clot formation and reduce the risk for heart attacks and strokes by reducing blood cholesterol and triglyceride levels and platelet aggregation, and increasing fibrinolytic activity. Although bell peppers are not as rich in these compounds as chili peppers,

WARNING: *If you are taking a prescription medication for lowering cholesterol, ask your doctor if you should avoid eating grapefruit or drinking grapefruit juice. Grapefruit reduces the activity of enzymes in the liver that your body uses to break down cholesterol-lowering "statin" drugs. If the drugs are not metabolized, they remain in the body in higher concentrations. This increases the risk of unwanted toxic effects, such as liver or muscle damage.*

they are still important in the diet of individuals with elevated cholesterol levels.

Diets rich in legumes, including peanuts, are being used to lower cholesterol levels, and soy protein has been shown in some studies to be able to lower total cholesterol levels by 30 percent and to lower LDL, or "bad," cholesterol levels by as much as 35 to 40 percent.

Nuts and seeds, particularly almonds and walnuts, are also quite useful in fighting against heart disease by lowering cholesterol through their fiber, monounsaturated oil, and essential fatty acid content. Hazelnuts have an exceptional concentration of copper, a key component in the intracellular form of an important antioxidant enzyme called superoxide dismutase, which disarms free radicals that would otherwise damage cholesterol and other lipids. Ground linseed lowers two cholesterol-carrying molecules, apolipoprotein A-1 and apolipoprotein B. Other foods that have shown beneficial effects on lowering cholesterol include avocados, cocoa butter, brewer's yeast, royal jelly, shiitake mushrooms, saffron, turmeric, honey, shellfish, and alfalfa sprouts.

Milk and cheese are often loaded with fat and cholesterol. However, milk fat also contains a number of bioactive components, including conjugated linoleic acid (CLA). Conjugated linoleic acid has been shown to possess activities that prevent cancer and the formation of cholesterol-containing plaques that contribute to heart disease.

Cheese provides many of the same nutritional benefits and health benefits attributed to milk, and it usually contains beneficial bacteria that produce propionic acid, which nourishes the cells of the colon and lowers blood cholesterol levels.

It is important to point out that while eggs are high in cholesterol (213 milligrams per egg) and many public health advocates have long recommended that individuals with high cholesterol levels avoid eggs, several recent studies have indicated that moderate egg consumption has little effect on cholesterol levels.

Other Recommendations

There are a number of specific natural medicines that effectively lower cholesterol levels. Since new ones come along all the time, it is easy to forget just how impressive the results with niacin (vitamin B3) have been.

The cholesterol-lowering activity of niacin was first described in the 1950s. It is now known that niacin does much more than lower total cholesterol. Specifically, niacin has been shown to lower LDL cholesterol, Lp(a) lipoprotein, triglyceride, and fibrinogen levels while simultaneously raising HDL cholesterol levels. Despite the fact that niacin has demonstrated better overall results in reducing risk factors for coronary heart disease than other cholesterol-lowering agents, physicians are often reluctant to prescribe niacin. The reason is a widespread perception that niacin is difficult to work with because of the bothersome side effect of flushing of the skin. In addition, since niacin is a widely available generic agent, no pharmaceutical company stands to earn the huge profits that the other lipid-lowering agents have generated. As a result, niacin does not benefit from the intensive advertising that focuses upon the statin drugs. Despite the advantages of niacin over other lipid-lowering drugs, it accounts for less than 10 percent of all cholesterol-lowering prescriptions.

Several studies have compared niacin to standard lipid-lowering drugs, including the statin drugs. These studies have shown significant advantages for niacin. For example, in one twenty-six-week study, patients were randomly assigned to receive treatment with either lovastatin (Mevacor) or niacin. The results indicated that while lovastatin produced a greater LDL cholesterol reduction, niacin provided better overall results despite the fact that fewer patients were able to tolerate a full dosage of niacin because of skin flushing. The percentage increase in HDL cholesterol, a more significant indicator for coronary heart disease, was dramatically in favor of niacin (33 percent versus 7 percent). Equally as impressive was the percentage decrease in Lp(a) for niacin. While niacin produced a 35 percent reduction in Lp(a) lipoprotein levels, lovastatin did not produce any effect. Other studies have shown that niacin can lower Lp(a) levels by an average of 38 percent.

The most recent comparative study involved niacin versus atorvastatin (Lipitor). The average dosage was 3,000 milligrams of niacin, and atorvastatin was used at 80 milligrams per day. The patients selected had abnormal LDL particle size in that the molecules were small and dense—these LDL molecules are considerably more atherogenic than larger, less dense LDL. The patients selected also had low levels (less than 40 percent) of a specific fraction of HDL associated with a greater protective effect than HDL alone. Although atorvastatin reduced total LDL cholesterol levels substantially more than niacin, niacin was more effective in increasing LDL particle size and raising HDL than the atorvastatin was.

Because taking niacin at higher dosages (3,000 milligrams or more) can impair glucose tolerance, many physicians have avoided niacin therapy for diabetics, but newer studies with slightly lower dosages (1,000–2,000 milligrams) of niacin have not been shown to adversely affect blood sugar regulation. For example, during a sixteen-week, double-blind, placebo-controlled trial, 148 type 2 diabetes patients were randomized to placebo or to 1,000 or 1,500 milligrams per day of niacin; in the niacin-treated groups, there was no significant loss in glycemic control, and the favorable effects on blood lipids were still apparent.

The side effect of skin flushing typically occurs twenty to thirty minutes after the niacin is taken and disappears in about the same time frame. Other occasional side effects of niacin include gastric irritation, nausea, and liver damage. To reduce the side effect of skin flushing, you can use some of the newer time-released formulas, including the prescription version Niaspan, or take the niacin just before going to bed. Most people sleep right through the flushing reaction. Taking cholesterol-lowering agents at night is best because most of the liver's manufacture of cholesterol happens at night. Another approach to reducing flushing is to use inositol hexaniacinate. This form of niacin has long been used in Europe to lower cholesterol levels and also to improve blood flow in intermittent claudication, a peripheral vascular disease that is quite common in diabetics. It yields slightly better clinical results than standard niacin and is much better tolerated in terms of both skin flushing and, more important, long-term side effects. If you start out by trying inositol hexaniacinate and it does not work, try regular niacin. Our experience is that some people respond only to the regular niacin.

If regular niacin or inositol hexaniacinate is being used, start with a dose of 500 milligrams before going to bed at night for one week. Increase the dosage to 1,000 milligrams the next week and 1,500 milligrams the following week. Stay at the 1,500 milligram dosage for two months before checking the response; dosage can be adjusted up or down depending upon the response. If you are using a time-release niacin product, such as Niaspan, start out at the full dosage of 1,500 milligrams at night. Regardless of the form of niacin being used, we strongly recommend periodic checking (minimum every three months) of cholesterol and liver function tests.

Cold, Common

The common cold is an upper respiratory tract infection that is caused by a virus.

Signs and Symptoms

Typically, an individual with a cold experiences general malaise, fever, headache, and upper respiratory tract congestion. The initial symptoms are usually a watery nasal discharge and sneezing, followed by thicker secretions containing mucus, white blood cells, and dead organisms. The throat may be red, sore, and quite dry. The common cold typically lasts anywhere from four to ten days.

Causes

We are all constantly exposed to many viruses, yet the majority of us experience the discomfort of a "cold" only once or twice a year at most. This scenario suggests that a decrease in resistance or immune function is the major factor in "catching" a cold.

Food Prescriptions

Increasing fluid consumption maintains a moist respiratory tract that can repel viral infection. Drinking plenty of liquids will also improve the function of white blood cells by decreasing the concentration of compounds that are in solution in the blood. The type of liquids you consume is very important. Studies have shown that consuming concentrated sources of sugars, such as glucose, fructose, sucrose, honey, or fruit juice, including orange juice, greatly reduces the ability of the white blood cells to kill bacteria. Before being consumed, fruit juices should be greatly diluted. Keep your daily intake of undiluted fruit juices to 4 to 8 ounces/125 to 240 milliliters.

Garlic also has a long history of use as an infection fighter. Its antimicrobial activity is due to allicin, the main pungent principle produced from raw garlic.

Jerusalem artichokes also have some immune-enhancing activity, as inulin has the ability to enhance a component of our immune system known as complement, which is responsible for increasing host defense mechanisms, such as neutralization of viruses.

Cinnamon-containing formulas are useful in cases of the common cold, influenza, and frostbite. Here is a great tea to have when you feel a cold coming on:

> One 1-inch/2½-centimetre slice of fresh ginger
> ¼ teaspoon cinnamon
> ¼ lemon
> 1 cup hot water

If you own a juice extractor, juice the ginger and lemon and add them to the water. If not, grind the ginger and squeeze the juice from ½ lemon and add them to the water.

Other Recommendations

Once a cold develops, there are several things that can speed up recovery. If you start soon enough, you may be able to shed the cold quickly. However, if the virus has already established a firm foothold, it may take you a couple of days to throw it off completely.

Do not expect immediate relief in most instances when using natural substances for cold symptom relief, since most natural therapies for colds involve assisting the body rather than the familiar drug action of suppressing the symptoms. In fact, the symptoms of the cold can temporarily worsen when using natural remedies. How can this be? Many of the symptoms of the cold are a result of our body's defense mechanisms. For example, the potent immune-stimulating compound interferon, released by our blood cells and other tissues during infections, is responsible for many flulike symptoms. Another example is the beneficial effect of fever on the course of infection. While an elevated body temperature can be uncomfortable, suppression of fever is thought to counteract a major defense mechanism and prolong the infection. In general, fever should not be suppressed during an infection unless it is dangerously high (>104 degrees F./40 degrees C.). For these and other reasons, it is not uncommon for the individual treating him- or herself for the common cold with natural medicines to experience a greater degree of discomfort due to the immune-enhancing effects of these compounds. On the plus side, though, the illness is generally much shorter-lived.

The most popular herbal treatment for the common cold is echinacea. Modern research has shown echinacea to exert significant effects on immune function in more than 300 scientific investigations. However, not all of the clinical studies have been positive. Mixed results from clinical studies with echinacea are most likely due to lack of, or insufficient quantity of, active compounds. What determines the effectiveness of any herbal product is its ability to deliver an effective dosage of active compounds. Chemical analysis of commercial echinacea preparations has demonstrated tremendous variation in the levels of key compounds even from batch to batch of the same product. Many manufacturers are not employing the necessary quality control tests required to ensure that the echinacea is being grown properly and is harvested at the exact time for maximal levels of all active compounds.

Since echinacea contains a wide assortment of chemical constituents with confirmed immune-enhancing effects, it is important for manufacturers to ensure sufficient levels of all these active compounds. The best assurance for consumers wanting the full benefit of echinacea is to use a product from a trusted manufacturer that guarantees the level of active ingredients. Many experts now consider Echinamide, a patented, superextracted echinacea product developed and marketed by Natural Factors, to be the ultimate echinacea product (this product is not currently available in the U.K.). Dr. Rudolf Bauer, of the University of Graz, Austria, has conducted and published more research on echinacea than any other person. His research has been critical not only to the understanding of echinacea but also to its growing acceptance as an immune-enhancing agent. According to Dr. Bauer, "Echinamide is unique in that it has certain standardized levels of polysaccharides, cichoric acid, and alkylamides." Double-blind clinical studies have validated the effectiveness of Echinamide. The proper dosage of Echinamide is clearly indicated on the bottle.

Constipation

Constipation is the inability to defecate. The frequency of defecation and the consistency and volume of stools vary so greatly from individual to individual that it is difficult to determine normal function. In general, most nutritionally oriented physicians recommend at least one bowel movement a day.

Signs and Symptoms

Hard, small, and difficult-to-pass stools are the most frequent complaint of those suffering from constipation. Also, elimination less than once daily indicates constipation. Associated symptoms can include wind, bloating, and abdominal pain.

Causes

There are a number of possible causes of constipation, but the most common is a low-fiber diet. Other common causes include inadequate fluid intake, lack of physical activity, various medications (e.g., anesthetics, antacids, and diuretics), low thyroid function, and irritable bowel syndrome.

Food Prescriptions

It is well established that a low-fiber diet causes constipation. Equally well established in treating chronic constipation is the efficacy of dietary changes that increase fiber intake. A high-fiber diet, plentiful fluid consumption, and exercise are an effective prescription in most cases of constipation. High levels of dietary fiber both increase the frequency and quantity of bowel movements and decrease the transit time of the stool (the amount of time between consumption of a food and its elimination in the faeces) and the absorption of toxins from the stool, and appear to be a preventive factor in several diseases. Particularly effective in relieving constipation are cereal bran, such as oat, rice, or wheat, radishes, and prunes. The typical recommendation for bran is ⅓ cup of bran cereal per day. When using bran, make sure to consume enough liquids; drink at least six to eight glasses of water per day. Whole prunes, as well as prune juice, also have good laxative effects. Eight ounces/240 grams per day is usually effective.

Cow's milk consumption was determined to be the cause of constipation in roughly two thirds of children with constipation, according to studies published in the prestigious *New England Journal of Medicine*. Presumably, the same holds for adults as well.

Other Recommendations

If you have been using stimulant laxatives, even natural ones, such as senna or *Cascara sagrada,* you will need to "retrain" your bowels to get them to function normally without them. Here is the programme that we recommend for reestablishing bowel regularity. It usually takes four to six weeks.

- Find and eliminate known causes of constipation.
- Never repress an urge to defecate.
- Add bran cereals to the diet and eat more high-fiber foods, such as whole grains, fruits, and vegetables.
- Drink six to eight glasses of fluid per day.
- Sit on the toilet at the same time every day (even when the urge to defecate is not present), preferably immediately after breakfast or exercise.

- Exercise for at least twenty minutes, three times per week.
- In the first week, every night before bed, take a stimulant laxative containing either *Cascara* or senna. Take the smallest amount necessary to ensure a bowel movement every morning.
- In each subsequent week, decrease the laxative dosage by half. If constipation recurs, go back to the previous week's dosage. Decrease the dosage if diarrhea occurs.

Depression

Depression is characterized by feelings of low self-esteem, pessimism, and despair. It can range from a transient "low mood" to a potentially life-threatening, severe clinical depression.

Signs and Symptoms

Clinical depression is more than feeling depressed. The official definition of clinical depression is based on the following eight primary criteria:

1. Poor appetite accompanied by weight loss, or increased appetite accompanied by weight gain.
2. Insomnia or excessive sleep habits (hypersomnia).
3. Physical hyperactivity or inactivity.
4. Loss of interest or pleasure in usual activities or decrease in sexual drive.
5. Loss of energy; feelings of fatigue.

6. Feelings of worthlessness, self-reproach, or inappropriate guilt.
7. Diminished ability to think or concentrate.
8. Recurrent thoughts of death or suicide.

The presence of five of these eight symptoms indicates clinical depression; an individual with four is probably depressed. The symptoms must be present for at least one month to be called clinical depression.

Causes

Depression can be the result of psychological or physiological factors. The most significant psychological theory is the "learned helplessness" model, which theorizes that depression is the result of habitual feelings of pessimism and hopelessness. The chief physiological theory is the "monoamine hypothesis," which stresses imbalances of monoamine neurotransmitters, such as serotonin, adrenaline/epinephrine, and noradrenaline/norepinephrine. Serotonin deficiency is the most common biochemical cause.

It is important to rule out simple organic factors that are known to contribute to depression, such as nutrient deficiency; drug use, including of many prescription and illicit drugs; consumption of alcohol, caffeine, and nicotine; hypoglycemia; hypothyroidism; and food allergy.

Food Prescriptions

A deficiency of any single nutrient can alter brain function and lead to depression, anxiety, and other mental disorders, especially deficiencies of vitamin B12, folic acid, other B vitamins, and omega-3 fatty acids. Alcohol utilizes many of these nutrients in its metabolism, and drinking alcohol regularly replaces calories one would otherwise get from food. In this case, nutrients are just not adequately consumed, and those that are consumed are often needed to rid the body of the alcohol. In the case of hypothyroidism, inadequate iodine intake can be a cause.

Since the brain requires a constant supply of blood sugar to function properly, hypoglycemia must be avoided. Symptoms of hypoglycemia can range from mild to severe and include depression, anxiety, irritability, and other psychological disturbances; fatigue; headache; blurred vision; excessive sweating; mental confusion; incoherent speech; bizarre behavior; and convulsions. Several studies have shown hypoglycemia to be very common in depressed individuals. Simply eliminating refined carbohydrates and caffeine (which can aggravate hypoglycemia) from the diet is sometimes all that is needed for effective therapy in patients whose depression results from reactive hypoglycemia.

Food allergy is also a significant factor in some people suffering from depression. Eliminating offending foods can bring about tremendous relief.

Other Recommendations

Saint John's wort (*Hypericum perforatum*) extract is a now well-known natural antidepressant. More than thirty double-blind studies involving more than 2,000 patients with mild to moderate depression have shown Saint John's wort extract to be very effective. However, while Saint John's wort extract appears to be as effective as or possibly even more effective than conventional antidepressant drugs in mild to moderate depression, it does not appear to be as effective as conventional drugs in severe depression.

No significant side effects have been reported in the numerous double-blind studies. In a large-scale safety study involving 3,250 patients conducted in Germany, undesired side effects were reported in 79 patients (2.43 percent). The most frequently noted side effects were gastrointestinal irritation (0.55 percent), allergic reactions (0.52 percent), fatigue (0.4 percent), and restlessness (0.26 percent).

People taking prescription drugs need to check with their doctor or pharmacist before taking Saint John's wort extract, as it appears to induce enzymes in the liver and gut that detoxify certain drugs. Drugs that are metabolized by these enzymes include cyclosporine; digoxin; indinavir; oral contraceptives; theophylline; tricyclic antidepressants, such as amitriptyline; and anticoagulants, such as warfarin (Coumadin). Do not use Saint John's wort if you are taking any of these drugs without consulting a physician first.

Saint John's wort extract may also potentiate prescription antidepressant and antianxiety drugs. There is one case report of simultaneous use of Saint John's wort and paroxetine (Aropax/Paxil) producing nausea, fatigue, lethargy, and weakness. Do not use Saint John's wort if you are taking a prescription antidepressant or antianxiety drug without consulting a physician first.

Diabetes Mellitus

Diabetes mellitus is a chronic disorder of carbohydrate, fat, and protein metabolism characterized by fasting elevations of blood sugar (glucose) levels and a greatly increased risk of heart disease, stroke, kidney disease, retinopathy, and loss of nerve function. Diabetes can occur when the pancreas does not secrete enough insulin or when the cells of the body become resistant to insulin. In either case, the blood sugar cannot get into the cells for storage, which then leads to serious complications.

Diabetes is divided into two major categories: type 1 and type 2. Type 1, or insulin-dependent, diabetes mellitus occurs most often in children and adolescents and is associated with complete destruction of the beta cells of the pancreas, which manufacture the hormone insulin. Type 1 diabetics require lifelong insulin for the control of blood sugar levels. Type 2, or non-insulin-dependent, diabetes mellitus (NIDDM), usually has an onset after forty years of age, although the incidence of type 2 diabetes in children and adolescents has increased dramatically in the last decade. About 90 percent of all diabetics are type 2. Initially, their insulin levels are typically elevated, indicating a loss of sensitivity to insulin by the cells of the body, otherwise known as insulin resistance.

Other types of diabetes include:

• Secondary diabetes, which is a form of diabetes that is secondary to other conditions, such as pancreatic disease, hormone disturbances, medication use, and malnutrition.

- Gestational diabetes, which is a form of glucose intolerance that occurs during pregnancy.
- Impaired glucose tolerance, which is a condition that includes prediabetic or borderline diabetes. Individuals with impaired glucose tolerance have blood glucose levels and glucose tolerance test (GTT) results that are intermediate between normal and clearly abnormal.

Signs and Symptoms

The classic symptoms of type 1 diabetes are frequent urination, excessive thirst, and excessive appetite. In type 2 diabetes, these symptoms may also be present but are usually much milder than in type 1. As a result, since these symptoms are not very serious, many people who have symptoms of diabetes do not seek medical care. In fact, of the more than 10 million Americans with diabetes, fewer than half know that they have diabetes or ever have consulted a physician. There are over 2 million people with diabetes in the U.K. and an estimated 1 million more with undiagnosed diabetes. The following criteria are used for diagnosing diabetes:

- Fasting (overnight): Serum glucose (blood sugar) concentration greater than or equal to 140 milligrams per deciliter/7.8 mmol/liter on at least two separate occasions.
- Following ingestion of 75 grams of glucose: Serum glucose concentration greater than or equal to 200 milligrams per deciliter/11.1 mmol/liter at two hours postingestion and at least one other sample during the two-hour test.

Causes

Although the exact cause of type 1 diabetes is unknown, current theory suggests that an autoimmune process leads to destruction of the insulin-producing beta cells in the pancreas. Antibodies to beta cells are present in 75 percent of all type 1 diabetics, compared to .5 to 2 percent of nondiabetics. The antibodies to the beta cells appear to develop in response to cell destruction due to other mechanisms, including chemical, free-radical, and viral, and food allergy.

In contrast, obesity is a major contributing factor to the development of insulin resistance in approximately 90 percent of individuals with type 2 diabetes. In most cases, achieving ideal body weight is associated with restoration of normal blood sugar levels in these patients.

Food Prescriptions

Diabetes, perhaps more than any other disease, is strongly associated with Western culture and diet, as it is uncommon in cultures consuming a more "primitive" diet. However, as cultures switch from their native diets to the "foods of commerce," their rate of diabetes increases, eventually reaching the same proportions seen in Western societies.

Dietary modification and treatment are fundamental to the successful treatment of both type 1 and type 2 diabetes. The dietary guidelines provided in chapter 2 are especially important to follow for prevention and treatment. All simple, processed, and concentrated carbohydrates must be avoided. Low-glycemic-load foods (see Appendix A) should be stressed, and saturated fats should be kept to a minimum.

Since diabetics have a higher incidence of death from cardiovascular disease (60 to 70 percent, versus 20 to 25 percent in people without diabetes), the dietary recommendations under "Atherosclerosis," page 691, are equally appropriate here. It may also be advisable for those with type 1 diabetes to avoid milk and wheat gluten (see page 585).

Weight loss, in particular a significant decrease in body fat percentage, is a prime objective in treating the majority of type 2 diabetics; it improves all aspects of diabetes and may result in cure. And for both type 1 and type 2 diabetics, there are some specific foods that have been shown to produce positive effects on blood sugar control. These foods include olives, soybeans and other legumes, nuts, artichokes, bitter melon, garlic, Jerusalem artichokes, mangoes, and onions. These foods all have a low glycemic index and glycemic load and are high in fiber. High-chromium brewer's yeast may also be helpful, since it contains chromium in the organic form of glucose tolerance factor. Please note that chromium-enriched brewer's yeast may affect blood glucose and insulin levels. Therefore people with diabetes or hypoglycemia should consult their doctors before using it as a supplement.

Cinnamon may also be helpful in controlling blood sugar levels. According to research, cinnamon may act as an insulin substitute in type 2 diabetes. A double-blind study of sixty people with type 2 diabetes revealed a significant decrease in fasting serum glucose (18 to 29 percent), triglyceride (23 to 30 percent), LDL cholesterol (7 to 27 percent), and total cholesterol (12 to 26 percent) levels after taking cinnamon for forty days. The effective dosage was as little as 1 gram (roughly ¼ teaspoon) per day.

Other Recommendations

Exercise is critical to achieving good blood sugar control. A graded exercise programme should be developed based on the individual's fitness level and interest, yet it should elevate the heart rate to at least 60 percent of maximum for a half hour, three times a week.

For more information, please consult *How to Prevent and Treat Diabetes with Natural Medicine.*

Diarrhea

Diarrhea is the excretion of extra fluid with a bowel movement. Diarrhea is usually a mild, temporary event. However, it may also be the first suggestion of a serious underlying disease or infection.

Signs and Symptoms

Diarrhea typically presents with loose or watery bowel movements that may be accompanied by undigested food or mucus. Urgency to defecate and lower abdominal pain can also occur with diarrhea. If an infection is present, there may also be a fever.

Causes

Diarrhea is divided into four major types: osmotic, secretory, exudative, and inadequate-contact.

- *Osmotic diarrhea* can be the result of carbohydrate malabsorption (e.g., lactose intolerance); magnesium salts; and excess vitamin C intake.

- *Secretory diarrhea* can be the result of toxin-producing bacteria; hormone-producing tumors; fat malabsorption (e.g., lack of bile output); laxative abuse; and surgical resection of the small intestine.

- *Exudative diarrhea* can be caused by inflammatory bowel disease (Crohn's disease or ulcerative colitis); pseudomembranous colitis (a postantibiotic diarrhea caused by an overgrowth of the bacterium *Clostridium difficile*); and bacterial infection by other organisms.

- *Inadequate-contact diarrhea* is the result of surgical removal of sections of the intestine.

Food Prescriptions

Here are the key dietary recommendations typically given people with any of the four types of diarrhea:

- Don't eat solid foods. During the acute phase of diarrhea, no solid foods should be consumed. Instead, the focus should be on liquid.

- Replace water and electrolytes by consuming herbal teas, vegetable broths, fruit juices, and electrolyte replacement drinks. An old naturopathic remedy is to sip a drink made of equal parts of sauerkraut and tomato juice.

- Avoid dairy products. Acute intestinal illnesses, such as viral or bacterial intestinal infections, frequently injure the cells that line the small intestine. This results in a temporary deficiency of lactase, the enzyme responsible for digesting the milk sugar (lactose) in dairy products. Avoid dairy products (with the possible exception of live-cultured yogurt) while experiencing diarrhea.

- Avoid food allergens. Food allergy is one of the most common causes of chronic diarrhea. The ingestion of an allergenic food can result in the release of histamine and other allergenic compounds from white blood cells, known as mast cells, that reside in the lining of the intestines. These allergenic compounds can produce a powerful laxative effect.

- During the chronic phase, to help solidify stools, pectin-rich fruits and vegetables, such as pears, apples, grapefruit, carrots, potatoes, and beetroot may offer some benefit. Also, fresh blueberries have a long historical use in treating diarrhea because of their tannins, which firm up a loose stool.

- Carob has been used medicinally as a treatment for diarrhea for centuries, and recent clinical studies have confirmed its clinical effectiveness, particularly for treating infants with diarrhea. Add 1 to 2 teaspoons of carob to stewed apple or other food, two to three times daily.

- Mango has been shown to afford protection against as well as eliminate *Giardia,* a parasite that can be encountered while traveling.

Other Recommendations

Since most acute diarrheal states are self-limited and are usually due to dietary indiscretions or mild gastrointestinal infections, simple dietary approaches should be used first. However, a physician should be consulted immediately if any of the following applies: diarrhea in a child under six years of age; severe or bloody diarrhea; diarrhea that lasts more than three days; and significant signs of dehydration, such as sunken eyes, severe dry mouth, and strong body odor.

Ear Infection (Otitis Media)

In acute ear infection *(otitis media),* the middle ear, including the eardrum, becomes inflamed and infected. Ear infection is usually preceded by an upper respiratory infection or allergy. Chronic ear infection *(serous otitis media)* includes a constant swelling of the middle ear, which can be a fertile breeding ground for an acute ear infection. Recurrent bouts of acute ear infection are responsible for more surgery visits by children to their GP than any other reason.

Signs and Symptoms

An acute ear infection is characterized by earache or irritability; history of recent upper respiratory infection or allergy; red, opaque, bulging eardrum; and fever and chills. Chronic inflammation of the middle ear is characterized by painless hearing loss and a dull, immobile eardrum (tympanic membrane). Since an ear infection can be quite serious, it is necessary for any individual with symptoms of either an acute or chronic ear infection to be seen by a physician.

Causes

The primary risk factors for an ear infection in children are day care attendance, wood-burning stoves, parental smoking (or exposure to other secondhand smoke), and not being breast-fed. Besides day care, where infection is contagious, all of the other factors have something in common: they lead to abnormal eustachian tube function, the underlying cause in virtually all cases of acute ear infection. The eustachian tube regulates air pressure in the middle ear, protects the middle ear from nose and throat secretions and bacteria, and clears fluids from the middle ear. Swallowing causes active opening of the eustachian tube due to the action of the surrounding muscles. Infants and small children are particularly susceptible to eustachian tube problems since theirs are smaller in diameter and more horizontal.

Abnormal eustachian tube function leads first to fluid buildup and then, if bacteria start to grow, bacterial infection. It results from collapse of the tube (due to weak tissues holding the tube in place and/or an abnormal opening mechanism), blockage with mucus in response to allergy or irritation, or infection.

Food Prescriptions

The role of allergy as the major cause of chronic ear infection has been firmly established in the medical literature. Elimination of food allergens has been shown to produce a dramatic effect in the treatment of chronic ear infection in more than 90 percent of children in some studies. Since it is usually not possible to determine the exact allergen during an acute attack, the most common allergenic foods should be eliminated from the diet: milk and dairy products, eggs, wheat, corn, oranges, and peanut butter. The diet should also eliminate concentrated simple carbohydrates, such as sugar, honey, dried fruit, and concentrated fruit juice, since they inhibit the immune system.

Recurrent ear infection is strongly associated with early bottle-feeding, while prolonged breast-feeding (for a minimum of six months) has a protective effect. Whether this is due to an allergy to formula or the protective effect of human milk against infection has not yet been determined. It is probably a combination of both. In addition, prolonged breast-feeding prevents food allergies, particularly if the mother avoids sensitizing foods (i.e., those to which she herself is allergic) during pregnancy and lactation. Also of value is excluding the foods to which children are most commonly allergic: wheat, egg, fowl, and dairy, particularly during the first nine months.

Other Recommendations

Locally applied heat is often very helpful in reducing discomfort. It can be applied as a hot pack, with warm oil (especially mullein oil), or by blowing hot air into the ear. Also of value is putting hygroscopic anhydrous glycerin (available at pharmacies) into the ear. This helps pull fluids out and reduces the pressure in the middle ear.

Eczema

Eczema is an allergic disorder of the skin, although the underlying allergy is often difficult to determine, as in atopic dermatitis or atopic eczema. In allergic contact dermatitis, eczema occurs as a response to an allergen touching the skin. Poison ivy would be a severe case of this condition. Irritant contact dermatitis is a milder form and often occurs with body care products, laundry products, and household cleaners, although other irritants may be implicated as well.

Signs and Symptoms

Eczema is characterized by chronically itchy, inflamed skin. The skin is very red and scaly and may blister and ooze. Scratching and rubbing lead to darkened and hardened areas of thickened skin with accentuated furrows, most commonly seen on the inside of the wrists and elbows, on the face, and on the backs of the knees. Secondary infections of the skin can occur due to repeated scratching. Eczema can resolve and return, but many children seem to simply outgrow eczema.

Causes

Food allergy is the most frequent cause of chronic eczema. Since allergies are often inherited, there is also a tendency for atopic dermatitis to be hereditary.

Food Prescriptions

Elimination of food allergy is the primary goal in dealing with eczema. Although any food or food additive can trigger eczema, eggs, fish, milk, peanuts, soy, and wheat appear to be the most common food allergens. In one study, eggs, milk, and peanuts accounted for roughly 81 percent of all cases of childhood eczema. For more information on dealing with food allergies, see "Food Allergy."

Patients with eczema also appear to have an essential fatty acid deficiency. This results in decreased synthesis of the anti-inflammatory prostaglandins. As a result, there is a relative increase in the prostaglandins that promote inflammation. Increasing the dietary intake of the omega-3 essential fatty acids, either by eating more fatty fish (e.g., mackerel, herring, and salmon) or through consuming linseed oil or fish oil supplements, can be of benefit. However, if fish allergy is suspected, a molecularly distilled fish oil product should be used.

Other Recommendations

A number of herbal substances have demonstrated an effect equal or superior to cortisone's when applied topically. *Glycyrrhiza glabra* (licorice) and *Matricaria chamomilla* (German chamomile) are the most active. Proprietary formulas containing these botanicals may be quite beneficial for the temporary relief of eczema.

It is also important to avoid rough-textured clothing; wash clothing with a mild soap and rinse it thoroughly; and avoid exposure to chemical irritants and any other agents that might cause skin irritation.

Fibrocystic Breast Disease

Fibrocystic breast disease (FBD), also known as cystic mastitis, is a benign breast condition associated with the presence of multiple cysts in the breast tissue. FBD is usually a component of premenstrual syndrome (PMS) and is considered a risk factor for breast cancer. It is not, however, as significant a factor as the classic breast cancer risk factors: family history, early onset of menstruation (menarche), and late or no first pregnancy.

Signs and Symptoms

FBD is characterized by the presence of multiple cysts of varying sizes, which give the breast a nodular consistency. Typically, FBD worsens premenstrually and may be associated with breast pain and tenderness.

Causes

FBD is apparently the result of an increased oestrogen-to-progesterone ratio. However, other hormones also play important roles. For example, the changes within the breast in FBD may be due to the hormone prolactin. Typically, significantly elevated levels of prolactin are found in women with FBD. The levels are higher than normal, but not so high as to cause loss of menstruation (amenorrhea). The increase in prolactin is thought to be the result of higher oestrogen levels.

Dietary Considerations

The diet should emphasize whole, unprocessed foods: whole grains, legumes, vegetables, fruits, nuts, and seeds. Emphasize foods high in vitamin B6, which helps detoxify oestrogen. Drink at least 48 ounces/1½ liters of water daily. These recommendations can help promote regular bowel movements. Women who have fewer than three bowel movements per week have a four and a half times greater rate of FBD than women who have at least one bowel movement a day. This association is probably due to the bacterial flora in the large intestine transforming excreted steroids into toxic derivatives or allowing these excreted steroids to be reabsorbed.

Eliminate caffeine. Population studies, experimental evidence, and clinical evaluations indicate a strong association between caffeine consumption and FBD. In one study, limiting consumption of coffee, tea, cola, chocolate, and caffeinated medications resulted in improvement in 97.5 percent of the forty-five women who completely abstained and in 75 percent of the twenty-eight who limited their consumption.

Other Recommendations

It is important to consult a physician immediately if you notice a lump of any kind. Although pain, cyclic variations in size, high mobility, and multiplicity of nodules are indicative of FBD, further steps are usually necessary to rule out breast cancer. Noninvasive procedures, such as ultrasound, can help to aid differentiation further, but at this time definitive diagnosis depends upon biopsy. It is better to be safe than sorry. The effective treatment for most types of breast cancer is dependent upon early diagnosis.

Several double-blind clinical studies have shown vitamin E to relieve many premenstrual symptoms, including FBD. The mode of action remains obscure, although vitamin E has been shown to normalize circulating hormones in PMS and FBD patients. Try taking 400 to 800 IU of mixed tocopherols per day.

Food Allergy

A food allergy or sensitivity occurs when there is an adverse reaction to the ingestion of a food. A classic food allergy occurs when an ingested food molecule acts as an antigen—a foreign substance that triggers the release of an antibody by white blood cells known as IgE (immunoglobulin E). An antigen may be a protein, starch, or other food component, or a food additive (e.g., coloring, flavoring agent, or preservative). When the IgE and food antigen bind to specialized cells known as mast cells or basophils, it causes the release of histamine and other allergic compounds leading to swelling and inflammation. Most food allergies are due to delayed hypersensitivity reactions of the immune system (as opposed to the IgE reaction of classical allergy) or neurological reactions that do not involve the immune system.

Signs and Symptoms

Food allergies are associated with a multitude of symptoms and health conditions:

- Gastrointestinal: celiac disease, chronic diarrhea, duodenal ulcer, gastritis, irritable bowel syndrome, malabsorption, mouth ulcers, ulcerative colitis.
- Genitourinary: Bed-wetting, chronic bladder infections, nephrosis.
- Immune: Chronic infections, frequent ear infections.
- Mental/emotional: Anxiety, depression, hyperactivity, inability to concentrate, insomnia, irritability, mental confusion, personality change, seizures.
- Musculoskeletal: Bursitis, joint pain, low back pain.
- Respiratory: Asthma, chronic bronchitis, wheezing.
- Skin: Acne, eczema, hives, itching, skin rash.
- Miscellaneous: Arrhythmia, oedema, fainting, fatigue, headache, hypoglycemia, itchy nose or throat, migraines, sinusitis.

Causes

Food allergy is often inherited. When both parents have allergies, there is a 67 percent chance that the children will also have allergies. Where only one parent is allergic, the chance of a child's being prone to allergies drops from 67 percent to 33 percent.

Repetitious exposure to a food, improper digestion, and poor integrity of the intestinal barrier are additional factors that can lead to the development and maintenance of food allergy.

Food Prescriptions

An allergy elimination diet is valuable in identifying food allergies. In an allergy elimination diet, many commonly eaten foods are eliminated and replaced with either hypoallergenic foods and foods that are rarely eaten, or special hypoallergenic formulas. The fewer the allergenic foods eaten, the greater the ease of establishing a diagnosis. The standard elimination diet consists of hypoallergenic foods, including lamb, chicken, potatoes, rice, bananas, apples, and cabbage-family vegetables, such as cabbage, Brussels sprouts, and broccoli. Variations of this diet may be suitable; the key point is that no allergenic foods be consumed.

The individual stays on the elimination diet for at least one week and up to one month. If the symptoms are related to food sensitivity, they will typically disappear by the fifth or sixth day of the diet. If the symptoms do not disappear, it is possible that a reaction to a food in the elimination diet is responsible. In that case, an even more restricted diet must be utilized. After the elimination diet period, methods range from reintroducing only a single food every two days to reintroducing a food every one or two meals. Usually, after the one-week "cleansing" period, the patient develops an increased sensitivity to offending foods.

Reintroduction of allergenic foods typically produces more severe or recognizable symptoms than before. A careful, detailed record must be kept describing when foods were reintroduced and what symptoms appeared upon reintroduction. It also can be very useful to track the wrist pulse during reintroduction, as changes in pulse rate—either faster or slower—may occur when an allergenic food is consumed.

Other Recommendations

Do not rely on the skin-prick test or skin-scratch test commonly employed by many allergists to determine food allergies. Skin-prick tests test only for IgE-mediated allergies. Since only about 10 to 15 percent of all food allergies are mediated by IgE, skin-prick tests are of little value in diagnosing most food allergies. If you don't want to do an elimination diet, most nutritionally oriented physicians now employ blood tests to diagnose food allergies. The best laboratory test appears to be the enzyme-linked immunosorbent assay (ELISA).

Common Allergenic Foods for Children

Citrus

Eggs

Fish and shellfish

Milk and dairy products

Nuts

Peanuts

Soy

Strawberries

Wheat and other gluten grains

Common Allergenic Foods for Adults

Citrus

Eggs

Milk and dairy products

Onions and garlic

Soy

Wheat and other gluten grains

Gallstones

Gallstones are round or oval, smooth or faceted lumps of solid matter found in the gallbladder, the sac under the liver where bile is stored and concentrated. They arise when there is an imbalance among the bile components. Bile is composed of bile salts; bilirubin; cholesterol, phospholipids, and fatty acids; water; electrolytes; and other substances. The most common stones are mixed, containing cholesterol and inorganic salts of calcium.

Signs and Symptoms

Gallstones may be without symptoms or may be associated with periods of intense pain in the abdomen that radiates to the upper back. Symptoms begin only when a gallstone gets stuck in the duct leading from the gallbladder to the intestine. An ultrasound exam provides definitive diagnosis of gallstones.

Causes

A low-fiber diet is one of the main causes of gallstones. Such a diet, which is typically high in refined carbohydrates and fat and low in fiber, leads to a reduction in the synthesis of bile acids by the liver, which in turn significantly reduces the solubility of the bile. A high intake of refined sugar is also a risk factor for gallstones.

The frequency of gallstones is two to four times as great in women as in men. Women are predisposed to gallstones because of either increased cholesterol synthesis or suppression of bile acids by oestrogens. Pregnancy, use of oral contraceptives, or other causes of elevated oestrogen levels greatly increase the incidence of gallstones. Obesity and constipation are also associated with a significant increase in risk.

Food Prescriptions

For prevention and treatment of gallstones, increase intake of vegetables, fruits, and dietary fiber, especially the gel-forming or mucilaginous fibers as found in linseed, oat bran, guar gum, and pectin; reduce consumption of saturated fats, cholesterol, sugar, and animal proteins; avoid all fried foods; and drink at least six eight-ounce/240-milliliter glasses of water each day to maintain the proper water content of the bile.

Radishes increase the flow of bile, helping to maintain a healthy gallbladder; however individuals with gallbladder disease should not consume large amounts of this vegetable.

Food allergies have long been known to trigger gallbladder attacks. A 1968 study revealed that 100 percent of a group of patients with gallstones were free of symptoms while they were on a basic elimination diet (consisting of beef, rye, soybean, rice, cherry, peach, apricot, beetroot, and spinach). Foods that induced symptoms of gallstones, in decreasing order of their occurrence, were egg, pork, onion, poultry, milk, coffee, citrus, corn, beans, and nuts. Adding eggs to the diet caused gallbladder attacks in 93 percent of the patients. *Note:* Coffee (both regular and decaffeinated) induces gallbladder contractions, so if you have gallstones, avoid consuming coffee until the stones are resolved.

A vegetarian diet has been shown to be protective against gallstone formation. While this may simply be a result of the increased fiber content of the vegetarian diet, other factors may be equally important. Animal proteins, such as casein from dairy products, have been shown to increase the formation of gallstones in animals, while vegetable proteins, such as soy, have been shown to be preventive against gallstone formation.

Other Recommendations

Achieving ideal body weight is an important goal in the treatment and prevention of gallstones. Obesity causes an increased secretion of cholesterol in the bile as a result of increased cholesterol synthesis. It is important to recognize that during active weight reduction, bile cholesterol saturation initially increases. The secretion of all bile components is reduced during weight loss, but the secretion of bile acids decreases more than that of cholesterol. Therefore, it is a good idea for people on weight loss programmes to support their liver function with high-fiber foods and plenty of liquids. Consumption of six to eight glasses of liquids is necessary each day to maintain the water content of bile. Pure water or fresh fruit and vegetable juices are the preferred ways to meet your body's water requirements.

Once the weight is stabilized, bile acid output returns to normal levels, while the cholesterol output remains low. The net effect of weight loss is a significant reduction in cholesterol saturation.

Gastroesophageal reflux disease: See Nonulcer Dyspepsia.

Gingivitis: See Periodontal Disease.

Glaucoma

Glaucoma refers to increased pressure within the eye (intraocular), which results from greater production than outflow of the fluid of the eye (the aqueous humor). The normal intraocular pressure (IOP) is about 10 to 21 mm Hg. In chronic glaucoma, the IOP is usually mildly to moderately elevated, at 22 to 40 mm Hg. In acute glaucoma, the IOP is greater than 40 mm Hg.

Signs and Symptoms

Since patients with the early stages of chronic glaucoma rarely have symptoms, regular eye exams are important—annually after the age of sixty. In the U.K., free eye tests are available to people with glaucoma or people over the age of forty with close relatives who have glaucoma. Chronic glaucoma can cause the gradual loss of peripheral vision, resulting in tunnel vision.

Signs and symptoms of acute glaucoma include extreme pain, blurring of vision, reddened eyes, and a fixed and dilated pupil. Acute glaucoma is a medical emergency. If you are showing any signs of acute glaucoma, consult an ophthalmologist immediately. Unless acute glaucoma is adequately treated within twelve to forty-eight hours, it results in permanent blindness within two to five days.

Causes

The cause of glaucoma appears to be an abnormality in the composition of the supportive structures of the eye. Specifically, structural changes reflecting poor collagen integrity and function are the hallmark features of glaucoma. These changes lead to blockage in the flow of the aqueous humour and result in elevated IOP readings. These changes can occur with aging and medication use, including of corticosteroids.

Food Prescriptions

For chronic glaucoma, a generally healthful diet is recommended, with a focus on foods high in vitamin C and flavonoids, such as fresh fruits and vegetables, particularly bilberries and blueberries. These foods prevent the connective tissue structure of the eye from oxidative damage, which can weaken these structures. In addition, regular consumption of cold-water fish, such as salmon, mackerel, and herring, is also encouraged due to their high content of omega-3 fatty acids. Animal studies have shown that increased consumption of omega-3 fatty acids can lower IOP.

Chronic glaucoma has been successfully treated by eliminating allergens. In one study, an immediate rise in IOP of up to 20 millimeters was noted in some people when they were exposed to a food- or airborne allergen. To treat glaucoma by eliminating food allergens, follow the guidelines given under "Food Allergy."

Other Recommendations

An individual with glaucoma should do everything possible to avoid corticosteroid drugs. Corticosteroid drugs, such as prednisone, that are used in severe allergic and inflammatory conditions, weaken collagen structures throughout the body, including the eyes. Use of corticosteroid drugs is a major risk for glaucoma. If you must take corticosteroids, it is advisable to supplement with vitamin C and flavonoids to support collagen integrity.

Gout

Gout is a common type of arthritis caused by an increased concentration of uric acid in biological fluids. Uric acid is created from the breakdown of purine, a molecule found in DNA and RNA. In gout, uric acid crystals are deposited in joints, tendons, kidneys, and other tissues, where they cause considerable inflammation and damage. Gout may lead to debilitation by the uric acid deposits around the joints and tendons, and deposits in the kidney may result in kidney failure.

Signs and Symptoms

The first attack of gout is characterized by intense pain, usually involving only one joint. The first joint of the big toe is affected in nearly half of all first attacks and is at some time affected in more than 90 percent of individuals with gout. If the attack progresses, fever and chills will appear. First attacks usually occur at night and are usually triggered by a specific event, such as dietary excess, alcohol ingestion, trauma, certain drugs (mainly chemotherapy drugs, certain diuretics, and high dosages of niacin), and surgery.

Causes

Gout is the result of increased synthesis of uric acid; reduced ability to excrete uric acid; or overproduction and underexcretion of uric acid. Several dietary factors are known to trigger gout, including consumption of alcohol, high-purine-content foods (such as organ meats, meat, yeast, and poultry), fats, refined carbohydrates, and excessive calories.

Food Prescriptions

The dietary treatment of gout involves the following, each of which will be briefly summarized:

1. Low-purine diet.
2. Elimination of alcohol intake.
3. Achievement of ideal body weight.
4. Liberal consumption of complex carbohydrates.
5. Low fat intake.
6. Low protein intake, alkaline diet.
7. Liberal fluid intake.
8. Liberal consumption of celery, cherries, and blueberries.

A low-purine diet has long been the mainstay of dietary therapy for gout. Foods with high purine levels should be omitted entirely. These include organ meats, yeast (brewer's and baker's), herring, sardines, mackerel, and anchovies. Intake of foods with moderate levels of purine should be reduced to one serving every two to three days as well. These include dried legumes, spinach, asparagus, fish, poultry, and mushrooms. Low-purine foods may be eaten in small amounts.

PURINE CONTENT RANKING

High-Purine Foods

Anchovies

Consommé

Herring

Mackerel

Meat extracts

Organ meats, including brain, kidney, and liver

Roe

Sardines

Yeast, including baker's and brewer's

Moderate-Purine Foods

Asparagus

Fish

Legumes

Meat

Mushrooms

Peas (dried)

Poultry

Shellfish

Spinach

Low-Purine Foods

Eggs

Fruit

Grains

Milk

Noodles

Nuts

Olives

Alcohol increases uric acid production by accelerating purine breakdown. It also reduces uric acid excretion by increasing lactate production, which impairs kidney function. For many individuals, elimination of alcohol is all that is needed to reduce uric acid levels and prevent gouty arthritis.

Obesity is associated with an increased rate of gout. Weight reduction in obese individuals significantly reduces serum uric acid levels. Weight reduction should involve the use of a high-fiber, low-fat diet, as this type of diet will help manage the elevated cholesterol and triglyceride levels that are also common in obesity.

Intake of refined carbohydrates, fructose, and saturated fat should be kept to a minimum. Simple sugars, such as refined sugar, honey, maple syrup, corn syrup, and fructose, increase uric acid production, while saturated fats decrease uric acid excretion. The diet should focus on complex carbohydrates, such as legumes, whole grains, and vegetables, rather than on simple sugars.

High-fat and high-protein foods are usually foods that are high in purines. High-fat animal foods also promote inflammation and should be avoided, regardless of purine content. High-protein foods that are not high in purines should be eaten only in small amounts to avoid taxing the kidneys, which are burdened with excreting excess uric acid. It is also important to eat an alkaline diet; see Appendix B for more information.

Liberal fluid intake keeps the urine diluted and promotes the excretion of uric acid. Furthermore, dilution of the urine reduces the risk of kidney stones. Drink at least 48 ounces/1½ liters of water each day.

Celery and cherries appear to be very effective in lowering uric acid levels and preventing attacks of gout. Celery contains the compound 3-*n*-butylphthalide, while cherries are a rich source of flavonoids. Both of these compounds are beneficial in gout via several mechanisms, including the ability to inhibit the formation of uric acid by inhibiting the enzyme xanthine oxidase.

Other Recommendations

The pain of an acute attack of gout is absolutely excruciating. In this situation, heroic measures are clearly appropriate. The standard medical treatment for acute gout is administration of colchicine, an anti-inflammatory drug. Colchicine has no effect on uric acid levels, but it does stop the inflammatory process. Studies indicate that more than 75 percent of patients with gout show major improvement in symptoms within the first twelve hours after receiving colchicine. Long-term treatment of gout with colchicine, however, is not appropriate, as colchicine can cause serious side effects with long-term use, such as bone marrow depression, hair loss, liver damage, depression, seizures, respiratory depression, and even death. Fortunately, most cases of gout can be adequately controlled with diet alone.

Hay Fever

Hay fever is characterized by a watery nasal discharge, sneezing, and itchy eyes and nose. It is usually associated with a particular season because of pollen or another allergen. As hay fever and asthma share similar causes and mechanisms as well as natural medicine treatments, see "Asthma" for more information.

Headache, Migraine

A migraine is a vascular-type headache characterized by a sharp, pounding pain, usually located on one side of the head.

Signs and Symptoms

The pain of a migraine is characterized as a throbbing or pounding, sharp pain. It is typically felt on just one side of the head. Although some migraines come on without warning, many migraine sufferers have warning symptoms or "auras" before the onset of pain. Typical auras last a few minutes and include blurring or bright spots in the vision, anxiety, fatigue, disturbed thinking, and numbness or tingling on one side of the body.

Causes

The mechanism of a migraine can be described as a three-stage process: initiation, prodrome (time between initiation and appearance of the headache), and headache. Although a particular stressor may be associated with the onset of a specific attack, it appears that initiation is dependent on the accumulation of several stressors over time. These stressors ultimately affect serotonin metabolism. Once a critical point of susceptibility is reached, a "cascade event" is initiated that sets in process a dominolike effect that ultimately produces a headache. Food allergies; histamine-releasing foods; alcohol, especially red wine; stress; hormonal changes, such as menstruation, ovulation, or use of birth control pills; and weather changes, especially barometric pressure changes, are examples of some common triggers of migraines. Considerable evidence supports an association between migraine headaches and instability of blood vessels. These stressors cause release of various chemicals, such as histamine, serotonin, and tyramine, that cause changes in the way blood vessels dilate and contract in migraine sufferers.

Food Prescriptions

Food allergy or sensitivity plays a primary role in many cases of tension and migraine headaches. Many double-blind, placebo-controlled studies have demonstrated that the detection and removal of allergenic foods will eliminate or greatly reduce headache symptoms in the majority of patients. Food allergy/intolerance induces a migraine attack largely as a result of platelets releasing serotonin and histamine. In addition, foods such as aged cheeses, beer, canned figs, chicken liver, chocolate, food additives, pickled fish, the pods of broad beans, wine, and brewer's yeast contain histamine, tyramine, and/or other compounds that can trigger migraines in sensitive individuals by causing blood vessels to expand. Red wine is much more likely than white wine to cause a headache because it contains higher levels of phenols and 20 to 200 times as much histamine. Hypoglycemia can also trigger a migraine.

Eating to prevent hypoglycemia also stabilizes blood vessels, preventing migraine attacks. Be sure to eat regularly, with small snacks between meals. Avoid sugar and refined carbohydrates, instead focusing on whole grains, legumes, fruits, and vegetables.

Other Recommendations

Biofeedback and relaxation training can also be helpful. The effectiveness of biofeedback and relaxation training in reducing the frequency and severity of recurrent migraine headaches has been the subject of more than thirty-five clinical studies. When the results of these studies were compared with those of studies using prescription drug therapy, it was apparent that the nondrug approach was as effective as the drug approach but without side effects. Ask your doctor about these therapies.

Headache, Tension

The two most common types of headache are tension and migraine. Tension headaches usually have a steady, constant, dull pain.

Signs and Symptoms

Tension headaches are characterized by a steady, constant, dull pain that starts at the back of the head or in the forehead and spreads over the entire head, giving the sensation of pressure or a feeling that a vise grip has been applied to the skull.

Causes

A tension headache is usually caused by tightening in the muscles of the face, neck, scalp, or shoulders as a result of stress or poor posture. These tight muscles pinch nerves or their blood supply, creating the sensation of pain and pressure. Relaxation of the muscles usually brings about immediate relief. Often a tension headache can be worsened (or improved) by applying hand pressure to trigger points on the neck muscles. A trigger point is the central area of tension in the muscle.

Food Prescriptions

Please see "Migraine Headache" above, as the recommendations there are also appropriate for tension headache.

Other Recommendations

Since tension headaches are primarily mechanical in nature, it is important to address any structural problems. Tension headaches often respond to physical treatments, such as acupuncture, manipulation, massage, and other forms of bodywork. Learning how to relax the muscles with progressive relaxation exercises or other technique has been shown in clinical studies to provide exceptional benefits without side effects.

Topical capsaicin preparations have also been shown in studies to be an effective treatment for cluster headaches, which occur repeatedly over a given period of time. If tension headaches are recurrent, topical capsaicin may be appropriate, as it needs to be applied four times for three to four days, then twice daily after that. Pain may increase in the first three to four days of treatment, as capsaicin works by depleting the pain-causing neurotransmitter substance P from the affected nerves.

Heart Disease

The general term "heart disease" is most often used to describe atherosclerosis (hardening of the artery walls due to a buildup of plaque, which contains cholesterol, fatty material, and cellular debris) of the coronary arteries, which are the blood vessels that supply the heart with oxygen and nutrients. See "Atherosclerosis" and "Cholesterol" for more information.

Heartburn: See "Nonulcer Dyspepsia."

Hemorrhoids

Hemorrhoids are enlarged or painful varicose veins in the anal/rectal area.

Signs and Symptoms

The symptoms most often associated with hemorrhoids include itching, burning, pain, inflammation, irritation, swelling, bleeding, and seepage. Pain is usually worse with defecation. A person with hemorrhoids may also notice bright red blood on the surface of the stool, on the toilet tissue, and/or in the toilet bowl.

Causes

The causes of hemorrhoids are similar to the causes of varicose veins (see "Varicose Veins"). Because the venous system that supplies the rectal area contains no valves, factors that increase venous congestion in the region can lead to hemorrhoid formation. These factors include increased intra-abdominal pressure, as caused by defecation, pregnancy, coughing, sneezing, vomiting, physical exertion, or cirrhosis of the liver; an increase in straining during defecation due to a low-fiber diet; diarrhea; and standing or sitting for prolonged periods of time.

Food Prescriptions

A low-fiber diet high in refined foods contributes greatly to the development of hemorrhoids. Individuals who consume a low-fiber diet tend to strain more during bowel movements, since their smaller, harder stools are more difficult to pass. This straining raises the pressure in the abdomen, which obstructs venous blood flow, increases pelvic congestion, and may significantly weaken the veins, causing hemorrhoids to form.

A high-fiber diet is perhaps the most important component in the prevention of hemorrhoids. A diet rich in vegetables, fruits, legumes, and whole grains promotes peristalsis, the normal rhythmic contractions of the intestines. Furthermore, many fiber components attract water to form gelatinous masses that keep the faeces soft, bulky, and easy to pass. The net effect of a high-fiber diet is significantly less straining during defecation; therefore, a significantly lower risk of developing hemorrhoids is achieved.

The diet should also contain liberal amounts of flavonoid-rich foods, such as bilberries, blackberries, blueberries, cherries, buckwheat, and citrus fruits to strengthen vein structures.

Other Recommendations

Several double-blind clinical trials have demonstrated that supplementing the diet with bulk-forming fibers can significantly reduce the symptoms of hemorrhoids and improve bowel habits. In general, psyllium seed husks are less irritating than wheat bran and other cellulose fiber products.

For temporary relief, topical therapy may be effective. Topical treatments involve the use of suppositories, ointments, and anorectal pads. Many over-the-counter products for hemorrhoids contain primarily natural ingredients, such as witch hazel (hamamelis water), shark liver oil, cod liver oil, cocoa butter, Peruvian balsam, zinc oxide, live yeast cell derivative, and allantoin. These products work by lubricating the intestine and providing some nutrients to repair the varicose veins and damaged surface tissue. Another useful treatment for temporary relief of hemorrhoids is a warm sitz bath, a partial-immersion bath of the pelvic region. The temperature of the water should be 100 to 105 degrees F./38–40 degrees C. Add 1 teaspoon of salt per liter of water.

Herpes Simplex

Herpes simplex is a virus that is responsible for cold sores and genital herpes. There are two types of herpes simplex viruses: type 1 (HSV-1) is most often responsible for cold sores (also referred to as fever blisters), while type 2 (HSV-2) is responsible for nearly 90 percent of cases of genital herpes (the remaining 10 percent are caused by HSV-1).

Signs and Symptoms

In some people (mostly children) an initial HSV-1 infection may cause fever, painful swelling, and open sores on the gums and inside the cheeks, or a painful sore throat. When these herpes symptoms do develop, they usually begin two to twelve days after exposure to someone with HSV-1.

Symptoms of a first episode of HSV-2 usually appear within two to ten days of exposure to the virus and last an average of two to three weeks. Early symptoms can include an itching or burning sensation; pain in the legs, buttocks, or genital area; vaginal discharge; or a feeling of pressure in the abdominal region. Within a few days, sores (lesions) appear at the site of infection. Lesions also can occur on the cervix in women or in the urinary passage in men. These small, red bumps may develop into blisters or painful open sores. Over a period of days, the sores become crusted and then heal without scarring. Other symptoms that may accompany a primary episode of genital herpes can include fever, headache, muscle aches, painful or difficult urination, vaginal discharge, and swollen glands in the groin area.

After the initial infection in the skin or mucous membranes, the virus travels to the sensory nerves at the end of the spinal cord and makes a home. In most people, the virus becomes dormant (inactive). In others, however, it can be reactivated by trauma or stress, or whenever else the immune system fails to keep it in check. When the virus becomes reactivated, it travels along the nerves to the skin, where it multiplies on the surface at or near the site of the original herpes sores, causing new sores to erupt. It can also reactivate without causing any visible sores.

Causes

Herpes is caused by an infection with the herpes simplex virus and is spread via direct contact with infected lesions.

Food Prescriptions

In general, the recommendations given under "Food Prescriptions" in "Immune System Depression," below, especially the avoidance of refined carbohydrates and food allergens, are appropriate here as well. There are also some special food prescriptions. A diet high in the amino acid lysine and low in the amino acid arginine can be effective in preventing HSV infections, especially if used in conjunction with lysine supplementation (1,500–3,000 milligrams daily). This dietary approach arose from research showing that lysine has antiviral activity in test-tube studies due to blocking arginine. HSV replication requires the manufacture of proteins rich in arginine, and arginine itself is suggested to be a stimulator of HSV replication. From a theoretical perspective, this approach should be effective, since *in vitro* studies have shown that HSV replication is dependent on adequate levels of arginine and low levels of lysine. Foods high in arginine are chocolate, peanuts, almonds, and other nuts and seeds. Foods high in lysine include most vegetables, milk, cheese, legumes, fish, turkey, and chicken.

Other Recommendations

Licorice root contains a compound, glycyrrhetinic acid, that inhibits both the growth and cell-damaging effects of herpes simplex. Regular consumption of licorice root tea should be encouraged in individuals prone to recurrent herpes infections. A particular form of bitter melon extract, called MAP 30, has also demonstrated powerful antiviral activity against the herpes simplex virus. Another antiviral compound is lauric acid, which is derived from coconut. Lauric acid can be used in doses of 12 to 25 grams per day during an active herpes infection.

Capsaicin-containing creams and gels applied topically are showing impressive results when applied to the skin in cases of postherpes pain (postherpetic neuralgia). These products should be applied four times daily for three to

---

TABLE 20.2

Arginine and Lysine Content of Selected Foods

Food	Serving Size	Arginine (milligrams)	Lysine (milligrams)
Almonds	70 nuts	2,730	580
Bacon	12 slices	2,100	2,000
Beans, green	¾ cup	80	80
Beans, lima	100 grams	1,170	1,470
Beans, mung	100 grams	1,320	1,930
Beans, red	½ cup	340	420
Beef chuck	100 grams	1,600	2,200
Brazil nut	100 grams	2,250	470
Bread, whole-wheat (wholemeal)	4 slices	510	290
Buckwheat	100 grams	1,200	460
Carob	100 grams	710	340
Cashews	40 nuts	1,990	740
Cheese, cheddar	100 grams	850	1,700
Chicken	100 grams	1,930	2,700
Chickpeas	100 grams	1,900	1,380
Chocolate	100 grams	4,500	2,000
Clams	½ cup	830	840

(continued on next page)

Food	Serving Size	Arginine (milligrams)	Lysine (milligrams)
Coconut	100 grams	470	148
Crustaceans	100 grams	1,330	1,260
Eggs	2 large	840	820
Fish fingers, breaded	4–5 sticks	940	1,400
Halibut	100 grams	140	2,220
Hazelnuts	100 grams	3,510	690
Lentils	100 grams	2,100	1,740
Linseeds	100 grams	2,030	810
Liver, ox	100 grams	1,590	1,950
Milk, whole	100 grams	130	280
Millet	100 grams	410	260
Oatmeal, cooked	⅓ cup	130	70
Oysters	5–8 medium	310	280
Peanuts, without skins	100 grams	3,240	1,090
Peas, green	⅝ cup	420	220
Pecans	100 grams	2,030	810
Pork, lean	100 grams	1,510	1,850
Prawns	100 grams	1,360	2,130
Rice, brown	⅔ cup	120	100
Salmon	100 grams	1,530	2,350
Sardines	7 medium	1,190	1,850
Sesame seeds	100 grams	2,590	580
Soybeans, boiled	⅔ cup	620	620
Sunflower	100 grams	1,190	540
Tuna	⅝ can	1,530	2,530
Turkey	100 grams	1,700	2,450
Walnuts, English	27 whole	2,250	490
Yeast	100 grams	1,940	3,510

four days, then twice daily for continued pain relief. See "Cayenne (Red) Pepper and Paprika," page 474, for more information.

High Blood Pressure (Hypertension)

Each time the heart beats, it sends blood coursing through the arteries. The peak reading of the pressure exerted by this contraction is the systolic pressure. Between beats the heart relaxes, and blood pressure drops. This lower reading is referred to as the diastolic pressure. Blood pressure readings are in millimeters of mercury (mm Hg). A normal blood pressure reading for adults is 120 (systolic)/80 (diastolic). Readings above this level are a major risk factor for heart attack and stroke. High blood pressure readings can be divided into the following levels:

Prehypertension (120–139/80–89)
Borderline (120–160/90–94)
Mild (140–160/95–104)
Moderate (140–180/105–114)
Severe (160+/115+)

Signs and Symptoms

Prehypertension to moderate hypertension is generally without symptoms. Severe hypertension may be associated with increased sleepiness, confusion, headache, nausea, and vomiting.

Causes

Although medical textbooks state that the cause is unknown in 95 percent of cases, hypertension is closely related to lifestyle and dietary factors, which have a direct effect on the health of the arteries. When the arteries become hard due to the buildup of cholesterol-containing plaque, blood pressure rises. Therefore, it is very important to prevent atherosclerosis (hardening of the arteries). See "Atherosclerosis."

Like that of other degenerative diseases, including atherosclerosis, the development of high blood pressure is closely related to lifestyle and dietary factors. Some of the important lifestyle factors that may cause high blood pressure include stress, lack of exercise, and smoking. Some of the dietary factors include obesity; a high sodium-to-potassium ratio; a low-fiber, high-sugar diet; high saturated fat and low omega-3 fatty acid intake; and a diet low in calcium, magnesium, and vitamin C. These same factors are known to impact the ability of the kidneys to regulate fluid volume and control blood pressure.

Food Prescriptions

Achieving ideal body weight is the most important recommendation for those with high blood pressure. However, overweight people who lose even modest amounts of weight experience a reduction in blood pressure.

Vegetarians generally have a lower incidence of high blood pressure and other cardiovascular diseases than do nonvegetarians. While dietary levels of sodium do not differ significantly between these two groups, a vegetarian's diet typically contains more potassium, complex carbohydrates, essential fatty acids, fiber, calcium, magnesium, and vitamin C, all of which have a favorable influence on blood pressure, and less saturated fat and refined carbohydrate.

A diet high in sodium and low in potassium is associated with high blood pressure. Conversely, a diet high in potassium and low in sodium can lower blood pressure. Numerous studies have shown that sodium restriction alone does not improve blood pressure control in most people; it must be accompanied by a high potassium intake. Most Americans have a potassium-to-sodium intake ratio of less than 1:2, meaning they ingest more than twice as much sodium as potassium. Researchers recommend a dietary potassium-to-sodium ratio of greater than 5:1 to maintain health. The easiest way to lower sodium intake is to avoid prepared foods and table salt, and use potassium chloride salt substitutes, such as the popular brands Solo and LoSalt, instead. The best way to boost potassium levels is to increase the intake of fruits, vegetables, whole grains, and legumes.

Two very large studies have shown quite clearly that diet can be effective in lowering blood pressure. These studies, the Dietary Approaches to Stop Hypertension (DASH), tested a diet rich in fruits, vegetables, and low-fat dairy foods, and low in saturated and total fat. The DASH diet was also low in cholesterol; high in dietary fiber, potassium, calcium, and magnesium; and moderately high in protein.

The first study showed that a diet rich in fruits, vegetables, and low-fat dairy products can reduce blood pressure in the general population and people with hypertension. The original DASH diet did not require either sodium restriction or weight loss—the two traditional dietary tools to control blood pressure—to be effective. The second study from the DASH research group found that coupling the original DASH diet with sodium restriction is more effective than dietary manipulation alone. In the first trial, the DASH diet produced a net blood pressure reduction of 11.4 and 5.5 mm Hg systolic and diastolic, respectively, in patients with hypertension. In the second trial, sodium intake was also quantified at a "higher" intake of 3,300 milligrams per day; an "intermediate" intake of 2,400 milligrams per day; and a "lower" intake of 1,500 milligrams per day. Compared to the control diet, the DASH diet was associated with a significantly lower systolic blood pressure at each sodium level. The DASH diet with the lower sodium level led to a mean systolic blood pressure that was 7.1 mm Hg lower in participants without hypertension, and 11.5 mm Hg lower in participants with hypertension. These results are clinically significant and indicate that a sodium intake below the recommended level of 2,400 milligrams daily can significantly and quickly lower blood pressure.

Special foods for people with high blood pressure include celery; garlic and onions, to lower cholesterol; nuts and seeds or their oils, for their essential fatty acid content; cold-water fish, e.g., salmon and mackerel; fish oil products concentrated, for the omega-3 fatty acids EPA and DHA; green leafy vegetables and sea vegetables, for their calcium and magnesium; whole linseeds and whole grains and legumes, for their fiber; and foods rich in vitamin C, such as broccoli and citrus fruits.

Other Recommendations

Caffeine, alcohol, and tobacco use should be eliminated. Stress reduction techniques, such as biofeedback, autogenics, meditation, yoga, hypnosis, and progressive muscle relaxation may offer some benefit in lowering blood pressure without the use of drugs. But even more importantly, regular aerobic exercise is extremely important to cardiovascular health.

The most effective natural products to lower blood pressure are anti-ACE peptides—purified mixtures of small peptides (proteins) derived from muscle of the fish bonito (a member of the tuna family) or sardines. Basically, these work to lower blood pressure by inhibiting ACE (angiotensin-converting enzyme). This enzyme converts angiotensin 1 to angiotensin 2, which is a compound that increases both the fluid volume and the degree of constriction of the blood vessels. If we use a garden hose model to illustrate the pressure in your arteries, the formation of angiotensin 2 would be similar to pinching off the hose while turning up the tap full blast. By inhibiting the formation of this compound, anti-ACE peptides relax the arterial walls and reduce fluid volume. Anti-ACE peptides exert the strongest inhibition of ACE reported for any naturally occurring substance available.

Five clinical studies have shown anti-ACE peptides from bonito and sardines to exert significant blood pressure-lowering effects in people with high blood pressure (hypertension). Anti-ACE peptides appear to be effective in about two thirds of people with high blood pressure—about the same percentage as with many prescription drugs. The degree of blood pressure reduction in these studies was quite significant, typically reducing the systolic by at least 10 mm Hg and the diastolic by 7 mm Hg in people with prehypertension and borderline hypertension. Greater reductions will be seen in people with higher initial blood pressure readings. (*Note:* People who do not respond to anti-ACE peptides after a two-month trial should try celery seed extract.)

Hives

Hives (urticaria) are an allergic reaction in the skin.

Signs and Symptoms

Hives are characterized by white or pink welts or bumps surrounded by redness. These welts are known as *wheals* and *flare lesions* and are caused primarily by the release of histamine (an allergic mediator) in the skin. They tend to be quite itchy. About 50 percent of patients with chronic hives develop *angioedema*—a deeper, more serious form of allergic reaction involving the tissue below the surface of the skin.

Causes

While the basic cause of hives involves the release of histamine from mast cells or basophils—white blood cells that play a key role in allergic reactions—what actually triggers this release can be a variety of factors, such as physical contact or pressure, heat (prickly heat rash), cold, water, autoimmune reactions, and allergies or sensitivities to drugs (especially antibiotics and aspirin), foods, food additives, and infectious organisms, such as hepatitis B, *Candida albicans*, and streptococcal bacteria. However, food allergy is the most common cause of hives, especially in chronic cases.

Food Prescriptions

The foods most commonly associated with triggering hives are milk, eggs, chicken, cured meat, alcoholic beverages, cheese, chocolate, citrus fruits, shellfish, and nuts. Food additives that trigger hives include colorants (azo dyes), flavorings (salicylates), artificial sweeteners (aspartame), preservatives (benzoates, nitrites, and sorbic acid), antioxidants (hydroxytoluene, sulphite, and gallate), and emulsifiers/stabilizers (polysorbates—E432–E436—and vegetable gums). Numerous clinical studies demonstrate that diets that are free of food allergens and/or food additives typically produce significant reductions in roughly 50 to 75 percent of people with chronic hives.

The best dietary recommendation appears to be an allergy elimination diet or, at the very least, a diet that excludes all common food allergens and all food additives. The strictest allergy elimination diet allows only water, lamb, rice, pears, and most vegetables. The individual stays on this limited diet for at least one week. If the hives are related to food allergy or food additives, they will typically disappear by the fifth or sixth day of the diet. After one week, individual foods are reintroduced at a rate of one new food every two days. Reintroduction of sensitive foods will typically produce more severe or recognizable hives than before.

Other Recommendations

Psychological stress is often reported as a triggering factor in patients with chronic hives. Stress may play an important role by decreasing the effectiveness of immune system mechanisms that block allergens. In a small study of fifteen patients with chronic hives, relaxation therapy and hypnosis were shown to provide significant benefit. Patients were given an audiotape and asked to use the relaxation techniques described on the tape at home. At a follow-up examination five to fourteen months after the initial session, six patients were free of hives and an additional seven reported improvement.

Hypoglycemia

Hypoglycemia is low blood sugar. Normally, the body maintains blood sugar levels within a narrow range through the coordinated effort of several glands and their hormones. If these control mechanisms are disrupted, hypoglycemia (low blood sugar) results. A few important causes of low blood sugar levels include stress and dietary factors, such as eating irregularly or having a diet high in refined carbohydrates. Chronic hypoglycemia can develop into diabetes (high blood sugar).

Signs and Symptoms

Symptoms of hypoglycemia can range from mild to severe, including headache; depression, anxiety, irritability, and other psychological disturbances; blurred vision; excessive sweating; mental confusion; incoherent speech; bizarre behavior; and convulsions.

The standard method of diagnosing hypoglycemia involves the measurement of blood glucose levels. The normal fasting blood glucose level is between 70 and 105 milligrams per deciliter/3.88 to 5.83 mmol/liter. At levels below

50 milligrams per deciliter/2.77 mmol/liter, the diagnosis is fasting hypoglycemia.

Causes

A tendency toward hypoglycemia can be hereditary, but dietary carbohydrates usually play a central role in its cause, prevention, and treatment. Simple carbohydrates, or sugars, are quickly absorbed by the body, resulting in a rapid elevation in blood sugar level; this stimulates a corresponding excessive elevation in serum insulin levels, which can then lead to hypoglycemia. Insulin is the hormone responsible for lowering blood sugar by taking sugar out of the blood and putting it into cells. High levels of insulin mean low levels of blood glucose.

Food Prescriptions

For best results in battling hypoglycemia, follow the recommendations given for diabetes (see page 716). In general, all simple, processed, and concentrated carbohydrates and high-glycemic-load foods must be avoided. When these refined carbohydrates are eaten, blood sugar levels rise quickly, producing a strain on blood sugar control. Eating foods high in simple sugars in any form—sucrose, honey, or maple syrup—can lead to hypoglycemia. Caffeine significantly worsens the effect.

Other Recommendations

Avoid alcohol, as its consumption severely stresses blood sugar control and is often a contributing factor to hypoglycemia. Alcohol induces reactive hypoglycemia by interfering with normal glucose utilization and increasing the secretion of insulin. The resultant drop in blood sugar produces a craving for food, particularly food that will quickly elevate blood sugar levels, as well as a craving for more alcohol. The increased sugar consumption aggravates the reactive hypoglycemia, particularly in the presence of more alcohol.

Exercise is critical to achieving good blood sugar control. A graded exercise programme should be developed related to the individual's fitness level and interest, yet it should elevate the heart rate to at least 60 percent of maximum for a half hour, three times a week.

Immune System Depression

Depressed immune system function increases the susceptibility to disease, from colds and flus to cancer. Support and enhancement of the immune system are perhaps the most important steps in achieving resistance to disease. Supporting the immune system involves a health-promoting lifestyle, stress management, exercise, diet, and the appropriate use of nutritional supplements and herbal medicines.

Signs and Symptoms

If you answer "yes" to any of the following questions, it is a sign that your immune system may need support:

Do you catch colds easily?
Do you get more than two colds a year?
Are you suffering from any chronic infection?

Do you get frequent cold sores or have recurrent genital herpes?

Are your lymph glands sore and swollen at times?

Do you have now or have you ever had cancer?

Recurrent or chronic infections—even very mild colds—occur only when the immune system is weakened. Under such circumstances, there is a repetitive cycle that makes it difficult to overcome the tendency toward infection: a weakened immune system leads to infection, infection causes damage to the immune system, which further weakens resistance. Enhancing the immune system can help to break the cycle.

Causes

The health of the immune system is greatly impacted by emotional state, level of stress, lifestyle, exercise and dietary habits, and nutritional status. Nutrient deficiency is the most frequent cause of a depressed immune system. An overwhelming number of clinical and experimental studies indicate that deficiency in any single nutrient can profoundly impair the immune system. Obesity is also associated with significant impairment of immune function.

Food Prescriptions

Optimal immune function requires a healthy diet that (1) is rich in whole, natural foods, such as fruits, vegetables, whole grains, beans, seeds, and nuts, (2) is low in fats and refined sugars, and (3) contains adequate, but not excessive, amounts of protein. On top of this, for optimal immune function, an individual should drink five or six 8-ounce/240-milliliter glasses of water (preferably pure) per day; take a basic multivitamin-mineral supplement; engage in a regular exercise programme of at least thirty minutes of aerobic exercise and five to ten minutes of passive stretching daily; perform daily deep breathing and relaxation exercises; take time each day to play and enjoy family and friends; and still get at least six to eight hours of sleep daily.

One of the food components most damaging to our immune system is sugar. In one study, the ingestion of 100 gram (3½-ounce) portions of carbohydrate as glucose, fructose, sucrose, honey, and pasteurized orange juice all significantly reduced the ability of white blood cells (neutrophils) to engulf and destroy bacteria. In contrast, the ingestion of 100 grams of starch had no effect. These effects started within less than thirty minutes after ingestion and lasted for more than five hours. Typically, there was at least a 50 percent reduction in neutrophil activity two hours after ingestion. Since neutrophils constitute 60 to 70 percent of the total circulating white blood cells, impairment of their activity leads to depressed immunity.

Other parameters of immune function are also undoubtedly affected by sugar consumption. For example, ingestion of 75 grams of glucose has been shown to depress lymphocyte activity. It has also been suggested that the ill effects of high glucose levels are a result of competition between blood glucose and vitamin C for membrane transport sites into the white blood cells. This is based on evidence that vitamin C and glucose appear to have opposite effects on immune function and the fact that both require insulin for membrane transport into many tissues.

Considering that the average American consumes 150 grams of sucrose (about 72 grams in the U.K.), plus other refined simple sugars, each day, the inescapable conclusion is that most Americans have chronically depressed immune systems. It is clear, particularly during an infection or chronic illness, such as cancer or AIDS, that the consumption of refined sugars is harmful to immune function.

On the other hand, some of the most important food components to enhance immune function are the carotenes. Many of the immune-enhancing effects of carotenes, as well as other antioxidants, are due to their ability to protect the thymus gland from damage. The thymus is the major gland of our immune system. It is composed of two soft, pinkish gray lobes lying in a biblike fashion just below the thyroid gland and above the heart. The thymus gland shows maximum development immediately after birth. During the aging process, the thymus gland undergoes a process of shrinkage, or involution. The reason for this involution is that the thymus gland is extremely susceptible to free-radical and oxidative damage caused by stress, drugs, radiation, infection, and chronic illness. When the thymus gland becomes damaged, its ability to control the immune system is severely compromised.

The thymus is responsible for many immune system functions, including the production of T lymphocytes, a type of white blood cell. The thymus gland also releases several hormones, such as thymosin, thymopoeitin, and serum thymic factor, which regulate many immune functions. Low levels of these hormones in the blood are associated with depressed immunity and an increased susceptibility to infection. Typically, thymic hormone levels are very low in the elderly; individuals prone to infection; cancer and AIDS patients; and when an individual is exposed to undue stress. Carotenes and other antioxidants may ensure optimal thymus gland activity by preventing damage to the thymus by free radicals and pro-oxidants.

Beyond protecting the thymus gland, carotenes have been shown to enhance the function of several types of white blood cells, as well as increase the antiviral and anticancer properties of our own immune system mediators, such as interferon. Simply stated, carotene-rich foods and drinks appear to be able to boost immunity.

Foods high in carotenes include highly colored vegetables, such as dark greens; yellow and orange squash, carrots, yams, and sweet potatoes; and red peppers and tomatoes. Also important for proper immune function, including protecting against cancer, is the inclusion of cabbage-family vegetables (broccoli, Brussels sprouts, cabbages, cauliflower, collards, kale, and greens from mustard, radish, and turnip), flavonoid-rich berries, garlic, and Jerusalem artichoke in the diet. For further information on these foods, see their respective segments in Part III.

Yogurt has an ability to boost immune function, particularly when made with large amounts (billions per serving) of *Bifidobacterium lactis* (see "Yogurt," page 593). Consuming yogurt with *Bifidobacterium lactis* increases the proportions of total, helper, and activated T lymphocytes and natural killer cells. Other effects include an increase in immune cells' ability to phagocytize or engulf and destroy invaders as well as the tumor cell-killing ability of their natural killer cells.

OTHER RECOMMENDATIONS

Numerous herbs and some nutrients have been shown to possess significant immune-enhancing properties. Perhaps the most popular herb used to enhance the immune system in the United States is echinacea. However, other inulin-containing herbs are also important for immune support (see page 76 for more information on inulin).

One application of herbs for immune support is making a soup as follows:

> *2 ounces/60 grams dried astragalus root*
> *2–4 ounces/60–125 grams shiitake*
>   *mushrooms, sliced*
> *2–4 ounces/60–125 grams reishi mushroom*
> *2 ounces/60 grams fresh burdock root, sliced*
>   *thin*
> *1–2 ounces/30–60 grams fresh ginger root*
> *4 ounces/125 grams chicken stock (optional)*

Combine all of the ingredients in 4 liters water and let soak for 30 minutes, then simmer for 45 minutes, covered. Remove the astragalus and reishi (you can tie these together in cheesecloth, as well as other ingredients you may not want to eat). Use as a base for soups or stews or to cook other foods in, such as grains.

Infections: See Immune System Depression.

Insomnia

Insomnia refers to difficulty in achieving or maintaining normal sleep.

Signs and Symptoms

There are two basic forms of insomnia. In sleep-onset insomnia, a person has a difficult time falling asleep. In sleep-maintenance insomnia, a person suffers from frequent or early awakening.

Causes

The most common causes of insomnia are psychological: depression, anxiety, and tension. If psychological factors do not seem to be the cause, various foods, drinks, and/or medications may be responsible. There are numerous compounds in foods and drinks that can interfere with normal sleep, most notably caffeine.

There are more than 300 drugs that interfere with normal sleep. Over-the-counter and prescription drugs can also cause abnormal sleep patterns. These are discussed below.

Food Prescriptions

In dealing with insomnia, it is essential that the diet be free of natural stimulants, such as the xanthines, including caffeine and other stimulants. Coffee, as well as less obvious caffeine sources, such as soft drinks, chocolate, coffee-flavored ice cream, hot cocoa, and tea, must all be eliminated. Even small amounts of caffeine, such as those found in decaffeinated coffee or chocolate, may be enough to cause insomnia in some people. Caffeine is also found in some over-the-counter cold and headache medications.

Other food compounds that can act as stimulants include some food colorings. Adverse food reactions such as food sensitivities and allergies can also cause insomnia. Although not considered stimulants, sugar and refined carbohydrates can interfere with sleep. Eating a diet high in sugar and refined carbohydrates and eating irregularly can cause a reaction in the body that triggers the "fight-or-flight" part of the nervous system, causing wakefulness.

Foods high in the amino acid tryptophan, such as turkey, milk, cottage cheese, chicken, eggs, and nuts, especially almonds, may help to promote sleep. In the brain, tryptophan is converted to serotonin and melatonin, which are natural sleep-inducing compounds.

Other Recommendations

Over-the-counter and prescription remedies for insomnia, while effective in the short term, can cause significant problems in the long term. Benzodiazepines and barbiturates (sleeping pills) are not designed to be used for the long term as they are addictive, have numerous side effects, and cause abnormal sleep patterns. As a result, people who take sleeping pills enter a vicious cycle. They take the drug to induce sleep, but the drug causes further disruption of normal sleep. In the morning, in an attempt to "get going," they typically drink large quantities of coffee, which further worsens their insomnia. Antihistamines also interfere with normal sleep patterns and should be avoided.

In comparison to medications, valerian root has historically been used for the relief of insomnia. Several recent clinical studies have substantiated this historical use. Unlike drugs, valerian actually improves sleep quality and sleep latency (the time required to go to sleep) but leaves no "hangover" the next morning. As a mild sedative, valerian may be taken in the following dose 30 to 45 minutes before retiring:

Dried root (or as tea): 2–3 grams.

Tincture (1:5): 5–7 milligrams (1–1½ teaspoons).

Fluid extract (1:1): 1–2 milligrams (½–1 teaspoon).

Valerian extract (0.8 percent valerenic acid): 150–300 milligrams.

Irritable Bowel Syndrome

Irritable bowel syndrome (IBS) is a functional disorder of the large intestine with no evidence of accompanying structural defect.

Signs and Symptoms

IBS is characterized by some combination of the following symptoms: abdominal pain or distension; altered bowel function, constipation, or diarrhea; hypersecretion of colonic mucus; dyspeptic symptoms, including flatulence, nausea, and anorexia; and varying degrees of anxiety or depression. If you have symptoms suggestive of IBS, please consult a physician for an accurate diagnosis.

Causes

There appear to be four main causes of IBS: stress, insufficient intake of dietary fiber, food allergies, and meals too high in sugar.

Stress increases the motility (the rhythmic contractions of the intestine that propel food through the digestive tract) of the colon and leads to abdominal pain and irregular bowel function. Stress can also cause spasm in the bowel, leading to constipation or diarrhea.

Insufficient intake of dietary fiber diminishes the ability of the colon to propel food through the digestive tract.

Food allergies also cause irritation and inflammation in the digestive tract, causing irregular bowel function. Food allergy as a cause of IBS has been recognized since the early 1900s. More recent studies have shown that the majority of patients with IBS (approximately two thirds) have at least one food allergy, and some have multiple food allergies. The most common allergens indicated to cause IBS are dairy products, at 40 to 45 percent, and grains, at 40 to 60 percent. Many patients have noted marked clinical improvement when using elimination diets (see "Food Allergy" for further discussion).

A diet high in refined sugar may be the key factor that makes IBS far more common in the United States than in other countries. Meals high in refined sugar can contribute to IBS by decreasing intestinal motility. Eating a diet high in sugar and refined carbohydrates usually means a diet low in fiber. Also, when blood sugar levels rise too rapidly, the normal rhythmic contractions of the gastrointestinal tract slow down and in some portions stop altogether. Also, excessive sugar and carbohydrates change the environment for organisms in the digestive tract, favoring organisms that can cause abnormal bowel function.

Food Prescriptions

Dietary fiber promotes proper colon function. Patients with constipation are much more likely to respond to dietary fiber than are those with diarrhea. Increasing intake of dietary fiber from fruit and vegetable sources, rather than cereal sources, may offer more benefit to some individuals. Increasing dietary fiber usually coincides with decreasing sugar and refined carbohydrates, as high-fiber foods are unrefined and low in sugar.

Ginger may also offer some relief. To those with IBS, ginger is an excellent carminative (a substance that promotes the elimination of intestinal wind) and intestinal spasmolytic (a substance that relaxes and soothes the intestinal tract). To gain the maximum benefit from ginger, add some fresh ginger (1-to-2¼-inch/2½-to-6-centimeter-thick slices) to fresh fruit or vegetable juice. Ginger can also be juiced and kept in the refrigerator for two to three days. Add ½ to 1 teaspoon of ginger juice to water and drink with each meal.

Other supportive information can be found in "Food Prescriptions" under "Constipation" and "Diarrhea."

Other Recommendations

Clinical studies have documented that psychological approaches, such as relaxation therapy, biofeedback, hypnosis, counseling, and stress management training, significantly improve the symptoms of IBS. Many people with IBS find that daily leisurely walks markedly reduce symptoms, probably due to the well-known stress reduction effects of exercise.

Several double-blind studies have also shown peppermint oil capsules to be quite helpful in the treatment of irritable bowel syndrome. In order to be most effective, peppermint oil should be enteric-coated to prevent the oil from being released in the stomach. Without enteric coating, peppermint oil tends to produce heartburn. With enteric coating, the peppermint oil travels to the small and large intestines, where it relaxes intestinal muscles as well as promotes the elimination of excess wind. The typical dosage is 1 to 2 capsules (0.2 milliliters per capsule) three times daily between meals.

Kidney Stones

Kidney stones are lumps of solid matter usually composed of calcium oxalate, uric acid, or other crystals. Approximately 1 in every 1,000 adults in the United States is hospitalized annually for kidney stones (renal calculi). In the U.K., three in twenty men and one in twenty women develop a kidney stone during their lifetime, often between the ages of twenty to forty. The problem recurs in half of these cases. However, surgery is necessary for only about 5 percent of people with kidney stones. Although kidney stones can be composed of different substances, more than 75 percent of the kidney stones in patients in the United States are made of calcium oxalate (80 percent in the U.K.). The information provided here applies to this form of kidney

stones. For uric acid kidney stones, follow these dietary recommendations in addition to those covered in "Food Prescriptions" under "Gout."

Signs and Symptoms

Kidney stones usually do not produce symptoms until a stone becomes dislodged. A dislodged stone can produce excruciating, intermittent, radiating pain originating in the flank or kidney; nausea, vomiting, and abdominal distension; and chills, fever, and urinary frequency.

Causes

Components in human urine, including calcium and oxalic acid, normally remain in solution due to pH control and the secretion of inhibitors of crystal growth. However, when an increase occurs in stone components (such as oxalate) or a decrease occurs in protective factors, kidney stones can develop. The high frequency of calcium-containing stones in affluent societies is directly associated with the following dietary patterns: low fiber, highly refined carbohydrates, high alcohol consumption, large amounts of animal protein, and high fat intake.

Food Prescriptions

A diet low in oxalates has been recommended by many physicians and is supported within the medical literature as effective. The ultimate goal is to reduce the level of oxalic acid being excreted in the diet. Researchers initially thought that the greater the oxalate level in a food, the more likely it was to increase the risk of forming a kidney stone. However, it is beginning to look as though only certain oxalate-containing foods are likely to significantly increase urinary oxalate. The foods reported to cause a significant increase in urinary oxalate include spinach, rhubarb, beets, nuts, chocolate, wheat bran, strawberries, peanuts, and almonds. However, there remains no universal consensus on which oxalate-containing foods belong on this list. Therefore it seems that the best approach in the prevention of recurrent kidney stones is simply to avoid all high-oxalate foods (see Appendix D). A low-oxalate diet is usually defined as containing less than 50 milligrams of oxalate per day, so foods in the moderate-oxalate category will have to be consumed with moderation.

It appears that people with recurrent kidney stones have a tendency to absorb higher levels of dietary oxalates than do normal subjects not prone to kidney stones, who absorb only 3 to 8 percent of dietary oxalate. Interestingly, for many years physicians cautioned against the use of calcium supplements by kidney stone patients, but now it looks as though calcium supplements are beneficial via their ability to bind the oxalate in the gut, thereby preventing oxalate absorption.

A low-oxalate diet is not always effective in reducing urinary oxalic acid levels because dietary oxalate contributes to less than 50 percent of the oxalate found in urine; the rest is made in the body and does not come from the diet. So the next approach involves trying to reduce the concentration of oxalic acid by other means, including a liberal water intake (3 to 4 liters per day).

Increase intake of fiber, complex carbohydrates, and green leafy vegetables, and decrease intake of simple and refined carbohydrates, as it has been shown that a simple, single change from white to whole-wheat (wholemeal) bread has resulted in lowering urinary calcium levels. Vegetarians have a decreased risk of developing stones. Studies have shown that even among meat eaters, those who ate higher amounts of fresh fruits and vegetables had a lower incidence of stones.

It is also important to increase your intake of high-magnesium-to-calcium-ratio foods, including barley, bran, corn, buckwheat, rye, soy, oats, brown rice, avocados, bananas, cashews, coconut, peanuts, sesame seeds, lima beans, and potatoes. If oxalate stones are present, reduce oxalate-containing foods, such as beet greens, black tea, cocoa and dark chocolate, aubergines, figs, plums, prunes, rhubarb, spinach, and Swiss chard. Foods that contain smaller amounts of oxalates and should be eaten only in moderation include berries, such as blueberries, cranberries, raspberries, and strawberries; cabbage-family greens, such as rocket, broccoli, Brussels sprouts, collards, kale, and mustard and turnip greens; leeks; nuts, such as cashews and peanuts; soy; summer squash; sweet potatoes; and tomatoes. However, it is not necessary to restrict calcium intake, as calcium actually inhibits oxalate absorption, according to recent studies. Calcium supplementation has also been shown to significantly reduce oxalate absorption.

Sugar consumption contributes to kidney stones. The ingestion of sucrose and other simple sugars causes an exaggerated increase in the urinary calcium oxalate content in approximately 70 percent of people with recurrent kidney stones. Also, salt (sodium chloride) consumption contributes to kidney stones by increasing calcium excretion. People who tend to form kidney stones have an even greater increase in urinary calcium with an increase in salt intake.

Cranberries may also help prevent kidney stones. Cranberries contain quinic acid, which, because it is not broken down in the body but is excreted unchanged in the urine, renders the urine mildly acid. This mild acidity prevents calcium and phosphate ions from forming insoluble stones. In patients with recurrent kidney stones, cranberry juice has also been shown to reduce the amount of ionized calcium by more than 50 percent. Since in the United States, 75 to 85 percent of kidney stones are composed of calcium salts (80 percent in the U.K.), cranberry's effects on calcium may provide significant protective benefit.

Other Recommendations

For prevention of kidney stones, increasing fluid consumption to dilute the urine is essential. A person with a history of kidney stones should consume enough fluids to produce a daily urinary volume of at least 2,000 milliliters (roughly 2 liters). Vitamin B6 (25 to 50 milligrams daily) reduces the formation of oxalate, and magnesium supplementation (250 to 500 milligrams daily) is also very important to balance calcium in the body.

Hair mineral analysis may be of value in patients with recurrent kidney stones, since many heavy metals, such as lead, mercury, aluminium, and cadmium, are toxic to the kidneys and may lead to stone formation. Hair mineral analysis will often, but not always, detect an increased body burden of heavy metals.

Macular Degeneration, Age-Related

The macula is the area of the retina where images are focused. It is the portion of the eye responsible for fine vision. Age-related macular degeneration (ARMD) is the leading cause of severe visual loss in the United States in persons aged fifty-five years and older. It is also the leading cause of sight loss in the U.K. where 500,000 people suffer from the condition.

Signs and Symptoms

Individuals with ARMD may experience blurred vision; see straight objects as distorted or bent; see a dark spot near or around the center of the visual field; and, while reading, may see parts of words missing. People with macular degeneration generally have good peripheral vision; they just can't see directly in front of them.

Causes

The major risk factors for ARMD are smoking, aging, atherosclerosis, and high blood pressure. Apparently, the degeneration is a result of free-radical damage, similar to the type of damage that induces cataracts. However, decreased blood and thus oxygen supply to the retina is the prelude to and key factor leading to ARMD.

The two most common types of ARMD are the atrophic ("dry") form, by far the more frequent, and the neovascular ("wet") form. Between 80 and 95 percent of people with ARMD have the dry form of the disease. The primary cause of dry ARMD is related to oxidative (free-radical) damage to the innermost layer of the retina. Wet ARMD is characterized by the growth of abnormal blood vessels.

Food Prescriptions

A diet rich in fruits and vegetables is associated with a lowered risk of ARMD. Presumably, this protection is the result of increased intake of antioxidant vitamins and minerals. However, various "nonessential" food components, such as the carotenes lutein, zeaxanthin, and lycopene, along with flavonoids, are proving to be even more significant in protecting against ARMD than traditional nutritional antioxidants, such as vitamin C, vitamin E, and selenium. The macula, especially the central portion (the fovea), owes its yellow color to its high concentration of lutein and zeaxanthin. These yellow carotenes function in preventing oxidative damage to the area of the retina responsible for fine vision and obviously play a central role in protecting against the development of macular degeneration. Focusing on dietary sources of these carotenes, such as leafy green and vibrantly colored vegetables, appears to be more practical than supplements. Good leafy green vegetables include those in the cabbage family, such as broccoli, Brussels sprouts, cabbages, collards, kale, and mustard and turnip greens. Some beneficial highly colored vegetables include red peppers and tomatoes for their lycopene and squash, sweet potatoes, and carrots for other carotenoids.

Bilberries and blueberries are also antioxidant-rich foods containing flavonoids that strengthen the macula. Regular consumption of these berries is beneficial for preventing and treating ARMD.

Other Recommendations

Wet ARMD can be treated quite effectively with laser photocoagulation therapy; dry ARMD cannot. Because wet ARMD can rapidly progress to a point where surgery cannot be utilized, the surgery should be performed as soon as possible. Anyone with any vision loss should see a physician for a complete evaluation, especially if the loss is progressing rapidly.

Menopause

Menopause is the cessation of menstruation in women, which on average occurs at the age of fifty but may occur as early as forty and as late as fifty-five years of age. Six to twelve months without a menstrual period is the commonly accepted rule for diagnosing menopause. The time period prior to menopause is referred to as perimenopause, while the time period after menopause is referred to as postmenopause. During the perimenopausal period, many women have irregular periods.

Signs and Symptoms

The most common complaints of perimenopause and menopause are hot flushes, headaches, atrophic vaginitis (vaginal dryness and irritation due to lack of oestrogen), frequent urinary tract infections, cold hands and feet, forgetfulness, and inability to concentrate. In the United States, 65 to 80 percent of menopausal women experience hot flushes to some degree. Hot flushes are also the most common symptom of menopause in the U.K., where 60 percent of women experience them.

Causes

Menopause occurs when there are no longer any active eggs left in the ovaries due to normal aging or as a result of chemotherapy or surgery. At birth, there are about 1 million eggs (ova). This number drops to around 300,000 or 400,000 at puberty, but only about 400 of these ova will actually mature during the reproductive years. By the time a woman reaches the age of 50, few eggs remain. With menopause, the absence of active follicles (the cellular housings of the eggs) results in reduced production of oestrogen and progesterone. In response to this drop in oestrogen, the pituitary gland increases secretion of follicle-stimulating hormone (FSH) and luteinizing hormone (LH). The fluctuation of hormones, particularly the decline in oestrogen and progesterone, is the cause of many perimenopausal and menopausal complaints.

Food Prescriptions

The key dietary recommendation to relieve menopausal symptoms is to increase the amount of plant foods, especially those high in phytoestrogens, while reducing the amount of animal foods in the diet. Phytoestrogens are plant compounds that are capable of binding to oestrogen receptors and can replace some of the effect of oestrogen that is no longer being made. Foods high in phytoestrogens include soybeans and soy foods, linseeds, nuts, whole grains, apples, fennel, celery, parsley, and alfalfa. A

high intake of phytoestrogens is thought to explain why hot flushes and other menopausal symptoms rarely occur in cultures in which people consume a predominantly plant-based diet. Increasing the intake of dietary phytoestrogens helps decrease hot flushes, increase maturation of vaginal cells, and inhibit osteoporosis. In addition, a diet rich in phytoestrogens results in a decreased frequency of breast, colon, and prostate cancers. Furthermore, it is important to increase the consumption of soy foods. Clinical studies have shown eating soy foods (the equivalent of ⅔ cup of soybeans daily) to be effective in relieving hot flushes and vaginal atrophy.

Cabbage-family foods, including broccoli, Brussels sprouts, cabbages, collards, kale, and mustard and turnip greens, are good food choices for women going through menopause, not only for their ability to protect against breast cancer and heart disease but also because of their high content of nutrients that are supportive of bone health, such as calcium, magnesium, and folic acid.

Other Recommendations

Black cohosh *(Cimicifuga racemosa)* a perennial herb native to North America, can help with menopausal symptoms, according to the results of double-blind studies. For example, in one study, when eighty patients were given either black cohosh extract (two tablets twice daily, providing 4 milligrams of 27-deoxyacteine daily) conjugated oestrogens (0.625 milligram daily), or placebo for twelve weeks, the black cohosh extract produced the best results. The number of hot flushes experienced each day dropped from an average of five to less than one in the black cohosh group. In comparison, the oestrogen group dropped only from five to three and a half. Even more impressive was the effect of black cohosh on building up the vaginal lining.

While an oestrogenic effect was noted in some early animal studies, more recent studies with black cohosh extracts have demonstrated no oestrogenic activity. In studies with various types of breast cancer cells, black cohosh has shown no stimulatory effects. Therefore, black cohosh does not increase the risk of breast cancer as conjugated oestrogens do.

Mouth Ulcers (Canker Sores)

Mouth ulcers or canker sores *(aphthous stomatitis)* are single or clustered shallow, painful ulcers found anywhere in the oral cavity. The ulcers usually resolve in seven to twenty-one days but are recurrent in many people.

Signs and Symptoms

Mouth ulcers are single or clustered shallow, painful ulcers, less than 1 centimeter in size, found anywhere in the oral cavity. They may be covered by a layer of white or gray skin or uncovered. In contrast to cold sores caused by the herpes virus, mouth ulcers occur only inside the mouth and are always flat, never creating fluid-filled bumps, or vesicles, like a cold sore.

Causes

Recurrent mouth ulcers appear to be related to trauma; food sensitivities, especially milk and gluten sensitivity; stress; and/or nutrient deficiency. Stress is often a precipitating factor in recurrent mouth ulcers.

Food Prescriptions

The association of recurrent mouth ulcers with food allergies is widely accepted, as a diet eliminating allergenic foods will most often prevent further recurrences. The most common offending foods are typically milk products and wheat. Gluten, a grain protein, appears to be a major causative factor for many individuals, as well. Withdrawing gluten from the diet results in complete remission of recurrent mouth ulcers in patients with celiac disease. It also usually produces some improvement in other patients. Underlying gluten sensitivity would also contribute to nutritional deficiencies.

The lining of the mouth and throat is often the first place where nutritional deficiency becomes visible because of the high turnover rate of the cells that line these epithelial surfaces. There are several studies that show nutrient deficiencies to be much more common among recurrent mouth ulcer sufferers than in the general population, especially deficiencies of thiamine, folic acid, vitamin B12, vitamin B6, and iron. When nutrient deficiencies were corrected, the majority of subjects with recurrent mouth ulcers experienced complete remission. Foods high in these nutrients include brewer's yeast, nuts, and whole grains for thiamine, folic acid, and vitamin B6; lean meats and fish for vitamins B12 and B6 as well as iron; and legumes and leafy green vegetables for folic acid.

Other Recommendations

Stress is often a precipitating factor in recurrent mouth ulcers, as stress greatly increases the development of allergies. During times of stress, it may be particularly important to make sure to avoid suspected allergens. Taking a high-potency multiple vitamin and mineral formula will ensure adequate intake of all nutrients linked to recurrent mouth ulcers as well as provide nutrients to help the body adapt to stress.

Multiple Sclerosis

Multiple sclerosis (MS) is a syndrome of progressive nerve disturbances that usually occurs early in adult life. It is caused by gradual loss of the myelin sheath that surrounds the nerve cell. This process is called demyelination. One of the key functions of the myelin sheath is to facilitate the transmission of the nerve impulse. Without the myelin sheath, nerve function is lost. Symptoms correspond to the nerves that have lost their myelin sheaths.

Signs and Symptoms

Symptoms of MS include sudden transient motor and sensory disturbances, such as blurred vision, dizziness, muscle weakness, and tingling sensations. Generally, only one or two symptoms present initially. As the disease progresses, the initial symptoms worsen and other symptoms can develop. The diagnosis is confirmed by the detection of evidence of demyelination on magnetic resonance imaging (MRI).

Causes

The cause of MS remains to be identified conclusively. It is thought that MS is an auto-immune disease, that is, a disease where the immune system attacks body tissues as if they were foreign proteins. What triggers this process in initiating or exacerbating MS is unknown.

Food Prescriptions

Dr. Roy Swank, professor of neurology at the University of Oregon Medical School, has provided convincing evidence that a diet low in saturated fats, maintained over a long period of time, tends to retard the disease process of MS and reduce the number of attacks. Swank, who began successfully treating patients with his low-fat diet in 1948, recommends:

- A saturated fat intake of no more than 10 grams per day.
- A daily intake of 40 to 50 grams of polyunsaturated oils (margarine, shortening, and hydrogenated oils are not allowed).
- At least 1 teaspoon of cod liver oil per day.
- A normal allowance of protein (0.8 gram per kilogram of body weight; see "Protein" in Part II).
- Consumption of cold-water fish (e.g., salmon, mackerel, and herring) three or more times per week in order to boost omega-3 fatty acids.

The Swank diet was originally thought to help patients with MS by overcoming an essential fatty acid deficiency. Currently, it is thought that the beneficial effects are probably a result of (1) decreasing platelet aggregation, (2) decreasing the autoimmune response, and (3) normalizing the decreased essential fatty acid levels found in patients with MS.

A high intake of saturated fatty acids and animal fat is linked to MS. Consumption of saturated fats increases the requirements for the essential fatty acids, creating a relative deficiency state. Making matters worse is that individuals with MS are also thought to have a defect in essential fatty acid absorption and/or transport, which results in a functional deficiency state. Without the essential fatty acids, the myelin sheath does not form or function properly.

Food allergy has been implicated in the progression of MS, in particular the consumption of two common allergens, gluten and milk. While there is no convincing clinical evidence that gluten-free or allergy elimination diets are universally beneficial in the management of MS, it certainly is generally healthful to eliminate food allergens as long as other dietary measures are also included, i.e., the Swank diet. There is anecdotal evidence that specific individuals have been helped by using this approach.

Other Recommendations

Synthetically produced beta-interferon (Avonex, Betaferon) is emerging as the most popular medical treatment for MS. However, alpha-interferon (Roferon-A, Intron) may prove to be a better choice. In preliminary studies, 83 percent of the patients receiving 5 million to 30 million IU of alpha-interferon per week improved or stabilized in the first year, and in year two, 76 percent remained improved or stabilized. The 83 percent remission rate with alpha-interferon is better than the 30 percent rate reported for beta-interferon. Further studies are needed, but if these preliminary results hold true, obviously alpha-interferon would be the better choice.

Nonulcer Dyspepsia

Nonulcer dyspepsia (NUD) is a medical term often used to label indigestion and/or heartburn that is not related to an ulcer. Another common term for similar symptoms is gastroesophageal reflux disease (GERD). The main symptoms of GERD are heartburn and/or upper abdominal pain.

Signs and Symptoms

Symptoms of NUD include symptoms of GERD (heartburn and/or upper abdominal pain), as well as difficulty swallowing, feelings of pressure or heaviness after eating, sensations of bloating after eating, stomach or abdominal pains and cramps, and all of the symptoms of irritable bowel syndrome (IBS). About three out of ten patients with NUD also meet the criteria for IBS.

Causes

NUD and GERD are caused by factors that increase intra-abdominal pressure, thereby causing the gastric contents to flow upward. Factors that increase intra-abdominal pressure include obesity and overeating. The other causes of NUD and GERD include factors that decrease the tone of the oesophageal sphincter, such as smoking, hiatal hernia, and consumption of chocolate, fried foods, carbonated beverages (soft drinks), tomatoes, mints, alcohol, and coffee.

Food Prescriptions

In most cases, simply eliminating or reducing the causative food(s) or beverage(s) is all that is necessary to relieve NUD and GERD. Other tips include decreasing the size of portions at mealtime, chewing food thoroughly and eating in a leisurely manner in a calm, relaxed atmosphere, and not eating within two hours of bedtime.

Other Recommendations

Cigarette smoking and use of other tobacco products is associated with an increased likelihood of experiencing NUD and GERD, so don't smoke.

Elevating the head of the bed on six-inch blocks or sleeping on a specially designed wedge (not propped up on pillows) reduces heartburn by allowing gravity to minimize reflux of stomach contents into the oesophagus.

Enteric-coated peppermint oil capsules have been shown to be of benefit in NUD and GERD (see page 496 for more information).

Obesity

Obesity is defined as a state of being more than 20 percent above "normal" weight or having a body fat percentage greater than 30 percent for women and 25 percent for men.

Signs and Symptoms

Obesity is divided into two categories based on how the fat is distributed in the body. Fat distributed primarily around the waist is referred to as male-pattern or android obesity, since it is typically seen in obese males. In android obesity, the waist is bigger around than the hips (apple-shaped). In gynecoid obesity, the hips are larger (pear-shaped). Android obesity carries with it a greater risk for cardiovascular disease and diabetes, while gynecoid obesity increases the risk of hormone-sensitive cancers, such as breast cancer.

Causes

Theories of the underlying causes of obesity are tied to genetics, low brain serotonin levels, impaired diet-induced thermogenesis (heat production), and the inner workings of fat cells. All of these models support the notion that obesity is not just a matter of overeating. They explain why some people can eat large quantities of food and not increase their weight substantially, while for others, just the reverse is true. For example, a certain amount of the food we consume is immediately converted to heat, which is known as diet-induced thermogenesis. Diet-induced thermogenesis is the method by which the body "wastes" calories. There is evidence that the level of diet-induced thermogenesis is what determines whether an individual is likely to be overweight. In lean individuals, a meal may stimulate up to a 40 percent increase in heat production. In contrast, overweight individuals often display only a 10 percent or less increase in heat production. The food energy is stored as fat instead of being converted to heat.

Food Prescriptions

There are literally hundreds of diets and diet

programmes that claim to be the answer to obesity. However, the basic equation for losing weight never changes. In order for an individual to lose weight, energy intake must be less than energy expenditure. This goal can be achieved by decreasing caloric intake (dieting) and/or by increasing the rate at which calories are burned (exercising). Of course, while reducing caloric intake, a person must follow the basic guidelines of constructing a health-promoting diet, as detailed in chapter 2. Most individuals will begin to lose weight if they decrease their caloric intake below 1,500 calories per day and do aerobic exercise for fifteen to twenty minutes, three to four times per week. Starvation and crash diets usually result in rapid weight loss (largely muscle and water) but cause rebound weight gain. The most successful approach to weight loss is gradual weight reduction (½ to 1 pound/¼ to ½ kilogram per week) through long-term dietary and lifestyle modifications.

Fiber supplements can be quite helpful in helping people lose weight. Fiber supplementation has been shown to enhance blood sugar control, decrease insulin levels, and reduce the number of calories absorbed by the body. The best fiber sources for promoting weight loss are those that are rich in water-soluble fibers, such as glucomannan (from konjac root), psyllium, guar gum, defatted fenugreek seed powder or fiber, seaweed fibers (alginate and carrageenan), and pectin.

When taken with water before meals, these fiber sources bind to the water in the stomach and small intestine to form a gelatinous, viscous mass that not only slows down the absorption of glucose but also induces a sense of satiety (fullness) and reduces the absorption of calories. In some of the clinical studies demonstrating weight loss, fiber supplements were shown to reduce the number of calories absorbed by 30 to 180 calories per day. While modest, this reduction in calories would, over the course of a year, result in a 3- to 18-pound/1½-to-8 kilogram weight loss.

TABLE 20.3

Examples of Clinical Studies with Dietary Fiber Supplements for Weight Loss

Fiber	Number of Subjects	Length of Study	Dosage (grams per day)	Calorie Restriction	Average Weight Loss (fiber, pounds/ kilograms)	Average Weight Loss (placebo, pounds/ kilograms)
Guar gum	33	2.5 months	15	None	5.5/2.5	0.9/0.4
Glucomannan	20	2 months	3	None	5.5/2.5	Weight gain of 1.5/0.7
Glucomannan	20	2 months	3	None	8.14/3.7	0.44/0.2
Mixture A*	60	3 months	5	Yes	18.7/8.5	14.7/6.7
Mixture B*	97	3 months	7	Yes	10.8/4.9	7.3/3.3
Mixture B*	52	6 months	7	Yes	12.1/5.5	6.1/2.8

* Mixture A: 80 percent fiber from grains, 20 percent fiber from citrus; mixture B: 90 percent insoluble and 10 percent soluble fiber from beet, barley, and citrus fibers.

The following two recommendations are important in choosing a fiber supplement:

- Avoid products that contain a lot of sugar or other sweeteners to camouflage the taste. The sugar provides more empty calories, which you are trying to avoid.
- Be sure to drink at least 12 ounces/350 milliliters of water when taking any fiber supplement, especially if it is in a dry form (pill, biscuit, capsule or bar).

As water-soluble fibers are fermented by intestinal bacteria, a great deal of wind can be produced, leading to increased flatulence and abdominal discomfort. Start out with a dosage of 1 to 2 grams before meals and at bedtime, and gradually increase the dosage to 5 grams before meals and bedtime to reach the full daily dosage of 15 grams. Generally, the digestive system adapts to fiber over a few days, and intestinal wind will become negligible.

Other Recommendations

A successful programme for weight loss is consistent with the basic tenets of good health: a positive mental attitude, a healthy lifestyle (especially important is regular exercise), a health-promoting diet, and supplementary measures. All of these components are interrelated, and no single component is more important than the others. Improvement in one may be enough to result in some improvement, but the best approach is one that is comprehensive.

That said, exercise is a critical component of any weight loss or weight maintenance programme. Here's why:

- When weight loss is achieved by dieting without exercise, a substantial portion of the total weight loss comes from the lean tissue, primarily as water loss.
- When exercise is included in a weight loss programme, there is usually an improvement in body composition due to a gain in lean body weight because of an increase in muscle mass and an accompanying decrease in body fat.
- Exercise helps counter the reduction in basal metabolic rate that usually accompanies calorie restriction alone.
- Exercise increases the basal metabolic rate for an extended period of time following the exercise session. Thus, extra calories are consumed for many hours after each exercise session.
- Moderate to intense exercise may have an appetite suppressant effect.
- Individuals who exercise during and after weight reduction are better able to maintain the weight loss than those who do not exercise.
- Exercise helps diminish anxiety, and it reduces depression—two major factors that often lead to stress-induced eating to find a sense of comfort.

Osteoarthritis

Osteoarthritis (OA), also known as degenerative joint disease, is a form of arthritis (inflammation of a joint) caused by degeneration of cartilage. Cartilage serves an important role in joint function. Its gellike nature provides protection to the ends of bones by acting as a shock absorber. Without the cartilage in the joint, bone literally rubs against bone, leading to pain, deformity, inflammation, and limitation of motion in the joint.

Signs and Symptoms

The onset of OA can be subtle. Morning joint stiffness is often the first symptom. As the disease progresses, there is pain on motion of the involved joint that is made worse by prolonged activity and relieved by rest. There are usually local tenderness, soft tissue swelling, joint crepitus (cracking sounds), bone swelling, restricted mobility, and bony nodules. X-ray findings show narrowing of the joint space (the area between the bones taken up by cartilage). The weight-bearing joints of the knees, hips, and spine, as well as those of the hands, are most often affected. These joints are under greater stress because of weight and use.

Causes

OA is divided into two categories, primary and secondary. In primary OA, the degenerative "wear-and-tear" process occurs after a person turns forty. The cumulative effects of decades of use lead to the degenerative changes by stressing the collagen matrix of the cartilage. Damage to the cartilage results in the release of enzymes that further destroy cartilage components. With aging, the ability to restore and manufacture normal cartilage structures decreases.

Secondary OA is associated with some predisposing factor that is responsible for the degenerative changes. Predisposing factors in secondary OA include inherited abnormalities in joint structure or function; trauma, including fractures along joint surfaces, surgery, and other injuries to the joint; presence of abnormal cartilage; and previous inflammatory disease of joints, such as rheumatoid arthritis and gout.

Food Prescriptions

Perhaps the most important dietary recommendation for individuals suffering from OA is that they achieve normal body weight. Being overweight means increasing the stress on weight-bearing joints affected with OA. Beyond that, it is critical that the diet be rich in fruits and vegetables because their natural plant compounds can protect against cellular damage, including damage to the joints. Foods especially beneficial for OA are flavonoid-rich fruits, such as cherries, blueberries, blackberries, and strawberries. Also important are sulphur-containing foods, such as garlic, onions, Brussels sprouts, and cabbage. The sulphur content in fingernails of arthritis sufferers is lower than that of healthy subjects without arthritis.

Ginger contains anti-inflammatory compounds called gingerols. These substances are believed to explain why so many people with osteoarthritis experience reduction in their pain levels and improvement in their mobility when they consume ginger regularly. Although most scientific studies have used powdered gingerroot, fresh gingerroot at an equivalent dosage is believed to yield even better results because it contains active enzymes. Most studies utilized 1 gram of powdered gingerroot. This would be equivalent to approximately 10 grams or ⅓ ounce of fresh gingerroot, roughly a ¼-inch/½-centimetre slice.

People with OA may want to avoid foods from the nightshade family. It appears that in genetically susceptible individuals, long-term, low-level consumption of the alkaloids found in tomatoes, potatoes, aubergine, peppers, and tobacco can worsen OA. Presumably these alkaloids inhibit normal collagen repair in the joints or promote the inflammatory degeneration of the joint. Although remaining to be proved, elimination of nightshade vegetables from the diet may offer some benefit to certain individuals and is certainly worth a try.

Other Recommendations

Various physical therapy modalities (exercise, heat, cold, diathermy, ultrasound, etc.) performed by physical therapists, naturopathic physicians, and chiropractors are often very beneficial in improving joint mobility and reducing pain in sufferers of OA. The importance of physical therapy appears to be quite significant, especially when administered regularly.

Beyond physical therapy, glucosamine sulphate is a very effective natural product for OA. Glucosamine is a simple molecule that can be manufactured in the body. The main function of glucosamine in joints is to stimulate the manufacture of molecules known as glycosaminoglycans (GAGs), which are the key structural components of cartilage. It appears that as some people age, they lose the ability to manufacture sufficient levels of glucosamine. The result is that cartilage loses its ability to act as a shock absorber. The inability to manufacture glucosamine has been suggested to be the major factor leading to OA.

Glucosamine sulphate has been the subject of more than 300 scientific investigations and more than twenty double-blind studies. Glucosamine sulphate has been used by millions of people worldwide and is registered as a drug in the treatment of OA in more than seventy countries.

The more than twenty published clinical trials with glucosamine sulphate have demonstrated an overall success rate of 72 to 95 percent in various forms of OA. In OA of the knee, the success rate is more than 80 percent. In addition to being shown to be more effective than a placebo in head-to-head, double-blind studies comparing glucosamine sulphate to nonsteroidal anti-inflammatory drugs (NSAIDs), glucosamine sulphate was shown to produce better results than NSAIDs in relieving the pain and inflammation of OA, despite the fact that glucosamine sulphate exhibits very little direct anti-inflammatory effect and no direct analgesic or pain-relieving effects. Glucosamine sulphate appears to address the cause of OA. By treating the root of the problem through the promotion of cartilage synthesis, glucosamine sulphate not only improves the symptoms, including pain, but also helps the body to repair damaged joints.

The double-blind studies indicate that with glucosamine sulphate supplementation, most people with OA will experience significant improvement within four weeks. However, the longer it is used the better the results, because the effects are cumulative and long-lasting.

The typical dosage of glucosamine sulphate is 1,500 milligrams per day.

Capsaicin-containing creams and gels applied topically are showing impressive results when applied to the skin in cases of osteoarthritis.

Capsaicin works by depleting the pain neuro-transmitter substance P. It should be applied four times daily for three to four days, during which time pain may actually be worse due to the depletion of substance P. After this time pain relief occurs and the applications can be reduced to twice daily.

Osteoporosis

Osteoporosis literally means "porous bone." While many people erroneously believe that osteoporosis is the result of the loss of calcium and other minerals of bone, it actually involves a loss of both the mineral (inorganic) and nonmineral (organic matrix, composed primarily of protein) components of bone. Bone is dynamic, living tissue that is constantly being broken down and rebuilt, even in adults. Osteoporosis occurs when there is more bone breaking down than being formed.

Signs and Symptoms

Osteoporosis is usually without symptoms until severe backache due to compression of the vertebrae or fracture occurs. It may also result in considerable loss of height. Osteoporosis is best diagnosed by dual-energy X-ray absorptiometry (DEXA), a technique that measures bone density.

Causes

Normal bone metabolism is dependent on an intricate interplay of many nutritional, lifestyle, and hormonal factors. Many dietary factors have been suggested as a cause of osteoporosis,

including low calcium intake, high phosphorus intake, high refined sugar intake, high-protein diet, high-acid-ash diet, high salt intake, and trace mineral deficiencies, to name a few. Other risk factors for osteoporosis include family history of osteoporosis; alcoholism; smoking; physical inactivity; short stature, low body mass, and/or small bones; and never having been pregnant. Osteoporosis is most common in postmenopausal Asian and white women.

Food Prescriptions

A high-protein diet is associated with increased excretion of calcium in the urine and increased risk of osteoporosis, too. Raising daily protein intake from 47 to 142 grams doubles the excretion of calcium in the urine. However, too little protein is also associated with an increased risk for osteoporosis.

In contrast, a vegetarian diet is associated with a lower risk of osteoporosis. Although bone mass in vegetarians does not differ significantly from that of omnivores in the third, fourth, and fifth decades of life, there are significant differences in the later decades. These findings indicate that the decreased incidence of osteoporosis among vegetarians is due not to increased initial bone mass, but rather to decreased bone loss.

A diet high in salt or acid ash also causes calcium removal from bones and increases calcium loss in the urine. Therefore, we recommend avoiding salt and eating an alkaline-based diet. Basically, an alkaline diet is one that focuses on vegetables, fruit, nuts, and legumes while avoiding overconsumption of meat and dairy products. See Appendix B for a complete table of the acid and alkaline natures of common foods.

Soft drinks containing phosphates (phosphoric acid) are definitely linked to osteoporosis because they lead to lower calcium levels and higher phosphate levels in the blood. When phosphate levels are high and calcium levels are low, calcium is pulled out of the bones. The phosphate content of soft drinks, such as Coca-Cola and Pepsi, is very high, and they contain virtually no calcium. If you are concerned about developing or are at risk of developing osteoporosis, you will want to eliminate soft drinks from your diet.

Refined sugar intake also increases the loss of calcium from the bone. Regular consumption of refined sugar increases loss of calcium from the blood through the urine. Calcium is then pulled from the bones to maintain blood calcium levels, as foods containing refined sugar generally do not contain calcium.

Calcium is not the only nutrient that is important for bone formation. Many trace minerals, such as copper, manganese, zinc, and boron, are also important. A deficiency in trace minerals can also predispose to osteoporosis.

Green leafy vegetables from the cabbage family, including broccoli, Brussels sprouts, kale, collards, and mustard greens, as well as green tea, offer significant protection against osteoporosis. These foods are rich sources of a broad range of vitamins and minerals that are important to maintaining healthy bones, including calcium, vitamin K1, and boron. Vitamin K1 is the form of vitamin K that is found in plants. A function of vitamin K1 is to convert inactive osteocalcin to its active form. Osteocalcin is an important protein in bone. Its role is to anchor calcium molecules and hold them in place within the bone.

In addition, soy foods, such as tofu, soy milk, roasted soybeans and soy extract powders, may be beneficial in preventing osteoporosis. In several double-blind studies, taking 40 grams of soy protein powder containing 80 to 90 milligrams of isoflavones increased bone mineral density of the spine and hips in postmenopausal women. Alfalfa is another isoflavone- and vitamin K-rich food that can be included in the diet.

However, while numerous clinical studies have demonstrated that calcium supplementation can help prevent bone loss, the data are inconclusive in regard to any link between a high dietary calcium intake from milk and prevention of osteoporosis and bone fractures. When reviewing the data from the Nurses' Health Study, a study involving 77,761 women, researchers found no evidence that higher intake of milk actually reduced fracture incidence. In fact, women who drank two or more glasses of milk per day had an increased relative risk of 45 percent for hip fracture compared to women consuming one glass or less per week. In other words, the more milk a woman consumed, the more likely she was to experience a hip fracture. This negative effect may turn out to be due to the vitamin A added to milk (at higher levels, vitamin A—but not beta-carotene—may interfere with bone formation). Interestingly, if you look at the rate of osteoporosis worldwide, it is much higher in countries where milk intake is highest.

Other Recommendations

Physical fitness is actually the major determinant of bone density. Physical exercise consisting of one hour of moderate activity three times a week has been shown to prevent bone loss. In fact, this type of exercise has actually been shown to increase the bone mass in post-menopausal women. Walking is probably the best exercise to start with. In contrast to exercise, immobility doubles the rate of calcium excretion, resulting in an increased likelihood of developing osteoporosis.

Coffee, alcohol, and smoking induce a negative calcium balance (more calcium is lost than absorbed) and are associated with an increased risk of developing osteoporosis. Obviously, these lifestyle factors should be eliminated.

Peptic Ulcer Disease

Peptic ulcer disease (PUD) refers to an ulcer that occurs in the stomach (gastric ulcer) or the first portion of the small intestine (duodenal ulcer). An ulcer is a small wound in the surface of these organs.

Signs and Symptoms

Although the symptoms of PUD may be absent or quite vague, most PUD is associated with abdominal discomfort noted forty-five to sixty minutes after meals or during the night. In the typical case, the pain is described as gnawing, burning, cramplike, or aching or as "heartburn." Eating virtually any food or using antacids usually results in great relief.

Causes

Even though duodenal and gastric ulcers occur at different locations, both appear to be the result of factors damaging the protective lining of

> **WARNING:** *Individuals experiencing any symptoms of PUD need competent medical care. PUD complications such as hemorrhage, perforation, and obstruction are medical emergencies that require immediate hospitalization. Individuals with PUD must be monitored by a physician.*

the stomach or duodenum. These factors include too much gastric acid, which can be caused by a low-fiber diet, the bacterium *Helicobacter pylori (H. pylori),* and various drugs, such as nonsteroidal anti-inflammatory drugs and prednisone.

Food Prescriptions

Food allergy appears to be a primary factor in many cases of PUD. A diet that eliminates food allergens has been used with great success in treating and preventing recurrent PUD (see "Food Allergy"). It is especially important to avoid milk and dairy products. Milk is one of the most common food allergens, and population studies show that the higher the milk consumption, the greater the likelihood of PUD. Milk, as well as coffee, significantly increases stomach acid production. Both should be avoided by individuals with PUD.

A high-fiber diet is associated with a reduced rate of PUD, as compared with a low-fiber diet, by decreasing prolonged stomach acidity. Fiber supplements (e.g., pectin, guar gum, oat bran, and psyllium) have been shown to produce beneficial effects as well.

In addition, raw cabbage juice is well documented as having remarkable success in treating

PUD. In one study, 1 liter of fresh raw cabbage juice per day, taken in divided amounts, resulted in total PUD healing in an average of only ten days. The beneficial effect is thought to be due to the amino acid glutamine, which is needed by the cells on the surface of the small intestine to regenerate. Broccoli and Brussels sprouts are in the same family as cabbage, and regular consumption is helpful in preventing recurrence of PUD, as these foods are rich in sulphoraphane, a compound that may be effective in helping the body get rid of *Helicobacter pylori*. This bacterium is responsible for most peptic ulcers and also increases a person's risk of getting gastric cancer three- to sixfold, and is also a causative factor in a wide range of other stomach disorders, including gastritis, oesophagitis, and acid indigestion.

Bananas, particularly plantains, may be of benefit due to their healing properties on the intestinal lining, while garlic, cayenne pepper, turmeric, and foods high in vitamin C may also be helpful due to their ability to inhibit the growth of *H. pylori*.

Other Recommendations

A special licorice extract known as "deglycyrrhizinated licorice," or DGL, is a remarkable anti-PUD agent. DGL's mode of action is different from that of the current medications used for the treatment of PUD. Rather than inhibit the release of acid, licorice stimulates the normal defense mechanisms that prevent PUD formation. In several head-to-head comparison studies, DGL has been shown to be more effective than Tagamet, Zantac, or antacids in both short-term treatment and maintenance therapy

of PUD. However, while these drugs are associated with significant side effects, DGL is extremely safe, and its cost is significantly less. The standard dose of DGL is two to four 380 milligram tablets between or twenty minutes before meals. DGL should be continued for eight to sixteen weeks, depending on the response.

Periodontal Disease

Periodontal disease is an inclusive term used to describe an inflammatory condition of the gums (gingivitis) and/or support structures (periodontitis). The periodontal disease process typically progresses from gingivitis to periodontitis.

Signs and Symptoms

Gingivitis is characterized by redness, contour changes, and bleeding of the gums. Periodontitis is characterized by localized pain, loose teeth, dental pockets, redness, swelling, and/or signs of infection. X-rays may reveal destruction of bone in the case of periodontitis.

Causes

Periodontal disease can be caused by poor dental hygiene or may be a manifestation of a more systemic condition, such as diabetes, collagen diseases, anemia, vitamin deficiency states, depressed immune system, or leukemia or other disorders of leukocyte function. An association with hardening of the arteries (atherosclerosis) has also been reported.

Food Prescriptions

The key dietary recommendation to prevent periodontal disease is to avoid sugar (sucrose). Sugar is known to significantly increase plaque accumulation while decreasing white blood cell function.

Foods high in zinc, such as nuts and seeds; vitamin C, such as green vegetables and citrus fruits; and high-flavonoid-content berries, such as blackberries, raspberries, and blueberries, provide important nutritional support to healthy gums. In particular, periodontal health is closely linked to vitamin C status.

Other Recommendations

In addition to proper dental care—brushing after meals, daily flossing, and regular dental cleaning—nutritional status and immune system function must be normalized if development and progression of periodontal disease are to be controlled. Bacterial plaque has long been considered the causative agent in most forms of periodontal disease. However, it is now widely accepted that people with poor nutritional status or depressed immune function are likely to develop periodontal disease even with the best possible oral hygiene.

Pneumonia: See Bronchitis and Pneumonia.

Premenstrual Syndrome

Premenstrual syndrome (PMS) is a recurrent condition in women, characterized by trouble-some symptoms seven to fourteen days before menstruation.

Signs and Symptoms

Typical symptoms of PMS include: acne, decreased energy level, tension, anxiety, irritability, depression, headache, altered sex drive, breast tenderness, fibrocystic breast disease, insomnia, backache, abdominal bloating, and oedema of the fingers and ankles. Severe PMS, with depression, irritability, and extreme mood swings, is referred to as premenstrual dysphoric disorder.

Causes

Although there is a wide spectrum of symptoms, common hormonal patterns are found among PMS patients compared to women who have no symptoms of PMS. The primary finding is that oestrogen levels are elevated and plasma progesterone levels are reduced five to ten days before the menses. In addition to this, hormonal abnormality, hypothyroidism, and/or elevated prolactin levels are common.

Food Prescriptions

Reduce or eliminate the amount of animal products in the diet, and increase consumption of fiber-rich plant foods, including fruits, vegetables, grains, and legumes. Vegetarian women have been shown to excrete two to three times more oestrogen in their faeces and have 50 percent lower levels of free oestrogen in their blood than omnivores. These differences are thought to be a result of the lower fat and higher fiber intake of vegetarians.

Considerable evidence suggests that caffeine consumption is strongly related to the presence and severity of PMS. Therefore, caffeine must also be avoided by women with PMS. The effect of caffeine is particularly significant in the psychological symptoms associated with PMS, such as anxiety, irritability, insomnia, and depression. If breast tenderness and fibrocystic breast disease are the major symptoms, it is very important to eliminate or greatly restrict caffeine intake as caffeine has an adverse effect on the way oestrogen stimulates breast tissue.

There is also evidence that phytoestrogens may exert a balancing effect when oestrogen levels are high, as is commonly seen in premenstrual syndrome (PMS). The consumption of soy foods is the most economical, and possibly the most beneficial, way to increase the intake of phytoestrogens. Vitamin B6 also has an effect on the metabolism of oestrogen. Vitamin B6 is high in yams, leafy green vegetables, and legumes.

Excessive salt (sodium chloride) consumption, coupled with diminished dietary potassium, greatly stresses the kidneys' ability to maintain proper fluid volume. As a result, some people are "salt-sensitive," in that high salt intake causes high blood pressure or, in other cases, water retention. In general, it is a good idea to avoid salt if you have PMS. If you tend to notice more water retention during the latter part of your menstrual cycle, reducing your salt intake is an absolute must.

Other Recommendations

Since 1975, more than a dozen double-blind studies have looked at the effect of vitamin B6 supplementation in the treatment of PMS. Most, but not all, of these studies have demonstrated a positive effect. For example, in one study, 84 percent of the subjects had fewer symptoms during the vitamin B6 treatment period. In another study, premenstrual acne flare-up was reduced in 72 percent of the 106 affected young women taking 50 milligrams of vitamin B6 daily for one week prior to and during the menstrual period.

Chasteberry *(Vitex agnus castus)* extract has also been shown to be effective in the treatment of PMS. Studies have shown that using chasteberry extract once in the morning over a period of several months helps normalize hormone balance and thus alleviates the symptoms of PMS. The typical dosage is 20 milligrams per day.

Prostate Enlargement

The prostate is a single, doughnut-shaped gland about the size of a walnut that lies below the bladder and surrounds the urethra in males. The muscular part of the prostate controls the release of urine. The prostate also secretes a thin, milky, alkaline fluid that increases sperm motility and lubricates the urethra to prevent infection. Prostate secretions are extremely important to successful fertilization of the egg in females.

Benign (nonmalignant) enlargement of the prostate gland is known medically as benign prostatic hyperplasia, or BPH.

BPH is an extremely common condition. Current estimates are that it affects more than

50 percent of men during their lifetime. The actual frequency increases with advancing age, from approximately 5 to 10 percent at age thirty to more than 90 percent in men over 85 years of age.

Signs and Symptoms

Because an enlarged prostate can pinch off the flow of urine, BPH is characterized by symptoms of bladder obstruction, such as increased urinary frequency, nighttime awakening to empty the bladder, and reduced force and caliber (speed of flow) of urination.

Causes

BPH is largely the result of age-associated hormonal changes. The ultimate effect of these changes is an increased concentration of testosterone within the prostate gland and an increased conversion of this testosterone to an even more potent form known as dihydrotestosterone (DHT). DHT is more stimulating to the growth and division of prostate cells than testosterone is.

Food Prescriptions

In trying to treat or prevent BPH, the diet should be as free as possible from pesticides and other contaminants (e.g., dioxin, polyhalogenated biphenyls, hexachlorobenzene, and dibenzofurans). It is quite possible that the tremendous increase in the occurrence of BPH in the last few decades reflects the ever-increasing effect that toxic chemicals have on our health. BPH is perhaps just one of many

> **WARNING:** Prostate disorders can be diagnosed only by a physician. Do not self-diagnose. If you are experiencing any symptoms associated with BPH, see your physician immediately for proper diagnosis.

health problems that may be due to these toxic substances. A diet rich in natural, whole foods may offer some protection against these toxins.

In particular, focus on whole, unprocessed foods, including whole grains, legumes, vegetables, fruits, nuts, and seeds in your diet. Eat ¼ cup of raw pumpkin seeds or sunflower seeds each day for zinc, which is used by prostate enzymes. These seeds are also good sources of phytosterols, clinically proven natural compounds shown to be effective in the improvement of BPH.

Consuming soy foods helps balance testosterone metabolism and should also be highlighted. Also, lycopene-rich vegetables, such as tomatoes, spinach, kale, mangoes, broccoli, and berries, when consumed daily, promote prostate health and play a role in preventing prostate cancer. It is also important to reduce the intake of alcohol (especially beer), caffeine, and sugar, all of which have an adverse effect on the way testosterone is metabolized and cleared from the body.

Other Recommendations

Numerous double-blind studies have shown an extract of saw palmetto berries to significantly improve the signs and symptoms of BPH. Roughly 90 percent of men with mild to moderate BPH experienced some improvement in symptoms during the first four to six weeks of therapy, and all major symptoms of BPH were improved, especially increased nighttime urination. The extract of saw palmetto berries works by improving the hormonal metabolism within the prostate gland. The typical dosage is 320 milligrams daily.

Psoriasis

Psoriasis is a common skin disorder characterized by the appearance of plaquelike, silvery scale lesions caused by a pileup of skin cells that have replicated too rapidly. In addition to affecting the skin, psoriasis can cause an inflammatory form of arthritis and affect the nails.

Signs and Symptoms

The lesions of psoriasis are usually sharply bordered reddened rashes or plaques covered with overlapping silvery scales, which can be itchy and/or painful. Psoriasis usually affects the wrists, elbows, knees, buttocks, and ankles; and sites of repeated trauma. Nail involvement results in a characteristic "oil drop" stippling or a thimblelike appearance. Psoriasis can also affect the joints, particularly the last joint of the fingers and toes, producing psoriatic arthritis.

Causes

Psoriasis is caused by a pileup of skin cells that have replicated too rapidly. The rate at which skin cells divide in psoriasis is roughly 1,000 times as great as in normal skin. This high rate

of replication is simply too fast for the cells to be shed, so they accumulate, resulting in the characteristic silvery scales of psoriasis. Although psoriasis has a significant genetic component, a number of factors appear to cause or contribute to psoriasis, including incomplete protein digestion, bowel toxemia, impaired liver function, alcohol consumption, excessive consumption of animal fats, and stress.

Food Prescriptions

Limit the consumption of sugar and increase the intake of high-fiber foods, such as vegetables, legumes, fruit, and whole grains. Dietary fiber helps bind gut-derived toxins that can otherwise be absorbed and trigger psoriasis. It appears that many psoriasis patients do well by avoiding sources of gluten, such as wheat. Finally, an allergy elimination diet can often help psoriasis. For instance, follow the recommendations given under "Food Allergy."

It is also important to limit the consumption of meat, animal fats, and dairy products while increasing the intake of cold-water fish, such as salmon, mackerel, herring, and halibut. In the skin of individuals who have psoriasis, the production of inflammatory compounds known as leukotrienes is many times greater than normal. These toxic compounds are produced from arachidonic acid. Since arachidonic acid is found only in animal tissues, it is necessary to limit intake of animal products, particularly meat, animal fats, and dairy products. At the same time, it is important to increase the intake of omega-3 fatty acids because of their favorable effects on reducing inflammation.

In addition, eliminate alcohol. Alcohol is

known to worsen psoriasis significantly because it increases the absorption of toxins from the gut that can stimulate psoriasis.

Other Recommendations

A number of natural herbal formulas for topical use can provide symptomatic relief of psoriasis. The best choices are products that contain one of the following: glycyrrhetinic acid from licorice *(Glycyrrhiza glabra),* chamomile *(Matricaria chamomilla),* and capsaicin from cayenne pepper *(Capsicum frutescens).* Of these three, preparations containing capsaicin are the easiest to find. Apply to affected areas of the skin two to three times per day.

Rheumatoid Arthritis

Rheumatoid arthritis (RA) is a chronic inflammatory condition that affects the entire body, but especially the joints. The joints typically involved are those in the hands, feet, wrists, ankles, and knees.

Signs and Symptoms

The onset of RA is usually gradual but occasionally is quite abrupt. Fatigue, low-grade fever, weakness, joint stiffness, and vague joint pain may precede the appearance of painful, swollen joints by several weeks. Several joints are usually involved at the onset, typically in a symmetrical fashion, i.e., both hands, wrists, or ankles. However, in about one third of persons with RA, initial involvement is confined to one or a few joints.

Involved joints are characteristically quite warm, tender, and swollen. The skin over the joint takes on a ruddy, purplish hue. X-ray findings usually show soft tissue swelling, erosion of cartilage, and joint-space narrowing. As the disease progresses, deformities develop in the joints of the hands and feet, although deformities can occur in the neck and shoulders.

Causes

Abundant evidence suggests that RA is an autoimmune reaction, in which antibodies formed by the immune system attack components of joint tissues. Yet what triggers this autoimmune reaction remains largely unknown. Speculation and investigation have centered around genetic factors, abnormal bowel permeability, lifestyle and nutritional factors, food allergies, impaired liver detoxification, and microorganisms. RA is a classic example of a multifactorial disease, wherein an assortment of genetic and environmental factors contributes to the disease process.

Food Prescriptions

Diet has been strongly implicated in RA for many years, in regard to both cause and cure. The major focus in dietary therapy is to eliminate food allergies, increase the intake of antioxidant nutrients, follow a vegetarian diet, and alter the intake of dietary fats and oils. A long-term study conducted in Norway at the Oslo Rheumatism Hospital showed that following these dietary principles can be "curative" in some individuals with RA and significantly reduce symptoms in others.

The first step is a therapeutic fast or an elimination diet (see "Food Allergy"), followed by careful reintroduction of foods to detect allergens. Virtually any food can aggravate RA, but the most common offenders are wheat, corn, milk and other dairy products, beef, nightshade-family foods (tomatoes, potatoes, aubergines, peppers, and tobacco), and coffee. After isolating and eliminating all allergens, a diet rich in whole foods, vegetables, and fiber and low in sugar, meat, refined carbohydrates, and animal fats is recommended.

The importance of a diet rich in fresh fruits and vegetables in the dietary treatment of RA cannot be overstated. These foods, including vitamin C, beta-carotene, vitamin E, and selenium, are the best sources of dietary antioxidants. Several studies have shown that the risk of RA is highest among people with the lowest levels of dietary antioxidants. Excellent sources of antioxidants include flavonoid-rich berries, such as cherries, cranberries, hawthorn berries, blueberries, blackberries, raspberries, and strawberries. Carotenoids are beneficial antioxidants found in yellow and green vegetables, including squashes, yams, carrots, and the cabbage-family vegetables.

Vegetarian diets are often beneficial in the treatment of inflammatory conditions such as RA, presumably as a result of decreasing the availability of arachidonic acid for conversion to inflammatory prostaglandins and leukotrienes. Another important way of decreasing the inflammatory response is the consumption of cold-water fish, such as mackerel, halibut, herring, sardines, and salmon. These fish are rich sources of the long-chain omega-3 fatty acids. In addition, supplementing the diet with 1.8 to 3 grams of omega-3 fatty acids from a pharmaceutical-grade fish oil product is recommended. Fish oils and olive oil, which acts as a neutral fat in the diet, should replace other dietary fats, such as saturated fats, animal fats, and omega-6 polyunsaturated fats, all of which promote the inflammatory process.

Another way in which a more vegetarian diet may be helpful in RA is that it has a higher alkalinity than a meat-based diet. The severity of RA has been shown to be inversely related to the pH of the joint fluid—the lower the pH (high acid) the greater the pain and inflammation.

There are many nutrients within a vegetarian diet that may also be responsible for the observed effect. For example, molybdenum is necessary for the production of an enzyme called sulphite oxidase, one of the most important enzymes in a liver detoxification pathway called sulphoxidation. Poor sulphoxidation is associated with inflammatory conditions including rheumatoid arthritis. A ½-cup serving of adzuki beans provides almost 200 percent of the daily recommended intake for molybdenum, and other legumes, cauliflower, brewer's yeast, and spinach are rich in molybdenum as well.

During flare-ups, fresh pineapple juice along with some fresh ginger or turmeric root may help to relieve symptoms of RA due to their anti-inflammatory activity. Ginger possesses anti-inflammatory action by inhibiting the manufacture of inflammatory compounds and by the presence of an anti-inflammatory enzyme similar to bromelain, which is found in pineapple. In one clinical study, seven patients with RA in whom conventional drugs had provided only temporary or partial relief were treated with ginger. One patient took 50 grams per day of lightly cooked ginger, while the remaining six took either 5 grams of fresh or 0.1 to 1 gram of powdered ginger daily. All patients reported substantial improvement, including pain relief, joint mobility, and decrease in swelling and morning stiffness.

Other Recommendations

Proteolytic enzymes (or proteases) refer to the various enzymes that digest protein. These enzymes include the pancreatic proteases chymotrypsin and trypsin, pancreatin, bromelain (pineapple enzyme), papain (papaya enzyme), fungal proteases, peptizyme SP, and *Serratia* peptidase (the "silkworm" enzyme). Preparations of proteolytic enzymes have been shown to be useful in RA and other inflammatory conditions. In order to get the most out of proteolytic enzymes, it is essential to use a high-quality product at an adequate dosage. Choose well-respected brands available through health food shops or natural pharmacies and take the product according to label instructions. For anti-inflammatory effects, proteolytic enzyme products should be taken on an empty stomach. In Europe, apart from papain and bromelain, proteolytic enzymes are only available as prescription drugs.

Capsaicin creams and gels can be helpful to relieve pain associated with RA. Applying the cream or gel four times daily for three to four days depletes the pain neurotransmitter substance P. Because substance P is being released,

pain may increase during these three to four days. After that time, substance P is depleted and the cream or gel can be used twice daily to maintain pain relief.

Ulcer: See Peptic Ulcer Disease.

Urinary Tract Infection

A urinary tract infection (UTI) occurs when bacteria invade any part of the urinary tract, particularly the urethra or urinary bladder. Bladder infections, also called cystitis, are very common in women because of their anatomy. In fact, 10 to 20 percent of all women have urinary tract discomfort at least once a year. In turn, men do not commonly get UTIs unless they have enlarged prostates. Recurrent UTIs are a significant problem and can cause progressive damage, resulting in scarring and, in rare cases, kidney failure.

Signs and Symptoms

Burning pain on urination; increased urinary frequency (especially at night); cloudy, foul-smelling, or dark urine; and lower abdominal pain are common symptoms of UTI. The urine of someone with a UTI will show a significant number of bacteria and white blood cells.

Causes

Most urinary tract infections are caused by the

> **WARNING:** *Although most urinary tract infections are not serious, it is important that you be properly diagnosed, treated, and monitored. If you have symptoms suggestive of a UTI, consult a physician immediately.*

E. coli bacterium. Many factors are associated with increased risk of UTI: pregnancy (twice as frequent); menopause; sexual intercourse (nuns have one tenth the incidence); mechanical trauma or irritation; and, perhaps most important, structural abnormalities of the urinary tract that block the free flow of urine, such as benign prostatic hyperplasia in men.

Food Prescriptions

The most important dietary recommendation for someone who suffers from a urinary tract infection is to increase the quantity of liquids consumed. Ideally, the liquids should be in the form of pure water, herbal teas, cranberry or blueberry juice, and fresh fruit and vegetable juices diluted with at least an equal amount of water. If you have a UTI, you should drink at least 64 ounces/2 liters of liquids from this group, with at least half of this amount being water and at least 16 ounces/½ liter being unsweetened cranberry or blueberry juice. You should also avoid such liquids as soft drinks, concentrated fruit drinks, coffee, and alcoholic beverages. (For more information about why cranberry and blueberry juice are particularly effective in combating UTIs, see page 271.)

Other Recommendations

One of the easiest and most cost-effective ways to take advantage of the benefits of cranberries in preventing or treating urinary tract infections is to take a cranberry extract in pill form. For example, CranMax is an extract made from 100 percent cranberry fruit solids through a proprietary process that intensifies the natural benefits of the whole cranberry, without the use of any solvents, preservatives, sugars, water, flavorings, or artificial color. It takes 34 pounds/15 kilograms of whole, fresh cranberries to produce 1 pound/½ kilogram of CranMax. It is more powerful and works faster in treating UTIs than cranberry juice not only because it is more concentrated but also because it uses a patented technology that protects the cranberry from destruction by gastric acid, delivering the nutrients to the lower gastrointestinal tract, where they can be absorbed through a time-release mechanism. The recommended dosage of CranMax is 500 milligrams daily for prevention and 500 milligrams three times per day during an active UTI.

Varicose Veins

Varicose veins are enlarged, dilated, tortuous, superficial veins in the legs. Veins are fairly frail structures. Defects in the wall of a vein lead to dilation of the vein and damage to the valves. Normally, these valves prevent blood from backing up, but when the valves become damaged, blood pools and causes the bulging veins known as varicose veins.

Signs and Symptoms

Varicose veins may be without symptoms or may be associated with fatigue, aching discomfort, feelings of heaviness, or pain in the legs. Fluid retention (oedema), discoloration, and ulceration of the skin may also develop. Hemorrhoids are also varicose veins.

Causes

The following factors can cause varicose veins: pregnancy; genetic weakness of the vein walls or their valves; excessive pressure within the vein due to a low-fiber-induced increase in straining during defecation; long periods of standing and/or heavy lifting; damage to the veins or venous valves resulting from inflammation; and weakness of the vein walls.

Food Prescriptions

A high-fiber diet is the most important component of the treatment and prevention of varicose veins. A diet rich in vegetables, fruits, legumes, and whole grains promotes peristalsis, and the many fiber components attract water to form gelatinous masses that keep the faeces soft, bulky, and easy to pass. Individuals who consume a low-fiber diet tend to strain more during bowel movements, since their smaller and harder stools are more difficult to pass. This straining increases the pressure in the abdomen, which obstructs the flow of blood up the legs and out of the rectum. The increased pressure may, over time, significantly weaken the vein walls, leading to the formation of varicose veins or hemorrhoids.

Flavonoid-rich foods, such as bilberries, blackberries, blueberries, cherries, and hawthorn berries, are beneficial in the prevention and treatment of varicose veins. These berries are very rich sources of proanthocyanidins and anthocyanidins, the bioflavonoids that give the berries their blue-red color and also improve the integrity of support structures of the veins and the entire vascular system. In addition, even drinking buckwheat tea, a rich source of flavonoids, has been shown to be quite effective in the prevention and treatment of varicose veins.

Individuals with varicose veins have a decreased ability to break down fibrin. When fibrin is deposited in the tissue near the varicose veins, the skin becomes hard and "lumpy" due to the presence of the fibrin and fat. In addition, a decreased ability to break down fibrin increases the risk of thrombus formation, which may result in thrombophlebitis, a heart attack, pulmonary embolism, or stroke. Foods that increase the fibrinolytic activity of the blood are therefore indicated. Cayenne pepper, garlic, onion, and ginger all increase fibrin breakdown. Liberal consumption of these spices in foods is recommended for individuals with varicose veins and other disorders of the cardiovascular system. In addition, bromelain, from fresh pineapple, promotes the breakdown of fibrin.

Other Recommendations

Extracts of several of the berries listed under "Food Prescriptions" are used widely in Europe as medications for various circulatory conditions, including varicose veins. However, horse chestnut seed extracts and the procyanidolic oligomers in grape seed extract and pine bark extract are the most popular and possibly the most effective.

While small "spider veins" may disappear entirely, do not expect well-formed, large varicose veins to go away magically. In these cases, elastic compression stockings are occasionally beneficial as they provide support to the weakened vein walls, which helps the flow of blood. Be sure to exercise and to avoid standing for long periods of time. Walking, bike riding, and jogging are particularly beneficial, as the contraction of the leg muscles pushes pooled blood back into circulation. In the case of severe varicose veins, the only real options are sclerotherapy and surgical excision.

Glycemic Index, Carbohydrate Content, and Glycemic Load of Selected Foods

A complete list of the glycemic index (GI) and glycemic load (GL) of all tested foods is beyond the scope of this book—it would be a book in itself. So we have selected the most common foods. This listing will give you a general sense of what are high- and low-GL foods. The glycemic index for this listing uses glucose, scored as 100.

We have listed the items by food groups. You may notice that certain food groups are not included. For example, you won't see nuts, seeds, fish, poultry, and meats listed because, individu-ally, these foods have little impact on blood sugar levels due to their low carbohydrate content. In fact, these foods, particularly fats and oils, can lower the glycemic index of carbohydrate-rich foods by delaying absorption. (For more information on glycemic index and glycemic load, see page 71.)

If you would like to see an even more complete listing, visit www.mendosa.com, a free website operated by medical writer David Mendosa. It is an excellent resource.

	Glycemic Load	Glycemic Index	Carbohydrates (grams)	Fiber (grams)
Beans (Legumes)				
Baked beans, canned in tomato sauce, ½ cup, 120 grams	10.0	48	21	8.8
Black beans, canned, ½ cup, 95 grams	5.7	45	15	7.0
Black-eyed beans, soaked, boiled, ½ cup, 120 grams	10.0	42	24	5.0

(continued on next page)

Food	Glycemic Load	Glycemic Index	Carbohydrates (grams)	Fiber (grams)
Beans (Legumes) (cont.)				
Broad beans, frozen, boiled, ½ cup, 80 grams	7.1	79	9	6.0
Chickpeas, canned, drained, ½ cup, 95 grams	6.3	42	15	5.0
Kidney beans, boiled, ½ cup, 90 grams	4.8	27	18	7.3
Kidney beans, canned and drained, ½ cup, 95 grams	6.7	52	13	7.3
Lentils, ½ cup, 100 grams	5.3	28	19	3.7
Lima beans, baby, ½ cup cooked, 85 grams	5.4	32	17	4.5
Peas, dried, boiled, ½ cup, 70 grams	8.0	22	4	4.7
Peas, green, fresh or frozen, boiled, ½ cup, 80 grams	2.0	48	5	2.0
Peas, split, yellow, boiled, ½ cup, 90 grams	5.1	32	16	4.7
Pinto beans, canned, ½ cup, 95 grams	5.8	45	13	6.7
Soybeans, cooked, ½ cup, 100 grams	1.6	14	12	7.0
White haricot beans, boiled, ½ cup, 90 grams	4.2	38	11	6.0
Bread				
Bagel, 1, 70 grams	25.0	72	35	0.4
Croissant, 1, 50 grams	18.0	67	27	0.2
Dark rye, black, 1 slice, 50 grams	16.0	76	21	0.4
French baguette, 30 grams	14.0	95	15	0.4
Gluten-free multigrain, 1 slice, 35 grams	12.0	79	15	1.8
Hamburger bun, 1 prepacked bun, 50 grams	15.0	61	24	0.5
Crusty roll, 1 roll, 50 grams	18.0	73	25	0.4
Light rye, 1 slice, 50 grams	16.0	68	23	0.4
Multigrain, unsweetened, 1 slice, 30 grams	4.0	43	9	1.4
Oat Bran and Honey Loaf, 1 slice, 40 grams	4.5	31	14	1.5
Pita, 1, 65 grams	22.0	57	38	0.4
Pumpernickel, 1 slice, 60 grams	8.6	41	21	0.5
Rye, 1 slice, 50 grams	15.0	65	23	0.4
Sourdough, rye, 1 slice, 30 grams	6.0	48	12	0.4
Sourdough, wheat, 1 slice, 30 grams	7.5	54	14	0.4
Stone-ground wholemeal, 1 slice, 30 grams	6.0	53	11	1.4
White (wheat flour), 1 slice, 30 grams	10.5	70	15	0.4
Whole wheat (wholemeal), 1 slice, 35 grams	9.6	69	14	1.4

Food	Glycemic Load	Glycemic Index	Carbohydrates (grams)	Fiber (grams)
Breakfast Cereals				
All-Bran, ½ cup, 40 grams	9.2	42	22	6.5
Bran flakes, ⅜ cup, 30 grams	18.0	74	24	2.0
Bran, ⅓ cup, 30 grams	8.0	58	14	14.0
Cheerios, ½ cup, 30 grams	15.0	74	20	2.0
Cocoa Pops, ⅜ cup, 30 grams	20.0	77	26	1.0
Corn flakes, 1 cup, 30 grams	21.8	84	26	0.3
Crunchy Nut Cornflakes (Kellogg's), 1 cup, 30 grams	18.0	72	25	2.0
Froot Loops, 1 cup, 30 grams	18.0	69	27	1.0
Frosties, ⅜ cup, 30 grams	15.0	55	27	1.0
Grape Nuts, ½ cup, 58 grams	33.3	71	47	2.0
Just Right, ⅜ cup, 30 grams	21.6	60	36	2.0
Oat bran, raw, 1 tablespoon, 10 grams	4.0	55	7	1.0
Oatmeal (cooked with water), 1 cup, 245 grams	10.0	42	24	1.6
Puffed wheat, 1 cup, 30 grams	17.6	80	22	2.0
Raisin Bran, 1 cup, 45 grams	25.5	73	35	4.0
Rice Krispies, 1 cup, 30 grams	22.0	82	27	0.3
Shredded wheat, ⅓ cup, 25 grams	12.0	67	18	1.2
Weetabix, 2 biscuits, 30 grams	13.0	69	19	2.0
Cake				
Cake, angel food, 1 slice, 30 grams	11.5	67	17	<1.0
Cake, banana, 1 slice, 80 grams	21.6	47	46	<1.0
Cake, chocolate fudge, mix (Betty Crocker), 1 slice cake, 73 grams cake + 33 grams icing	20.5	38	54	<1.0
Cake, cupcake, with icing and cream filling, 1 cake, 38 grams	19.0	73	26	<1.0
Cake, pound, 1 slice, 80 grams	22.6	54	42	<1.0
Cake, scone, made from mix, 1 scone, 40 grams	83.0	92	90	<1.0
Cake, sponge, 1 slice, 60 grams	14.7	46	32	<1.0

(continued on next page)

Food	Glycemic Load	Glycemic Index	Carbohydrates (grams)	Fiber (grams)
Crackers				
Crackers, Corn Thins, puffed corn cake, 2, 12 grams	7.8	87	9	<1.0
Crackers, graham, 1, 30 grams	16.0	74	22	1.4
Crackers, rice cake, 2, 25 grams	17.0	82	21	0.4
Crackers, Ryvita or Wasa, 2, 20 grams	11.0	69	16	3.0
Crackers, water biscuits, 5, 25 grams	14.0	78	18	0.0
Fruit				
Apple, 1 medium, 150 grams	6.8	38	18	3.5
Apple, dried, 30 grams	6.9	29	24	3.0
Apricots, canned, light syrup, ½ cup, 125 grams	8.3	64	13	1.5
Apricots, dried, 5–6 pieces, 30 grams	4.0	31	13	2.2
Apricots, fresh, 3 medium, 100 grams	4.0	57	7	1.9
Banana, raw, 1 medium, 150 grams	17.6	55	32	2.4
Cherries, 20 cherries, 80 grams	2.2	22	10	2.4
Dates, dried, 5, 40 grams	27.8	103	27	3.0
Figs, dried, tenderized (water added), 50 grams	13.4	61	22	3.0
Fruit cocktail, canned in natural juice, ½ cup, 125 grams	8.25	55	15	1.5
Grapes, green, 1 cup, 100 grams	6.9	46	15	2.4
Kiwi, 1 raw, peeled, 80 grams	4.0	52	8	2.4
Mango, 1 small, 150 grams	10.4	55	19	2.0
Orange, 1 medium, 130 grams	4.4	44	10	2.6
Peach, fresh, 1 large, 110 grams	3.0	42	7	1.9
Peaches, canned, light syrup, ½ cup, 125 grams	9.4	52	18	1.5
Peaches, canned, natural juice, ½ cup, 125 grams	4.5	38	12	1.5
Pear, fresh, 1 medium, 150 grams	8.0	38	21	3.1
Pears, canned in pear juice, ½ cup, 125 grams	5.5	43	13	1.5
Pineapple, fresh, 2 slices, 125 grams	6.6	66	10	2.8
Plums, 3–4 small, 100 grams	2.7	39	7	2.2
Prunes, pitted, 6 prunes, 40 grams	7.25	29	25	3.0
Raisins, ¼ cup, 40 grams	18.0	64	28	3.1
Sultanas, ¼ cup, 40 grams	16.8	56	30	3.1
Watermelon, 1 cup, 150 grams	5.7	72	8	1.0

Food	Glycemic Load	Glycemic Index	Carbohydrates (grams)	Fiber (grams)
Grains				
Barley, pearl, boiled, ½ cup, 80 grams	4.25	25	17	6.0
Brown rice, steamed, 1 cup, 150 grams	16.0	50	32	1.0
Buckwheat, cooked, ½ cup, 80 grams	30.0	54	57	3.5
Bulgur, cooked, ⅔ cup, 120 grams	10.6	48	22	3.5
Couscous, cooked, ⅔ cup, 120 grams	18.0	65	28	1.0
Millet, cooked, ½ cup, 120 grams	8.52	71	12	1.0
Rice bran, extruded, 1 tablespoon, 10 grams	0.57	19	3	1.0
Rice, arborio, white, boiled, 100 grams	29.0	69	35	0.2
Rice, Basmati, white, boiled, 1 cup, 180 grams	29.0	58	50	0.2
Rice, instant, cooked, 1 cup, 180 grams	33.0	87	38	0.2
Rice, jasmine, white, long-grain, steamed, 1 cup, 180 grams	42.5	109	39	0.2
Rice, white, boiled, 1 cup, 150 grams	26.0	72	36	0.2
Tapioca (boiled with milk), 1 cup, 265 grams	41.0	81	51	<1.0
Tapioca (steamed 1 hour), 1 cup, 100 grams	38.0	70	54	<1.0
Ice Cream				
Ice cream, full fat, 2 scoops, 50 grams	6.1	61	10	0
Ice cream, low-fat French vanilla, 2 scoops, 50 grams	5.7	38	15	0
Jam				
Jam, no sugar, 1 tablespoon, 25 grams	6.0	55	11	<1.0
Jam, sweetened, 1 tablespoon, 25 grams	8.0	48	17	<1.0
Milk, Soy Milk, and Juices				
Apple juice, unsweetened, 1 cup, 250 milliliters	13.2	40	33	1.0
Coca-Cola, 375 milliliters	25.2	63	40	0.0
Cranberry juice cocktail, 240 milliliters	23.0	68	34	0.0
Gatorade, 1 cup, 250 milliliters	11.7	78	15	0.0
Grapefruit juice, unsweetened, 1 cup, 250 milliliters	7.7	48	16	1.0
Milk, chocolate-flavored, lowfat, 1 cup, 250 milliliters	7.8	34	23	0.0
Milk, full fat, 1 cup, 250 milliliters	3.0	27	12	0.0
Milk, skim, 1 cup, 250 milliliters	4.0	32	13	0.0

(continued on next page)

Food	Glycemic Load	Glycemic Index	Carbohydrates (grams)	Fiber (grams)
Milk, Soy Milk, and Juices (cont.)				
Milk, sweetened condensed, ½ cup, 160 grams	55.0	61	90	0.0
Nesquik chocolate powder, 3 teaspoons in 250 milliliters	7.7	55	14	0.0
Orange juice, 1 cup, 250 milliliters	9.7	46	21	1.0
Pineapple juice, unsweetened, canned, 250 milliliters	12.4	46	27	1.0
Soft drinks, 375 milliliters	34.7	68	51	0.0
Soy milk, 1 cup, 250 milliliters	3.7	31	12	0.0
Muffins and Pancakes				
Muffin, apple, 1, 80 grams	19.0	44	44	1.5
Muffin, apple, oat and sultana, 1, 50 grams	15.0	54	28	1.0
Muffin, apricot, coconut and honey, 1, 50 grams	16.0	60	27	1.5
Muffin, banana, oat and honey, 1, 50 grams	18.0	65	28	1.5
Muffin, blueberry, 1, 80 grams	24.0	59	41	1.5
Muffin, bran, 1, 80 grams	20.0	60	34	2.5
Muffin, chocolate butterscotch, 1, 50 grams	15.0	53	28	1.0
Pancake, buckwheat, 1, 40 grams	30.0	102	30	2.0
Pancake, enriched wheat, 1 large, 80 grams	39.0	67	58	1.0
Pasta				
Pasta, fettucini, cooked, 1 cup, 180 grams	18.2	32	57	2.0
Pasta, macaroni cheese, packaged, cooked, 1 cup, 220 grams	19.2	64	30	2.0
Pasta, ravioli, meat-filled, cooked, 1 cup, 220 grams	11.7	39	30	2.0
Pasta, rice noodles, fresh, boiled, 1 cup, 176 grams	17.6	40	44	0.4
Pasta, rice pasta, brown, cooked, 1 cup, 180 grams	52.0	92	57	2.0
Pasta, spaghetti, gluten-free, in tomato sauce, 1 cup, 220 grams	18.5	68	27	2.0
Pasta, spaghetti, white, cooked, 1 cup, 180 grams	23.0	41	56	2.0
Pasta, spaghetti, wholemeal, cooked, 1 cup, 180 grams	17.75	37	48	3.5
Pasta, star pastina, cooked, 1 cup, 180 grams	21.0	38	56	2.0
Pasta, tortellini, cheese, cooked, 1 cup, 180 grams	10.5	50	21	2.0
Pasta, vermicelli, cooked, 1 cup, 180 grams	15.7	35	45	2.0

Food	Glycemic Load	Glycemic Index	Carbohydrates (grams)	Fiber (grams)
Sugars				
Fructose, 2 teaspoons, 10 grams	2.3	23	10	0.0
Glucose, 2 teaspoons, 10 grams	10.2	102	10	0.0
Honey, ½ tablespoon, 10 grams	4.6	58	16	0.0
Lactose, 2 teaspoons, 10 grams	4.6	46	10	0.0
Maltose, 2 teaspoons, 10 grams	10.5	105	10	0.0
Sucrose, 2 teaspoons, 10 grams	6.5	65	10	0.0
Snacks				
Corn chips, Doritos original, 50 grams	13.9	42	33	<1.0
Mars bar, 60 grams	26.6	65	41	0.0
Pretzels, 50 grams	18.3	83	22	<1.0
Real Fruit bar, strawberry, 20 grams	15.3	90	17	<1.0
Skittles, 62 grams	38.5	70	55	0.0
Snickers, 59 grams	14.3	41	35	0.0
Tofu frozen dessert (nondairy), 100 grams	15.0	115	13	<1.0
Twix bar (caramel), 59 grams	16.2	44	37	<1.0
Soups				
Black bean, 1 cup, 220 milliliters	6.0	64	9	3.4
Lentil, canned, 1 cup, 220 milliliters	6.0	44	14	3.0
Split pea, canned, 1 cup, 220 milliliters	8.0	60	13	3.0
Tomato, canned, 1 cup, 220 milliliters	6.0	38	15	1.5
Vegetables				
Beetroot, canned, drained, 2–3 slices, 60 grams	3.0	64	5	1.0
Carrots, peeled, boiled, ½ cup, 70 grams	1.5	49	3	1.5
Carrots, raw, ½ cup, 80 grams	1.0	16	6	1.5
Corn on the cob, sweet, boiled 20 minutes, 1 medium cob, 80 grams	8.0	48	14	2.9
Corn, canned and drained, ½ cup, 80 grams	8.5	55	15	3.0
Cornmeal (polenta), ⅓ cup, 40 grams	20	68	30	2.0
Gnocchi, cooked, 1 cup, 145 grams	48	68	71	1.0

(continued on next page)

Food	Glycemic Load	Glycemic Index	Carbohydrates (grams)	Fiber (grams)
Vegetables *(cont.)*				
Low-glycemic vegetables:	≈ 1.4	≈ 20	≈ 7	≈ 1.5
Asparagus, 1 cup cooked or raw				
Aubergine, 1 cup cooked				
Bell peppers, 1 cup cooked or raw				
Broccoli, 1 cup cooked or raw				
Brussels sprouts, 1 cup cooked or raw				
Cabbage, 1 cup cooked or raw				
Cauliflower, 1 cup cooked or raw				
Celery, 1 cup cooked or raw				
Courgettes, 1 cup cooked or raw				
Cucumber, 1 cup				
Green beans, 1 cup cooked or raw				
Kale, 1 cup cooked, 2 cups raw				
Lettuce, 2 cups raw				
Mushrooms, 1 cup cooked or raw				
Spinach, 1 cup cooked, 2 cups raw				
Tomatoes, 1 cup cooked or raw				
Parsnips, boiled, ½ cup, 75 grams	8.0	97	8	3.0
Potatoes, baked in oven (no fat), 1 medium, 120 grams	14	93	15	2.4
Potatoes, French fries, fine cut, ½ cup, 120 grams	36	75	49	1.0
Potatoes, instant, prepared, ½ cup, 120 grams	15	83	18	1.0
Potatoes, mashed, ½ cup, 120 grams	14	91	16	1.0
Potatoes, new, unpeeled, boiled, 5 small (cocktail), 175 grams	20	78	25	2.0
Potatoes, peeled, boiled, 1 medium, 120 grams	10	87	13	1.4
Potatoes, with skin, boiled, 1 medium, 120 grams	11	79	15	2.4
Pumpkin, peeled, boiled, ½ cup, 85 grams	4.5	75	6	3.4
Sweet corn, ½ cup boiled, 80 grams	10.0	55	18	3.0
Sweet potato, peeled, boiled, 1 medium, 80 grams	8.6	54	16	3.4
Yam, boiled, 1 medium, 80 grams	13	51	26	3.4
Yogurt				
Yogurt, low-fat, artificial sweetener, 1 cup, 200 grams	2.0	14	12	0.0
Yogurt, low-fat, 1 cup, 200 grams	8.5	33	26	0.0
Yogurt, with fruit, 1 cup, 200 grams	8.0	26	30	0.0

Acid–Alkaline Values of Selected Foods

One of the basic necessities for the body to function properly is maintaining the proper balance of acidity and alkalinity (pH) in the blood and other body fluids. The acid–alkaline theory of disease is an oversimplification, but it basically states that many diseases are caused by excess acid accumulation in the body. There is accumulating evidence that certain disease states, such as osteoporosis, rheumatoid arthritis, gout, and many others, may be influenced by the dietary acid–alkaline balance. For example, osteoporosis may be the result of a chronic intake of acid-forming foods consistently outweighing the intake of alkaline foods, leading to the bones being constantly forced to give up their alkaline minerals (calcium and magnesium) in order to buffer the excess acid.

The dietary goal for good health is simple: make sure you consume more alkaline-producing foods than acid-producing foods.

Keep in mind that there is a difference between between acidic foods and acid-forming foods. For example, while foods such as lemons and citrus fruits are acidic, they actually have an alkalizing effect on the body. What determines the pH nature of the food in the body is the metabolic end products when it is digested. For example, the citric acid in citrus fruit is metabolized in the body to its alkaline form (citrate) and may even be converted to bicarbonate, another alkaline compound.

The following food table was prepared by Professor Jürgen Vormanne of the Institute for Prevention and Diet in Ismaning, Germany (used with permission). Foods with a negative value exert a base (B) or alkaline effect, foods with a positive value an acid (A) effect. Neutral foodstuffs are labeled with N. The calculation is based upon the potential acid load to the kidneys in milliequivalents per 100 gram serving.

Food	A, B, or N	Potential Acidic Load	Food	A, B, or N	Potential Acidic Load
Beverages			**Fats, Oils, and Nuts (cont.)**		
Apple juice, unsweetened	B	−2.2	Peanuts, plain	A	8.3
Beer, draft	B	−0.2	Pistachio	A	8.5
Beer, pale	A	0.9	Sunflower seed oil	N	0.0
Beer, stout	B	−0.1	Walnuts	A	6.8
Beetroot juice	B	−3.9			
Carrot juice	B	−4.8	**Fish and Seafood**		
Coca-Cola	A	0.4	Carp	A	7.9
Cocoa, made with semiskimmed milk	B	−0.4	Cod, fillets	A	7.1
			Eel, smoked	A	11.0
Coffee, infusion, 5 minutes	B	−1.4	Haddock	A	6.8
Espresso	B	−2.3	Halibut	A	7.8
Fruit tea, infusion	B	−0.3	Herring	A	7.0
Grape juice	B	−1.0	Mussels	A	15.3
Grape juice, unsweetened	B	−1.0	Prawns (large)	A	15.5
Green tea, infusion	B	−0.3	Prawns (small)	A	7.6
Herbal tea	B	−0.2	Rosefish	A	10.0
Lemon juice	B	−2.5	Salmon	A	9.4
Mineral water (Apollinaris)	B	−1.8	Salted matje (herring)	A	8.0
Mineral water (Volvic)	B	−0.1	Sardines in oil	A	13.5
Orange juice, unsweetened	B	−2.9	Sole	A	7.4
Red wine	B	−2.4	Tiger prawn	A	18.2
Tea, Indian, infusion	B	−0.3	Trout, steamed	A	10.8
Tomato juice	B	−2.8	Zander	A	7.1
Vegetable juice (tomato, beetroot, carrot)	B	−3.6	**Fruits**		
White wine, dry	B	−1.2	Apples	B	−2.2
			Apricots	B	−4.8
Fats, Oils, and Nuts			Bananas	B	−5.5
Almonds	A	4.3	Black currants	B	−6.5
Butter	A	0.6	Cherries	B	−3.6
Hazelnuts	B	−2.8	Figs, dried	B	−18.1
Margarine	B	−0.5	Grapefruit	B	−3.5
Olive oil	N	0.0	Grapes	B	−3.9

Food	A, B, or N	Potential Acidic Load	Food	A, B, or N	Potential Acidic Load
Fruits (cont.)			**Pasta**		
Kiwifruit	B	−4.1	Macaroni	A	6.1
Lemon	B	−2.6	Noodles	A	6.4
Mango	B	−3.3	Spaetzle (German sort of pasta)	A	9.4
Orange	B	−2.7			
Peach	B	−2.4	Spaghetti, white	A	6.5
Pear	B	−2.9	Spaghetti, wholemeal	A	7.3
Pineapple	B	−2.7	**Bread**		
Raisins	B	−21.0	Bread, rye flour	A	4.1
Strawberries	B	−2.2	Bread, rye flour, mixed	A	4.0
Watermelon	B	−1.9	Bread, wheat flour, mixed	A	3.8
Grains and Flour			Bread, wheat flour, wholemeal	A	1.8
Amaranth	A	7.5	Bread, white wheat	A	3.7
Barley (wholemeal)	A	5.0	Coarse wholemeal bread	A	5.3
Buckwheat (whole grain)	A	3.7	Crispbread, rye	A	3.3
Corn (whole grain)	A	3.8	Pumpernickel	A	4.2
Cornflakes	A	6.0	Wholemeal bread	A	7.2
Dried unripe spelt grains (wholemeal)	A	8.8	**Legumes**		
Millet (whole grain)	A	8.6	Beans, green/French	B	−3.1
Oat flakes	A	10.7	Lentils, green and brown, whole, dried	A	3.5
Rice, brown	A	12.5			
Rice, white	A	4.6	Peas	A	1.2
Rice, white, boiled	A	1.7	Soybeans	B	−3.4
Rye flour	A	4.4	Soy milk	B	−0.8
Rye flour, wholemeal	A	5.9	Tofu	B	−0.8
Wheat flour, white	A	6.9	**Meat and Sausages**		
Wheat flour, wholemeal	A	8.2	Beef, lean only	A	7.8
			Cervelat sausage	A	8.9
			Chicken, meat only	A	8.7

(continued on next page)

Food	A, B, or N	Potential Acidic Load	Food	A, B, or N	Potential Acidic Load
Meat and Sausages (cont.)			**Milk, Dairy Products, and Eggs (cont.)**		
Corned beef, canned	A	13.2	Egg, yolk	A	23.4
Duck	A	4.1	Emmenthal, full fat	A	21.1
Duck, lean only	A	8.4	Fresh cheese (quark)	A	11.1
Frankfurters	A	6.7	Full-fat soft cheese	A	4.3
Goose, lean only	A	13.0	Gouda	A	18.6
Jagdwurst sausage	A	7.2	Hard cheese	A	19.2
Lamb, lean only	A	7.6	Ice cream, dairy, vanilla	A	0.6
Liver (veal)	A	14.2	Ice cream, fruit, mixed	B	−0.6
Liver sausage	A	10.6	Kefir cheese, full fat	N	0.0
Luncheon meat, canned	A	10.2	Milk, skimmed	A	0.7
Ox liver	A	15.4	Milk, whole, evaporated	A	1.1
Pig's liver	A	15.7	Milk, whole, pasteurized and sterilized	A	0.7
Pork sausage	A	7.0			
Pork sausage (wiener)	A	7.7	Parmesan	A	34.2
Pork, lean only	A	7.9	Processed cheese, plain	A	28.7
Rabbit, lean only	A	19.0	Rich creamy full-fat cheese	A	13.2
Rump steak, lean and fat	A	8.8	Whey	B	−1.6
Salami	A	11.6	Yogurt, whole milk, fruit	A	1.2
Slicing sausage containing ham	A	8.3	Yogurt, whole milk, plain	A	1.5
Turkey, meat only	A	9.9			
Veal, fillet	A	9.0	**Sweets**		
			Chocolate, bitter	A	0.4
Milk, Dairy Products, and Eggs			Chocolate, milk	A	2.4
Buttermilk	A	0.5	Honey	B	−0.3
Camembert	A	14.6	Madeira cake	A	3.7
Cheddar-type cheese, reduced fat	A	26.4	Marmalade	B	−1.5
			Nougat hazelnut cream	B	−1.4
Cottage cheese, plain	A	8.7	Sugar, brown	B	−1.2
Cream, fresh, sour	A	1.2	Sugar, white	N	0.0
Curd cheese	A	0.9			
Edam, full fat	A	19.4			
Egg, chicken, whole	A	8.2			
Egg, white	A	1.1			

Food	A, B, or N	Potential Acidic Load	Food	A, B, or N	Potential Acidic Load
Vegetables			**Vegetables (cont.)**		
Asparagus	B	−0.4	Lettuce	B	−2.5
Aubergine	B	−3.4	Lettuce, iceberg	B	−1.6
Broccoli, green	B	−1.2	Mushrooms, common	B	−1.4
Brussels sprouts	B	−4.5	Onions	B	−1.5
Carrots	B	−4.9	Peppers, green bell	B	−1.4
Cauliflower	B	−4.0	Potatoes	B	−4.0
Celery	B	−5.2	Radish, red	B	−3.7
Chicory	B	−2.0	Rocket	B	−7.5
Courgette	B	−4.6	Sauerkraut	B	−3.0
Cucumber	B	−0.8	Spinach	B	−14.0
Fennel	B	−7.9	Tomato	B	−3.1
Garlic	B	−1.7			
Gherkin, pickled	B	−1.6	**Herbs and Vinegar**		
Kale	B	−7.8	Apple vinegar	B	−2.3
Kohlrabi	B	−5.5	Basil	B	−7.3
Lamb's lettuce	B	−5.0	Chives	B	−5.3
Leeks	B	−1.8	Parsley	B	−12.0
			Wine vinegar, balsamic	B	−1.6

Pesticide Content of Popular Fruits and Vegetables

The Environmental Working Group (EWG) is a nonprofit consumer advocate group in the U.S.A. composed of professionals in various areas, e.g., scientists, engineers, policy experts, lawyers, and computer programmers, bound together to expose threats to our health and the environment and to find solutions.

One of the documents that this organization has put together is "The Shopper's Guide to Pesticides in Produce." In this report, the EWG ranked pesticide contamination for forty-seven popular fruits and vegetables based on an analysis of more than 100,000 tests for pesticides on these foods, conducted from 1992 to 2001 by the U.S. Department of Agriculture and the Food and Drug Administration. Contamination was measured in six different ways, and crops were ranked based on a composite score from all categories. The six measures of contamination used were:

- Percentage of the samples tested with detectable pesticides.

- Percentage of the samples with two or more pesticides.
- Average number of pesticides found on a sample.
- Average amount (level in parts per million) of all pesticides found.
- Maximum number of pesticides found on a single sample.
- Number of pesticides found on the food in total.

The guide does not present a complex assessment of pesticide risks but instead simply reflects the overall load of pesticides found on commonly eaten fruits and vegetables. The produce listed in the guide was chosen after an analysis of USDA food consumption data.

Most Contaminated: The Dirty Dozen

The EWG designated the top twelve foods in the pesticide ranking "the dirty dozen." Eight fruits represented twelve of the most contaminated foods. Among these eight fruits:

- Nectarines had the highest percentage of samples test positive for pesticides (97.3 percent), followed by pears (94.4 percent) and peaches (93.7 percent).
- Nectarines also had the highest likelihood of multiple pesticides on a single sample—85.3 percent had two or more pesticide residues—followed by peaches (79.9 percent) and cherries (75.8 percent).
- Peaches and raspberries had the most pesticides detected on a single sample with nine pesticides on a single sample, followed by strawberries and apples, where eight pesticides were found on a single sample.
- Peaches had the most pesticides overall, with some combination of up to forty-five pesticides found on the samples tested, followed by raspberries with thirty-nine pesticides and apples and strawberries, both with thirty-six.

Among vegetables, spinach, celery, potatoes, and sweet bell peppers are the most likely to expose consumers to pesticides. Among these four vegetables:

- Celery had the highest percentage of samples test positive for pesticides (94.5 percent), followed by spinach (83.4 percent) and potatoes (79.3 percent).

- Celery also had the highest likelihood of multiple pesticides on a single vegetable (78 percent of samples), followed by spinach (51.8 percent) and sweet bell peppers (48.5 percent).
- Spinach was the vegetable with the most pesticides detected on a single sample (ten found on one sample), followed by celery and sweet bell peppers (both with nine).
- Sweet bell pepper was the vegetable with the most pesticides overall with thirty-nine, followed by spinach with thirty-six and celery and potatoes, both with twenty-nine.

Least Contaminated: Consistently Clean

The five fruits least likely to have pesticide residues on them are pineapples, mangoes, bananas, kiwis, and papaya.

- Fewer than 10 percent of pineapple and mango samples had detectable pesticides on them, and fewer than 1 percent of samples had more than one pesticide residue.
- Though 53 percent of bananas had detectable pesticides, multiple residues are rare, with only 4.7 percent of samples containing more than one residue. Kiwi and papaya had residues on 23.6 percent and 21.7 percent of samples, respectively, and just 10.4 percent and 5.6 percent of samples, respectively, had multiple pesticide residues.

The vegetables least likely to have pesticides on them are sweet corn, avocado, cauliflower, asparagus, onions, peas, and broccoli.

- Nearly three-quarters (73 percent) of the pea and broccoli samples had no detectable pesticides. Among the other vegetables on the least-contaminated list, there were no detectable residues on 90 percent or more of the samples.
- Multiple pesticide residues are extremely rare on any of these least-contaminated vegetables. Broccoli had the highest likelihood, with a 2.6 percent chance of more than one pesticide when ready to eat. Avocado and corn both had the lowest chance, with zero samples containing more than one pesticide when eaten.
- The largest number of pesticides detected on a single sample of any of these low-pesticide vegetables was three as compared to ten found on spinach, the most contaminated crop with the most residues.
- Broccoli and onions both had the most pesticides found on a single vegetable crop, at up to seventeen pesticides, but far fewer than the most contaminated vegetable, sweet bell peppers, on which thirty-nine were found.

Rank	Food	Combined Score
1	Peaches	100
2	Strawberries	89
3	Apples	88
4	Spinach	85
5	Nectarines	85
6	Celery	83
7	Pears	80
8	Cherries	76
9	Potatoes	67
10	Sweet bell peppers	66

Rank	Food	Combined Score
11	Raspberries	66
12	Grapes, north S.	64
13	Carrots	57
14	Green beans	57
15	Hot peppers	55
16	Oranges	53
17	Apricots	51
18	Cucumbers	51
19	Tomatoes	48
20	Collard greens	48
21	Grapes, U.S.	47
22	Turnip greens	41
23	Honeydew melons	40
24	Lettuce	40
25	Kale	39
26	Mushrooms	36
27	Cantaloupe melon	36
28	Sweet potatoes	35
29	Grapefruit	34
30	Winter squash	34
31	Blueberries	30
32	Watermelon	27
33	Plums	26
34	Tangerines	25
35	Cabbage	25
36	Papaya	23
37	Kiwi	23
38	Bananas	19
39	Broccoli	18
40	Onions	17
41	Asparagus	16
42	Sweet peas	13
43	Mango	12
44	Cauliflower	10
45	Pineapples	6
46	Avocado	4
47	Sweet corn	1

Oxalate Content of Selected Foods

A low-oxalate diet is a common prescription for recurrent calcium oxalate kidney stones. The ultimate goal is to reduce the level of oxalic acid being excreted. It appears that people with recurrent kidney stones have a tendency to absorb higher levels of dietary oxalates compared to normal subjects not prone to kidney stones, who absorb only 3 to 8 percent of dietary oxalate. A low-oxalate diet is usually defined as containing less than 50 milligrams of oxalate per day, so foods in the high- and moderate-oxalate category will have to be curtailed.

The list below is designed to provide an estimate of the oxalate content of food as it is so highly variable. The level of oxalate in a particular food in published reports can vary two- to fifteen-fold. Differences in climate, soil quality, state of ripeness, and even which part of the plant is analyzed will affect the value. We have grouped the foods into broad ranges based on the higher values reported for each food.

In using this list, it is very important to realize that it is based upon the amount of oxalate in a typical serving of the food.

VEGETABLES

High-Oxalate (> 10 milligrams per serving)
Aubergine
Beets, greens or root*
Celery
Collards
Dandelion greens
Escarole
Green beans
Kale
Leeks
Okra†
Parsley
Parsnips
Peppers, green
Potatoes
Pumpkin
Spinach*
Squash, yellow summer

Sweet potatoes
Swiss chard *
Tomato sauce, canned
Turnip greens
Watercress

Moderate-Oxalate (<10 milligrams per serving)
Artichokes
Asparagus
Broccoli
Brussels sprouts
Carrots
Cucumber
Garlic
Lettuce
Mangetout
Mushrooms
Mustard greens
Onions
Peppers, green
Potato crisps
Potato salad (¼ cup)
Pumpkin
Radishes
Tomato, fresh ‡
Tomato sauce, canned (¼ cup)

Low-Oxalate (2–5 milligrams per serving)
Acorn squash
Courgette
Ketchup (1 tablespoon)
Onions
Pepper, red
Rocket

FRUITS
High-Oxalate (>10 milligrams per serving)
Concord grapes
Figs, dried †
Kiwi
Lemon peel
Lime peel
Orange peel
Rhubarb *

Moderate-Oxalate (<10 milligrams per serving)
Apples
Apricots
Berries (¼ cup)
Blackberries
Blueberries
Cherries, red, sour
Cranberries, dried
Currants, black
Oranges
Peaches
Pears
Pineapple
Plums
Prunes, Italian
Raspberries, red
Tangerines

Low-Oxalate (2–5 milligrams per serving)
Apples, peeled
Avocado
Cantaloupe melon
Cherries, bing
Cranberries
Grapes
Lemon juice (1 cup)

Lemons
Lime juice (1 cup)
Raisins

GRAINS

High-Oxalate (>10 milligrams per serving)
Bread, whole wheat (wholemeal)
Buckwheat ‡
Oatmeal
Popcorn
Spelt
Stone-ground flour
Wheat bran
Wheat germ
Whole-wheat (wholemeal) flour

*Moderate-Oxalate (<10 milligrams
per serving)*
Bagel (1 medium)
Barley, cooked
Bread, white (2 slices)
Corn
Cornbread
Cornmeal (polenta), yellow (1 cup dry)
Cornflour (¼ cup)
Corn tortilla (1 medium)
Pasta
Rice, brown
Spaghetti
Wheat, white flour

Low-Oxalate (2–5 milligrams per serving)
Rice, white
Rice, wild
Rye bread

LEGUMES

High-Oxalate (>10 milligrams per serving)
Chickpeas
Lentils
Soy and all soy products

*Moderate-Oxalate (<10 milligrams
per serving)*
Lima beans
Split peas

Low-Oxalate (2–5 milligrams per serving)
Peas, green

NUTS AND SEEDS

High-Oxalate (>10 milligrams per serving)
Almonds †
Brazil nuts
Hazelnuts
Peanut butter ‡
Peanuts ‡
Pecans
Sesame seeds *
Sunflower seeds

*Moderate-Oxalate (<10 milligrams
per serving)*
Cashews
Linseed
Walnuts

Low-Oxalate (2–5 milligrams per serving)
Coconut

HERBS AND SPICES

High-Oxalate (>10 milligrams per serving)
None

Moderate-Oxalate (<10 milligrams per serving)
Cinnamon, ground (1½ teaspoons)
Ginger, powdered (1 tablespoon)
Pepper, black (1 teaspoon)
Thyme, dried (1 teaspoon)

Low-Oxalate (2–5 milligrams per serving)
Basil, fresh (1 tablespoon)
Dill (1 tablespoon)
Ginger, raw, sliced (1 teaspoon)
Malt, powder (1 tablespoon)
Mustard, Dijon (1½ cup)
Nutmeg (1 tablespoon)
Pepper (1 teaspoon)

MISCELLANEOUS
High-Oxalate (>10 milligrams per serving)
Beer
Chocolate
Cocoa
Soy sauce (1 tablespoon)
Tea, black
Tea, green

Moderate-Oxalate (<10 milligrams per serving)
Coffee
Tea, rose hip
Red wine
Sardines

Low-Oxalate (2–5 milligrams per serving)
Beef
Chicken
Corned beef, canned
Eggs
Fish, haddock, plaice, and flounder
Ham
Hamburger
Lamb
Pork
Turkey
Venison

* More than 50 milligrams per serving.
† More than 100 milligrams per serving.
‡ More than 200 milligrams per serving.

Food–Drug Interactions

A food–drug interaction is simply the modulation of the pharmacologic activity of a drug (i.e., the object drug) by a food or dietary component. The interaction can cause the drug to have an enhanced action or a decreased action. For example, simply taking some drugs with meals can decrease a drug's rate of absorption and/or decrease the extent of absorption significantly. On the flip side, the absorption of some drugs is enhanced when taken with food. There are also other, more complex interactions, such as a food component directly antagonizing the action of the drug. Food ingredients can also either increase or decrease the body's ability to get rid of a drug, thereby either increasing or decreasing its effectiveness and toxicity. Table E.1 summarizes some specific food–drug interactions. The key point that we want to make here is that if you are taking any prescription medication it is essential to ask your physician or pharmacist about food–drug interactions.

High-Risk Patients and Drug Interactions

The problem of food–drug interactions increases significantly in certain patient populations, especially the elderly. The elderly population is at high risk because of the number of medications consumed, complicated drug regimens, and more severe illnesses being dealt with. About 80 percent of elderly patients routinely take more than one prescription and nonprescription medication concurrently. As many as 39 percent are taking at least eight drugs simultaneously. According to Help the Aged, in the U.K., about 80 percent of older people take at least one prescribed drug, and a third take four or more medicines every day.

TABLE E.1

Examples of Food–Drug Interactions

Drugs	Effect(s) of Food*
Acetaminophen, aspirin, digoxin	Decreased/delayed drug absorption
ACE inhibitors (captopril and moexipril)	Significant decrease in serum drug levels
Tetracycline, fluoroquinolones (ciprofloxacin, levofloxacin, ofloxacin, trovafloxacin)	Avoid taking with antacids (especially magnesium and aluminium types) and iron products; significantly decrease drug absorption
Didanosine or DDI	Food in general and acidic foods/juices significantly decrease drug absorption
Saquinavir, griseofulvin, itraconazole, lovastatin, spironolactone	Food, especially high-fat meals, improves drug absorption; take with food, or within two hours of a meal
Famotidine	Decreased/delayed drug absorption
Ketoconazole	Acidic foods/juices and sodas (e.g., cola) significantly increase drug absorption
Iron, levodopa, penicillins (most), tetracycline, erythromycin	High-carbohydrate meals decrease drug absorption

* When the increased or decreased absorption effects of food are undesirable, take the drug on an empty stomach, either one hour before or two hours after meals.

PATIENTS AT HIGH RISK FOR DRUG INTERACTIONS

High Risk Associated with the Severity of Disease State Being Treated

Aplastic anemia
Asthma
Cardiac arrhythmia
Critical care/intensive care patients
Diabetes
Epilepsy
Hepatic disease
Hypothyroid

High Risk Associated with Drug Interaction Potential of Related Therapy

Autoimmune disorders

Cardiovascular disease
Gastrointestinal disease
Infection
Psychiatric disorders
Respiratory disorders
Seizure disorders

High-Risk Drugs

Certain drugs carry with them an increased risk of food–drug interactions. Most often, severe food–drug interactions are the result of the drug's producing a toxic effect at a dose that may be only slightly above the therapeutic dose. A slight increase in the dose may produce a large increase in drug blood level and clinical effect. Conversely, a slight decrease in the blood level of drugs may result in a significant loss of therapeutic effect. Examples of drugs that have a narrow therapeutic index include Coumadin (discussed more fully below); see the following list for more examples.

EXAMPLES OF DRUGS WITH A NARROW THERAPEUTIC INDEX

Aminoglycoside antibiotics (gentamicin, tobramycin)

Anticoagulants (Coumadin [warfarin], heparins)

Aspirin

Carbamazepine

Conjugated oestrogens

Cyclosporin

Digoxin

Esterified oestrogens

Hypoglycemic agents

Levothyroxine sodium

Lithium

Phenytoin

Procainamide

Quinidine sulphate/gluconate

Theophylline

Tricyclic antidepressants

Valproic acid

The Special Case of Coumadin

Perhaps one of the best-known food–drug interactions is the one between the drug Coumadin (warfarin) and vitamin K. Coumadin blocks the action of vitamin K in the clotting of blood and is used as the primary drug in conditions where blood clots are likely to form, such as certain cardiovascular diseases (e.g., deep-vein thrombosis, atrial fibrillation). In order for Coumadin to be effective, certain dietary safeguards must be followed. The most important fact that you must be aware of is that your specific dose of Coumadin will be determined according to the results of a blood test known as the International Normalized Ratio (INR). Most often, physicians and pharmacists will counsel patients taking Coumadin to avoid all dietary sources of vitamin K. The reality is that what is most important is that you do not increase or decrease your consumption. Simply eat the same levels you're accustomed to. Your physician will monitor your blood using the INR test to be sure the Coumadin is working and to change your dose (up or down) as needed. The key is consistency. Given the importance of vitamin K-containing foods in your diet, if you want to include them in your diet and you take Coumadin, it is absolutely essential that you eat the same-sized serving of green leafy vegetables every day and monitor your INR closely. Rich sources of vitamin K are dark green leafy vegetables, green tea, spinach, broccoli, lettuce, and cabbage. Good sources are asparagus, oats, whole wheat, and fresh green peas.

Nutrient Content of Selected Foods per 100 Gram Serving

		General						Fatty Acids									
Unit	Calories	Carbohydrates	Fat	Protein	Fiber	Water	Stearic acid	Oleic acid	Linoleic acid	Linolenic acid	Arachidonic acid	EPA	DHA	Cholesterol	Monounsaturated fat	Polyunsaturated fat	Saturated fat
	kcal	g	g	g	g	g	g	g	g	g	g	g	g	mg	g	g	g
Vegetables																	
Artichoke, boiled	50	11.18	0.16	3.48	5.4	83.97	0.003	0.005	0.049	0.018	0	0	0	0	0.005	0.068	0.037
Asparagus, boiled	24	4.23	0.31	2.59	1.6	92.2	0.004	0.009	0.129	0.007	0	0	0	0	0.01	0.136	0.071
Aubergine, boiled	28	6.64	0.23	0.83	2.5	91.77	0.012	0.018	0.078	0.015	0	0	0	0	0.02	0.093	0.044
Beetroot, boiled	44	9.96	0.18	1.68	2	87.06	0.001	0.035	0.058	0.005	0	0	0	0	0.035	0.064	0.028
Bell peppers, sweet, red, raw	27	6.43	0.19	0.89	2	92.19	0.007	0.011	0.093	0.009	0	0	0	0	0.013	0.102	0.028
Bitter melon, boiled	19	4.32	0.18	0	2	93.95	0.004	0.033	0.078	0	0	0	0	0	0.033	0.078	0.014
Broccoli, boiled	28	5.06	0.35	2.98	2.9	90.69	0.007	0.024	0.038	0.129	0	0	0	0	0.024	0.167	0.054
Brussels sprouts, boiled	39	8.67	0.51	2.55	2.6	87.32	0.005	0.033	0.077	0.168	0.002	0	0	0	0.039	0.26	0.105
Cabbage	27	6.12	0.26	1.39	2	91.55	0.001	0.018	0.051	0.067	0.001	0	0	0	0.019	0.125	0.034
Carrots, raw	43	10.14	0.19	1.03	3	87.79	0.001	0.006	0.067	0.01	0	0	0	0	0.008	0.077	0.03
Cauliflower, boiled	23	4.11	0.45	1.84	2.7	93	0.008	0.032	0.05	0.167	0	0	0	0	0.032	0.217	0.07
Celery, raw	16	3.65	0.14	0.75	1.7	94.64	0.003	0.026	0.069	0	0	0	0	0	0.027	0.069	0.037
Cucumbers, with peel, raw	13	2.76	0.13	0.69	0.8	96.01	0.003	0.003	0.022	0.03	0	0	0	0	0.003	0.053	0.034
Dandelion greens, boiled	33	6.4	0.6	2	2.9	89.8	0.006	0.012	0.224	0.038	0	0	0	0	0.012	0.262	0.146
Endive, raw	17	3.35	0.2	1.25	3.1	93.79	0.002	0.004	0.075	0.013	0	0	0	0	0.004	0.087	0.048
Fennel, bulb, raw	31	7.29	0.2	1.24	3.1	90.21								0			
Garlic, raw	149	33.07	0.5	6.36	2.1	58.58	0	0.011	0.229	0.02	0	0	0	0	0.011	0.249	0.089
Jerusalem artichokes (sunchokes), raw	76	17.44	0.01	2	1.6	78.01	0	0.004	0.001	0	0	0	0	0	0.004	0.001	0
Jicama, raw	38	8.82	0.09	0.72	4.9	90.07	0.002	0.005	0.029	0.014	0	0	0	0	0.005	0.043	0.021
Kale/collards, raw	50	10.01	0.7	3.3	2	84.46	0.004	0.049	0.138	0.18	0.002	0	0	0	0.052	0.338	0.091
Leeks, boiled	31	7.62	0.2	0.81	1	90.8	0.001	0.003	0.045	0.066				0	0.003	0.111	0.027
Lettuce, looseleaf, raw	18	3.5	0.3	1.3	1.9	94	0.004	0.009	0.047	0.113	0	0	0	0	0.012	0.159	0.039
Mustard greens, boiled	15	2.1	0.24	2.26	2	94.46	0.002	0.018	0.024	0.022	0	0	0	0	0.11	0.046	0.012
Onions, raw	38	8.63	0.16	1.16	1.8	89.68	0.002	0.023	0.059	0.003	0	0	0	0	0.023	0.062	0.026
Parsley, raw	36	6.33	0.79	2.97	3.3	87.71	0.039	0.287	0.115	0.008	0	0	0	0	0.295	0.124	0.132
Parsnips, boiled	81	19.53	0.3	1.32	4	77.72	0.014	0.102	0.041	0.003	0	0	0	0	0.112	0.047	0.05
Potatoes, baked, with skin	93	21.15	0.13	2.5	2.2	74.89	0.005	0.001	0.043	0.013	0	0	0	0	0.003	0.058	0.035
Radish, raw	20	3.59	0.54	0.6	1.6	94.84	0.004	0.016	0.016	0.029	0	0	0	0	0.017	0.045	0.03
Rocket, raw	25	3.65	0.66	2.58	1.6	91.71	0.004	0.046	0.13	0.17	0.002	0	0	0	0.049	0.319	0.086
Spinach, raw	22	3.5	0.35	2.86	2.7	91.58	0.003	0.004	0.022	0.115	0	0	0	0	0.01	0.146	0.056
Squash, pumpkins, gourds, boiled	20	4.89	0.07	0.72	1.1	93.69	0.002	0.005	0.002	0.002	0	0	0	0	0.009	0.004	0.037
Squash, summer, boiled	20	4.31	0.31	0.91	1.4	93.7	0.006	0.021	0.049	0.082	0	0	0	0	0.023	0.131	0.064
Squash, winter, baked	39	8.75	0.63	0.89	2.8	89.02	0.013	0.043	0.099	0.165	0	0	0	0	0.047	0.265	0.13
Sweet potato, baked	103	24.27	0.11	1.72	3	72.85	0.002	0.004	0.041	0.008	0	0	0	0	0.004	0.049	0.024
Swiss chard, boiled	20	4.14	0.08	1.88	2.1	92.65	0	0.016	0.025	0.003	0	0	0	0	0.016	0.028	0.012
Tomatoes, red, raw	21	4.64	0.33	0.85	1.1	93.76	0.013	0.049	0.13	0.005	0	0	0	0	0.05	0.135	0.045
Turnips, boiled	21	4.9	0.08	0.71	2	93.6	0.001	0.004	0.009	0.032	0	0	0	0	0.005	0.042	0.008

Minerals   Vitamins

Calcium mg	Copper mg	Iron mg	Magnesium mg	Manganese mg	Phosphorus mg	Potassium mg	Selenium mg	Sodium mg	Zinc mg	Folic acid mcg	Niacin mg	Pantothenic acid mg	Riboflavin mg	Thiamine mg	Vitamin A IU	Vitamin B12 mcg	Vitamin B6 mg	Vitamin C mg	Vitamin E mg	Vitamin K mcg
45	0.233	1.29	60	0.259	86	354	0.2	95	0.49	0	1.001	0.342	0.066	0.065	177	0	0.111	10	0.19	
20	0.112	0.73	10	0.152	54	160	1.7	11	0.42	0	1.082	0.161	0.126	0.123	539	0	0.122	10.8	0.38	
6	0.108	0.35	13	0.136	22	248	0.4	3	0.15	0	0.6	0.075	0.02	0.076	64	0	0.086	1.3	0.03	
16	0.074	0.79	23	0.326	38	305	0.7	77	0.35	0	0.331	0.145	0.04	0.027	35	0	0.067	3.6	0.3	
9	0.065	0.46	10	0.116	19	177	0.3	2	0.12	0	0.509	0.08	0.03	0.066	5700	0	0.248	190	0.69	
9	0.033	0.38	16	0.086	36	319	0.2	6	0.77	0	0.28	0.193	0.053	0.051	113	0	0.041	33	0.7	
46	0.043	0.84	24	0.218	59	292	1.9	26	0.38	0	0.574	0.508	0.113	0.055	1388	0	0.143	74.6	1.69	270
36	0.083	1.2	20	0.227	56	317	1.5	21	0.33	0	0.607	0.252	0.08	0.107	719	0	0.178	62	0.85	
51	0.097	0.49	15	0.18	42	206	0.9	11	0.21	0	0.3	0.324	0.03	0.05	40	0	0.21	57	0.105	44
27	0.047	0.5	15	0.142	44	323	1.1	35	0.2	0	0.928	0.197	0.059	0.097	28129	0	0.147	9.3	0.46	5
16	0.027	0.33	9	0.138	32	142	0.5	15	0.18	0	0.41	0.508	0.052	0.042	17	0	0.173	44.3	0.04	10
40	0.034	0.4	11	0.102	25	287	0.9	87	0.13	0	0.323	0.186	0.045	0.046	134	0	0.087	7	0.36	12
14	0.033	0.26	11	0.076	20	144	0	2	0.2	0	0.221	0.178	0.022	0.024	215	0	0.042	5.3	0.079	19
140	0.115	1.8	24	0.23	42	232	0.3	44	0.28	0	0.514	0.057	0.175	0.13	11700	0	0.16	18	2.5	
52	0.099	0.83	15	0.42	28	314	0.2	22	0.79	0	0.4	0.9	0.075	0.08	2050	0	0.02	6.5	0.44	231
49	0.066	0.73	17	0.191	50	414	0.7	52	0.2	0	0.64	0.232	0.032	0.01	134	0	0.047	12		
181	0.299	1.7	25	1.672	153	401	14.2	17	1.16	0	0.7	0.596	0.11	0.2	0	0	1.235	31.2	0.01	
14	0.14	3.4	17	0.06	78	429	0.7	4	0.12	0	1.3	0.397	0.06	0.2	20	0	0.077	4	0.19	
12	0.048	0.6	12	0.06	18	150	0.7	4	0.16	0	0.2	0.135	0.029	0.02	21	0	0.042	20.2	0.457	
135	0.29	1.7	34	0.774	56	447	0.9	43	0.44	0	1	0.091	0.13	0.11	8900	0	0.271	120	0.8	817
30	0.062	1.1	14	0.247	17	87	0.5	10	0.06	0	0.2	0.072	0.02	0.026	46	0	0.113	4.2		
68	0.044	1.4	11	0.75	25	264	0.2	9	0.29	0	0.4	0.2	0.08	0.05	1900	0	0.055	18	0.44	210
	0.084	0.7	15	0.274	41	202	0.6	16	0.11	0	0.433	0.12	0.063	0.041	3031	0	0.098	25.3	2.01	
20	0.06	0.22	10	0.137	33	157	0.6	3	0.19	0	0.148	0.106	0.02	0.042	0	0	0.116	6.4	0.31	2
138	0.149	6.2	50	0.16	58	554	0.1	56	1.07	0	1.313	0.4	0.098	0.086	5200	0	0.09	133	1.79	540
37	0.138	0.58	29	0.294	69	367	1.7	10	0.26	0	0.724	0.588	0.051	0.083	0	0	0.093	13	1	
15	0.118	1.08	28	0.219	70	535	0.4	10	0.36	0	1.41	0.376	0.048	0.064	10	0	0.311	9.6	0.045	4
21	0.04	0.29	9	0.07	18	232	0.7	24	0.3	0	0.3	0.088	0.045	0.005	8	0	0.071	22.8	0.001	0.1
160	0.076	1.46	47	0.321	52	369	0.3	27	0.47	0	0.305	0.437	0.086	0.044	2373	0	0.073	15	0.427	
99	0.13	2.71	79	0.897	49	558	1	79	0.53	0	0.724	0.065	0.189	0.078	6715	0	0.195	28.1	1.89	400
15	0.091	0.57	9	0.089	30	230	0.2	1	0.23	0	0.413	0.201	0.078	0.031	1082	0	0.044	4.7	1.06	
27	0.103	0.36	24	0.213	39	192	0.2	1	0.39	0	0.513	0.137	0.041	0.044	287	0	0.065	5.5	0.12	
14	0.095	0.33	8	0.211	20	437	0.4	1	0.26	0	0.701	0.35	0.024	0.085	3557	0	0.072	9.6	0.12	
28	0.208	0.45	20	0.56	55	348	0.7	10	0.29	0	0.604	0.646	0.127	0.073	21822	0	0.241	24.6	0.28	
58	0.163	2.26	86	0.334	33	549	0.9	179	0.33	0	0.36	0.163	0.086	0.034	3139	0	0.085	18	1.89	
5	0.074	0.45	11	0.105	24	222	0.4	9	0.09	0	0.628	0.247	0.048	0.059	623	0	0.08	19.1	0.38	6
22	0.064	0.22	8	0.1	19	135	0.6	50	0.2	0	0.299	0.142	0.023	0.027	0	0	0.067	11.6	0.03	

	General						Fatty Acids										
	Calories	Carbohydrates	Fat	Protein	Fiber	Water	Stearic acid	Oleic acid	Linoleic acid	Linolenic acid	Arachidonic acid	EPA	DHA	Cholesterol	Monounsaturated fat	Polyunsaturated fat	Saturated fat
Unit	kcal	g	g	g	g	g	g	g	g	g	g	g	g	mg	g	g	g
Vegetables (cont.)																	
Turnip greens, boiled	20	4.36	0.23	1.14	3.5	93.2	0.007	0.004	0.028	0.064	0	0	0	0	0.015	0.091	0.053
Yams, boiled	116	27.6	0.14	1.49	3.9	70.13	0.003	0.005	0.05	0.009	0	0	0	0	0.005	0.06	0.029
Fruits																	
Apple, raw, with skin	59	15.25	0.36	0.19	2.7	83.93	0.007	0.014	0.087	0.018	0	0	0	0	0.015	0.105	0.058
Apricot, raw	48	11.12	0.39	1.4	2.4	86.35	0.003	0.17	0.077	0	0	0	0	0	0.17	0.077	0.027
Avocado, raw	161	7.39	15.32	1.98	5	74.27	0.027	8.965	1.84	0.111	0.004	0	0	0	9.608	1.955	2.437
Bananas, raw	92	23.43	0.48	1.03	2.4	74.26	0.006	0.027	0.056	0.033	0	0	0	0	0.041	0.089	0.185
Blueberries, raw	56	14.13	0.38	0.67	2.7	84.61	0.007	0.052	0.099	0.067	0	0	0	0	0.054	0.166	0.032
Cantaloupe, muskmelon, raw	35	8.36	0.28	0.88	0.8	89.78	0.007	0.004	0.047	0.063	0	0	0	0	0.007	0.11	0.071
Cherries, raw	72	16.55	0.96	1.2	2.3	80.76	0.052	0.259	0.147	0.142	0	0	0	0	0.262	0.289	0.216
Cranberries, raw	49	12.68	0.2	0.39	4.2	86.54	0.003	0.028	0.053	0.035	0	0	0	0	0.028	0.088	0.017
Dates, dry	275	73.51	0.45	1.97	7.5	22.5	0.009	0.148	0.028	0.002	0	0	0	0	0.149	0.031	0.191
Figs, raw	74	19.18	0.3	0.75	3.3	79.11	0.012	0.066	0.144	0	0	0	0	0	0.066	0.144	0.06
Grapefruit, raw, pink and red	30	7.68	0.1	0.55		91.38	0.001	0.012	0.019	0.005				0	0.013	0.024	0.014
Grapes, red or green, raw	71	17.77	0.58	0.66	1	80.56	0.022	0.023	0.13	0.039	0	0	0	0	0.023	0.169	0.189
Honeydew melon, raw	35	9.18	0.1	0.46	0.6	89.66	0.002	0.002	0.017	0.022	0	0	0	0	0.002	0.039	0.025
Kiwifruit, raw	61	14.88	0.44	0.99	3.4	83.05	0.01	0.039	0.206	0.035	0	0	0	0	0.039	0.241	0.029
Lemon, raw, without peel	29	9.32	0.3	1.1	2.8	88.98	0.002	0.01	0.063	0.026	0	0	0	0	0.011	0.089	0.039
Lime juice, raw	27	9.01	0.1	0.44	0.011	90.21	0	0.008	0.018	0.009	0	0	0	0		0.01	0.027
Mango, raw	65	17	0.27	0.51	1.8	81.71	0.003	0.054	0.014	0.037	0	0	0	0	0.101	0.051	0.066
Orange, raw	47	11.75	0.12	0.94	2.4	86.75	0	0.02	0.018	0.007	0	0	0	0	0.023	0.025	0.015
Papaya	39	9.81	0.14	0.61	1.8	88.83	0.002	0.018	0.006	0.025	0	0	0	0	0.038	0.031	0.043
Peaches and nectarines, raw	43	11.1	0.09	0.7	2	87.66	0.001	0.034	0.044	0.001	0	0	0	0	0.034	0.045	0.01
Pear, raw	59	15.11	0.4	0.39	2.4	83.81	0.003	0.081	0.093	0.001	0	0	0	0	0.084	0.094	0.022
Pineapple, raw	49	12.39	0.43	0.39	1.2	86.5	0.011	0.045	0.084	0.062	0	0	0	0	0.048	0.146	0.032
Plums, raw	55	13.01	0.62	0.79	1.5	85.2	0.009	0.4	0.134	0	0	0	0	0	0.406	0.134	0.049
Prunes, dried, uncooked	239	62.73	0.52	2.61	7.1	32.39	0.007	0.335	0.112	0	0	0	0	0	0.34	0.112	0.041
Raisins, seedless	300	79.13	0.46	3.22	4	15.42	0.018	0.018	0.104	0.031	0	0	0	0	0.018	0.135	0.15
Raspberries, raw	49	11.57	0.55	0.91	6.8	86.57	0.003	0.049	0.208	0.105	0	0	0	0	0.053	0.313	0.019
Strawberries, raw	30	7.02	0.37	0.61	2.3	91.57	0.004	0.051	0.108	0.078	0	0	0	0	0.052	0.186	0.02
Watermelon, raw	32	7.18	0.43	0.62	0.5	91.51	0.018	0.107	0.146	0	0	0	0	0	0.107	0.146	0.048
Grains																	
Amaranth	374	66.17	6.51	14.45	15.2	9.84	0.22	1.433	2.834	0.057				0	1.433	2.891	1.662
Barley, pearl, cooked	123	28.22	0.44	2.26	3.8	68.8	0.003	0.047	0.193	0.021	0	0	0	0	0.057	0.214	0.093
Buckwheat	343	71.5	3.4	13.25	10	9.75	0.047	0.988	0.961	0.078	0	0	0	0	1.04	1.039	0.741
Corn (cornmeal/polenta)	362	76.89	3.59	8.12	7.3	10.26	0.057	0.945	1.589	0.049	0	0	0	0	0.948	1.638	0.505
Millet, cooked	119	23.67	1	3.51	1.3	71.41	0.037	0.176	0.48	0.028	0	0	0	0	0.184	0.508	0.172

				Minerals											Vitamins					
Calcium mg	Copper mg	Iron mg	Magnesium mg	Manganese mg	Phosphorus mg	Potassium mg	Selenium mg	Sodium mg	Zinc mg	Folic acid mcg	Niacin mg	Pantothenic acid mg	Riboflavin mg	Thiamine mg	Vitamin A IU	Vitamin B12 mcg	Vitamin B6 mg	Vitamin C mg	Vitamin E mg	Vitamin K mcg
137	0.253	0.8	22	0.337	29	203	0.9	29	0.14	0	0.411	0.274	0.072	0.045	5498	0	0.18	27.4	1.721	
14	0.152	0.52	18	0.371	49	670	0.7	8	0.2	0	0.552	0.311	0.028	0.095	0	0	0.228	12.1	0.16	
7	0.041	0.18	5	0.045	7	115	0.3	0	0.04	0	0.077	0.061	0.014	0.017	53	0	0.048	5.7	0.32	
14	0.089	0.54	8	0.079	19	296	0.4	1	0.26	0	0.6	0.24	0.04	0.03	2612	0	0.054	10	0.89	
11	0.262	1.02	39	0.226	41	599	0.4	10	0.42	0	1.921	0.971	0.122	0.108	612	0	0.28	7.9	1.34	40
6	0.104	0.31	29	0.152	20	396	1.1	1	0.16	0	0.54	0.26	0.1	0.045	81	0	0.578	9.1	0.27	0.5
6	0.061	0.17	5	0.282	10	89	0.6	6	0.11	0	0.359	0.093	0.05	0.048	100	0	0.036	13	1	
11	0.042	0.21	11	0.047	17	309	0.4	9	0.16	0	0.574	0.128	0.021	0.036	3224	0	0.115	42.2	0.15	1
15	0.095	0.39	11	0.092	19	224	0.6	0	0.06	0	0.4	0.127	0.06	0.05	214	0	0.036	7	0.13	
7	0.058	0.2	5	0.157	9	71	0.6	1	0.13	0	0.1	0.219	0.02	0.03	46	0	0.065	13.5	0.1	
32	0.288	1.15	35	0.298	40	652	1.9	3	0.29	0	2.2	0.78	0.1	0.09	50	0	0.192	0	0.1	
35	0.07	0.37	17	0.128	14	232	0.6	1	0.15	0	0.4	0.3	0.05	0.06	142	0	0.113	2	0.89	
11	0.044	0.12	8	0.01	9	129		0	0.07	0	0.191	0.283	0.02	0.034	259	0	0.042	38.1		
11	0.09	0.26	6	0.058	13	185	0.2	2	0.05	0	0.3	0.024	0.057	0.092	73	0	0.11	10.8	0.7	3
6	0.041	0.07	7	0.018	10	271	0.4	10	0.07	0	0.6	0.207	0.018	0.077	40	0	0.059	24.8	0.15	
26	0.157	0.41	30		40	332	0.6	5	0.17	0	0.5		0.05	0.02	175	0	0.09	98	1.12	25
26	0.037	0.6	8	0.03	16	138	0.4	2	0.06	0	0.1	0.19	0.02	0.04	29	0	0.08	53	0.24	0.2
9	0.03	0.03	6	0.008	7	109	0.1	1	0.06	8	0.1	0.138	0.01	0.02	10	0	0.043	29.3	0.09	
10	0.11	0.13	9	0.027	11	156	0.6	2	0.04	0	0.584	0.16	0.057	0.058	3894	0	0.134	27.7	1.12	
40	0.045	0.1	10	0.025	14	181	0.5	0	0.07	0	0.282	0.25	0.04	0.087	205	0	0.06	53.2	0.24	0.1
24	0.016	0.1	10	0.011	5	257	0.6	3	0.07	0	0.338	0.218	0.032	0.027	284	0	0.019	61.8	1.12	
5	0.068	0.11	7	0.047	12	197	0.4	0	0.14	0	0.99	0.17	0.041	0.017	535	0	0.018	6.6	0.7	3
11	0.113	0.25	6	0.076	11	125	1	0	0.12	0	0.1	0.07	0.04	0.02	20	0	0.018	4	0.5	
7	0.11	0.37	14	1.649	7	113	0.6	1	0.08	0	0.42	0.16	0.036	0.092	23	0	0.087	15.4	0.1	0.1
4	0.043	0.1	7	0.049	10	172	0.5	0	0.1	0	0.5	0.182	0.096	0.043	323	0	0.081	9.5	0.6	12
51	0.43	2.48	45	0.22	79	745	2.3	4	0.53	0	1.961	0.46	0.162	0.081	1987	0	0.264	3.3	1.45	
49	0.309	2.08	33	0.308	97	751	0.7	12	0.27	0	0.818	0.045	0.088	0.156	8	0	0.249	3.3	0.7	
22	0.074	0.57	18	1.013	12	152	0.6	0	0.46	0	0.9	0.24	0.09	0.03	130	0	0.057	25	0.45	
14	0.049	0.38	10	0.29	19	166	0.7	1	0.13	0	0.23	0.34	0.066	0.02	27	0	0.059	56.7	0.14	
8	0.032	0.17	11	0.037	9	116	0.1	2	0.07	0	0.2	0.212	0.02	0.08	366	0	0.144	9.6	0.15	
153	0.777	7.59	266	2.26	455	366		21	3.18	0	1.286	1.047	0.208	0.08	0	0	0.223	4.2	1.03	
11	0.105	1.33	22	0.259	54	93	8.6	3	0.82	0	2.063	0.135	0.062	0.083	7	0	0.115	0	0.05	
18	1.1	2.2	231	1.3	347	460	8.3	1	2.4	0	7.02	1.233	0.425	0.101	0	0	0.21	0	1.03	
6	0.193	3.45	127	0.498	241	287	15.5	35	1.82	0	3.632	0.425	0.201	0.385	469	0	0.304	0	0.67	
3	0.161	0.63	44	0.272	100	62	0.9	2	0.91	0	1.33	0.171	0.082	0.106	0	0	0.108	0	0.056	

	General						Fatty Acids											
Unit	Calories	Carbohydrates	Fat	Protein	Fiber	Water	Stearic acid	Oleic acid	Linoleic acid	Linolenic acid	Arachidonic acid	EPA	DHA	Cholesterol	Monounsaturated fat	Polyunsaturated fat	Saturated fat
	kcal	g	g	g	g	g	g	g	g	g	g	g	g	mg	g	g	g
Grains *(cont.)*																	
Oats	389	66.27	6.9	16.89	10.6	8.22	0.065	2.165	2.424	0.111				0	2.178	2.535	1.217
Quinoa	374	68.9	5.8	13.1	5.9	9.3	0.049	1.525	2.214	0.133				0	1.535	2.347	0.59
Rice, brown, cooked	112	23.51	0.83	2.32	1.8	72.96	0.015	0.297	0.283	0.013				0	0.3	0.296	0.165
Rye flour, dark	324	68.74	2.69	14.03	22.6	11.07	0.01	0.301	1.031	0.169	0	0	0	0	0.326	1.2	0.309
Sorghum (not common in the U.K.)	339	74.63	3.3	11.3		9.2	0.035	0.964	1.305	0.065				0	0.993	1.37	0.457
Triticale flour, whole grain (not common in the U.K.)	338	73.14	1.81	13.18	14.6	10.01	0.027	0.154	0.741	0.053				0	0.183	0.794	0.318
Wheat flour, whole grain	339	72.57	1.87	13.7	12.2	10.27	0.015	0.219	0.738	0.038	0.002	0	0	0	0.232	0.779	0.322
Legumes (Beans)																	
Adzuki, boiled	128	24.77	0.1	7.52	7.3	66.29		0.009	0.021					0			0.036
Broad, fava, boiled	110	19.65	0.4	7.6	5.4	71.54	0.008	0.078	0.152	0.012	0	0	0	0	0.079	0.164	0.066
Carob flour	222	88.88	0.65	4.62	39.8	3.58	0.014	0.194	0.212	0.004	0	0	0	0	0.197	0.216	0.09
Chickpeas, garbanzos, boiled	164	27.41	2.59	8.86	7.6	60.21	0.037	0.578	1.113	0.043	0	0	0	0	0.583	1.156	0.269
Haricot, boiled	142	26.31	0.57	8.7	6.4	63.18	0.05	0.134	0.112					0	0.05	0.246	0.148
Kidney, boiled	127	22.81	0.5	8.67	7.4	66.94	0.008	0.039	0.107	0.168	0	0	0	0	0.039	0.275	0.072
Lentils, boiled	116	20.14	0.38	9.02	7.9	69.64	0.005	0.061	0.137	0.037	0	0	0	0	0.064	0.175	0.053
Lima, boiled	115	20.89	0.38	7.8	7	69.79	0.018	0.029	0.118	0.052	0	0	0	0	0.034	0.171	0.089
Miso																	
Mung, boiled	105	19.14	0.38	7.02	7.6	72.66	0.024	0.054	0.119	0.009	0	0	0	0	0.054	0.128	0.116
Pinto, boiled	137	25.65	0.52	8.21	8.6	64.27	0.002	0.106	0.078	0.109	0	0	0	0	0.106	0.188	0.109
Peas, boiled	118	21.11	0.39	8.34	8.3	69.49	0.01	0.077	0.137	0.028	0	0	0	0	0.081	0.165	0.054
Soybeans, boiled	173	9.92	8.97	16.64	6	62.55	0.32	1.956	4.465	0.598	0	0	0	0	1.981	5.064	1.297
Soy milk	33	1.81	1.91	2.75	1.3	93.27	0.053	0.322	0.735	0.098	0	0	0	0	0.326	0.833	0.214
Tempeh	193	9.39	10.8	18.54		59.65	0.6	2.75	3.591	0.22	0			0	3	3.827	2.22
Tofu (bean curd), raw, firm	145	4.28	8.72	15.78	2.3	69.83	0.311	1.901	4.339	0.582				0	1.925	4.921	1.261
String beans, raw	31	7.14	0.12	1.82	3.4	90.27	0.004	0.004	0.023	0.036	0	0	0	0	0.005	0.059	0.026
Nuts, Seeds, and Their Oils																	
Almond	578	19.74	50.64	21.26	11.8	5.25	0.683	31.921	12.214	0	0	0	0	0	32.155	12.214	3.881
Brazil	656	12.8	66.22	14.34	5.4	3.34	5.679	22.382	23.807	0.062	0	0	0	0	23.016	24.129	16.154
Cashew	553	30	44	18	3	4	3.22	23.5	7.787	0.06	0	0	0	0	23.02	7.8	7.8
Chestnut, roasted	245	52.96	2.2	3.17	5.1	40.48	0.021	0.728	0.776	0.093	0	0	0	0	0.759	0.869	0.414
Coconut, raw	354	15.23	33.49	3.33	9	46.99	1.734	1.425	0.366	0	0	0	0	0	1.425	0.366	29.698
Hazelnut (filbert)	628	16.7	60.75	14.95	9.7	5.31	1.265	45.405	7.833	0.087	0	0	0	0	45.652	7.92	4.464
Linseed (flaxseed)	492	34.25	34	19.5	27.9	8.75	1.394	6.868	4.318	18.122	0	0	0	0	6.868	22.44	3.196
Macadamia, roasted	718	13.38	76.08	7.79	8		2.28	44.377	1.303	0.196	0	0	0	0	59.275	1.498	11.947
Olives, ripe, canned	115	6.26	10.68	0.84	3.2	79.99	0.236	7.77	0.847	0.064	0	0	0	0	7.888	0.911	1.415
Peanut, dry roasted	585	21.51	49.66	23.68	8	1.55	1.109	23.961	15.69	0.003	0	0	0	0	24.64	15.694	6.893
Pecan	691	13.86	71.97	9.17	9.6	3.52	1.745	40.594	20.628	0.986	0	0	0	0	40.801	21.614	6.18

Minerals / Vitamins

Calcium mg	Copper mg	Iron mg	Magnesium mg	Manganese mg	Phosphorus mg	Potassium mg	Selenium mg	Sodium mg	Zinc mg	Folic acid mcg	Niacin mg	Pantothenic acid mg	Riboflavin mg	Thiamine mg	Vitamin A IU	Vitamin B12 mcg	Vitamin B6 mg	Vitamin C mg	Vitamin E mg	Vitamin K mcg
54	0.626	4.72	177	4.916	523	429	0.75	2	3.97	0	0.961	1.349	0.139	0.763	0	0	0.119	0	0.7	
60	0.82	9.25	210	2.26	410	740	0.484	21	3.3	0	2.93	1.047	0.396	0.198	0	0	0.223	0		
10	0.081	0.53	44	1.097	77	79	0.12	1	0.62	0	1.33	0.392	0.012	0.102	0	0	0.149	0		
56	0.75	6.45	248	6.73	632	730	35.7	1	5.62	0	4.27	1.456	0.251	0.316	0	0	0.443	0	2.58	
28		4.4			287	350	0.462	6				2.927	0.546	0.142	0.237	0	0		0		
35	0.559	2.59	153	4.185	321	466	0.599	2	2.66	0	2.86	2.167	0.132	0.378	0	0	0.403	0	0.9	
34	0.382	3.88	138	3.799	346	405	70.7	5	2.93	0	6.365	1.008	0.215	0.447	0	0	0.341	0	1.23	
28	0.298	2	52	0.573	168	532	1.2	8	1.77	0	0.717	0.43	0.064	0.115	6	0	0.096	0		
36	0.259	1.5	43	0.421	125	268	2.6	5	1.01	0	0.711	0.157	0.089	0.097	15	0	0.072	0.3	0.09	
348	0.571	2.94	54	0.508	79	827	5.3	35	0.92	0	1.897	0.047	0.461	0.053	14	0	0.366	0.2	0.63	
49	0.352	2.89	48	1.03	168	291	3.7	7	1.53	0	0.526	0.286	0.063	0.116	27	0	0.139	1.3	0.35	
70	0.295	2.48	59	0.556	157	368	5.8	1	1.06	0	0.531	0.255	0.061	0.202	2	0	0.164	0.9		
28	0.242	2.94	45	0.477	142	403	1.2	2	1.07	0	0.578	0.22	0.058	0.16	0	0	0.12	1.2	0.08	
19	0.251	3.33	36	0.494	180	369	2.8	2	1.27	0	1.06	0.638	0.073	0.169	8	0	0.178	1.5	0.11	
17	0.235	2.39	43	0.516	111	508	4.5	2	0.95	0	0.421	0.422	0.055	0.161	0	0	0.161	0	0.18	
27	0.156	1.4	48	0.298	99	266	2.5	2	0.84	0	0.577	0.41	0.061	0.164	24	0	0.067	1	0.51	
48	0.257	2.61	55	0.556	160	468	7.1	2	1.08	0	0.4	0.285	0.091	0.186	2	0	0.155	2.1	0.94	
14	0.181	1.29	36	0.396	99	362	0.6	2	1	0	0.89	0.595	0.056	0.19	7	0	0.048	0.4	0.39	
102	0.407	5.14	86	0.824	245	515	7.3	1	1.15	0	0.399	0.179	0.285	0.155	9	0	0.234	1.7	1.95	
4	0.12	0.58	19	0.17	49	141	1.3	12	0.23	0	0.147	0.048	0.07	0.161	32	0	0.041	0	0.01	3
111	0.56	2.7	81	1.3	266	412	0	9	1.14	0	2.64	0.278	0.358	0.078	0	0.08	0.215	0		
683	0.378	2.66	58	1.181	190	237	17.4	14	1.57	0	0.381	0.133	0.102	0.158	166	0	0.092	0.2		
37	0.069	1.04	25	0.214	38	209	0.6	6	0.24	0	0.752	0.094	0.105	0.084	668	0	0.074	16.3	0.41	47
248	1.11	4.3	275	2.535	474	728	4.4	1	3.36	0	3.925	0.349	0.811	0.241	10	0	0.131	0	26.179	
176	1.77	3.4	225	0.774	600	600	2960	2	4.59	0	1.622	0.236	0.122	1	0	0	0.251	0.7	7.6	
37	2.2	6.7	292	1.7	593	660	19.9	12	5.8	35	1.1	0.9	0.1	0.4	0	0	0.4	0.5	0.9	34
29	0.507	0.91	33	1.18	107	592	1.2	2	0.57	0	1.342	0.554	0.175	0.243	24	0	0.497	26	1.2	
14	0.435	2.43	32	1.5	113	356	10.1	20	1.1	0	0.54	0.3	0.02	0.066	0	0	0.054	3.3	0.73	
114	1.725	4.7	163	6.175	290	680	4	0	2.45	0	1.8	0.918	0.113	0.643	40	0	0.563	6.3	15.188	
199	1.041	6.22	362	3.281	498	681	5.5	34	4.17	0	1.4	1.53	0.16	0.17	0	0	0.927	1.3	5	
70	0.57	2.65	118	3.036	198	363	3.6	4	1.29	0	2.274	0.603	0.087	0.71	0	0	0.359	0.7	0.569	
88	0.251	3.3	4	0.02	3	8	0.9	872	0.22	0	0.037	0.015	0	0.003	403	0	0.009	0.9	3	
54	0.671	2.26	176	2.083	358	658	7.5	6	3.31	0	13.525	1.395	0.098	0.438	0	0	0.256	0	7.8	
70	1.2	2.53	121	4.5	277	410	6	0	4.53	0	1.167	0.863	0.13	0.66	77	0	0.21	1.1	4.05	

	General						Fatty Acids										
Unit	Calories	Carbohydrates	Fat	Protein	Fiber	Water	Stearic acid	Oleic acid	Linoleic acid	Linolenic acid	Arachidonic acid	EPA	DHA	Cholesterol	Monounsaturated fat	Polyunsaturated fat	Saturated fat
	kcal	g	g	g	g	g	g	g	g	g	g	g	g	mg	g	g	g
Nuts, Seeds, and their Oils (cont.)																	
Pine nut	566	14.22	50.7	24	4.5	6.69	1.672	17.9	20.689	0.654	0	0	0	0	19.076	21.343	7.797
Pistachio, dry roasted	571	27.65	45.97	21.35	10.3	1.99	0.514	23.583	13.636	0.262	0	0	0	0	24.216	13.899	5.555
Pumpkin seed, dried	541	17.81	45.85	24.54	3.9	6.92	2.811	14.146	20.702	0.181	0	0	0	0	14.258	20.904	8.674
Sesame seed, dried, hulled	588	9.39	54.78	26.38	11.6	4.81	2.305	20.425	23.572	0.415	0	0	0	0	20.687	24.011	7.672
Sesame seed, dried, whole	573	23.45	49.67	17.73	11.8	4.69	2.09	18.521	21.375	0.376	0	0	0	0	18.759	21.773	6.957
Sunflower seed, dry roasted	582	24.07	49.8	19.33	11.1	1.2	2.212	9.399	32.782	0.069	0	0	0	0	9.505	32.884	5.219
Walnut	618	9.91	59	24.06	6.8	4.56	1.445	14.533	33.072	2.006	0	0	0	0	15.004	35.077	3.368
Common Herbs and Spices																	
Basil, fresh	27	4.34	0.61	2.54	3.9	90.96	0.005	0.088	0.073	0.316	0	0	0	0	0.088	0.389	0.041
Cardamom	311	68.47	6.7	10.76	28	8.28	0.06	0.85	0.31	0.12				0	0.87	0.43	0.68
Cayenne (red) pepper and paprika	314	54.66	16.76	12.26	34.2	7.79	0.847	3.33	6.727	0.731	0	0	0	0	3.574	7.458	2.953
Cinnamon	261	79.85	3.19	3.89	54.3	9.52	0.005	0.45	0.53	0	0	0	0	0	0.48	0.53	0.65
Cloves	323	61.21	20.07	5.98	34.2	6.86	0.344	1.337	2.586	4.257	0.045	0	0	0	1.471	7.088	5.438
Coriander, leaf	279	52.1	4.78	21.93	10.4	7.3	0.009	2.216	0.328	0	0	0	0	0	2.232	0.328	0.115
Cumin	375	44.24	22.27	17.81	10.5	8.06	0.14	13.618	3.103	0.176	0	0	0	0	14.04	3.279	1.535
Dill	43	7.02	1.12	3.46	2.1	85.95	0.021	0.798	0.082	0.013				0	0.802	0.095	0.06
Ginger	347	70.79	5.95	9.12	12.5	9.38	0.025	1	1.02	0.29	0	0	0	0	1	1.31	1.94
Horseradish	48	11.29	0.69	1.18	3.3	85.08	0.25	0.127	0.285	0.053	0	0	0	0	0.13	0.339	0.09
Mint (peppermint)	70	14.89	0.94	3.75	8	78.65	0.17	0.029	0.069	0.435				0	0.033	0.508	0.246
Mustard seeds	469	34.94	28.76	24.94	14.7	6.86	0.58	5.9	2.59	2.68	0	0	0	0	19.83	5.39	1.46
Nutmeg	525	49.29	36.31	5.84	20.8	6.23	0	1.59	0.35	0	0	0	0	0	3.22	0.35	25.94
Oregano and marjoram	306	64.43	10.25	11	42.8	7.16	4.991	0.51	1.05	4.18	0	0	0	0	0.67	5.23	2.66
Pepper, black	255	64.81	3.26	10.95	26.5	10.51	0.247	1.01	0.97	0.16	0	0	0	0	1.01	1.13	0.98
Rosemary	331	64.06	15.22	4.88	42.6	9.31	1.25	2.66	1.16	1.076	0	0	0	0	3.014	2.339	7.371
Saffron	310	65.37	5.85	11.43	3.9	11.9	0.41	0.39	0.754	1.242	0.013	0	0	0	0.429	2.067	1.586
Sage	315	60.73	12.75	10.63	40.3	7.96	0.28	1.75	0.53	1.23	0	0	0	0	1.87	1.76	7.03
Tarragon	295	50.22	7.24	22.77	7.4	7.74	0.232	0.361	0.742	2.955	0	0	0	0	0.474	3.698	1.881
Thyme	276	63.94	7.43	9.11	37	7.79	0.036	0.47	0.5	0.69	0	0	0	0	0.47	1.19	2.73
Turmeric	354	64.93	9.88	7.83	21.1	11.36	0.012	1.66	1.694	0.482	0	0	0	0	1.66	2.18	3.12
Fish and Shellfish																	
Clams, steamed	148	5.13	1.95	25.55	0	63.64	0.019	0.068	0.032	0.008	0.082	0.138	0.146	67	0.172	0.552	0.188
Cod	82	0	0.63	17.9	0	81.28	0.063	0.051	0.006	0.002	0.017	0.08	0.135	37	0.082	0.244	0.081
Crab, steamed	97	0	1.54	19.35	0	77.55	0.02	0.089	0.02	0.014	0.043	0.295	0.118	53	0.185	0.536	0.133
Halibut	140	0	2.94	26.69	0	71.69	0.059	0.463	0.038	0.083	0.178	0.091	0.374	41	0.967	0.94	0.417
Lobster	98	1.28	0.59	20.5	0	76.03	0.142	0.095	0.005	0	0	0.053	0.031	72	0.16	0.091	0.107
Mahimahi	109	0	0.9	23.72	0	71.22	0.137	0.11	0.046	0.006	0.003	0.026	0.113	94	0.155	0.211	0.241
Oysters, steamed	163	9.9	4.6	18.9	0	64.12	0.011	0.382	0.064	0.064	0.076	0.876	0.5	100	0.716	1.788	1.02

				Minerals											**Vitamins**					
Calcium	Copper	Iron	Magnesium	Manganese	Phosphorus	Potassium	Selenium	Sodium	Zinc	Folic acid	Niacin	Pantothenic acid	Riboflavin	Thiamine	Vitamin A	Vitamin B12	Vitamin B6	Vitamin C	Vitamin E	Vitamin K
mg	mg	mg	mg	mg	mg	mg	mg	mg	mg	mcg	mg	mg	mg	mg	IU	mcg	mg	mg	mg	mcg
26	1.026	9.2	233	4.298	508	599	16.6	4	4.25	0	3.57	0.208	0.19	0.81	29	0	0.11	1.9	3.5	
110	1.325	4.2	120	1.275	485	1042	8	10	2.3	0	1.425	0.513	0.158	0.84	533	0	1.7	2.3	4.263	
43	1.387	14.97	535	3.021	1174	807	5.6	18	7.46	0	1.745	0.339	0.32	0.21	380	0	0.224	1.9	1	
131	1.46	7.8	347	1.43	776	407	1.7	40	10.25	0	4.682	0.681	0.085	0.722	66	0	0.146	0	2.27	
975	4.082	14.55	351	2.46	629	468	5.7	11	7.75	0	4.515	0.05	0.247	0.791	9	0	0.79	0	2.27	8
70	1.83	3.8	129	2.11	1155	850	79.3	3	5.29	0	7.042	7.042	0.246	0.106	0	0	0.804	1.4	50.27	
61	1.36	3.12	201	3.896	513	523	17	2	3.37	0	0.47	1.66	0.13	0.057	40	0	0.583	1.7	4.691	
154	0.29	3.17	81	1.446	69	462	0.3	4	0.85	0	0.925	0.238	0.073	0.026	3864	0	0.129	18	0.26	
383	0.383	13.97	229	28	178	1119		18	7.47	0	1.102		0.182	0.198	0	0	0.23	21		
278	0.429	14.25	170	2.165	303	1916	8.6	1010	2.7	0	7.893		0.794	0.349	34927	0	3.67	64.1	1.03	
1228	0.233	38.07	56	16.667	61	500	1.1	26	1.97	0	1.3		0.14	0.077	260	0	0.31	28.5	0.01	
646	0.347	8.68	264	30.033	105	1102	5.9	243	1.09	0	1.458		0.267	0.115	530	0	1.29	80.8	1.69	
1246	1.786	42.46	694	6.355	481	4466	29.3	211	4.72	0	10.707		1.5	1.252	5850	0	0.61	566.7	1.03	
931	0.867	66.36	366	3.333	499	1788	5.2	168	4.8	0	4.579		0.327	0.628	1270	0	0.435	7.7	1.03	
208	0.146	6.59	55	1.264	66	738	0.158	61	0.91	0	1.57	0.397	0.296	0.058	7718	0	0.185	85		
116	0.48	11.52	184	26.5	148	1343	38.5	32	4.72	0	5.155		0.185	0.046	147	0	0.84	7	0.28	
56	0.058	0.42	27	0.126	31	246	2.8	314	0.83	0	0.386	0.093	0.024	0.008	2	0	0.073	24.9	0.01	
243	0.329	5.08	80	1.176	73	569	0.146	31	1.11	0	1.706	0.338	0.266	0.082	4248	0	0.129	31.8	0.34	
521	0.41	9.98	298	1.767	841	682	133.6	5	5.7	0	7.89		0.381	0.543	62	0	0.43	3	2.5	
184	1.027	3.04	183	2.9	213	350	1.6	16	2.15	0	1.299		0.057	0.346	102	0	0.16	3	2.5	
1576	0.943	44	270	4.667	200	1669	5.9	15	4.43	0	6.22		0.32	0.341	6903	0	1.21	50	1.69	
437	1.127	28.86	194	5.625	173	1259	3.1	44	1.42	0	1.142		0.24	0.109	190	0	0.34	21	1.03	
1280	0.55	29.25	220	1.867	70	955	4.6	50	3.23	0	1		0.428	0.514	3128	0	1.74	61.2	2.03	
111	0.328	11.1	264	28.408	252	1724	5.6	148	1.09	0	1.46		0.267	0.115	530	0	1.01	80.8	1.69	
1652	0.757	28.12	428	3.133	91	1070	3.7	11	4.7	0	5.72		0.336	0.754	5900	0	2.69	32.4	1.69	
1139	0.677	32.3	347	7.967	313	3020	4.4	62	3.9	0	8.95		1.339	0.251	4200	0	2.41	50	1.69	
1890	0.86	123.6	220	7.867	201	814	4.6	55	6.18	0	4.94		0.399	0.513	3800	0	0.55	50	1.69	
183	0.603	41.42	193	7.833	268	2525	4.5	38	4.35	0	5.14		0.233	0.152	0	0	1.8	25.9	0.07	
92	0.688	27.96	18	1	338	628	64	112	2.73	0	3.354	0.68	0.426	0.15	570	98.89	0.11	22.1		
7	0.026	0.26	24	0.012	174	403	36.5	71	0.4	0	2.04	0.14	0.042	0.022	28	0.9	0.4	2.9	0.23	
59	1.182	0.76	63	0.04	280	262	40	1072	7.62	0	1.34	0.4	0.055	0.053	29	11.5	0.18	7.6		
60	0.035	1.07	107	0.02	285	576	46.8	69	0.53	0	7.123	0.38	0.091	0.069	179	1.37	0.397	0	1.09	
61	1.94	0.39	35	0.061	185	352	42.7	380	2.92	0	1.07	0.285	0.066	0.007	87	3.11	0.077	0	1	
19	0.053	1.45	38	0.019	183	533	46.8	113	0.59	0	7.429	0.865	0.085	0.023	208	0.69	0.462	0		
16	2.679	9.2	44	1.222	243	302	154	212	33.24	0	3.618	0.9	0.443	0.127	486	28.8	0.09	12.8		

	General						Fatty Acids											
Unit	Calories kcal	Carbohydrates g	Fat g	Protein g	Fiber g	Water g	Stearic acid g	Oleic acid g	Linoleic acid g	Linolenic acid g	Arachidonic acid g	EPA g	DHA g	Cholesterol mg	Monounsaturated fat g	Polyunsaturated fat g	Saturated fat g

Fish and Shellfish (cont.)

Prawns, steamed	99	0	1.08	20.91	0	77.28	0.271	0.114	0.021	0.012	0.071	0.171	0.144	195	0.197	0.44	0.289
Salmon	116	0	3.45	19.94	0	76.35	0.096	0.546	0.05	0.034	0.078	0.419	0.586	52	0.934	1.353	0.558
Scallops	88	2.36	0.76	16.78	0	78.57	0.07	0.017	0.004	0	0.023	0.09	0.108	33	0.037	0.261	0.079
Snapper, red	128	0	1.72	26.3	0	70.35	0.394	0.123	0.025	0.044			0.273	47	0.322	0.588	0.365
Swordfish	155	0	5.14	25.39	0	68.75	0.405	1.392	0.037	0.238	0.087	0.138	0.681	50	1.981	1.182	1.406
Tuna	184	0	6.28	29.91	0	59.09	4.007	1.185	0.068		0.055	0.363	1.141	49	2.053	1.844	1.612

Dairy Products

Cheese, cheddar	403	1.28	33.14	24.9	0	36.75	0.441	7.905	0.577	0.365	0	0	0	105	9.391	0.942	21.092
Cow's milk, whole	61	4.66	3.34	3.29	0	87.99	0.151	0.84	0.075	0.049	0	0	0	14	0.965	0.124	2.079
Goat's milk	69	4.45	4.14	3.56	0	87.03	1.6	0.977	0.109	0.04	0	0	0	11	1.109	0.149	2.667
Yogurt, lowfat	63	7.04	1.55	5.25	0	85.07	3.86	0.354	0.031	0.013	0	0	0	6	0.426	0.044	1

Meats

Beef	405	0	33.82	23.4	0	42.62	0.74	13.02	0.83	0.39	0.04	0	0	92	15.15	1.28	14.01
Calf's liver	217	7.85	8	26.72	0	55.68	2.226	1.57	1	0	0.33	0	0.29	482	1.62	1.71	2.67
Chicken	223	0	13.39	23.97	0	62.1	2.84	4.45	2.55	0.12	0.11	0.01	0.03	76	5.4	2.92	3.74
Eggs, chicken	149	1.22	10.02	12.49	0	75.33	2.04	3.473	1.148	0.033	0.142	0.004	0.037	425	3.809	1.364	3.1
Lamb	294	0	20.94	24.52	0	53.72	1	8	1.14	0.3	0.07	0	0	97	8.82	1.51	8.83
Pork	273	0	17.18	27.57	0	54.55	0.67	6.92	1.28	0.05	0.07	0	0	91	7.64	1.45	6.22
Turkey	243	0	14.38	26.59	0	57.94	0.06	4.05	3.18	0.19	0.23	0	0.04	91	5	3.7	4.18
Venison	158	0	3.19	30.21	0	65.23	9.47	0.83	0.4	0.09	0.13			112	0.88	0.62	1.25

Miscellaneous Foods

Blackstrap molasses	235	0	0	0	0	28.7									0	0	0
Brewer's yeast	105	18.1	1.9	8.4	8.1	69	0	0.491	0.004	0	0	0	0	0	1.047	0.004	0.243
Chocolate, semisweet	479	63.1	30	4.2	5.9	0.7		9.89	0.91	0.06	0	0	0	0	9.97	0.97	17.75
Honey	304	82.4	0	0.3	0.2	17.1	0.002	0	0	0	0	0	0	0	0	0	0
Maple syrup	318	71.3	0	6.2	0	21.1	0.011								0	0	0
Mushrooms, button/crimini	22	4.12	0.1	2.5	0.6	92.3	0.086	0.002	0.04	0	0	0	0	0	0.002	0.042	0.014
Mushrooms, shiitake	55	14.28	0.22	1.56	2.1	83.48	0	0.031	0.028	0.003	0	0	0	0	0.068	0.031	0.055
Sea vegetables	43	9.57	0.56	1.68	1.3	81.58		0.086	0.02	0.004	0.012	0.004	0	0	0.098	0.047	0.247
Tea	1	0.3	0	0	0	99.7		0	0.001	0.003	0	0	0	0	0.001	0.004	0.002

	Minerals										Vitamins										
Calcium	Copper	Iron	Magnesium	Manganese	Phosphorus	Potassium	Selenium	Sodium	Zinc	Folic acid	Niacin	Pantothenic acid	Riboflavin	Thiamine	Vitamin A	Vitamin B12	Vitamin B6	Vitamin C	Vitamin E	Vitamin K
mg	mg	mg	mg	mg	mg	mg	mg	mg	mg	mcg	mg	mg	mg	mg	IU	mcg	mg	mg	mg	mcg
39	0.193	3.09	34	0.034	137	182	39.6	224	1.56	0	2.59	0.34	0.032	0.031	219	1.49	0.127	2.2	0.51	
13	0.077	0.77	26	0.015	230	323	44.6	67	0.55	0	7	0.75	0.06	0.17	118	3	0.2	0	1	0.4
24	0.053	0.29	56	0.09	219	322	22.2	161	0.95	0	1.15	0.143	0.065	0.012	50	1.53	0.15	3	1	
40	0.046	0.24	37	0.017	201	522	49	57	0.44	0	0.346	0.87	0.004	0.053	115	3.5	0.46	1.6		
6	0.162	1.04	34	0.02	337	369	61.7	115	1.47	0	11.79	0.38	0.116	0.043	137	2.02	0.381	1.1		
10	0.11	1.31	64	0.02	326	323	46.8	50	0.77	0	10.54	1.37	0.306	0.278	2520	10.88	0.525	0		
721	0.031	0.68	28	0.01	512	98	13.9	621	3.11	0	0.08	0.413	0.375	0.027	1059	0.83	0.074	0	0.36	3
119	0.01	0.05	13	0.004	93	152	2	49	0.38	0	0.084	0.314	0.162	0.038	126	0.36	0.042	0.9	0.1	0.3
134	0.046	0.05	14	0.018	111	204	1.4	50	0.3	0	0.277	0.31	0.138	0.048	185	0.07	0.046	1.3	0.09	
183	0.013	0.08	17	0.004	144	234	3.3	70	0.89	0	0.114	0.591	0.214	0.044	66	0.56	0.049	0.8	0.042	0.3
10	0.102	2.44	19	0.013	179	269	24.1	57	5.04	0	3.252	0.316	0.198	0.074	0	2.31	0.29	0		
11	4.466	6.28	23	0.423	461	364	57	106	5.45	0	14.44	5.92	4.14	0.21	36105	111.8	1.43	23	0.635	
12	0.058	1.26	20	0.018	179	211	23.6	73	1.45	0	7.418	0.918	0.143	0.057	83	0.27	0.35	0	0.265	
49	0.014	1.44	10	0.024	178	121	30.8	126	1.1	0	0.073	1.255	0.508	0.062	635	1	0.139	0	1.05	
17	0.119	1.88	23	0.022	188	310	26.4	72	4.46	0	6.66	0.66	0.25	0.1	0	2.55	0.13	0	0.14	
25	0.067	1.1	24	0.01	232	354	40.6	62	2.9	0	4.926	0.665	0.328	0.77	8	0.77	0.394	0.3	0.26	
33	0.142	2.19	22	0.023	189	260	37.8	73	3.92	0	3.446	1.073	0.224	0.054	0	0.34	0.3	0	0.587	
7	0.3	4.47	24	0.046	226	335	12.9	54	2.75		6.71		0.6	0.18	0			0		
60.8	2.04	17.5	215	2.61	40	2492	17.8	55	1	0	1.08	0.88	0.052	0.033	0	0	0.7	0	0	
19	0.148	3.25	40	0.2	336	601	8.1	30	9.97	0	12.3	4.9	1.13	1.88	0	0.01	0.43	0.1	0.08	
32	0.7	3.13	115	0.8	132	365	3.1	11	1.62	0	0.427	0.105	0.09	0.055	21	0	0.035	0	1.19	
6	0.036	0.42	2	0.08	4	52	0.8	4	0.22	0	0.121	0.068	0.038	0	0	0	0.024	0.5	0	0.02
61	0.2	0.96	72	0.1	236	320	12.3	35	0.14	0	8.12	0.171	0.393	0.011	0	0	0.5	0	0	
18	0.5	0.4	9	0.142	120	448	26	6	1.1	0	3.8	1.5	0.49	0.095	0	0.1	0.11	0	0.113	
3	0.896	0.44	14	0.204	29	117	24.8	4	1.33	0	1.5	3.594	0.17	0.037	0	0	0.159	0.3	0.12	
168	0.13	2.85	121	0.2	42	89	0.7	233	1.23	0	0.47	0.642	0.15	0.05	116	0	0.002	3	0.87	
0	0.01	0.02	3	0.219	1	37	0	3	0.02	0	0	0.011	0.014	0	0	0	0	0	0	0.05

RESOURCES

The following websites represent a small selection rather than an exhaustive list of useful sources for foods not easily found in supermarket chains or on the high street, and for information and help. It is worth surfing for other sites too.

www.baldwins.co.uk Source of organic foods, including amaranth seeds, and supplements.

www.bhf.org.uk Website of the British Heart Foundation.

www.bodykind.com Supplies natural health products including royal jelly, bee pollen and propolis products.

www.brogdale.org Home of the National Fruit Collection.

www.cancerresearchuk.org Information about cancer and living with cancer.

www.cancerhelpuk.org Information about cancer and living with cancer.

www.coeliac.co.uk Website offering information, support and resources for celiacs.

www.dietaryneedsdirect.co.uk Supplies foods suitable for allergy sufferers and celiacs and others with special dietary needs, including rice bran and amaranth flakes.

www.dwi.gov.uk Website of the Drinking Water Inspectorate of England and Wales.

www.dwqr.org.uk Website of the Drinking Water Quality Regulator of Scotland.

www.ehsni.gov.uk Website of the Northern Ireland Environment Agency and Heritage Service that regulates drinking water in Ulster.

www.environment-agency.gov.uk Website of the Environment Agency, responsible for watercourse, underground and coastal water quality. A good site to consult about fishing.

www.foodstandards.gov.uk Information on many aspects of food safety, regulations, etc.

www.goodnessdirect.co.uk Good general site for organic foods and supplements. Also stocks Veggi Wash vegetable cleanser.

www.healthy.co.uk Supplies natural health products including xylitol.

www.hollandandbarrett.com Suppliers of vitamins, minerals and food supplements.

www.lactolite.co.uk Supplies reduced-lactose milk.

www.mammathonian.co.uk Website selling a variety of seeds, including different types of squash.

www.nickys-nursery.co.uk Source of a wide variety of seeds to grow your own vegetables and herbs.

www.nutrition.org.uk Website of the British Nutrition Foundation containing lots of information on many aspects of nutrition including Reference Nutrient Intakes (RNIs).

www.oakleaf-european.co.uk and www.simply-thai-uk.com Stock various exotic vegetables, herbs and spices including bitter melon, jicama and whole turmeric plus other Thai vegetables.

www.pan-uk.org Information on pesticides.

www.pesticides.gov.uk Website of the Pesticides Safety Directorate.

www.rivercottage.net Hugh Fearnley-Whittingstall's website containing lots of information about fresh, organic, locally produced food including how to source it in your own area.

www.saffronspecialist.co.uk Supplies a variety of saffrons.

www.seeds-by-size.co.uk Website selling a variety of seeds, including different types of chard.

www.seedfest.co.uk Website selling a variety of seeds, including different types of chard.

www.seedsofitaly.sagenet.co.uk Website selling a variety of seeds, including different types of squash.

www.soilassociation.org The principal certification body for organic food producers in the U.K. Information on many aspects of organic food production.

www.vivaverde.co.uk Website selling a variety of seeds, including different types of squash and amaranth.

REFERENCES

The primary resources for the materials presented in this book are from the personal files of the authors. Over the past thirty years, we have painstakingly collected thousands of scientific articles from medical journals on the healing powers of foods and food components. The references provided are by no means a complete list of all of the studies reviewed or mentioned in *The Encyclopaedia of Healing Foods*. Instead, we have chosen to focus on key studies and comprehensive review articles that readers may find helpful.

We also encourage interested parties to visit the website of the National Library of Medicine (NLM) at http://gateway.nlm.nih.gov for additional studies.

The NLM Gateway is a Web-based system that lets users search simultaneously in multiple retrieval systems at the NLM. From this site you can access all of the NLM databases, including the PubMed database. The PubMed database was developed in conjunction with publishers of biomedical literature as a search tool for accessing literature citations and linking to full-text journal articles at websites of participating publishers.

Publishers participating in PubMed supply NLM with their citations electronically prior to or at the time of publication. If the publisher has a website that offers full-text versions of its journals, PubMed provides links to the site, as well as sites with other biological data, sequence centers, and so on. User registration, a subscription fee, or some other type of fee may be required to access the full text of articles in some journals.

PubMed provides access to bibliographic information, including MEDLINE, the NLM's premier bibliographic database, covering the fields of medicine, nursing, dentistry, veterinary medicine, the health care system, and the preclinical sciences. MEDLINE contains bibliographic citations and author abstracts from more than 4,000 medical journals published in the United States and seventy other countries. The file contains more than 11 million citations dating back to the mid-1960s. Coverage is worldwide, but most records are from English-language sources or have English abstracts (summaries). Conducting a search is quite easy, and the site has a link to a tutorial that fully explains the search process.

Chapter I: Human Nutrition

Cordain, L., S. B. Eaton, J. B. Miller, N. Mann, and K. Hill. "The Paradoxical Nature of Hunter-Gatherer Diets: Meat-Based, Yet Non-atherogenic." *Eur J Clin Nutr* 2002;56(Suppl. 1): S42–S52.

Eaton, S. B., and S. B. Eaton III. "Paleolithic vs. Modern Diets—Selected Pathophysiological Implications." *Eur J Nutr* 2000;39: 67–70.

Milton, K. "Nutritional Characteristics of Wild Primate Food: Do the Diets of Our Closest Living Relatives Have Lessons for Us?" *Nutrition* 15 (1999): 488–498.

Ryde, D. "What Should Humans Eat?" *Practitioner* 1985;232: 415–418.

Simopoulos, A. P. "Genetic Variation and Nutrition." *Nutr Rev* 1999;57: S10–S19.

Trowell, H., and D. Burkitt. *Western Diseases: Their Emergence and Prevention.* Cambridge, Mass.: Harvard University Press, 1981.

Chapter 2: Designing a Healthy Diet

Eat a "Rainbow" Assortment of Fruits and Vegetables

La Vecchia, C., and A. Taviani. "Fruit and Vegetables, and Human Cancer." *Eur J Cancer Prev* 1998;7: 3–8.

Steinmetz, K. A., and J. D. Potter. "Vegetables, Fruit, and Cancer Prevention: A Review." *Journal of the American Dietetic Association* 1996;96: 1027–1039.

Steinmetz, K. A., and J. D. Potter. "Vegetables, Fruit, and Cancer. II. Mechanisms." *Cancer Causes and Control* 1991;2: 427–42.

Van Duyn, M. A., and E. Pivonka. "Overview of the Health Benefits of Fruit and Vegetable Consumption for the Dietetics Professional: Selected Literature." *Journal of the American Dietetic Association* 2000;100(12): 1511–1521.

Reduce Your Exposure to Pesticides

Aronson, K. J., A. B. Miller, C. G. Woolcott, et al. "Breast Adipose Tissue Concentrations of Polychlorinated Biphenyls and Other Organochlorines and Breast Cancer Risk." *Cancer Epidemiology Biomarkers and Prevention* 2000;9: 55–63.

Baris, D., and S. H. Zahm. "Epidemology of Lymphomas." *Curr Opin Oncol* 2000;12(5): 383–394.

Blair, A., and S. H. Zahm. "Agricultural Exposures and Cancer." *Environ Heath Perspect* 1995; 103(Suppl. 8): 205–208.

Jaga, K., and D. Brosius. "Pesticide Exposure: Human Cancers on the Horizon." *Rev Environ Health* 1999;14(1): 39–50.

Mao, Y., J. Hu, A. M. Ugnat, and K. White. "Non-Hodgkin's Lymphoma and Occupational Exposure to Chemicals in Canada. Canadian Cancer Registries Epidemiology Research Group." *Ann Oncol* 2000;11(Suppl. 1): 69–73.

Zhang, S. M., D. J. Hunter, B. A. Rosner, et al. "Intakes of Fruits, Vegetables, and Related Nutrients and the Risk of Non-Hodgkin's Lymphoma Among Women." *Cancer Epidemiology Biomarkers and Prevention* 2000;9(5): 477–485.

Eat to Support Blood Sugar Control

Jenkins, D. J., C. W. Kendall, L. S. Augustin, et al. "Glycemic Index: Overview of Implications in Health and Disease." *The American Journal of Clinical Nutrition* 2002 Jul;76(1): S266–S273.

Liu, S., W. C. Willett, M. J. Stampfer, F. B. Hu, et al. "A Prospective Study of Dietary Glycemic Load, Carbohydrate Intake, and Risk of Coronary Heart Disease in U.S. Women." *The American Journal of Clinical Nutrition* 2000;71: 1455–1461.

Willett, W., J. Manson, and S. Liu. "Glycemic Index, Glycemic Load, and Risk of Type 2 Diabetes." *The American Journal of Clinical Nutrition* 2002;76: S274–S280.

Reduce Your Intake of Meat and Other Animal Foods

Bingham, S. A. "High-Meat Diets and Cancer Risk." *Proc Nutr Soc* 1999;58(2): 243–248.

Blot, W. J., B. E. Henderson, and J. D. Boice, Jr. "Childhood Cancer in Relation to Cured Meat Intake: Review of the Epidemiological Evidence." *Nutr Cancer* 1999;34: 111–118.

Preston-Martin, S., J. M. Pogoda, B. A. Mueller, et al. "Maternal Consumption of Cured Meats and Vitamins in Relation to Pediatric Brain Tumors." *Cancer Epidemiology Biomarkers and Prevention* 1996;5: 599–605.

Whigham, L. D., M. E. Cook, and R. L. Atkinson. "Conjugated Linoleic Acid: Implications for Human Health." *Pharmacol Res* 2000;42: 503–510.

Zheng, W., D. R. Gustafson, R. Sinha, et al. "Well-Done Meat Intake and the Risk of Breast Cancer." *Journal of the National Cancer Institute* 1998;90: 1724–1729.

Eat the Right Types of Fats

Alarcon de la Lastra, C., M. D. Barranco, V. Motilva, and J. M. Herrerias. "Mediterranean Diet and Health: Biological Importance of Olive Oil." *Curr Pharm Des* 2001;7: 933–950.

Bougnoux, P. "N-3 Polyunsaturated Fatty Acids and Cancer." *Curr Opin Clin Nutr Metab Care* 1999;2: 121–126.

Bucher, H. C., P. Hengstler, C. Schindler, and G. Meier. "N-3 Polyunsaturated Fatty Acids in Coronary Heart Disease: A Meta-Analysis of Randomized Controlled Trials." *Am J Med* 2002;112: 298–304.

Fraser, G. E. "Nut Consumption, Lipids, and Risk of a Coronary Event." *Clin Cardiol* 1999;22(Suppl. 7): 11–5.

Jiang, R., J. E. Manson, M. J. Stampfer, et al. "Nut and Peanut Butter Consumption and Risk of Type 2 Diabetes in Women." *Journal of the American Medical Association* 2002;288(20): 2554–2560.

Keep Salt Intake Low, Potassium Intake High

Jansson, B. "Potassium, Sodium, and Cancer: A Review." *J Env Pathol Toxicol Oncol* 1996;15: 65–73.

Khaw, K. T., and E. Barrett-Connor. "Dietary Potassium and Stroke-Associated Mortality." *The New England Journal of Medicine* 1987;316: 235–240.

Langford, H. G. "Dietary Potassium and Hypertension: Epidemiological Data." *Annals of Internal Medicine* 1990;98: 770–772.

Sacks, F. M., L. P. Svetkey, W. M. Vollmer, et al. "Effects on Blood Pressure of Reduced Dietary Sodium and the Dietary Approaches to Stop Hypertension (DASH) Diet. DASH-Sodium Collaborative Research Group." *The New England Journal of Medicine* 2001;344: 3–10.

Whelton, P. K., and J. He. "Potassium in Preventing and Treating High Blood Pressure." *Semin Nephrol* 1999;19: 494–499.

Drink Sufficient Amounts of Water Each Day

Kleiner, S. M. "Water: An Essential but Overlooked Nutrient." *Journal of the American Dietetic Association* 1999;99: 200–206.

A Quick Look at Some Popular Diets

ATKINS DIET

Foster, G. D., H. R. Wyatt, J. O. Hill, et al. "A Randomized Trial of a Low-Carbohydrate Diet for Obesity." *The New England Journal of Medicine* 2003;348: 2082–2090.

Hays, N. P., R. D. Starling, X. Liu, et al. "Effects of an *ad libitum* Low-fat, High-Carbohydrate Diet on Body Weight, Body Composition, and Fat Distribution in Older Men and Women." *Arch Intern Med* 2004;164: 210–217.

Stern, L., N. Iqbal, P. Seshadri, et al. "The Effects of Low-Carbohydrate Versus Conventional Weight Loss Diets in Severely Obese Adults: One-year Follow-up of a Randomized Trial." *Annals of Internal Medicine* 2004;140: 769–777.

Yancy, W. S., M. K. Olsen, J. R. Guyton, et al. "A Low-Carbohydrate, Ketogenic Diet Versus a Low-Fat

Diet to Treat Obesity and Hyperlipidemia."
Annals of Internal Medicine 2004;140: 769–777.

BLOOD TYPE DIET

Cordain, L., L. Toohey, M. J. Smith, and M. S. Hickey. "Modulation of Immune Function by Dietary Lectins in Rheumatoid Arthritis." *Br J Nutr* 2000;83(3): 207–217.

ORNISH DIET

Gould, K. L., D. Ornish, L. Scherwitz, et al. "Changes in Myocardial Perfusion Abnormalities by Positron Emission Tomography After Long-Term, Intense Risk Factor Modification." *Journal of the American Medical Association* 1995;274: 894–901.

Koertge, J., G. Weidner, M. Elliott-Eller, et al. "Improvement in Medical Risk Factors and Quality of Life in Women and Men with Coronary Artery Disease in the Multicenter Lifestyle Demonstration Project." *Am J Cardiol* 2003;91(11): 1316–1322.

Ornish. D. "Can Lifestyle Changes Reverse Coronary Heart Disease?" *The Lancet* 1990;336: 129–133.

MACROBIOTIC DIET

Dagnelie, P. C., et al. "Macrobiotic Nutrition and Child Health: Results of a Population-Based, Mixed-Longitudinal Cohort Study in the Netherlands." *American Journal of Clinical Nutrition* 1994;59: S1187–S1196.

Kushi, L. H., J. E. Cunningham, J. R. Hebert, et al. "The Macrobiotic Diet in Cancer." *The Journal of Nutrition* 2001;131(Suppl. 11): S3056–S3064.

VEGETARIAN DIET

Key, T. J., G. K. Davey, and P. N. Appleby. "Health Benefits of a Vegetarian Diet." *Proc Nutr Soc* 1999;58(2): 271–275.

Resnicow, K., J. Barone, A. Engle, et al. "Diet and Serum Lipids in Vegan Vegetarians: A Model for Risk Reduction." *Journal of the American Dietetic Association* 1991;91(4): 447–453.

Segasothy, M., and P. A. Phillips. "Vegetarian Diet: Panacea for Modern Lifestyle Diseases?" *QJM* 1999;92(9): 531–544.

ZONE DIET

Grundy, S. M. "The Optimal Ratio of Fat-to-Carbohydrate in the Diet." *Annu Rev Nutr* 1999;19: 325–341.

Sears, B. "The Zone Diet and Athletic Performance." *Sports Med* 2000;29(4): 289–294.

Chapter 3: Safe Eating

Foodborne Illness

Bryan, F. L. "Where We Are in Retail Food Safety, How We Got to Where We Are, and How Do We Get There?" *J Environ Health* 2002;65(2): 29–36.

Lasky T. "Foodborne Illness—Old Problem, New Relevance." *Epidemiology* 2002;13(5): 593–598.

Sivapalasingam, S., C. R. Friedman, L. Cohen, and R. V. Tauxe. "Fresh Produce: A Growing Cause of Outbreaks of Foodborne Illness in the United States, 1973 Through 1997." *J Food Prot* 2004;67(10): 2342–2453.

Tauxe, R. V. "Emerging Foodborne Pathogens." *Int J Food Microbiol* 2002;78(1–2): 31–41.

Food Irradiation

Farkas, J. "Irradiation as a Method for Decontaminating Food. A Review." *Int J Food Microbiol* 1998;44(3): 189–204.

Frenzen, P. D., E. E. DeBess, K. E. Hechemy, et al. "Consumer Acceptance of Irradiated Meat and Poultry in the United States." *J Food Prot* 2001;64(12): 2020–2026.

Genetically Modified Food

Atherton, K. T. "Safety Assessment of Genetically Modified Crops." *Toxicology* 2002;181–182: 421–426.

Bakshi, A. "Potential Adverse Health Effects of Genetically Modified Crops." (Critical review.) *J Toxicol Environ Health B* 2003;6(3): 211–325.

Lack, G., M. Chapman, N. Kalsheker, et al. "Report on the Potential Allergenicity of Genetically

Modified Organisms and Their Products." *Clin Exp Allergy* 2002;32(8): 1131–1143.

Food Additives

Boris, M., and F. S. Mandel. "Foods and Additives Are Common Causes of the Attention Deficit Hyperactive Disorder in Children." *Ann Allergy* 1994;72(5): 462–468.

Groten, J. P., W. Butler, V. J. Feron, G. Kozianowski, et al. "An Analysis of the Possibility for Health Implications of Joint Actions and Interactions Between Food Additives." *Regul Toxicol Pharmacol* 2000;31(1): 77–91.

Kinghorn, A. D., N. Kaneda, N. I. Baek, E. J. Kennelly, and D. D. Soejarto. "Noncariogenic Intense Natural Sweeteners." *Med Res Rev* 1998;18: 347–360.

Lessof, M. H. "Reactions to Food Additives." *Clin Exp Allergy* 1995;25(Suppl. 1): 27–28.

Simon, R. A. "Adverse Reactions to Food Additives." *Curr Allergy Asthma Rep* 2003;3(1): 62–66.

Chapter 4: Protein

General

Bowman, B. A., and R. M. Russell (eds.). *Present Knowledge in Nutrition.* 8th ed. Washington, D.C.: International Life Sciences Institute, Nutrition Foundation, 2001.

Shils, M. E., J. A. Olson, M. Shike, and A. C. Ross (eds.). *Modern Nutrition in Health and Disease.* 9th ed. Baltimore: Lippincott, Williams & Wilkins, 1999.

Protein Requirements

Fielding, R. A., and J. Parkington. "What Are the Dietary Protein Requirements of Physically Active Individuals? New Evidence on the Effects of Exercise on Protein Utilization During Post-Exercise Recovery." *Nutr Clin Care* 2002;5(4): 191–196.

Millward, D. J. "Protein and Amino Acid Requirements of Adults: Current Controversies." *Can J Appl Physiol* 2001;26(Suppl.): S130–S140.

Arginine

Appleton, J. "Arginine: Clinical Potential of a Semi-essential Amino Acid." *Altern Med Rev* 2002;7(6): 512–522.

Tapiero, H., G. Mathe, P. Couvreur, and K. D. Tew. "Arginine." *Biomed Pharmacother* 2002;56(9): 439–445.

Branched-Chain Amino Acids

Freund, H. R., and M. Hanani. "The Metabolic Role of Branched-Chain Amino Acids." *Nutrition* 2002;18(3): 287–288.

Glutamine

Neu, J., V. DeMarco, and N. Li. "Glutamine: Clinical Applications and Mechanisms of Action." *Curr Opin Clin Nutr Metab Care* 2002;5(1): 69–75.

Tapiero, H., G. Mathe, P. Couvreur, and K. D. Tew. "Glutamine and Glutamate." *Biomed Pharmacother* 2002;56(9): 446–457.

Lysine

Flodin, N. W. "The Metabolic Roles, Pharmacology, and Toxicology of Lysine." *Journal of the American College of Nutrition* 1997;16(1): 7–21.

Methionine and Cysteine

Bottiglieri, T. "*S*-Adenosyl-l-Methionine (SAMe): From the Bench to the Bedside—Molecular Basis of a Pleiotrophic Molecule." *The American Journal of Clinical Nutrition* 2002;76(5): S1151–S1157.

Taurine

Lourenco, R., and M. E. Camilo. "Taurine: A Conditionally Essential Amino Acid in Humans? An Overview in Health and Disease." *Nutr Hosp* 2002;17(6): 262–270.

Tryptophan

Riedel, W. J., T. Klaassen, and J. A. Schmitt. "Tryptophan, Mood, and Cognitive Function." *Brain Behav Immun* 2002;16(5): 581–589.

Chapter 5: Carbohydrates and Dietary Fiber

General

Bowman, B. A., and R. M. Russell (eds.). *Present Knowledge in Nutrition.* 8th ed. Washington, D.C.: International Life Sciences Institute, Nutrition Foundation, 2001.

Shils M. E., J. A. Olson, M. Shike, and A. C. Ross (eds.). *Modern Nutrition in Health and Disease.* 9th ed. Baltimore: Lippincott, Williams & Wilkins, 1999.

Fiber

Andoh, A., T. Tsujikawa, and Y. Fujiyama. "Role of Dietary Fiber and Short-Chain Fatty Acids in the Colon." *Curr Pharm Des* 2003;9(4): 347–358.

Brown, L., B. Rosner, W. W. Willett, and F. M. Sacks. "Cholesterol-Lowering Effects of Dietary Fiber: A Meta-Analysis." *The American Journal of Clinical Nutrition* 1999;69: 30–42.

Kim, Y. I. "AGA Technical Review: Impact of Dietary Fiber on Colon Cancer Occurrence." *Gastroenterology* 2000;118(6): 1235–1257.

Marlett, J. A., M. I. McBurney, and J. L. Slavin. American Dietetic Association. "Position of the American Dietetic Association: Health Implications of Dietary Fiber." *Journal of the American Dietetic Association* 2002;102(7): 993–1000.

Inositol

Jariwalla, R. J. "Inositol Hexaphosphate (IP6) as an Anti-Neoplastic and Lipid-Lowering Agent." *Anticancer Res* 1999;19(5A): 3699–3702.

Levine, J. "Controlled Trials of Inositol in Psychiatry." *Eur Neuropsychopharmacol* 1997;7(2): 147–155.

Palatnik, A., K. Frolov, M. Fux, and J. Benjamin. "Double-Blind, Controlled, Crossover Trial of Inositol Versus Fluvoxamine for the Treatment of Panic Disorder." *J Clin Psychopharmacol* 2001;21(3): 335–339.

Lignans

Ford, J. D., L. B. Davin, N. G. Lewis. "Plant Lignans and Health: Cancer Chemoprevention and Biotechnological Opportunities." *Basic Life Sci* 1999;66: 675–694.

Fructooligosaccharides

Carabin, I. G., and W. G. Flamm. "Evaluation of Safety of Inulin and Oligofructose as Dietary Fiber." *Regul Toxicol Pharmacol* 1999;30(3): 268–282.

Davidson, M. H., C. Synecki, and K. C. Maki, and K. B. Drennen. "Effects of Dietary Inulin in Serum Lipids in Men and Women with Hypercholesterolaemia." *Nutr Res* 1998;3: 503–517.

Flamm, G., W. Glinsmann, D. Kritchevsky, L. Prosky, and M. Roberfroid. "Inulin and Oligofructose as Dietary Fiber: A Review of the Evidence." *Crit Rev Food Sci Nutr* 2001;41(5): 353–362.

Jackson, K. G., G. R. J. Taylor, A. M. Clohessy, C. M. Williams. "The Effect of the Daily Intake of Inulin on Fasting Lipid, Insulin and Glucose Concentrations in Middle-Aged Men and Women." *Br J Nutr* 1999;82: 23–30.

Roberfroid, M. "Dietary Fibre, Inulin and Oligofructose. A Review Comparing Their Physiological Effects." *Crit Rev Food Sci Nutr* 1993;33: 103–148.

van Dokkum, W., B. Wezendonk, T. S. Srikumar, and E. G. van den Heuvel. "Effect of Nondigestible Oligosaccharides on Large-Bowel Functions, Blood Lipid Concentrations and Glucose Absorption in Young Healthy Male Subjects." *Eur J Clin Nutr* 1999;53: 1–7.

Chapter 6: Fats

Saturated Fats

Cater, N. B., and A. Garg. "Serum Low-Density Lipoprotein Cholesterol Response to Modification of Saturated Fat Intake: Recent Insights." *Curr Opin Lipidol* 1997;8(6): 332–336.

Holmes, M. D., D. J. Hunter, G. A. Colditz, M. J. Stampfer, S. E. Hankinson, F. E. Speizer, B. Rosner, and W. C. Willett. "Association of Dietary Intake of Fat and Fatty Acids with Risk of Breast

Cancer." *Journal of the American Medical Association* 1999;281(10): 914–920.

Hum, F. B., M. J. Stampfer, J. E. Manson, et al. "Dietary Saturated Fats and Their Food Sources in Relation to the Risk of Coronary Heart Disease in Women." *The American Journal of Clinical Nutrition* 1999;70(6): 1001–1008.

Salmeron, J., F. B. Hu, J. E. Manson, et al. "Dietary Fat Intake and Risk of Type 2 Diabetes in Women." *The American Journal of Clinical Nutrition* 2001;73(6): 1019–1026.

Monounsaturated Fats

Alarcon de la Lastra, C., M. D. Barranco, V. Motilva, and J. M. Herrerias. "Mediterranean Diet and Health: Biological Importance of Olive Oil." *Curr Pharm Des* 2001;7: 933–950.

Fraser, G. E. "Nut Consumption, Lipids, and Risk of a Coronary Event.: *Clin Cardiol* 1999;22(Suppl. 7): 11–15.

Jiang, R., J. E. Manson, M. J. Stampfer, et al. "Nut and Peanut Butter Consumption and Risk of Type 2 Diabetes in Women." *Journal of the American Medical Association* 2002;288(20): 2554–2560.

Omega-6 Fatty Acids

Simopoulos, A. P. "The Importance of the Ratio of Omega-6/Omega-3 Essential Fatty Acids." *Biomed Pharmacother* 2002;56(8): 365–379.

Omega-3 Fatty Acids

Albert, C. M., H. Campos, M. J. Stampfer, et al. "Blood Levels of Long-Chain *N*-3 Fatty Acids and the Risk of Sudden Death." *The New England Journal of Medicine* 2002;346: 1113–1118.

Bougnoux, P. "*N*-3 Polyunsaturated Fatty Acids and Cancer." *Curr Opin Clin Nutr Metab Care* 1999;2: 121–126.

Bucher, H. C., P. Hengstler, C, Schindler, and G. Meier. "*N*-3 Polyunsaturated Fatty Acids in Coronary Heart Disease: A Meta-Analysis of Randomized Controlled Trials." *Am J Med* 2002;112: 298–304.

Hum F. B., L. Bronner, W. C. Willett, et al. "Fish and Omega-3 Fatty Acid Intake and Risk of Coronary Heart Disease in Women." *Journal of the American Medical Association* 2002;287: 1815–1821.

Simopoulos, A. P. "Omega-3 Fatty Acids in Inflammation and Autoimmune Diseases." *Journal of the American College of Nutrition* 2002;21(6): 495–505.

Wu, D., and S. N. Meydani. "*N*-3 Polyunsaturated Fatty Acids and Immune Function." *Proc Nutr Soc* 1998;57: 503–509.

Phospholipids

Canty, D. J., and S. H. Zeisel. "Lecithin and Choline in Human Health and Disease." *Nutr Rev* 1994;52(10): 327–339.

Monograph. "Phosphatidylcholine." *Altern Med Rev* 2002;7(2): 150–154.

Cholesterol

McNamara, D. J. "Dietary Cholesterol and Atherosclerosis." *Biochim Biophys Acta* 2000(December 15);1529(1–3): 310–320.

Conjugated Linoleic Acid

Gaullier, J. M., J. Halse, K. Hoye, K. Kristiansen, et al. "Conjugated Linoleic Acid Supplementation for 1 y Reduces Body Fat Mass in Healthy Overweight Humans." *The American Journal of Clinical Nutrition* 2004;79(6): 1118–1125.

Whigham, L. D., M. E. Cook, and A. Atkinson. "Conjugated Linoleic Acid: Implications for Human Health." *Pharmacol Res* 2000;42: 503–510.

Ferulic Acid Derivatives

Cicero, A. F., and A. Gaddi. "Rice Bran Oil and Gamma-oryzanol in the Treatment of Hyperlipoproteinaemias and Other Conditions." *Phytother Res* 2001;15(4): 277–289.

Sugano, M., K. Koba, and E. Tsuji. "Health Benefits of Rice Bran Oil." *Anticancer Res* 1999;19(5A): 3651–3657.

Octacosanol

Gouni-Berthold, I., and H. K. Berthold. "Policosanol: Clinical Pharmacology and Therapeutic Significance of a New Lipid-Lowering Agent." *Am Heart J* 2002;143(2): 356–365.

Saint-John, M., and L. McNaughton. "Octacosanol Ingestion and Its Effects on Metabolic Responses to Submaximal Cycle Ergometry, Reaction Time and Chest and Grip Strength." *Int Clin Nutr Rev* 1986;6(2): 81–87.

Chapter 7: Vitamins

General

Bowman, B. A., and R. M. Russell (eds.). *Present Knowledge in Nutrition.* 8th ed. Washington, D.C.: International Life Sciences Institute, Nutrition Foundation, 2001.

Shils, M. E., J. A. Olson, M. Shike, and A. C. Ross (eds.). *Modern Nutrition in Health and Disease.* 9th ed. Baltimore: Lippincott, Williams & Wilkins, 1999.

Vitamin A and Beta-carotene

Dawson, M. I. "The Importance of Vitamin A in Nutrition." *Curr Pharm Des* 2000;6(3): 311–325.

Russell, R. M. "The Vitamin A Spectrum: From Deficiency to Toxicity." *The American Journal of Clinical Nutrition* 2000;71(4): 878–884.

Stephensen, C. B. "Vitamin A, Infection, and Immune Function." *Annu Rev Nutr* 2001;21: 167–192.

West, C. E. "Meeting Requirements for Vitamin A." *Nutr Rev* 2000;58(11): 341–345.

Vitamin D

Holick, M. F. "Vitamin D: A Millenium Perspective." *J Cell Biochem* 2003;88(2): 296–307.

Suda, T., Y. Ueno, K. Fujii, and T. Shinki. "Vitamin D and Bone." *J Cell Biochem* 2003;88(2): 259–266.

Zella, J. B., and H. F. DeLuca. "Vitamin D and Autoimmune Diabetes." *J Cell Biochem* 2003(February 1);88(2): 216–222.

Vitamin E

Azzi, A., R. Ricciarelli, and J. M. Zingg. "Non-antioxidant Molecular Functions of Alphatocopherol (Vitamin E)." *FEBS Lett* 2002;519(1–3): 8–10.

Brigelius-Flohe, R., F. J. Kelly, et al. "The European Perspective on Vitamin E: Current Knowledge and Future Research." *The American Journal of Clinical Nutrition* 2002;76(4): 703–716.

Herrera, E., and C. Barbas. "Vitamin E: Action, Metabolism and Perspectives." *J Physiol Biochem* 2001;57(2): 43–56.

Meydani, M. "Vitamin E and Atherosclerosis: Beyond Prevention of LDL Oxidation." *The Journal of Nutrition* 2001;131(2): S366–S368.

Vitamin K

Berkner, K. L. "The Vitamin K-Dependent Carboxylase." *The Journal of Nutrition* 2000;130(8): 1877–1880.

Weber, P. "Vitamin K and Bone Health." *Nutrition* 2001;17(10): 880–887.

Thiamine (Vitamin B1)

Suter, P. M., and W. Vetter. "Diuretics and Vitamin B1: Are Diuretics a Risk Factor for Thiamin Malnutrition?" *Nutr Rev* 2000;58(10): 319–323.

Biotin

McMahon, R. J. "Biotin in Metabolism and Molecular Biology." *Annu Rev Nutr* 2002;22: 221–239.

Pacheco-Alvarez, D., R. S. Solorzano-Vargas, and A. L. Del Rio. "Biotin in Metabolism and Its Relationship to Human Disease." *Arch Med Res* 2002;33(5): 439–447.

Said, H. M. "Biotin: The Forgotten Vitamin." *The American Journal of Clinical Nutrition* 2002;75(2): 179–180.

Riboflavin (Vitamin B2)

Powers, H. J. "Riboflavin (Vitamin B-2) and Health." *The American Journal of Clinical Nutrition* 2003;77(6): 1352–1360.

Niacin (Vitamin B3)

Jonas, W. B., C. P. Rapoza, and W. F. Blair. "The Effect of Niacinamide on Osteoarthritis: A Pilot Study." *Inflamm Res* 1996;45: 330–334.

Kamanna, V. S., and M. L. Kashyap. "Mechanism of Action of Niacin on Lipoprotein Metabolism." *Curr Atheroscler Rep* 2000;2(1): 36–46.

Folic Acid

Bailey, L. B., G. C. Rampersaud, and G. P. Kauwell. "Folic Acid Supplements and Fortification Affect the Risk for Neural Tube Defects, Vascular Disease and Cancer: Evolving Science." *The Journal of Nutrition* 2003;133(6): S1961–S1968.

Reynolds, E. H. "Folic Acid, Ageing, Depression, and Dementia." *British Medical Journal* 2002;324 (7352): 1512–1515.

Stanger, O. "Physiology of Folic Acid in Health and Disease." *Curr Drug Metab* 2002;3(2): 211–223.

Vitamin B6 (Pyridoxine)

Bender, D. A. "Non-nutritional Uses of Vitamin B6." *Br J Nutr* 1999;81(1): 7–20.

Vitamin B12

Oh, R., and D. L. Brown. "Vitamin B12 Deficiency." *Am Fam Physician* 2003(March 1);67(5): 979–986.

Pantothenic Acid

Prisco, D., P. G. Rogasi, M. Matucci, et al. "Effect of Oral Treatment with Pantethine on Platelet and Plasma Phospholipids in IIa Hyperlipoproteinemia." *Angiology* 1987;38(3): 241–247.

Tahiliani, A. G., and C. J. Beinlich. "Pantothenic Acid in Health and Disease." *Vitam Horm* 1991;46: 165–228.

Vitamin C

Carr, A. C., and B. Frei. "Toward a New Recommended Dietary Allowance for Vitamin C Based on Antioxidant and Health Effects in Humans." *The American Journal of Clinical Nutrition* 1999;69(6): 1086–1107.

Jacob, R. A., and G. Sotoudeh. "Vitamin C Function and Status in Chronic Disease." *Nutr Clin Care* 2002;5(2): 66–74.

Hemila, H., and R. M. Douglas. "Vitamin C and Acute Respiratory Infections." *Int J Tuberc Lung Dis* 1999;3(9): 756–761.

Padayatty, S. J., A. Katz, Y. Wang, et al. "Vitamin C as an Antioxidant: Evaluation of Its Role in Disease Prevention." *Journal of the American College of Nutrition* 2003;22(1): 18–35.

Chapter 8: Minerals

General

Bowman, B. A., and R. M. Russell (eds.). *Present Knowledge in Nutrition.* 8th ed. Washington, D.C.: International Life Sciences Institute, Nutrition Foundation, 2001.

Shils M. E., J. A. Olson, M. Shike, and A. C. Ross (eds.). *Modern Nutrition in Health and Disease.* 9th ed. Baltimore: Lippincott, Williams & Wilkins, 1999.

Calcium

Bronner, F. "Calcium Nutrition and Metabolism." *Dent Clin North Am* 2003;47(2): 209–224.

Cashman, K. D. "Calcium Intake, Calcium Bioavailability and Bone Health." *Br J Nutr* 2002;87 (Suppl. 2): S169–S177.

Power, M. L., R. P. Heaney, H. J. Kalkwarf, et al. "The Role of Calcium in Health and Disease." *Am J Obstet Gynecol* 1999;181(6): 1560–1569.

Resnick, L. M. "The Role of Dietary Calcium in Hypertension: A Hierarchical Overview." *Am J Hypertens* 1999;12(1): 99–112.

Phosphorus

Sax, L. "The Institute of Medicine's 'Dietary Reference Intake' for Phosphorus: A Critical Perspective." *Journal of the American College of Nutrition* 2001;20(4): 271–278.

Potassium, Sodium, and Chloride

Jansson, B. "Potassium, Sodium, and Cancer: A Review." *J Env Pathol Toxicol Oncol* 1996;15: 65–73.

Sacks, F. M., L. P. Svetkey, W. M. Vollmer, et al. "Effects on Blood Pressure of Reduced Dietary Sodium and the Dietary Approaches to Stop Hypertension (DASH) Diet. DASH-Sodium Collaborative Research Group." *The New England Journal of Medicine* 2001;344: 3–10.

Whelton, P. K., and J. He. "Potassium in Preventing and Treating High Blood Pressure." *Semin Nephrol* 1999;19: 494–499.

Magnesium

Fox, C., D. Ramsoomair, and C. Carter. "Magnesium: Its Proven and Potential Clinical Significance." *South Med J* 2001;94(12): 1195–1201.

Saris, N. E., E. Mervaala, H. Karppanen, J. A. Khawaja, and A. Lewenstam. "Magnesium. An Update on Physiological, Clinical and Analytical Aspects." *Clin Chim Acta* 2000;294(1–2): 1–26.

Vaquero, M. P. "Magnesium and Trace Elements in the Elderly: Intake, Status and Recommmendations." *J Nutr Health Aging* 2002;6(2): 147–153.

Sulphur

Komamisky, L. A., R. J. Christopherson, and T. K. Basu. "Sulfur: Its Clinical and Toxicologic Aspects." *Nutrition* 2003;19(1): 54–61.

Boron

Devirian, T. A., and S. L. Volpe. "The Physiological Effects of Dietary Boron." *Crit Rev Food Sci Nutr* 2003;43(2): 219–231.

Naghii, M. R. "The Significance of Dietary Boron, with Particular Reference to Athletes." *Nutr Health* 1999;13(1): 31–7.

Nielsen, F. H. "The Emergence of Boron as Nutritionally Important Throughout the Life Cycle." *Nutrition* 2000(July–August);16(7–8): 512–524.

Chromium

Anderson, R.A. "Chromium in the Prevention and Control of Diabetes." *Diabetes Metab* 2000; 26(1): 22–27.

Ryan, G. J., N. S. Wanko, A. R. Redman, and C. B. Cook. "Chromium as Adjunctive Treatment for Type 2 Diabetes." *Ann Pharmacother* 2003;37(6): 876–885.

Steams, D. M. "Is Chromium a Trace Essential Metal?" *Biofactors* 2000;11(3): 149–162.

Vincent, J. B. "The Biochemistry of Chromium." *The Journal of Nutrition* 2000;130(4): 715–718.

Copper

Ford, E. S. "Serum Copper Concentration and Coronary Heart Disease Among U.S. Adults." *American Journal of Epidemiology* 2000;151: 1182–1188.

Sandstead, H. H. "Requirements and Toxicity of Essential Trace Elements, Illustrated by Zinc and Copper." *The American Journal of Clinical Nutrition* 1995;61(Suppl.): S62–S64.

Iodine

Burman, K. D., and L. Wartofsky. "Iodine Effects on the Thyroid Gland: Biochemical and Clinical Aspects." *Rev Endocr Metab Disord* 2000;1(1–2): 19–25.

Iron

Beard, J. "Iron Deficiency Alters Brain Development and Functioning." *The Journal of Nutrition* 2003;133(5 Suppl. 1): S1468–S1472.

Hallberg, L. "Perspectives on Nutritional Iron Deficiency." *Annu Rev Nutr* 2001;21: 1–21.

Ross, E. M. "Evaluation and Treatment of Iron Deficiency in Adults." *Nutr Clin Care* 2002(September–October);5(5): 220–224.

Shah, S. V., and M. G. Alam. "Role of Iron in Atherosclerosis." *Am J Kidney Dis* 2003;41(3 Suppl. 2): S80–S83.

Manganese

Freeland-Graves, J. H. "Manganese: An Essential Nutrient for Humans." *Nutr Today* 1989;23: 13–19.

Molybdenum

Turnlund, J. R. "Molybdenum Metabolism and Requirements in Humans." *Met Ions Biol Syst* 2002;39: 727–739.

Selenium

Arthur, J. R., R. C. McKenzie, and G. J. Beckett. "Selenium in the Immune System." *The Journal of Nutrition.* 2003 May;133(5 Suppl. 1): S1457–S1459.

Combs, G. F., Jr., L. C. Clark, and B. W. Turnbull. "Reduction of Cancer Risk with an Oral Supplement of Selenium." *Biomed Environ Sci* 1997;10: 227–234.

Combs, G. F., and W. P. Gray: "Chemopreventive Agents: Selenium." *Pharmacol Ther* 1998;79: 179–192.

Ip, C., Y. Dong, and H. E. Ganther. "New Concepts in Selenium Chemoprevention." *Cancer Metastasis Rev* 2002;21(3–4): 281–289.

Silicon

Lassus, A. "Colloidal Silicic Acid for Oral and Topical Treatment of Aged Skin, Fragile Hair and Brittle Nails in Females." *J Int Med Res* 1993;21: 209–215.

Vanadium

Cam, M. C., R. W. Brownsey, and J. H. McNeill. "Mechanisms of Vanadium Action: Insulin-Mimetic or Insulin-Enhancing Agent?" *Can J Physiol Pharmacol* 2000(October);78(10): 829–847.

Sakurai, H. "A New Concept: The Use of Vanadium Complexes in the Treatment of Diabetes Mellitus." *Chem Rec* 2002;2(4): 237–248.

Zinc

Camara, F, and M. A. Amaro. "Nutritional Aspect of Zinc Availability." *Int J Food Sci Nutr* 2003;54(2): 143–151.

Ibs, K. H., and L. Rink. "Zinc-Altered Immune Function." *The Journal of Nutrition* 2003;133(5 Suppl. 1): S1452–S1456.

Prasad, A. S., and O. Kucuk. "Zinc in Cancer Prevention." (Review.) *Cancer Metastasis Rev* 2002;21 (3–4): 291–295.

Salgueiro, M. J., M. B. Zubillaga, A. E. Lysionek, R. A. Caro, R. Weill, and J. R. Boccio. "The Role of Zinc in the Growth and Development of Children." *Nutrition* 2002;18(6): 510–519.

Salgueiro, M. J., N. Krebs, M. B. Zubillaga, et al. "Zinc and Diabetes Mellitus: Is There a Need of Zinc Supplementation in Diabetes Mellitus Patients?" *Biol Trace Elem Res* 2001;81(3): 215–228.

Chapter 9: Accessory Nutrients and Phytochemicals

Betaine

Barak, A. J., H. C. Beckenhauer, and D. J. Tuma. "Betaine, Ethanol, and the Liver: A Review." *Alcohol* 1996;13: 395–398.

Barak, A. J., H. C. Beckenhauer, S. Badakhsh, and D. J. Tuma. "The Effect of Betaine in Reversing Alcoholic Steatosis." *Alcohol Clin Exp Res* 1997; 21: 1100–1102.

Craig, S. A. "Betaine in Human Nutrition." *The American Journal of Clinical Nutrition* 2004; 80(3): 539–549.

Selhub, J. "Homocysteine Metabolism." *Annu Rev Nutr* 1999;19: 217–246.

van Guldener, C., M. J. Janssen, K. de Meer, et al. "Effect of Folic Acid and Betaine on Fasting and Postmethionine-Loading Plasma Homocysteine and Methionine Levels in Chronic Haemodialysis Patients." *J Intern Med* 1999;245: 175–183.

Carnitine

Brass, E. P. "Supplemental Carnitine and Exercise." *The American Journal of Clinical Nutrition* 2000;72(Suppl. 2): S618–S623.

Evangeliou, A., and D. Vlassopoulos. "Carnitine Metabolism and Deficit—When Supplementation Is Necessary?" *Curr Pharm Biotechnol* 2003;4(3): 211–219.

Kelly, G. S. "l-Carnitine: Therapeutic Applications of a Conditionally-Essential Amino Acid." *Altern Med Rev* 1998;3(5): 345–360.

Pettegrew, J. W., J. Levine, and R. J. McClure. "Acetyl-l-Carnitine Physical-Chemical, Metabolic, and Therapeutic Properties: Relevance for Its Mode of Action in Alzheimer's Disease and Geriatric Depression." *Mol Psychiatry* 2000;5(6): 616–632.

Carnosine

Bonfanti, L., P. Peretto, S. De Marchis, and A. Fasolo. "Carnosine-Related Dipeptides in the Mammalian Brain." *Prog Neurobiol* 1999;59: 333–353.

Gardner, M. L., K. M. Illingworth, J. Kelleher, and D. Wood. "Intestinal Absorption of the Intact Peptide Carnosine in Man, and Comparison with Intestinal Permeability to Lactulose." *J Physiol* 1991;439: 411–422.

Hipkiss, A. R. "Carnosine, a Protective, Anti-Ageing Peptide?" *Int J Biochem Cell Biol* 1998;30: 863–868.

Quinn, P. J., A. A. Boldyrev, and V. E. Formazuyk. "Carnosine: Its Properties, Functions and Potential Therapeutic Applications." *Mol Aspects Med* 1992;13: 379–444.

Carotenes

Argarwal, S., and A. V. Rao. "Tomato Lycopene and Low Density Lipoprotein Oxidation: A Human Dietary Intervention Study." *Lipids* 1998;33: 981–984.

Cooper, D. A., A. L. Eldridge, and J. C. Peters. "Dietary Carotenoids and Lung Cancer: A Review of Recent Research." *Nutr Rev* 1999;57: 133–145.

Kohlmeier, L., J. D. Kark, and E. Gomez-Gracia, et al. "Lycopene and Myocardial Infarction Risk in the EURAMIC Study." *American Journal of Epidemiology* 1997;146: 618–626.

Krinsky, N. I. "The Antioxidant and Biological Properties of the Carotenoids." *Ann NY Acad Sci* 1998;854: 443–447.

Kritchevsky, S. B. "Beta-carotene, Carotenoids and the Prevention of Coronary Heart Disease." *The Journal of Nutrition* 1999;129: 5–8.

Landrum, J. T., R. A. Bone, and M. D. Kilburn. "The Macular Pigment: A Possible Role in Protection from Age-Related Macular Degeneration." *Adv Pharmacol* 1997;38: 537–556.

Mares-Perlman, J. A., A. E. Millen, T. L. Ficek, and S. E. Hankinson. "The Body of Evidence to Support a Protective Role for Lutein and Zeaxanthin in Delaying Chronic Disease." *The Journal of Nutrition* 2002;132(3): S518–S524.

Rao, A. V., and S. Agarwal. "Role of Antioxidant Lycopene in Cancer and Heart Disease." *Journal of the American College of Nutrition* 2000;19(5): 563–569.

Russell, R. M. "Physiological and Clinical Significance of Carotenoids." (Review.) *Int J Vitam Nutr Res* 1998;68(6): 349–353.

Weisburger, J. H. "Lycopene and Tomato Products in Health Promotion." *Exp Biol Med* 2002;227 (10): 924–927.

Chlorophyll

Chernomorsky, S. A., and A. B. Segelman. "Biological Activities of Chlorophyll Derivatives." *N J Med* 1988;85: 669–673.

Sarkar, D., A. Sharma, and G. Talukder. "Chlorophyll and Chlorophyllin as Modifiers of Genotoxic Effects." *Mutat Res* 1994;318(3): 239–247.

Choline

Shronts, E. P. "Essential Nature of Choline with Implications for Total Parenteral Nutrition." *Journal of the American Dietetic Association* 1997;97 (6): 639–646, 649.

Zeisel, S. H. "Choline: An Essential Nutrient for Humans." *Nutrition* 2000;16(7–8): 669–671.

Zeisel, S. H. "Choline: Needed for Normal Development of Memory." *Journal of the American College of Nutrition* 2000;19(Suppl. 5): S528–S531.

Ellagic Acid

Barch, D. H., L. M. Rundhaugen, G. D. Stoner, et al. "Structure-Function Relationships of the Dietary Anticarcinogen Ellagic Acid." *Carcinogenesis* 1996;17(2): 265–269.

de Ancos, B., E. M. Gonzalez, and M. P. Cano. "Ellagic Acid, Vitamin C, and Total Phenolic Contents and Radical Scavenging Capacity Affected by Freezing and Frozen Storage in Raspberry Fruit." *J Agric Food Chem* 2000;48(10): 4565–4570.

Lin, S. S., C. F. Hung, C. C. Ho, et al. "Effects of Ellagic Acid by Oral Administration on *N*-Acetylation and Metabolism of 2-Aminofluorene in Rat Brain Tissues." *Neurochem Res* 2000;25(11): 1503–1508.

Enzymes

Maurer, H. R. "Bromelain: Biochemistry, Pharmacology and Medical Use." *Cell Mol Life Sci* 2001;58: 1234–1245.

Flavonoids

Di Carlo, G., N. Mascolo, A. A. Izzo, and F. Capasso. "Flavonoids: Old and New Aspects of a Class of Natural Therapeutic Drugs." *Life Sci* 1999;65: 337–353.

Kuhnau, J. "The Flavonoids: A Class of Semiessential Food Components: Their Role in Human Nutrition." *World Review of Nutrition and Diet* 1976;24: 117–191.

Middleton, E., Jr., C. Kandaswami, and T. C. Theoharides. "The Effects of Plant Flavonoids on Mammalian Cells: Implications for Inflammation, Heart Disease, and Cancer." *Pharmacol Rev* 2000;52: 673–751.

Nijveldt, R. J., E. van Nood, D. E. van Hoorn, et al. "Flavonoids: A Review of Probable Mechanisms of Action and Potential Applications." *The American Journal of Clinical Nutrition* 2001;74: 418–425.

Pietta, P. G. "Flavonoids as Antioxidants." *J Nat Prod* 2000;63: 1035–1942.

Glutathione

Jones, D. P., R. J. Coates, E. W. Flagg, et al. "Glutathione in Foods Listed in the National Cancer Institutes Health Habits and History Food Frequency Questionnaire." *Nutr Cancer* 1995;17: 57–75.

Lenzi, A., F. Culasso, L. Gandini, et al. "Placebo-Controlled, Double-Blind, Cross-over Trial of Glutathione Therapy in Male Infertility." *Hum Reprod* 1993;8(10): 1657–1662.

Flagg, E. W., R. J. Coates, D. P. Jones, et al. "Dietary Glutathione Intake and the Risk of Oral and Pharyngeal Cancer." *American Journal of Epidemiology* 1994;139: 453–465.

Sen, C. K. "Nutritional Biochemistry of Cellular Glutathione." *Nutr Biochem* 1997;8: 660–672.

Smyth, J. F., A. Bowman, T. Perren, et al. "Glutathione Reduces the Toxicity and Improves Quality of Life of Women Diagnosed with Ovarian Cancer Treated with Cisplatin: Results of a Double-Blind, Randomised Trial." *Ann Oncol* 1997;8(6): 569–573.

Witschi, A., S. Reddy, B. Stofer, and B. H. Lauterburg. "The Systemic Availability of Oral Glutathione." *Eur J Clin Pharmacol* 1992;43(6): 667–669.

Terpenes

Crowell, P. L., A. Siar Ayoubi, and Y. D. Burke. "Antitumorigenic Effects of Limonene and Perillyl Alcohol Against Pancreatic and Breast Cancer." *Adv Exp Med Biol* 1996;401: 131–136.

Whysner, J., and G. M. Williams. "d-Limonene Mechanistic Data and Risk Assessment: Absolute Species-Specific Cytotoxicity, Enhanced Cell Proliferation, and Tumor Promotion." Pharmacol Ther. 1996;71(1–2): 127–136.

Chapter 10: Vegetables

How Should We Eat Vegetables?

Cheng, K. K., N. E. Day, S. W. Duffy, et al. "Pickled Vegetables in the Aetiology of Oesophageal Cancer in Hong Kong Chinese." *The Lancet* 1992;339: 1314–1318.

Sen NP, S. W. Seaman, P. A. Baddoo, C. Burgess, and D. Weber. "Formation of *N*-Nitroso-*N*-Methylurea in Various Samples of Smoked/Dried Fish, Fish Sauce, Seafoods, and Ethnic

Fermented/Pickled Vegetables Following Incubation with Nitrite Under Acidic Conditions." *J Agric Food Chem* 2001;49(49): 2096–2103.

Artichoke

Gebhardt, R. "Antioxidative and Protective Properties of Extracts from Leaves of the Artichoke (*Cynara scolymus* L.) Against Hydroperoxide-Induced Oxidative Stress in Cultured Rat Hepatocytes." *Toxicol Appl Pharmacol* 1997;144(2): 279–286.

Gebhardt, R. "Inhibition of Cholesterol Biosynthesis in Primary Cultured Rat Hepatocytes by Artichoke (*Cynara scolymus* L.) Extracts." *J Pharmacol Exp Ther* 1998;286(3): 1122–1128.

Lupattelli, G., S. Marchesi, R. Lombardini, et al. "Artichoke Juice Improves Endothelial Function in Hyperlipemia." *Life Sci* 2004;76(7): 775–782.

Montini, M., P. Levoni, A. Angoro, and G. Pagani. "Controlled Trial of Cynarin in the Treatment of the Hyperlipemic Syndrome." *Arzneim Forsch* 1975;25: 1311–1314.

Pristautz, H. "Cynarin in the Modern Treatment of Hyperlipemias." *Wiener Medizinische Wochenschrift* 1975;1223: 705–709.

Asparagus

Jang, D. S., M. Cuendet, H. H. Fong, J. M. Pezzuto, and A. D. Kinghorn. "Constituents of *Asparagus officinalis* Evaluated for Inhibitory Activity Against Cyclooxygenase-2." *J Agric Food Chem* 2004;52(8): 2218–2222.

Wiboonpun, N., P. Phuwapraisirisan, and S. Tippyang. "Identification of Antioxidant Compound from *Asparagus racemosus.*" *Phytother Res* 2004;18(9): 771–773.

Aubergine

Jorge, P. A., L. C. Neyra, R. M. Osaki, et al. "Effect of Eggplant on Plasma Lipid Levels, Lipidic Peroxidation and Reversion of Endothelial Dysfunction in Experimental Hypercholesterolemia." *Arq Bras Cardiol* 1998;70(2): 87–91.

Kimura, Y., Y. Araki, A. Takenaka, and K. Igarashi. "Protective Effects of Dietary Nasunin on Paraquat-Induced Oxidative Stress in Rats." *Biosci Biotechnol Biochem* 1999;63(5): 799–804.

Noda, Y., T. Kneyuki, K. Igarashi, et al. "Antioxidant Activity of Nasunin, an Anthocyanin in Eggplant Peels." *Toxicology* 2000;148(2–3): 119–123.

Beets

Bobek, P., S. Galbavy, and M. Mariassyova. "The Effect of Red Beet (*Beta vulgaris* var. *rubra*) Fiber on Alimentary Hypercholesterolemia and Chemically Induced Colon Carcinogenesis in Rats." *Nährung* 2000;44(3): 184–187.

Gallaher, D. D., P. Locket, and C. M. Gallaher. "Bile Acid Metabolism in Rats Fed Two Levels of Corn Oil and Brans of Oat, Rye, and Barley and Sugar Beet Fiber." *The Journal of Nutrition* 1992;122: 473–481.

Ilnitskii, A. P., and V. A. Iurchenko. "Effect of Fruit and Vegetable Juices on the Changes in the Production of Carcinogenic *N*-nitroso Compounds in Human Gastric Juice." *Vopr Pitan* 1993;(4): 44–46.

Manousos, O., N. E. Day, D. Trichopoulus, et al. "Diet and Colorectal Cancer: A Case-Control Study in Greece." *Int J Cancer* 1983;32: 1–5.

Nagai, T., S. Ishizuka, H. Hara, and Y. Aoyama. "Dietary Sugar Beet Fiber Prevents the Increase in Aberrant Crypt Foci Induced by Gamma-Irradiation in the Colorectum of Rats Treated with an Immunosuppressant." *The Journal of Nutrition* 2000;130(7): 1682–1687.

Bell (Sweet) Peppers

Gonzaez de Mejia, E, A. Quintanar-Hernandez, and G. Loarca-Pina. "Antimutagenic Activity of Carotenoids in Green Peppers Against Some Nitroarenes." *Mutat Res* 1998;416(1–2) 11–19.

Kaneyuki, T., Y. Noda, M. G. Traber, et al. "Superoxide Anion and Hydroxyl Radical Scavenging Activities of Vegetable Extracts Measured Using Electron Spin Resonance." *Biochem Mol Biol Int* 1999;47(6): 979–989.

Bitter Melon

Ahmad, N., M. R. Hassan, H. Halder, and K. S. Bennoor. "Effect of *Momordica charantia* (Karolla) Extracts on Fasting and Postprandial Serum Glucose Levels in NIDDM Patients." *Bangladesh Med Res Counc Bull* 1999;25(1): 11–13.

Ahmed, I., E. Adeghate, A. K. Sharma, D. J. Pallot, and J. Singh. "Effects of *Momordica charantia* Fruit Juice on Islet Morphology in the Pancreas of the Streptozotocin-Diabetic Rat." *Diabetes Res Clin Pract* 1998;40(3): 145–151.

Claflin, A. J., D. L. Vesely, J. L. Hudson, C. B. Bagwell, D. C. Lehotay, T. M. Lo, M. A. Fletcher, N. L. Block, and G. S. Levey. "Inhibition of Growth and Guanylate Cyclase Activity of an Undifferentiated Prostate Adenocarcinoma by an Extract of the Balsam Pear *(Momardica charantia abbreviata)*." *Proc Natl Acad Sci U S A* 1978;75(2): 989–993.

Foa-Tomasi, L., G. Campadelli-Fiume, L. Barbieri, and F. Stirpe. "Effect of Ribosome-Inactivating Proteins on Virus-Infected Cells. Inhibition of Virus Multiplication and of Protein Synthesis." *Arch Virol* 1982;71(4): 323–332.

Miura, T., C. Itoh, N. Iwamoto, M. Kato, M. Kawai, S. R. Park, and I. Suzuki. "Hypoglycemic Activity of the Fruit of the *Momordica charantia* in Type 2 Diabetic Mice." *J Nutr Sci Vitaminol* 2001; 47(5): 340–344.

Broccoli

Fahey, J. W., X. Haristoy, P. M. Dolan, et al. "Sulforaphane Inhibits Extracellular, Intracellular, and Antibiotic-Resistant Strains of *Helicobacter pylori* and Prevents Benzo[a]pyrene-Induced Stomach Tumors." *Proc Natl Acad Sci U S A* 2002; 99(11): 7610–7615.

Fahey, J. W., Y. Zhang, and P. Talalay. "Broccoli Sprouts: An Exceptionally Rich Source of Inducers of Enzymes That Protect Against Chemical Carcinogens." *Proc Natl Acad Sci U S A* 1997;94 (19): 10367–10372.

Faulkner, K., et al. "Selective Increase of the Potential Anticarcinogen Methylsulphonylbutyl Glucosinolate in Broccoli." *Carcinogenesis* 1998;19(4): 605–609.

Gao, X., A. T. Dinkova-Kostova, and P. Talalay. "Powerful and Prolonged Protection of Human Retinal Pigment Epithelial Cells, Keratinocytes, and Mouse Leukemia Cells Against Oxidative Damage: The Indirect Antioxidant Effects of Sulforaphane." *Proc Natl Acad Sci U S A* 2001; 98(26): 15221–15226.

Meng, Q., I. D. Goldberg, E. M. Rosen, and S. Fan. "Inhibitory Effects of Indole-3-Carbinol on Invasion and Migration in Human Breast Cancer Cells." *Breast Cancer Res Treat* 2000;63(2): 147–152.

Nestle, M. "Broccoli Sprouts as Inducers of Carcinogen-Detoxifying Enzyme Systems: Clinical, Dietary, and Policy Implications." *Proc Natl Acad Sci USA* 1997;94(21): 11149–11151.

van Poppel, G., D. T. Verhoeven, H. Verhagen, and R. A. Goldbohm. "Brassica Vegetables and Cancer Prevention. Epidemiology and Mechanisms." *Adv Exp Med Biol* 1999;472: 159–168.

Brussels Sprouts

Beecher, C. "Cancer Preventive Properties of Varieties of *Brassica oleracea*: A Review." *The American Journal of Clinical Nutrition* 1994;59 (Suppl.): S1166–S1170.

Kawamori, T., T. Tanaka, M. Ohnishi, et al. "Chemoprevention of Azoxymethane-Induced Colon Carcinogenesis by Dietary Feeding of *S*-Methyl Methane Thiosulfonate in Male F344 Rats." *Cancer Res* 1995;55(18): 4053–4058.

Stoewsand, G. S. "Bioactive Organosulfur Phytochemicals in *Brassica oleracea* Vegetables—A Review." *Food Chem Toxicol* 1995;33(6): 537–543.

Stoewsand, G. S., J. L. Anderson, and L. Munson. "Protective Effect of Dietary Brussels Sprouts Against Mammary Carcinogenesis in Sprague-Dawley Rats." *Cancer Lett* 1988;39(2): 199–207.

Verhagen, H., H. E. Poulsen, S. Loft, et al. "Reduction of Oxidative DNA-Damage in Humans by Brussels Sprouts." *Carcinogenesis* 1995;16(4): 969–970, 1995.

Cabbage

Cheney, G. "Anti-Peptic Ulcer Dietary Factor." *Journal of the American Dietetic Association* 1950;26: 668–672.

Cheney, G. "Rapid Healing of Peptic Ulcers in Patients Receiving Fresh Cabbage Juice." *Cal Med* 1949;70: 10–14.

Kwak, M. K., P. A. Egner, P. M. Dolan, et al. "Role of Phase 2 Enzyme Induction in Chemoprotection by Dithiolethiones." *Mutat Res* 2001;480–481: 305–315.

Michnovicz, J. J., and H. L. Bradlow. "Altered Estrogen Metabolism and Excretion in Humans Following Consumption of Indole-3-Carbinol." *Nutr Cancer* 1991;16(1): 59–66.

Steinkellner, H., S. Rabot, C. Freywald, et al. "Effects of Cruciferous Vegetables and Their Constituents on Drug Metabolizing Enzymes Involved in the Bioactivation of DNA-Reactive Dietary Carcinogens." *Mutat Res* 2001;480–481: 285–297.

Stoewsand, G. S. "Bioactive Organosulfur Phytochemicals in *Brassica oleracea* Vegetables—A Review." *Food Chem Toxicol* 1995;33(6): 537–543.

van Poppel, G., D. T. Verhoeven, H. Verhagen, and R. A. Goldbohm. "Brassica Vegetables and Cancer Prevention. Epidemiology and Mechanisms." *Adv Exp Med Biol* 1999;472: 159–168.

Verhoeven, D. T., R. A. Goldbom, G. van Poppel, et al. "Epidemiological Studies on Brassica Vegetables and Cancer Risk." *Cancer Epidemiology Biomarkers and Prevention* 1996;5(9): 773–748.

Carrots

Kritchevsky, S. B. "Beta-carotene, Carotenoids and the Prevention of Coronary Heart Disease." *The Journal of Nutrition* 1999;129(1): 5–8.

Matthews-Roth, M. M. "Amenorrhea Associated with Carotenemia." *Journal of the American Medical Association* 1983;250: 731.

Mathews-Roth, M. M. "Neutropenia and Beta-carotene." *The Lancet* 1982;2: 222.

Michaud, D. S., D. Feskanich, E. B. Rimm, et al. "Intake of Specific Carotenoids and Risk of Lung Cancer in 2 Prospective U.S. Cohorts." *The American Journal of Clinical Nutrition* 2000;72 (4): 990–997.

Cauliflower

Beecher, C. "Cancer Preventive Properties of Varieties of *Brassica oleracea:* A Review." *The American Journal of Clinical Nutrition* 1994;59 (Suppl.): S1166–S1170.

Verhoeven, D., et al. "A Review of Mechanisms Underlying Anticarcinogenicity by Brassica Vegetables." *Chemico-Biological Interactions* 1997;103 (2): 79–129, 1997.

Celery

Finkelstein, E., U. Afek, E. Gross, et al. "An Outbreak of Phytophotodermatitis Due to Celery." *Int J Dermatol* 1994;33(2): 116–118.

Khaw, K. T., S. Bingham, A. Welch, et al. "Relation Between Plasma Ascorbic Acid and Mortality in Men and Women in EPIC-Norfolk Prospective Study: A Prospective Population Study. European Prospective Investigation into Cancer and Nutrition." *The Lancet* 2001;357(9257): 657–663.

Tsi, D., and B. K. Tan. "The Mechanism Underlying the Hypocholesterolaemic Activity of Aqueous Celery Extract, Its Butanol and Aqueous Fractions in Genetically Hypercholesterolaemic RICO Rats." *Life Sci* 2000;66(8): 755–767.

Dandelion

Ahmad, V. U., S. Yasmeen, Z. Ali, M. A. Khan, M. I. Choudhary, F. Akhtar, G. A. Miana, and M. Zahid. "Taraxacin, a New Guaianolide from *Taraxacum wallichii.*" *J Nat Prod* 2000;63(7): 1010–1011.

Cho, S. Y., J. Y. Park, E. M. Park, M. S. Choi, M. K. Lee, S. M. Jeon, M. K. Jang, M. J. Kim, and Y. B. Park. "Alternation of Hepatic Antioxidant Enzyme Activities and Lipid Profile in Streptozocin-Induced Diabetic Rats by Supplementation of Dandelion Water Extract." *Clin Chim Acta* 2002;317(1–2): 109–117.

Maliakal, P. P., and S. Wanwimolruk. "Effect of

Herbal Teas on Hepatic Drug Metabolizing Enzymes in Rats." *J Pharm Pharmacol* 2001;53(10): 1323–1329.

Zhu, M., P. Y. Wong, and R. C. Li. "Effects of *Taraxacum mongolicum* on the Bioavailability and Disposition of Ciprofloxacin in Rats." *J Pharm Sci* 1999;88(6): 632–634.

Fennel

Chainy, G. B., S. K. Manna, M. M. Chaturvedi, and B. B. Aggarwal. "Anethole Blocks Both Early and Late Cellular Responses Transduced by Tumor Necrosis Factor: Effect on NF-kappaB, AP-1, JNK, MAPKK and Apoptosis." *Oncogene* 2000; 19(25): 2943–2950.

Javidnia, K., L. Dastgheib, S. Mohammadi Samani, and A. Nasiri. "Antihirsutism Activity of Fennel (fruits of *Foeniculum vulgare*) Extract. A Double-Blind Placebo Controlled Study." *Phytomedicine* 2003;10(6–7): 455–458.

Ostad, S. N., M. Soodi, M. Shariffzadeh, et al. "The Effect of Fennel Essential Oil on Uterine Contraction as a Model for Dysmenorrhea, Pharmacology and Toxicology Study." *J Ethnopharmacol* 2001;76(3): 299–304.

Ruberto, G., M. T. Baratta, S. G. Deans, and H. J. Dorman. "Antioxidant and Antimicrobial Activity of *Foeniculum vulgare* and *Crithmum maritimum* Essential Oils." *Planta Med* 2000;66(8): 687–693.

Garlic

Ali, M., M. Thomson, and M. Afzal. "Garlic and Onions: Their Effect on Eicosanoid Metabolism and Its Clinical Relevance." *Prostaglandins Leukot Essent Fatty Acids* 2000;62(2): 55–73.

Augusti, K. T. "Therapeutic Values of Onion (*Allium cepa* L.) and Garlic (*Allium sativum* L.)." *Indian J Exp Biol* 1996;34(7): 634–640.

Challier, B., J. M. Perarnau, and J. F. Viel. "Garlic, Onion and Cereal Fibre as Protective Factors for Breast Cancer: A French Case-Control Study." *Eur J Epidemiol* 1998;14(8): 737–747.

Dorant, E., P. A. van den Brandt, and R. A. Goldbohm. "Allium Vegetable Consumption, Garlic Supplement Intake, and Female Breast Carcinoma Incidence." *Breast Cancer Res Treat* 1995;33(2): 163–170.

Fukushima, S., N. Takada, T. Hori, and H. Wanibuchi. "Cancer Prevention by Organosulfur Compounds from Garlic and Onion. *J Cell Biochem* 1997;27(Suppl.): 100–105.

Riley, D. M., F. Bianchini, and H. Vainio. "Allium Vegetables and Organosulfur Compounds: Do They Help Prevent Cancer?" *Environ Health Perspect* 2001;109(9): 893–902.

Sainani, G. S., D. B. Desai, N. H. Gohre, et al. "Effect of Dietary Garlic and Onion on Serum Lipid Profile in Jain Community." *Ind J Med Res* 1979;69: 776–780.

Silagy, C. A., and A. W. Neil. "A Meta-Analysis of the Effect of Garlic on Blood Pressure." *J Hypertens* 1994;12: 463–468.

Spigelski, D., and P. J. Jones. "Efficacy of Garlic Supplementation in Lowering Serum Cholesterol Levels." *Nutr Rev* 2001(July);59(7): 236–241.

Jerusalem Artichoke

Kleessen, B., B. Sykura, H. J. Zunft, and M. Blaut. "Effects of Inulin and Lactose on Fecal Microflora, Microbial Activity, and Bowel Habit in Elderly Constipated Persons." *The American Journal of Clinical Nutrition* 1997;65(5): 1397–1402.

Kolida, S., K. Tuohy, and G. R. Gibson. "Prebiotic Effects of Inulin and Oligofructose." *Br J Nutr* 2002;87(Suppl. 2): S193–S197.

Roberfroid, M. "Functional Food Concept and Its Application to Prebiotics." *Dig Liver Dis* 2002; 34(Suppl. 2): S105–S110.

Rumessen, J. J., S. Bode, O. Hamberg, and E. Hoyer. "Fructans of Jerusalem Artichokes: Intestinal Transport, Absorption, Fermentation, and Influence on Blood Glucose, Insulin, and C-Peptide Responses in Healthy Subjects." *The American Journal of Clinical Nutrition* 1990;52: 675–681.

Onions

Ali, M., M. Thomson, and M. Afzal. "Garlic and Onions: Their Effect on Eicosanoid Metabolism and Its Clinical Relevance." *Prostaglandins Leukot Essent Fatty Acids* 2000;62(2): 55–73.

Augusti, K. T. "Therapeutic Values of Onion (*Allium cepa* L.) and Garlic (*Allium sativum* L.)." *Indian J Exp Biol.* 1996;34(7): 634–640.

Challier, B., J. M. Perarnau, and J. F. Viel. "Garlic, Onion and Cereal Fibre as Protective Factors for Breast Cancer: A French Case-Control Study." *Eur J Epidemiol* 1998;14(8): 737–747.

Dorant, E., P. A. van den Brandt, and R. A. Goldbohm. "A Prospective Cohort Study on the Relationship Between Onion and Leek Consumption, Garlic Supplement Use and the Risk of Colorectal Carcinoma in the Netherlands." *Carcinogenesis* 1996;17(3): 477–484.

Dorsch, W., M. Ettl, G. Hein, et al. "Antiasthmatic Effects of Onions. Inhibition of Platelet-Activating Factor-Induced Bronchial Obstruction by Onion Oils." *Int Arch Allergy Appl Immunol* 1987;82(3–4): 535–536.

Fukushima, S., N. Takada, T. Hori, and H. Wanibuchi. "Cancer Prevention by Organosulfur Compounds from Garlic and Onion." *J Cell Biochem* 1997(Suppl.);27: 100–105.

Knekt, P., J. Kumpulainen, R, Jarvinen, H. Rissanen, M. Heliovaara, A. Reunanen, T. Hakulinen, and A. Aromaa. "Flavonoid Intake and Risk of Chronic Diseases." *The American Journal of Clinical Nutrition* 2002;76(3): 560–568.

Moon, J. H., R. Nakata, S. Oshima, et al. "Accumulation of Quercetin Conjugates in Blood Plasma After the Short-Term Ingestion of Onion by Women." *Am J Physiol Regul Integr Comp Physiol* 2000;279(2): R461–R467.

Riley, D. M., F. Bianchini, and H. Vainio. "Allium Vegetables and Organosulfur Compounds: Do They Help Prevent Cancer?" *Environ Health Perspect* 2001;109(9): 893–902.

Sheela, C. G., K. Kumud, and K. T. Augusti. "Antidiabetic Effects of Onion and Garlic Sulfoxide Amino Acids in Rats." *Planta Med* 1995;61(4): 356–357.

Wagner, H., W. Dorsch, T. Bayer, et al. "Antiasthmatic Effects of Onions: Inhibition of 5-Lipoxygenase and Cyclooxygenase *in vitro* by Thiosulfinates and Cepaenes." *Prostaglandins Leukot Essent Fatty Acids* 1990;39(1): 59–62.

Potatoes

Keswani, M. H., A. M. Vartak, A. Patil, and J. W. L. Davies: "Histological and Bacteriological Studies of Burn Wounds Treated with Boiled Potato Peel Dressings." *Burns* 1990;16: 137–143.

Spinach

Edenharder, R., G. Keller, K. L. Platt, and K. K. Unger. "Isolation and Characterization of Structurally Novel Antimutagenic Flavonoids from Spinach (*Spinacia oleracea*)." *J Agric Food Chem* 2001;49(6): 2767–2773.

He, T., C. Y. Huang, H. Chen, and Y. H. Hou. "Effects of Spinach Powder Fat-Soluble Extract on Proliferation of Human Gastric Adenocarcinoma Cells." *Biomed Environ Sci* 1999;12(4): 247–252.

Joseph, J. A., B. Shukitt-Hale, N. A. Denisova, et al. "Reversals of Age-Related Declines in Neuronal Signal Transduction, Cognitive, and Motor Behavioral Deficits with Blueberry, Spinach, or Strawberry Dietary Supplementation." *J Neurosci* 1999;19(18): 8114–8121.

Longnecker, M. P., P. A. Newcomb, R. Mittendorf, et al. "Intake of Carrots, Spinach, and Supplements Containing Vitamin A in Relation to Risk of Breast Cancer." *Cancer Epidemiology Biomarkers and Prevention* 1997;6(11): 887–892.

Nyska, A., L. Lomnitski, J. Spalding, et al. "Topical and Oral Administration of the Natural Water-Soluble Antioxidant from Spinach Reduces the Multiplicity of Papillomas in the Tg. AC Mouse Model." *Toxicol Lett* 2001;122(1): 33–44.

Squash, Summer

Edenharder, R., P. Kurz, K. John, et al. *"In vitro* Effect of Vegetable and Fruit Juices on the Mutagenicity of 2- Amino-3-Methylimidazo[4,5-f] Quinoline, 2-Amino-3, 4-Dimethylimidazo [4,5-f]Quinoline and 2-Amino-3,8-Dimethylimidazo[4,-f]Quinox." *Food Chem Toxicol* 1994; 32(5): 443–459.

Squash, Winter

Edenharder, R., P. Kurz, K. John, et al. *"In vitro* Effect of Vegetable and Fruit Juices on the Mutagenicity of 2- Amino-3-Methylimidazo[4,5-f] Quinoline, 2-Amino-3, 4-Dimethylimidazo [4,5-f]Quinoline and 2-Amino-3,8-Dimethylimidazo[4,-f]Quinox." *Food Chem Toxicol* 1994; 32(5): 443–459.

Suzuki, K., Y. Ito, S. Nakamura, J. Ochiai, and K. Aoki. "Relationship Between Serum Carotenoids and Hyperglycemia: A Population-Based Cross-sectional Study." *J Epidemiol* 2002;12: 357–366.

Wilt, T. J., A. Ishani, I. Rutks, and R. MacDonald. "Phytotherapy for Benign Prostatic Hyperplasia." *Public Health Nutr* 2000;3(4A): 459–472.

Sweet Potato

Hou, W. C., Y. C. Chen, H. J. Chen, et al. "Antioxidant Activities of Trypsin Inhibitor, a 33 KDa Root Storage Protein of Sweet Potato (*Ipomoea batatas* (L.) Lam cv. Tainong 57)." *J Agric Food Chem* 2001;49(6): 2978–2981.

Kusano, S., and H. Abe. "Antidiabetic Activity of White Skinned Sweet Potato (*Ipomoea batatas* L.) in Obese Zucker Fatty Rats." *Biol Pharm Bull* 2000;23(1): 23–26.

Terahara, N., I. Konczak-Islam, M. Nakatani, et al. "Anthocyanins in Callus Induced from Purple Storage Root of *Ipomoea batatas* L." *Phytochemistry* 2000;54(8): 919–922.

Wallerstein, C. "New Sweet Potato Could Help Combat Blindness in Africa." *British Medical Journal* 200030;321(7264): 786.

Tomatoes

Giovannucci, E., E. B. Rimm, Y. Liu, M. J. Stampfer, and W. C. Willett. "A Prospective Study of Tomato Products, Lycopene, and Prostate Cancer Risk." *Journal of the National Cancer Institute* 2002;94(5): 391–398.

Khachik, F., L. Carvalho, P. S. Bernstein, et al. "Chemistry, Distribution, and Metabolism of Tomato Carotenoids and Their Impact on Human Health." *Exp Biol Med* 2002;227(10): 845–851.

Kohlmeyer, L., J. D. Kark, E. Gomez-Gracia, et al. "Lycopene and Myocardial Infarction Risk in the EUROMIC Study." *American Journal of Epidemiology* 1997;146: 618–626.

Weisburger, J. H. "Lycopene and Tomato Products in Health Promotion." *Exp Biol Med* 2002;227 (10): 924–927.

Chapter II: Fruits

Crapo, P. A., O. G. Kolterman, and J. M. Olefsky. "Effect of Oral Fructose in Normal, Diabetic, and Impaired Glucose Tolerance Subjects." *Diab Care* 1980;3: 575–582.

Gregersen, S., O. Rasmussen, S. Larsen, and K. Hermansen. "Glycaemic and Insulinaemic Responses to Orange and Apple Compared with White Bread in Non-Insulin Dependent Diabetic Subjects." *Eur J Clin Nutr* 1992;46: 301–303.

Rodin, J. "Comparative Effects of Fructose, Aspartame, Glucose, and Water Preloads on Calorie and Macronutrient Intake." *The American Journal of Clinical Nutrition* 1990;51: 428–435.

Rodin, J. "Effects of Pure Sugar vs. Mixed Starch Fructose Loads on Food Intake." *Appetite* 1992; 17: 213–219.

Spitzer, L., and J. Rodin. "Effects of Fructose and Glucose Preloads on Subsequent Food Intake." *Appetite* 1987;8: 135–145.

Apple

Boyer, J., and R. H. Liu. "Apple Phytochemicals and Their Health Benefits." *Nutr J* 2004;3(1): 5.

El-Shebini, S. M., L. M. Hanna, S. T. Topouzada, et al. "The Role of Pectin as a Slimming Agent." *J Clini Biochem Nutr* 1988;4: 255–262.

Fernandez, M. L. "Soluble Fiber and Nondigestible Carbohydrate Effects on Plasma Lipids and Cardiovascular Risk." *Curr Opin Lipidol* 2001;12(1): 35–40.

Knekt, P., R. Jarvinen, A. Reunanen, J. Maatela. "Flavonoid Intake and Coronary Mortality in Finland: A Cohort Study." *British Medical Journal* 1996;312(7029): 478–481.

Knekt, P., J. Kumpulainen, R. Jarvinen, H. Rissanen, M. Heliovaara, A. Reunanen, T. Hakulinen, and A. Aromaa. "Flavonoid Intake and Risk of Chronic Diseases." *The American Journal of Clinical Nutrition* 2002;76(3): 560–568.

Pearson, D. A., C. H. Tan, J. B. German, et al. "Apple Juice Inhibits Low Density Lipoprotein Oxidation." *Life Sci* 1999;64(21): 1913–1920.

Sable-Amplis, R., R. Sicart, and R. Agid. "Further Studies on the Cholesterol-Lowering Effect of Apple in Humans. Biochemical Mechanisms Involved." *Nutr Res* 1983;3: 325–383.

Apricot

Olszewska, M., R. Glowacki, M. Wolbis, and E. Bald. "Quantitative Determination of Flavonoids in the Flowers and Leaves of *Prunus spinosa* L." *Acta Pol Pharm* 2001;58(3): 199–203.

Wills, R. B., F. M. Scriven, and H. Greenfield. "Nutrient Composition of Stone Fruit (*Prunus* spp.) Cultivars: Apricot, Cherry, Nectarine, Peach and Plum." *J Sci Food Agric* 1983;34(12): 1383–1389.

Avocado

Lopez, L., R. Ledesma, A. C. Frati Munari, B. C. Hernandez Dominguez, et al. "Monounsaturated Fatty Acid (Avocado) Rich Diet for Mild Hypercholesterolemia." *Arch Med Res* 1996;27(4): 519–523.

Perkin, J. E. "The Latex and Food Allergy Connection." *Journal of the American Dietetic Association* 2000;100(11): 1381–1384.

Sanchez-Monge, R., C. Blanco, A. D. Perales, et al. "Class I Chitinases, the Panallergens Responsible for the Latex-Fruit Syndrome, Are Induced by Ethylene Treatment and Inactivated by Heating." *J Allergy Clin Immunol* 2000;106(1 Part 1): 190–195.

Banana

Beezhold, D. H., G. L. Sussman, G. M. Liss, and N. S. Chang. "Latex Allergy Can Induce Clinical Reactions to Specific Foods." *Clin Exp Allergy* 1996;26(4): 416–422.

Best, R., D. A. Lewis, and N. Nasser. "The Antiulcerogenic Activity of the Unripe Plantain Banana (*Musa* Species)." *Br J Pharmacol* 1984;82: 107–116.

Delbourg, M. F., L. Guilloux, D. A. Moneret-Vautrin, and G. Ville. "Hypersensitivity to Banana in Latex-Allergic Patients. Identification of Two Major Banana Allergens of 33 and 37 kD." *Ann Allergy Asthma Immunol* 1996;76(4): 321–326.

Dunjic, B. S., I. Svensson, J. Axelson, et al. "Green Banana Protection of Gastric Mucosa Against Experimentally Induced Injuries in Rats. A Multicomponent Mechanism?" *Scand J Gastroenterol* 1993;28(10): 894–898.

Ercan, N., F. Q. Nuttall, et al. "Plasma Glucose and Insulin Responses to Bananas of Varying Ripeness in Persons with Noninsulin-Dependent Diabetes Mellitus." *Journal of the American College of Nutrition* 1993;12(6): 703–709.

Hills, B. A., and C. A. Kirwood. "Surfactant Approach to the Gastric Mucosal Barrier: Protection of Rats by Banana Even When Acidified." *Gastroenterology* 1989;97: 294–303.

Rao, N. M. "Protease Inhibitors from Ripened and Unripened Bananas." *Biochem Int* 1991;24(1): 13–22.

Sanchez-Monge, R., C. Blanco, A. Diaz-Perales, et al. "Isolation and Characterization of Major

Banana Allergens: Identification as Fruit Class I Chitinases." *Clin Exp Allergy* 1999;29(5): 673–680.

Blueberries

Amouretti, M. "Therapeutic Value of *Vaccinium myrtillus anthocyanosides* in an Internal Medicine Department." *Thérapeutique* 1972;48: 579–581.

Bickford, P. C., T. Gould, L. Briederick, et al. "Antioxidant-Rich Diets Improve Cerebellar Physiology and Motor Learning in Aged Rats." *Brain Res* 2000;866(1–2): 211–217.

Caselli, L. "Clinical and Electroretinographic Study on Activity of Anthocyanosides." *Arch Med Int* 1985;37: 29–35.

Galli, R. L., B. Shukitt-Hale, K. A. Youdim, and J. A. Joseph. "Fruit Polyphenolics and Brain Aging: Nutritional Interventions Targeting Age-Related Neuronal and Behavioral Deficits." *Ann NY Acad Sci* 2002;959: 128–132.

Joseph, J. A., B. Shukitt-Hale, N. A. Denisova, et al. "Reversals of Age-Related Declines in Neuronal Signal Transduction, Cognitive, and Motor Behavioral Deficits with Blueberry, Spinach, or Strawberry Dietary Supplementation." *J Neurosci* 1999;19(18): 8114–8121.

Ofek, I., and J. Goldhar. "Anti-escherichia Activity of Cranberry and Blueberry Juices." *The New England Journal of Medicine* 1991;324: 1599.

Prior, R. L., S. A. Lazarus, G. Cao, et al. "Identification of Procyanidins and Anthocyanins in Blueberries and Cranberries (*Vaccinium* spp.) Using High-Performance Liquid Chromatography/Mass Spectrometry." *J Agric Food Chem* 2001; 49(3): 1270–1276.

Youdim, K. A., B. Shukitt-Hale, S. MacKinnon, et al. "Polyphenolics Enhance Red Blood Cell Resistance to Oxidative Stress: *In vitro* and *in vivo*." *Biochim Biophys Acta* 2000;1523(1): 117–122.

Cherries

Blau, L. W. "Cherry Diet Control for Gout and Arthritis." *Tex Rep Biol Med* 1950;8: 309–311.

Burkhardt, S., D. X. Tan, L. C. Manchester, R. Hardeland, and R. J. Reiter. "Detection and Quantification of the Antioxidant Melatonin in Montmorency and Balaton Tart Cherries (*Prunus cerasus*)." *J Am Chem Soc* 2001;49: 4898–4902.

Jacob, R. A., G. M. Spinozzi, V. A. Simon, et al. "Consumption of Cherries Lowers Plasma Urate in Healthy Women." *The Journal of Nutrition* 2003;133(6): 1826–1829.

Llewellyn, G. C., T. Eadie, and W. V. Dashek. "Susceptibility of Strawberries, Blackberries, and Cherries to *Aspergillus* Mold Growth and Aflatoxin Production." *J Assoc Off Anal Chem* 1982;65(3): 659–664.

Seeram, N. P., R. A. Momin, M. G. Nair, and L. D. Bourquin. "Cyclooxygenase Inhibitory and Antioxidant Cyanidin Glycosides in Cherries and Berries." *Phytomedicine* 2001;8(5): 362–369.

Olszewska, M., R. Glowacki, M. Wolbis, and E. Bald. "Quantitative Determination of Flavonoids in the Flowers and Leaves of *Prunus spinosa* L." *Acta Pol Pharm* 2001;58(3): 199–203.

Wang, H., M. G. Nair, G. M. Strasburg, et al. "Cyclooxygenase Active Bioflavonoids from Balaton Tart Cherry and Their Structure Activity Relationships." *Phytomedicine* 2000;7(1): 15–19.

Cranberries

Allison, D. G., M. A. Cronin, J. Hawker, and S. Freeman. "Influence of Cranberry Juice on Attachment of *Escherichia coli* to Glass." *J Basic Microbiol* 2000;40(1): 3–6.

Avorn, J., M. Monane, J. H. Gurwitz, R. J. Glynn, et al. "Reduction of Bacteriuria and Pyruia After Using Cranberry Juice." *Journal of the American Medical Association* 1994;272: 590.

Jepson, R. G., L. Mihaljevic, and J. Craig. "Cranberries for Preventing Urinary Tract Infections." *Cochrane Database Syst Rev* 2001;3: CD001321.

Kiel, R. J., J. Nashelsky, and B. Robbins. "Does Cranberry Juice Prevent or Treat Urinary Tract Infection?" *J Fam Pract* 2003;52(2): 154–155.

Reed, J. "Cranberry Flavonoids, Atherosclerosis and

Cardiovascular Health." *Crit Rev Food Sci Nutr* 2002;42(Suppl. 3): 301–316.

Reid, G. "The Role of Cranberry and Probiotics in Intestinal and Urogenital Tract Health." *Crit Rev Food Sci Nutr* 2002;42(Suppl. 3): 293–300.

Sobota, A. E. "Inhibition of Bacterial Adherence by Cranberry Juice: Potential Use for the Treatment of Urinary Tract Infections." *J Urology* 1984;131: 1013–1016.

Vinson, J. A., X. Su, L. Zubik, and P. Bose. "Phenol Antioxidant Quantity and Quality in Foods: Fruits." *J Agric Food Chem* 2001;49(11): 5315–5321.

Wang, S. Y., and H. Jiao. "Scavenging Capacity of Berry Crops on Superoxide Radicals, Hydrogen Peroxide, Hydroxyl Radicals, and Singlet Oxygen." *J Agric Food Chem* 2000;48(11): 5677–5684.

Yan, X., B. T. Murphy, G. B. Hammond, J. A. Vinson, and C. C. Neto. "Antioxidant Activities and Antitumor Screening of Extracts from Cranberry Fruit *(Vaccinium macrocarpon).*" *J Agric Food Chem* 2002;50(21): 5844–5849.

Dates

Ishurd, O., C. Sun, P. Xiao, A. Ashour, and Y. Pan. "A Neutral Beta-d-Glucan from Dates of the Date Palm, *Phoenix dactylifera* L." *Carbohydr Res* 2002;337(14): 1325–1328.

Kwaasi, A. A., H. A. Harfi, R. S. Parhar, S. T. Al-Sedairy, K. S. Collison, R. C. Panzani, and F. A. Al-Mohanna. "Allergy to Date Fruits: Characterization of Antigens and Allergens of Fruits of the Date Palm (*Phoenix dactylifera* L.)." *Allergy* 1999;54(12): 1270–1277.

Kwaasi, A. A., H. A. Harfi, R. S. Parhar, S. Saleh, K. S. Collison, R. C. Panzani, S. T. Al-Sedairy, and F. A. Al-Mohanna. "Cross-reactivities Between Date Palm (*Phoenix dactylifera* L.) Polypeptides and Foods Implicated in the Oral Allergy Syndrome." *Allergy* 2002;57(6): 508–518.

Vayalil, P. K. "Antioxidant and Antimutagenic Properties of Aqueous Extract of Date Fruit (*Phoenix dactylifera* L." *Arecaceae). J Agric Food Chem* 2002;50(3): 610–617.

Figs

Canal, J. R., M. D. Torres, A. Romero, and C. Perez. "A Chloroform Extract Obtained from a Decoction of *Ficus carica* Leaves Improves the Cholesterolaemic Status of Rats with Streptozotocin-Induced Diabetes." *Acta Physiol Hung* 2000;87 (1): 71–76.

de Amorin, A., H. R. Borba, J. P. Carauta, et al. "Anthelmintic Activity of the Latex of *Ficus* Species." *J Ethnopharmacol* 1999;64(3): 255–258.

Perez, C., J. R. Canal, J. E. Campillo, et al. "Hypotriglyceridaemic Activity of *Ficus carica.* Leaves in Experimental Hypertriglyceridaemic Rats." *Phytother Res* 1999;13(3): 188–191.

Rubnovk, S., Y. Kashman, R. Rabinowitz, et al. "Suppressors of Cancer Cell Proliferation from Fig *(Ficus carica)* Resin: Isolation and Structure Elucidation." *J Nat Prod* 2001;64(7): 993–996.

Serraclara, A., F. Hawkins, C. Perez, et al. "Hypoglycemic Action of an Oral Fig-Leaf Decoction in Type-I Diabetic Patients." *Diabetes Res Clin Pract* 1998;39(1): 19–22.

Grapefruit

Cerda, J. J., S. J. Normann, M. P. Sullivan, et al. "Inhibition of Atherosclerosis by Dietary Pectin in Microswine with Sustained Hypercholesterolemia." *Circulation* 1994;89(3): 1247–1253.

Cerda, J., F. L. Robbins, C. W. Burgin, et al. "The Effects of Grapefruit Pectin on Patients at Risk for Coronary Heart Disease Without Altering Diet or Lifestyle." *Clin Cardiol* 1988;11: 589–594.

Robbins, R. C., F. G. Martin, and J. M. Roe. "Ingestion of Grapefruit Lowers Elevated Hematocrits in Human Subjects." *Int J Vit Nutr Res* 1988;58: 414–417.

Grapes

Day, A. P., H. J. Kemp, C. Bolton C, et al. "Effect of Concentrated Red Grape Juice Consumption on Serum Antioxidant Capacity and Low-Density Lipoprotein Oxidation." *Ann Nutr Metab* 1997; 41(6): 353–357.

Freedman, J. E., C. Parker 3rd, L. Li, et al. "Select Flavonoids and Whole Juice from Purple Grapes Inhibit Platelet Function and Enhance Nitric Oxide Release." *Circulation* 2001;103(23): 2792–2798.

Miyagi, Y., K. Miwa, and H. Inoue. "Inhibition of Human Low-Density Lipoprotein Oxidation by Flavonoids in Red Wine and Grape Juice." *Am J Cardiol* 1997;80(12): 1627–1631.

Potter, G. A., L. H. Patterson, E. Wanogho, P. J. Perry, P. C. Butler, T. Ijaz, K. C. Ruparelia, J. H. Lamb, P. B. Farmer, L. A. Stanley, and M. D. Burke. "The Cancer Preventative Agent Resveratrol Is Converted to the Anticancer Agent Piceatannol by the Cytochrome P450 Enzyme CYP1B1." *Br J Cancer* 2002;86(5): 774–778.

Kiwifruit

Collins, B. H., A. Horska, P. M. Hotten, et al. "Kiwifruit Protects Against Oxidative DNA Damage in Human Cells and *in vitro.*" *Nutr Cancer* 2001;39(1): 148–153.

Ikken, Y., P. Morales, A. Martinez, et al. "Antimutagenic Effect of Fruit and Vegetable Ethanolic Extracts Against *N*-nitrosamines Evaluated by the Ames Test." *J Agric Food Chem* 1999;47(8): 3257–3264.

Sommerburg, O., J. E. Keunen, A. C. Bird, and F. J. van Kuijk. "Fruits and Vegetables That Are Sources for Lutein and Zeaxanthin: The Macular Pigment in Human Eyes." *Br J Ophthalmol* 1998;82(8): 907–910.

Lemon

Kawaii, S., Y. Tomono, E. Katase, et al. "Antiproliferative Effects of the Readily Extractable Fractions Prepared from Various Citrus Juices on Several Cancer Cell Lines." *J Agric Food Chem* 1999;47(7): 2509–2512.

Kodama, R., T. Yano, Furukawa, et al. Studies on the Metabolism of d-Limonene *Xenobiotica* 1976;6: 377–389.

Misra, N., S. Batra, and D. Mishra. "Fungitoxic Properties of the Essential Oil of *Citrus limon* (L.) *Burm.* Against a Few Dermatophytes." *Mycoses* 1988;31(7): 380–382.

Miyake, Y., A. Murakami, Y. Sugiyama, et al. "Identification of Coumarins from Lemon Fruit *(Citrus limon)* as Inhibitors of *in vitro* Tumor Promotion and Superoxide and Nitric Oxide Generation." *J Agric Food Chem* 1999;47(8): 3151–3157.

Ogata, S., Y. Miyake, K. Yamamoto, et al. "Apoptosis Induced by the Flavonoid from Lemon Fruit *(Citrus limon* BURM. f.) and Its Metabolites in HL-60 Cells." *Biosci Biotechnol Biochem* 2000;64(5): 1075–1078.

Lime

Berhow, M. A., R. D. Bennett, S. M. Poling, et al. "Acylated Flavonoids in Callus Cultures of *Citrus aurantifolia.*" *Phytochemistry* 1994;36(5): 1225–1227.

Gharagozloo, M., and A. Ghaderi. "Immunomodulatory Effect of Concentrated Lime Juice Extract on Activated Human Mononuclear Cells." *J Ethnopharmacol* 2001;77(1): 85–90.

Kawaii, S., Y. Tomono, E. Katase, et al. "Antiproliferative Effects of the Readily Extractable Fractions Prepared from Various Citrus Juices on Several Cancer Cell Lines." *J Agric Food Chem* 1999;47(7): 2509–2512.

Mata, L., C. Vargas, D. Saborio, and M. Vives. "Extinction of *Vibrio cholerae* in Acidic Substrata: Contaminated Cabbage and Lettuce Treated with Lime Juice." *Rev Biol Trop* 1994;42(3): 487–492.

Rodrigues, A., H. Brun, and A. Sandstrom. "Risk Factors for Cholera Infection in the Initial Phase of an Epidemic in Guinea-Bissau: Protection by Lime Juice." *Am J Trop Med Hyg* 1997;57(5): 601–604.

Rodrigues, A., A. Sandstrom, T. Ca, et al. "Protection from Cholera by Adding Lime Juice to Food—Results from Community and Laboratory Studies in Guinea-Bissau, West Africa." *Trop Med Int Health* 2000;5(6): 418–422.

Mango

Bates, C. J., N. Matthews, B. West, L. Morison, and G. Walraven. "Plasma Carotenoid and Vitamin E Concentrations in Women Living in a Rural West African (Gambian) Community." *Int J Vitam Nutr Res* 2002;72(3): 133–141.

Calvert, M. L., I. Robertson, and H. Samaratunga. "Mango Dermatitis: Allergic Contact Dermatitis to *Mangifera indica*." *Australas J Dermatol* 1996; 37(1): 59–60.

Drammeh, B. S., G. S. Marquis, E. Funkhouser, C. Bates, I. Eto, and C. B. Stephensen. "A Randomized, 4-Month Mango and Fat Supplementation Trial Improved Vitamin A Status Among Young Gambian Children." *The Journal of Nutrition* 2002;132(12): 3693–3699.

Fernandez, C., A. Fiandor, A. Martinez-Garate, and J. Martinez Quesada. "Allergy to Pistachio: Crossreactivity Between Pistachio Nut and Other Anacardiaceae." *Clin Exp Allergy* 1995;25 (12): 1254–1259.

Ponce-Macotela, M., I. Navarro-Alegria, M. N. Martinez-Gordillo, and R. Alvarez-Chacon. "*In vitro* Effect Against Giardia of 14 Plant Extracts." *Rev Invest Clin* 1994;46(5): 343–347.

Rodriguez-Amaya, D. B. "Latin American Food Sources of Carotenoids." *Arch Latinoam Nutr* 1999;49(3 Suppl. 1): S74–S84.

Roongpisuthipong, C., S. Banphotkasem, S. Komindr, and V. Tanphaichitr V. "Postprandial Glucose and Insulin Responses to Various Tropical Fruits of Equivalent Carbohydrate Content in Non-Insulin-Dependent Diabetes Mellitus." *Diabetes Res Clin Pract* 1991;14(2): 123–131.

Thurnham, D. I., C. A. Northrop-Clewes, F. S. McCullough, B. S. Das, and P. G. Lunn. "Innate Immunity, Gut Integrity, and Vitamin A in Gambian and Indian Infants." *J Infect Dis* 2000; 182(Suppl. 1): S23–S28.

Orange

Galati, E. M., A. Trovato, S. Kirjavainen, et al. "Biological Effects of Hesperidin, a Citrus Flavonoid. (Note III): Antihypertensive and Diuretic Activity in Rat." *Farmaco* 1996;51(3): 219–221.

Rapisarda P, A. Tomaino, R. Lo Cascio, et al. "Antioxidant Effectiveness as Influenced by Phenolic Content of Fresh Orange Juices." *J Agric Food Chem* 1994;74(11): 4718–4723.

Stange, R. R., Jr., S. L. Midland, J. W. Eckert, J. J. Sims. "An Antifungal Compound Produced by Grapefruit and Valencia Orange After Wounding of the Peel." *J Nat Prod* 1993;56(9): 1627–1629.

Peaches

Tomas-Barberan, F. A., M. I. Gil, P. Cremin, A. L. Waterhouse, B. Hess-Pierce, and A. A. Kader. "HPLC-DAD-ESIMS Analysis of Phenolic Compounds in Nectarines, Peaches, and Plums." *J Agric Food Chem* 2001;49(10): 4748–4760.

Pineapple

Maurer, H. R. "Bromelain: Biochemistry, Pharmacology and Medical Use." *Cell Mol Life Sci* 2001; 58(9): 1234–1245.

Plums

Ballot, D., R. D. Baynes D, T. H. Bothwell, et al. "The Effects of Fruit Juices and Fruits on the Absorption of Iron from a Rice Meal." *Br J Nutr* 1987;57(3): 331–343.

Egbekun, M. K., J. I. Akowe, and R. J. Ede. "Physico-Chemical and Sensory Properties of Formulated Syrup from Black Plum *(Vitex doniana)* Fruit." *Plant Foods Hum Nutr* 1996;49(4): 301–306.

Nakatani, N., S. Kayano, H. Kikuzaki, et al. "Identification, Quantitative Determination, and Antioxidative Activities of Chlorogenic Acid Isomers in Prune *(Prunus domestica* L.)." *J Agric Food Chem* 2000;48(11): 5512–5516.

Tomas-Barberan, F. A., M. I. Gil, P. Cremin, A. L. Waterhouse, B. Hess-Pierce, and A. A. Kader. "HPLC-DAD-ESIMS Analysis of Phenolic Compounds in Nectarines, Peaches, and Plums." *J Agric Food Chem* 2001;49(10): 4748–4760.

Prunes

Ballot, D., R. D. Baynes, T. H. Bothwell, et al. "The Effects of Fruit Juices and Fruits on the Absorption of Iron from a Rice Meal." *Br J Nutr* 1987;57(3): 331–343.

Stacewicz-Sapuntzakis, M., P. E. Bowen PE, E. A. Hussain, B. I. Damayanti-Wood, N. R. Farnsworth. "Chemical Composition and Potential Health Effects of Prunes: A Functional Food?" *Crit Rev Food Sci Nutr* 2001;41(4): 251–286.

Raisins

Karadeniz, F., R. W. Durst, and R. E. Wrolstad. "Polyphenolic Composition of Raisins." *J Agric Food Chem* 2000;48(11): 5343–5350.

Karakaya, S., S. N. El, and A. A. Tas. "Antioxidant Activity of Some Foods Containing Phenolic Compounds." *Int J Food Sci Nutr* 2001;52(6): 501–508.

Rainey, C. J., L. A. Nyquist, R. E. Christensen, et al. "Daily Boron Intake from the American Diet." *Journal of the American Dietetic Association* 1999;99(3): 335–340.

Raspberries

Rauha, J. P., S. Remes, M. Heinonen, et al. "Antimicrobial Effects of Finnish Plant Extracts Containing Flavonoids and Other Phenolic Compounds." *Int J Food Microbiol* 2000;56(1): 3–12.

Seeram, N. P., R. A. Momin, M. G. Nair, and L. D. Bourquin. "Cyclooxygenase Inhibitory and Antioxidant Cyanidin Glycosides in Cherries and Berries." *Phytomedicine* 2001;8(5): 362–369.

Wang, S. Y., and H. Jiao. "Scavenging Capacity of Berry Crops on Superoxide Radicals, Hydrogen Peroxide, Hydroxyl Radicals, and Singlet Oxygen." *J Agric Food Chem* 2000;48(11): 5677–5684.

Wang, S. Y., and H. S. Lin. "Antioxidant Activity in Fruits and Leaves of Blackberry, Raspberry, and Strawberry Varies with Cultivar and Development Stage." *J Agric Food Chem* 2000;48(2): 140–146.

Strawberries

Kahkonen, M. P., A. I. Hopial, M. Heinonen. "Berry Phenolics and Their Antioxidant Activity." *J Agric Food Chem* 2001;49(8): 4076–4082.

Kalt, W., C. F. Forney, A. Martin, and R. L. Prior. "Antioxidant Capacity, Vitamin C, Phenolics, and Anthocyanins After Fresh Storage of Small Fruits." *J Agric Food Chem* 1999;47(11): 4638–4644.

Zhang, W., M. F. Jin, X. J. Yu, Q. Yuan. "Enhanced Anthocyanin Production by Repeated-Batch Culture of Strawberry Cells with Medium Shift." *Appl Microbiol Biotechnol* 2001;55(2): 164–169.

Chapter 12: Grains

Fung, T. T., F. B. Hu, M. A. Pereira, et al. "Whole-Grain Intake and the Risk of Type 2 Diabetes: A Prospective Study in Men." *The American Journal of Clinical Nutrition* 2002;76: 535–540.

Jacobs, D. R., M. A. Pereira, K. A. Meyer, and L. H. Kushi. "Fiber from Whole Grains, but Not Refined Grains, Is Inversely Associated with All-Cause Mortality in Older Women: The Iowa Women's Health Study." *Journal of the American College of Nutrition* 2000;19(Suppl. 3): S326–S330.

Montonen, J., P. Knekt, R. Jarvinen, A. Aromaa, and A. Reunanen. "Whole-Grain and Fiber Intake and the Incidence of Type 2 Diabetes." *The American Journal of Clinical Nutrition* 2003;77: 622–629.

Pereira, M. A., D. R. Jacobs, Jr., J. J. Pins, S. K. Raatz, M. D. Gross, J. L. Slavin, and E. R. Seaquist. "Effect of Whole Grains on Insulin Sensitivity in Overweight Hyperinsulinemic Adults." *The American Journal of Clinical Nutrition* 2002;75 (5): 848–855.

Wheat

Ferguson, L. R., and P. J. Harris. "Protection Against Cancer by Wheat Bran: Role of Dietary Fibre and Phytochemicals." *Eur J Cancer Prev* 1999;8: 17–25.

McIntosh, G. H., M. Noakes, P. J. Royle, and P. R. Foster. "Whole-Grain Rye and Wheat Foods and

Markers of Bowel Health in Overweight Middle-Aged Men." *The American Journal of Clinical Nutrition* 2003;77(4): 967–974.

Rice

Sugano, M., K. Koba, and E. Tsuji. "Health Benefits of Rice Bran Oil." *Anticancer Res* 1999;19(5A): 3651–3657.

Corn

Bucchini, L., and L. R. Goldman. "Starlink Corn: A Risk Analysis." *Environ Health Perspect* 2002; 110: 5–13.

Oats

Ripsin, C. M., J. M. Keenan, D. R. Jacobs, et al. "Oat Products and Lipid Lowering, a Meta-Analysis." *Journal of the American Medical Association* 1992;267: 3317–3325.

Amaranth

Chaturvedi, A., G. Sarojini, and N. L. Devi. "Hypocholesterolemic Effect of Amaranth Seeds (*Amaranthus esculantus*)." *Plant Foods Hum Nutr* 1993;44: 63–70.

Chaturvedi, A., G. Sarojini, G. Nirmala, N. Nirmalamma, D. Satyanarayana. "Glycemic Index of Grain Amaranth, Wheat and Rice in NIDDM Subjects." *Plant Foods Hum Nutr* 1997;50:171–178.

Escudero, N. L., G. Albarracin, S. Fernandez, L. M. De Arellano, and S. Mucciarelli. "Nutrient and Antinutrient Composition of *Amaranthus muricatus*." *Plant Foods Hum Nutr* 1999;54: 327–336.

Grajeta, H. "Effect of Amaranth and Oat Bran on Blood Serum and Liver Lipids in Rats Depending on the Kind of Dietary Fats." *Nährung* 1999;43: 114–117.

Qureshi, A. A., J. W. Lehmann, and D. M. Peterson. "Amaranth and Its Oil Inhibit Cholesterol Biosynthesis in 6-Week-Old Female Chickens." *The Journal of Nutrition* 1996;126: 1972–1978.

Yadav, S. K., and S. Sehgal. "Effect of Domestic Processing and Cooking Methods on Total, HCl

Extractable Iron and *in vitro* Availability of Iron in Spinach and Amaranth Leaves." *Nutr Health* 2002;16: 113–120.

Barley

Bansal, H. C., K. N. Strivastava, B. O. Eggum, and S. L. Mehta. "Nutritional Evaluation of High Protein Genotypes of Barley." *J Sci Food Agric* 1977;28: 157–160.

Jood, S., and S. Kalra. "Chemical Composition and Nutritional Characteristics of Some Hull Less and Hulled Barley Cultivars Grown in India." *Nährung* 2001;45: 35–39.

Norbaek, R., K. Brandt, and T. Kondo. "Identification of Flavone C-glycosides Including a New Flavonoid Chromophore from Barley Leaves (*Hordeum vulgare* L.) by Improved NMR Techniques." *J Agric Food Chem* 2000;48: 1703–1707.

Buckwheat

Gabrovska, D., V. Fiedlerova, M. Holasova, et al. "The Nutritional Evaluation of Underutilized Cereals and Buckwheat." *Food Nutr Bull* 2002; 23(Suppl. 3): 246–249.

He, J., M. J. Klag, P. K. Whelton, et al. "Oats and Buckwheat Intakes and Cardiovascular Disease Risk Factors in an Ethnic Minority of China." *The American Journal of Clinical Nutrition* 1995;61: 366–372.

Skrabanja, V., H. G. Liljeberg Elmstahl, I. Kreft, and I. M. Bjorck. "Nutritional Properties of Starch in Buckwheat Products: Studies *in vitro* and *in vivo*." *Agric Food Chem* 2001;49(1): 490–496.

Millet

Gabrovska, D., V. Fiedlerova, M. Holasova, et al. "The Nutritional Evaluation of Underutilized Cereals and Buckwheat." *Food Nutr Bull* 2002;23 (Suppl. 3): 246–249.

Quinoa

Ogungbenle, H. N. "Nutritional Evaluation and Functional Properties of Quinoa (*Chenopodium quinoa)* Flour." *Int J Food Sci Nutr* 2003;54: 153–158.

Rye

Grasten, S. M., K. S. Juntunen, K. Poutanen, H. K. Gylling, T. A. Miettinen, and H. M. Mykkanen. "Rye Bread Improves Bowel Function and Decreases the Concentrations of Some Compounds That Are Putative Colon Cancer Risk Markers in Middle-Aged Women and Men." *The Journal of Nutrition* 2000;130: 2215–2221.

McIntosh, G. H., M. Noakes, P. J. Royle, P. R. Foster. "Whole-Grain Rye and Wheat Foods and Markers of Bowel Health in Overweight Middle-Aged Men." *The American Journal of Clinical Nutrition* 2003;77(4): 967–974.

Sorghum

Hamaker, B. R., A. W. Kirleis, E. T. Mertz, and J. D. Axtell. "Effect of Cooking on *in vitro* Digestibility of Sorghum and Maize." *J Agric Food Chem* 1986;34: 647–649.

Rooney, T. K., L. W. Rooney, and J. R. Lupton. "Physiological Characteristics of Sorghum and Millet Brans in the Rat Model." *Cereal Foods World* 37(10): 782–786.

Spelt

Gabrovska, D., V. Fiedlerova, M. Holasova, et al. "The Nutritional Evaluation of Underutilized Cereals and Buckwheat." *Food Nutr Bull* 2002;23 (Suppl. 3): 246–249.

Triticale

Adom, K. K., and R. H. Liu. "Antioxidant Activity of Grains." *J Agric Food Chem* 2002;50(21): 6182–6187.

Sikka, K. C., S. K. Duggal, R. Singh, D. P. Gupta, M. G. Joshi. "Comparative Nutritive Value and Amino Acid Content of Triticale, Wheat, and Rye." *J Agric Food Chem* 1978;26: 788–791.

Chapter 13: Legumes (Beans)

Messina, M. J. "Legumes and Soybeans: Overview of Their Nutritional Profiles and Health Effects." *The American Journal of Clinical Nutrition* 1999;70(Suppl. 3): S439–S450.

Wu, X., G. R. Beecher, J. Holden, et al. "Lipophilic and Hydrophilic Antioxidant Capacities of Common Foods in the United States." *J Agric Food Chem* 2004;52: 4026–4037.

Soy

Allred, C. D., K. F. Allred, Y. H. Ju, S. M. Virant, and W. G. Helferich. "Soy Diets Containing Varying Amounts of Genistein Stimulate Growth of Estrogen-Dependent (MCF-7) Tumors in a Dose-Dependent Manner." *Cancer Res* 2001;61: 5045–5050.

Carrol, K. K. "Review of Clinical Studies on Cholesterol-Lowering Response to Soy Protein." *Journal of the American Dietetic Association* 1991;91: 820–827.

Davis, J. N., O. Kucuk, Z. Djuric, and F. H. Sarkar. "Soy Isoflavone Supplementation in Healthy Men Prevents NF-kappa B Activation by TNF-alpha in Blood Lymphocytes." *Free Radic Biol Med* 2001;30(11): 1293–1302.

Jacobsen, B. K., S. F. Knutsen, and G. E. Fraser. "Does High Soy Milk Intake Reduce Prostate Cancer Incidence? The Adventist Health Study (United States)." *Cancer Causes and Control* 1998;9: 553–557.

Martini, M. C., B. B. Dancisak, C. J. Haggans, W. Thomas, and J. L. Slavin. "Effects of Soy Intake on Sex Hormone Metabolism in Premenopausal Women." *Nutr Cancer* 1999;34: 133–139.

Messina, M. J. "Legumes and Soybeans: Overview of Their Nutritional Profiles and Health Effects." *The American Journal of Clinical Nutrition* 1999; 70(Suppl. 3): S439–S450.

Messina, M. "Soy, Soy Phytoestrogens (Isoflavones), and Breast Cancer." *The American Journal of Clinical Nutrition* 1999;70: 574–575.

Shu, X. O., F. Jin, Q. Dai, et al. "Soyfood Intake During Adolescence and Subsequent Risk of Breast Cancer Among Chinese Women." *Cancer Epidemiology Biomarkers and Prevention* 2001;10: 483–488.

Sirtori, C. R. "Risks and Benefits of Soy Phytoestrogens in Cardiovascular Diseases, Cancer, Climacteric Symptoms and Osteoporosis." *Drug Safety* 2001;24: 665–682.

Young, V. R. "Soy Protein in Relation to Human Protein and Amino Acid Nutrition." *Journal of the American Dietetic Association* 1991;91: 828–835.

Alfalfa

Abd El-Gawad, H. M., A. E. Khalifa, H. M. Abd El-Gawad, and E. Khalifa E. "Quercetin, Coenzyme Q10, and l-Canavanine as Protective Agents Against Lipid Peroxidation and Nitric Oxide Generation in Endotoxin-Induced Shock in Rat Brain." *Pharmacol Res* 2001;43: 257–263.

Alcocer-Varela, J., A. Iglesias, L. Llorente, and D. Alarcon-Segovia. "Effects of l-Canavanine on T Cells May Explain the Induction of Systemic Lupus Erythematosus by Alfalfa." *Arthritis Rheum* 1985;28: 52–57.

Bence, A. K., V. R. Adams, and P. A. Crooks. "l-Canavanine as a Radiosensitization Agent for Human Pancreatic Cancer Cells." *Mol Cell Biochem* 2003;244: 37–43.

Bence, A. K., D. R. Worthen, V. R. Adams, and P. A. Crooks. "The Antiproliferative and Immunotoxic Effects of l-Canavanine and l-Canaline." *Anticancer Drugs* 2002;13: 313–320.

Kurzer, M. S., and X. Xu. "Dietary Phytoestrogens." *Annu Rev Nutr* 1997;17: 353–381.

Powell, J. J., J. Van de Water J, and M. E. Gershwin. "Evidence for the Role of Environmental Agents in the Initiation or Progression of Autoimmune Conditions." *Environ Health Perspect* 1999;107 (Suppl. 5): S667–S672.

Story, J. A., S. L. LePage, M. S. Petro, L. G. West, M. M. Cassidy, F. G. Lightfoot, and G. V. Vahouny. "Interactions of Alfalfa Plant and Sprout Saponins with Cholesterol *in vitro* and in Cholesterol-Fed Rats." *The American Journal of Clinical Nutrition* 1984;39: 917–929.

Suzuki, N., A. Sakamoto, and R. Ogawa. "Effect of l-Canavanine, an Inhibitor of Inducible Nitric Oxide Synthase, on Myocardial Dysfunction During Septic Shock." *J Nippon Med Sch* 2002; 69: 13–18.

Carob

Greally, P., F. J. Hampton, U. M. MacFadyen, and H. Simpson. "Gaviscon and Carobel Compared with Cisapride in Gastroesophageal Reflux." *Arch Dis Child* 1992;67: 618–621.

Hostettler, M., R. Steffen, and A. Tschopp. "Efficacy of Tolerability of Insoluble Carob Fraction in the Treatment of Travellers' Diarrhea." *J Diarr Dis Res* 1995;13: 155–158.

Leob, H., Y. Vandenplas, P. Wursch, and P. Guesry. "Tannin-Rich Carob Pod for the Treatment of Acute-Onset Diarrhea." *J Pediatr Gastroent Nutr* 1989;8: 480–485.

Chickpeas

Chavan, J. K., S. S. Kadam, and D. K. Salunkhe. "Biochemistry and Technology of Chickpea (*Cicer arietinum* L.) Seeds." *Crit Rev Food Sci Nutr* 1986;25: 107–158.

el-Adawy, T. A. "Nutritional Composition and Antinutritional Factors of Chickpeas (*Cicer arietinum* L.) Undergoing Different Cooking Methods and Germination." *Plant Foods Hum Nutr* 2002;57: 83–97.

Common Beans

Adebamowo, C. A., E. Cho, L. Sampson, et al. "Dietary Flavonols and Flavonol-Rich Foods Intake and the Risk of Breast Cancer." *Int J Cancer* 2004;114(4): 628–633.

Kidney Beans

McIntosh, M., and C. Miller. "A Diet Containing Food Rich in Soluble and Insoluble Fiber

Improves Glycemic Control and Reduces Hyperlipidemia Among Patients with Type 2 Diabetes Mellitus." *Nutr Rev* 2001;59(2): 52–55.

Menotti, A., D. Kromhout, H. Blackburn, et al. "Food Intake Patterns and 25-Year Mortality from Coronary Heart Disease: Cross-Cultural Correlations in the Seven Countries Study. The Seven Countries Study Research Group." *Eur J Epidemiol* 1999;15: 507–515.

Lentil

Adebamowo, C. A., E. Cho, L. Sampson, et al. "Dietary Flavonols and Flavonol-Rich Foods Intake and the Risk of Breast Cancer." *Int J Cancer* 2004;114(4): 628–633.

Lin, H. C., N. A. Moller, M. M. Wolinsky, et al. "Sustained Slowing Effect of Lentils on Gastric Emptying of Solids in Humans and Dogs." *Gastrology* 1992;102: 787–792.

McIntosh, M., and C. Miller. "A Diet Containing Food Rich in Soluble and Insoluble Fiber Improves Glycemic Control and Reduces Hyperlipidemia Among Patients with Type 2 Diabetes Mellitus." *Nutr Rev* 2001;59: 52–55.

Menotti, A., D. Kromhout, H. Blackburn, et al. "Food Intake Patterns and 25-Year Mortality from Coronary Heart Disease: Cross-Cultural Correlations in the Seven Countries Study. The Seven Countries Study Research Group." *Eur J Epidemiol* 1999;15: 507–515.

Tempeh

Davis, J. N., O. Kucuk, Z. Djuric, F. H. Sarkar. "Soy Isoflavone Supplementation in Healthy Men Prevents NF-kappaB Activation by TNF-alpha in Blood Lymphocytes." *Free Radic Biol Med* 2001;30(11): 1293–1302.

Shen, J. C., R. D. Klein, Q. Wei, et al. "Low-Dose Genistein Induces Cyclin-Dependent Kinase Inhibitors and G(1) Cell-Cycle Arrest in Human Prostate Cancer Cells." *Mol Carcinog* 2000;29(2): 92–102.

Chapter 14: Nuts, Seeds, and Oils

Albert, C. M., J. M. Gaziano, W. C. Willett, and J. E. Manson. "Nut Consumption and Decreased Risk of Sudden Cardiac Death in the Physicians' Health Study." *Arch Intern Med* 2002;162(12): 1382–1387.

Flynn, N. E., C. J. Meininger, T. E. Haynes, and G. Wu. "The Metabolic Basis of Arginine Nutrition and Pharmacotherapy." *Biomed Pharmacother* 2002;56(9): 427–438.

Fraser, G. E., J. Sabate, W. L. Beeson, and T. M. Strahan. "A Possible Protective Effect of Nut Consumption on Risk of Coronary Heart Disease." *Arch Intern Med* 152: 1416–1424, 1992.

Hu, F. B., and M. J. Stampfer. "Nut Consumption and Risk of Coronary Heart Disease: A Review of Epidemiologic Evidence." *Curr Atheroscler Rep* 1999;1(3): 204–209.

Jiang, R., J. E. Manson, M. J. Stampfer, et al. "Nut and Peanut Butter Consumption and Risk of Type 2 Diabetes in Women." *Journal of the American Medical Association* 2002;288(20): 2554–2560.

Rivellese, A. A., C. De Natale, S. Lilli. "Type of Dietary Fat and Insulin Resistance. *Ann N Y Acad Sci* 2002;967: 329–335.

Weller, D. P., J. D. Zaneveld, and N. R. Farnsworth. "Gossypol: Pharmacology and Current Status as a Male Contraceptive." *Econ Med Plant Res* 1985;1: 87–112.

Almond

Abbey, M., M. Noakes, G. B. Belling, P. J. Nestel. "Partial Replacement of Saturated Fatty Acids with Almonds or Walnuts Lowers Total Plasma Cholesterol and Low-Density-Lipoprotein Cholesterol." *The American Journal of Clinical Nutrition* 1994;59(5): 995–999.

Centers for Disease Control and Prevention (CDC). "Outbreak of *Salmonella* Serotype Enteritidis Infections Associated with Raw Almonds—United States and Canada, 2003–2004." *MMWR Morb Mortal Wkly Rep* 2004;53(22): 484–487.

Durlach, J. "Commentary on Recent Clinical Advances: Almonds, Monounsaturated Fats, Magnesium and Hypolipidaemic Diets." *Magnes Res* 1992;5(4): 315.

Griffith, R., D. DeLong, and J. Nelson. "Relation of Arginine-Lysine Antagonism to Herpes Simplex Growth in Tissue Culture." *Chemotherapy* 1981; 27: 209–213.

Hu, F. B., and M. J. Stampfer. "Nut Consumption and Risk of Coronary Heart Disease: A Review of Epidemiologic Evidence." *Curr Atheroscler Rep* 1999;1(3): 204–209.

Zittlau, E. "Effect of Sweet Almonds on the Stress Ulcer in Rats." *Dtsch Tierarztl Wochenschr* 1985;92(4): 151–154.

Brazil

Chang, J. C., W. H. Gutenmann, C. M. Reid, and D. J. Lisk. "Selenium Content of Brazil Nuts from Two Geographic Locations in Brazil." *Chemosphere* 1995;30(4): 801–802.

Dutau, G., J. L. Rittie, F. Rance, A. Juchet, and F. Bremont. "New Food Allergies." *Presse Med* 1999;28 (28): 1553–1559.

Freire, F. C., Z. Kozakiewicz, and R. R. Paterson. "Mycoflora and Mycotoxins in Brazilian Black Pepper, White Pepper and Brazil Nuts." *Mycopathologia* 2000;149(1): 13–19.

Kannamkumarath, S. S., K. Wrobel, K. Wrobel, A. Vonderheide, and J. A. Caruso. "HPLC-ICP-MS Determination of Selenium Distribution and Speciation in Different Types of Nut." *Anal Bioanal Chem* 2002;373(6): 454–460.

Macfarlane, B. J., W. R. Bezwoda, T. H. Bothwell, et al. "Inhibitory Effect of Nuts on Iron Absorption." *The American Journal of Clinical Nutrition* 1988;47(2): 270–274.

Mobius, M. E., B. E. Lauderdale, S. R. Nagel, and H. M. Jaeger. "Size Separation of Granular Particles." *Nature* 2001;414: 270.

Coconut

Bach, A. C., et al. "Clinical and Experimental Effects of Medium Chain Triglyceride Based Fat Emulsions—A Review." *Clin Nutr* 1989;8: 223.

Bakker, N., P. Van't Veer, P. L. Zock. "Adipose Fatty Acids and Cancers of the Breast, Prostate and Colon: An Ecological Study. EURAMIC Study Group." *International Journal of Cancer* 1997;72: 587–591.

Bergsson, G., J. Arnfinnsson, S. M. Karlsson, O. Steingrimsson, and H. Thormar. "*In vitro* Inactivation of *Chlamydia trachomatis* by Fatty Acids and Monoglycerides." *Antimicrobial Agents and Chemotherapy* 1998;42: 2290–2294.

Blackburn, G. L., G. Kater, E. A. Mascioli, M. Kowalchuk, V. K. Babayan, and B. R. Bistrian. "A Reevaluation of Coconut Oil's Effect on Serum Cholesterol and Atherogenesis." *The Journal of the Philippine Medical Association* 1989;65: 144–152.

Bray, G. A., et al. "Weight Gain of Rats Fed Medium-Chain Triglycerides Is Less Than Rats Fed Long-Chain Triglycerides." *Int J Obes* 1980;4: 27–32.

Clevidence, B. A., J. T. Judd, E. J. Schaefer, J. L. Jenner, A. H. Lichtenstein, R. A. Muesing, J. Wittes, and M. E. Sunkin. "Plasma Lipoprotein (a) Levels in Men and Women Consuming Diets Enriched in Saturated, Cis-, or Trans-monounsaturated Fatty Acids." *Arterioscler Thromb Vasc Biol* 1997;17: 1657–1661.

Ellis, R. W. "Infection and Coronary Heart Disease." *J Med Microbiol* 1997;46: 535–539.

Felton, C. V., D. Crook, M. J. Davies, and M. F. Oliver. "Dietary Polyunsaturated Fatty Acids and Composition of Human Aortic Plaques." *The Lancet* 1994;344: 1195–1196.

Florentino, R. F., and A. R. Aguinaldo. "Diet and Cardiovascular Disease in the Philippines." *The Philippine Journal of Coconut Studies* 1987;12: 56–70.

Garfinkel, M., S. Lee, E. C. Opara, and O. E. Akkwari. "Insulinotropic Potency of Lauric Acid: A Metabolic Rational for Medium Chain

Fatty Acids (MCF) in TPN Formulation." *J Surg Research* 1992;52: 328–333.

Geliebter, A. "Overfeeding with a Diet Containing Medium Chain Triglycerides Impedes Accumulation of Body Fat." *Clin Research* 1980;28: 595A.

Geliebter, A. "Overfeeding with Medium-Chain Triglycerides Diet Results in Diminished Deposition of Fat." *The American Journal of Clinical Nutrition* 1983;37: 1–4.

Gerster, H. "Can Adults Adequately Convert Alpha-linolenic Acid (18:3n-3) to Eicosapentaenoic Acid (20:5n-3) and Docosahexaenoic Acid (22:6n-3)?" *Int J Vitamin and Nutrition Research* 1998;68: 159–173.

Grundy, S. M. "Cholesterol Metabolism in Man." *Western J Med* 1978;128: 13.

Halden, V. W., and H. Lieb. "Influence of Biologically Improved Coconut Oil Products on the Blood Cholesterol Levels of Human Volunteers." *Nutr Dieta* 1961;3: 75–88.

Hashim, S. A., R. E. Clancy, D. M. Hegsted, and F. J. Stare. "Effect of Mixed Fat Formula Feeding on Serum Cholesterol Level in Man." *The American Journal of Clinical Nutrition* 1959;7: 30–34.

Hasihim, S. A., and P. Tantibhedyangkul. "Medium Chain Triglyceride in Early Life: Effects on Growth of Adipose Tissue." *Lipids* 1987;22: 429.

Hill, J. O., J. C. Peters, D. Yang, T. Sharp, M. Kaler, N. N. Abumrad, H. L. Greene. "Thermogenesis in Humans During Overfeeding with Medium-Chain Triglycerides." *Metabolism* 1989;38: 641.

Hornstra, G., A. C. van Houwelingen, A. D. Kester, and K. Sundram. "A Palm Oil-enriched Diet Lowers Serum Lipoprotein(a) in Normocholesterolemic Volunteers." *Atherosclerosis* 1991;90: 91–93.

Hornung, B., E. Amtmann, and G. Sauer. "Lauric Acid Inhibits the Maturation of Vesicular Stomatitis Virus." *J Gen Virology* 1994;75: 353–361.

Hostmark, A. T., O. Spydevold, and E. Eilertsen. "Plasma Lipid Concentration and Liver Output of Lipoproteins in Rats Fed Coconut Fat or Sunflower Oil." *Artery* 1980;7: 367–383.

Isaacs, C. E., K. S. Kim, and H. Thormar. "Inactivation of Enveloped Viruses in Human Bodily Fluids by Purified Lipids." *Annals NY Acad Sci* 1994;724: 457–464.

Isaacs, C. E., R. E. Litov, P. Marie, and H. Thormar. "Addition of Lipases to Infant Formulas Produces Antiviral and Antibacterial Activity." *J Nutr Biochem* 1992;3: 304–308.

Jones, P. J. H. "Regulation of Cholesterol Biosynthesis by Diet in Humans." *The American Journal of Clinical Nutrition* 1997;66: 438–446.

Kaunitz, H., C. S. Dayrit. "Coconut Oil Consumption and Coronary Heart Disease." *Philippine Journal of Internal Medicine* 1992;30: 165–171.

Ng, T. K. W., K. Hassan, J. B. Lim, M. S. Lye, and R. Ishak. "Nonhypercholesterolemic Effects of a Palm-Oil Diet in Malaysian Volunteers." *The American Journal of Clinical Nutrition* 1991;53: S1015–S1020.

Oh, D. H., and D. L. Marshall. "Antimicrobial Activity of Ethanol, Glycerol Monolaurate or Lactic Acid Against *Listeria monocytogenes*." *Int J Food and Microbiol* 1993;20: 239–246.

Petschow, B. W., R. P. Batema, and L. L. Ford. "Susceptibility of *Helicobacter pylori* to Bactericidal Properties of Medium-Chain Monoglycerides and Free Fatty Acids." *Antimicrobial Agents and Chemotherapy* 1996;40: 302–306.

Sircar, S., and U. Kansra. "Choice of Cooking Oils—Myths and Realities." *J Indian Med Assoc* 1998; 96: 304–307.

Seaton, T. B., et al. "Thermic Effect of Medium-Chain and Long-Chain Triglycerides in Man." *The American Journal of Clinical Nutrition* 1986;44: 630.

Smit, M. J., H. Wolters, A. M. Temmerman, F. Kuipers, A. C. Beynen, and R. J. Vonk. "Effects of Dietary Corn and Olive Oil Versus Coconut Fat on Biliary Cholesterol Secretion in Rats." *Internatl J Vitamin and Nutr Res* 1994;64: 75–80.

Sundram, K., K. C. Hayes, and O. H. Siru. "Dietary Palmitic Acid Results in Lower Serum

Cholesterol Than Does a Lauric-Myristic Acid Combination in Normolipemic Humans." *The American Journal of Clinical Nutrition* 1994;59: 841–846.

Thormar, H., E. C. Isaacs, H. R. Brown, M. R. Barshatzky, and T. Pessolano. "Inactivation of Enveloped Viruses and Killing of Cells by Fatty Acids and Monoglycerides." *Antimicrob Agents and Chemother* 1987;31: 27–31.

Hazelnut (Filbert)

Balkan, J., A. Hatipoglu, G. Aykac-Toker, and M. Uysal. "Influence on Hazelnut Oil Administration on Peroxidation Status of Erythrocytes and Apolipoprotein B 100-Containing Lipoproteins in Rabbits Fed on a High Cholesterol Diet." *J Agric Food Chem* 2003;51(13): 3905–3909.

Hansen, K. S., B. K. Ballmer-Weber, D. Luttkopf, P. S. Skov, B. Wuthrich, C. Bindslev-Jensen, S. Vieths, and L. K. Poulsen. "Roasted Hazelnuts—Allergenic Activity Evaluated by Double-Blind, Placebo-Controlled Food Challenge." *Allergy* 2003;58(2): 132–138.

Schafer, T., E. Bohler, S. Ruhdorfer, L. Weigl, D. Wessner, J. Heinrich, B. Filipiak, H. E. Wichmann, and J. Ring. "Epidemiology of Food Allergy/Food Intolerance in Adults: Associations with Other Manifestations of Atopy." *Allergy* 2001;56(12): 1172–1179.

Straumann, F., and B. Wuthrich. "Food Allergies Associated with Birch Pollen: Comparison of Allergodip and Pharmacia CAP for Detection of Specific IgE Antibodies to Birch Pollen Related Foods." *J Investig Allergol Clin Immunol* 2000; 10(3): 135–141.

Wensing, M., A. H. Penninks, S. L. Hefle, et al. "The Range of Minimum Provoking Doses in Hazelnut-Allergic Patients as Determined by Double-Blind, Placebo-Controlled Food Challenges." *Clin Exp Allergy* 2002;32(12): 1757–1762.

Linseed (Flax)

Adlercreutz, H., T. Fotsis, C. Bannwart C, et al. "Determination of Urinary Lignans and Phytoestrogen Metabolites, Potential Antiestrogens and Anticarcinogens, in Urine of Women in Various Habitual Diets." *J Steroid Biochem* 1986;25: 791–797.

Allman, M. A., M. M. Pena, and D. Pang. "Supplementation with Flaxseed Oil Versus Sunflowerseed Oil in Healthy Young Men Consuming a Lowfat Diet: Effects on Platelet Composition and Function." *Eur J Clin Nutr* 1995;49(3): 169–178.

Berry, E. M. and J. Hirsch. "Does Dietary Linolenic Acid Influence Blood Pressure?" *The American Journal of Clinical Nutrition* 1986;44: 336–340.

Chan, J. K., V. M. Bruce, and B. E. McDonald. "Dietary-Alpha-Linolenic Acid Is as Effective as Oleic Acid and Linoleic Acid in Lowering Blood Cholesterol in Normolipidemic Men." *The American Journal of Clinical Nutrition* 1991;53: 1230–1234.

Cunnane, S. C., M. J. Hamadeh, A. C. Liede, et al. "Nutritional Attributes of Traditional Flaxseed in Healthy Young Adults." *The American Journal of Clinical Nutrition* 1995;61(1): 62–68.

Demark-Wahnefried, W., D. T. Price, T. J. Polascik TJ, et al. "Pilot Study of Dietary Fat Restriction and Flaxseed Supplementation in Men with Prostate Cancer Before Surgery: Exploring the Effects on Hormonal Levels, Prostate-Specific Antigen, and Histopathologic Features." *Urology* 2001;58: 47–52.

Haggans, C. J., A. M. Hutchins, B. A. Olson BA, et al. "Effect of Flaxseed Consumption on Urinary Estrogen Metabolites in Postmenopausal Women." *Nutr Cancer* 1999;33: 188–195.

Leaf, A., and P. C. Weber. "Cardiovascular Effects of N-3 Fatty Acids." *The New England Journal of Medicine* 1988;318: 549–557.

Lucas, E. A., R. D. Wild, L. J. Hammond, A. D. A. Khalil, S. Juma, B. P. Daggy, B. J. Stoecker, and B. H. Arjmandi. "Flaxseed Improves Lipid Profile Without Altering Biomarkers of Bone Metabolism in Postmenopausal Women." *J Clin Endocrinol Metab* 2002;87(4): 1527–1532.

Mantzioris, E., M. J. James, R. A. Gibson, and L. G. Cleland. "Nutritional Attributes of Dietary Flaxseed Oil." *The American Journal of Clinical Nutrition* 1995;62(4): 841–842.

Nesbitt, P. D., L. U. Thompson. "Lignans in Home-made and Commercial Products Containing Flaxseed." *Nutr Cancer* 1997;29(3): 222–227.

Newcomer, L. M., I. B. King, K. G. Wicklund, and J. L. Stanford. "The Association of Fatty Acids with Prostate Cancer Risk." *Prostate* 2001;47: 262–268.

Serraino, M., and L. U. Thompson. "The Effect of Flaxseed Supplementation on Early Risk Markers for Mammary Carcinogenesis." *Cancer Letters* 1991;60: 135–142.

Singer, P. "Alpha-linolenic Acid vs. Long-Chain Fatty Acids in Hypertension and Hyperlipidemia." *Nutr* 1992;8: 133–135.

Thompson, L. U., S. E. Rickard, L. J. Orcheson, and M. M. Seidl. "Flaxseed and its Lignan and Oil Components Reduce Mammary Tumor Growth at a Late Stage of Carcinogenesis." *Carcinogenesis* 1996;17: 1373–1376.

Thompson, L. U., M. M. Seidl, S. E. Rickard, L. J. Orcheson, and H. H. Fong. "Antitumorigenic Effect of a Mammalian Lignan Precursor from Flaxseed." *Nutr Cancer* 1996;26: 159–165.

Ward, W. E., F. O. Jiang, and L. U. Thompson. "Exposure to Flaxseed or Purified Lignan During Lactation Influences Rat Mammary Gland Structures." *Nutr Cancer* 2000;37: 187–192.

Olives and Olive Oil

Alarcon de la Lastra, C., M. D. Barranco, V. Motilva, and J. M Herrerias. "Mediterranean Diet and Health: Biological Importance of Olive Oil." *Curr Pharm Des* 2001;7: 933–950.

Martinez-Dominguez, E., R. de la Puerta, V. Ruiz-Gutierrez. "Protective Effects upon Experimental Inflammation Models of a Polyphenol-Supplemented Virgin Olive Oil Diet." *Inflamm Res* 2001;50(2): 102–106.

Visioli, F., A. Romani, N. Mulinacci, et al. "Antioxidant and Other Biological Activities of Olive Mill Waste Waters." *J Agric Food Chem* 1999(August);47(8): 3397–3401.

Peanut

Albert, C. M., J. M. Gaziano, W. C. Willett, and J. E. Manson. "Nut Consumption and Decreased Risk of Sudden Cardiac Death in the Physicians' Health Study." *Arch Intern Med* 2002;162(12): 1382–1387.

Caster, W. O., T. A. Burton, T. R. Irvin, and M. A. Tanner. "Dietary Aflatoxins, Intelligence and School Performance in Southern Georgia." *Inter J Vit Nutr Res* 1986;56: 291–295.

Flynn, N. E., C. J. Meininger, T. E. Haynes, G. Wu. "The Metabolic Basis of Arginine Nutrition and Pharmacotherapy." *Biomed Pharmacother* 2002; 56(9): 427–438.

Jiang, R., J. E. Manson, M. J. Stampfer, et al. "Nut and Peanut Butter Consumption and Risk of Type 2 Diabetes in Women." *Journal of the American Medical Association* 2002;288(20): 2554–2560.

Kris-Etherton, P. M., T. A. Pearson, Y. Wan, R. L. Hargrove, K. Moriarty, V. Fishell, and T. D. Etherton. "High-Monounsaturated Fatty Acid Diets Lower Both Plasma Cholesterol and Triacylglycerol Concentrations." *The American Journal of Clinical Nutrition* 1999;70(6): 1009–1015.

Sicherer, S. H., and H. A. Sampson. "Peanut and Tree Nut Allergy." *Curr Opin Pediatr* 2000;12(6): 567–573.

Pecan

Morgan, W. A., and B. J. Clayshulte. "Pecans Lower Low-Density Lipoprotein Cholesterol in People with Normal Lipid Levels." *Journal of the American Dietetic Association* 2000;100(3): 312–318.

Rajaram, S., K. Burke, B. Connell, T. Myint, and J. Sabate. "A Monounsaturated Fatty Acid-Rich Pecan-Enriched Diet Favorably Alters the Serum Lipid Profile of Healthy Men and Women." *The Journal of Nutrition* 2001;131(9): 2275–2279.

Pine Nut

Maselli, J. P., Sanz ML, and M. Fernandez-Benitez. "Allergy to Pine Nut." *Allergol Immunopathol* (Madrid) 2002;30(2): 104–108.

Pistachio

Edwards, K., I. Kwaw, J. Matud, and I. Kurtz. "Effect of Pistachio Nuts on Serum Lipid Levels in Patients with Moderate Hypercholesterolemia." *Journal of the American College of Nutrition* 1999;18(3): 229–232.

Erario, M., J. N. Cooper, and M. J. Sheridan. "Effect of Daily Pistachio Nut Consumption on Serum Lipid Levels." *FASEB J* 2001;15(4): 327.4A.

Giner-Larza, E. M., S. Manez, M. C. Recio, R. M. Giner, J. M. Prieto, M. Cerda-Nicolas, and J. L. Rios. "Oleanonic Acid, a 3-oxotriterpene from *Pistacia*, Inhibits Leukotriene Synthesis and Has Anti-inflammatory Activity." *Eur J Pharmacol* 2001;428(1): 137–143.

Janakat, S., H. Al-Merie. "Evaluation of Hepatoprotective Effect of *Pistacia lentiscus, Phillyrea latifolia* and *Nicotiana glauca*." *J Ethopharmacol* 2002;83(1–2): 135–138.

Pumpkin Seeds

Berges, R. R., J. Windeler, H. J. and Trampisch. "Randomised, Placebo-Controlled, Double-Blind Clinical Trial of Beta-sitosterol in Patients with Benign Prostatic Hyperplasia." *The Lancet* 1995; 345: 1529–1532.

Bombardelli, E., and P. Morazzoni. "*Cucurbita pepo* L." *Fitoterapia* 1997;68: 291–302.

Carbin, B. E., B. Larsson, and O. Lindahl. "Treatment of Benign Prostatic Hyperplasia with Phytosterols." *Br J Urol* 1990;66: 639–641.

Schiebel-Schlosser, G., and M. Friederich. "Phytotherapy of BPH with Pumpkin Seeds—A Multicenter Clinical Trial." *Zeis Phytother* 1998;19: 71–76.

Sesame Seeds

Fukuda, YM, T. Osawa, and M. Namike. "Studies on Antioxidative Substances in Sesame Seed." *Agric Biol Chem* 1985;49: 301–306.

Hirata, F., K. Fujita, Y. Ishikura, et al. "Hypocholesterolemic Effect of Sesame Lignan in Humans." *Atherosclerosis* 1996;122(1): 135–136.

Hirose, N., T. Inoue, K. Nishihara, et al. "Inhibition of Cholesterol Absorption and Synthesis in Rats by Sesamin." *J Lipid Res* 1991;32: 629–638.

Kamal-Eldin, A., D. Pettersson, and L. A. Appelqvist. "Sesamin (a Compound from Sesame Oil) Increases Tocopherol Levels in Rats Fed *ad libitum*." *Lipids* 1995;30(6): 499–505.

Kita, S., Y. Matsumura, S. Morimoto, et al. "Antihypertensive Effect of Sesamin. II. Protection Against Two-Kidney, One-Clip Renal Hypertension and Cardiovascular Hypertrophy." *Biol Pharm Bull* 1995;18(9): 1283–1285.

Matsumura, Y., S. Kita, S. Morimoto, et al. "Antihypertensive Effect of Sesamin. I. Protection Against Deoxycorticosterone Acetate-Salt-Induced Hypertension and Cardiovascular Hypertrophy." *Biol Pharm Bull* 1995;18(7): 1016–1019.

Matsumura, Y., S. Kita, R. Ohgushi, and T. Okui. "Effects of Sesamin on Altered Vascular Reactivity in Aortic Rings of Deoxycorticosterone Acetate-Salt-Induced Hypertensive Rat." *Biol Pharm Bull* 2000;23(9): 1041–1045.

Nonaka, M., K. Yamashita, Y. Iizuka, et al. "Effects of Dietary Sesaminol and Sesamin on Eicosanoid Production and Immunoglobulin Level in Rats Given Ethanol." *Biosci Biotechnol Biochem* 1997; 61(5): 836–839.

Ogawa, H., S. Sasagawa, T. Murakami, and H. Yoshizumi. "Sesame Lignans Modulate Cholesterol Metabolism in the Stroke-Prone Spontaneously Hypertensive Rat." *Clin Exp Pharmacol Physiol* 1995;22(Suppl. 1): S310–S312.

Sirato-Yasumoto, S., M. Katsuta, Y. Okuyama, et al. "Effect of Sesame Seeds Rich in Sesamin and Sesamolin on Fatty Acid Oxidation in Rat Liver." *J Agric Food Chem* 2001;49(5): 2647–2651.

Walnut

Almario, R. U., V. Vonghavaravat, R. Wong, and S. E. Kasim-Karakas. "Effects of Walnut Consumption on Plasma Fatty Acids and Lipoproteins in Combined Hyperlipidemia." *The American Journal of Clinical Nutrition* 2001;74 (1): 72–79.

Anderson, K. J., S. S. Teuber, A. Gobeille, P. Cremin, A. L. Waterhouse, and F. M. Steinberg. "Walnut Polyphenolics Inhibit *in vitro* Human Plasma and LDL Oxidation." *The Journal of Nutrition* 2001;131(11): 2837–2842.

Munoz, S., M. Merlos, D. Zambon, C. Rodriguez, J. Sabate, E. Ros, J. C. Laguna. "Walnut-Enriched Diet Increases the Association of LDL from Hypercholesterolemic Men with Human HepG2 Cells." *J Lipid Res* 2001;42(12): 2069–2076.

Zambon, D., J. Sabate, S. Munoz, B. Campero, E. Casals, M. Merlos, J. C. Laguna, and E. Ros. "Substituting Walnuts for Monounsaturated Fat Improves the Serum Lipid Profile of Hypercholesterolemic Men and Women. A Randomized Crossover Trial." *Annals of Internal Medicine* 2000;132(7): 538–546.

Chapter 15: Herbs and Spices

Basil

Elgayyar, M., F. A. Draughon, D. A. Golden, and J. R. Mount. "Antimicrobial Activity of Essential Oils from Plants Against Selected Pathogenic and Saprophytic Microorganisms." *J Food Prot* 2001;64(7): 1019–1024.

Orafidiya, L. O., A. O. Oyedele, A. O. Shittu, and A. A. Elujoba. "The Formulation of an Effective Topical Antibacterial Product Containing *Ocimum gratissimum* Leaf Essential Oil." *Int J Pharm* 2001;224(1–2): 177–183.

Uma Devi, P. "Radioprotective, Anticarcinogenic and Antioxidant Properties of the Indian Holy Basil, *Ocimum sanctum* (Tulasi)." *Indian J Exp Biol* 2001;39(3): 185–190.

Vrinda, B., and P. Uma Devi. "Radiation Protection of Human Lymphocyte Chromosomes *in vitro* by Orientin and Vicenin." *Mutat Res* 2001;498 (1–2): 39–46.

Cayenne Pepper

Attal, N. "Chronic Neuropathic Pain: Mechanisms and Treatment." *Clin J Pain* 2000;16(Suppl. 3): S118–S130.

Bortolotti, M., G. Coccia, and G. Grossi. "Red Pepper and Functional Dyspepsia." *The New England Journal of Medicine* 2002;346: 947–948.

Gonzalez, R., R. Dunkel, B. Koletzko, et al. "Effect of Capsaicin-Containing Red Pepper Sauce Suspension on Upper Gastrointestinal Motility in Healthy Volunteers." *Dig Dis Sci* 1998;43(6): 1165–1171.

Hautkappe, M., M. F. Roizen, A. Toledano, S. Roth, J. A. Jeffries, and A. M. Ostermeier. "Review of the Effectiveness of Capsaicin for Painful Cutaneous Disorders and Neural Dysfunction." *Clin J Pain* 1998;14(2): 97–106.

Joe, B., and B. R. Lokesh. "Prophylactic and Therapeutic Effects of *N*-3 Polyunsaturated Fatty Acids, Capsaicin and Curcumin on Adjuvant Induced Arthritis in Rats." *Nutr Biochem* 1997;8: 397–407.

Robbins, W. "Clinical Applications of Capsaicinoids." *Clin J Pain* 2000;16(Suppl. 2): S86–S89.

Rodriguez-Stanley, S., K. L. Collings, M. Robinson, W. Owen, and P. B. Miner, Jr. "The Effects of Capsaicin on Reflux, Gastric Emptying and Dyspepsia." *Aliment Pharmacol Ther* 2000;14(1): 129–134.

Sambaiah, K., and M. N. Satyanarayana. "Hypocholesterolemic Effect of Red Pepper & Capsaicin." *Indian J Exp Biol* 1980;18(8): 898–899.

Visudhiphan, S., S. Poolsuppasit, O. Piboonnakarintr, and S. Tumliang. "The Relationship Between High Fibrinolytic Activity and Daily Capsicum Ingestion in Thais." *The American Journal of Clinical Nutrition* 1982;35: 1452–1458.

Cinnamon

Broadhurst, C. L., M. M. Polansky, and R. A. Anderson. "Insulin-like Biological Activity of Culinary and Medicinal Plant Aqueous Extracts *in vitro*." *J Agric Food Chem* 2000;48(3): 849.

Ouattara, B., R. E. Simard, R. A. Holley, et al. "Antibacterial Activity of Selected Fatty Acids and Essential Oils Against Six Meat Spoilage Organisms." *Int J Food Microbiol* 1997;37(2–3): 155–162.

Quale, J. M., D. Landman, M. M. Zaman, et al. *"In vitro* Activity of *Cinnamomum zeylanicum* Against Azole Resistant and Sensitive *Candida* Species and a Pilot Study of Cinnamon for Oral Candidiasis." *Am J Chin Med* 1996;24(2): 103–109.

Takenaga, M., A. Hirai, T. Terano, et al. *"In vitro* Effect of Cinnamic Aldehyde, a Main Component of *Cinnamomi cortex,* on Human Platelet Aggregation and Arachidonic Acid Metabolism." *J Pharmacobiodyn* 1987;10(5): 201–208.

Cloves

Ghelardini, C., N. Galeotti, L. Di Cesare Mannelli, et al. "Local Anaesthetic Activity of Beta-caryophyllene." *Farmaco* 2001;56(5–7): 387–389.

Meeker, H. G., and H. A. Linke. "The Antibacterial Action of Eugenol, Thyme Oil, and Related Essential Oils Used in Dentistry." *Compendium* 1988;9(1): 32, 34–5, 38.

Coriander (Cilantro)

Chithra, V., and S. Leelamma. *"Coriandrum sativum* Changes the Levels of Lipid Peroxides and Activity of Antioxidant Enzymes in Experimental Animals." *Indian J Biochem Biophys* 1999;36(1): 59–61.

Chithra V, and S. Leelamma. "Hypolipidemic Effect of Coriander Seeds *(Coriandrum sativum)*: Mechanism of Action." *Plant Foods Hum Nutr* 1997;51(2): 167–172.

Cortes-Eslava, J., S. Gomez-Arroyo, R. Villalobos-Pietrini, and J. J. Espinosa-Aguirre. "Antimuta-genicity of Coriander *(Coriandrum sativum)* Juice on the Mutagenesis Produced by Plant Metabolites of Aromatic Amines." *Toxicol Lett* 2004;153(2): 283–292.

Gray, A. M., and P. R. Flatt. "Insulin-Releasing and Insulin-like Activity of the Traditional Anti-diabetic Plant *Coriandrum sativum* (Coriander)." *Br J Nutr* 1999;81(3): 203–209.

Dill

Zheng, G. Q., P. M. Kenney, and L. K. Lam. "Anetho-furan, Carvone, and Limonene: Potential Cancer Chemopreventive Agents from Dill Weed Oil and Caraway Oil." *Planta Med* 1992;58(4):338–341.

Ginger

Fischer-Rasmussen, W., S. K. Kjaer, C. Dahl, et al. "Ginger Treatment of Hypereesis Gravidarum." *Eur J Obstet Gynecol Reprod Biol* 1990;38: 19–24, 1990.

Srivastava, K. C., and T. Mustafa. "Ginger *(Zingiber officinale)* and Rheumatic Disorders." *Med Hypothesis* 1989;29:25–28.

Srivastava, K. C., and T. Mustafa. "Ginger *(Zingiber officinale)* in Rheumatism and Musculoskeletal Disorders." *Med Hypothesis* 1992;39: 342–348.

Horseradish

Morimitsu, Y., K. Hayashi, Y. Nakagawa, et al. "Antiplatelet and Anticancer Isothiocyanates in Japanese Domestic Horseradish, Wasabi." *Biofactors* 2000;13(1–4): 271–276.

Shofran, B. G., S. T. Purrington, F. Breidt, and H. P. Fleming. "Antimicrobial Properties of Sinigrin and Its Hydrolysis Products." *J Food Sci* 1998;63.

Mint (Peppermint)

Briggs, C. "Peppermint. Medicinal Herb and Flavoring Agent." *Can Pharm J* 1993 (March): 89–92.

Nutmeg

Broadhurst, C. L., M. M. Polansky, and R. A. Anderson. "Insulin-like Biological Activity of Culinary and Medicinal Plant Aqueous Extracts *in vitro.*" *J Agric Food Chem* 2000;48(3): 849–852.

De, M., A. Krishna De, and A. B. Banerjee. "Antimicrobial Screening of Some Indian Spices." *Phytother Res* 1999;13(7): 616–618.

Dorman, H. J., and S. G. Deans. "Antimicrobial Agents from Plants: Antibacterial Activity of Plant Volatile Oils." *J Appl Microbiol* 2000;88(2): 308–316.

Grover, J. K., S. Khandkar, V. Vats, Y. Dhunnoo, and D. Das. "Pharmacological Studies on *Myristica fragrans*—Antidiarrheal, Hypnotic, Analgesic and Hemodynamic (Blood Pressure) Parameters." *Methods Find Exp Clin Pharmacol* 2002; 24(10): 675–680.

Olajide, O. A., F. F. Ajayi, A. I. Ekhelar, S. O. Awe, J. M. Makinde, and A. R. Alada. "Biological Effects of *Myristica fragrans* (Nutmeg) Extract." *Phytother Res* 1999;13(4): 344–345.

Sangalli, B. C., and W. Chiang. "Toxicology of Nutmeg Abuse." *J Toxicol Clin Toxicol* 2000;38(6): 671–678.

Stein, U., H. Greyer, and H. Hentschel. "Nutmeg (Myristicin) Poisoning—Report on a Fatal Case and a Series of Cases Recorded by a Poison Information Centre." *Forensic Sci Int* 2001;118(1): 87–90.

Oregano and Marjoram

Akgul, A., and M. Kivanc. "Inhibitory Effects of Selected Turkish Spices and Oregano Components on Some Foodborne Fungi." *Int J Food Microbiol* 1988;6(3): 263–268.

Lagouri, V., and D. Boskou. "Nutrient Antioxidants in Oregano." *Int J Food Sci Nutr* 1996;47(6): 493–497.

Lambert, R. J., P. M. Skandamis, P. J. Coote, G. J. Nychas GJ. "A Study of the Minimum Inhibitory Concentration and Mode of Action of Oregano Essential Oil, Thymol and Carvacrol." *J Appl Microbiol* 2001;91(3): 453–462.

Martinez-Tome, M., A. M. Jimenez, S. Ruggieri, N. Frega, R. Strabbioli, and M. A. Murcia. "Antioxidant Properties of Mediterranean Spices

Compared with Common Food Additives." *J Food Prot* 2001;64(9): 1412–1419.

Zheng, W., and S. Y. Wang. "Antioxidant Activity and Phenolic Compounds in Selected Herbs." |*J Agric Food Chem* 2001;49(11): 5165–5170.

Pepper, Black

Abila, B., A. Richens, and J. A. Davies. "Anticonvulsant Effects of Extracts of the West African Black Pepper, *Piper guineense.*" *J Ethnopharmacol* 1993; 39(2): 113–117.

Ao, P., S. Hu, and A. Zhao. "[Essential Oil Analysis and Trace Element Study of the Roots of *Piper nigrum* L.J." *Zhongguo Zhong Yao Za Zhi* 1998; 23(1): 42–43, 63.

Dorman, H. J., S. G. Deans. "Antimicrobial Agents from Plants: Antibacterial Activity of Plant Volatile Oils." *J Appl Microbiol* 2000;88(2): 308–316.

Mujumdar, A. M., J. N. Dhuley, V. K. Deshmukh, et al. "Anti-inflammatory Activity of Piperine." *Jpn J Med Sci Biol* 1990;43(3): 95–100.

Rosemary

Kelm, M. A., M. G. Nair, G. M. Strasburg, and D. L. DeWitt. "Antioxidant and Cyclooxygenase Inhibitory Phenolic Compounds from *Ocimum sanctum* Linn." *Phytomedicine* 2000;7(1): 7–13.

Saffron

Abe, K., and H. Saito. "Effects of Saffron Extract and Its Constituent Crocin on Learning Behaviour and Long-Term Potentiation." *Phytother Res* 2000;14(3): 149–152.

Escribano, J., G. L. Alonso, M. Coca-Prados, and J. A. Fernandez. "Crocin, Safranal and Picrocrocin from Saffron (*Crocus sativus* L.) Inhibit the Growth of Human Cancer Cells *in vitro.*" *Cancer Lett* 1996;100(1–2): 23–30.

Garcia-Olmo, D. C., H. H. Riese, J. Escribano, J. Ontanon, J. A. Fernandez, M. Atienzar, D. and Garcia-Olmo. "Effects of Long-Term Treatment of Colon Adenocarcinoma with Crocin, a Carotenoid from Saffron (*Crocus sativus* L.): An

Experimental Study in the Rat." *Nutr Cancer* 1999;35(2): 120–126.

Lucas, C. D., J. B. Hallagan, S. L. and Taylor. "The Role of Natural Color Additives in Food Allergy." *Adv Food Nutr Res* 2001;43: 195–216.

Martinez-Tome, M., A. M. Jimenez, S. Ruggieri, N. Frega, R. Strabbioli, and M. A. Murcia. "Antioxidant Properties of Mediterranean Spices Compared with Common Food Additives." *J Food Prot* 2001;64(9): 1412–1419.

Nair, S. C., S. K. Kurumboor, and J. H. Hasegawa. "Saffron Chemoprevention in Biology and Medicine: A Review." *Cancer Biother* 1995;10(4): 257–264.

Nair, S. C., M. J. Salomi, C. D. Varghese, B. Panikkar, K. R. Panikkar. "Effect of Saffron on Thymocyte Proliferation, Intracellular Glutathione Levels and Its Antitumor Activity." *Biofactors* 1992;4 (1): 51–54.

Nair, S. C., B. Pannikar, and K. R. Panikkar. "Antitumour Activity of Saffron *(Crocus sativus)*." *Cancer Lett* 1991 1;57(2): 109–114.

Premkumar, K., S. K. Abraham, S. T. Santhiya, P. M. Gopinath, and A. Ramesh. "Inhibition of Genotoxicity by Saffron (*Crocus sativus* L.) in Mice." *Drug Chem Toxicol* 2001;24(4): 421–428.

Sannohe, S., Y. Makino, T. Kita, N. Kuroda, and T. Shinozuka. "Colchicine Poisoning Resulting from Accidental Ingestion of Meadow Saffron *(Colchicum autumnale)*." *J Forensic Sci* 2002;47 (6): 1391–1396.

Verma, S. K., and A. Bordia. "Antioxidant Property of Saffron in Man." *Indian J Med Sci* 1998;52(5): 205–207.

Sage

Kelm, M. A., M. G. Nair, G. M. Strasburg, and D. L. DeWitt. "Antioxidant and Cyclooxygenase Inhibitory Phenolic Compounds from *Ocimum sanctum* Linn." *Phytomedicine* 2000;7(1): 7–13.

Malencic, D., O. Gasic, M. Popovic, and P. Boza. "Screening for Antioxidant Properties of *Salvia reflexa hornem.*" *Phytother Res* 2000;14(7): 546–548.

Tarragon

Meepagala, K. M., G. Sturtz, and D. E. Wedge. "Antifungal Constituents of the Essential Oil Fraction of *Artemisia dracunculus* L. var. *dracunculus.*" *J Agric Food Chem* 2002;50(24): 6989–6992.

Parejo, I., F. Viladomat, J. Bastida, A. Rosas-Romero, N. Flerlage, J. Burillo, and C. Codina. "Comparison Between the Radical Scavenging Activity and Antioxidant Activity of Six Distilled and Nondistilled Mediterranean Herbs and Aromatic Plants." *J Agric Food Chem* 2002;50(23): 6882–6890.

Swanston-Flatt, S. K., C. Day, C. J. Bailey, and P. R. Flatt. "Evaluation of Traditional Plant Treatments for Diabetes: Studies in Streptozotocin Diabetic Mice." *Acta Diabetol Lat* 1989;26(1): 51–55.

Thyme

Cosentino, S., C. I. Tuberoso, B. Pisano, et al. "*In-vitro* Antimicrobial Activity and Chemical Composition of Sardinian *Thymus* Essential Oils." *Lett Appl Microbiol* 1999;29(2): 130–135.

Kelm, M. A., M. G. Nair, G. M. Strasburg, and D. L. DeWitt. "Antioxidant and Cyclooxygenase Inhibitory Phenolic Compounds from *Ocimum sanctum* Linn." *Phytomedicine* 2000;7(1): 7–13.

Kulevanova, S., A. Kaftandzieva, A. Dimitrovska, et al. "Investigation of Antimicrobial Activity of Essential Oils of Several Macedonian *Thymus* L. Species (Lamiaceae)." *Boll Chim Farm* 2000;139 (6): 276–280.

Meeker, H. G., H. A. Linke. "The Antibacterial Action of Eugenol, Thyme Oil, and Related Essential Oils Used in Dentistry." *Compendium* 1988;9(1): 32, 34–35, 38.

Turmeric

Arbiser, J. L., N. Klauber, R. Rohan, et al. "Curcumin Is an *in vivo* Inhibitor of Angiogenesis." *Mol Med* 1998;4(6): 376–383.

Asai, A., and T. Miyazawa. "Dietary Curcuminoids Prevent High-Fat Diet-Induced Lipid

Accumulation in Rat Liver and Epididymal Adipose Tissue." *The Journal of Nutrition* 2001;131(11): 2932–2935.

Asai, A., K. Nakagawa, and T. Miyazawa. "Antioxidative Effects of Turmeric, Rosemary and Capsicum Extracts on Membrane Phospholipid Peroxidation and Liver Lipid Metabolism in Mice." *Biosci Biotechnol Biochem* 1999;63(12): 2118–2122.

Chen, H., Z. S. Zhang, Y. L. Zhang, and D. Y. Zhou. "Curcumin Inhibits Cell Proliferation by Interfering with the Cell Cycle and Inducing Apoptosis in Colon Carcinoma Cells." *Anticancer Res* 1999;19: 3675–3680.

Dorai, T., Y. C. Cao, B. Dorai, et al. "Therapeutic Potential of Curcumin in Human Prostate Cancer. III. Curcumin Inhibits Proliferation, Induces Apoptosis, and Inhibits Angiogenesis of LNCaP Prostate Cancer Cells *in vivo.*" *Prostate* 2001;47 (4): 293–303.

Gururaj, A., M. Belakavadi, D. Venkatesh, D. Marme, B. Salimath. "Molecular Mechanisms of Anti-angiogenic Effect of Curcumin." *Biochem Biophys Res Commun* 2002;297(4): 934.

Li, J. K., and S. Y. Lin-Shia. "Mechanisms of Cancer Chemoprevention by Curcumin." *Proc Natl Sci Counc Repub China B* 2001;25: 59–66.

Lim, G. P., T. Chu, F. Yang, et al. "The Curry Spice Curcumin Reduces Oxidative Damage and Amyloid Pathology in an Alzheimer Transgenic Mouse." *J Neurosci* 2001;21(21): 8370–8377.

Natarajan, C., and J. J. Bright. "Curcumin Inhibits Experimental Allergic Encephalomyelitis by Blocking IL-12 Signaling Through Janus Kinase-STAT Pathway in T Lymphocytes." *J Immunol* 2002;168(12): 6506–6513.

Natarajan, C., and J. J. Bright. "Peroxisome Proliferator-Activated Receptor-Gamma Agonists Inhibit Experimental Allergic Encephalomyelitis by Blocking IL-12 Production, IL-12 Signaling and Th1 Differentiation." *Genes Immun* 2002;3 (2): 59–70.

Navis, I., P. Sriganth, and B. Premalatha. "Dietary Curcumin with Cisplatin Administration Modulates Tumour Marker Indices in Experimental Fibrosarcoma." *Pharmacol Res* 1999;39: 175–179.

Olszewska, M., R. Glowacki, M. Wolbis, E. Bald. "Quantitative Determination of Flavonoids in the Flowers and Leaves of *Prunus spinosa* L." *Acta Pol Pharm* 2001;58(3): 199–203.

Phan, T. T., P. See, S. T. Lee, S. Y. Chan. "Protective Effects of Curcumin Against Oxidative Damage on Skin Cells *in vitro:* Its Implication for Wound Healing." *J Trauma* 2001(November);51(5): 927–931.

Polasa, K., T. C. Raghuram, T. P. Krishna, K. Krishnaswamy. "Effect of Turmeric on Urinary Mutagens in Smokers." *Mutagenesis* 1992;7: 107–109.

Rinaldi, A. L., M. A. Morse, H. W. Fields, D. A. Rothas, P. Pei, K. A. Rodrigo, R. J. Renner, and S. R. Mallery. "Curcumin Activates the Aryl Hydrocarbon Receptor yet Significantly Inhibits (−)-Benzo(a)Pyrene-7R-Trans-7, 8-Dihydrodiol Bioactivation in Oral Squamous Cell Carcinoma Cells and Oral Mucosa." *Cancer Res* 2002;62(19): 5451–5456.

Shah, B. H., Z. Nawaz, S. A. Pertani, et al. "Inhibitory Effect of Curcumin, a Food Spice from Turmeric, on Platelet-Activating Factor-and Arachidonic Acid-Mediated Platelet Aggregation Through Inhibition of Thromboxane Formation and Ca2+ Signa." Biochem Pharmacol 1999;58(7): 1167–1172.

Shankar, T. N. B., N. V. Shantha, H. P. Ramesh, et al. "Toxicity Studies on Turmeric (*Curcuma longa*). Acute Toxicity Studies in Rats, Guinea Pigs & Monkeys." *Indian J Exp Biol* 1980;18: 73–75.

Shao, Z. M., Z. Z. Shen, C. H. Liu, M. R. Sartippour, V. L. Go, D. Heber, and M. Nguyen. "Curcumin Exerts Multiple Suppressive Effects on Human Breast Carcinoma Cells." *Int J Cancer* 2002 (March 10);98(2): 234–240.

Srinivas, L., and V. K. Shalini. "DNA Damage by Smoke. Protection by Turmeric and Other Inhibitors of ROS." *Free Radical Biol Med* 1991;11: 277–283.

Chapter 16: Fish and Shellfish

Fish

Albert, C. M., H. Campos, M. J. Stampfer, et al. "Blood Levels of Long-Chain *N*-3 Fatty Acids and the Risk of Sudden Death." *The New England Journal of Medicine* 2002;346: 1113–1118.

Bucher, H. C., P. Hengstler, C. Schindler, and G. Meier. *N*-3 "Polyunsaturated Fatty Acids in Coronary Heart Disease: A Meta-Analysis of Randomized Controlled Trials." *Am J Med* 2002; 112: 298–304.

Cho, E., S. Hung, W. C. Willett, et al. "Prospective Study of Dietary Fat and the Risk of Age-Related Macular Degeneration." *The American Journal of Clinical Nutrition* 2001;73(2): 209–218.

Easton, M. D., D. Luszniak, and G. E. Von der, "Preliminary Examination of Contaminant Loadings in Farmed Salmon, Wild Salmon and Commercial Salmon Feed." *Chemosphere* 2002; 46(7): 1053–1074.

Fernandez, E., L. Chatenoud, C. La Vecchia, et al. "Fish Consumption and Cancer Risk." *The American Journal of Clinical Nutrition* 1999;70 (1): 85–90.

Guallar, E., M. I. Sanz-Gallardo, P. van't Veer, P. Bode, et al. "Mercury, Fish Oils, and the Risk of Myocardial Infarction." *The New England Journal of Medicine* 2002;347: 1747–1754.

Hightower, J. M., and D. Moore. "Mercury Levels in High-End Consumers of Fish." *Environ Health Perspect* 2003;111(4): 604–608.

Hu, F. B., L. Bronner, W. C. Willett, et al. "Fish and Omega-3 Fatty Acid Intake and Risk of Coronary Heart Disease in Women." *Journal of the American Medical Association* 2002;287: 1815–1821.

Crustaceans

de Oliveira e Silva, E. R., C. E. Seidman, J. J. Tian, et al. "Effects of Shrimp Consumption on Plasma Lipoproteins." *The American Journal of Clinical Nutrition* 1996;64(5): 712–717.

Mollusks

Childs, M. T., C. S. Dorsett, I. B. King, J. G. Ostrander, and W. K. Yamanaka. "Effects of Shellfish Consumption on Lipoproteins in Normolipidemic Men." *The American Journal of Clinical Nutrition* 1990;51(6): 1020–1027.

King, I., M. T. Childs, C. Dorsett, J. G. Ostrander, and E. R. Monsen. "Shellfish: Proximate Composition, Minerals, Fatty Acids, and Sterols." *Journal of the American Dietetic Association* 1990;90 (5): 677–685.

Tanaka, K., M. Fukuda, I. Ikeda, and M. Sugano. "Effects of Dietary Short-Necked Clam, *Tapes japonica,* on Serum and Liver Cholesterol Levels in Mice." *J Nutr Sci Vitaminol* (Tokyo). 1994;40 (4): 325–333.

Chapter 17: Milk and Other Dairy Products

Cow's Milk

Beynen, A. C., R. Van der Meer, and C. E. West CE. "Mechanism of Casein-Induced Hypercholesterolemia: Primary and Secondary Features." *Atherosclerosis* 1986;60: 291–293.

Feskanich, D., V. Singh, W. C. Willett, and G. A. Colditz. "Vitamin A Intake and Hip Fractures Among Postmenopausal Women." *Journal of the American Medical Association* 2002;287(1): 47–54.

Feskanich, D., W. C. Willett, and G. A. Colditz. "Calcium, Vitamin D, Milk Consumption, and Hip Fractures: A Prospective Study Among Postmenopausal Women." *The American Journal of Clinical Nutrition* 2003;77(2): 504–511.

Jiang, J., A. Wolk, and B. Vessby. "Relation Between the Intake of Milk Fat and the Occurrence of Conjugated Linoleic Acid in Human Adipose Tissue." *The American Journal of Clinical Nutrition* 1999;70(1): 21–27.

Weinsier, R. L., and C. L. Krumdieck. "Dairy Foods and Bone Health: Examination of the Evidence." *The American Journal of Clinical Nutrition* 2000; 72: 681–689.

Goat's Milk

Pellerin, P. "Goat's Milk in Nutrition." *Ann Pharm Fr* 2001;59(1): 51–62.

Yogurt

Fortes, C., F. Forastiere, S. Farchi, et al. "Diet and Overall Survival in a Cohort of Very Elderly People." *Epidemiology* 2000;11(4): 440–445.

Gill, H. S., K. J. Rutherfurd, M. L. Cross, and P. K. Gopal. "Enhancement of Immunity in the Elderly by Dietary Supplementation with the Probiotic *Bifidobacterium lactis* HN019." *The American Journal of Clinical Nutrition* 2001;74 (6): 833–839.

Hilton, E., H. D. Isenberg, P. Alperstein, et al. "Ingestion of Yogurt Containing *Lactobacillus acidophilus* as Prophylaxis for Candidal Vaginitis." *Annals of Internal Medicine* 1992;116(5): 353–357.

Meydani, S. N., and W. K. Ha. "Immunologic Effects of Yogurt." *The American Journal of Clinical Nutrition* 2000;71(4): 861–872.

Chapter 18: Meat, Poultry, and Eggs

Beef

Bingham, S. A. "High-Meat Diets and Cancer Risk." *Proc Nutr Soc* 1999;58(2): 243–248.

Chao, A., M. J. Thun, C. J. Connell, et al. "Meat Consumption and Risk of Colorectal Cancer." *Journal of the American Medical Association* 2005;293(2): 172–182.

Davidson, M. H., D. Hunninghake, K. C. Maki, et al. "Comparison of the Effects of Lean Red Meat vs Lean White Meat on Serum Lipid Levels Among Free-Living Persons with Hypercholesterolemia: A Long-Term, Randomized Clinical Trial." *Arch Intern Med* 1999;159(12): 1331–1338.

Zheng, W., D. R. Gustafson, R. Sinha, et al. "Well-Done Meat Intake and the Risk of Breast Cancer." *Journal of the National Cancer Institute* 1998;90: 1724–1729.

Eggs

Howell, W. H., D. J. McNamara, M. A. Tosca, et al. "Plasma Lipid and Lipoprotein Responses to Dietary Fat and Cholesterol: A Meta-Analysis." *The American Journal of Clinical Nutrition* 1997;65 (6): 1747–1764, 1997.

Hu, F. B., M. J. Stampfer, E. B. Rimm, J. E. Manson, A. Ascherio, G. A. Colditz, B. A. Rosner, D. Spiegelman, F. E. Speizer, F. M. Sacks, C. H. Hennekens, and W. C. Willett. "A Prospective Study of Egg Consumption and Risk of Cardiovascular Disease in Men and Women." *Journal of the American Medical Association* 1999;281(15): 1387–1394.

Chapter 19: Miscellaneous Foods

Blackstrap Molasses

Aslan, Y., E. Erduran, H. Mocan, et al. "Absorption of Iron from Grape-Molasses and Ferrous Sulfate: A Comparative Study in Normal Subjects and Subjects with Iron Deficiency Anemia." *Turk J Pediatr* 1997;39(4): 465–471.

Brewer's Yeast

Bahijiri, S. M., S. A. Mira, A. M. Mufti, and M. A. Ajabnoor. "The Effects of Inorganic Chromium and Brewer's Yeast Supplementation on Glucose Tolerance, Serum Lipids and Drug Dosage in Individuals with Type 2 Diabetes." *Saudi Med J* 2000;21(9): 831–837.

Clausen, J., and S. A. Nielsen. "Comparison of Whole Blood Selenium Values and Erythrocyte Glutathione Peroxidase Activities of Normal Individuals on Supplementation with Selenate, Selenite, L-Selenomethionine, and High Selenium Yeast." *Biol Trace Elem Res* 1988;15: 125–138.

Elwood, J. C., D. T. Nash, and D. H. Streeten. "Effect of High-Chromium Brewer's Yeast on Human Serum Lipids." *Journal of the American College of Nutrition* 1982;1(3): 263–274.

Grossowicz, N., M. Rachmilewitz, and G. Izak. "Utilization of Yeast Polyglutamate Folates in Man." *Proc Soc Exp Biol Med* 1975;150(1): 77–79.

Konig, D., J. Keul, H. Northoff, M. Halle, and A. Berg. "Effect of 6-Week Nutritional Intervention with Enzymatic Yeast Cells and Antioxidants on Exercise Stress and Antioxidant Status." *Wien Med Wochenschr* 1999;149(1): 13–18.

Korhola, M., A. Vainio, and K. Edelmann. "Selenium Yeast." *Ann Clin Res* 1986;18(1): 65–68.

Li, Y. C. "Effects of Brewer's Yeast on Glucose Tolerance and Serum Lipids in Chinese Adults." *Biol Trace Elem Res* 1994;41(3): 341–347.

McCarthy, M. "High Chromium Yeast for Acne?" *Med Hypoth* 1984;14: 307–310.

Offenbacher, E. G., and F. X. Pi-Sunyer. "Beneficial Effect of Chromium-Rich Yeast on Glucose Tolerance and Blood Lipids in Elderly Subjects." *Diabetes* 1980;29(11): 919–925.

Weber G., A. Adamczyk, S. Freytag. "Treatment of Acne with a Yeast Preparation." *Fortschr Med* 1989;107(26): 563–566.

Chocolate

Bruinsma, K., and D. L. Taren. "Chocolate: Food or Drug?" *Journal of the American Dietetic Association* 1999;99(10): 1249–1256.

C. de O G Mendonca, L. A. Martini, A. C. Baxmann, J. L. Nishiura, L. Cuppari, D. M. Sigulem, and I. P. Heilberg. "Effects of an Oxalate Load on Urinary Oxalate Excretion in Calcium Stone Formers." *J Ren Nutr* 2003;13(1): 39–46.

Dillinger, T. L., and L. E. Grivetti. "Food of the Gods: Cure for Humanity? A Cultural History of the Medicinal and Ritual Use of Chocolate." *Journal of Nutrition* 2000;130: S2057–S2072.

Hannum, S. M., H. H. Schmitz, and C. L. Keen. "Chocolate: A Heart-Healthy Food? Show Me the Science!" *Nutr Today.* 2002;37(3): 103–109.

Hatano, T., H. Miyatake, M. Natsume, et al. "Proanthocyanidin Glycosides and Related Polyphenols from Cacao Liquor and Their Antioxidant Effects." *Phytochemistry* 2002;59(7): 749–758.

Hollman, P. C., and M. B. Katan. "Dietary Flavonoids: Intake, Health Effects and Bioavailability." *Food Chem Toxic* 1999;37: 937–942.

Hurst, W. J., S. M. Tarka, Jr., T. G. Powis, F. Valdez, Jr., and T. R. Hester. "Cacao Usage by the Earliest Maya Civilization." *Nature* 2002;418(6895): 289–290.

Kris-Etherton, P. M., and C. L. Keen. "Evidence That the Antioxidant Flavonoids in Tea and Cocoa Are Beneficial for Cardiovascular Health." *Curr Opin Lipidol* 2002;13(1): 41–49.

Lee, I. M., and R. Paffenbarger. "Life Is Sweet: Candy Consumption and Longevity." *British Medical Journal* 1998;317: 1683–1684.

Mathur, S., S. Devaraj, S. M. Grundy, and I. Jialal. "Cocoa Products Decrease Low Density Lipoprotein Oxidative Susceptibility but Do Not Affect Biomarkers of Inflammation in Humans." *The Journal of Nutrition* 2002;132(12): 3663–3667.

Murphy, K. J., A. K. Chronopoulos, I. Singh, M. A. Francis, H. Moriarty, M. J. Pike, A. H. Turner, N. J. Mann, and A. J. Sinclair. "Dietary Flavanols and Procyanidin Oligomers from Cocoa *(Theobroma cacao)* Inhibit Platelet Function." *The American Journal of Clinical Nutrition* 2003;77 (6): 1466–1473.

Osakabe, N., C. Sanbongi, M. Yamagishi, T. Takizawa, and T. Osawa. "Effects of Polyphenol Substances Derived from *Theobroma cacao* on Gastric Mucosal Lesion Induced by Ethanol." *Biosci Biotechnol Biochem* 1998;62: 1535–1538.

Planells, E., M. Rivero, J. Mataix, J. Llopis. "Ability of a Cocoa Product to Correct Chronic Mg Deficiency in Rats." *Int J Vitam Nutr Res* 1999;69(1): 52–60.

Rios, L. Y., M. P. Gonthier, C. Remesy, et al. "Chocolate Intake Increases Urinary Excretion of Polyphenol-Derived Phenolic Acids in Healthy Human Subjects." *The American Journal of Clinical Nutrition* 2003;77(4): 912–918.

Steinberg, F., M. Bearden, C. Keen. "Cocoa and Chocolate Flavonoids: Implications for Cardiovascular Health." *Journal of the American Dietetic Association* 2003;103: 215–223.

Zurer, P. "Chocolate May Mimic Marijuana in Brain." *Chemical and Engineering News* 1996; 74: 31.

Honey and Other Bee Products

Burdock, G. A. "Review of the Biological Properties and Toxicity of Bee Propolis (Propolis)." *Food Chem Toxicol* 1998;36: 347–363.

Crisan, I., C. N. Zaharia, F. Popovici, et al. "Natural Propolis Extract NIVCRISOL in the Treatment of Acute and Chronic Rhinopharyngitis in Children." *Rom J Virol* 1995;46: 115–133.

Gheldof, N., and N. J. Engeseth. "Antioxidant Capacity of Honeys from Various Floral Sources Based on the Determination of Oxygen Radical Absorbance Capacity and Inhibition of *in vitro* Lipoprotein Oxidation in Human Serum Samples." *J Agric Food Chem* 2002;50(10): 3050–3055.

Gheldof, N., X. H. Wang, and N. J. Engeseth. "Identification and Quantification of Antioxidant Components of Honeys from Various Floral Sources." *J Agric Food Chem* 2002;50(21): 5870–5877.

Hove, A., Sr., P. S. Dimick, and A. W. Benton. "Composition of Freshly Harvested and Commercial Royal Jelly." *J Apic Res* 1985;24: 52–61.

Khayyal, M. T., M. A. El-Ghazaly, and A. S. El-Khatib. "Mechanisms Involved in the Antiinflammatory Effect of Propolis Extract." *Drugs Exptl Clin Res* 1993;29: 197–203.

Lin, S. C., Y. H. Lin, C. F. Chen, C. Y. Chung, and S. H. Hsu. "The Hepatoprotective and Therapeutic Effects of Propolis Ethanol Extract on Chronic Alcohol-Induced Liver Injuries." *Am J Chin Med* 1997;25: 325–332.

Szanto, E., D. Gruber, M. Sator, W. Knogler, and J. C. Huber. "Placebo-Controlled Study of Melbrosia in Treatment of Climacteric Symptoms." *Wien Med Wochenschr* 1994;144: 130–133.

Vittek, J. "Effect of Royal Jelly on Serum Lipids in Experimental Animals and Humans with Atherosclerosis." *Experentia* 1995;51: 927–935.

Mushrooms, Crimini

Bobek, P., S. Galbavy, L. Ozdin L. "Effect of Oyster Mushroom *(Pleurotus ostreatus)* on Pathological Changes in Dimethylhydrazine-Induced Rat Colon Cancer." *Oncol Rep* 1998;5(3): 727–730.

Grube, B. J., E. T. Eng, Y. C. Kao, et al. "White Button Mushroom Phytochemicals Inhibit Aromatase Activity and Breast Cancer Cell Proliferation." *The Journal of Nutrition* 2001;131(12): 3288–3293.

Kidd, P. M. "The Use of Mushroom Glucans and Proteoglycans in Cancer Treatment." *Altern Med Rev* 2000;5(1): 4–27.

Shiitake, Maitake, and Reishi Mushrooms

Borchers, A. T., J. S. Stern, R. M. Hackman, et al. "Mushrooms, Tumors, and Immunity." *Proc Soc Exp Biol Med* 1999;221: 281–293.

Fukushima, M., T. Ohashi, Y. Fujiwara, et al. "Cholesterol-Lowering Effects of Maitake *(Grifola frondosa)* Fiber, Shiitake *(Lentinus edodes)* Fiber, and Enokitake *(Flammulina velutipes)* Fiber in Rats." *Exp Biol Med* 2001;226(8): 758–765.

Gordon, M., B. Bihari, E. Goosby, et al. "A Placebo-Controlled Trial of the Immune Modulator, Lentinan, in HIV-Positive Patients: A Phase I/II Trial." *J Med* 1998;29(5–6): 305–330.

Jong, S. C., and J. M. Birmingham. "Medicinal and Therapeutic Value of the Shiitake Mushroom." *Adv Appl Microbiol* 1993;39: 153–184.

Kabir, Y., M. Yamaguchi, and S. Kimura. "Effect of Shiitake *(Lentinus edodes)* and Maitake *(Grifola frondoza)* Mushrooms on Blood Pressure and Plasma Lipids of Spontaneously Hypertensive Rats." *J Nutr Sci Vitaminol* (Tokyo) 1987;33(5): 341–346.

Nanba, H., and H. Kuroda. "Antitumor Mechanisms of Orally Administered Shiitake Fruit Bodies." *Chem Pharm Bull* (Tokyo) 1987;35(6): 2459–2464.

Nanba, H., K. Mori, T. Toyomasu, and H. Kuroda. "Antitumor Action of Shiitake *(Lentinus edodes)* Fruit Bodies Orally Administered to Mice." *Chem Pharm Bull* (Tokyo) 1987;35(6): 2453–2458.

Takehara, M., K. Mori, K. Kuida, and M. A. Hanawa. "Antitumor Effect of Virus-like Particles from *Lentinus edodes* (Shiitake) on Ehrlich Ascites Carcinoma in Mice." *Arch Virol* 1981;68(3–4): 297–301.

Sea Vegetables

Blondin, C., F. Chaubet, A. Nardella, et al. "Relationships Between Chemical Characteristics and Anticomplementary Activity of Fucans." *Biomaterials* 1996;17(6): 597–603.

Blondin, C., E. Fischer, C. Boisson-Vidal, et al. "Inhibition of Complement Activation by Natural Sulfated Polysaccharides (fucans) from Brown Seaweed." *Mol Immunol* 1994;31(4): 247–253.

Tea

Gupta, S., N. Ahmad, and H. Mukhtar. "Prostate Cancer Chemoprevention by Green Tea." *Semin Urol Oncol* 1999;17: 70–76.

Imai, K., K. Suga, and K. Nakachi. "Cancer-Preventive Effects of Drinking Tea Among a Japanese Population." *Prev Med* 1997;26: 769–775.

Inoue, M., K. Tajima, M. Mizutani, et al. "Regular Consumption of Green Tea and the Risk of Breast Cancer Recurrence: Follow-up Study from the Hospital-Based Epidemiologic Research Program at Aichi Cancer Center (HERPACC), Japan." *Cancer Lett* 2001;167: 175–182.

Nakachi, K., S. Matsuyama, S. Miyake, M. Suganuma, and K. Imai. "Preventive Effects of Drinking Green Tea on Cancer and Cardiovascular Disease: Epidemiological Evidence for Multiple Targeting Prevention." *Biofactors* 2000;13: 49–54.

Nakachi, K., K. Suemasu, K. Suga, et al. "Influence of Drinking Green Tea on Breast Cancer Malignancy Among Japanese Patients." *Jpn J Cancer Res* 1998;89: 254–261.

Nihal, A., and M. Hasan. "Green Tea Polyphenols and Cancer: Biological Mechanisms and Practical Implications." *Nutr Rev* 1999;57: 78–83.

Setiawan, V. W., Z. F. Zhang, G. P. Yu, et al. "Protective Effect of Green Tea on the Risks of Chronic Gastritis and Stomach Cancer." *Int J Cancer* 2001;92: 600–604.

Chapter 20: Promoting Health and Healing

Note: In an effort to reduce duplication and save space, references are provided only where a new statement is made. For example, under the acne discussion we mention again that brewer's yeast was shown to be effective in the treatment of acne. Since the references were provided under "Brewer's Yeast" on page 855 we will not duplicate the citation under acne. Conversely, since the role of zinc in acne treatment was not mentioned previously, a reference is provided under "Acne."

Acne

Fulton, J. E., Jr., G. Plewig, and A. M. Kligman. "Effect of Chocolate on Acne Vulgaris." *Journal of the American Medical Association* 1969;210: 2071–2074.

Michaelson, G., L. Juhlin, K. Ljunghall. "A Double Blind Study of the Effect of Zinc and Oxytetracycline in Acne Vulgaris." *Br J Dermatol* 1977;97: 561–565.

Michaelsson, G., A. Vahlquist, and L. Juhlin. "Serum Zinc and Retinol-Binding Protein in Acne." *Br J Dermatol* 1977;96: 283–286.

AIDS and HIV Infection

Gilbert, C. L., D. A. Wheeler, G. Collins G, et al. "Randomized, Controlled Trial of Caloric Supplements in HIV Infection." *J Acquir Immune Defic Syndr* 1999;22: 253–259.

Shabert, J. K., C. Winslow, J. M. Lacey, D. W. Wilmore. "Glutamine-Antioxidant Supplementation Increases Body Cell Mass in AIDS Patients with Weight Loss: A Randomized, Double-Blind Controlled Trial." *Nutrition* 1999;15: 860–864.

Alcoholism

Biery, J. R., J. H. Williford, and E. A. McMullen. "Alcohol Craving in Rehabilitation: Assessment of

Nutrition Therapy." *Journal of the American Dietetic Association* 1991;91: 463–466.

Guenther, R. M. "Role of Nutritional Therapy in Alcoholism Treatment." *Int J Biosoc Res* 1983;4: 5–18.

Alzheimer's Disease

Clarke, R., D. Smith, K. A. Jobst, et al. "Folate, Vitamin B12, and Serum Total Homocysteine Levels in Confirmed Alzheimer Disease." *Arch Neurol* 1998;55: 1449–1455.

Ebly, E. M., J. P. Schaefer, N. R. Campbell, and D. B. Hogan. "Folate Status, Vascular Disease and Cognition in Elderly Canadians." *Age Ageing* 1998;27: 485–491.

Grant, W. B. "Dietary Links to Alzheimer's Disease." *Alzheimer Dis Rev* 1997;2: 42–55.

Smith, M. A., G. J. Petot, and G. Perry. "Diet and Oxidative Stress: A Novel Synthesis of Epidemiological Data on Alzheimer's Disease." *Alzheimer Dis Rev* 1997;2: 58–59.

Tully, A. M., H. M. Roche, R. Doyle, et al. "Low Serum Cholesteryl Ester-Docosahexaenoic Acid Levels in Alzheimer's Disease: A Case-Control Study." *Br J Nutr* 2003;89(4): 483–489.

Anemia

Little, D. R. "Ambulatory Management of Common Forms of Anemia." *Am Fam Physician* 1999;59: 1598–1604.

Anxiety

Bruce, M., et al. "Anxiogenic Effects of Caffeine in Patients with Anxiety Disorders." *Arch Gen Psychiatry* 1992;49: 867–869.

Asthma

Burney, P. G., J. E. Neild, C. H. Twort, et al. "Effect of Changing Dietary Sodium on the Airway Response to Histamine." *Thorax* 1989;44: 36–41.

Carey, O. J., C. Locke C, and J. B. Cookson. "Effect of Alterations of Dietary Sodium on the Severity of Asthma in Men." *Thorax* 1993;48: 714–718.

Fogarty, A., and J. Britton. "The Role of Diet in the Aetiology of Asthma." *Clin Exp Allergy* 2000;30: 615–627.

Forastiere, F., R. Pistelli, P. Sestini, et al. "Consumption of Fresh Fruit Rich in Vitamin C and Wheezing Symptoms in Children. SIDRIA Collaborative Group, Italy (Italian Studies on Respiratory Disorders in Children and the Environment)." *Thorax* 2000;55: 283–288.

Genton, C., P. C. Frei, and A. Pecoud. "Value of Oral Provocation Tests to Aspirin and Food Additives in the Routine Investigation of Asthma and Chronic Urticaria." *J Asthma* 1985;76: 40–45.

Gotshall, R. W., T. D. Mickleborough, and L. Cordain. "Dietary Salt Restriction Improves Pulmonary Function in Exercise-Induced Asthma." *Med Sci Sports Exerc* 2000;32: 1815–1819.

Javaid, A., M. J. Cushley, M. F. Bone. "Effect of Dietary Salt on Bronchial Reactivity to Histamine in Asthma." *British Medical Journal* 1988;297: 454.

Lindahl, O., L. Lindwall, A. Spangberg, et al. "Vegan Regimen with Reduced Medication in the Treatment of Bronchial Asthma." *J Asthma* 1985;22: 45–55.

Medici, T. C., A. Z. Schmid, M. Hacki, and W. Vetter. "Are Asthmatics Salt-Sensitive? A Preliminary Controlled Study." *Chest* 1993;104: 1138–1143.

Neuman, I., H. Nahum, and A. Ben-Amotz. "Reduction of Exercise-Induced Asthma Oxidative Stress by Lycopene, a Natural Antioxidant." *Allergy* 2000;55: 1184–1189.

Roberts, G., and G. Lack. "Food Allergy and Asthma—What Is the Link?" *Paediatr Respir Rev* 2003;4(3): 205–212.

Stenius-Aarniala, B., T. Poussa, J. Kvamstrom, et al. "Immediate and Long Term Effects of Weight Reduction in Obese People with Asthma: Randomised Controlled Study." *British Medical Journal* 2000;320: 827–832.

Atherosclerosis

Albert, C. M., H. Campos, M. J. Stampfer, et al. "Blood Levels of Long-Chain *N*-3 Fatty Acids and the Risk of Sudden Death." *The New England Journal of Medicine* 2002;346: 1113–1118.

Bougnoux, P. "*N*-3 Polyunsaturated Fatty Acids and Cancer." *Curr Opin Clin Nutr Metab Care* 1999; 2: 121–126.

Bucher, H. C., P. Hengstler, C. Schindler, and G. Meier. "*N*-3 Polyunsaturated Fatty Acids in Coronary Heart Disease: A Meta-Analysis of Randomized Controlled Trials." *Am J Med* 2002; 112: 298–304.

De Lorgeril, M., P. Salen, J.-L. Martin, et al. "Mediterranean Diet, Traditional Risk Factors, and the Rate of Cardiovascular Complications After Myocardial Infarction. Final Report of the Lyon Diet Heart Study." *Circulation* 1999;99: 779–785.

Fernandez, M. L. "Soluble Fiber and Nondigestible Carbohydrate Effects on Plasma Lipids and Cardiovascular Risk." *Curr Opin Lipidol* 2001;12(1): 35–40.

Hu, F. B., L. Bronner, W. C. Willett, et al. "Fish and Omega-3 Fatty Acid Intake and Risk of Coronary Heart Disease in Women." *Journal of the American Medical Association* 2002;287: 1815–1821.

Knekt, P., J. Kumpulainen, R. Jarvinen, H. Rissanen, M. Heliovaara, A. Reunanen, T. Hakulinen, and A. Aromaa. "Flavonoid Intake and Risk of Chronic Diseases." *The American Journal of Clinical Nutrition* 2002;76(3): 560–568.

Kromhout, D., A. Menotti, B. Bloemberg, et al. "Dietary Saturated and Trans Fatty Acids and Cholesterol and 25-Year Mortality from Coronary Heart Disease: The Seven Countries Study." *Prev Med* 1995;24: 308–315.

Nelson, G. J. "Dietary Fat, Trans Fatty Acids, and Risk of Coronary Heart Disease." *Nutr Rev* 1998;250–252.

Bladder Infection (Cystitis)

Stothers, L. "A Randomized Trial to Evaluate Effectiveness and Cost Effectiveness of Naturopathic Cranberry Products as Prophylaxis Against Urinary Tract Infection in Women." *Can J Urol* 2002;9(3): 1558–1562.

Bronchitis and Pneumonia

Cohen, G. A., G. Hartman, R. N. Hamburger, and R. D. O'Connor. "Severe Anemia and Chronic Bronchitis Associated with a Markedly Elevated Specific IgG to Cow's Milk Protein." *Ann Allergy* 1985;55: 38–40.

Hide, D. W., and B. M. Guyer. "Clinical Manifestations of Allergy Related to Breast and Cows' Milk Feeding." *Arch Dis Child* 1981;56: 172–175.

La Vecchia, C., A. Decarli, and R. Pagano. "Vegetable Consumption and Risk of Chronic Disease." *Epidemiology* 1998;9: 208–210.

Cancer

Barber, M. D., D. C. McMillan, T. Preston, et al. "Metabolic Response to Feeding in Weight-Losing Pancreatic Cancer Patients and Its Modulation by a Fish-Oil-Enriched Nutritional Supplement." *Clin Sci* 2000;98: 389–399.

Barber, M. D., J. A. Ross, A. C. Voss, M. J. Tisdale, and K. C. Fearon. "The Effect of an Oral Nutritional Supplement Enriched with Fish Oil on Weight-Loss in Patients with Pancreatic Cancer." *Br J Cancer* 1999;81: 80–86.

Bounous, G. "Whey Protein Concentrate (WPC) and Glutathione Modulation in Cancer Treatment." *Anticancer Res* 2000;20: 4785–4792.

Calder, P. C., and P. Yaqoob. "Glutamine and the Immune System." *Amino Acids* 1999;17: 227–241.

Grogan, M., L. Tabar, B. Chua, H. H. Chen, and J. Boyages. "Estimating the Benefits of Adjuvant Systemic Therapy for Women with Early Breast Cancer." *Br J Surg* 2001;88: 1513–1518.

Kennedy, R. S., G. P. Konok, G. Bounous, S. Baruchel, T. D. Lee. "The Use of a Whey Protein Concentrate in the Treatment of Patients with Metastatic Carcinoma: A Phase I–II Clinical Study." *Anticancer Res* 1995;15: 2643–2649.

Kimmick, G. G., and H. B. Muss. "Systematic Therapy for Older Women with Breast Cancer." *Oncology* 2001;15: 280–291.

Medina, M. A. "Glutamine and Cancer." *The Journal of Nutrition* 2001;131(Suppl.9): S2539–S2542.

Sirtori, C. R. "Risks and Benefits of Soy Phyto-estrogens in Cardiovascular Diseases, Cancer, Climacteric Symptoms and Osteoporosis." *Drug Safety* 2001;24: 665–682.

Candidiasis, Chronic

Kroker, G. F. "Chronic Candidiasis and Allergy." In *Food Allergy and Intolerance,* ed. J. Brostoff and S. J. Challacombe. Philadelphia: W. B. Saunders, 1987, pp. 850–872.

Truss, C. O. "The Role of *Candida albicans* in Human Illness." *J Orthomol Psychiatry* 1981,10: 228–238.

Weig, M., E. Werner, M. Frosch, and H. Kasper. "The Limited Effect of Refined Carbohydrate Dietary Supplementation on Colonization of the Gastrointestinal Tract of Healthy Subjects by *Candida albicans." The American Journal of Clinical Nutrition* 1999;69: 1170–1173.

Carpal Tunnel Syndrome

Bernstein, A. L., and J. S. Dinesen. "Brief Communication: Effect of Pharmacologic Doses of Vitamin B6 on Carpal Tunnel Syndrome, Electronencephalographic Results, and Pain." *Journal of the American College of Nutrition* 1993;12: 73–76.

Ellis, J. M. "Treatment of Carpal Tunnel Syndrome with Vitamin B6." *Southern Med J* 1987;80(7): 882–884.

Jacobson, M. D., K. D. Plancher, and W. B. Kleinman. "Vitamin B6 (Pyridoxine) Therapy for Carpal Tunnel Syndrome." *Hand Clin* 1996;12 (2): 253–257

Cataracts

Jacques, P. F. "The Potential Preventive Effects of Vitamins for Cataract and Age-Related Macular Degeneration." *Int J Vitam Nutr Res* 1999;69(3): 198–205.

Lyle, B. J., J. A. Mares-Perlman, B. E. Klein, et al. "Antioxidant Intake and Risk of Incident Age-Related Nuclear Cataracts in the Beaver Dam Eye Study." *American Journal of Epidemiology* 1999;149: 801–809.

Tavani, A., E. Negri, and C. LaVecchia. "Food and Nutrient Intake and Risk of Cataract." *Ann Epidem* 1996;6: 41–46.

Cervical Dysplasia

Butterworth, C. E., Jr., K. D. Hatch, M. Macaluso, et al. "Folate Deficiency and Cervical Dysplasia." *Journal of the American Medical Association* 1992;267: 528–533.

Kantesky, P. A., M. D. Gammon, J. Mandelblatt, et al. "Dietary Intake and Blood Levels of Lycopene: Association with Cervical Dysplasia Among Non-Hispanic, Black Women." *Nutr Cancer* 1998;31: 31–40.

Kwasniewska, A., J. Charzewska, A. Tukendorf, and M. Semczuk M. "Dietary Factors in Women with Dysplasia Colli Uteri Associated with Human Papillomavirus Infection." *Nutr Cancer* 1998;30: 39–45.

Romney, S. L., P. R. Palan, J. Basu, and M. Mikhail. "Nutrient Antioxidants in the Pathogenesis and Prevention of Cervical Dysplasias and Cancer." *J Cell Biochem* 1995;23(Suppl.): 96–103.

Cholesterol

El-Enein, A. M. A. "The Role of Nicotinic Acid and Inositol Hexaniacinate as Anticholesterolemic and Antilipemic Agents." *Nutr Rep Intl* 1983;28: 899–911.

Illingworth, D. R., et al. "Comparative Effects of Lovastatin and Niacin in Primary Hypercholesterolemia." *Arch Intern Med* 1994;154: 1586–1595.

Pan, J., M. Lin, R. L. Kesala, J. Van, M. A. Charles. "Niacin Treatment of the Atherogenic Lipid Profile and Lp(a) in Diabetes." *Diabetes Obes Metab* 2002;4: 255–261.

Common Cold

Ringsdorf, W. M., E. Cheraskin, R. R. Ramsay. "Sucrose, Neutrophilic Phagocytosis and Resistance to Disease." *Dent Survey* 1976;52(12): 46.

Sanchez, A., J. L. Reeser, H. S. Lau, et al. "Role of Sugars in Human Neutrophilic Phagocytosis." *The American Journal of Clinical Nutrition* 1973;26: 1180–1184.

Constipation

Daher, S., D. Solé, M. B. De Morias. "Cow's Milk and Chronic Constipation in Children." *The New England Journal of Medicine* 1999;340: 891.

Iacono, G., F. Cavataio, G. Montalto, et al. "Intolerance of Cow's Milk and Chronic Constipation in Children." *The New England Journal of Medicine* 1998;339: 1100–1104.

Müller-Lissner, S. A. "Effect of Wheat Bran on Weight of Stool and Gastrointestinal Transit Time: A Meta Analysis." *British Medical Journal* 1988;296: 615–617.

Depression

Christensen, L. "Psychological Distress and Diet-Effects of Sucrose and Caffeine." *J Applied Nutr* 1988;40: 44–50.

Gettis, A. "Food Sensitivities and Psychological Disturbance: A Review." *Nutr Health* 1989;6: 135–146.

Maes, M., A. Christophe, J. Delanghe J, et al. "Lowered Omega-3 Polyunsaturated Fatty Acids in Serum Phospholipids and Cholesteryl Esters of Depressed Patients." *Psychiatry Res* 1999;85: 275–291.

Penninxm B. W., J. M. Guralnik, L. Ferrucci L, et al. "Vitamin B(12) Deficiency and Depression in Physically Disabled Older Women: Epidemiologic Evidence from the Women's Health and Aging Study." *Am J Psychiatry* 2000;157: 715–721.

Schrader, D. "Equivalence of St. John's Wort Extract (ZE 117) and Fluoxetine: A Randomized, Controlled Study in Mild-Moderate Depression." *International Clin Psychopharmacol* 2000;15: 61–68.

Stoll, A. L., W. E. Severus, M. P. Freeman, et al. "Omega 3 Fatty Acids in Bipolar Disorder. A Preliminary Double-Blind, Placebo-Controlled Trial." *Arch Gen Psychiatry* 1999;56: 407–412.

Volz, H. P., and P. Laux. "Potential Treatment

for Subthreshold and Mild Depression: A Comparison of St. John's Wort Extracts and Fluoxetine." *Compr Psychiatry* 2000;41(2 Suppl. 1): 133–137.

Weber, B., U. Schweiger, M. Deuschle, I. Heuser. "Major Depression and Impaired Glucose Tolerance." *Exp Clin Endocrinol Diabetes* 2000;108: 187–190.

Woelk, H. "Comparison of St. John's Wort and Imipramine for Treating Depression: Randomized Controlled Trial." *British Medical Journal* 2000;321: 536–539.

Diabetes

Brynes, A. E., J. L. Lee, R. E. Brighton=, et al. "A Low Glycemic Diet Significantly Improves the 24-h Blood Glucose Profile in People with Type 2 Diabetes, as Assessed Using the Continuous Glucose MiniMed Monitor." *Diabetes Care* 2003;26: 548–549.

Chandalia, M., A. Garg, D. Lutjohann, et al. "Beneficial Effects of High Dietary Fiber Intake in Patients with Type 2 Diabetes Mellitus." *The New England Journal of Medicine* 2000;342: 1392–1398.

Giacco, R., M. Parillo, A. A. Rivellese, et al. "Long-Term Dietary Treatment with Increased Amounts of Fiber-Rich Low-Glycemic Index Natural Foods Improves Blood Glucose Control and Reduces the Number of Hypoglycemic Events in Type 1 Diabetic Patients." *Diabetes Care* 2000;23: 1461–1466.

Hung, T., J. L. Sievenpiper, A. Marchie, C. W. Kendall, D. J. Jenkins. "Fat Versus Carbohydrate in Insulin Resistance, Obesity, Diabetes and Cardiovascular Disease." *Curr Opin Clin Nutr Metab Care* 2003;6: 165–176.

Jarvi, A. E., B. E. Karlstrom, Y. E. Granfeldt, et al. "Improved Glycemic Control and Lipid Profile and Normalized Fibrinolytic Activity on a Low-Glycemic Index Diet in Type 2 Diabetic Patients." *Diabetes Care* 1999;22: 10–18.

Khan, A., M. Safdar, M. M. Ali Khan, K. N. Khattak, and R. A. Anderson. "Cinnamon Improves Glucose and Lipids of People with Type 2 Diabetes." *Diabetes Care* 2003;26(12): 3215–3218.

Diarrhea

James, J. M., and A. W. Burks. "Food-Associated Gastrointestinal Disease." *Curr Opin Pediatr* 1996;8: 471–475.

Ear Infections

Juntti, H., S. Tikkanen, J. Kokkonen, et al. "Cow's Milk Allergy Is Associated with Recurrent Otitis Media During Childhood." *Acta Otolaryngol* 1999;119: 867–873.

Nsouli, T. M., S. M. Nsouli, R. E. Linde, et al. "Role of Food Allergy in Serous Otitis Media." *Ann Allerg* 1994;73: 215–219.

Eczema (Atopic Dermatitis)

Berth-Jones, J., and R. A. C. Graham-Brown. "Placebo-Controlled Trial of Essential Fatty Acid Supplementation in Atopic Dermatitis." *The Lancet* 1993;341: 1557–1560.

Niggemann, B., B. Sielaff, K. Beyer, et al. "Outcome of Double-Blind, Placebo-Controlled Food Challenge Tests in 107 Children with Atopic Dermatitis." *Clin Exp Allergy* 1999;29: 91–96.

Søyland, E., J. Funk, G. Rajka, et al. "Dietary Supplementation with Very Long-Chain *N*-3 Fatty Acids in Patients with Atopic Dermatitis. A Double-Blind Multicentre Study." *Br J Dermatol* 1994;130: 757–764.

Worm, M., I. Ehlers, W. Sterry, and T. Zuberbier. "Clinical Relevance of Food Additives in Adult Patients with Atopic Dermatitis." *Clin Exp Allergy* 2000;30: 407–414.

Fibrocystic Breast Disease

Allen, S., D. G. Froberg DG. "The Effect of Decreased Caffeine Consumption on Benign Proliferative Breast Disease: A Randomized Clinical Trial." *Surgery* 1987;101: 720–730.

Boyd, N. F., V. McGuire, P. Shannon, et al. "Effect of a Low-Fat High-Carbohydrate Diet on Symp-

toms of Cyclical Mastopathy." *The Lancet* 1988;2: 128–132.

Lubin, F., E. Ron, Y. Wax Y, et al. "A Case-Control Study of Caffeine and Methylxanthines in Benign Breast Disease." *Journal of the American Medical Association* 1985;253(16): 2388–2392.

Marshall, J. M., S. Graham, and M. Swanson. "Caffeine Consumption and Benign Breast Disease: A Case-Control Comparison." *Am J Publ Health* 1982;72(6): 610–612.

Rose, D. P., A. P. Boyar, C. Cohen, L. E. Strong. "Effect of a Low-Fat Diet on Hormone Levels in Women with Cystic Breast Disease. I. Serum Steroids and Gonadotropins." *Journal of the National Cancer Institute* 1987;78: 623–626.

Food Allergy

Bahna, S. L. "Clinical Expressions of Food Allergy." *Ann Allergy Asthma Immunol* 2003;90(6 Suppl. 3): S41–S44.

David, T. J. "Adverse Reaction and Intolerance to Foods." (Review). *Br Med Bull* 2000;56: 34–50.

Fiocchi, A, A. Martelli, A. De Chiara, et al. "Primary Dietary Prevention of Food Allergy." *Ann Allergy Asthma Immunol* 2003;91(1): 3–12.

Fogg, M. I., and J. M. Spergel. "Management of Food Allergies." *Expert Opin Pharmacother* 2003;4(7): 1025–1037.

"Bibliography. Current World Literature. Food Allergy." *Curr Opin Allergy Clin Immunol* 2003;3 (3): 226–233. (No abstract available.)

Sabra, A., J. A. Bellanti, J. M. Rais, et al. "IgE and Non-IgE Food Allergy." *Ann Allergy Asthma Immunol* 2003;90(6 Suppl. 3): S71–S76.

Gallstones

Breneman, J. C. "Allergy Elimination Diet as the Most Effective Gallbladder Diet." *Ann Allerg* 1968;26: 83–87.

Halsted, C. H. "Obesity: Effects on the Liver and Gastrointestinal System." *Curr Opin Clin Nutr Metab Care* 1999;2(5): 425–9.

Misciagna, G., S. Centonze, C. Leoci, et al. "Diet, Physical Activity, and Gallstones—A

Population-Based, Case-Control Study in Southern Italy." *The American Journal of Clinical Nutrition* 1999;69: 120–126.

Glaucoma

McGuire, R. "Fish Oil Cuts Lower Ocular Pressure." *Med Tribune* 1991(September 19): 25.

Richer, S. "Nutritional Influences on Eye Health." *Optometry* 2000;71(10): 657–666.

Gout

Schlesinger, N., and H. R. Schumacher, Jr. "Gout: Can Management Be Improved?" *Curr Opin Rheumatol* 2001;13(3): 240–244.

Hay Fever (see Asthma)

Headache (see Migraine)

Heart Disease (see Atherosclerosis)

Hemorrhoids

Moesgaard, F., M. L. Nielsen, J. B. Hansen, and J. T. Knudsen. "High-Fiber Diet Reduces Bleeding and Pain in Patients with Hemorrhoids." *Dis Colon Rectum* 1982;25: 454–456.

Herpes Simplex

Algert, S. J., N. E. Stubblefield, B. J. Grasse, et al. "Assessment of Dietary Intake of Lysine and Arginine in Patients with Herpes Simplex." *Journal of the American Dietetic Association* 1987;87: 1560–1561.

Flodin, N. W. "The Metabolic Roles, Pharmacology, and Toxicology of Lysine." (Review.) *Journal of the American College of Nutrition* 1997;16: 7–21.

Griffith, R. S., A. L. Norins, C. Kagan C. "A Multicentered Study of Lysine Therapy in Herpes Simplex Infection." *Dermatologica* 1978;156: 257–267.

Griffith, R. S., D. E. Walsh, K. H. Myrmel, et al. "Success of l-lysine Therapy in Frequently Recurrent Herpes Simplex Infection." *Dermatologica* 1987; 175: 183–190.

Milman, N., J. Scheibel, and O. Jessen. "Lysine Pro-

phylaxis in Recurrent Herpes Simplex Labialis: A Double Blind, Controlled Crossover Study." *Acta Derm Venereol* 1980;60: 85–87.

High Blood Pressure

Appel, L. J., T. J. Moore, E. Obarzanek, et al. "A Clinical Trial of the Effects of Dietary Patterns on Blood Pressure. DASH Collaborative Research Group." *The New England Journal of Medicine* 1997;336: 1117–1124.

Fujita, H., T. Yamagami, K. Ohshima. "Effect of an ACE-Inhibitory Agent, Katuobishi Oligopeptide, in the Spontaneously Hypertensive Rat and in Borderline and Mildly Hypertensive Subjects." *Nutr Res* 2001;21: 1149–1158.

Fujita, H., R. Yasumoto, M. Hasegawa, K. Ohsima. "Antihypertensive Activity of 'Katsuobushi Oligopeptide' in Hypertensive and Borderline Hypertensive Subjects." *Jpn Pharmacol Ther* 1997;25: 147–151.

Moore, T. J., P. R. Conlin, Ard J, and L. P. Svetkey. "DASH (Dietary Approaches to Stop Hypertension) Diet Is Effective Treatment for Stage 1 Isolated Systolic Hypertension." *Hypertension* 2001;38: 155–158.

Sacks, F. M., L. P. Svetkey, V. M. Vollmer, et al. "Effects on Blood Pressure of Reduced Dietary Sodium and the Dietary Approaches to Stop Hypertension (DASH) Diet. DASH-Sodium Collaborative Research Group." *The New England Journal of Medicine* 2001;344: 3–10.

Whelton, P. K., and J. He. "Potassium in Preventing and Treating High Blood Pressure." *Semin Nephrol* 1999;19: 494–499.

Hives (Urticaria)

Henz, B. M., and T. Zuberbier. "Most Chronic Urticaria Is Food-Dependent, Not Idiopathic." *Exp Dermatol* 1998;7: 139–142.

Lessof, M. H. "Reactions to Food Additives." *Clin Exp Allergy* 1995;25(Suppl. 1): 27–28.

Juhlin L. "Additives and Chronic Urticaria." *Ann Allergy* 1987;59: 119–123.

Hypoglycemia

Sanders, L. R., F. D. Hofeldt, M. C. Kirk, and J. Levin. "Refined Carbohydrate as a Contributing Factor in Reactive Hypoglycemia." *South Med J* 1982;75: 1072–1075.

Watson, J. M., E. J. Jenkins, P. Hamilton, et al. "Influence of Caffeine on the Frequency and Perception of Hypoglycemia in Free-Living Patients with Type 1 Diabetes." *Diabetes Care* 2000;23: 455–459.

Immune Support

Chandra, R. K. "Nutrition and the Immune System: An Introduction." *The American Journal of Clinical Nutrition* 1997;66: 460–3S.

Nieman, D. C., D. A. Henson, and S. L. Nehlsen-Cannarella. "Influence of Obesity on Immune Function." *Journal of the American Dietetic Association* 1999;99: 294–249.

Ringsdorf, W. M., E. Cheraskin, and R. R. Ramsay. "Sucrose, Neutrophilic Phagocytosis and Resistance to Disease." *Dent Survey* 1976;52(12): 46.

Sanchez, A., J. L. Reeser, H. S. Lau, et al. "Role of Sugars in Human Neutrophilic Phagocytosis." *The American Journal of Clinical Nutrition* 1973;26: 1180–1184.

Insomnia

Donath, F., S. Quispe, K. Diefenbach, et al. "Critical Evaluation of the Effect of Valerian Extract on Sleep Structure and Sleep Quality." *Pharmacopsychiatry* 2000;33: 47–53.

Leathwood, P. D., F. Chauffard, E. Heck, R. Munoz-Box. "Aqueous Extract of Valerian Root (*Valeriana officinalis* L.) Improves Sleep Quality in Man." *Pharmacol Biochem Behav* 1982;17: 65–71.

Irritable Bowel Syndrome

Bohmer, C. J., and H. A. Tuynman. "The Clinical Relevance of Lactose Malabsorption in Irritable Bowel Syndrome." *Eur J Gastroenterol Hepatol* 1996;8: 1013–1016.

Fernandez-Banares, F., M. Esteve-Pardo, R. de Leon R, et al. "Sugar Malabsorption in Functional Bowel Disease: Clinical Implications." *Am J Gastroenterol* 1993;88: 2044–2050.

Francis, C. Y., and P. J. Whorwell. "Bran and Irritable Bowel Syndrome: Time for Reappraisal." *The Lancet* 1994;344: 39–40.

Hotz, J., and K. Plein. "Effectiveness of Plantago Seed Husks in Comparison with Wheat Bran on Stool Frequency and Manifestations of Irritable Colon Syndrome with Constipation." *Med Klin* 1994;89: 645–651.

Liu, J.-H., G.-H. Chen, H.-Z. Yeh, et al. "Enteric-Coated Peppermint-Oil Capsules in the Treatment of Irritable Bowel Syndrome: A Prospective, Randomized Trial." *J Gastroenterol* 1997;32: 765–768.

Niec, A. M., B. Frankum, and N. J. Talley. "Are Adverse Food Reactions Linked to Irritable Bowel Syndrome?" *Am J Gastroenterol* 1998;93: 2184–2190.

Parker, T. J., S. J. Naylor, A. M. Riordan, and J. O. Hunter. "Management of Patients with Food Intolerance in Irritable Bowel Syndrome: The Development and Use of an Exclusion Diet." *J Hum Nutr Diet* 1995;8: 159–166.

Kidney Stones

Hassapidou, M. N., S. T. Paraskevopoulos, P. A. Karakoltsidis, et al. "Dietary Habits of Patients with Renal Stone Disease in Greece." *J Human Nutr Dietet* 1999;12: 47–51.

Hiatt, R. A., B. Ettinger, B. Caan, et al. "Randomized Controlled Trial of a Low Animal Protein, High Fiber Diet in the Prevention of Recurrent Calcium Oxalate Kidney Stones." *American Journal of Epidemiology* 1996;144: 25–33.

Hughes, J., and R. W. Norman. "Diet and Calcium Stones." *Can Med Assoc J* 1992;146: 137–143.

Martini, L. A., and R. J. Wood. "Should Dietary Calcium and Protein Be Restricted in Patients with Nephrolithiasis?" *Nutr Rev* 2000;58: 111–117.

Massey, L. K. "Dietary Influences on Urinary Oxalate and Risk of Kidney Stones." *Front Biosci* 2003;8: S584–S594.

Macular Degeneration

Gale, C. R., N. F. Hall, D. I. Phillips, and C. N. Martyn. "Lutein and Zeaxanthin Status and Risk of Age-Related Macular Degeneration." *Invest Ophthalmol Vis Sci* 2003;44(6): 2461–2465.

Jacques, P. F. "The Potential Preventive Effects of Vitamins for Cataract and Age-Related Macular Degeneration." *Int J Vitam Nutr Res* 1999;69(3): 198–205.

Seddon, J. M., U. A. Ajani, R. D. Sperduto, et al. "Dietary Carotenoids, Vitamins A, C, and E, and Advanced Age-Related Macular Degeneration." *Journal of the American Medical Association* 1994;272: 1413–1420.

Smith, W., P. Mitchell, and S. R. Leeder. "Dietary Fat and Fish Intake and Age-Related Maculopathy." *Arch Ophthalmol* 2000;118: 401–404.

Menopause

Baird, D. D., D. M. Umbach, L. Landsedell, et al. "Dietary Intervention Study to Assess Estrogenicity of Dietary Soy Among Postmenopausal Women." *J Clin Endocrinol Metab* 1995;80: 1685–1690.

Knight, D. C., and J. A. Eden. "A Review of the Clinical Effects of Phytoestrogens." *Obstet Gynecol* 1996;87: 897–904.

Lieberman, S. "A Review of the Effectiveness of *Cimicifuga racemosa* (Black Cohosh) for the Symptoms of Menopause." *J Womens Health* 1998;7: 525–529.

Liske, E. "Therapeutic Efficacy and Safety of *Cimicifuga racemosa* for Gynecological Disorders." *Advances Therapy* 1998;15: 45–53.

Migraine Headache

Dexter, J. D., J. Roberts, and J. A. Byer. "The Five Hour Glucose Tolerance Test and Effect of Low Sucrose Diet in Migraine." *Headache* 1978;18: 91–94.

Egger, J., C. M. Carter, J. F. Soothill, and J. Wilson. "Oligoantigenic Diet Treatment of Children with Epilepsy and Migraine." *J Pediatr* 1989;114: 51–58.

Koehler, S. M., and A. Glaros. "The Effect of Aspartame on Migraine Headache." *Headache* 1988;28: 10–13.

Wilkinson, C. F., Jr. "Recurrent Migrainoid Headaches Associated with Spontaneous Hypoglycemia." *Am J Med* Sci 1949;218: 209–212.

Mouth Ulcers

Hunter, I. P., M. M. Ferguson, C. Scully, et al. "Effects of Dietary Gluten Elimination in Patients with Recurrent Minor Aphthous Stomatitis and No Detectable Gluten Enteropathy." *Oral Surg Oral Med Oral Pathol* 1993;75: 595–598.

Nolan, A., P. J. Lamey, K. A. Milligan, and A. Forsyth. "Recurrent Aphthous Ulceration and Food Sensitivity." *J Oral Pathol Med* 1991;20: 473–475.

Nolan, A., W. B. McIntosh, B. F. Allam, P. J. Lamey. "Recurrent Aphthous Ulceration: Vitamin B1, B2 and B6 Status and Response to Replacement Therapy." *J Oral Pathol Med* 1991;20: 389–391.

O'Farrelly, C., C. O'Mahony, F. Graeme-Cook, et al. "Gliadin Antibodies Identify Gluten-Sensitive Oral Ulceration in the Absence of Villous Atrophy." *J Oral Pathol Med* 1991;20: 476–478.

Olson, J. A., I. Feinberg, S. Silverman, et al. "Serum Vitamin B12, Folate, and Iron Levels in Recurrent Aphthous Ulceration." *Oral Surg Oral Med Oral Pathol* 1982;54: 517–520.

Wray, D., M. M. Ferguson, W. A. Hutcheon, and J. H. Dagg. "Nutritional Deficiencies in Recurrent Aphthae." *J Oral Pathol* 1978;7: 418–423.

Multiple Sclerosis

Ghadirian, P., M. Jain, S. Ducic, et al. "Nutritional Factors in the Aetiology of Multiple Sclerosis: A Case-Control Study in Montreal, Canada." *Int J Epidemiol* 1998;5: 845–852.

Kidd, P. M. "Multiple Sclerosis, an Autoimmune Inflammatory Disease: Prospects for Its Integrative Management." *Altern Med Rev* 2001;6(6): 540–566.

Mayer, M. "Essential Fatty Acids and Related Molecular and Cellular Mechanisms in Multiple Sclerosis: New Looks at Old Concepts." *Folia Biol* 1999;45(4): 133–141.

Nordvik, I., K. M. Myhr, H. Nyland, K. S. Bjerve. "Effect of Dietary Advice and N-3 Supplementation in Newly Diagnosed MS Patients." *Acta Neurol Scand* 2000;102: 143–149.

Simopoulos, A. P. "Omega-3 Fatty Acids in Inflammation and Autoimmune Diseases." *Journal of the American College of Nutrition* 2002;21(6): 495–505.

Swank, R. L. "Multiple Sclerosis: Twenty Years on Lowfat Diet." *Arch Neurol* 1970;23: 460–474.

Nonulcer Dyspepsia

Friese, J., and S. Köhler. "Peppermint/Caraway Oil-Fixed Combination in Non-ulcer Dyspepsia: Equivalent Efficacy of the Drug Combination in an Enteric Coated or Enteric Soluble Formula." *Pharmazie* 1999;54: 210–215.

Madisch, A., C. J. Heydenreich, V. Wieland, et al. "Treatment of Functional Dyspepsia with a Fixed Peppermint Oil and Caraway Oil Combination Preparation as Compared to Cisapride." *Arzneim Forsch* 1999;49: 925–932.

May, B., H. D. Kuntz, M. Kieser, and S. Köhler. "Efficacy of a Fixed Peppermint/Caraway Oil Combination in Non-ulcer Dyspepsia." *Arzneimittelforschung* 1996;46: 1149–1153.

Obesity

Howarth, N. C., E. Saltzman, and S. B. Roberts. "Dietary Fiber and Weight Regulation." *Nutr Rev* 2001;59(5): 129–139.

Osteoarthritis

Childers, N. F., and M. S. Margoles. "An Apparent Relation of Nightshades (Solanaceae) to Arthritis." *J Neurol Orthop Med Surg* 1993;14: 227–231.

Felson, D. T., Y. Zhang, J. M. Anthony, et al. "Weight Loss Reduces the Risk for Symptomatic Knee Osteoarthritis in Women. The Framingham Study." *Annals of Internal Medicine* 1992;116: 535–539.

Reginster, J. Y., R. Deroisy, L. Rovati, et al. "Long-Term Effects of Glucosamine Sulphate on Osteoarthritis Progression: A Randomised, Placebo-Controlled Clinical Trial." *The Lancet* 2001;357: 251–256.

Osteoporosis

Dawson-Hughes, B. "Interaction of Dietary Calcium and Protein in Bone Health in Humans." *The Journal of Nutrition* 2003;133(3): S852–S854.

Evans, C. E., A. Y. Chughtai, A. Blumsohn, et al. "The Effect of Dietary Sodium on Calcium Metabolism in Premenopausal and Postmenopausal Women." *Eur J Clin Nutr* 1997;51: 394–349.

Feskanich, D., W. C. Willett, M. J. Stampfer, and G. A. Colditz. "Protein Consumption and Bone Fractures in Women." *American Journal of Epidemiology* 1996;143: 472–479.

Hernandez-Avila M., G. A. Colditz, M. J. Stampfer, et al. "Caffeine, Moderate Alcohol Intake, and Risk of Fractures of the Hip and Forearm in Middle-Aged Women." *The American Journal of Clinical Nutrition* 1991;54: 157–163.

Hunt, I. F., N. J. Murphy, C. Henderson, et al. "Bone Mineral Content in Postmenopausal Women: Comparison of Omnivores and Vegetarians." *The American Journal of Clinical Nutrition* 1989;50: 517–523.

Kerstetter, J. E., and L. H. Allen. "Dietary Protein Increases Urinary Calcium." *The Journal of Nutrition* 1990;120: 134–136.

Kerstetter, J. E., A. C. Looker, and K. L. Insogna. "Low Dietary Protein and Low Bone Density." *Calcif Tissue Int* 2000;66: 313.

Kim, S. H., D. J. Morton, E. L. Barrett-Connor. "Carbonated Beverage Consumption and Bone Mineral Density Among Older Women: The Rancho Bernardo Study." *Am J Public Health* 1997;87: 276–279.

Mannan, M. T., K. Tucker, B. Dawson-Hughes, et al. "Effect of Dietary Protein on Bone Loss in

Elderly Men and Women: The Framingham Osteoporosis Study." *J Bone Mineral Res* 2000;15: 2504–2512.

Mazariegos-Ramos, E., F. Guerrero-Romero, F. Rodriguez-Moran, et al. "Consumption of Soft Drinks with Phosphoric Acid as a Risk Factor for the Development of Hypocalcemia in Children: A Case-Control Study." *J Pediatr* 1995;126: 940–942.

Moriguti, J. C., E. Ferriolli, and J. S. Marchini. "Urinary Calcium Loss in Elderly Men on a Vegetable:Animal (1:1) High-Protein Diet." *Gerontology* 1999;45: 274–278.

Potter, S. M., J. A. Baum, H. Teng, et al. "Soy Protein and Isoflavones: Their Effects on Blood Lipids and Bone Density in Postmenopausal Women." *The American Journal of Clinical Nutrition* 1998;68(Suppl.): S1375–S1379.

Tesar, R., M. Notelovitz, E. Shim, et al. "Axial and Peripheral Bone Density and Nutrient Intakes of Postmenopausal Vegetarian and Omnivorous Women." *The American Journal of Clinical Nutrition* 1992;56: 699–704.

Wyshak, G., R. E. Frisch. "Carbonated Beverages, Dietary Calcium, the Dietary Calcium/Phosphorus Ratio, and Bone Fractures in Girls and Boys." *J Adolescent Health* 1994;15: 210–215.

Peptic Ulcer Disease

Bardhan, K. D., D. C. Cumberland, R. A. Dixon, C. D. Holdsworth. "Clinical Trial of Deglycyrrhizinised Liquorice in Gastric Ulcer." *Gut* 1978;19: 779–782.

Cohen, S., and G. H. Booth, Jr. "Gastric Acid Secretion and Lower-Esophageal-Sphincter Pressure in Response to Coffee and Caffeine." *The New England Journal of Medicine* 1975;293: 897–899.

Graham, D. Y., S. Y. Anderson, T. Lang. "Garlic or Jalapeño Peppers for Treatment of *Helicobacter pylori* Infection." *Am J Gastroenterol* 1999;94: 1200–1202.

Harju, E., and T. K. Larme. "Effect of Guar Gum Added to the Diet of Patients with Duodenal Ulcers." *J Parenteral Enteral Nutr* 1985;9: 496–500.

Kang, J. Yl, H. H. Tay, R. Guan. "Dietary Supplementation with Pectin in the Maintenance Treatment of Duodenal Ulcer." *Scand J Gastroenterol* 1988;23: 95–99.

Katchinski, B. D., R. F. A. Logan, M. Edmond, and M. J. S. Langman. "Duodenal Ulcer and Refined Carbohydrate Intake: A Case-Control Study Assessing Dietary Fiber and Refined Sugar Intake." *Gut* 1990;31: 993–996.

Kern, R. A., G. Stewart. "Allergy in Duodenal Ulcer: Incidence and Significance of Food Hypersensitivities as Observed in 32 Patients." *J Allergy* 1931;3: 51.

Kumar, N., A. Kumar, S. L. Broor, et al. "Effect of Milk on Patients with Duodenal Ulcers." *British Medical Journal* 1986;293: 666.

Morgan, A. G., C. Pacsoo, and W. A. F. McAdam. "Maintenance Therapy: A Two Year Comparison Between Caved-S and Cimetidine Treatment in the Prevention of Symptomatic Gastric Ulcer Recurrence." *Gut* 1985;26: 599–602.

Reimann, H. J., and J. Lewin. "Gastric Mucosal Reactions in Patients with Food Allergy." *Am J Gastroenterol* 1988;83: 1212–1219.

Sivam, G. P., J. W. Lampe, B. Ulness, et al. "*Helicobacter pylori—in vitro* Susceptibility to Garlic (*Allium sativum*) Extract." *Nutr Cancer* 1997;27: 118–121.

Yan, R., Y. Sun, R. Sun. "Early Enteral Feeding and Supplement of Glutamine Prevent Occurrence of Stress Ulcer Following Severe Thermal Injury." *Chung Hwa Cheng Hsing Shao Shang Wai Ko Tsa Chih* 1995;11: 189–192.

Periodontal Disease

Vaananen, M. K., H. A. Markkanen, V. J. Tuovinen, et al. "Periodontal Health Related to Plasma Ascorbic Acid." *Proc Finn Dent Soc* 1993;89: 51–59.

Premenstrual Syndrome

Fenster, L., C. Quale, K. Waller K, et al. "Caffeine Consumption and Menstrual Function." *American Journal of Epidemiology* 1999;149: 550–557.

Kleijnen, J., G. T. Riet, P. Knipschild. "Vitamin B6 in

the Treatment of the Premenstrual Syndrome—A Review." *Br J Obstet Gynaecol* 1990;97: 847–852.

Schellenberg, R. "Treatment for the Premenstrual Syndrome with *Agnus castus* Fruit Extract: Prospective, Randomized, Placebo Controlled Study." *British Medical Journal* 2001;20: 134–137.

Prostate Enlargement (BPH)

Wilt, T. J., A. Ishani, G. Stark, et al. "Saw Palmetto Extracts for Treatment of Benign Prostatic Hyperplasia. A Systematic Review." *Journal of the American Medical Association* 1998;280: 1604–1609.

Psoriasis

Bittiner, S. B., W. F. G. Tucker, I. Cartwright, S. S. Bleehen. "A Double-Blind, Randomised, Placebo-Controlled Trial of Fish Oil in Psoriasis." *The Lancet* 1988;1: 378–380.

Kojima, T., T. Terano, E. Tanabe, et al. "Long-Term Administration of Highly Purified Eicosapentaenoic Acid Provides Improvement of Psoriasis." *Dermatologica* 1991;182: 225–230.

Michäelsson, G., B. Gerdén, E. Hagforsen, et al. "Psoriasis Patients with Antibodies to Gliadin Can Be Improved by a Gluten-Free Diet." *Br J Dermatol* 2000;142: 44–51.

Poikolainen, K., T. Reunala, J. Karvonen, et al. "Alcohol Intake: A Risk Factor for Psoriasis in Young and Middle Aged Men?" *British Medical Journal* 1990;300: 780–783.

Soyland, E., J. Funk, G. Rajka, et al. "Effect of Dietary Supplementation with Very-Long-Chain N-3 Fatty Acids in Patients with Psoriasis." *The New England Journal of Medicine* 1993;328: 1812–1816.

Rheumatoid Arthritis

Hafstrom, I., B. Ringertz, and A. Spangberg. "A Vegan Diet Free of Gluten Improves the Signs and Symptoms of Rheumatoid Arthritis: The Effects on Arthritis Correlate with a Reduction in Antibodies to Food Antigens." *Rheumatology* 2001;40(10): 1175–1179.

Heliövaara, M., K. Aho, P. Knekt P, et al. "Coffee Consumption, Rheumatoid Factor, and the Risk of Rheumatoid Arthritis." *Ann Rheum Dis* 2000;59: 631–635.

Kjeldsen-Kragh, J. "Rheumatoid Arthritis Treated with Vegetarian Diets. *The American Journal of Clinical Nutrition* 1999;70(Suppl. 3): S594–S600.

Linos, A., V. G. Kaklamani, Y. Koukmantaki, et al. "Dietary Factors in Relation to Rheumatoid Arthritis: A Role for Olive Oil and Cooked Vegetables." *The American Journal of Clinical Nutrition* 1999;70: 1077–1082.

Mangge, H., J. Hermann, K. Schauenstein. "Diet and Rheumatoid Arthritis—A Review." *Scand J Rheumatol* 1999;28(4): 201–209.

Muller, H., F. W. de Toledo, and K. L. Resch. "Fasting Followed by Vegetarian Diet in Patients with Rheumatoid Arthritis: A Systematic Review." *Scand J Rheumatol* 2001;30(1): 1–10.

Simopoulos, A. P. "Omega-3 Fatty Acids in Inflammation and Autoimmune Diseases." *Journal of the American College of Nutrition* 2002;21(6): 495–505.

Varicose Veins

Diehm, C. "Comparison of Leg Compression Stocking and Oral Horse-Chestnut Seed Extract Therapy in Patients with Chronic Venous Insufficiency." *The Lancet* 1996;347: 292–294.

Ihme, N., H. Kieswetter, F. Jung F, et al. "Leg Edema Protection from Buckwheat Herb Tea in Patients with Chronic Venous Insufficiency: A Single-Center, Randomized, Double-Blind, Placebo-Controlled Clinical Trial." *Eur J Clin Pharmacol* 1995;50: 443–447.

INDEX

abdominal pain, 754–5
acesulphame K, 46
acetate, 79
acetylcholine, 76, 113, 629, 684
acid–alkaline values of foods, 783–7
acidifiers, 41
acidophilus cultured milk, 575
acne, 136, 638, 680–1
acorns, 418
acorn squash, 236–8
adaptogenic effect, 280
addiction, to chocolate, 650
additives:
    acidifiers, 41
    antioxidants to prevent spoilage,
      46, 512
    artificial flavors, 41, 43
    color, 42–3, 512–13, 745
    Feingold hypothesis, 43
    preservatives, 41, 43, 46–7
    sweeteners, 43–46, 69–70
adenosine, 264
adequate intake (AI), 97
adrenal glands, 299
adrenaline (epinephine), 60, 715
Adriatic figs, 277
adzuki (aduki) beans, 383–5
    cooking, 369, 384–5
    history, 383–4
    nutrition and health, 384, 769
    preparation tips, 384–5
    quick serving ideas, 385

    safety issues, 385
    selection and storage, 384
aflatoxin, 270, 410, 443, 503
agar, 75
Agriculture Department, U.S.
    (USDA):
    dietary guidelines, 7, 10
    grading system for fruits and
      vegetables, 155–6
AIDS, 682–3
alachlor, 50
alanine, 140
Alaskan king crab, 550–1, 552
alcohol, 29
    and depression, 715
    as diuretic, 699
    and hypoglycemia, 741
    and liver damage, 139
    and osteoporosis, 762
    and prostate, 766
    and psoriasis, 767–8
alcoholism, 683–4
aldehyde oxidase, 133
alder pollen, allergy to, 431
aldicarb, 48–9
aldosterone, 123
aldrin, 48
ale and beer, 634, 635
aleurone, 322, 323
Alexander the Great, 333
alfalfa, 385–9
    history, 386

    nutrition and health, 386–7, 761
    quick serving ideas, 387–8
    safety issues, 388–9
    selection and storage, 387
algal polysaccharides, 73, 75
alginates, 75
alkaline–acid values of foods, 783–7
alkaline foods, 274, 277, 760
allergies, 723–5
    and anaphylaxis (shock), 443,
      554, 660
    to citrus peels, 281, 291, 293
    and daisy family, 161, 195, 206
    and diarrhea, 719
    and ear infections, 720–1
    to fish and shellfish, 535, 554
    and flavonoids, 147, 149
    and food coloring, 43
    and gallbladder attacks, 726
    and hay fever, 496, 730
    and hives, 793
    and hypoallergenic fruit, 305,
      306, 308
    and immune function, 724
    and irritable bowel syndrome, 746
    and multiple sclerosis, 754
    to nuts, 408, 410, 443
    to pollens, 276, 431
    symptoms, 337, 723–4
    and ulcers, 762
    to wheat, 337
allicin, 200–1

ACKNOWLEDGMENTS

First of all, it is important for us to acknowledge all the researchers, physicians, and scientists who over the years have sought to better understand the role of diet and natural medicines in the prevention and treatment of disease. Without their work, this book would certainly not exist. Next, we must acknowledge the important role that our agent, Bonnie Solow, played in linking us up with Tracy Behar and Atria Books. We are indebted to everyone on the team for having the perseverance to make our book as reader-friendly and practical as possible.

Michael T. Murray, N.D.: Most of all, I would like to acknowledge my wife, Gina. Her love, support, and patience are the major blessings in my life, along with our wonderful children, Alexa, Zachary, and Addison.

Joseph E. Pizzorno, N.D.: In appreciation of my wonderful family, who blesses my life: Lara, my beloved spouse; Raven, my dear daughter; and Galen, my brilliant son. Thank you to Dr. Michael Murray, whose keen intelligence and remarkable ability to communicate have dramatically increased the public understanding of natural medicine.

Lara Pizzorno, M.A. (Divinity), M.A. (Lit.), LMT: It's lovely to be able to publicly acknowledge my sweet soul mate and husband, Joe; Galen, our most dear son; Raven, the daughter of my heart; and our two faithful felines, Catnip, who will always live in our hearts, and Smidge, who worked late with me many nights. A special thanks to Juan San Mames for sharing his expertise on saffron, and to Dr. Jeff Dahlberg, Dr. Lloyd Rooney, and Dr. Ronald Prior for sharing their research on sorghum. Finally, I would like to thank Dr. Michael Murray; without his vision, encyclopaedic knowledge, and hard work, this book would not exist.